READINGS IN
HEALTH CARE
ETHICS

→ Principles
Both discussed → used to argue
for euthanasia

* Euthanasia   (321 - 344) ✓
    → Fundamental issues
    → Self - determination   (345 - 349)

* Therapeutic Relationships   (3-13) ✓
    → 4 models of the Physician-Patient
    → Relational approach to autonomy   (14-32) ✓   ✓

* Consent   (89-92) ✓
    → Competency
    → Proxy Consent   (98 - 104)* ✓   ✓
      → Brans argues that it is acceptable
       to performed medical research
        on incapable of consenting.
         "common good"

* Cloning   (195 - 210) ✓ ✓
    → Wisdom of Repugnance
    → Cloning, ethics, & Religion   (571 - 4) ✓
    → On Cloning Humans   (575 - 584) ✓

* Abortion
    → Abortion immoral   (213 - 224) ✓
    → Moral Significance of birth   (225 - 237)
    → Abortion through Feminism   (238 - 250) ✓

READINGS
IN HEALTH CARE
ETHICS

second edition

edited by
Elisabeth (Boetzkes) Gedge and Wilfrid J. Waluchow

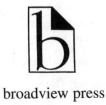

broadview press

Library and Archives Canada Cataloguing in Publication

Readings in health care ethics / edited by Elisabeth (Boetzkes) Gedge and Wilfrid J. Waluchow.—2nd ed.

Includes bibliographical references.
ISBN 978-1-55481-038-3

1. Medical ethics.   I. Boetzkes, Elisabeth Airini   II. Waluchow, Wilfrid J., 1953-

R724.R435 2012   174.2   C2011-907559-8

Broadview Press is an independent, international publishing house, incorporated in 1985.

We welcome comments and suggestions regarding any aspect of our publications—please feel free to contact us at the addresses below or at broadview@broadviewpress.com.

North America
Post Office Box 1243, Peterborough, Ontario, Canada K9J 7H5
2215 Kenmore Avenue, Buffalo, NY, USA 14207
Tel: (705) 743-8990; Fax: (705) 743-8353
email: customerservice@broadviewpress.com

UK, Europe, Central Asia, Middle East, Africa, India, and Southeast Asia
Eurospan Group, 3 Henrietta St., London WC2E 8LU, United Kingdom
Tel: 44 (0) 1767 604972; Fax: 44 (0) 1767 601640
email: eurospan@turpin-distribution.com

Australia and New Zealand
NewSouth Books
c/o TL Distribution, 15-23 Helles Ave., Moorebank, NSW, Australia 2170
Tel: (02) 8778 9999; Fax: (02) 8778 9944
email: orders@tldistribution.com.au

www.broadviewpress.com

Copy-edited by Martin Boyne

Broadview Press acknowledges the financial support of the Government of Canada through the Canada Book Fund for our publishing activities.

The interior of this book is printed on paper containing 100% post-consumer fibre.

Typesetting and assembly: True to Type Inc., Claremont, Canada.

PRINTED IN CANADA

CONTENTS

CHAPTER NINE: GENETICS

PREFACE

Health care ethics is a diverse field of rapid change whose norms may have general application or may vary under differing legal or distributive schemes. Our revised edition of *Readings in Health Care Ethics* reflects this complexity. As in the first edition, we offer an overview of theoretical resources, but we have updated it to include a new direction in feminist naturalized ethics. Recognizing the growing significance for bioethics of policy documents and legal decisions, we have included links to a number of national and international policies, such as Canada's Tri-Council Statement on the Ethical Conduct for Research Involving Humans and the 2005 UNESCO Universal Declaration on Bioethics and Human Rights. Supreme Court of Canada cases with particular relevance to clinical ethics and health rights have been summarized and links provided to the rulings.

Chapter 1 on relationships preserves the emphasis on the clinical context but has been expanded to include articles on the ethics of industry-university partnerships and industry-clinician relationships.

A new chapter (Chapter 2) is dedicated to health care in Canada, reflecting the urgency of addressing the sustainability of health care delivery, our commitment to and interpretation of the Canada Health Act, and the ethical implications of a move toward increased privatization. The Supreme Court decision in *Chaoulli v. The Attorney General of Quebec and the Attorney General of Canada* (2005) is important here, and it is referenced and discussed in this chapter.

Under "Consent" (Chapter 3) we have added ethical analysis of the novel procedure of face transplantation, which raises rich philosophical issues about identity while highlighting the epistemic uncertainties surrounding consent to such new procedures.

The chapter on reproduction (Chapter 4) reflects recent debates on the use of human embryos and the choice of "surgical birth." Under "Fetuses and Newborns" in Chapter 5 we include a discussion of "saviour siblings," and the chapter on research (Chapter 7) extends our previous treatment to include a debate over therapeutic misconception in clinical trials, as well as a critical look at evidence-based medicine and women's health.

In the wake of SARS and Hurricane Katrina we believed a section on ethics in catastrophic situations was called for, so we have expanded the section on scarce resources to include discussion in Chapter 8 of the limits of the duty to treat. Finally, we have updated the chapter on genetics (Chapter 9) to reflect recent trends, such as gene banking and genetic enhancement.

Readings in Health Care Ethics is aimed primarily at an undergraduate readership and presupposes only an interest in the bioethical issues that are shaping our world. We are confident that the second edition contains sufficient material of general interest to engage non-Canadian students, but we are also pleased to offer a distinctive Canadian focus on many of the issues covered. Finally, profound thanks must go to our wonderful research assistants, Mike Hinds and Chris Morano, for their cheerful industry and sound philosophical instincts.

INTRODUCTION

ETHICAL RESOURCES FOR DECISION-MAKING

Wilfrid J. Waluchow and Elisabeth Gedge

Moral Philosophy

The current prominence enjoyed by health care ethics is due, in no small measure, to the impact of biochemistry and improved technology. There is much more that can be done for (or to) patients than could ever be done before. New technological possibilities raise all sorts of questions which never had to be faced in the past. At one time the question "What *should* be done?" may have been more or less equivalent to the question "What *can* be done?" Whether or not this was true in the past, it is clearly not true now. To take one example: medicine is now able to keep people alive on respirators and other life-support mechanisms in situations where many question the propriety of doing so. If someone is irreversibly comatose, it may be that we *can* keep her alive. But whether we *should* utilize scarce resources to do so is another question altogether. This is only one example of the many decisions that arise in health care ethics. How can philosophy help?

Decision-making has always had a moral dimension, and many ethical decisions are extremely difficult. Moral philosophers are not moral experts capable of providing ready-made answers when difficult or intransigent moral conflicts arise. Rather, they perform more modest tasks: clarifying the terms of moral debate, scrutinizing distinctions to see if they stand up to rational examination, assessing the validity and cogency of arguments, and examining the fit between moral practice and moral principles and values.

Moral philosophers are of course also concerned sometimes with defending their own moral theories and convictions, particularly when they detect unwarranted, dogmatic beliefs. But a student unaccustomed to the ways of the moral philosopher will often find the philosopher's arguments a trifle strange. The moral philosopher will often seek to defend or justify the obvious—e.g., that it is morally wrong intentionally to deceive a patient about the dangerous side-effects of an experimental drug the patient is being asked to take, or that it is wrong deliberately to enrol mentally competent patients in clinical trials without their consent. At other times the moral philosopher will offer arguments which *question* the obvious. She might even try to defend a position which strikes others as patently false— e.g., that elderly people have less right to scarce medical resources than younger people or that other animals have less claim to moral consideration than do humans. The main reason for these strange activities of the moral philosopher lies in his chief motivation, expressed in a maxim propounded by the ancient Greek philosopher Socrates. According to Socrates (Plato, *Apology*, 37e-38a), the unexamined life is not worth living. Socrates and other moral philosophers always want to know *why* we should believe the things we do, even those things which we firmly and passionately believe to be true. Many of our moral beliefs just seem right to us. We've never had occasion to question them or to ask ourselves why we hold them. Yet if pushed to articulate the grounds or bases of our moral beliefs, we are often unable to provide them. And even if we do manage to come up with something, we often find that our grounds do not stand up well to critical scrutiny. It may seem obvious that no patient should be enroled in a clinical drug trial without the prior consent of the patient or a person entitled to give consent on the patient's behalf. This principle, P, helps to explain why we would condemn a physician/experimenter who, without first gaining informed consent, tried out a new drug on a group of patients in their thirties who had lung cancer but were otherwise normal adults.

But now ask whether principle P stands up to rational scrutiny. Imagine that you are on an Ethics Review Board at a University Hospital and that a project in which principle P seems to be compromised comes before the Board for approval. The situation is as follows.

Babies are sometimes born with a hypotensive condition for which potentially life-saving medication is immediately required. Your hospital has routinely used two types of medication to combat this condition, some physicians preferring the one drug, X, others the second, Y. Both X and Y seem effective, but they operate in different ways. It is also unclear whether X or Y is preferable in terms of degree of efficacy or severity of potential side-effects. The doctors want to clear up these uncertainties and ascertain whether X or Y is better. A trial is proposed in which all new-born babies with hypotension will be randomly allocated to receive either X or Y. The study protocol calls for "double blinding." That is, no one, including the doctors and nurses in the neonatal ward who will be administering the medication, will know to which group any particular baby has been assigned. There is only one hitch. Hypotension is not a condition which can be predicted before birth. Therefore it is not feasible to gain consent from parents before their baby is born. It is also not feasible, in most cases, to gain consent after birth when it becomes apparent that medication for hypotension is immediately required. As a consequence, the researcher suggests the following. If the parents are available, they will be asked to consent to enrolment of their baby in the study. If they object, their baby will then receive whichever of X or Y the attending physician happens to prefer. If they consent to their baby's participation, then the baby will be enrolled in the study and assigned, randomly and blindly, either to the group receiving X or to the group receiving Y. As for those babies whose parents are unavailable when the necessity for immediate medication becomes apparent, they will be enrolled in the study *without consent*. The parents of these babies will be contacted, however, as soon as possible and asked for consent to the con-

tinued enrolment of their baby. Should there be any objections at this stage, the choice of the baby's medication will then fall into the hands of the attending physician who will exercise his discretion in choosing X or Y.

Given that both X and Y are standard drugs in common use at the hospital, that parents are given the choice of opting out as soon as they can be reached, and that the proposed procedure for gaining consent is the only feasible one under the circumstances, it seems reasonable, and ethical, to permit temporary enrolment in the study without the parents' consent. But then doesn't this show that principle P must be rejected, or at least modified in some way? If so, what might the alternative be? We need to develop a moral theory for distinguishing cases where *prior* consent is vital from special cases in which it may not be necessary. It is here that the moral philosopher might be of some help. He might be able to supply an ethical theory upon the basis of which it is possible to support a reasonable alternative to P.

The family of activities pursued by the moral philosopher is prompted largely by a desire for clarity of thought and integrity of action—by Socrates' maxim that the unexamined life is not worth living. The student of moral philosophy must be prepared to approach the subject with the correct frame of mind, with a willingness to challenge the obvious and to consider seriously both the questionable and the unfamiliar. Should she do so, there is much of value that can be gleaned from the study of health care ethics.

One final point about the role of the moral philosopher. Moral philosophy is not the moral conscience of society. On the contrary, moral philosophers should be viewed as partners with the rest of the citizenry in worrying through troublesome moral questions. Moral philosophers are not out simply to criticize for moral failure—except perhaps when blind dogma rules moral practice, where the lives we lead do remain largely unexamined. Most important of all, perhaps, is the following point. To raise or consider a moral question is not necessarily to imply that there is something inherently immoral or unethical going on. The questions which arise in health care ethics are difficult ones, and those who disagree with us or are generally perplexed do not necessarily have any less moral integrity than we do.

Morality versus Ethics

Moral persons are equally distributed in all walks of life. As noted earlier, morality is always of relevance, but no one can claim to be a moral expert. Ethics or ethical theory is another matter. Ethical theory, as opposed to morality, is the systematic, critical study of the basic underlying principles, values, and concepts utilized in thinking about moral life. Ethics, so understood, is something the average person concerns himself with only infrequently, if ever. But this is not true of moral philosophers or ethicists. They are primarily concerned with ethical theory. They have developed concepts, theories, and techniques of argument which can often be of use to non-philosophers in finding their way through the tangled moral issues to which the practice of medicine often gives rise. We would do well, then, to consider the general ethical theories of some of the most influential moral philosophers of Western civilization. This we will do in later sections. First, a few thoughts on the nature and role of ethical theories.

Levels of Moral Response

Consider the question "Why do you oppose abortion?" As put to an opponent of abortion, this question can trigger different types of responses.

The Expressive Level

At the most primitive level the answer is likely to be: "Because abortion is repugnant" or "I hate the very thought of killing a fetus." These responses are unanalyzed expressions or feelings which, in themselves, do not constitute any kind of justification or reason for opposing abortion. This is not to deny that feelings are relevant to morality or that moral convictions are often accompanied by strong emotions. It is simply to say that the mere fact that one feels a certain way about an action or practice in no way constitutes an adequate justification for making moral pronouncements on it.

The Pre-Reflective Level

At the next level of response, justification is offered by reference to values, rules, and principles—i.e., norms—accepted uncritically. Most often it is offered by reference to what we will call, somewhat loosely, a "conventional" norm. Such a standard may be expressed in a legal rule, in one of society's conventionally accepted values, in a religious pronouncement, or in a professional code of ethics. At this level of response one's opposition to abortion might take the following form: "I disapprove of abortion because my priest informs me that it is morally wrong" or "I disapprove of treating patients without their consent because this is prohibited by the professional code governing my national Medical Association."

It is a defining feature of the pre-reflective level of response that its conventional norms are uncritically accepted and acted upon. We don't stop to think why we should act or base our judgments upon the conventional norms or if they are good standards to adopt. Assuming that the conventional norms are good ones, any ensuing behaviour may be classified as conventionally moral or ethical, but it is important to realize that it is a species of externally directed behaviour. It is the blind following of standards or norms set by someone else. As noted, this is not necessarily bad. Sometimes conventional norms are capable of reasoned defence and can be fully justified morally. Sometimes there is even good moral reason to follow conventional rules just because they are conventionally accepted. Conventional norms can help to foster common understandings and serve to ground justified expectations in others concerning how we will conduct ourselves. Sometimes it is crucial to know that other people will be playing by the same rules that we are. Imagine what it would be like if there were no conventionally agreed rules governing the making of promises. We would never be certain whether a promise had been made or whether its author considered it binding.

It is a serious mistake, however, to think that morality is exhausted by conventional norms alone or that moral justification *ends* with the invocation of a conventional rule. The norms must always be subject to critical moral scrutiny. Perhaps there are much better rules which we should try to persuade others to adopt. Or perhaps existing conventions are morally objectionable. That X is generally accepted as morally right never, in itself, entails that X is morally right. Slavery was at one time widely accepted as morally correct. Slavery was, and always will be, morally wrong nonetheless. It is quite possible that practices currently sanctioned by conventional morality should likewise be modified or rejected. Morality requires eternal vigilance: we must always be prepared to think about the justification of what we are about to do.

The Reflective Level

At this level of response our moral judgments are not based entirely on conventional norms blindly accepted, but on principles, rules, and values to which we ourselves consciously subscribe and with regard to which we, as rational moral agents, are prepared to offer reasoned moral defence. It is possible of course that the norms to which we subscribe at the reflective level are in fact norms conventionally accepted as well. They might, for instance, be those which have found their way into a professional code (e.g., the Canadian Nurses Association [CNA] or Canadian Medical Association [CMA] Codes of Ethics) by which one is expected to abide. The point is that at the reflective level of moral response we must be prepared to consider questions of justification. We must not blindly accept the conventional norms but be prepared to consider for ourselves whether they are justified, or whether other, perhaps wholly novel, norms are those by which people should lead their lives.

At the reflective level, opposition to abortion may now take the form: "I oppose abortion because the fetus's right to life takes precedence over the woman's right to control her own reproductive processes." Here a reason is given—a basis or ground for the moral judgment is provided. The complexity and sophistication of the reflective level of response is evident from the presence of competing judgments and the plausible bases for them. One can imagine, as a reply to the above, the following retort: "Abortion is morally permissible because the rights of *actual* persons (pregnant women) take precedence over the rights of *potential* persons (fetuses)." As this example illustrates, ethics at the reflective level admits of few easy answers!

Of the three levels considered, the reflective level is the one at which most of the discussion in the present book takes place. This is so despite grounds for misgivings about the possibilities for full resolution of moral controversies at the reflective level. Reflection does not guarantee agreement. As will be evident throughout this book, moral reflection often yields *a* defensible position, but rarely yields the *only* defensible position. Not only do people feel differently at the expressive level, and uncritically favour different conventional rules at the pre-reflective level, they also often reach different conclusions at the reflective level. It is important to stress, once again, that there are no moral experts and that at each level, including the reflective one, we are often met with genuine dilemmas and competing bases for moral belief. Arriving at unassailable moral judgments is difficult, and some think impossible, not only because there are different levels of moral response, but also because people approach moral questions with very different perspectives.

A Variety of Perspectives

The different approaches that moral agents take to moral questions may be illustrated by distinguishing between three ways in which the term "know" can be used.

(i) Sometimes the claim to know amounts to nothing more than a claim to feel sure or certain. This yields no more than a subjective, psychological criterion. While emotionally reassuring, a feeling of certainty is not a reliable mark of bona fide moral judgments. Others with different, even opposing, moral views may feel just as strongly that they are right. One who claims to know, and tries to add as a warrant that he just feels certain about what he believes, offers no warrant at all. His certainty is no more a warrant than the certainty with which many people at one time believed slavery to be morally justified.

(ii) Next the claim to know may be reduced to: "The position I hold is the one for which the best reasoned justification seems possible." Such a claim acknowledges the requirement of reasoned defence and that the position held may not be the only defensible one. It recognizes that rational people of good will and integrity may reasonably disagree about moral matters and that no one can claim, with absolute certainty, to have *the right* answer.

(iii) The third use of "know" is much stronger than the second and, according to many moral philosophers, quite unwarranted. It is equivalent to: "I know my view is the right one, and anyone who disagrees with me suffers from moral blindness, error, or misunderstanding." Leaving aside the question of whether, in moral life, there are ever uniquely correct solutions to moral issues, the degree of self-assurance echoed in the above claim amounts to sheer audacity and arrogance. Even a commitment to the notion that there is "a final truth" in ethics should be accompanied by the acknowledgment that in practice we must often operate in humility with only partial knowledge and approximations to the truth. Moral progress is possible at both the social and the personal levels. Just as we believe that a society's practices can improve morally, as when slavery was abandoned, we should always believe that our own personal practices and beliefs can be improved, usually by listening to what others, whose opinions we respect, have to say.

Misgivings about the ethical enterprise may go even deeper than the foregoing comments suggest. There are profound philosophical disputes about the status of ethics itself—about whether moral judgments are in the end capable of full justification. Three of the more extreme difficulties are as follows.

The Issue of Verification

The problem of verification in the context of moral judgments may be illustrated by reference to the following scenario. Apple Mary is sitting in the downtown Hamilton market selling her produce. Suddenly a furtive-looking character sneaks up behind her and clubs her. As she falls to the ground, her assailant scoops up her purse and vanishes.

Imagine two witnesses commenting as follows:

A. Did you see that?
B. I did.

A. What a dreadful thing to happen in our town.
B. I agree.
A. What that man did was terribly wrong.
B. I didn't see anything wrong.
A. How can you possibly say that?
B. Easily. Let's go over carefully what happened.
A. Let's do that.
B. I saw Apple Mary sitting at her stall. I saw a man creep up behind her. I saw him lift a club and bring it down on her head. I saw Mary slump to the ground and her assailant take off with her purse. I didn't see anything wrong.

The clue to the dispute between A and B is to be found in the ambiguity of the word "see." Of course B is correct if by "see" we mean physical seeing. We do not see the wrong in the way we see arms raised, clubs wielded, and purses snatched. Moral seeing is more like "seeing that" (making a judgment) than seeing with our eyes. We see that assault is wrong. We see that stealing is wrong. Moral insights are expressed in the form of judgments which are not verifiable empirically in the way that observational statements are. Rather they are substantiated by reference to principles, rules, or values which serve as their ground or warrant. According to the first ethical theory we will examine, as well as one version of the second, we justify our actions in terms of the following schemata:

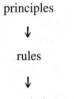

principles

↓

rules

↓

actions or judgments

The contemplated action, or a moral judgment concerning it, falls under a rule, and the rule, in turn, conforms to a higher-order principle. By contrast, the third routine we will consider involves identifying principles specifying "prima facie duties," and in situations of conflicting prima facie duties, determining which takes precedence. But more on this later. The point to be stressed at this stage is that we do not see moral properties in the way we see the club which hit Apple Mary. Moral judgments are not open to empirical verification—indeed, they cannot be substantiated by way of a universally agreed routine or procedure. There is a plurality of competing theories on how our moral judgments are to be substantiated. Most, but not all, may be mapped onto the above schemata.

A Plurality of Ethical Systems

The existence of a plurality of different approaches to the justification of moral judgments may be a cause for dismay. It is one thing to be made aware that the morality of our actions is not open to empirical verification; it is quite another to learn that different ethical theories prescribe quite different routines to be utilized in moral reasoning. It would certainly be simpler if there were only one theory and one routine. The only problems then remaining would be problems of casuistry (i.e., application of rules or principles to particular cases). But philosophers have yet to discover an ethical theory upon which all reasonable people agree, and as we have already seen, there are those who believe that no such theory will ever be found. As the understanding we have of ourselves and the world around us increases, we should expect our ethical theories to change, and we hope, progress. In this particular respect, ethics is no different from science where change and progress are routinely accepted as inevitable. The best we can do at present is to engage in the pursuit of a defensible ethical theory and try to learn as much as we can from those who have done so in the past. There is much to be learned from the theorists whose views will be outlined below.

The Limits of Justification

If one were to adopt, for example, a rule-based moral stance, the prescribed routine for justifying moral judgments would be more or less clear. It might be difficult to tell precisely what action the theory required of us in a particular case, but it would be reasonably clear how to go about trying to answer that question. Two rule-based approaches are discussed below—that of Immanuel Kant, and that of an important strain of utilitarianism. For Kant, as we

shall see, an action is morally obligatory if it conforms to a rule and the rule, in turn, conforms to a principle which Kant calls the Categorical Imperative. For a rule-utilitarian there is an analogous procedure. Our actions must conform to a rule, and the rule must conform to the principle of utility: actions must facilitate the greatest possible degree of good for the greatest possible number. For fully committed utilitarians or Kantians, justification is limited to judgments made within the prescribed framework. We inquire, "Does the action in question conform to the rule and the rule to the (appropriate) principle?" If the answer is affirmative, the morality of the action is settled and we know what the theory prescribes as the right thing to do.

It is possible, of course, for a rule-utilitarian to raise questions about Kant's Categorical Imperative or for a Kantian to challenge the principle of utility. This involves raising questions concerning the validity of the frameworks themselves. In such cases what we have is a deeply philosophical dispute, the kind of dispute which is a primary concern of ethical theorists. Utilitarians and Kantians will marshal philosophical arguments which challenge the validity of the other's ethical theory. They will do so even when it is clear what actions the opposing frameworks require of us in particular cases, or even when the different frameworks prescribe exactly the same actions. The two theorists may agree on *what* we should do but disagree about *why* we should do it. Again, the reason is clear: the philosopher is concerned to understand why we should do certain things and refrain from doing others.

External philosophical questions concerning the validity of ethical frameworks are best dealt with in books devoted exclusively to ethical theory. This is not such a book. In what follows we shall outline five competing frameworks and only briefly mention some of the many external, philosophical questions which have been raised about them. Some students will likely feel a strong affinity for one of the five theories discussed below, but most will find something of value in each one. This is not surprising. Four of the theories to be examined reflect currents of thought which have dominated western culture in recent centuries, and the fifth is expressive of a powerful contemporary movement of thought. For those strongly inclined to think that one of the theories represents the truth of the matter, the old adage should be borne in mind: "Those who live in glass houses should not throw stones." External challenges to other systems should be seasoned with a measure of caution and humility and the recognition that questions of morality and ethics are ones upon which reasonable people of good will and integrity do often disagree.

They should also be informed by the wisdom of John Stuart Mill's observation that "conflicting doctrines, instead of one being true and the other false, [often] share the truth between them, and the non-conforming opinion is needed to supply the remainder of the truth of which the received doctrine embodies only a part."[1]

Given these profound difficulties with the ethical enterprise, the student may wonder why we should bother at all with an introduction to ethical theory. Why not just get on with an analysis of the various specific, moral issues that arise in the practice of health care, issues like prescribing birth control pills to minors or screening fetuses for genetic defects? One response is that we are not warranted in dropping ethical theory altogether simply because it has difficulties. Quantum physics is fraught with theoretical difficulties too, but it would be silly to give it up entirely because of this. Another response is that there are valuable lessons to be learned from the ways in which some of the greatest thinkers within our cultural history have seriously and systematically approached ethical issues. These are thinkers whose formulations have been extremely influential and whose theories provide the frameworks within which current ethical disputes are argued. One cannot get too far in modern moral debate without encountering some appeal to the concept of utility or to the value of individual autonomy. These concepts are the cornerstones of the theories of Mill and Kant respectively.

Some Basic Concepts

Before turning to examine the theories of Kant, Mill, Ross, Aristotle, and the feminists, let us consider some basic terminology that is employed by ethical theorists. This terminology will be introduced by way of noting several distinctions.

First we should distinguish between *judgments of obligation* and *judgments of value*. Judgments of obligation concern what we ought to do. In expressing such judgments, we use sentences like: "You *ought* to take all steps to save human life"; "Your overriding *duty* was to protect the interests of your patient, not her fetus"; "You were under an obligation to honour your patient's wishes"; "It wasn't right to proceed without consent"; "He had a right to your best clinical judgment." All these judgments have to do directly with our conduct, with how we should behave.

Judgments of value, by contrast, are not directly related to action. These are judgments not about the right thing to do but about what is *good* or has *value*. For instance the judgments that freedom is a good thing for human beings to enjoy, and that pleasure is the only thing of ultimate or intrinsic worth are judgments of value. They don't tell us what is right to do. For this we need a judgment of obligation. Under some ethical theories a judgment of obligation is dependent on, and follows directly from, a judgment of value. If an ethical theory does hold that judgments of obligation are dependent in this way, then it is what philosophers call a *teleological* or *consequentialist* theory of obligation. A teleological theory of obligation posits one and only one fundamental obligation and that is to maximize the good consequences and minimize the bad consequences of our actions. Insofar as we need to know, under such theories, which consequences are good so that we can maximize them and which are bad so that we can minimize them, it is easy to see why a teleological theory of obligation presupposes a *theory of value*. Such a theory will provide us with the basis for justifying our judgments of value and thus ultimately our judgments of obligation.

The duty to maximize the good and minimize the bad consequences of our actions is the only fundamental duty under a teleological theory of obligation. On such a theory, then, any other obligations by which we feel bound, such as the obligation to honour our agreements or to tell the truth, are secondary and derivable from this one primary obligation. Mill's utilitarianism, as we shall see, is a teleological theory of obligation. In his view, all questions concerning what we ought to do are ultimately based on

[handwritten margin notes: "Judgement of obligation examples" and "Judgement of value"]

the principle of utility which requires that we maximize what is intrinsically good, namely, happiness or pleasure, and minimize what is intrinsically bad, unhappiness or pain. We have a duty to tell the truth, Mill would argue, but only because truth-telling is (normally) prescribed by the principle of utility.

In contrast to teleological theories of obligation there are those which are non-teleological. These we call *deontological theories* of obligation. Deontological theories of obligation essentially deny what teleological theories assert. They deny that we have one and only one fundamental duty, which is to maximize the good and minimize the bad consequences of our actions. There are basically two forms which this denial can take. First, a theory may suggest that the good and bad consequences of our actions have absolutely no bearing whatsoever on whether they are morally right or wrong. Such a strong deontological theory of obligation can operate wholly independently of any theory of value. We needn't know, as we do with teleological theories of obligation, what the good is if we are to know what we ought to do. The reason is simple: our obligation does not in any way involve the maximization of good consequences. Our duty is not to maximize what is ultimately of value and so we needn't have a theory of value which tells us what that is. Kant, as we shall see, appears to have held a strong deontological theory. Kant is notorious for suggesting that the rightness or wrongness of our actions is totally independent of whether or not they maximize good consequences. According to Kant, a judgment of obligation, like the judgment that health-care professionals must never withhold the truth from their patients, is in no way justified in terms of consequences. It is justified if and only if it meets the Categorical Imperative test which ignores consequences altogether.

A deontological theory of obligation need not, however, follow Kant's lead and claim that the consequences of our actions are completely irrelevant to their rightness or wrongness. There is a second kind of deontological theory which makes the weaker claim that good and bad consequences are not always the only things of moral importance. We have other ultimate obligations in addition to our duty to maximize the good and minimize the bad conse-

quences of our actions. According to Ross, for example, the principle of beneficence, which requires promoting the good of others in our actions, is only one of many ultimate principles defining our moral obligations. Others include the obligation to be grateful for benefits given and the duty to be fair to other people. In Ross's view, we sometimes have a duty to be grateful even when neglecting this duty would on that occasion lead to the best consequences overall. Some actions, such as displays of gratitude are right, regardless of their consequences. Other actions, such as instances of unfairness, are sometimes wrong, even when they lead to good consequences.

Unlike Kant and Mill, then, Ross suggests that we have many fundamental obligations. The duty to be grateful and the duty to be fair are ultimate obligations which are not based on any moral basic principle of obligation. This clearly separates Ross from Kant and Mill. We frequently have a duty to be fair, Mill would urge, but this is because being fair normally maximizes the balance of good over bad consequences. Ross will have none of this. For him the duty to be fair is just as ultimate as the duty to maximize good consequences. We have many basic obligations and these cannot be reduced to any of the others. Ross's theory of obligation, insofar as it is not based on a single, fundamental principle defining a single, fundamental obligation is a *pluralist theory of obligation*. A pluralist theory of obligation, put simply, is one which does not posit a single, fundamental obligation upon which all other secondary obligations are based. A *monistic theory of obligation*, by contrast, does posit one such obligation. A utilitarian will be happy to talk of obligations to tell the truth or to be fair to others in our dealings with them. He will simply add that we have these obligations because fairness and truth-telling usually lead, in the end and all things considered, to the best consequences. Hence his theory is monistic. So too is Kant's.

To sum up, teleological theories of obligations are all logically dependent on theories of value. Some deontological theories of obligation are also dependent on a theory of value. Strong deontological theories such as Kant's exclude, as irrelevant, questions about the good or bad consequences of our actions (i.e., the value or disvalue to be realized in them). They therefore have no need of a theory of value. But most deontological theories do have such a need, since most deontological theories are pluralistic. Most are like Ross's in espousing principles which direct us, but not exclusively, to the good and bad consequences of our actions.

When we turn to theories of value, we find that these too may be categorized as either monistic or pluralistic. A monistic theory of value, as one might expect, posits one and only one thing, or characteristic of things, as being of value for its own sake. It posits, in other words, only one thing or characteristic as intrinsically valuable. Hedonism is one influential type of monistic theory of value. On this view, pleasure is the only thing which is valuable for its own sake. Anything else we value, say money or health, is valuable only instrumentally, as a means to the pleasure it brings. Classical utilitarianism, of the form espoused by Mill and his teacher Jeremy Bentham, is hedonistic. But it needn't be. Utilitarians who agree on a theory of obligation may divide on their theories of value. G.E. Moore, for instance, was a utilitarian like Mill. But unlike Mill, Moore espoused a pluralistic theory of value which saw pleasure as only one of many things of intrinsic value. Knowledge and aesthetic experience are among many other things worthy of pursuit for their own sakes.[2] If one holds a pluralistic theory of value, then one is faced with a difficulty: what to do in situations where two or more values conflict or cannot be pursued together. If freedom from manipulation and freedom from disease are both intrinsically valuable, then doctors may have to decide somehow between allowing their patients complete freedom of choice concerning their own medical treatment (thus risking bad decisions) and leading their patients to make what they, the doctors, think is the right choice. The question arises, however, whether it is possible to compare such very different values. Is comparing freedom from manipulation with freedom from disease, so as to see which is of greater value or importance in the circumstances, something that can be done rationally? Is an attempt to compare these two values a bit like trying to compare apples with oranges?

If, on the other hand, we adopt a monistic theory of value, we may seem to rid ourselves of such problems. We only have to compare, say, one pleasure with the next. But there are serious difficulties even here. How does one compare one person's pleasure with that of another, especially if those persons are as different as Bill Clinton and Pope John Paul II?

Monistic theories of value face another objection of some importance. According to many people there are numerous things in the world of ultimate, irreducible value. Friendship, for example, seems to be compromised if an attempt is made to reduce its value to the pleasure it brings. As will be seen, the attempt to place "value" on human lives and welfare is fraught with such difficulties. Some of these will be explored later in discussions concerning the propriety of utilizing "quality of life" as a criterion for decisions involving health care.

Five Types of Ethical Theory ~This

Here follows a brief survey of five major types of ethical theory. The main reason for including the theories of Kant and Mill is that their contributions have dominated western moral thought since the scientific revolution. Kant strove to establish ethics as a purely rational enterprise, while Mill believed that an objective standard of right and wrong could be discovered in the methods of the empirical sciences. If the rightness of our actions depends on the pleasure and pain they produce, then we ought to be able to estimate their rightness by empirical observation, measurements, and induction. Mill's utilitarianism is an ancestor of modern theories of cost-benefit analysis, which are assuming an ever-increasing role in controversies surrounding the allocation of money to various forms of health care.

Between them Kant and Mill zero in on the roles played respectively by intention and consequences in shaping our moral responses. One cannot get very far in discussions of ethics without paying deference to the Kantian notions of autonomy and universalizability, or the injunction to treat human beings as ends in themselves and not merely as means. Similarly one cannot ignore Mill's emphasis on protecting and promoting human happiness or well-being.

W.D. Ross's contribution to ethics is invaluable not only for its reaction to Kant and Mill, but because, in certain crucial respects, it seems more accurately to reflect the ordinary thinking and practice of moral agents than the more systematic reflections of professional moral philosophers. This is particularly evident in Ross's opposition to Kant's and Mill's reductionism in moral theory. Ross was unwilling to subscribe to a monistic theory of obligation. While acknowledging the powerful contributions of Kant and Mill to ethical theory, Ross resists elevating either the Categorical Imperative or the principle of utility to the status of a foundational first principle from which all other moral principles, rules, and judgments follow. In coming to grips with the moral issues considered in this text, it will be difficult to escape making reference to Ross's notion of *prima facie* duty.

Contemporary ethical theorists have expressed renewed interest in the ethical writings of the ancient Greek philosopher, Aristotle. Among Aristotle's many contributions to the history of ethical thought is his doctrine of the mean. As we will see below, Aristotle attempts to isolate a number of virtues which we can more or less express or display in our lives when we aim for the *golden mean* between undesirable extremes. For example, we display the virtue courage when, in conducting our lives, we successfully steer clear of the extremes of cowardliness and foolhardiness. Courage is the mean between these two vices, and a courageous person is one whose character and (developed) dispositions lead him to act in neither a foolhardy nor a cowardly manner.

Those who are impressed with the immense complexity of moral life, and with the difficulties encountered when we try to articulate rules and principles to cover all cases, may find enormous potential in the Aristotelian approach. It is a consequence of Aristotle's conception of the moral life that there are no hard and fast rules or principles to tell us whether and to what extent our conduct approximates the relevant mean and is therefore virtuous. There are also no hard and fast rules to tell us what to do when our situation involves more than one virtue, as when our beneficence inclines us towards treating someone who would object were she informed about the matter, but our wish to be an honest person leads us in the other direction. In addressing moral questions we are not asking for rules

which tell us what to do on some particular occasion. Rather, we are asking ourselves what kind of person we would be, what kinds of virtues we would display, were we to conduct our lives in a particular manner. And to these types of questions there are almost never uniquely correct answers. Perhaps in this respect Aristotle's theory more accurately reflects our moral experience, and the humility of which we have spoken above.

Finally, we have included a section on feminist perspectives. Feminist writings in health care ethics have been characterized as much by the *approach* taken to ethical theory as by any distinctive set of principles, rules, or values. Most varieties of feminist ethics are marked by a heightened concern for the personal and social *contexts* in which ethical decisions are made, and by the ways in which traditional ethical theory, with its attempt to discover universal, and therefore necessarily abstract, moral norms, ignores the context in which decisions are made. Of particular concern to most feminists is the perceived failure of mainstream ethical theory to appreciate the context of oppressed individuals, like women and the socially vulnerable, and the various ways in which their legitimate concerns and interests are ignored, undervalued, or suppressed.

Utilitarianism

As noted above, utilitarianism is an ethical theory founded on the belief that the right action is that which facilitates the greatest possible degree of good for all those affected by the action. It is a monistic theory in that it posits a single fundamental obligation upon which all other secondary obligations are based; and it is a teleological theory in that it rests on a theory of value. In the context of this introduction we will largely ignore the different theories of value espoused by utilitarians, and concentrate instead on what they have to say about obligation.

Essentially there are two different kinds of utilitarianism, act and rule utilitarianism. Act utilitarianism (AU) defines the rightness or wrongness of individual actions in terms of the good or bad consequences realized by those actions themselves. In other words, AU defines the rightness or wrongness of an action in terms of its "utility" and "disutility." The term "utility" stands for whatever it is that is intrinsically valuable under the utilitarian's theory of value, "disutility" for whatever is thought to be intrinsically bad. According to John Stuart Mill, "actions are right in proportion as they tend to promote happiness; wrong as they tend to produce the reverse of happiness."[3] For him "utility" means happiness, and "disutility" unhappiness. Mill went on to identify happiness with pleasure and unhappiness with pain. Hence, Mill may be characterized as a *hedonistic* utilitarian, one on whose theory of value pleasure is the only thing of intrinsic worth. But a utilitarian need not make this identification, nor need he define utility in terms of happiness. Some utilitarians think it best to define utility in terms of the satisfaction of our actual preferences, while others would have us look to satisfy preferences we would have were we fully informed and rational. Regardless of the theory of value with which it is associated, however, AU always makes the following claim:

AU: An act is right if and only if there is no other action I could have done instead which either (a) would have produced a greater balance of utility over disutility; or (b) would have produced a smaller balance of disutility over utility

We must add (b) to account for those unfortunate situations where whatever we do we seem to cause more disutility than utility—where we're damned if we do and damned if we don't. In short, AU tells us to act always so as to bring about the best consequences we can, and sometimes that means trying to make the best of a bad situation.

AU was made famous in modern times by Mill and Bentham, at a time when it was quite natural for many people to think that some individuals simply count more than others. There were some who thought that members of the aristocracy, the Church, or a particular race were in some sense more worthy or superior than others and were therefore deserving of special consideration or privilege. The utilitarians were part of a social revolution which would have none of this. In the famous words of Bentham, "each is to count for one, none to count for more than one." In other words, according to utilitarians, *all* those affected by my actions should count *equally* in my

deliberations concerning my moral obligations. The happiness of the King is to count equally with the equal happiness of the shop clerk. Mill put this important point in the following way:

I must again repeat what the assailants of utilitarianism seldom have the justice to acknowledge, that the happiness which forms the utilitarian standard of what is right in conduct is *not* the agent's own happiness but that of all concerned. As between others, utilitarianism requires him to be as *strictly impartial as a disinterested benevolent spectator*.[4]

So built into AU is a commitment to equality and impartiality. We are to be concerned equally and impartially with the happiness or welfare, i.e., utility, of all those, including ourselves, who might be affected by our actions. On these grounds alone, AU is a very appealing theory. What could be better than to be sure that I always maximize, not my own happiness or that of my friends, but the happiness of all those people affected by my actions whoever they might be? What more could morality require?

Despite its inherently desirable features, many philosophers have come to find serious difficulties with AU. These have led some utilitarians to opt for an alternative form of the theory. One of the more serious difficulties for AU revolves around *special duties* and *special relationships*. These include duties of loyalty, of fidelity, and familial obligations. The latter rest in part on the special relationships which arise out of family ties and require some degree of partiality and special concern towards family members. It would be wrong, some think, to be impartial between friends and family, on the one hand, and perfect strangers on the other. It would be equally wrong to be impartial between one's patient and others who might benefit from the knowledge to be gained from using one's patient in an experiment. The importance of personal relationships in the moral evaluation of conduct is often stressed by feminists who reject the "impartiality" required by utilitarianism. In their view, treating everyone the same would be equivalent to treating them all as strangers.

Let us centre on promises to illustrate some of the most serious difficulties facing AU. Suppose I am a doctor and that a dear friend, Monica, comes to my clinic concerned that she might have AIDS. Monica has been unfaithful to her husband, Jack, whom I have also known for years. Our friendships go a long way back and are a continual source of happiness for all of us. However, nervousness about the possibility of HIV infection has got Monica worried. In order to ease her concern, I run the appropriate tests and determine that Monica has not been exposed to the HIV virus (the cause of AIDS). She is extremely relieved. Now she can continue her affair without worry. Her partner had a similar test done recently and so they are both clean. As Monica leaves my office she announces with a smile that of course she fully expects me to keep quiet about the test and the on-going affair. Under no circumstances must Jack ever find out. She points out that as her physician I owe her a duty of confidentiality, a duty which is even stronger in this case, given our long friendship.

Upon reflection, however, I begin to wonder whether my duty does ultimately lie in confidentiality. I add up the utilities and disutilities involved for all affected by my decision, including not only Jack and Monica but their two young children and Monica's sexual partner as well. I correctly conclude that overall utility would be maximized, on balance, if I told Jack about the affair. He's a very reasonable and forgiving person and would likely be able to keep the marriage on track, something which would be of benefit to the entire family. As for Monica's partner, he will likely experience no difficulty in finding another sexual partner. As a consequence of my valid, act-utilitarian reasoning, I betray the confidence, despite my apparent duty as a physician and a friend. I consider it my moral obligation to maximize utility, even at the expense of harming a dear friend and violating a trust which has been placed in me.

Some philosophers believe that examples such as this show that AU takes promises, commitments, special relationships of trust, and so on, far too lightly. Indeed, some think it makes such factors totally irrelevant. This is because AU is a monistic theory of obligation which posits one and only one obligation—to maximize utility. Future consequences are all that count. Past commitments and special relationships are irrelevant.

A defender of AU, on the other hand, will likely reply that I have simply failed to consider all the relevant consequences. Of crucial importance here is not simply the fact that a marriage may be saved and a potentially destructive affair stopped, but also that my action will almost certainly destroy at least one valuable relationship (my friendship with Monica) which, in the long run, would add significantly to the utility I am able to bring about in my future actions. There is also the possibility that my betrayal will become common knowledge, thus threatening my role as a physician who can be trusted. Without my patients' trust, how can I practice medicine effectively? And if I cannot practice medicine effectively, how am I going to promote utility in my role as a doctor? Of course there's also the possibility that my action will weaken the public's trust of physicians in general—an even more disastrous possibility, viewed from the perspective of AU. All of these indirect consequences of breaking the agreement, when put into the balance, tip the scales in favour of keeping quiet. Those who think that AU takes special relationships and commitments far too lightly have simply ignored all the long-range, indirect effects of doing so.

So the defender of AU has a fairly forceful reply to such counter-examples to his theory of obligation. We should always be sure to ask, when a critic provides such an example: Have all the relevant consequences, long-range and indirect as well as immediate and direct, been accounted for? In all likelihood, they have not been. This is true whether we are talking about breaking confidences or violating autonomy.

Philosophers are fairly industrious when it comes to thinking up counter-examples to ethical theories. Having met replies such as the above, they have altered their counter examples to get rid of those convenient indirect, long-range effects upon which the defence is based. Some have dreamt up the *Desert Island Promise Case*, a version of which now follows.

You and a friend are alone on a deserted island. Your friend is dying and asks you to see to it when you are rescued that the elder of her two children receives the huge sum of money your friend has secretly stashed away. You now are the only other person who knows of its existence. You solemnly promise to fulfil your friend's final request and she passes away secure in the knowledge that her last wish is in good hands. Upon rescue you are faced with a dilemma. The elder child turns out to be a lazy lout who squanders to no good end—even his own pleasure—whatever money he has. Even when he has lots of money to spend he still ends up being miserable and causing misery to other people. Your friend's younger child, however, is an aspiring researcher in dermatology. She is on the brink of uncovering a solution to the heartache of psoriasis, but will fail unless she receives financial backing. All her applications for grants have unjustly been denied and she has been left in desperation. As a good act utilitarian, you reason that utility would obviously be maximized if your solemn word to your dying friend were broken and you gave the money to the younger daughter. Think of all the utility that would be realized, all the suffering that would be alleviated! Compare this with the very little utility and considerable disutility that would result were you to give the money to the elder son.

Notice that in this case all the indirect, long-range consequences to which appeal was made in Monica's case are absent. No one will know that the promise is being broken and there are no valuable, utility-enhancing relationships in jeopardy. Your friend is dead. There seems little doubt in this situation that the promise should be broken according to AU—this is your moral obligation. But surely, the opponent will argue, this cannot be so. Solemn promises to dying friends, regardless of the good consequences which might be realized by breaking them, must be kept, except perhaps where disaster would result from keeping them. That it seems in such cases to give no weight at all to such promises shows that AU is a faulty theory of obligation. Solemn promises should weigh heavily—and independently of good consequences. Hence AU cannot be an adequate theory.

So promises and other such special commitments pose difficulties for AU. Free riders do too. Suppose there is a temporary but serious energy shortage in your community. All private homes and businesses have been requested to conserve electricity and gas. Private homes are to keep their thermostats no higher than 15 degrees centigrade and all businesses are temporarily to cut production by one-half. If everyone helps out in this way an overload which would prove disastrous will be avoided. Being a good act utilitarian, and knowing the tendencies of your neighbours, you reason as follows: "I know that everyone else will pay scrupulous attention to the government's request. So the potential disaster will be averted regardless of what I do. It will make no difference whatsoever if I run my production lines at two-thirds capacity. The little bit of extra electricity we use will have no negative effect at all. Of course if everyone ran at two-thirds, then disaster would result, but I know this is not going to happen and so the point is irrelevant. As for my employees, they will see a reduction and assume that the cut was to one-half, so no one will know but me. Using two-thirds, then, will in no way prove harmful, but it will make a considerable amount of difference to my balance sheet. The extra production will enable the company to show a much higher profit this year. All things considered, then, it is morally permissible, indeed, my moral obligation, to run at two-thirds. This is what AU tells me that I should do."

Imagine the moral outrage which would result were your acting on this line of reasoning to become common knowledge. If the case seems far-fetched, consider how an analogous line of reasoning could be employed to justify extra diagnostic tests for a patient. Were you to pursue the recommended conduct, you would be labelled a "free rider," one who rides freely while others shoulder the burdens necessary for all to prosper. Your actions would be thought most unfair to all those who had willingly sacrificed their best interests, or the interests of their patients, for the good of everyone concerned. All this despite your efforts to maximize the utility of your actions.

In response to these (and similar) sorts of objections, some utilitarians have developed an alternative to AU. Consider further what would be said if your free riding came to light. The likely response would be to say: "Sure, no one is harmed if you use the extra electricity or prescribe the extra diagnostic tests. But imagine what would happen if everyone did what you are doing. Imagine if that became the norm. Disaster would result!" This request: "Imagine what would happen if everybody did that" has great probative force for many people. If *not everyone* could do what I propose to do without serious harm resulting, then many are prepared to say that it would be wrong for *anyone* to do it, and hence wrong for me to do it. In response to the force of this intuition, some utilitarians have developed a very different variety of their theory called *rule utilitarianism* (RU). On this version the rightness or wrongness of an action is not to be judged by its consequences. Rather, it is to be judged by the consequences of everyone's adopting a *general rule* under which the action falls.

As an introduction to RU, consider a case outlined by John Rawls in his famous paper "Two Concepts of Rules."[5] Rawls has us imagine that we are a sheriff in the deep American south. The rape of a white woman has taken place and although the identity of the rapist is unknown, it is clear that the offender was black. The predominantly white and racially bigoted community is extremely agitated over the incident and great social unrest is threatening. Riots are about to break out and many innocent, and possibly some not so innocent, people will be killed. If you were able to identify and arrest the rapist, the unrest would undoubtedly subside; but unfortunately you have no leads, other than the fact that the rapist was black. It occurs to you that you do not really need the actual culprit to calm things down. Why not simply concoct a case against a randomly chosen black man who has no alibi and have him arrested? The crowd will be placated, and although one innocent man will suffer, many innocent lives will be saved.

Rawls uses this example to illustrate an apparent weakness in AU and how RU allows one to overcome it. The consequences of framing the (possibly) innocent black are far better (or less bad), in terms of utility, than allowing the riot to occur. Hence, AU seems to require the frame, a course of action which is clearly unjust. Of course the defender of AU has several tricks up his sleeve at this point. He can once again appeal to the possible indirect effects of the frame. Suppose the lie came to light. Terrible social paranoia and unrest would result; people would no longer trust the judicial system and would wonder

constantly whether they might be next. Indirect consequences such as these, the defender of AU will argue, clearly outweigh any short-term, direct benefits. But Rawls suggests that we consider a different question than the one AU would have us ask. We are to consider whether a general rule which permits the framing of innocent persons could possibly figure in a moral code general acceptance of which would result in the maximization of utility. If it could not (which is surely the case), then the proposed frame is morally impermissible. Since no such general rule could find its way into an acceptable moral code, largely for the reasons mentioned above in the parenthetical aside, an action in accordance with that rule would be morally wrong. Hence it would be morally wrong on RU to frame the possibly innocent black, even if the consequences of that particular action would be better than those of the alternatives. We are not morally required, on RU, to perform actions which individually would maximize utility. Rather we are to perform actions which accord with a set of rules whose general observance would maximize utility. Actions are judged according to whether they conform with acceptable rules; only the rules themselves are judged in terms of utility. The essence of RU is expressed in the following claim:

RU: An act is morally right if and only if it conforms with a set of rules whose general observance would maximize utility.

One extremely important difference between RU and AU is worth stressing. It is quite possible, on RU, to be required to perform an action which does not, on that particular occasion, maximize utility. Observance of the best set of general rules does not, on each individual occasion, always lead to the best consequences. Of course it *generally* does, but there are exceptions. This is something the defender of RU seems willing to live with for the sake of overall, long-term utility gains and the ability to deal with desert-island promises, free riders, and so on.

RU is not without its difficulties, however. Some utilitarians claim, for example, that RU really does violate the spirit of utilitarianism and amounts to "rule worship."[6] If the ideal behind utilitarianism is the maximization of utility, then should we not be able to deviate from the generally acceptable rules when doing so will serve to maximize utility? If the defender of RU allows exceptions to be made in such cases, then he runs the risk of collapsing his RU into AU. The rules would no longer hold any special weight or authority in our moral decisions. We would end up following the rules when it is best to do so and depart from them when that seems best.[7] In each case we seem led to do what AU requires, namely, maximize the utility of our individual actions. If, on the other hand, the defender of RU holds fast and says we must *never* deviate from rules which generally advance utility but sometimes do not, then the charge of rule worship comes back to plague the utilitarian.

A second problem facing RU can be summed up in an example. Suppose it were true that the best set of rules for the circumstances of our society would place an obligation on first-born children to provide for their elderly parents. I, the younger of two sons, reason that I therefore have no obligation whatsoever to provide for my elderly parents, even though I know that my elder brother is unwilling to provide more than the 50 per cent he thinks we each ought to provide. My parents end up living a life of abject poverty on only 50 per cent of what they need to sustain themselves. Something seems clearly wrong here. Our obligations, it would seem, cannot be entirely a function of an *ideal code* which may never in fact be followed by anyone except me. We seem to require, in an acceptable moral theory, some recognition of how other people are behaving, what rules they are in fact following. The rules they are following may be perfectly acceptable but not ideal, in which case I should perhaps follow them too. This is as true in medicine as it is elsewhere. Serious harm might result were an idealistic physician to act according to an ideal code, general observance of which would maximize utility, when no one else was prepared to do so. Perhaps here the excuse, "But no one else is willing to do it" carries some weight.

To sum up, there are significant differences between AU and RU and neither theory is free from difficulty. AU requires that we always seek, on each particular occasion, to maximize utility. It has difficulties with, among other things, free riders, desert-

island promises, and sheriffs tempted by good consequences to commit injustice. RU tells us to perform actions that conform to a set of rules general observance of which would lead to the best consequences overall. This theory seems to provide solutions to many of the problems plaguing AU but it does so only at the expense of introducing new puzzles of its own. It must somehow provide a bridge between the best ideal code and the actual beliefs, practices, and accepted rules of one's society, all the while steering a course between rule worship and a straightforward reduction to AU.

Deontological Ethics: Immanuel Kant

Kant, like Mill, proposes a monistic theory of obligation. Unlike that of Mill, however, the theory is thoroughly non-consequentialist. It denies that the possible consequences of our actions are what determine their rightness or wrongness. According to Kant,

> An action done from duty has its moral worth, not in *the purpose* [i.e., the consequences] to be attained by it, but in the maxim in accordance with which it is decided upon; it depends, therefore, not on the realization of the object of the action, but solely on the *principle of volition* [the maxim] in accordance with which, irrespective of all objects of the faculty of desire [i.e., pleasure, happiness, preferences] the action has been performed.[8]

In this remark we see clearly that Kant espouses a deontological theory of obligation. The morality of an action is determined not by its consequences but by the maxim, the general principle, to which it conforms. Its moral worth lies not in the happiness or pleasure it produces, but in the kind of action it is. Let's try to clarify this point.

A key notion in Kant's theory is that of a maxim. By this technical term Kant means a general rule or principle which specifies what it is I conceive myself as doing and my reason for doing it. For example, suppose I decide to tell a lie in order to avoid distress to my patient. The maxim of my action could be expressed in the following way: "Whenever I am able to avoid distress to my patient by lying, I shall do so." This maxim makes plain that I conceive myself as lying and that my reason is the avoidance of a patient's distress. It makes plain that I consider the avoidance of such distress as a *sufficient reason* to lie. Were I to act on my maxim I would in effect be expressing my commitment to a general rule which extends in its scope beyond the particular situation in which I find myself. In supposing that the avoidance of patient distress is a sufficient reason in that situation to lie, I commit myself to holding that in any other situation just like it, i.e., any other case in which a lie would serve to avoid a patient's distress, I should tell a lie. This *generalizability of reasons* and maxims can perhaps be illustrated through an example involving a non-moral judgment.

Suppose you and I are baseball fans.

I say to you, "The Toronto Blue Jays are a good baseball team because their team batting average is about .260 and the average ERA among their starting pitchers is under 3.50."

You reply, "What is your opinion of the Philadelphia Phillies?"

I say, "They are a lousy team."

You reply, "But their team batting average is also about .260 and the average ERA among their starters is 3.40."

I am stuck here in a logical inconsistency. I must either modify my earlier assessment of the Blue Jays—say that they too are a lousy team—or admit that the Phillies are also a good team. By citing my reasons for judging the Blue Jays a good ball team, I commit myself to a general maxim that *any* baseball team with a team batting average of over .260 and whose starting rotation has an ERA of below 3.50 is a good baseball team. If I don't agree with the implications of that general maxim, e.g., I still think the Phillies are a bad ball team, then logical consistency demands that I reject or modify the maxim. Perhaps I will add that in addition to a team batting average of over .260 and an ERA among starting pitchers of under 3.50, a good baseball team must have several "clutch" players. I would add this if I thought that the absence of clutch players explains why the Phillies, unlike the Blue Jays, are not a good team. Of course I could make this alteration only if I thought the Blue Jays did have at least a few clutch players.

So my maxim that whenever I can avoid distress to my patient by lying I shall do so, insofar as it expresses a general reason, applies to other situations similar to the one in which I initially act upon it. But this is not the full extent of my commitment. If avoiding patient distress really is a sufficient reason for *my* telling a lie, then it must also be a sufficient reason for *anyone else* who finds herself in a situation just like mine. According to Kant, and virtually all moral philosophers, acting upon a maxim commits me, as a rational moral agent, to a *universal* moral rule governing all persons in situations just like mine (in the relevant respects). I must be prepared to accept that a sufficient reason for me is a sufficient reason for anyone else in precisely my situation. This is the force of the first formulation of Kant's Categorical Imperative we are about to consider. If I think some other person in a position to avoid patient distress by lying should not tell the lie, then I must either retract my earlier maxim or specify some relevant difference between our situations, as I did when I tried to show that the Expos are a bad baseball team despite their strong team batting average and pitching staff.

The Categorical Imperative, First Formation: Logical Consistency

Acting for reasons, that is, acting rationally (which is required, according to Kant if we are to be moral), commits me to universal rules or maxims which I must be prepared to accept. Kant expresses this point in terms of my capacity to will that my personal maxim should become a *universal law*. According to the first formulation of the Categorical Imperative, the fundamental principle of obligation in Kant's monistic system, "I ought never to act except in such a way that *I can also will that my maxim should become a universal law*."[9] Later he writes, "*Act as if the maxim of your action were to become through your will a universal law of nature*."[10] According to Kant, immoral maxims and the immoral actions based upon them can never, under any conceivable circumstances, pass the Categorical Imperative test. This is not, as we shall now see, because the consequences of general observance of an immoral maxim would be undesirable in terms of utility. Rather it is because the state of affairs in which the maxim is observed as a universal law is *logically impossible* or *inconceivable*—it involves us in contradiction.

Some states of affairs simply cannot exist, in the strongest sense of "cannot." The state of affairs in which I am, at one and the same time, Rob's father *and* Rob's son is logically impossible. It cannot exist. Were I for some strange reason to will that this state of affairs exist, my will, Kant would say, would contradict itself. It would be willing inconsistent, contradictory things: that I am Rob's father and son at one and the same time. Now consider a case actually discussed by Kant. Suppose that a man

> finds himself driven to borrowing money because of need. He well knows that he will not be able to pay it back; but he sees too that he will get no loan unless he gives a firm promise to pay it back within a fixed time. He is inclined to make such a promise; but he has still enough conscience to ask "Is it not unlawful and contrary to duty to get out of difficulties in this way?" Supposing, however, he did resolve to do so, the maxim of his action would run thus, "Whenever I believe myself short of money, I will borrow money and promise to pay it back, though I know that this will never be done." Now this principle of self-love or personal advantage is perhaps quite compatible with my own entire future welfare; only there remains the question "Is it right?" I therefore transform the demand of self love into a universal law and frame my question thus, "How would things stand if my maxim became a universal law?" I then see straight away that this maxim can never rank as a universal law of nature and be self-consistent, but must necessarily contradict itself. For the universality of a law that every one believing himself to be in need can make any promise he pleases with the intention not to keep it would make promising, and the very purpose of promising, itself impossible, since no one would believe he was being promised anything, but would laugh at utterances of this kind as empty shams.[11]

It is important to be clear exactly what Kant is saying in this passage. He is not objecting to insincere promises on the ground that they will cause oth-ers to lose confidence in us and mean that we will jeopardize the valuable consequences of future promises. Nor is he arguing that false promises contribute to a general mistrust of promises and the eventual collapse of a valuable social practice. These are all *consequentialist* considerations which, according to the deontologist Kant, are totally irrelevant to questions of moral obligation. His point is a very different one. He is suggesting that a state of affairs in which everyone in need makes false promises is incoherent. There is a *contradiction* because, on the one hand, everyone in need *would* borrow on false promises. They would be following the maxim "as a law of nature," with the same regularity as the planets observe Kepler's laws of planetary motion. Yet on the other hand, in this very same state of affairs no one *could* borrow on a false promise, because if such promises were always insincere, no one would be stupid enough to lend any money. Promising requires trust on the part of the promisee, but in the state of affairs contemplated there just couldn't be any, and so promises of the sort in question would simply be impossible. Hence, any attempt to will, as a universal law of nature, the maxim "Whenever I believe myself short of money, I will borrow money and promise to pay it back, though I know that this will never be done," lands us in contradiction. "I ... see straight away that this maxim can never rank as a universal law of nature and be self-consistent, but must necessarily contradict itself."[12]

With Kant, then, we have a moral test of our actions which does not lie in an assessment of their consequences. Nor does the test lie in weighing the consequences of adopting a general rule which licences those actions. Rather, the test considers the logical coherence of the universalized maxim upon which I personally propose to act. Whether this test successfully accounts for all of our moral obligations is highly questionable. Is there anything incoherent in the state of affairs in which everyone kills his neighbour if she persists in playing her stereo at ear-piercing levels? Such a state of affairs might be highly *undesirable* (though some days I really do wonder) but it seems perfectly possible or conceivable. Yet killing off annoying neighbours seems hardly the right thing to do.

The Categorical Imperative, Second Formulation:
Don't Just Use People

Kant provided two further formulations of his Categorical Imperative. He thought these versions equivalent to the first, though it is difficult to see why
Kant thought this to be so. The equivalence question
needn't concern us here however. The additional formulations bring to light two important principles
which many people find highly appealing and which
may prove helpful in dealing with some of the problems discussed later in this text.

According to Kant, if I act only on maxims
which could, without contradiction, serve as universal laws I will never treat people as *mere means*
to my ends. The Categorical Imperative requires
that I "Act in such a way that [I] always treat
humanity, whether in [my] own person or in the
person of any other, never simply as a means, but
always at the same time as an end."[13] In more common terms, we should never just *use* people. The
emphasis here is on the *intrinsic worth* and *dignity*
of rational creatures. I treat rational beings as ends
in themselves if I respect in them the same value I
discover in myself, namely, my freedom to determine myself to action and to act for reasons which
I judge for myself. As Kant observes, there can be
nothing more dreadful to a rational creature than
that his actions should be subject to the will of
another. I treat others as mere things rather than as
persons, subject them to my will in the way I do a
tool, if I fail to respect their dignity. This principle
has an important role to play in assessing, for
example, the therapeutic relationship, the requirement of informed, valid consent to medical experimentation, and requests for physician-assisted
suicide.

The Categorical Imperative, Third Formulation:
Autonomous Agents

Kant's third formulation of the Categorical Imperative seems closely tied to the second. In effect, it
spells out what it is in rational agents which gives
them their dignity and worth. It requires that we treat
others as *autonomous* agents, capable of self-directed, rational action. The capacity to rise above the

compelling forces of desire, self-interest, and physical necessity, to act freely on the basis of *reasons*, is
what gives rational beings their dignity and worth. To
treat a person as an end in herself, then, is to respect
her autonomy and freedom. It rules out various kinds
of manipulative practices and paternalistically motivated behaviours. In a case involving asbestos poi-
soning at Johns Manville,[14] company doctors
neglected to tell workers the alarming results of their
medical tests. This was rationalized on the ground
that there was nothing that could be done to curb the
disease anyway, and so the workers were better off
not knowing. Such paternalistic conduct clearly violated Kant's Categorical Imperative. It failed to
respect the autonomy and dignity of the asbestos
workers. Of course the conduct might have been fully
justified by AU, though this point is open to argument. Whether in the long run such deceptions serve
to maximize utility is perhaps questionable.

With Kant we have a clear alternative to the
monistic, teleological theory of obligation provided
by the act and rule utilitarians. Kant's theory is clearly deontological and is at the very least monistic in
its intent. Kant attempts to ground all our obligations
on one fundamental principle: the Categorical
Imperative. As we have seen, Kant provides three
formulations of this principle, though it is difficult to
see how they are exactly equivalent. In any event, we
may view Kant as requiring that we ask the following three questions:

1. Could I consistently will, as a universal law, the
   personal maxim upon which I propose to act?
2. Would my action degrade other rational agents or
   myself by treating them or myself as a mere
   means?
3. Would my action violate the autonomy of some
   rational agent, possibly myself?

Should any of these three questions yield the wrong
answer, my moral obligation is to refrain from acting
on my personal maxim.

Ethical Pluralism: W.D. Ross

As we noted above, W.D. Ross's contribution to
ethics is valuable both for its reaction to what some

see as the reductionism of Kant and Mill, and because it seems more accurately to reflect the ordinary thinking and practice of moral agents than the more systematic reflections of professional moral philosophers.

Ross's theory of obligation arose mainly out of his dissatisfaction with utilitarian theories. While Ross's main target was G.E. Moore, his criticisms are relevant to utilitarianism in general, particularly AU. According to Ross, utilitarianism in all of its guises grossly oversimplifies the moral relationships between people. As we have seen, utilitarianism is, in the end, concerned solely with the maximization of utility. Our concern should rest exclusively with the overall consequences of our actions, or the rules under which we perform them. In Ross's view, morality should acknowledge the importance of consequences, but not exclusively. Utilitarianism errs in thinking that consequences are all that matter, in thinking that "the only morally significant relationship in which my neighbours stand to me is that of being possible beneficiaries [or victims] of my action."[15] It errs, in other words, in being a monistic, teleological theory of obligation. Ross proposes instead a pluralistic theory of obligation which recognizes several, irreducible moral relationships and principles. In addition to their role as possible beneficiaries of my actions, my fellow human beings "may also stand to me in the relation of promisee to promiser, of creditor to debtor, of wife to husband, of child to parent, of friend to friend, of fellow countryman to fellow countryman, and the like."[16] "The like" no doubt includes the relation of doctor to patient, doctor to nurse, experimenter to subject and so on, relationships which are integral to the health-care professions and which are ignored only at the cost of moral confusion.

In Ross's view, utilitarianism not only oversimplifies the moral relationships in which we stand to others, it also distorts the whole basis of morality by being thoroughly teleological in orientation. On utilitarian theories we must always be *forward-looking* to the future consequences of our actions or rules. But sometimes, Ross urges, morality requires that we look *backwards* to what has occurred in the past. There is significance, for example, in the sheer fact that a promise has been made, a promise which has moral force independent of any future good consequences that might arise from keeping it. This moral force explains why we should normally keep promises made to dying friends even if utility would be maximized were we to break them. A promise itself, because of the *kind* of action it is, has a moral force which is totally independent of its consequences. Teleological theories, because they ignore such features and are entirely forward-looking, distort morality. *Promises*, *contracts*, *commitments* to serve a certain role, *agreements*, *loyalty*, *friendship*, and so on, all have moral force, and all can give rise to obligations and responsibilities independently of good or bad consequences.

Ross provides us, then, with a pluralistic, deontological theory of obligation. In this theory we find a plurality of ultimate principles, only some of which are consequentialist in orientation. According to Ross, each of these principles specifies a *prima facie* duty or obligation. These are duties which we must fulfil *unless* we are also, in the circumstances, subject to another, competing prima facie duty of greater weight. We have a prima facie duty to tell the truth, which means that we must always tell the truth unless a more stringent duty applies to us and requires a falsehood. An example from Kant helps to illustrate this feature nicely.

Kant is notorious for arguing that the Categorical Imperative establishes an unconditional duty always to tell the truth. He has us consider a case where a murderer comes to our door asking for the whereabouts of his intended victim. Should we tell him the truth, that the victim is seeking refuge in our house, and thereby become accomplices in his murder? Both AU and RU would undoubtedly license a lie under such extraordinary circumstances, but according to Kant the Categorical Imperative does not. The duty to tell the truth is unconditional, despite the consequences of its observance. "To be truthful (honest) in all declarations ... is a sacred and absolutely commanding decree of reason, limited by no expediency."[17] According to Ross's theory this is not so. Kant's case is clearly one where our prima facie duty to be truthful is overridden or outweighed by more stringent duties to our friend.

Ross's list of prima facie duties provides a helpful classification of some of the various duties and morally significant relationships recognized in our everyday moral thinking. There are:

1. Duties resting on previous actions of our own. These include:
   (a) duties of *fidelity* arising from explicit or implicit promises;
   (b) duties of *reparation*, resting on previous wrongful acts of ours and requiring that we compensate, as best we can, the victims of our wrongful conduct.
2. Duties resting on the services of others; duties of gratitude which require that we return favour for favour.
3. Duties involving the *fair* distribution of goods; duties of *justice*, which require fair sharing of goods to be distributed.
4. Duties to improve the condition of others; duties of *beneficence* (which in part form the basis of utilitarian theories of obligation).
5. Duties to improve our own condition; duties of *self-improvement*.
6. Duties not to injure others; duties of *non-maleficence*.[18]

Ross's list of duties is by no means exhaustive, and no doubt many would quarrel with some of the duties Ross has included. For instance, it might be questioned whether duties of self-improvement belong on a list of *moral* duties. It is plausible to suppose that moral duties arise only in our relationships with other people; that the demands of morality govern inter-personal relationships only. Allowing one's talents to lie unused or allowing one's health to deteriorate may be imprudent or foolish, but is it immoral? Perhaps it is if others, say our children, are depending on us. But in this case it is not a moral duty of self-improvement which is violated but rather the duty of beneficence and possibly that of non-maleficence.

Another questionable entry on Ross's list is the duty to be grateful. If someone does me a favour, is it true that I am required, as a matter of duty, to be grateful? Is gratitude something that can be subject to duty, or is it rather something that must be freely given, given not out of a sense of duty but out of genuine, heartfelt goodwill? If a favour is done with the sense that something is *owing* as a result, then perhaps it is not really a favour at all, but an investment.

According to Ross, that we have the prima facie duties he mentions is simply *self-evident* to any rational human being who thinks seriously about the requirements of morality. The existence of these duties, and the validity of the principles which describe them, are known through *moral intuition*. To say that a principle is self-evident and known through intuition is to say that its truth is evident to an attentive mind, that it neither needs supporting evidence nor needs to be deduced from other propositions. It stands alone as something obviously true. In this instance, it stands alone as something whose truth is known directly through *moral* intuition.

This feature of Ross's theory is very controversial among philosophers, who are generally suspicious of "self-evident principles" and "intuition." In the case of morality, the apparent obviousness of some principles, and the certainty with which many believe them, seem better explained by such things as uniform moral upbringing and common experiences. And then there is the problem of disagreement. If a principle truly is self-evident, then should not everyone agree on its validity? Yet this is seldom, if ever, the case with moral principles, including those on Ross's list.

This is not the place to discuss further the reasons behind the philosopher's suspicions concerning self-evidence and moral intuition, except to add the following. One who claims self-evidence for his views has little to say to those holding conflicting self-evident claims. He can ask that we think again, but he cannot undertake to prove his claims to us. If his claims truly are self-evident and known through intuition, they are in need of no proof. Perhaps more importantly, none can be given. So if, after careful reflection, you continue to disagree with some of the principles on Ross's list, he has little recourse but to accuse you of moral blindness. He must view you as equivalent to a person who cannot see the difference between red and blue; your moral blindness is on a par with his colour blindness. One might ask whether this is a satisfactory response to serious moral disagreements among reasonable people of good will and integrity.

Ross believes that his self-evident principles articulate prima facie moral obligations. These are obligations which hold unless overridden in individual cases by a more stringent or weightier duty. As for how we are to determine which of two or more prima facie duties has greater weight in a given case, Ross simply says that we must use our best judgment. This is of little help because it fails to tell us the considerations upon which our judgments are to be based. Ross is fully aware that in most cases of conflicting obligations it is far from clear which duty is more stringent. Reasonable people of moral integrity will disagree. We therefore seem left with a serious gap in the theory and must either accept that in cases of conflict there is no one right thing to do, that the best we can do is fulfil one of our conflicting duties and violate the other; or we must continue to look for a *criterion* in terms of which conflicts can be resolved.

It is at this point that the utilitarian will be more than happy to offer assistance. In his view, Ross has isolated the basis for a set of rules which are indeed important in everyday moral thinking. According to the defender of AU, these Rossian rules are useful guidelines or rules of thumb which we are well advised in most cases to follow. If we follow them regularly, our actions will in the long run end up maximizing utility. The act of promising usually does maximize utility, as does a display of gratitude. But in those cases in which a conflict in the rules arises, or where an applicable rule seems inappropriate for good utilitarian reasons, we must resort directly to the AU criterion and decide which action will maximize utility. As for the proponent of RU, he will likely claim that Ross's rules will almost certainly figure in the set of rules general observance of which, within a modern society, will maximize utility. He too is likely to claim that in cases in which the rules conflict direct recourse must be made to the principle of utility. We must follow the rule which in the circumstances will lead to the maximization of utility. Of course Ross must reject the utilitarian's offer of rescue. Were he to follow the utilitarian's lead he would in effect be adopting the principle of utility as defining a single, ultimate obligation, and this would be to deny Ross's central claim that each of his prima facie duties is ultimate and irreducible.

But then it is far from clear how this plurality of irreducible duties is to be dealt with in cases of conflict. We seem truly left with a serious gap. Without a means of adjudicating among conflicting prima facie duties, we are left short just where we need guidance the most.

Virtue Ethics: Aristotle

What Should We Be? versus What Ought We to Do?

Despite their many differences, the theories of Kant, Ross, and the utilitarians had at least one thing in common: they were all designed to answer directly the question "What ought I to do?" In other words, these theories were designed to help us determine what action(s) we should perform in particular circumstances. The concern, in short, was with the rightness of actions, with determining wherein our duty lies. According to Kant, the question "What ought I to do?" is answered by determining whether the maxim of one's action can be universalized. For rule utilitarians the answer lies in whether the rule(s) under which one acts maximize(s) overall utility. Although act utilitarians believe that rules have no role in our moral reasoning, except as rules of thumb, the question remains: "What is the right thing for me to do in these circumstances?" According to act utilitarians, we answer this question by determining which of the actions open to us would maximize utility. Ross too was concerned to help us determine what we should do in particular circumstances, with determining the course of (right) action wherein our moral duty lies. Modern theories sometimes transform the questions of Mill, Ross, and Kant into questions about our rights, but still the emphasis is on the evaluation of actions, on determining what we have or do not have rights to do.

Much earlier in the history of moral philosophy, the Greek philosopher Aristotle sought to cast ethics in an entirely different mould. This is a mould which some contemporary moral philosophers find highly appealing partly because it allows us to avoid many of the difficulties encountered by the traditional deontological and utilitarian theories, but also because it is thought to provide a much better understanding of our moral lives, what it is we strive to be in pursuing the moral life and why the moral life is important to us. The fundamental ethical question for Aristotle is not "What should I *do*?" but "What should I *be*?" As one similarly minded theorist put it,

> ... morality is internal. The moral law ... has to be expressed in the form, "be this," not in the form "do this." ... the true moral law says "hate not," instead of "kill not." ... the only mode of stating the moral law must be as a rule of character.[19]

For Aristotle, moral behaviour expresses virtues or qualities of character. There is a much greater emphasis on "character traits" and "types of persons," than on rules, obligations, duties, and rights. Aristotle is interested in questions such as these: Should we be stingy or generous? Hateful or benevolent? Cowardly or courageous? Over-indulgent or temperate? In what do these traits consist? How are they cultivated? And how do they figure in a life well lived? In discussing these questions about the character traits integral to moral life, Aristotle offered exemplars of virtue to emulate and vices to avoid rather than rules or principles to be obeyed or disobeyed. In short, for Aristotle, morality is character-oriented rather than rule-driven. Aristotle would no doubt have frowned on modern ethical theories which divorce actions and questions about them from the character of moral (or immoral) agents who perform them. Praiseworthy and blameworthy actions are not those which match up to a particular template of rules or principles, but rather ones which flow from and reveal a certain type of character. Moral agency is not merely a matter of which rules to follow; it flows from a whole way of life which requires a unity of thought and feeling characteristic of what Aristotle called "virtue."

Theoretical and Practical Reason

Aristotle divided knowledge into the theoretical and the practical. *Episteme* is concerned with speculative or theoretical inquiries, and its object is knowledge of the truth. This he contrasted with *phronesis* or practical knowledge which focuses on what is "*doable*" rather than on what is *knowable* for its own sake.

Without *phronesis*, particular virtues of character (e.g., courage, moderation, and generosity) would not be achievable by human beings, and the conduct which flows from and expresses these virtues would not be likely. It is central to Aristotle's view of human knowledge and moral excellence that whereas the intellectual virtues associated with *episteme* can be acquired through teaching, the virtues of character achievable via *phronesis* require practice until they become "second nature." Moral virtue cannot just be taught; it requires "training" and "habituation," the doing of virtuous actions. In order to be a virtuous person one must develop the disposition to be virtuous; and this requires training and the doing of virtuous actions till this becomes a settled disposition.

Human Good

Aristotle's ethical theory is teleological. "Every art and every inquiry, every action and choice, seems to aim at some good; whence the good has rightly been defined as that at which all things aim."[20] There are different goods corresponding to the various arts and modes of inquiry. Navigation aims at safe voyages, the musical arts at the creation of beautiful music, and the medical arts aim at health. Is there, Aristotle asks, a good for human beings as such? If so, then perhaps we can begin to understand what we might call the art of living well by considering what is necessary to the achievement of that end? Just as we can understand proper medical practice in relation to the good which medicine strives to achieve, perhaps we can also understand moral life in relation to the good for humans which moral life strives to achieve. So Aristotle is interested in action insofar as it contributes to the good for human beings. The right thing to do is best understood in relation to what is conducive to the good for human beings, just as a "proper prescription" is best understood in relation to what is conducive to the patient's health.

In his classic work, the *Nicomachean Ethics*, Aristotle confines his discussion of the good, that at which all things aim, to human good. The good aimed at by human beings is *eudaemonia*, usually translated as "happiness" or "well-being."[21] Some people identify human good with such things as wealth, pleasure, and honour, but Aristotle quickly shows that these people cannot be right. Wealth, for example, is at best a (very unreliable) means to happiness, not happiness itself. Pleasure is not the good for human beings even though it is true, as Aristotle's teacher Plato argued, that the good person takes pleasure in virtuous activity. Pleasure is not itself the good, but only an external sign of the presence of goodness. One will experience pleasure when one does things well; doing well does not consist of the achievement of pleasure. In Aristotle's sense of the term, happiness or well-being is something enjoyed over a lifetime in the exercise of virtues such as courage, moderation, and generosity of spirit. In one sense the exercise of the virtues is a means to the achievement of happiness or well-being. In a deeper sense it is not. The exercise of virtue is integral to the achievement of happiness, constitutive of it, not merely a pre-payment of dues to insure happiness. In short, the virtuous life is not a means to the end of well-being; it *is* the life of well-being.

Virtue

Central to the Aristotelian conception of ethics and the good life is, as we have seen, the notion of "virtue." Aristotle's definition of this key notion is as follows. Virtue is "a state of character concerned with choice, lying in a mean, i.e., the mean relative to us, this being determined by rational principle, that principle by which the man [sic] of practical wisdom would determine it ..."[22] The key notions in this definition need to be clarified.

A central element in Aristotle's conception of virtue is "disposition." Virtue, as we will see, is a kind of disposition. William Frankena summarizes the nature of dispositions as follows:

> ... dispositions or traits ... are not wholly innate; they must all be acquired, at least in part, by teaching and practice, or, perhaps by grace. They are also traits of "character," rather than traits of "personality" like charm or shyness, and they all involve a tendency to do certain kinds of action in certain kinds of situations, not just to think or feel in certain ways. They are not just abilities or skills, like intelligence or carpentry, which one may have without using.[23]

Linguistically, terms describing dispositions are often contrasted with "occurrence" terms. A dispositional term like "timid" tells us a good deal more about a person than the occurrence word "frightened." The former tells us something about the character of the individual, whereas the latter may tell us nothing more than that the person was in a particular state on some occasion or other. It is possible that the state we might call "Tom's being frightened" occurred on some occasion even though Tom has no disposition to be frightened. Very little future behaviour can be predicted from being told that someone is frightened or angry, even if we know the reasons why he is frightened or angry. On the other hand, if we are told that Sue is timid or irascible, then we can predict that she will tend to get frightened or angry in circumstances that would not frighten or anger other people with a more courageous or gentler disposition. Having such dispositions does not, of course, rule out the possibility of sometimes acting "out of character." There are provocations that would try even the patience of Job, some tasks so dangerous as to deter the most courageous and resolute persons, and some offers that even the most conscientious person cannot refuse. Dispositions, as tendencies, have an elasticity about them.

Aristotle's definition of virtue begins with virtue as a disposition, but it does not end there. Virtue is a disposition *to choose well*. Commenting on the etymology of the Greek word for choice, *prohairesis*, Aristotle writes: "the very term *prohairesis* ... denotes something chosen before other things."[24] Choosing something before other things requires (a) the presence of alternatives. Without alternatives there can be no choice. It also requires (b) deliberation about the relative merits of the alternatives open to the agent. Virtuous actions are principled and thoughtful. They are responses rather than reactions. Deliberation about the alternatives open to the agent requires (c) ranking of those alternatives. One alternative is preferred to another and chosen. Finally, *prohairesis* presupposes (d) voluntarism. Virtue requires that we are responsible for our own actions. We are the begetters or efficient causes of our own actions, agents not patients. Our actions must be "self-caused," i.e., "in our power and voluntary."[25]

Aristotle emphasizes that primarily choice is restricted to means and not ends. The ultimate and remote end of our choosing, *eudaemonia* or happiness, is fixed by human nature.

Human Nature, Essentialism, Relativism

Just as all things within the universe have an essential nature (understood by Aristotle in terms of a unique function the thing serves) in relation to which their "good" can be understood, human nature provides a natural basis for understanding the good for human beings. This particular feature of Aristotle's view allows him to avoid arbitrariness in his ethics; ethics is not based on variable social norms or customs, or on the personal predilections of individuals or groups of individuals. Ethics is not "culturally relative" or "subjective" on this account; it is grounded in nature and to that extent "objective." Although the "objectivity" of the Aristotelian schema allows Aristotle to avoid relativism, it is a serious source of concern for some. Many critics see danger in the idea that there is a largely fixed, essential human nature in terms of which the moral life, and the requirements it places upon us, are to be understood. Some followers of Aristotle have argued that procreation is "natural" to human beings (as it is to all organisms) and that so-called "artificial" means of reproduction are therefore inherently suspicious and perhaps even immoral. Others take a similar line of argument in supporting the view that homosexuality is immoral. Whether such views follow from the Aristotelian system is highly questionable. But there is, nevertheless, cause to be concerned about a theory which seeks to define the moral in terms of what is "natural" for human beings. All too often what is thought to be "natural" is really only the conventional. And as feminists and other social critics point out, the conventional is often the result of bias, misunderstanding, and oppression.

If the ultimate end of our choosing is fixed by human nature, and the alternatives open to us when we seek to be virtuous are alternative ways of promoting this end, i.e., alternative ways of promoting *eudaemonia*, then the following question arises. Is Aristotle in fact advocating what we might call the *principle of eudaemonia*, as opposed to the principle of utility? And is this not a principle which can be applied, either directly or indirectly, to our actions in such a way that we have a means of determining morally right actions? For example, particular virtues like truth-telling, promise-keeping, and their ilk could be viewed as means toward achieving the ultimate end of *eudaemonia* or happiness. If this is so, then in actual fact there may be little to distinguish Aristotle's so-called "virtue ethics" from the action-centred "duty ethics" of Kant, Mill, and Ross.

The Aristotelian Mean

Although there is some truth in this assessment of Aristotle's ethics, it would be a mistake to exaggerate it. This is because, for Aristotle, virtuous action is not action which accords with a principle, but rather action which springs from a disposition to choose a way which lies between two extremes, the one an excess and the other a deficiency. Virtuous action lies in choosing *the mean* between extremes of behaviour one of which is a vice through excess, the other of which is a vice through deficiency. And Aristotle is clear that there is no arithmetical formula which allows us to determine with precision what lies at the mean in a particular set of circumstances. This is one reason why he says that the mean must be determined "relatively to us," and as determined not by a rule universally applicable and established in advance, but by a rule "by which a practically wise man [sic] would determine it." On Aristotle's account, there is a kind of indeterminacy in moral judgments when it comes to deciding on particular courses of action. The variable contexts of moral life prevent us from fashioning hard-and-fast rules or procedures for settling what we ought to do. The best we can do is rely on *phronesis*, our virtuous dispositions, and the examples set by paragons of virtue. We must, in other words, try under the circumstances to act as "the man [sic] of practical reason would act." This is the best that we can do. Whether this is a weakness in Aristotle's account of moral life is a good question. Perhaps this inherent indeterminacy better reflects moral reality and the perplexing dilemmas with which we are often faced, than theories which purport to provide ready-made answers which fail to emerge when we seek to apply the theories to concrete circumstances. Is it any more helpful to be told that one must maximize utility, or seek to treat humanity as an end in itself, than it is to be told that one must seek a mean between deficiency and excess? In explicitly acknowledging that moral theory can provide only a limited amount of help, Aristotle's theory may in fact be the more honest one.

Virtue lies at the mean between the vices of excess and deficiency. The virtues of courage and moderation (or temperance) are among those chosen by Aristotle to elucidate his doctrine of the mean. The accounts are perhaps dated, but they nevertheless serve to illustrate the main lines of Aristotle's thought. For Aristotle, courage is primarily a virtue of soldiers and his examples are culled entirely from the battlefield. Courage is located between the defect of fear and the excess of over-spiritedness or brashness. When the occasion arises, a courageous soldier can be counted on to subdue fear and enter bravely into the fray even in the face of death. Cowardice is the vice (defect) associated with fear. In more modern parlance, we may link it with the instinct of "flight" in the face of danger. But rashness is also a vice, in this case an excess associated with spiritedness. This vice we may link with the instinct of "fight" in the face of danger. But one can be too spirited. Soldiers emboldened by anger may rush impulsively into the fray, "blind to the dangers that await them."[26] "Right reason" moderates fear, and courage emerges as fear tempered by spirit.

The application of Aristotle's model of course need not be limited. One may as readily look for displays of courage in the more familiar domains of sickness and death. These domains are also "battlefields" of sorts, in which individuals face handicap, major surgery, debilitating illness, and prolonged and painful dying. Aristotle's ethics-of-virtue may prove helpful in such circumstances. While it may prove impossible to determine a hard-and-fast rule to answer our moral questions in such instances, it may be possible to answer the question: "What kind of people do we wish to *be* when we are faced with such circumstances?" Do we wish, for example, to be cowardly, cringing in fear in the face of death, demanding that everything conceivable be done to prolong our lives regardless of quality? Or is this an option which would not be pursued by the person of courage? Is this how the person "of practical wisdom" would act, lacking in regard for others, insensitive to the fact that the resources used to prop up his life might be of more benefit to others with a more favourable prognosis? Or do we want to be courageous, moderating our fear of death and insensitivity to the needs of others as much as it lies within us to do so? In another context the relevant question might be: What kind of people do we want to be in the face of severe handicap or disability? Cowardly, living each moment in fear; or brash—at the opposite extreme from fear—living in denial, masking our true feelings from others and conducting ourselves in an unwarranted display of over-confidence or *bravado* rather than bravery? Or will we try to avoid both extremes and be courageous, striving to temper fear of death or handicap with a more reasonably nuanced and spirited response, trying to live life to the fullest within our disability, even though such daring involves risk? To these questions we may find reasonable answers, even if there are no rules by which they can be determined, and even if we must in the end still choose for ourselves that course of action which best exemplifies the virtuous mean.

The second virtue upon which Aristotle focuses is temperance—the trait which moderates our appetites for food, drink, and sex. One can eat too little or too much food. Aristotle designates health as the goal of eating. Gluttons are guilty of excess. They live to eat rather than eat to live. They dig their graves with their teeth. They imperil rather than preserve their health by over-eating. This is a vice of excess. The vice of defect or deficiency involves eating insufficient food in circumstances where there is enough to go around. In time of scarcity and famine, failure to eat sufficient food is not morally blameworthy. Strictly speaking, in such circumstances eating insufficient food does not qualify as a voluntary activity. Although Aristotle does not mention it, malnutrition can be caused by eating the wrong foods, not just by failing to eat enough food. One can be malnourished on a diet of soda pop and chips, or with fad diets motivated by a perceived need to be slim. In such cases, Aristotle would attribute malnutrition to vice rather than misfortune or famine.

To be clear on Aristotle's ordering of values in this context, it must be borne in mind that while health is an immediate end of eating, it is not good in itself. Rather it is a means to happiness or well-being, i.e., *eudaemonic*, and is properly conceived only in this way. Relative to moderation in partaking of food and drink, health is a proximate end, but relative to the final end, happiness, it is *usually* a necessary means. This last point must be kept clearly in mind in medical contexts where there is sometimes a tendency to confuse means with ends. Life and "health" are important ends of human action, including medical action, but only if and to the extent that they contribute to what really counts: *eudaemonia*. When they do not, the person of practical reason and virtue will no longer see them as worthy of pursuit. The implications of this point for decisions concerning the "saving" of people who judge their lives no longer worth living are apparent and profound. Life and "health" are goods which confer rightness on the means for their achievement, but only when these contribute to *eudaemonia*.

Feminist Perspectives

Many contemporary women and not a few men find all the approaches to ethics outlined above to be in many respects unsatisfactory and alienating. These theories were all developed by men who, it is claimed, inadvertently brought to bear upon their theoretical positions a number of biases and ways of viewing the world which skew the results of their analyses. The resultant theories do little justice to the moral concerns and experiences of women. Indeed, in the view of most feminist ethicists, the traditional theories "do not constitute the objective, impartial theories that they are claimed to be; rather, most theories reflect and support explicitly gender-biased and often blatantly misogynist values."[27] It would be impossible to provide a complete and fully accurate account of the important, multi-faceted themes pursued by feminist ethicists. Instead, we will attempt, in what follows, to sketch two of the most common concerns of feminists regarding traditional ethical theories.

First, there is the issue of power relationships, for which the health-care context provides an obvious set of examples. Built right into most medical situations is a power imbalance between, on the one hand, vulnerable patients in need of assistance, and on the other hand, health-care workers whose knowledge, skill, and special privileges often place them in a superior position. But for women the inherent power imbalance has traditionally been all the more difficult to overcome because of a further factor: gender imbalance. According to many theorists, evidence shows that male physicians (which is to say, until recently, the overwhelming majority of doctors) have tended to treat female patients with condescension or disdain—and that the medical system itself has been heavily biased towards taking male afflictions much more seriously than female ones. In similar fashion, the role of (primarily male) doctors was often the near-exclusive focus of attention, and the role of (primarily female) nurses was often ignored. Such systemic gender-based imbalances have been a major focus of feminist attention.

Many feminists share a broader concern with power imbalances—between men and women, certainly, but also between other advantaged and oppressed groups such as adults and children, the able and the disabled, and the rich and the poor. Many feminists have pointed out that the field of ethical theory (like most fields) has historically been dominated by men whose perspectives may have been biased against women. Some traditional ethicists, e.g., Kant and Aristotle, thought that women have a decidedly different character from men, and are to a much greater extent than men moved by emotion as opposed to reason. In the view of these theorists, this tendency towards the emotional serves as a barrier to the level of abstract reasoning required for satisfactory moral thought. Feminist ethicists are concerned to undermine these stereotypes and to assert the equal ability of women to engage in moral thought.

More widely, one strain of feminist thought is opposed to the search for abstract, universalizable principles and rules (or even virtues) with which to answer everyone's moral questions. The theories of Kant and Mill are often cited as illustrative of the insufficiency of traditional ethical theory. In the view of many feminist critics, Kant's theory rejects the emotional, personal component of moral life in favour of the rational universalizability of individual maxims. In seeking rationally to universalize our maxims, we are inescapably led to ignore or sub-merge our concern for all those complex factors which *individuate* our situations and the relation-ships in which we find ourselves. Most importantly perhaps, in seeking such abstractions, we are led to ignore or abstract away all that makes us individual persons enmeshed in inter-personal relationships involving caring and trust. Among the factors so eliminated are the emotional bonds between people and the special concerns they have for one another, as parents, friends, siblings, and colleagues. In seek-ing to universalize we are, it is claimed, led to forget that most of the time we approach one another—and believe ourselves right in doing so—not as strangers subject to the same set of universalized maxims or rights, but as unique individuals in highly personal, context-specific relationships in which we have much invested emotionally. These are relationships which, by their very nature, cannot be reduced to universalized rules and principles. According to Susan Sherwin, a leading feminist philosopher:

Because women are usually charged with the responsibility of caring for children, the elderly, and the ill as well as the responsibility of physi-cally and emotionally nurturing men, both at work and at home, most women experience the world as a complex web of interdependent relationships, where responsible caring for others is implicit in their moral lives. The abstract reasoning of moral-ity that centres on the rights [and duties] of inde-pendent agents is inadequate for the moral reality in which they live. Most women find that a differ-ent model for ethics is necessary; the traditional ones are not persuasive.[28]

The feminist concern for the importance of con-text leads in another direction as well. Many feminist philosophers argue not only for the importance of appreciating the factors which individuate one case from the other, and tie us to one another in a variety of personal ways; they also stress the importance of appreciating the wider context of decision-making. This is a context which, more often than not, pro-foundly influences the options available, or the options thought available, to us. Feminists look beyond the individual situations in which decisions are made and question the social and political insti-tutions, practices, and beliefs that create those situa-tions and define the available options. Consider, for example, the case of reproductive technologies. Here a plethora of ethical questions arises whenever a woman requests reproductive assistance in the face of infertility. Should any woman who asks for such aid be accommodated? What if she is unmarried, a lesbian, or already has children of her own? Is it per-missible to create multiple fertilized eggs when only a few will actually be implanted at any one time? If so, may some of the extra eggs be used for purposes of medical research? These questions, and many oth-ers like them, are ones which everyone agrees deserve attention.

But many feminist ethicists want to dig much deeper. They want to uncover for discussion the vari-ety of social, political, and environmental factors which give rise to such questions and possibly frame the available answers. They wish to expose certain social factors which arguably lead many women to request treatment despite the negligible chance of success and the profound disappointment which often accompanies failure. Many argue that the con-ventionally accepted view of women's social role, as fundamentally involving the production and rearing of offspring, encourages infertile women to see themselves as defective and lacking in value. As a consequence, they are in effect "coerced" into seek-ing biomedical interventions to correct themselves. And they suffer great feelings of inadequacy and worthlessness if, as is all too common, such inter-ventions fail to bring about the desired result. Simi-lar points are made in relation to cosmetic surgery which, it is argued, is often pursued by women only because of the force of socially generated stereo-types of femininity which ground a woman's value in her good looks.

To sum up, many feminist approaches to ethics are marked by their rejection of traditional ethical theo-ry as far too abstract and concerned with universal-ized rules and principles. As such, traditional ethical theory misses out on two fronts. First, it renders irrelevant a host of individuating factors which inform our moral lives and which most of us, women in particular, consider integral to moral assessment. These include the importance of personal relationships and the emotional bonds which exist between individuals who care for one another. Second, traditional ethical theory often ignores the wider social, political, and environmental contexts in which moral questions are shaped and the available options are defined.

For much of the 1980s and 1990s a great deal of attention was paid to a strain of feminist thought that we have not yet mentioned—care ethics. According to theories put forward by Carol Gilligan and others, women had particular claims to ethical insight as a result of their being (whether from nature or from nurture) predisposed to an ethic of caring and concern for their fellow creatures. While this theory has attracted a great deal of attention, it has attracted considerable criticism as well, not least of all from feminists of a different stamp, who have seen in care ethics unfortunate echoes of nineteenth-century views of women's "special role"—views that supported restrictions against women becoming involved in society outside the home or the "helping professions" of teacher, governess, nurse.

Care ethics may have helped to raise the level of esteem in which such professions are held. But it has proved to be only one current of feminist thought, and not the main stream. This last is an important point in that it illustrates that there are many feminisms rather than one. Within the discipline of philosophy it is now broadly recognized that there are many varieties of feminist thought—and that they provide a range of challenges to traditional moral theory.

Naturalized Feminist Bioethics

A recent development in feminist approaches to bioethics is naturalized feminist bioethics, most often associated with the philosopher Margaret Urban Walker.[29] Like other feminist commentators, Walker is critical of theoretical approaches that abstract from the contexts of ethical decision-making and that model ethical knowledge on the understandings of knowledge and method in science. Walker views attempts to deduce ethical judgments from an overarching principle, such as the principle

of utility or the Categorical Imperative, as mistaken. Labelling such approaches *theoretical-juridical*, Walker offers instead an *expressive-collaborative* approach, which emphasizes the negotiations that take place in moral communities when arriving at norms of conduct. In the expressive-collaborative approach *responsibilities* (the central ethical notion) are seen as a product of negotiation and as the basis of calling agents to account for their actions or inactions.

Theoretical Approach

In the expressive-collaborative approach there is no overarching principle from which to derive good decisions or to identify virtues or values. Rather, moral agents are considered to be already engaged in dynamic moral communities which relate to one another in a "moral medium" of understandings about right and wrong, good and bad, duties and aspirations. Individual agents assess their own responsibilities in the context of their self-understanding, their relationships with others (including special relationships such as patient-provider), and the moral norms already recognized by the group as operating amongst them. Within that context individuals may be held accountable; but they can contest their accountability. Take the example of Hurricane Katrina. Whereas the responsibilities of health-care providers are fairly well understood in clinics, hospitals, and educational settings, and even in everyday life, where health professionals are expected to come to the aid of those in need, in catastrophic situations their responsibilities are not so clear. As the waters were rising around a health centre in New Orleans, health workers were faced with difficult choices: should they attempt to rescue dying patients when the rescue itself might kill the patients? If not, should they administer drugs that could speed patients' deaths? Should the health providers stay with their dying patients, and risk death themselves? The usual norms of professional conduct seem inappropriate in this setting, and there are no straightforward answers from doctors' or nurses' codes of ethics. According to the expressive-collaborative approach, health providers may contest the applicability of the usual norms of conduct, and offer the best justifications they can provide for their conduct. Through the ensuing discussion new norms will emerge within the community.

Walker is not naïve about the role of status and authority in ethical debates, and as a feminist she recognizes the need to make space for the voices of those who have lacked authority. A satisfactory moral norm—whether an agreed-upon rule of conduct or a particular moral judgment or an ascription of responsibility—should be viewed as more authoritative the more transparent the process by which it was reached and the more inclusive the negotiation. Strong objectivity, on this feminist understanding, is achieved when as a regular matter we bring a critical perspective to bear on our conclusions, and provide for contestation and discussion. Where the voices of important stakeholders are excluded, relationships and institutions will be unstable, and moral communities less *habitable*. Collaboration through transparency, inclusion, and critical contestation should generate habitable moral relationships, institutions and communities.

Interdisciplinarity and Naturalized Bioethics

As we have noted, the expressive-collaborative approach recognizes the importance of including diverse perspectives in moral debate. In the preceding section we spoke of diversity in relation to the social position of collaborators—whether they have authoritative social status or are socially marginalized. But diversity can also refer to the range of disciplines that should inform bioethics. Naturalized bioethics recognizes that the context of decision-making and policy-making in bioethics is complex, and insights into its complexities can come from many disciplinary perspectives. Sociologists, economists, psychologists, historians and others can all contribute to an understanding of our motivations, resources, self-understandings, and options, thus filling out the contexts—broad and narrow—of moral decision-making. Naturalized bioethics recognizes that diverse disciplinary perspectives not only enrich the content of moral decision-making; they position bioethics as one among many relevant disciplines, thus calling bioethics to account for itself as a source of knowledge and prescriptivity.

Commenting on the methodology of naturalized bioethics and its relation to other disciplines, Margaret Urban Walker said,

> Our conception of naturalism ... renders reflective equilibrium very wide, with relevant beliefs encompassing natural and social scientific findings; discursive and epistemological analysis of our frames of thought in particular times and places; ethnographic perspectives on institutions and social environments; experiential and third-person narratives that capture the detail of lives and situations; literary studies of how narratives are shaped by contexts and, in turn, shape our understandings; political and organizational analyses of the constraints on dialogue, deliberation, and decision; and more. In addition, our socially critical and power-sensitive approach to naturalizing ethics asks about the terms of reflective equilibrium not only among beliefs but among *people* who are parties to, and subjects of, moral decision-making and who should be intelligible and accountable to each other."[30]

Thus, interdisciplinarity not only informs and enriches bioethical reflection; it also calls bioethicists to account by reminding them of the situatedness—personal and professional—of their own perspective, and the need to take responsibility for the judgments and recommendations they make.

Guiding Questions

As a theoretical approach to bioethical decision-making, naturalized feminist bioethics shares with earlier feminist approaches a particular attention to voice and privilege. Feminists ask, "Whose voices have been heard in this decision or policy? Whose interests will be served by this outcome?" The naturalized feminist bioethicist asks "How transparent have the processes leading to a decision or policy been, and to whom?" "Has there been an opportunity for contestation?" and "How habitable and stable is the resulting state of affairs?" Together these questions provide a framework for moral decision-making that, when accompanied by the insights of utilitarianism, deontology, and virtue ethics, render moral decision-making more grounded, more democratic, and more accountable.

The Language of Rights

An introduction to the basic theories and concepts of ethics would be radically incomplete without some mention of "rights." At one time it was quite natural to express moral requirements using concepts such as *ought*, *duty*, and *obligation*. It was in terms of the latter three concepts that the ethical theories just discussed were presented by their authors. Today, however, our moral vocabulary is dominated by the notion of rights. Instead of saying "You ought not to have done that," or "Your responsibility was to have done this rather than that," a modern person is more apt to remark "You had no *right* to do that." But rights come in a variety of different forms which are often confused with one another. In order to facilitate discussion of the moral issues raised in this book, a brief analysis of these differences follows. The conceptual map sketched is largely derivative from the theory proposed early in the twentieth century by the American legal scholar, Wesley Hohfeld and from the more recent account developed by the contemporary moral philosopher Joel Feinberg.[31]

Claim-Rights

What is a "right?" Where does it come from? On what does it rest? Strictly speaking, Hohfeld thought, a right is an enforceable claim to someone else's action or non-action. If one has a right to X, then one can demand X as one's due. It is not merely good, desirable, or preferable that one should have X: one is entitled to it and another person, or group of persons, has a correlative duty or obligation to respect your entitlement to X. For instance, I have a right not to be assaulted by you. This entails that you are under an obligation of non-action, that is, a duty *not* to assault me. This kind of right, a claim against other people, is what Hohfeld called a *claim-right*. A claim-right is always paired with a corresponding duty or obligation which applies to at least one other person. Violation of my claim-right is always the violation by someone else of his or her duty towards me.

Claim-rights come in a variety of different forms. In sorting these out, Joel Feinberg develops three important distinctions:

(i)   in personam versus in rem rights
(ii) positive versus negative rights
(iii) passive versus active rights.

In personam rights are said to hold against one or more determinate, specifiable persons. These are determinate persons who are under corresponding or correlative obligations. For example, if Bill owes Jean a weekend at Camp David, then there is a specific person, Bill, against whom Jean enjoys his claim-right. Other examples are rights under contract, rights of landlords to payment of rent from their tenants, the right against one's employer to a safe and healthy working environment, the right against one's doctor to her best professional judgment about one's medical care, and so on. Many of the duties on Ross's list of prima facie duties could easily be expressed in terms of the correlative claim-rights. Paired with a Rossian duty of fidelity, for example, will be a claim-right against a person with whom one has made an agreement to the honouring of that agreement. That person has a duty to perform his end of the deal; you have a correlative claim-right to his performance.

Not all claim-rights, however, are held against specifiable persons. Some hold against people generally. These kinds of rights, called *in rem rights*, are said to hold against "the world at large." For instance, my right not to be assaulted holds not against any particular person or group of persons, but against anyone and everyone who might be in a position to commit such an offence against me. This includes my neighbours, people at bus stops, and surgeons who might be tempted to operate on me in a non-emergency situation without first obtaining my consent. All such persons have a correlative duty not to assault me. This latter, correlative duty, would no doubt fall under Ross's duties of non-maleficence.

Positive and negative rights form another subclass of claim-rights. A positive right is a right to someone else's positive action. A negative right, on the other hand, is a right to another person's non-action or forbearance. If I have a positive right to something, this means that there is at least one other person who has an obligation actually to do something, usually something for my benefit. By contrast, I have a negative right when there is at least one other person who has a duty to refrain from doing something, usually something which would harm me. Depending on what it is that the other person(s) must refrain from doing, my negative right can be either passive or active.

Active rights are negative rights to go about one's own business free from the interference of others. Paired with active claim rights are duties of non-interference. Health-care professionals who complain that governments should allow them to practice medicine free from bureaucratic interference are usually asserting active claim-rights not to be interfered with or hindered in their medical pursuits. Corresponding to such rights would be a duty on the part of a government to allow health-care professionals a measure of freedom and autonomy—even when this involves such things as "extra-billing" patients over and above what is provided by a government-sponsored Medicare program.

Passive negative rights are rights not to have certain things done to us. We might, for convenience, call them "security rights." Obvious examples are the right not to be killed or assaulted, and the right not to be inflicted with disease and injury by negligent or reckless medical staff. Health care workers who assert a right not to be exposed to the AIDS virus also have in mind a negative, passive right. In this case it is the right not to be infected by AIDS victims. Passive rights are not rights against interference with one's own activities. Rather they are rights not to have certain unwanted or harmful things done to us.

It is worth noting that typically active rights of non-interference can be protected only at the expense of other people's passive security rights. The active right of a manufacturer to pursue a livelihood within the capitalist system often competes with the passive, in personam, security rights of workers. It also competes with the passive, in rem rights of the community or world at large not to have its environment fouled by industrial activities. In general, a key problem of moral, legal, and political philosophy is how to balance active freedom rights against passive security rights. Different theories will place differing emphases on the competing rights. The resolution of such conflicts is as difficult as the resolution of conflicts among Ross's prima facie duties.

To sum up, claim rights can be either in personam or in rem, positive or negative, and if they are negative, they can be either passive or active. Correlated with any one of these rights is always a duty or obligation on the part of at least one other individual. Such rights are claims against others who are under duty to respect them.

Liberties or Privileges

Sometimes the situations in which people assert rights do not involve claims against others who are under correlative obligations. Rather they involve what Hohfeld called "privileges" or "liberties." My having a privilege does not entail that others are under obligation towards me. Rather it entails only the *absence* of an obligation on *my* part. If I enjoy the privilege of doing something, then I am free or at liberty to do it (or not do it) and I do no wrong should I exercise my privilege. In short, a privilege is "freedom from duty." An example from law may help to clarify the nature of privileges.

In most legal systems there is a standing duty to provide the court with whatever information it requests. One must provide that information even if one would prefer not to. However, many jurisdictions also recognize a special area in which this standing duty does not apply. They recognize a right—a privilege—against self-incrimination. What this means is that in this special area—i.e., evidence which may implicate them in a crime—citizens are at liberty to decline the court's request. Here they enjoy an absence of duty. If the testimony in question may incriminate them, they don't have to testify if they don't want to. But notice, if I have no *claim-right* against self-incrimination, but only a privilege, then if a sharp lawyer somehow gets me to incriminate myself, he has in no way violated my rights. This would be true only if my right were a claim-right against him. Were it a claim-right, then the lawyer would be under a corresponding duty or obligation to respect a claim I would then have against him. But with privileges there are no such corresponding duties—only the absence of duty on my part. I have a freedom to act (or not to act), but it is not a freedom which enjoys the protection afforded by corresponding duties on the part of other people to respect my freedom. There is no requirement on their part that they refrain from interfering with my action or non-action.

Situations in health care where the notion of a privilege or liberty arises are not entirely obvious at first glance. Examples can be found, however, in any situation in which some people are exempt from duties to which they would otherwise be held. Certain health care professionals, for example, are privileged with respect to confidential information about your medical history. Access to such private, confidential information is something from which the general public is barred. The general public is under a duty to respect the confidentiality of your medical records. They have no right to these privileged items. Those who are privileged, however, enjoy a freedom from this duty. They are exempt from the general duty to keep away or to mind their own business which applies to the public at large.

Privileges also figure prominently in the therapeutic relationship. By providing consent to surgery, for example, a patient waives his claim-right not to be "touched" by the surgeon, thereby relieving or freeing the latter from his standing duty not to touch the patient. In short, he grants the surgeon a privilege without which any act of touching would amount to assault or battery.

It is perhaps worth stressing once again that privileges are *unprotected* freedoms. Contrast a situation in which a patient grants me the privilege of examining his confidential medical records with a situation involving the Medical Officer of Health. If the Medical Officer has a claim-right to examine the files, say for purposes of tracking an infectious disease, then the hospital (and the patient) must respect that right. They have a duty to turn the files over and do wrong if they should fail to do so. If, on the other hand, the patient simply forgets to arrange for his records to reach my hands, he has in no way violated my rights. This is because I have been granted a mere privilege, not a claim-right with its corresponding duty.

Powers

Sometimes the terminology of rights is used to describe neither a claim-right nor a privilege. In some situations we have the capacity to alter existing legal or moral relationships involving rights and duties. In such cases we enjoy what Hohfeld called a normative *power*. In law, for example, we find powers of attorney which enable an agent to bring about changes in the legal relationships of his client. An agent may, for instance, be empowered to sign a contract on behalf of his client. In exercising this power, the agent imposes on his client a duty to honour his part of the agreement with the third party. He also, of course, invests in his client a right that the third party do the same. In these ways, then, the agent alters the existing normative relationships between his client and the third party.

Powers also enter into the practice of medicine. A surrogate is one empowered to act on behalf of a patient. He is able, for example, to alter the legal/moral relationship between patient and physician by consenting to surgery. In so doing the surrogate grants the surgeon the privilege of operating, relieving her of her otherwise standing duty not to invade the patient's body. Put another way, the surrogate *waives* the patient's claim-right not to be "touched." Without the exercise of this power by the surrogate on the patient's behalf, the surgeon's actions would, strictly speaking, amount to assault or battery. Of course in most cases patients themselves exercise the power of consent. But when for some reason a patient is unable to do so, the power and its exercise may fall to the surrogate, who must act on the patient's behalf. The surrogate is empowered to alter certain of the patient's normative relationships, but only when this is in the best interests of the patient.

The power to waive claim-rights will serve as a focus of attention in many of the cases that follow. In some instances, the question of who has the legal or moral power to waive patients' rights arises. In others, the issue will be whether such a power exists at all. Does anyone, patient included, have the power to waive someone's right to life?

Further Reflections on Rights

While, nowadays, the rights approach to morality and ethics is most prominent, it offers no panacea for resolving moral conflicts. Instead of presenting the abortion dispute as a conflict of obligations, the obligation to protect human life (of the fetus) versus the obligation to respect human freedom (of the woman), now the tension is located in a conflict between the fetus's right to life and the woman's right to exercise control over her own reproductive processes, as it arguably distorts the moral relationship between the woman and her fetus while failing to resolve this tension.

One should be careful when encountering talk of "rights." It is always important to ask whether the right being asserted is a claim-right or a privilege, or possibly even a power. These are different conceptually and have very different implications. If the right is a claim-right, then one should ask whether it is in rem or in personam. In particular it may be crucial to determine whether the right is negative or positive. Does it require only that others *refrain* from doing something, or does it require positive action(s)? This is an important difference which figures prominently in many public debates. One famous case in which the difference proved crucial was the United States Supreme Court's decision in *Roe v. Wade*. The Court ruled that every woman has a right to abort a fetus within specified limits. This was interpreted by some to mean that the Court had recognized a positive right to abortion which entailed aid and financial assistance from the government. A 1977 ruling, however, made it clear that while it was unconstitutional to prevent a woman from having an elective abortion, within the prescribed limits, women did not have a right to aid or financial assistance. In other words, *Roe v. Wade* had granted only a *negative*, not a *positive*, right to an abortion.

Concluding Thoughts

We have now looked at numerous moral theories and different vocabularies with which to express them. How may the insights of ethical theory be applied to actual practice? The strategies one could adopt in linking moral theory to practice are numerous and varied. Nevertheless, it is possible to isolate three basic patterns of response.

(i) *Make decisions on an ad hoc, case-by-case, basis, ignoring ethical theories altogether.*
Despite the undeniable importance of individual context, this is neither a promising nor an inviting option. Although there is some measure of truth in the adage that "no two cases are ever alike," it would be a mistake to exaggerate it. Any two cases will necessarily be unlike one another in many respects, but it fails to follow that they will be unlike one another *in the relevant respects*. No two murders are completely similar, but they are alike in what is often the only relevant respect: an innocent human being has been killed. If cases can be classified as being similar to one another in a limited number of relevant respects, and these cases are familiar and recurring ones, then the possibility arises of discovering moral rules and principles to govern them. We are able to fashion workable legal rules governing murder because there are a limited number of recurring, relevant aspects of murder cases which can be dealt with in simple, general rules. The same is often true with moral rules and principles. So while we must be sensitive to the importance of varying contexts, to what individuates us in our personal relationships with others, and to the dangers inherent in Aristotle's attempt to ground morality on a fixed human nature, we should also be sensitive to the importance of similarities. My relationship with my daughter is unique and special to me. It may also be very different from the relationship shared by fathers and daughters in other, more patriarchal cultures. But the relationship I share with my daughter may yet be in many ways relevantly similar to the unique, special relationships many fathers have with their daughters.

If the possibility of moral norms, and ethical theories to support and explain them, exists, then it would be counter-productive to ignore them entirely. We would have to "start from scratch" every time we had to make a difficult moral decision. This would be inefficient, to say the least, and would be a hindrance to moral understanding. Understanding the world involves recognizing similarities and differences among situations and people. Without moral rules, principles, values and virtues, and theories to generate them, we make it difficult, if not impossible, to gain moral understanding. So long as we do not claim too much for it, working with an admittedly limited theory is better than working with no theory at all.

(ii) *Make a firm and irrevocable commitment to a particular ethical theory.*

While this option promotes single-mindedness, and simplifies our moral deliberations, it has the serious disadvantage of ignoring the possible insights of other ethical theories and approaches. It compels one to resolve all moral quandaries within the boundaries of the theory chosen and this smacks of artificiality and arbitrariness. This will be so unless one is convinced that one "knows the truth" with absolute certainty, an unlikely possibility for someone willing to ascend to the reflective level of moral thinking (see above). Blindly committing oneself to an ethical theory or approach is no better than blindly committing oneself to a conventional rule. It is to descend to the pre-reflective level where blind acceptance replaces critical reflection and the possibility of moral progress.

(iii) *Allow for both fixity and flexibility.*

This is clearly the preferred option. The fixity is provided by acknowledging that moral conflicts need not, and perhaps should not, be resolved within a moral vacuum, and that the application of an ethical theory with which one is not entirely happy can nevertheless shed light on the issues in dispute. It may at the very least bring some of the important considerations into relief where they may be more easily examined and discussed reasonably. Flexibility arises in acknowledging that competing theories and approaches may well offer insight as well and that one's own favoured theory is always open to improvement or, at some point, rejection. Reasonable flexibility may even lead us judiciously to extract rules, principles, or values from competing systems as determined by their apparent relevance to the case in question. It may be true that sometimes Mill provides a better answer than Kant—and that the tables are reversed at other times. Sometimes

feminist theorists may be right in stressing the individuating features of a moral situation, features which might in some instance render the relevant issue incapable of resolution by way of a universalizable moral principle. This is not necessarily a cause for dismay, as Ross seemed to appreciate. Consider an analogous case in physics. Sometimes the wave theory provides a better account of the properties and behaviour of light than the particle theory does. At other times the reverse is true. A single, unified theory would no doubt be preferable. But until such time as one becomes available, it would be imprudent to ignore the existing theories altogether, or to subscribe to one and forget about the other(s). The same is true in moral philosophy. We must not let our failures to achieve completeness, or our failures to appreciate in all cases the full range of factors at play in particular contexts, blind us to the incremental gains in knowledge that have been made. Perhaps we would do well, in the end, to heed Aristotle's caution that "precision is not to be sought alike in all discussions. We must be content, in speaking of such subjects [as ethics and politics], to indicate the truth roughly and in outline."[32]

Notes

1   John Stuart Mill, *On Liberty*, Shields ed. (Indianapolis: Bobbs-Merrill, 1956), 56.

2   See G.E. Moore, *Principia Ethica* (London: Cambridge University Press, 1903).

3   John Stuart Mill, *Utilitarianism* (New York: Bobbs Merrill, 1957), 10.

4   Mill, *Utilitarianism*, 22.

5   John Rawls, "Two Concepts of Rules," *The Philosophical Review* (January 1955), 3-13.

6   See J.J.C. Smart and Bernard Williams, *Utilitarianism: For and Against* (London: Cambridge University Press, 1973), 10.

7   See David Lyons, *The Forms and Limits of Utilitarianism* (Oxford: Oxford University Press, 1965), where it is argued that any version of RU faithful to the utilitarian credo collapses logically into AU.

8   Immanuel Kant, *Groundwork of the Metaphysics of Morals*, trans. H.J. Paton (New York: Harper and Row, 1964), 67-68.

9   Kant, 70.

10　Kant, 89.

11　Kant, 89-90.

12　Kant, 90.

13　Kant, 96.

14　See Lloyd Tataryn, "From Dust to Dust," in D. Poff and W. Waluchow, eds., *Business Ethics in Canada* (Scarborough: Prentice Hall Canada, 1987), 122-25.

15　W.D. Ross, *The Right and the Good* (Oxford: Clarendon Press, 1930), 21.

16　Ross, 13.

17　Immanuel Kant, "On a Supposed Right to Lie from Altruistic Motives," in Lewis White Beck, ed. and trans., *Critique of Practical Reason and Other Writings in Moral Philosophy* (Chicago: University of Chicago Press, 1949), 346-50.

18　Ross, 21.

19　Leslie Stephen, *The Science of Ethics* (New York: G.P. Putnam's Sons, 1882), 155, 158.

20　Aristotle, *Nicomachean Ethics*, trans. J.L. Ackrill (New York: Humanities Press, 1973), 1094.

21　Aristotle, 1095 a16-20.

22　Aristotle, 1106 b36-1107 a2.

23　William Frankena, *Ethics*, 2nd ed. (Englewood Cliffs, NJ: Prentice-Hall, 1973), 63.

24　Aristotle, 1112 a16-17.

25　Aristotle, 1113 b20.

26　Aristotle, 1116 b37.

27　Susan Sherwin, "Ethics, 'Feminine Ethics,' and Feminist Ethics," in Debra Shogan, ed., *A Reader in Feminist Ethics* (Toronto: Canadian Scholars' Press, 1993), 10.

28　Sherwin, 14.

29　Margaret Urban Walker, *Moral Understandings: A Feminist Study in Ethics*, 2nd ed. (Oxford: Oxford University Press, 2007).

30　Margaret Urban Walker, "Groningen Naturalism in Bioethics," in Hilde Lindemann, Marian Verkerk, and Margaret Urban Walker, *Naturalised Bioethics: Toward Responsible Knowing and Practice* (Cambridge: Cambridge University Press, 2009).

31　See W. Hohfeld, *Fundamental Legal Conceptions* (New Haven, CT: Yale University Press, 1919), and Joel Feinberg, "Duties Rights and Claims," in *Rights, Justice and the Bounds of Liberty* (Princeton, NJ: Princeton University Press, 1980).

32　Aristotle, 1094 b12, 18.

CHAPTER ONE

RELATIONSHIPS IN
HEALTH CARE

Web Links

(1) Link to the Canadian Medical Association (CMA) Code of Ethics.

http://policybase.cma.ca/dbtw-wpd/PolicyPDF/PD04-06.pdf

The CMA code of ethics delineates the standards of *ethical* behaviour for physicians in Canada. It sets out ethical standards, which may or may not coincide with legal standards.

(2) Steven Lewis et al., "Dancing with the Porcupine: Rules for Governing the University-Industry Relationship"

http://pubmedcentralcanada.ca/articlerender.cgi?accid=PMC81459&tool=pmcentrez

(3) Elaine Gibson et al., "Dances with the Pharmaceutical Industry"

http://pubmedcentralcanada.ca/articlerender.cgi?accid=PMC99354&tool=pmcentrez

* For an up-to-date list of the web links in this book, please visit: http://sites.broadviewpress.com/healthcare.

1.
FOUR MODELS OF THE PHYSICIAN-PATIENT RELATIONSHIP

Ezekiel J. Emanuel and Linda L. Emanuel

SOURCE: *Journal of the American Medical Association* 267.16 (1992): 2212-26.

During the last two decades or so, there has been a struggle over the patient's role in medical decision making that is often characterized as a conflict between autonomy and health, between the values of the patient and the values of the physician. Seeking to curtail physician dominance, many have advocated an ideal of greater patient control.[1] Others question this ideal because it fails to acknowledge the potentially imbalanced nature of this interaction when one party is sick and searching for security, and when judgments entail the interpretation of technical information.[2] Still others are trying to delineate a more mutual relationship.[3] This struggle shapes the expectation of physicians and patients as well as the ethical and legal standards for the physician's duties, informed consent, and medical malpractice. This struggle forces us to ask, What should be the ideal physician-patient relationship?

We shall outline four models of physician-patient interaction, emphasizing the different understanding of (1) the goals of the physician-patient interaction, (2) the physician's obligations, (3) the role of patient values, and (4) the conception of patient autonomy. To elaborate the abstract description of these four models, we shall indicate the types of response the models might suggest in a clinical situation. Third, we shall also indicate how these models inform the current debate about the ideal physician-patient relationship. Finally, we shall evaluate these models and recommend one as the preferred model.

As outlined, the models are Weberian ideal types. They may not describe any particular physician-patient interaction but highlight, free from complicating details, different visions of the essential characteristics of the physician-patient interaction.[4] Consequently, they do not embody minimum ethical or legal standards, but rather constitute relative ideals that are "higher than the law" but not "above the law."[5]

The Paternalistic Model

First is the *paternalistic* model, sometimes called the parental[6] or priestly[7] model. In this model, the physician-patient interaction ensures that patients receive the interventions that best promote their health and well-being. To this end, physicians use their skills to determine the patient's medical condition and his or her stage in the disease process and to identify the medical tests and treatments most likely to restore the patient's health or ameliorate pain. Then the physician presents the patient with selected information that will encourage the patient to consent to the intervention the physician considers best. At the extreme, the physician authoritatively informs the patient when the intervention will be initiated.

The paternalistic model assumes that there are shared objective criteria for determining what is best. Hence the physician can discern what is in the patient's best interest with limited patient participation. Ultimately, it is assumed that the patient will be thankful for decisions made by the physician even if he or she would not agree to them at the time.[8] In the tension between the patient's autonomy and well-being, between choice and health, the paternalistic physician's main emphasis is toward the latter.

In the paternalistic model, the physician acts as the patient's guardian articulating and implementing what is best for the patient. As such, the physician has obligations, including that of placing the patient's interest above his or her own and soliciting the views of others when lacking adequate knowledge. The conception of patient autonomy is patient assent, either at the time or later, to the physician's determinations of what is best.

The Informative Model

Second is the *informative* model, sometimes called the scientific,[9] engineering,[10] or consumer model. In this model, the objective of the physician-patient interaction is for the physician to provide the patient with all relevant information, for the patient to select the medical interventions he or she wants, and for the physician to execute the selected interventions. To this end, the physician informs the patient of his or her disease state, the nature of possible diagnostic and therapeutic interventions, the nature and probability of risks and benefits associated with the intervention, and any uncertainties of knowledge. At the extreme, patients could come to know all medical information relevant to their disease and available interventions and select the interventions that best realize their values.

The informative model assumes a fairly clear distinction between facts and values. The patient's values are well defined and known; what the patient lacks is facts. It is the physician's obligation to provide all the available facts, and the patient's values then determine what treatments are to be given. There is no role for the physician's values, the physician's understanding of the patient's values, or his or her judgment of the worth of the patient's values. In the informative mode, the physician is a purveyor of technical expertise, providing the patient with the means to exercise control. As technical experts, physicians have important obligations to provide truthful information, to maintain competence in their area of expertise, and to consult others when their knowledge or skills are lacking. The conception of patient autonomy is patient control over medical decision making.

The Interpretive Model

The third model is the *interpretive* model. The aim of the physician-patient interaction is to elucidate the patient's values and what he or she actually wants, and to help the patient select the available medical interventions that realize these values. Like the informative physician, the interpretive physician provides the patient with information on the nature of the condition and the risks and benefits of possible interventions.

Beyond this, however, the interpretive physician assists the patient in elucidating and articulating his or her values and in determining what medical interventions best realize the specified values, thus helping to interpret the patient's values for the patient. According to the interpretive model, the patient's values are not necessarily fixed and known to the patient. They are often inchoate, and the patient may only partially understand them; they may conflict when applied to specific situations. Consequently, the physician working with the patient must elucidate and make coherent these values. To do this, the physician works with the patient to reconstruct the patient's goals and aspirations, commitments and character. At the extreme, the physician must conceive the patient's life as a narrative whole, and from this specify the patient's values and their priority.[11] Then the physician determines which tests and treatments best realize these values. Importantly, the physician does not dictate to the patient; it is the patient who ultimately decides which values and course of action best fit who he or she is. Neither is the physician judging the patient's values; he or she helps the patient to understand and use them in the medical situation.

In the interpretive model, the physician is a counselor, analogous to a cabinet minister's advisory role to a head of state, supplying relevant information, helping to elucidate values and suggesting what medical interventions realize these values. Thus the physician's obligations include those enumerated in the informative model but also require engaging the patient in a joint process of understanding. Accordingly, the conception of patient autonomy is self-understanding; the patient comes to know more clearly who he or she is and how the various medical options bear on his or her identity.

The Deliberative Model

Fourth is the *deliberative* model. The aim of the physician-patient interaction is to help the patient determine and choose the best health-related values

Table x.1   Comparing the Four Models

	Informative	*Interpretive*	*Deliberative*	*Paternalistic*
Patient values	Defined, fixed, and known to the patient	Inchoate and conflicting, requiring elucidation	Open to development and revision through moral discussion	Objective and shared by physician and patient
Physician's obligation	Providing relevant factual information and implementing patient's selected intervention	Elucidating and interpreting relevant patient values as well as informing the patient and implementing the patient's selected intervention	Articulating and persuading the patient of the most admirable values as well as informing the patient and implementing the patient's selected intervention	Promoting the patient's well-being independent of the patient's current preferences
Conception of patient's autonomy	Choice of, and control over, medical care	Self-understanding relevant to medical care	Moral self-development relevant to medical care	Assenting to objective values
Conception of physician's role	Competent technical expert	Counselor or advisor	Friend or teacher	Guardian

that can be realized in the clinical situation. To this end, the physician must delineate information on the patient's clinical situation and then help elucidate the types of values embodied in the available options. The physician's objectives include suggesting why certain health-related values are more worthy and should be aspired to. At the extreme, the physician and patient engage in deliberation about what kind of health-related values the patient could and ultimately should pursue. The physician discusses only health-related values, that is, values that affect or are affected by the patient's disease and treatments; he or she recognizes that many elements of morality are unrelated to the patient's disease or treatment and beyond the scope of their professional relationship. Further, the physician aims at no more than moral persuasion; ultimately, coercion is avoided, and the patient must define his or her life and select the ordering of values to be espoused. By engaging in moral deliberation, the physician and patient judge the worthiness and importance of the health-related values.

In the deliberative model, the physician acts as a teacher or friend,[12] engaging the patient in dialogue on what course of action would be best. Not only does the physician indicate what the patient could do, but, knowing the patient and wishing what is best, the physician indicates what the patient should do, what decision regarding medical therapy would be admirable. The conception of patient autonomy is moral self-development; the patient is empowered not simply to follow unexamined preferences or examined values, but to consider, through dialogue, alternative health-related values, their worthiness, and their implications for treatment.

Comparing the Four Models

Table x.1 compares the four models on essential points. Importantly, all models have a role for patient autonomy; a main factor that differentiates the models is their particular conception of patient autonomy. Therefore, no single model can be endorsed because it alone promotes patient autonomy. Instead the models must be compared and evaluated, at least in part, by evaluating the adequacy of their particular conceptions of patient autonomy.

The four models are not exhaustive. At a minimum there might be added a fifth: the *instrumental* model. In this model, the patient's values are irrelevant; the physician aims for some goal independent of the patient, such as the good of society or furtherance of scientific knowledge. The Tuskegee syphilis experiment[13] and the Willowbrook hepatitis study,[14] are examples of this model. As the moral condemnation of these cases reveals, this model is not an ideal but an aberration. Thus we have not elaborated it herein.

A Clinical Case

To make tangible these abstract descriptions and to crystallize essential differences among the models, we will illustrate the responses they suggest in a clinical situation, that of a 43-year-old premenopausal woman who has recently discovered a breast mass. Surgery reveals a 3.5 cm ductal carcinoma with no lymph node involvement that is estrogen receptor positive. Chest roentgenogram, bone scan, and liver function tests reveal no evidence of metastatic disease. The patient was recently divorced and has gone back to work as a legal aide to support herself. What should the physician say to this patient?

In the paternalistic model a physician might say, "There are two alternative therapies to protect against recurrence of cancer in your breast: mastectomy or radiation. We now know that the survival with lumpectomy combined with radiation therapy is equal to that with mastectomy. Because lumpectomy and radiation offers the best survival and the best cosmetic result, it is to be preferred. I have asked the radiation therapist to come and discuss radiation treatment with you. We also need to protect you against the spread of cancer to other parts of your body. Even though the chance of recurrence is low, you are young, and we should not leave any therapeutic possibilities untried. Recent studies involving chemotherapy suggest improvements in survival without recurrence of breast cancer. Indeed, the National Cancer Institute [NCI] recommends chemotherapy for women with your type of breast cancer. Chemotherapy has side effects. Nevertheless, a few months of hardship now are worth the potential added years of life without cancer."

In the informative model a physician might say, "With node-negative breast cancer there are two issues before you: local control and systemic control. For local control, the options are mastectomy or lumpectomy with or without radiation. From many studies we know that mastectomy and lumpectomy

with radiation result in identical overall survival, about 80% 10-year survival. Lumpectomy without radiation results in a 30% to 40% chance of tumor recurrence in the breast. The second issue relates to systemic control. We know that chemotherapy prolongs survival for premenopausal women who have axillary nodes involved with tumor. The role for women with node-negative breast cancer is less clear. Individual studies suggest that chemotherapy is of no benefit in terms of improving overall survival, but a comprehensive review of all studies suggests that there is a survival benefit. Several years ago, the NCI suggested that for women like yourself, chemotherapy can have a positive therapeutic impact. Finally, let me inform you that there are clinical trials, for which you are eligible, to evaluate the benefits of chemotherapy for patients with node-negative breast cancer. I can enroll you in a study if you want. I will be happy to give you any further information you feel you need."

The interpretive physician might outline much of the same information as the informative physician, then engage in discussion to elucidate the patient's wishes, and conclude, "It sounds to me as if you have conflicting wishes. Understandably, you seem uncertain how to balance the demands required for receiving additional treatment, rejuvenating your personal affairs, and maintaining your psychological equilibrium. Let me try to express a perspective that fits your position. Fighting your cancer is important, but it must leave you with a healthy self-image and quality time outside the hospital. This view seems compatible with undergoing radiation therapy but not chemotherapy. A lumpectomy with radiation maximizes your chance of surviving while preserving your breast. Radiotherapy fights your breast cancer without disfigurement. Conversely, chemotherapy would prolong the duration of therapy by many months. Further, the benefits of chemotherapy in terms of survival are smaller and more controversial. Given the recent changes in your life, you have too many preoccupations to undergo months of chemotherapy for a questionable benefit. Do I understand you? We can talk again in a few days."

The deliberative physician might begin by outlining the same factual information, engage in a conversation to elucidate the patient's values, but continue, "It seems clear that you should undergo radiation therapy. It offers maximal survival with minimal risk, disfigurement, and disruption of your life. The issue of chemotherapy is different, fraught with conflicting data. Balancing all the options, I think the best one for you is to enter a trial that is investigating the potential benefit of chemotherapy for women with node-negative breast cancer. First, it ensures that you receive excellent medical care. At this point, we do not know which therapy maximizes survival. In a clinical study the schedule of follow-up visits, tests, and decisions is specified by leading breast cancer experts to ensure that all the women receive care that is the best available anywhere. A second reason to participate in a trial is altruistic: it allows you to contribute something to women with breast cancer in the future who will face difficult choices. Over decades, thousands of women have participated in studies that inform our current treatment practices. Without those women, and the knowledge they made possible, we would probably still be giving you and all other women with breast cancer mastectomies. By enrolling in a trial you participate in a tradition in which women of one generation receive the highest standard of care available but also enhance the care of women in future generations because medicine has learned something about which interventions are better. I must tell you that I am not involved in the study; if you elect to enroll in this trial, you will initially see another breast cancer expert to plan your therapy. I have sought to explain our current knowledge and offer my recommendation so you can make the best possible decision."

Lacking the normal interchange with patients, these statements may seem contrived, even caricatures. Nevertheless, they highlight the essence of each model and suggest how the objectives and assumptions of each inform a physician's approach to his or her patients. Similar statements can be imagined for other clinical situations such as an obstetrician discussing prenatal testing or a cardiologist discussing cholesterol-reducing interventions.

The Current Debate and the Four Models

In recent decades there has been a call for greater patient autonomy or, as some have called it, "patient

sovereignty,"[15] conceived as patient *choice* and *control* over medical decisions. This shift toward the informative model is embodied in the adoption of business terms for medicine, as when physicians are described as health care providers and patients as consumers. It can also be found in the propagation of patient rights statements,[16] in the promotion of living will laws, and in rules regarding human experimentation. For instance, the opening sentences of one law state: "The Rights of the Terminally Ill Act authorizes an adult person to *control* decisions regarding administration of life-sustaining treatment.... The Act merely provides one way by which a terminally-ill patient's *desires* regarding the use of life-sustaining procedures can be legally implemented" (emphasis added).[17] Indeed, living will laws do not require or encourage patients to discuss the issue of terminating care with their physicians before signing such documents. Similarly, decisions in "right-to-die" cases emphasize patient control over medical decisions. As one court put it:[18]

> The right to refuse medical treatment is basic and fundamental.... Its exercise requires no one's approval.... *[T]he controlling decision belongs to a competent informed patient*.... It is not a medical decision for her physicians to make.... *It is a moral and philosophical decision that, being a competent adult, is [the patient's] alone.* (emphasis added)

Probably the most forceful endorsement of the informative model as the ideal inheres in informed consent standards. Prior to the 1970s, the standard for informed consent was "physician based."[19] Since 1972 and the *Canterbury* case, however, the emphasis has been on a "patient-oriented" standard of informed consent in which the physician has a "duty" to provide appropriate medical facts to empower the patient to use his or her values to determine what interventions should be implemented.[20]

> True consent to what happens to one's self is the informed exercise of a choice, and that entails an opportunity to evaluate knowledgeably the options available and the risks attendant upon each.... *[I]t is the prerogative of the patient, not*

the physician, to determine for himself the direction in which his interests seem to lie. To enable the patient to chart his course understandably, some familiarity with the therapeutic alternatives and their hazards become essential.[21] (emphasis added)

Shared Decision Making

Despite its dominance, many have found the informative mode "arid."[22] The President's Commission and others contend that the ideal relationship does not vest moral authority and medical decision-making power exclusively in the patient but must be a process of shared decision making constructed around "mutual participation and respect."[23] The President's Commission argues that the physician's role is "to help the patient understand the medical situation and available courses of action, and the patient conveys his or her concerns and wishes."[24] Brock and Wartman[25] stress this fact-value "division of labor"—having the physician provide information while the patient makes value decisions—by describing "shared decision making" as a collaborative process

in which both physicians and patients make active and essential contributions. Physicians bring their medical training, knowledge, and expertise—including an understanding of the available treatment alternatives—to the diagnosis and management of patients' condition. Patients bring knowledge of their own subjective aims and values, through which risks and benefits of various treatment options can be evaluated. With this approach, selecting the best treatment for a particular patient requires the contribution of both parties.

Similarly, in discussing ideal medical decision making, Eddy[26] argues for this fact-value division of labor between the physician and patient as the ideal:

It is important to separate the decision process into these two steps.... The first step is a question of facts. The anchor is empirical evidence.... [T]he second step is a question not of facts but of personal values or preferences. The thought process is not analytic but personal and subjective.... [I]t is the patient's preferences that should determine the decision.... Ideally, you and I [the physicians] are not in the picture. What matters is what Mrs. Smith thinks.

This view of shared decision making seems to vest the medical decision-making authority with the patient while relegating physicians to technicians "transmitting medical information and using their technical skills as the patient directs."[27] Thus, while the advocates of "shared decision making" may aspire toward a mutual dialogue between physician and patient, the substantive view informing their ideal re-embodies the informative model under a different label.

Other commentators have articulated more mutual models of the physician-patient interaction.[28] Prominent among these efforts is Katz' *The Silent World of the Doctor and Patient*.[29] Relying on a Freudian view in which self-knowledge and self-determination are inherently limited because of unconscious influences, Katz views dialogue as a mechanism for greater self-understanding of one's values and objectives. According to Katz, this view places a duty on physicians and patients to reflect and communicate so that patients can gain a greater self-understanding and self-determination. Katz' insight is also available on grounds other than Freudian psychological theory and is consistent with the interpretive model.[30]

Objections to the Paternalistic Model

It is widely recognized that the paternalistic model is justified during emergencies when the time taken to obtain informed consent might irreversibly harm the patient.[31] Beyond such limited circumstances, however, it is no longer tenable to assume that the physician and patient espouse similar values and views of what constitutes a benefit. Consequently, even physicians rarely advocate the paternalistic model as an ideal for routine physician-patient interactions.[32]

Objections to the Informative Model

The informative model seems both descriptively and prescriptively inaccurate. First, this model seems to have no place for essential qualities of the ideal physician-patient relationship. The informative physician cares for the patient in the sense of competently implementing the patient's selected interventions. However, the informative physician lacks a caring approach that requires understanding what the patient values or should value and how his or her illness impinges on these values. Patients seem to expect their physician to have a caring approach; they deem a technically proficient but detached physician as deficient, and properly condemned. Further, the informative physician is proscribed from giving a recommendation for fear of imposing his or her will on the patient and thereby competing for the decision making control that has been given to the patient.[33] Yet, if one of the essential qualities of the ideal physician is the ability to assimilate medical facts, prior experience of similar situations, and intimate knowledge of the patient's view into a recommendation designed for the patient's specific medical and personal condition,[34] then the informative physician cannot be ideal.

Second, in the informative model the ideal physician is a highly trained subspecialist who provides detailed factual information and competently implements the patient's preferred medical intervention. Hence, the informative model perpetuates and accentuates the trend toward specialization and impersonalization within the medical profession.

Most importantly, the informative model's conception of patient autonomy seems philosophically untenable. The informative model presupposes that persons possess known and fixed values, but this is inaccurate. People are often uncertain about what they actually want. Further, unlike animals, people have what philosophers call "second-order desires," that is, the capacity to reflect on their wishes and to revise their own desire and preferences. In fact, freedom of the will and autonomy inhere in having "second-order desires"[35] and being able to change our preferences and modify our identity. Self-reflection and the capacity to change what we want often

require a "process" of moral deliberation in which we assess the value of what we want. And this is a process that occurs with other people who know us well and can articulate a vision of who we ought to be that we can assent to.[36] Even though changes in health or implementation of alternative interventions can have profound effects on what we desire and how we realize our desires, self-reflection and deliberation play no essential role in the informative physician-patient interaction. The informative model's conception of autonomy is incompatible with a vision of autonomy that incorporates second-order desires.

Objections to the Interpretive Model

The interpretive model rectifies this deficiency by recognizing that persons have second-order desires and dynamic value structures and placing the elucidation of values in the context of the patient's medical condition at the center of the physician-patient interaction. Nevertheless, there are objections to the interpretive model.

Technical specialization militates against physicians cultivating the skills necessary to the interpretive model. With limited interpretive talents and limited time, physicians may unwittingly impose their own values under the guise of articulating the patient's values. And patients, overwhelmed by their medical condition and uncertain of their own views, may too easily accept this imposition. Such circumstances may push the interpretive model towards the paternalistic model in actual practice.

Further, autonomy viewed as self-understanding excludes evaluative judgment of the patient's values or attempts to persuade the patient to adopt other values. This constrains the guidance and recommendations the physician can offer. Yet in practice, especially in preventive medicine and risk-reduction interventions, physicians often attempt to persuade patients to adopt particularly health-related values. Physicians frequently urge patients with high cholesterol levels who smoke to change their dietary habits, quit smoking, and begin exercise programs before initiating drug therapy. The justification given for these changes is that patients should value their health more than they do. Similarly, physicians are encouraged to persuade their human immunodeficiency virus (HIV)-infected patients who might be engaging in unsafe sexual practices either to abstain or, realistically, to adopt "safer sex" practices. Such appeals are not made to promote the HIV-infected patient's own health, but are grounded on an appeal for the patient to assume responsibility for the good of others. Consequently, by excluding evaluative judgments, the interpretive model seems to characterize inaccurately ideal physician-patient interactions.

Objection to the Deliberative Model

The fundamental objections to the deliberative model focus on whether it is proper for physicians to judge patients' values and promote particular health-related values. First, physicians do not possess privileged knowledge of the priority of health-related values relative to other values. Indeed, since ours is a pluralistic society in which people espouse incommensurable values, it is likely that a physician's values and view of which values are higher will conflict with those of other physicians and those of his or her patients.

Second, the nature of the moral deliberation between physician and patient, the physician's recommended interventions, and the actual treatments used will depend on the values of the particular physician treating the patient. However, recommendations and care provided to patients would not depend on the physician's judgment of the worthiness of the patient's values or on the physician's particular values. As one bioethicist put it:[37]

> The hand is broken, the physician can repair the hand; therefore the physician must repair the hand—as well as possible—without regard to personal values that might lead the physician to think ill of the patient or of the patient's values.... [A]t the level of clinical practice, medicine should be value-free in the sense that the personal values of the physician should not distort the making of medical decisions.

Third, it may be argued that the deliberative model misconstrues the purpose of the physician-patient interaction. Patients see their physicians to receive health care, not to engage in moral deliberation or to revise their values. Finally, like the interpretive model, the deliberative model may easily metamorphose into unintended paternalism, the very practice that generated the public debate over the proper physician-patient interaction.

The Preferred Model
and the Practical Implications

Clearly, under different clinical circumstances different models may be appropriate. Indeed, at different times all four models may justifiably guide physicians and patients. Nevertheless, it is important to specify one model as the shared, paradigmatic reference; exceptions to use other models would not be automatically condemned, but would require justification based on the circumstances of a particular situation. Thus, it is widely agreed that in an emergency where delays in treatment to obtain informed consent might irreversibly harm the patient, the paternalistic model correctly guides physician-patient interactions. Conversely, for patients who have clear but conflicting values, the interpretive model is probably justified. For instance, a 65-year-old woman who has been treated for acute leukemia may have clearly decided against reinduction chemotherapy if she relapses. Several months before the anticipated birth of her first grandchild, the patient relapses. The patient becomes torn about whether to endure the risks of reinduction chemotherapy in order to live to see her first grandchild or whether to refuse therapy, resigning herself to not seeing her grandchild. In such cases, the physician may justifiably adopt the interpretive approach. In other circumstances, where there is only a one-time physician-patient interaction without an ongoing relationship in which the patient's values can be elucidated and compared with ideals, such as in a walk-in center, the informative model may be justified.

Descriptively and prescriptively, we claim that the ideal physician-patient relationship is the deliberative model. We will adduce six points to justify this claim. First, the deliberative model more nearly embodies our ideal of autonomy. It is an oversimplification and distortion of the Western tradition to view respecting autonomy as simply permitting a person to select, unrestricted by coercion, ignorance, physical interference, and the like, his or her preferred course of action from a comprehensive list of available options.[38] Freedom and control over medical decisions alone do not constitute patient autonomy. Autonomy requires that individuals critically assess their own values and preferences; determine whether they are desirable; affirm, upon reflection, these values as ones that should justify their actions; and then be free to initiate action to realize the values. The process of deliberation integral to the deliberative model is essential for realizing patient autonomy understood in this way.

Second, our society's image of an ideal physician is not limited to one who knows and communicates to the patient relevant factual information and competently implements medical interventions. The ideal physician—often embodied in literature, art, and popular culture—is a caring physician who integrates the information and relevant values to make a recommendation and, through discussion, attempts to persuade the patient to accept this recommendation as the intervention that best promotes his or her overall well-being. Thus, we expect the best physicians to engage their patients in evaluating discussions of health issues and related values. The physician's discussion does not invoke values that are unrelated or tangentially related to the patient's illness and potential therapies. Importantly, these efforts are not restricted to situations in which patients might make "irrational and harmful" choices[39] but extend to all health care decisions.

Third, the deliberative model is not a disguised form of paternalism. Previously there may have been category mistakes in which instances of the deliberative model have been erroneously identified as physician paternalism. And no doubt, in practice, the deliberative physician may occasionally lapse into paternalism. However, like the ideal teacher, the deliberative physician attempts to persuade the patient of the worthiness of certain values, not to impose those values paternalistically; the physician's aim is not to subject the patient to his or her will, but to persuade the patient of a course of action as desirable. In the Laws, Plato[40] characterizes this funda-

mental distinction between persuasion and imposition for medical practice that distinguishes the deliberative from the paternalistic model:

> A physician to slaves never gives his patients any account of his illness ... the physician offers some order gleaned from experience with an air of infallible knowledge, in the brusque fashion of a dictator.... The free physician, who usually cares for free men, treats their disease first by thoroughly discussing with the patient and his friends his ailment. This way he learns something from the sufferer and simultaneously instructs him. Then the physician does not give his medications until he has persuaded the patient; the physician aims at complete restoration of health by persuading the patient to comply with his therapy.

Fourth, physician values are relevant to patients and do inform their choice of a physician. When a pregnant woman chooses an obstetrician who does not routinely perform a battery of prenatal tests or, alternatively, one who strongly favors them; when a patient seeks an aggressive cardiologist who favors procedural interventions or one who concentrates therapy on dietary changes, stress reduction, and life-style modifications, they are, consciously or not, selecting a physician based on the values that guide his or her medical decisions. And, when disagreements between physicians and patients arise, there are discussions over which values are more important and should be realized in medical care. Occasionally, when such disagreements undermine the physician-patient relationship and a caring attitude, a patient's care is transferred to another physician. Indeed, in the informative model the grounds for transferring care to a new physician is either the physician's ignorance or incompetence. But patients seem to switch physicians because they do not "like" a particular physician or that physician's attitude or approach.

Fifth, we seem to believe that physicians should not only help fit therapies to the patients' elucidated values, but should also promote health-related values. As noted, we expect physicians to promote certain values, such as "safer sex" for patients with HIV or abstaining from or limiting alcohol use. Similarly, patients are willing to adjust their values and actions to be more compatible with health-promoting values.[41] This is in the nature of seeking a caring medical recommendation.

Finally, it may well be that many physicians currently lack the training and capacity to articulate the values underlying their recommendations and persuade patients that these values are worthy. But, in part, this deficiency is a consequence of the tendencies toward specialization and the avoidance of discussion of values by physicians that are perpetuated and justified by the dominant informative model. Therefore, if the deliberative model seems most appropriate, then we need to implement changes in medical care and education to encourage a more caring approach. We must stress understanding rather than mere provisions of factual information in keeping with the legal standards of informed consent and medical malpractice; we must educate physicians not just to spend more time in physician-patient communication but to elucidate and articulate the values underlying their medical care decisions, including routine ones; we must shift the publicly assumed conception of patient autonomy that shapes both the physician's and the patient's expectations from patient control to moral development. Most important, we must recognize that developing a deliberative physician-patient relationship requires a considerable amount of time. We must develop a health care financing system that properly reimburses—rather than penalizes—physicians for taking the time to discuss values with their patients.

Conclusion

Over the last few decades, the discourse regarding the physician-patient relationship has focused on two extremes: autonomy and paternalism. Many have attacked physicians as paternalistic, urging the empowerment of patients to control their own care. This view, the informative model, has become dominant in bioethics and legal standards. This model embodies a defective conception of patient autonomy, and it reduces the physician's role to that of a technologist. The essence of doctoring is a fabric of knowledge, understanding, teaching, and action, in which the caring physician integrates the patient's medical con-

dition and health-related values, makes a recommendation on the appropriate course of action, and tries to persuade the patient of the worthiness of this approach and the values it realizes. The physician with a caring attitude is the ideal embodied in the deliberative model, the ideal that should inform laws and policies that regulate the physician-patient interaction.

Finally, it may be worth noting that the four models outlined herein are not limited to the medical realm: they may inform the public conception of other professional interactions as well. We suggest that the ideal relationships between lawyer and client,[42] religious mentor and laity, and educator and student are well described by the deliberative model, at least in some of their essential aspects.

Acknowledgements

We would like to thank Robert Mayer, MD, Craig Henderson, MD, Lynn Peterson, MD, and John Stoeckle, MD, as well as Dennis Thompson, PhD, Arthur Applebaum, PhD, and Dan Brock, PhD, for their critical reviews of the manuscript. We would also like to thank the "ethics and the professions" seminar participants, especially Robert Rosen, JD, Francis Kamm, PhD, David Wilkins, JD, and Oliver Avens, who enlightened us in discussions.

Notes

1   R.M. Veatch, *A Theory of Medical Ethics* (New York: Basic Books, 1981); also R. Macklin, *Mortal Choices* (New York: Pantheon Books Inc., 1987).

2   F.J. Ingelfinger, "Arrogance," *N Engl J Med* 304 (1980): 1507; also P.M. Marzuk, "The right kind of paternalism," *N Engl J Med* 313 (1985): 1474-76.

3   M. Siegler, "The progression of medicine: from physician paternalism to patient autonomy to bureaucratic parsimony" *Arch Intern Med* 145 (1985): 713-15; also T.S. Szasz and M.H. Hollender, "The basic models of the doctor-patient relationship," *Arch Intern Med* 97 (1956): 585-92.

4   M. Weber and T. Parsons, ed. *The Theory of Social and Economic Organization* (New York: The Free Press, 1974).

5   H.T. Ballantine, "Annual discourse—the crisis in ethics, anno domini 1979," *N Engl J Med* 301 (1979): 634-38.

6   G. Burke, "Ethics and medical decision-making," *Prim Care* 7 (1980): 615-24.

7   R.M. Veatch, "Models for ethical medicine in a revolutionary age," *Hastings Cent Rep* 2 (1975): 3-5.

8   A.A. Stone, *Mental Health and Law: A System in Transition* (New York: Jason Aronson Inc., 1976).

9   Burke, "Ethics."

10 Veatch, "Models for ethical medicine."

11 A. MacIntyre, *After Virtue* (South Bend, IN: University of Notre Dame Press, 1981); M.J. Sandel, *Liberalism and the Limits of Justice* (New York: Cambridge University Press, 1982).

12 C. Fried, "The lawyer as friend: the moral foundations of the lawyer client relationship," *Yale Law J* 85 (1976): 1060-89.

13 J.H. Jones, *Bad Blood* (New York: Free Press, 1981); *Final Report of the Tuskegee Syphilis Study Ad Hoc Advisory Panel* (Washington, DC: Public Health Service, 1973); A.M. Brandt, "Racism and research: the case of the Tuskegee Syphilis Study," *Hastings Cent Rep* 8 (1978): 21-29.

14 S. Krugman and J.P. Giles, "Viral hepatitis: new light on an old disease," *JAMA* 212 (1970): 1019-29; also F.J. Ingelfinger, "Ethics of experiments on children," *N Engl J Med* 288 (1973): 791-92.

15 President's Commission for the Study of Ethical Problems in Medicine and Biomedical and Behavioral Research, *Making Health Care Decisions* (Washington, DC: US Government Printing Office, 1982).

16 *Statement of a Patient's Bill of Rights* (Chicago: American Hospital Association, 17 November 1972).

17 "Uniform Rights of the Terminally Ill Act," in *Handbook of Living Will Laws* (New York: Society for the Right to Die, 1987), 135-47.

18 *Bouvia v Superior Court*, 225 Cal Rptr. 297 (1986).

19 *Natanson v Kline*, 350 P2d 1093 (Kan 1960); also P.S. Applebaum, C.W. Lidz, and A. Meisel, *Informed Consent: Legal Theory and Clinical Practice* (New York: Oxford University Press, 1987), ch. 3; R.R. Faden·and T.L. Beauchamp, *A History and Theory of Informed Consent* (New York: Oxford University Press, 1986).

20 Applebaum et al., *Informed Consent,* ch. 3; also Faden and Beauchamp, *A History and Theory of Informed Consent*; *Canterbury v Spence*, 464 F2d 772 (DC Cir 1972).

21 *Canterbury v Spence.*

22 *Statement of a Patient's Bill of Rights.*

23 President's Commission, *Making Health Care Decisions*; also D. Brock, "The ideal of shared decision making between physicians and patients," *Kennedy Institute J Ethics* 1 (1991): 28-47.

24 *Statement of a Patient's Bill of Rights.*

25 D.W. Brock and S.A. Wartman, "When competent patients make irrational choices," *N Engl J Med* 322 (1990): 1595-99.

26 D.M. Eddy, "Anatomy of a decision" *JAMA* 263 (1990): 441-43.

27 President's Commission, *Making Health Care Decisions*; Brock, "The ideal of shared decision making."

28 Siegler, "The progression of medicine"; also Szasz and Hollender, "The basic models"; Applebaum et al., *Informed Consent,* ch. 3.

29 J. Katz, *The Silent World of Doctor and Patient* (New York: Free Press, 1984).

30 Sandel, *Liberalism.*

31 Veatch, *A Theory of Medical Ethics;* Macklin, *Mortal Choices.*

32 I.F. Tannock and M. Boyer, "When is a cancer treatment worthwhile?" *N Engl J Med* 322 (1990): 989-90.

33 Applebaum et al., *Informed Consent,* ch. 3.

34 Ingelfinger, "Arrogance"; Marzuk, "The right kind of paternalism"; Siegler, "The progression of medicine."

35 H. Frankfurt, "Freedom of the will and the concept of a person," *J Philosophy* 68 (1971): 5-20; C. Taylor, *Human Agency and Language* (New York: Cambridge University Press, 1985), 15-44; G. Dworkin, *The Theory and Practice of Autonomy* (New York: Cambridge University Press, 1988), ch. 1.

36 Sandel, *Liberalism.*

37 S. Gorovitz, *Doctors' Dilemmas: Moral Conflict and Medical Care* (New York: Oxford University Press, 1982), ch. 6.

38 Taylor, *Human Agency and Language,* 15-44; also Dworkin, *The Theory and Practice of Autonomy,* ch. 1.

39 Brock and Wartman, "When competent patients."

40 E. Hamilton and H. Cairns, eds., *Plato: The Collected Dialogues* (Princeton, NJ: Princeton University Press, 1961), 720 c-e; trans. E.J. Emanuel.

41 D.C. Walsh, R.W. Hingson, D.M. Merrigan, et al., "The impact of a physician's warning on recovery after alcoholism treatment," *JAMA* 267 (1992): 663-67.

42 Fried, "The lawyer as friend."

2.
A RELATIONAL APPROACH TO AUTONOMY IN HEALTH CARE

Susan Sherwin

SOURCE: The Feminist Health Care Ethics Research Network, *The Politics of Women's Health: Exploring Agency and Autonomy* (Philadelphia: Temple University Press, 1998).

Respect for patient autonomy (or self-direction) is broadly understood as recognition that patients have the authority to make decisions about their own health care. The principle that insists on this recognition is pervasive in the bioethics literature: it is a central value within virtually all the leading approaches to health care ethics, feminist and other. It is not surprising, then, that discussions of autonomy constantly emerged within our own conversations in the Network [on Feminist Health Care Ethics]; readers will recognize that autonomy is woven throughout the book in our various approaches to the issues we take up. It is, however, an ideal that we felt deeply ambivalent about, and, therefore, we judged it to be in need of a specifically feminist analysis.

In this chapter, I propose a feminist analysis of autonomy, making vivid both our attraction to and distrust of the dominant interpretation of this concept. I begin by reviewing some of the appeal of the autonomy ideal in order to make clear why it has achieved such prominence within bioethics and feminist health care discussions. I then identify some difficulties I find with the usual interpretations of the concept, focusing especially on difficulties that arise from a specifically feminist perspective. In response to these problems, I propose an alternative conception of autonomy that I label "relational" though the terms *socially situated* or *contextualized* would describe it equally well. To avoid confusion, I explicitly distinguish my use of the term *relational* from that of some other feminist authors, such as Carol Gilligan (1982), who reserve it to refer only to the narrower set of interpersonal relations. I apply the term to the full range of influential human relations, personal and public. Oppression permeates both per-

sonal and public relationships; hence, I prefer to politicize the understanding of the term *relational* as a way of emphasizing the political dimensions of the multiple relationships that structured an individual's selfhood, rather than to reserve the term to protect a sphere of purely private relationships that may appear to be free of political influence.[1] I explain why I think the relational alternative is more successful than the familiar individualistic interpretation at addressing the concerns identified. Finally, I briefly indicate some of the implications of adopting a relational interpretation of autonomy with respect to some of the issues discussed elsewhere in this book, and I identify some of the changes that this notion of relational autonomy suggests for the delivery of health services.

The Virtues of a Principle of Respect for Patient Autonomy

It is not hard to explain the prominence of the principle of respect for patient autonomy within the field of health care ethics in North America: respect for personal autonomy is a dominant value in North American culture and it plays a central role in most of our social institutions. Yet, protection of autonomy is often at particular risk in health care settings because illness, by its very nature, tends to make patients dependent on the care and good will of others; in so doing, it reduces patients' power to exercise autonomy and it also makes them vulnerable to manipulation and even to outright coercion by those who provide them with needed health services. Many patients who are either ill or at risk of becoming ill are easily frightened into overriding their own preferences and following expert advice rather than risking abandonment by their caregivers by rejecting that advice. Even when their health is not immediately threatened, patients may find themselves compelled to comply with the demands of health care providers in order to obtain access to needed services from health professionals who are, frequently, the only ones licensed to provide those services (e.g., abortion, assistance in childbirth, legitimate excuses from work, physiotherapy).[2]

Without a strong principle of respect for patient autonomy, patients are vulnerable to abuse or exploitation, when their weak and dependent position makes them easy targets to serve the interests (e.g., financial, academic, or social influence) of others. Strong moral traditions of service within medicine and other health professions have provided patients with some measure of protection against such direct harms, though abuses nonetheless occur.[3] Most common is the tendency of health care providers to assume that by virtue of their technical expertise they are better able to judge what is in the patient's best interest than is the patient. For example, physicians may make assumptions about the advantages of using fetal heart monitors when women are in labor without considering the ways in which such instruments restrict laboring-women's movement and the quality of the birthing experience from their perspective. By privileging their own types of knowledge over that of their patients (including both experiential knowledge and understanding of their own value scheme), health care providers typically ignore patients' expressed or implicit values and engage in paternalism[4] (or the overriding of patient preferences for the presumed benefit of the patient) when prescribing treatment.

Until very recently, conscientious physicians were actually trained to act paternalistically toward their patients, to treat patients according to the physician's own judgment about what would be best for their patients, with little regard for each patient's own perspectives or preferences. The problem with this arrangement, however, is that health care may involve such intimate and central aspects of a patient's life—including, for example, matters such as health, illness, reproduction, death, dying, bodily integrity, nutrition, lifestyle, self-image, disability, sexuality, and psychological well-being—that it is difficult for anyone other than the patient to make choices that will be compatible with that patient's personal value system. Indeed, making such choices is often an act of self-discovery or self-definition and as such it requires the active involvement of the patient. Whenever possible, then, these types of choices should be made by the person whose life is central to the treatment considered. The principle of respect for patient autonomy is aimed at clarifying and protecting patients' ultimate right to make up their own minds about the specific health services they receive (so long as they are competent to do so). It also helps to ensure that patients have full access to relevant information about their health status so that they can make informed choices about related aspects of their lives. For example, information about a terminal condition may affect a person's decisions to reproduce, take a leave of absence from work, seek a reconciliation from estranged friends or relatives, or revise a will.

Although theorists disagree about the precise definition of *autonomy*,[5] there are some common features to its use within bioethics. In practice, the principle of respect for patient autonomy is usually interpreted as acknowledging and protecting competent patients' authority to accept or refuse whatever specific treatments the health care providers they consult find it appropriate to offer them (an event known as informed choice). Since everyone can imagine being in the position of patient, and most can recognize the dangers of fully surrendering this authority to near strangers, it is not surprising that the principle of respect for patient autonomy is widely endorsed by nearly all who consider it. Despite different theoretical explanations, the overwhelming majority of bioethicists insist on this principle as a fundamental moral precept for health care. Support is especially strong in North America, where it fits comfortably within a general cultural milieu in which attention to the individual and protection of individual rights are granted (at least rhetorical) dominance in nearly all areas of social and political policy.[6] Both Canadian and U.S. Courts have underlined the importance of protection of individual rights as a central tenet of patient-provider interactions, making it a matter of legal as well as moral concern.

Further, the principle requiring respect for patient autonomy helps to resolve problems that arise when health care providers are responsible for the care of patients who have quite different experiences, values, and world views from their own; under such circumstances, it is especially unlikely that care givers can accurately anticipate the particular needs and interests of their patients. This problem becomes acute when there are significant differences in power between patients and the health care professionals who care for them. In most cases, the relevant interactions are between patients and physicians, where, typically, patients have less social power than their physicians: doctors are well educated and they tend to be (relatively) healthy and affluent, while the patients they care for are often poor, and lacking in education and social authority. In fact, according to most of the standard dichotomies supporting dominance in our culture—gender, class, race, ability status—odds are that if there is a difference between the status of the physician and the patient, the physician is likely to fall on the dominant side of that distinction and the patient on the subordinate side. The tendency of illness to undermine patients' autonomy is especially threatening when the patients in question face other powerful barriers to the exercise of their autonomy, as do members of groups subject to systemic discrimination on the basis of gender, race, class, disability, age, sexual preference, or any other such feature. A principle insisting on protection of patient autonomy can be an important corrective to such overwhelming power imbalances.

Moreover, physician privilege and power is not the only threat to patient autonomy. Increasingly, the treatment options available to both patients and physicians are circumscribed by the policies of governments and other third-party payers. In the current economic climate, those who fund health care services are insisting on ever more stringent restrictions on access to specific treatment options; physicians find themselves asked to perform gate-keeping functions to keep costs under control. In such circumstances, where patient care may be decided by general guidelines that tend to be insensitive to the particular circumstances of specific patients, and where the financial interests of the institution being billed for the patient's care may take priority over the patient's needs or preferences, the principle of respect for patient autonomy becomes more complicated to interpret even as it takes on added importance.

The principle of respect for patient autonomy can also be seen as an attractive ideal for feminists because of its promise to protect the rights and interests of even the most socially disadvantaged patients. Feminist medical historians, anthropologists, and sociologists have documented many ways in which health care providers have repeatedly neglected and misperceived the needs and wishes of the women they treat.[7] The ideal of respect for patient autonomy seems a promising way to correct much that is objectionable in the abuses that feminist researchers have documented in the delivery of health services to women and minorities. Most feminists believe that the forces of systematic domination and oppression work together to limit the autonomy of women and members of other oppressed groups; many of their political efforts can be seen as aimed at disrupting those forces and promoting greater degrees of autonomy (often represented as personal "choice") for individuals who fall victim to oppression. For example, many feminists appeal at least implicitly to the moral norm of autonomy in seeking to increase the scope of personal control for women in all areas of their reproductive lives (especially with respect to birth control, abortion, and childbirth, often discussed under a general rubric of "reproductive freedom" or "reproductive choice").

In a world where most cultures are plagued by sexism, which is usually compounded by other deeply entrenched oppressive patterns, fundamental respect for the humanity, dignity, and autonomy of members of disadvantaged groups, though extremely fragile, seems very important and in need of strong ethical imperatives. Feminists strive to be sensitive to the ways in which gender, race, class, age, disability, sexual orientation, and marital status can undermine a patient's authority and credibility in health care contexts and most are aware of the long history of powerful medical control over women's lives. They have good reason, then, to oppose medical domination through paternalism. Promotion of patient autonomy appears to be a promising alternative.[8] Understood in its traditional sense as the alternative to heteronomy (governance by others), auton-omy (self-governance) seems to be an essential fea-ture of any feminist strategy for improving health services for women and achieving a nonoppressive society.

Problems with the Autonomy Ideal

Nonetheless, despite this broad consensus about the value of a principle of respect for patient autonomy in health care, there are many problems with the princi-ple as it is usually interpreted and applied in health care ethics. As many health critics have observed, we need to question how much control individual patients really have over the determination of their treatment within the stressful world of health care ser-vices. Even a casual encounter with most modern hospitals reveals that wide agreement about the moral importance of respect for patient autonomy does not always translate into a set of practices that actually respect and foster patient autonomy in any meaning-ful sense. Ensuring that patients meet some measure of informed choice—or, more commonly, informed consent[9]—before receiving or declining treatment has become accepted as the most promising mechanism for insuring patient autonomy in health care settings, but, in practice, the effectiveness of the actual proce-dures used to obtain informed consent usually falls short of fully protecting patient autonomy. This gap is easy to understand: attention to patient autonomy can be a time-consuming business and the demands of identifying patient values and preferences are often sacrificed in the face of heavy patient loads and staff shortages. In addition, health care providers are often constrained from promoting and responding to patients' autonomy in health care because of pres-sures they experience to contain health care costs and to avoid making themselves liable to lawsuits. More-over, most health care providers are generally not well trained in the communication skills necessary to ensure that patients have the requisite understanding to provide genuine informed consent. This problem is compounded within our increasingly diverse urban communities where differences in language and cul-ture between health care providers and the patients they serve may create enormous practical barriers to informed choice.

There are yet deeper problems with the ideal of autonomy invoked in most bioethical discussions. The paradigm offered for informed consent is built on a model of articulate, intelligent patients who are accustomed to making decisions about the course of their lives and who possess the resources necessary to allow them a range of options to choose among. Decisions are constructed as a product of objective calculation on the basis of near perfect information. Clearly, not all patients meet these ideal conditions (perhaps none does), yet there are no satisfactory guidelines available about how to proceed when dealing with patients who do not fit the paradigm.

Feminist analysis reveals several problems inher-ent in the very construction of the concept of auton-omy that is at the heart of most bioethics discus-sions.[10] One problem is that autonomy provisions are sometimes interpreted as functioning indepen-dently of and outweighing all other moral values. More specifically, autonomy is often understood to exist in conflict with the demands of justice because the requirements of the latter may have to be imposed on unwilling citizens. Autonomy is fre-quently interpreted to mean freedom from interfer-ence; this analysis can be invoked (as it frequently is) to oppose taxation as coercive and, hence, a vio-lation of personal autonomy. But coercive measures like taxation are essential if a society wants to reduce inequity and provide the disadvantaged with access to the means (e.g., basic necessities, social respect, education, and health care) that are necessary for meaningful exercise of their autonomy. In contrast to traditional accounts of autonomy that accept and indeed presume some sort of tension between auton-omy and justice, feminism encourages us to see the connections between these two central moral ideals.

In fact, autonomy language is often used to hide the workings of privilege and to mask the barriers of oppression. For example, within North America it seems that people who were raised in an atmos-phere of privilege and respect come rather easily to think of themselves as independent and self-governing; it feels natural to them to conceive of themselves as autonomous. Having been taught that they need only to apply themselves in order to take advantage of the opportunities available to them, most learn to think of their successes as self-created and deserved. Such thinking encourages them to be oblivious to the barriers that oppression and disadvantage create, and it allows them to see the failures of others as evidence of the latter's unwillingness to exercise their own presumed autonomy responsibly. This individualistic approach to autonomy makes it very easy for people of privilege to remain ignorant of the social arrangements that support their own sense of independence, such as the institutions that provide them with an exceptionally good education and a relatively high degree of personal safety. Encouraged to focus on their own sense of individual accomplishment, they are inclined to blame less well-situated people for their lack of comparable success rather than to appreciate the costs of oppression. This familiar sort of thinking tends to interfere with people's ability to see the importance of supportive social conditions for fostering autonomous action. By focusing instead on the injustice that is associated with oppression, feminism helps us to recognize that autonomy is best achieved where the social conditions that support it are in place. Hence, it provides us with an alternative perspective for understanding a socially grounded notion of autonomy.

Further, the standard conception of autonomy, especially as it is invoked in bioethics, tends to place the focus of concern quite narrowly on particular decisions of individuals; that is, it is common to speak of specific health care decisions as autonomous, or, at least, of the patient as autonomous with respect to the decision at hand. Such analyses discourage attention to the context in which decisions are actually made. Patient decisions are considered to be autonomous if the patient is (1) deemed to be sufficiently competent (rational) to make the decision at issue, (2) makes a (reasonable) choice from a set of available options, (3) has adequate information and understanding about the available choices, and (4) is free from explicit coercion toward (or away from) one of those options. It is assumed that these criteria can be evaluated in any particular case, simply by looking at the state of the patient and her deliberations in isolation from the social conditions that structure her options. Yet, each of these conditions is more problematic than is generally recognized.

The competency criterion threatens to exclude people who are oppressed from the scope of autonomy provisions altogether. This is because competency is often equated with being rational,[11] yet the rationality of women and members of other oppressed groups is frequently denied. In fact, as Genevieve Lloyd (1984) has shown, the very concept of rationality has been constructed in opposition to the traits that are stereotypically assigned to women (e.g., by requiring that agents demonstrate objectivity and emotional distance),[12] with the result that women are often seen as simply incapable of rationality.[13] Similar problems arise with respect to stereotypical assumptions about members of racial minorities, indigenous peoples, persons with disabilities, welfare recipients, people from developing countries, those who are nonliterate, and so on. Minimally, then, health care providers must become sensitive to the ways in which oppressive stereotypes can undermine their ability to recognize some sorts of patients as being rational or competent.

Consider, also, the second condition, which has to do with making a (reasonable) choice from the set of available options. Here, the difficulty is that the set of available options is constructed in ways that may already seriously limit the patient's autonomy by prematurely excluding options the patient might have preferred. There is a whole series of complex decisions that together shape the set of options that health care providers are able to offer their patients: these can involve such factors as the forces that structure research programs, the types of results that journals are willing to publish, curriculum priorities in medical and other professional schools, and funding policies within the health care system.[14] While all patients will face limited choices by virtue of these sorts of institutional policy decisions, the consequences are especially significant for members of oppressed groups because they tend to be underrepresented on the bodies that make these earlier decisions, and therefore their interests are less likely to be reflected in each of the background decisions that are made. In general, the sorts of institutional decisions in question tend to reflect the biases of discriminatory values and practices. Hence, the outcomes of these multiple earlier decisions can have a significant impact on an oppressed patient's ultimate autonomy by disproportionately and unfairly restricting the choices available to her. Nevertheless, such background conditions are seldom visible within discussions of patient autonomy in bioethics.

The third condition is also problematic in that the information made available to patients is, inevitably, the information that has been deemed worthy of study and that is considered relevant by the health care providers involved. Again, research, publication, and education policies largely determine what sorts of data are collected and, significantly, what questions are neglected; systemic bias unquestionably influences these policies. Further, the very large gap in life experience between physicians, who are, by virtue of their professional status, relatively privileged members of society, and some of their seriously disadvantaged patients makes the likelihood of the former anticipating the specific information needs of the latter questionable. While an open consent process will help reduce this gap by providing patients with the opportunity to raise questions, patients often feel too intimidated to ask or even formulate questions, especially when they feel socially and intellectually inferior to their physicians and when the physicians project an image of being busy with more important demands. Often, one needs some information in order to know what further questions to ask, and large gaps in perspective between patients and their health care providers may result in a breakdown in communication because of false assumptions by either participant.

The fourth condition, the one that demands freedom from coercion in exercising choice, is extremely difficult to evaluate when the individual in question is oppressed. The task becomes even trickier if the choice is in a sphere that is tied to her oppression. The condition of being oppressed can be so fundamentally restrictive that it is distorting to describe as autonomous some specific choices made under such conditions. For example, many women believe they have no real choice but to seek expensive, risky cosmetic surgery because they accurately perceive that their opportunities for success in work or love depend on their more closely approximating some externally defined standard of beauty. Similar sorts of questions arise with respect to some women's choice of dangerous, unproven experiments in new reproductive technologies because continued childlessness can be expected to have devastating consequences for their lives. In other cases, women sometimes choose to have abortions because they fear that giving birth will involve them in unwanted and lifelong relationships with abusive partners. Some women have little access to contraceptives and find themselves choosing sterilization as the most effective way of resisting immediate demands of their partners even if they might want more children in the future. Or, some women seek out prenatal diagnosis and selective abortion of cherished fetuses because they realize that they cannot afford to raise a child born with a serious disability, though they would value such a child themselves. Many middle-class Western women choose hormone replacement therapy at menopause because they recognize that their social and economic lives may be threatened if they appear to be aging too quickly. When a woman's sense of herself and her range of opportunities have been oppressively constructed in ways that (seem to) leave her little choice but to pursue all available options in the pursuit of beauty or childbearing, or when she is raised in a culture that ties her own sense of herself to external norms of physical appearance or fulfillment associated with childbearing or, conversely, when having a(nother) child will impose unjust and intolerable costs on her, it does not seem sufficient to restrict our analysis to the degree of autonomy associated with her immediate decision about a particular treatment offered. We need a way of acknowledging how oppressive circumstances can interfere with autonomy, but this is not easily captured in traditional accounts.

Finally, there are good reasons to be wary of the ways in which the appearance of choice is used to mask the normalizing powers of medicine and other health-related institutions. As Michel Foucault (1979, 1980b) suggests, in modern societies the illusion of choice can be part of the mechanism for controlling behavior. Indeed, it is possible that bioethical efforts to guarantee the exercise of individual informed choice may actually make the exercise of medical authority even more powerful and effective than it would be under more traditionally paternalistic models. In practice, the ideal of informed choice amounts to assuring patients of the opportunity to consent to one of a limited list of relatively similar, medically encouraged procedures. Thus, informed consent procedures aimed simply at protecting autonomy in the narrow sense of specific choice among preselected options may ultimately serve to secure the compliance of docile patients who operate under the illusion of autonomy by virtue of being invited to consent to procedures they are socially encouraged to choose. Unless we find a way of identifying a deeper sense of autonomy than that associated with the expression of individual preference in selecting among a limited set of similar options, we run the risk of struggling to protect not patient autonomy but the very mechanisms that insure compliant medical consumers, preoccupied with the task of selecting among a narrow range of treatments.

Focus on the Individual

A striking feature of most bioethical discussions about patient autonomy is their exclusive focus on individual patients; this pattern mirrors medicine's consistent tendency to approach illness as primarily a problem of particular patients.[15] Similar problems are associated with each discipline. Within the medical tradition, suffering is located and addressed in the individuals who experience it rather than in the social arrangements that may be responsible for causing the problem. Instead of exploring the cultural context that tolerates and even supports practices such as war, pollution, sexual violence, and systemic unemployment—practices that contribute to much of the illness that occupies modern medicine—physicians generally respond to the symptoms troubling particular patients in isolation from the context that produces these conditions. Apart from population-based epidemiological studies (which, typically, restrict their focus to a narrow range of patterns of illness and often exclude or distort important social dimensions), medicine is primarily oriented toward dealing with individuals who have become ill (or pregnant, [in] fertile, or menopausal). This orientation directs the vast majority of research money and expertise toward the things that can be done to change the individual, but it often ignores key elements at the source of the problems.

For example, physicians tend to respond to infertility either by trivializing the problem and telling women to go home and "relax," or by prescribing hormonal and surgical treatment of particular women, rather than by demanding that research and public health efforts be aimed at preventing pelvic inflammatory disease, which causes many cases of infertility, or by encouraging wide public debate (or private reflections) on the powerful social pressures to reproduce that are directed at women. In similar fashion, the mainstream scientific and medical communities respond to the growth of breast cancer rates by promoting individual responsibility for self-examination and by searching for the gene(s) that makes some women particularly susceptible to the disease; when it is found in a patient, the principal medical therapy available is to perform "prophylactic" double mastectomies. Few physicians demand examination of the potential contributory role played by the use of pesticides or chlorine, or the practice of feeding artificial hormones to agricultural animals. Or they deal with dramatically increased skin cancer rates by promoting the personal use of sunscreens while resigning themselves to the continued depletion of the ozone layer. In another area, health care professionals generally deal with the devastating effects of domestic violence by patching up its victims, providing them with medications to relieve depression and advice to move out of their homes, and devising pathological names for victims who stay in violent relationships ("battered woman syndrome" and "self-defeating personality disorder"), but few actively challenge the sexism that accepts male violence as a "natural" response to frustration and fears of abandonment.

Some qualifications are in order. Clearly, these are crude and imprecise generalizations. They describe a general orientation of current health practices, but they certainly do not capture the work of all those involved in medical research and practice. Fortunately, there are practitioners and researchers engaged in the very sorts of investigation I call for, but they are exceptional, not typical. Moreover, I do not want to imply that medicine should simply abandon its concern with treating disease in individuals. I understand that prevention strategies will not eliminate all illness and I believe that personalized health care must continue to be made available to those who become ill. Further, I want to be clear that my critique does not imply that physicians or other direct care providers are necessarily the ones who ought to be assuming the task of identifying the social and environmental causes of disease. Health care training, and especially the training of physicians, is directed at developing the requisite skills for the extremely important work of caring for individuals who become ill. The responsibility for investigating the social causes of illness and for changing hazardous conditions is a social one that is probably best met by those who undertake different sorts of training and study. The problem is that medicine, despite the limits of its expertise and focus, is the primary agent of health care activity in our society and physicians are granted significant social authority to be the arbiters of health policy. Hence, when medicine makes the treatment of individuals its primary focus, we must understand that important gaps are created in our society's ability to understand and promote good health.

In parallel fashion, autonomy-focused bioethics concentrates its practitioners' attention on the preferences of particular patients, and it is, thereby, complicit in the individualistic orientation of medicine. It asks health care providers to ensure that individual patients have the information they need to make rational decisions about their health care, yet it does not ask the necessary questions about the circumstances in which such decisions are made. The emphasis most bioethicists place on traditional, individualistic understandings of autonomy reinforces the tendency of health care providers and ethicists to neglect exploration of the deep social causes and conditions that contribute to health and illness. Moreover, it encourages patients to see their own health care decisions in isolation from those of anyone else, thereby increasing their sense of vulnerability and dependence on medical authority.

The narrow individual focus that characterizes the central traditions within both medicine and bioethics obscures our need to consider questions of power, dominance, and privilege in our interpretations and responses to illness and other health-related matters as well as in our interpretations of the ideal of autonomy. These ways of structuring

thought and practice make it difficult to see the political dimensions of illness, and, in a parallel way, they obscure the political dimensions of the conventional criteria for autonomous deliberation. As a result, they interfere with our ability to identify and pursue more effective health practices while helping to foster a special environment that ignores and tolerates oppression. In both cases, a broader political perspective is necessary if we are to avoid the problems created by restricting our focus to individuals apart from their location.

Feminism offers just such a broader perspective. In contrast to the standard approaches in bioethics, feminism raises questions about the social basis for decisions about health and health care at all levels. Here, as elsewhere, feminists are inclined to ask whose interests are served and whose are harmed by the traditional ways of structuring thought and practice. By asking these questions, we are able to see how assumptions of individual-based medicine help to preserve the social and political status quo. For example, the current taxonomy in Canada designates certain sorts of conditions (e.g., infertility, cancer, heart disease, anxiety) as appropriate for medical intervention, and it provides grounds for ensuring that such needs are met. At the same time, it views other sorts of conditions (e.g., malnutrition, fear of assault, low self-esteem) as falling beyond the purview of the health care system and, therefore, as ineligible to draw on the considerable resources allocated to the delivery of health services.[16] In this way, individualistic assumptions support a system that provides expert care for many of the health complaints of those with greatest financial privilege while dismissing as outside the scope of health care many of the sources of illness that primarily affect the disadvantaged. A more social vision of health would require us to investigate ways in which nonmedical strategies, such as improving social and material conditions for disadvantaged groups, can affect the health status of different segments of the community.[17]

None of the concerns I have identified argues against maintaining a strong commitment to autonomy in bioethical deliberations. In fact, I have no wish to abandon this ideal (just as I have no desire to abandon patient-centered medical care). I still believe that a principle of respect for patient autonomy is an important element of good patient care. Moreover, I believe that appeal to a principle of respect for autonomy can be an important instrument in challenging oppression and it can actually serve as the basis for many of the feminist criticisms I present with respect to our current health care system.[18]

What these criticisms do suggest, however, is that we must pursue a more careful and politically sensitive interpretation of the range of possible restrictions on autonomy than is found in most of the nonfeminist bioethics literature. We need to be able to look at specific decisions as well as the context that influences and sometimes limits such decisions. Many of the troublesome examples I review above are entirely compatible with traditional conceptions of autonomy, even though the patients in question may be facing unjust barriers to care or may be acting in response to oppressive circumstances; traditional conceptions are inadequate to the extent that they make invisible the oppression that structures such decisions. By focusing only on the moment of medical decision making, traditional views fail to examine how specific decisions are embedded within a complex set of relations and policies that constrain (or, ideally, promote) an individual's ability to exercise autonomy with respect to any particular choice.

To understand this puzzle it is necessary to distinguish between agency and autonomy. To exercise agency, one need only exercise reasonable choice.[19] The women who choose some of the controversial practices discussed (e.g., abortion to avoid contact with an abusive partner, cosmetic surgery to conform to artificial norms of beauty, use of dangerous forms of reproductive technology) are exercising agency; clearly they are making choices, and, often, those choices are rational under the circumstances.[20] They also meet the demands of conventional notions of autonomy that ask only that anyone contemplating such procedures be competent, or capable of choosing (wisely), have available information current practice deems relevant, and be free of direct coercion. But insofar as their behavior accepts and adapts to oppression, describing it as autonomous seems inadequate. Together, the habits of equating agency (the making of a choice) with autonomy (self-gover-

nance) and accepting as given the prevailing social arrangements have the effect of helping to perpetuate oppression: when we limit our analysis to the quality of an individual's choice under existing conditions (or when we fail to inquire why some people do not even seek health services), we ignore the significance of oppressive conditions. Minimally, autonomous persons should be able to resist oppression—not just act in compliance with it—and be able to refuse the choices oppression seems to make nearly irresistible. Ideally, they should be able to escape from the structures of oppression altogether and create new options that are not defined by these structures either positively or negatively.

In order to ensure that we recognize and address the restrictions that oppression places on people's health choices, then, we need a wider notion of autonomy that will allow us to distinguish genuinely autonomous behavior from acts of merely rational agency. This conception must provide room to challenge the quality of an agent's specific decision-making ability and the social norms that encourage agents to participate in practices that may be partially constitutive of their oppression.[21] A richer, more politically sensitive standard of autonomy should make visible the impact of oppression on a person's choices as well as on her very ability to exercise autonomy fully. Such a conception has the advantage of allowing us to avoid the trap of focusing on the supposed flaws of the individual who is choosing under oppressive circumstances (e.g., by dismissing her choices as "false consciousness"), for it is able to recognize that such choices can be reasonable for the agent. Instead, it directs our attention to the conditions that shape the agent's choice and it makes those conditions the basis of critical analysis.

The problems that I identify with the conventional interpretation of patient autonomy reveal a need to expand our understanding of the types of forces that interfere with a patient's autonomy. On nonfeminist accounts, these are irrationality, failure to recognize that a choice is called for, lack of necessary information, and coercion (including psychological compulsion). Since each of these conditions must be reinterpreted to allow for the ways in which oppression may be operating, we must add to this list recognition of the costs and effects of oppression and of the particular ways in which oppression is manifested. But we must do more than simply modify our interpretation of the four criteria reviewed above. We also need an understanding of the ways in which a person can be encouraged to develop (or discouraged from developing) the ability to exercise autonomy. For this task, we need to consider the presence or absence of meaningful opportunities to build the skills required to be able to exercise autonomy well (Meyers 1989), including the existence of appropriate material and social conditions. In addition, our account should reflect the fact that many decision makers, especially women, place the interests of others at the center of their deliberations. Such an analysis will allow us to ensure that autonomy standards reflect not only the quality of reasoning displayed by a patient at the moment of medical decision making but also the circumstances that surround this decision making.

A Relational Alternative

A major reason for many of the problems identified with the autonomy ideal is that the term is commonly understood to represent freedom of action for agents who are paradigmatically regarded as independent, self-interested, and self-sufficient. As such, it is part of a larger North American cultural ideal of competitive individualism in which every citizen is to be left "free" to negotiate "his" way through the complex interactions of social, economic, and political life.[22] The feminist literature is filled with criticism of such models of agency and autonomy: for example, many feminists object that this ideal appeals to a model of personhood that is distorting because, in fact, no one is fully independent. As well, they observe that this model is exclusionary because those who are most obviously dependent on others (e.g., because of disability or financial need) seem to be disqualified from consideration in ways that others are not. Many feminists object that the view of individuals as isolated social units is not only false but impoverished: much of who we are and what we value is rooted in our relationships and affinities with others. Also, many feminists take issue with the common assumption that agents are single-mindedly self-interested, when so much of our experience is devoted to building or maintaining personal relationships and communities.[23]

If we are to effectively address these concerns, we need to move away from the familiar Western understanding of autonomy as self-defining, self-interested, and self-protecting, as if the self were simply some special kind of property to be preserved.[24] Under most popular interpretations, the structure of the autonomy-heteronomy framework (governance by self or by others) is predicated on a certain view of persons and society in which the individual is thought to be somehow separate from and to exist independently of the larger society; each person's major concern is to be protected from the demands and encroachment of others. This sort of conception fails to account for the complexity of the relations that exist between persons and their culture. It idealizes decisions that are free from outside influence without acknowledging that all persons are, to a significant degree, socially constructed, that their identities, values, concepts, and perceptions are, in large measure, products of their social environment.

Since notions of the self are at the heart of autonomy discussions, alternative interpretations of autonomy must begin with an alternative conception of the self. Curiously, despite its focus on individuals, standard interpretations of autonomy have tended to think of selves as generic rather than distinctive beings. In the traditional view, individuals tend to be treated as interchangeable in that no attention is paid to the details of personal experience. Hence, there is no space within standard conceptions to accommodate important differences among agents, especially the effects that oppression (or social privilege) has on a person's ability to exercise autonomy. In order to capture these kinds of social concerns, some feminists have proposed turning to a relational conception of personhood that recognizes the importance of social forces in shaping each person's identity, development, and aspirations.[25] Following this suggestion, I now explore a relational interpretation of autonomy that is built around a relational conception of the self that is explicitly feminist in its conception.

Under relational theory, selfhood is seen as an ongoing process, rather than as something static or fixed. Relational selves are inherently social beings that are significantly shaped and modified within a web of interconnected (and sometimes conflicting) relationships. Individuals engage in the activities that are constitutive of identity and autonomy (e.g., defining, questioning, revising, and pursuing projects) within a configuration of relationships, both interpersonal and political, by including attention to political relationships of power and powerlessness, this interpretation of relational theory provides room to recognize how the forces of oppression can interfere with an individual's ability to exercise autonomy by undermining her sense of herself as an autonomous agent and by depriving her of opportunities to exercise autonomy. Thus, it is able to provide us with insight into why it is that oppressed people often seem less autonomous than others even when offered a comparable range of choices. Under a relational view, autonomy is best understood to be a capacity or skill that is developed (and constrained) by social circumstances. It is exercised within relationships and social structures that jointly help to shape the individual while also affecting others' responses to her efforts at autonomy.[26]

Diana Meyers (1989) has developed one such theory of personal autonomy. She argues that autonomy involves a particular competency that requires the development of specific skills. As such, it can be either enhanced or diminished by the sort of socialization the agent experiences. Meyers shows how the specific gender socialization most (Western) women undergo trains them in social docility and rewards them for defining their interests in terms of others, thereby robbing them of the opportunity to develop the essential capacity of self-direction. Such training relegates most women to a category she labels "minimally autonomous" (as distinct from her more desirable categories of medially autonomous and fully autonomous). Relational theory allows us to appreciate how each relationship a person participates in plays a role in fostering or inhibiting that individual's capacity for autonomous action by encouraging or restricting her opportunities to understand herself as an autonomous agent and to practice exercising the requisite skills. Such a conception makes clear the importance of discovering the ways in which oppression often reduces a person's ability to develop and exercise the skills that are necessary for achieving a reasonable degree of autonomy.

For instance, relational theory allows us to see the damaging effects on autonomy of internalized oppression. Feminists have long understood that one of the most insidious features of oppression is its tendency to become internalized in the minds of its victims. This is because internalized oppression diminishes the capacity of its victims to develop self-respect, and, as several feminists have argued, reduced (or compromised) self-respect undermines autonomy by undermining the individual's sense of herself as capable of making independent judgments (Meyers 1989; Dillon 1992; Benson 1991, 1994). Moreover, as Susan Babbitt (1993, 1996) has argued, these oppression-induced barriers to autonomy cannot necessarily be rectified simply by providing those affected with more information or by removing explicit coercive forces (as the traditional view assumes). When the messages of reduced self-worth are internalized, agents tend to lose the ability even to know their own objective interests. According to Babbitt, in such cases transformative experiences can be far more important to autonomy than access to alternative information. Feminist theory suggests, then, that women and members of other oppressed groups can be helped to increase their autonomy skills by being offered more opportunities to exercise those skills and a supportive climate for practicing them (Meyers 1989), by being provided with the opportunity to develop stronger senses of self-esteem (Benson 1994; Dillon 1992; Meyers 1989), by having the opportunity for transformative experiences that make visible the forces of oppression (Babbitt 1993, 1996), and by having experiences of making choices that are not influenced by the wishes of those who dominate them (Babbitt 1993, 1996).

Autonomy requires more than the effective exercise of personal resources and skills, however; generally, it also demands that appropriate structural conditions be met. Relational theory reminds us that material restrictions, including very restricted economic resources, ongoing fear of assault, and lack of educational opportunity (i.e., the sorts of circumstances that are often part of the condition of being oppressed), constitute real limitations on the options available to the agent. Moreover, it helps us to see how socially constructed stereotypes can reduce both society's and the agent's sense of that person's ability to act autonomously. Relational theory allows us to recognize how such diminished expectations readily become translated into diminished capacities.

The relational interpretation I favor is feminist in that it takes into account the impact of social and political structures, especially sexism and other forms of oppression, on the lives and opportunities of individuals. It acknowledges that the presence or absence of a degree of autonomy is not just a matter of being offered a choice. It also requires that the person had the opportunity to develop the skills necessary for making the type of choice in question, the experience of being respected in her decisions, and encouragement to reflect on her own values. The society, not just the agent, is subject to critical scrutiny under the rubric of relational autonomy.

It is important, however, to avoid an account that denies any scope for autonomy on the part of those who are oppressed. Such a conclusion would be dangerous, since the widespread perception of limited autonomy can easily become a self-fulfilling prophecy. Moreover, such a conclusion would be false. Many members of oppressed groups do manage to develop autonomy skills and, thus, are able to act autonomously in a wide variety of situations, though the particular demands of acting autonomously under oppression are easily overlooked (Benson 1991). Some feminists, such as bell hooks (1990) and Sarah Hoagland (1992), have observed that the marginality associated with being oppressed can sometimes provide people with better opportunities than are available to more well-situated citizens for questioning social norms and devising their own patterns of resistance to social convention. Because those who are especially marginalized (e.g., those who are multiply oppressed or who are "deviant" with respect to important social norms) may have no significant social privilege to lose, they are, sometimes, freer than others to demand changes in the status quo. They may be far more likely to engage in resistance to the norms of oppression than are those who derive some personal benefits from oppressive structures (e.g., middle-class, able-bodied, married women).

Still, we must not make the mistake of romanticizing the opportunities available to the oppressed.

An adequate conception of autonomy should afford individuals more than the opportunity to resist oppression; it should also ensure that they have opportunities to actively shape their world. A relational conception of autonomy seems better suited than the traditional models to handle the complexities of such paradoxes because it encourages us to attend to the complex ways in which the detailed circumstances of an individual's social and political circumstances can affect her ability to act in different kinds of contexts.

When relational autonomy reveals the disadvantage associated with oppression in terms of autonomy, the response should not be that others are thereby licensed to make decisions for those who are oppressed; this response would only increase their powerlessness. Rather, it demands attention to ways in which oppressed people can be helped to develop the requisite autonomy skills. The best way of course to help oppressed people to develop autonomy skills is to remove the conditions of their oppression. Short of that, long-term social projects can help to provide educational opportunities to counter the psychological burdens of oppression. In the short term, it may be necessary to spend more time than usual in supporting patients in the deliberative process of decision making and providing them with access to relevant political as well as medical information when they contemplate controversial procedures (e.g., information about the social dimensions of hormone replacement therapy).

Relational autonomy is not only about changing the individual, however. It also demands attention to ways in which the range of choices before those who belong to oppressed groups can be modified to include more nonoppressive options, that is, options that will not further entrench their existing oppression (as often happens, for example, when women choose cosmetic surgery or the use of many reproductive technologies). Whereas in traditional autonomy theory only the mode and quality of specific decisions are evaluated, feminist relational autonomy regards the range and nature of available and acceptable options as being at least as important as the quality of specific decision making. Only when we understand the ways in which oppression can infect the background or baseline conditions under which choices are to be made will we be able to modify those conditions and work toward the possibility of greater autonomy by promoting nonoppressive alternatives.

As in health matters, it is important in relational discussions not to lose sight of the need to continue to maintain some focus on the individual. Relational autonomy redefines autonomy as the social project it is, but it does not deny that autonomy ultimately resides in individuals. Our attention to social and political contexts helps deepen and enrich the narrow and impoverished view of autonomy available under individualistic conceptions, but it does not support wholesale neglect of the needs and interests of individuals in favor of broader social and political interests. Rather, it can be seen as democratizing access to autonomy by helping to identify and remove the effects of barriers to autonomy that are created by oppression. A relational approach can help to move autonomy from the largely exclusive preserve of the socially privileged and see that it is combined with a commitment to social justice in order to ensure that oppression is not allowed to continue simply because its victims have been deprived of the resources necessary to exercise the autonomy required to challenge it.

Implications of a Relational Interpretation of Autonomy for Health Care

Let us now consider what a relational interpretation of autonomy offers when we consider some of the subjects explored elsewhere in this book [*The Politics of Women's Health*]. Many of the concerns we raise in Chapter 10 regarding the ethics of research with human subjects stem from the fact that ordinary criteria of informed consent are often insufficient to ensure that proper attention is paid to all the morally relevant circumstances; we seek ethical norms that will be concerned with relational autonomy and not merely individual consent to some predetermined research project. Whereas traditional bioethics relies on the familiar individualistic understanding of autonomy, and, hence, focuses on the ability of potential research subjects to refuse to participate in a proposed project, our relational conception leads us to a variety of broader concerns. Rather than just

asking whether research subjects truly understand all relevant details about their involvement (a question we still consider important), we argue that questions must also be asked about who is invited to participate and who is not and how the specific research questions were selected. Our recommendations that new research ethics guidelines provide members of oppressed groups a larger say in the planning, structure, and conduct of research are intended to counteract the ways in which existing power relations foster research that selectively serves the interests of those with privilege at the expense of those who are oppressed.

Margaret Lock's discussion of how women's aging bodies are culturally constructed in North American and Japanese societies (Chapter 8) helps to make vivid the limitations of traditional autonomy conceptions when evaluating women's personal choices regarding the use of hormone replacement therapy at menopause. She explains how different cultural expectations about women's aging bodies seem to produce important differences not only in medical practices but also in the experience of aging for women in these two cultures. Women in North America are far more likely than their Japanese counterparts to be offered hormone replacement therapy as either relief from menopausal symptoms or as prevention of heart disease or osteoporosis (or, perhaps, Alzheimer's disease). Most women, however, find the decision extremely difficult to make. The problem is not merely one of insufficient data—there is an overwhelming amount of data available, but much of it is inconclusive or contradictory and, very frequently, the data come from studies sponsored by the pharmaceutical companies that market these products and do not address questions of significance to women. Nor is it a problem of coercion—even though some women feel quite strong pressure from their physicians, most doctors are themselves sufficiently ambivalent about the risks and benefits of long-term hormone use that they are happy to leave the decision to their patients. Rather, the problem women face is trying to weigh up their discomfort about the visible signs of aging in a culture that prefers its women young against the uncertain risks of long-term artificial hormone use, their lifelong training to avoid being a burden on others as background to their fears of becoming disabled, their lack of experience in evaluating competing and incommensurable risks, and the background condition of having their whole prior reproductive lives subject to medical surveillance and intervention. What makes hormone replacement therapy a difficult choice for the mostly middle-class, middle-aged Western women who are wrestling with this decision are the social expectations (both external and internal) that women confront as they approach menopause, combined with their own habits of deferring to medical expertise to monitor and regulate their bodies' changes.[27] Relational autonomy makes visible the importance of considering how such social factors affect women's decision making, and it invites us to consider how the burden of unjust social demands might be made explicit so that it can be separated out of the calculations. It allows us to help reshape the considerations that should be operative in this type of choice and to seek political changes that will challenge those influential factors that are discriminatory; at the same time, it warns us of the need to help ensure that women have the necessary autonomy skills before confronting such decisions. And it makes clear the need to ensure that if hormone replacement therapy is of benefit to some women, it be made available to all who can be expected to benefit from it and not simply to those who can afford it or who find themselves in a society that considers medical intervention an appropriate response to women's aging.

Wendy Mitchinson invites us to consider the complexity of the relationships between women and their doctors in Canada between 1850 and 1950 (Chapter 6). She reminds us that power is seldom a straightforward relation where one party holds it all and the other is fully subservient. In the past, as in the present, physicians enjoyed a great deal of social and personal power relative to most of their women patients. But they have never been in full control. Women patients always make choices and thereby exercise agency. Further, patients often make demands and pressure physicians into offering services (e.g., twilight sleep at childbirth) that the physicians might initially resist. Perhaps the modern equivalent is the tendency of many women to demand access to reproductive technologies in order to try to fulfill their reproductive aspirations. As patients, women demand as well as comply; when sufficient numbers make similar demands, they may well affect the course of medical practice. But, for the reasons reviewed above, it is not clear that we should count such influence as full autonomy as long as the conditions of choice are restricted and oppressive.

Both patients and physicians recognize that the options they may reasonably consider are limited by economic and legal restrictions and by the force of professional standards of acceptable practice. Evaluating autonomous decision making in medical encounters, then, requires us to attend to the circumstances of particular physicians and patients and to the nature of their interactions. Increasing autonomy for patients is a matter not just of increasing their power relative to their physicians but of increasing patients' social power more broadly and restructuring the health care system to ensure that it is responsive to an appropriate range of women's needs by removing discriminatory attitudes and barriers and by promoting the necessary knowledge base. It is necessary to avoid simplistic understandings of the patient-physician (or, more generically, the patient-health care worker) relationship as a contractual agreement between two fully independent parties (as is often suggested in the nonfeminist bioethics literature). We need to attend to ways in which those involved in delivering health care participate in social understandings of women, and of specific groups of women, when offering women a predefined set of treatment options. Relational autonomy invites us to appreciate that both physicians and patients are socially situated and the options each considers, like the choices each makes, are a reflection of social expectations that may well be oppressive.

Consider also what a relational ideal of autonomy might mean in some of the concrete circumstances of health care services. First, under relational as under individualistic conceptions of autonomy, it is important for health care workers to continue their efforts to explore the needs, interests, and concerns of their patients at all stages of treatment—to seek informed choice in the fullest sense possible. Under both relational and individualistic understandings, informed consent must be understood as an ongoing process; a relational interpretation can make it clearer that the pursuit of informed consent is also an interactive process in which both parties may be transformed. Also, both interpretations provide support for insisting that, apart from emergencies, health care providers should not presume to know what is best for their patients because they cannot have access to all of the relevant facts and values associated with the complexities of their patients' lives and interests.

A relational view helps us to understand how the specific social location of patients can affect their autonomy status. It explains why requiring health care providers to disclose relevant information and seek the permission of patients is a necessary, but not a sufficient, criterion for protecting patient autonomy. Because oppressive norms can undermine a patient's opportunities to develop the experience and skills necessary to practice autonomy, we need to explore ways of reversing such deficiencies and fostering greater autonomy skills. Clearly, this task extends far beyond the boundaries of health care and calls for social changes that will provide the oppressed with opportunities to develop autonomy skills that are comparable to the opportunities of the more privileged. Within health care, it is important to keep in mind that patients who have had little opportunity to exercise autonomy in other areas of their lives may need more time and more counseling than others before they are asked to give their decisions on health matters, in order to be sure that the patient understands that a choice is genuinely in her hands.

Moreover, a relational interpretation of autonomy should call into question health care orientations that view health-related services simply as consumer options, to be made available to anyone who chooses them. Policy questions about what health care procedures are developed and what services health professionals are trained to provide and encouraged to offer involve social and political values that should be subject to public debate and widespread ethical reflection. For example, each society needs to determine if it wants its medical researchers and practitioners occupied with the full range of emerging new reproductive technologies or if it wishes to set some restrictions;[28] each must also decide

whether it supports massive genetic screening and testing efforts to reduce health problems associated with genetic variations, or whether it will focus its resources on other sorts of preventative initiatives and on strategies for relieving the burdens of genetic variations that now fall on individuals. It should not be the sole responsibility of physicians and researchers to determine whether to meet the demands of individuals who seek such procedures as assisted reproduction, cosmetic surgery, organ transplants, prenatal genetic testing, or diet aids.

The need for more sophisticated analyses and public policy is especially urgent when the services in question reflect and reinforce oppressive social norms that are difficult for those who are oppressed to resist. Individualistic interpretations of autonomy seem to suggest that medical consumers should be provided with whatever services are voluntarily chosen (i.e., in the absence of explicit coercion), but a relational understanding of autonomy requires that we raise questions about the context of those choices. It encourages us to explore whether the growth of practices such as cosmetic surgery and prenatal diagnosis contribute to a climate in which these practices become so normalized that future patients may find themselves unable to refuse such services. Just as home births became virtually impossible to arrange once the majority of women in North America chose hospital births, there is a real risk that the current wide acceptance and popularity of prenatal genetic testing may soon make it nearly impossible for pregnant women to refuse. Because the autonomy of some may well be affected by the choices of others, we need to recognize the interpersonal implications of current practices on the autonomy of future patients.

In addition, because a relational conception highlights rather than obscures the roles played by social and material conditions, it helps us see the importance of ensuring that material constraints do not unduly restrict the options that are actually available to socially disadvantaged patients. This implies a duty on the part of each citizen to join the political fight to retain a commitment to the principles of universality and equal access in the Canadian health care system and other countries where these principles are now threatened and to seek to have such principles endorsed in the United States. It also suggests that we consider broadening the definition of health services to make certain that nonmedical services that improve health are also covered by public funding.

And, finally, a relational theory can show the importance of demanding that health care providers become sensitive to their own biases and assumptions so that they can better resist the common tendency to deny authority to patients with less social status. By disrupting norms that validate the experiences and perceptions of the powerful while dismissing those of the oppressed, relational ideals reveal the need for health care workers to listen carefully to the concerns and priorities of patients who belong to groups that are systematically oppressed. Health professionals must learn to stop assuming total expertise on health matters. They must broaden their understanding of their responsibilities; rather than seeing their task as simply one of educating and persuading patients to accept their learned advice, they need to develop the skills necessary to find out how the condition in question is experienced by the patient and what constraints on treatment options face the patient. Such a shift in orientation should lead to more effective, patient-centered health care. It may also help to transform the historical pattern in which health-related research and practice have focused on the specific needs and experiences of privileged members of society at the expense of less advantaged people whose distinctive health needs are largely neglected.

If we are truly to respect patient autonomy, we, as a society, need to develop a health care system that is more attentive to the actual needs of the diverse variety of citizens who depend on its services. That task will require that policy makers and providers learn to respond more appropriately to patients who are differently situated. A relational approach to autonomy allows us to maintain a central place for autonomy within bioethics, but it requires an interpretation that is both deeper and more complicated than the traditional conception acknowledges—one that sets standards that involve political as well as personal criteria of adequacy. It examines patient autonomy in the social and political dimensions within which it resides and provides us with theoretical resources that we need for restructuring health care practices in ways that will genuinely expand the autonomy of *all* patients.

Acknowledgments

This chapter has evolved over the course of the Network interactions and has benefited enormously from Network discussions. I am grateful to all Network members for careful readings of many earlier drafts and stimulating comments. In addition to input from Network members, I have also benefited from the generous attention paid by Keith Burgess-Jackson, Sue Campbell, Richmond Campbell, Carmel Forde, Jody Graham, Carl Matheson, Barbara Secker, and Eldon Soifer.

Notes

1 Some Network members prefer the terms "contextual" or "situated" as a way of avoiding all confusion with those feminists who reserve the term "relational" to refer exclusively to interpersonal relations. I feel that this usage perpetuates the misleading sense that interpersonal relations are themselves "apolitical." I have, therefore, chosen to insist on a thoroughly political reading of the term "relational" that applies to both interpersonal and more public sorts of relations.

2 While questions of patient autonomy arise in interactions with all health care providers, North American health care delivery is largely structured around provision of medical services; moreover, physicians control most of the decision making that determines provision of health care services. Hence, much of the subsequent discussion focuses explicitly on patient autonomy in relation to physician authority, even though many of the concerns raised also extend to other (nonmedical) types of health care practice.

3 The most vivid examples appear in distressing history of medical research with human subjects. See, for example, Katz (1972).

4 I deliberately retain the gendered term in this particular instance since it accurately reflects the connection to the traditional gendered role of patriarchal father who presumes authority to make decisions on behalf of all other family members. Traditional stereotypes

of mothering and gender-neutral parenting do not retain this hierarchical flavor.

5　For a review of most of the common interpretations, see Dworkin (1988).

6　Interest in respect for patient autonomy is hardly unique to North America, however. See note 20.

7　See, for example, Corea (1985a); Ehrenreich and English (1979); Fisher (1986); Perales and Young (1988); and White (1990). This is not a straightforward history of constant abuse or one-sided power, however; as Wendy Mitchinson documents in Chapter 6 [of the book from which this extract is taken], the relationship between women and their doctors has long been complex and ambiguous.

8　At the very least, we need a more complex analysis of the options for decision making than is provided by the familiar dichotomous structure of patient autonomy versus medical paternalism. See Mahowald (1993) for development of the idea of maternalism as an alternative that is aimed at capturing both these aspects of medical responsibility; see also Sherwin (1992) for a brief proposal of "amicalism."

9　*Informed choice* suggests a wider scope for patient autonomy than *informed consent* in that it includes the possibility of patients' initiating treatment suggestions where *informed consent* implies that the role of the patient is merely to consent to the treatment proposed by the physician; further, *informed choice* makes more explicit that patients ought also to be free to refuse recommended treatments as well as to accept them.

10　Many of these concerns are not exclusive to feminists; several have also been raised by other sorts of critics. I call them feminist because I came to these concerns through a feminist analysis that attends to the role in society of systems of dominance and oppression, especially those connected with gender.

11　This reduction may be a result of a tendency to collapse the ideal of personal autonomy central to bioethics discussions with the concept of moral autonomy developed by Immanuel Kant.

12　It is often taken as a truism in our culture that emotional involvement constitutes irrationality, that emotions are direct threats to rationality. It is hard to see, however, how decisions about important life decisions are improved if they are made without any emotional attachment to the outcomes.

13　Susan Babbitt (1996) argues that the traditional conception of rationality is defined in terms of propositional understanding in ways that obscure the experiences and needs of oppressed people.

14　For example, research priorities have led to the situation where birth control pills are available only for women and this increases the pressure on women seeking temporary protection against pregnancy to take the pill even when it endangers their health.

15　I focus primarily on medicine since it is the dominant health profession and is responsible for the organization of most health services in developed countries. Most health professions involve a similar bias toward treatment of individuals, though some (e.g., social work) pride themselves on attending to social structures as well as individual need, and most health professions, including medicine, include subspecialties concerned with matters of public health.

16　Because health care is a provincial responsibility, there are differences in the precise services offered from province to province and from one administration to the next within provinces. The examples here are broad generalizations.

17　Such considerations do play a role in health care planning at a governmental level where the focus shifts from medical interventions to the idea of *health determinants*, but here, too, there is excessive attention paid to what the individual can and should be doing ("healthism") and insufficient concern about promoting egalitarian social conditions. [...]

18　When I read an early version of this section of the paper to the Second World Congress of the International Association of Bioethics in Buenos Aires, Argentina, in November 1994, I was struck by how passionately committed local feminists were to retaining a version of the respect for autonomy principle. They felt that most women in their country had very little authority over decisions about their health care, and so they were struggling to reverse a strongly paternalistic bias on the part of physicians by appeal to the principle of respect for autonomy. While they acknowledged that this principle was not as well-entrenched in their society as it is in North America, they considered it very important to their own feminist health agenda. They see respect for patient autonomy as having profoundly liberatory potential in their own society; this perspective provides clear reason not to dismiss this principle lightly, flawed though it may be.

19 The language of agency and autonomy is quite varied within feminist (and other) discourse. For example, the term *agency* is used throughout the collection *Provoking Agents: Gender and Agency in Theory and Practice* (Gardiner 1995) in ways that sometimes appear to overlap with my usage of *relational autonomy*. Susan Babbitt (1996), on the other hand, seems to use the two terms in ways analogous to the use here.

20 The notion of agency is itself highly contested within current feminist theory. Postmodern accounts seem to deny the possibility of subjectivity in any familiar sense; since agency is traditionally assigned to a single subject, once the subject is eliminated, the possibility of agency seems to disappear as well. I do not address this complex theoretical issue here but continue to rely on common sense understandings of both subjectivity and agency. Readers interested in understanding the feminist debates around agency may consult Gardiner (1995).

21 In addition, we need the conceptual space to be able to acknowledge that restrictive definitions of health sometimes preempt autonomy analysis by limiting the opportunity of some people even to enter the relatively well-funded health care system for assistance with problems (e.g., poverty) that affect their health.

22 The agent imagined in such cases is always stereotypically masculine.

23 Feminist discussion of these and other critiques can be found in Gilligan (1982); Baier (1985b); Code (1991); and Held (1993).

24 See Nedelsky (1989) for discussion of this view and its limitations.

25 For example, Baier (1985b); Code (1991); and Held (1993).

26 An alternative feminist conception of a relational view of autonomy is provided by Anne Donchin (1998). I see her account as complementary to, not competitive with, this one.

27 This cohort includes half of our research Network, so it is a question whose urgency we feel strongly.

28 For example, Canada funded the four-year Royal Commission on New Reproductive Technologies (1989-1993) to advise on public policy regarding these technologies. In June 1996, Bill C-47, which involves restrictions on commercialization of any aspects of human reproduction, including the buying or selling of gametes or embryos, prohibits human cloning and other sorts of technologies on the horizon and restricts the use of prenatal sex selection to medical conditions, was introduced to the House of Commons in Canada.

References

Babbitt, Susan. 1993. "Feminist and Objective Interests." In *Feminist Epistemologies*, ed. Linda Alcoff and Elizabeth Potter. New York: Routledge.

——. 1996. *Impossible Dreams: Rationality, Integrity, and Moral Indignation*. Boulder, CO: Westview Press.

Baier, Annette. 1985. "What do Women Want in a Moral Theory?" *Nous* 19(1): 53-63.

Benson, Paul. 1991. "Autonomy and Oppressive Socialization." *Social Theory and Practice* 17(3): 385-408.

——. 1994. "Free Agency and Self-Worth." *Journal of Philosophy* 91(12): 650-68.

Code, Lorraine. 1991. *What Can She Know? Feminist Theory and the Construction of Knowledge*. Ithaca, NY: Cornell University Press.

Corea, Gena. 1985. *The Hidden Malpractice: How American Medicine Mistreats Women*. New York: Harper Colophon Books.

Dillon, Robin. 1992. "Toward a Feminist Conception of Self-Respect." *Hypatia* 7(1) 52-69.

Donchin, Anne. 2001. "Understanding Autonomy Relationally: Toward a Reconfiguration of Bioethical Principles." *Journal of Medicine and Philosophy* 26(4): 365-386.

Dworkin, Gerald. 1988. *The Theory and Practice of Autonomy*. Cambridge: Cambridge University Press.

Ehrenreich, Barbara, and Deirdre English. 1972. *Witches, Midwives, and Nurses: A History of Women Healers*. Glass Mountain Pamphlet, no. 1. Old Westbury, NY: The Feminist Press.

Fisher, Sue. 1986. *In the Patient's Best Interests: Women and the Politics of Medical Decisions*. New Brunswick, NJ: Rutgers University Press.

Foucault, Michel. 1979. *Discipline and Punish*. New York: Vintage.

——. 1980. *Power/Knowledge*. Ed. Colin Gordon. Brighton: Harvester.

Gardiner, Judith Kegan. 1995. *Provoking Agents: Gender*

and Agency in Theory and Practice. Chicago: University of Illinois Press.

Gilligan, Carol. 1982. *In a Different Voice: Psychological Theory and Women's Moral Development*. Cambridge, MA: Harvard University Press.

Held, Virginia. 1993. *Feminist Morality: Transforming Culture, Society, and Politics*. Chicago: University of Chicago Press.

Hoagland, Sarah Lucia. 1992. "Lesbian Ethics and Female Agency." In *Explorations in Feminist Ethics: Theory and Practice*. Ed. Susan Browning Cole and Susan Coultrap-McQuin. Bloomington: Indiana University Press.

hooks, bell. 1990. *Yearning: Race, Gender, and Cultural Politics*. Toronto: Between the Lines.

Katz, Jay, ed. 1972. *Experimentation with Human Beings: The Authority of the Investigator, Subject, Professions, and State in the Human Experimentation Process*. New York: Russell Sage Foundation.

Lloyd, Genevieve. 1984. *The Man of Reason: "Male" and "Female" in Western Philosophy*. Minneapolis: University of Minnesota Press.

Mahowald, Mary Briody. 1993. *Women and Children in Health Care: An Unequal Majority*. New York: Oxford University Press.

Meyers, Diana. 1989. *Self, Society, and Personal Choice*. New York: Columbia University Press.

Nedelsky, Jennifer. 1989. "Reconceiving Autonomy." *Yale Journal of Law and Feminism* 1(1): 7-36.

Perales, Cesar A., and Lauren S. Young, eds. 1988. *Too Little, Too Late: Dealing with the Health Needs of Women in Poverty*. New York: Harrington Park Press.

Sherwin, Susan. 1992. *No Longer Patient: Feminist Ethics and Health Care*. Philadelphia: Temple University Press.

White, Evelyn C., ed. 1990. *The Black Women's Health Book: Speaking for Ourselves*. Seattle, WA: Seal Press.

3.
THE PHYSICIAN AS THERAPIST AND INVESTIGATOR

John E. Thomas

Source: *Medical Ethics and Human Life* (Toronto: Samuel Stevens, 1993).

Moral dilemmas posed by experimenting with human subjects cluster around a tension between the need for scientific investigation to improve the effectiveness of treatment and the patient's claim to care. Two values underlie this tension—scientific freedom and individual inviolability; the right of scientists to inquire and the rights of human beings to be respected as persons and not to be treated as experimental materials. Over a wide range of intri-·cate interactions these values are compatible, even complementary. Sometimes, however, they are in conflict, and when that happens we need to be reassured that patients' rights will not be sacrificed to scientific inquiry.

Formerly the researcher's and the physician's roles seldom overlapped. In recent years, however, particularly in teaching and research centres, doctors increasingly sport two hats—that of investigator and that of physician. The differences between them can be brought out in three ways: by reference to

(i) the different models underpinning the roles of physician and experimenter;
(ii) the divergence of the avowed goals of physician and researcher; and
(iii) the disparity in the knowledge to which the physician and investigator respectively lay claim.

First, consider the different models underpinning the roles of the physician and researcher. In its simplest form the physician-patient relationship may be diagrammed as follows:

THE THERAPEUTIC MODEL

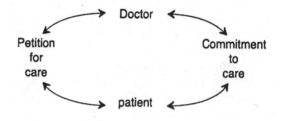

This contract or covenant is an agreement to which each party brings its own expectations. The primary thrust of the doctor-patient relationship, as the first model indicates, is *therapeutic*—the operative word is "care." In this relationship the doctor is the agent of the patient alone.

Contrast with this the different roles into which the doctor and patient are cast by the very nature of the experimental setting. Now the doctor confronts his subject as a scientist.

THE RESEARCH MODEL

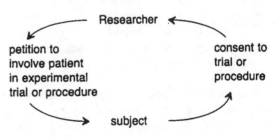

This contract is also an agreement to which each party brings its own expectations. Notice, in an experimental setting the doctor becomes a researcher and the patient a subject. The shift in the terms of the contract as well as in the roles of the parties to it are sufficiently radical to warrant disclosure to the patient. This is not to deny that the subject in the experimental situation will continue to receive care, perhaps even superior care to the recipients of standard or conventional treatment, but that fact in itself does not warrant withholding information about the change in the terms of the contract and the roles of the participants. Failure to keep these two models distinct may give rise to two serious misunderstandings. First, the patient is likely still to think of the researcher as a doctor (which, of course, he may be, but not in the sense relevant to this context). Second, the patient may mistake experiment for therapy.

Another undesirable consequence of the blurring of the distinction between physician and researcher is that the researcher may be tempted to claim for himself privileges that properly belong to the therapeutic model. This occurred in the notorious Brooklyn Jewish Hospital case. Ethically "the stone of stumbling and rock of offence" in the Brooklyn case was *not* that the procedure of injecting live cancer cells into geriatric patients was a particularly hazardous procedure (on the contrary, I have been assured it was a relatively harmless procedure). In court the researchers appealed to the physicians' right to withhold information from patients in certain circumstances. At this point in the trial the defence took a peculiar twist. The researchers defended their actions on the ground that the patients would *not* have agreed to the experiment if they had been told they were to be injected with live cancer cells—a curious justification for the waiver of the consent regulation that the court justifiably discounted.

In summing up their judgment of this case, the Board of Regents of the Brooklyn hospital put the whole matter in proper perspective:

> The physician when he is acting as an experimenter, has no claim to the doctor-patient relationship that, in a therapeutic situation would give him the generally acknowledged right to withhold information if he judged it in the best interest of the patient.[1]

So a shift in the roles of the parties to the contract radically affects the terms of the contract. Hence the investigator, even though also a physician, may not presume that the privileges accruing to the therapeutic model are automatically transferrable to the research model.

Second, not only do we witness a radical shift in the roles of the parties to the doctor-patient relationship as one moves from therapy to experimentation, there is also a *divergence in the goals* of the doctor and researcher. Primarily, the doctor is concerned to restore the patient to health, or where that proves impossible, to ameliorate his/her condition. These things the physician attempts to do as quickly and as efficiently as possible. By contrast the goal of the researcher is different. His objective is medical reconnaissance in which the emphasis now shifts from cure or amelioration of the subject's condition to a focus on *learning* more about the disease. This objective is accomplished by testing for more effective forms of treatment, which in turn hold promise of benefitting future sufferers if the present subjects are beyond hope. Getting clear about our goals in these situations need not cripple *bona fide* research. What it promises to do is to facilitate more intelligent and informed participation in the experiment.

Third, consider the disparity in the knowledge to which the physician and investigator, respectively, lay claim. In the experimental context the labels "researcher" and "subject" signal that the "patient" is no longer in the standard situation in which "the doctor knows best." In the standard setting the physician offers the most effective treatment consistent with the current state of the medical art. The scientific investigator, by his own admission, does *not* know best. Rather he is unsure whether the conventional treatment for the patient's malady is effective. Indeed it is this uncertainty that inspires the project and furnishes the moral imperative to undertake the clinical testing calculated to resolve the doubt. Because of this uncertainty the researcher is unable to say "This is the more effective treatment form." Instead, having acquainted the "patient" of the change in the terms of the contract or covenant signalled by the shift from the therapeutic to the research model and having informed the patient of the risks and potential benefits, he issues the invitation "While we don't know which treatment form is effective will you consent to being a party to finding out?"

The observation was made earlier that acquainting the patient-subject with such facts as we have been considering need not cripple *bona fide* research. It must be acknowledged, however, that it may slow down the pace of research. This is so for the following reasons. First, once the patient has an understanding of these factors he/she may decline to participate in an experimental procedure. I accept this as one of the risks associated with disclosure. Secondly, because the patients' physician performs a dual role—that of colleague of the investigator and that of patient advocate—tensions may arise in situations where there is a conflict between the patients' wishes and the experimenter's advice. In such cases, since I view the advocate's role of the patient as primary, again some refusals to participate may be forthcoming.

Another consideration involves some potentially coercive elements in a nontherapeutic experimental situation, that is, in a situation where the subject and benefittee are not identical.

The following imaginary conversation is put by Professor Hans Jonas into the mouth of a researcher:

> There is nothing more I can do for you. But you can do something for me. Speaking no longer as your physician but on behalf of medical science, we could learn a great deal about future cases of this kind if you would permit me to perform certain experiments on you. It is understood that you yourself would not benefit from any knowledge we might gain: but future patients would.[2]

One interesting thing about Jonas' example is that even though the experimental procedures envisaged hold no promise of direct benefit to the patient, they are nevertheless related to his disease, that is, they are potentially therapeutic from the researcher's standpoint, but not from the standpoint of the subject. The invitation to participate in such activities, however, poses an interesting ethical problem. Do patients have an obligation to acquiesce to such requests? If patients do have an obligation to participate in experimental procedures what is the source of this obligation? Frequently there are actions we feel obliged to perform from motives of gratitude. Are experimental procedures among such actions?

After all, couldn't it be argued that the patients in question have been recipients of the physician's efforts on their behalf? What could be more natural than to claim that the sufferer now owes medicine a debt of gratitude? All other things being equal such a claim has some force. But all things are not equal in such circumstances, for the patient is already in an extremely disadvantageous and vulnerable position. Can we add to his/her burden by imposing yet another burden—the repayment of a debt of gratitude that might well involve further risk, discomfort, inconvenience and suffering? I think not. The patient's plight nullifies the obligation in this case. At most, sufferers at this kind of disadvantage may be "allowed to volunteer for" as opposed to "be expected to endure" such additional discomfort and risks as these experimental procedures are likely to incur. But, and this point is crucial, if such participation falls into the category of moral obligation, then it falls into the category of unenforceable rather than enforceable obligation. In the case of proposals where the interests of the investigator are strongly in favour of research, special consideration and sensitivity are essential lest the patient be made to feel guilty if he/she refuses to acquiesce to experiments geared to the worthy goal of possibly benefitting future sufferers from the same complaint. The investigator must resist exploiting the motive of gratitude for services rendered or the worthy objective of possibly benefitting others. Indeed, in conjunction, gratitude and service may serve as powerful clubs to coerce participation in experimental procedures against the patient's wishes and better judgment.

Pressures on the subject to participate in experimental procedures, while often subtle, are nevertheless relentless. We have focussed on the temptation to exploit the motive of gratitude and incentive for service. Yet other patients respond from fear—the fear that if they refuse to acquiesce in the researcher's request that they will not receive proper treatment. A groundless fear from the researcher's viewpoint, especially since "patients" who are in an experiment "are likely to be more carefully observed and cared for than if they were not research subjects." But as groundless as the fear is from the researcher's vantage point, it may be so real from the patient's perspective as to count as duress. Not infrequently "patients" respond affirmatively to the invitation of the researcher to participate in an experimental procedure out of sheer physical weakness. Rendered less than sovereign by suffering, consent is marred by lowered resistance.

Sometimes even subtler influences brought to bear on the patient necessitate vigilance. These are the pressures resulting from pressures. The compulsion to do research easily translates itself into recruiting subjects for the project. After all, this is the *researcher's*, not the *subject's* project and its successful outcome will have a profound effect on his career. Medical schools and university hospitals are dominated by scientific investigations. Every young researcher knows that his/her professional career is contingent upon his/her ability as investigator as measured by publications.[3] Ramsey makes the same point: "it is not only that medical benefits are attained by research, but also that a man rises to the top in medicine by the success and significance of his research."[4] So, both the potential medical benefits to society as well as the investigator's promotion hinge upon conducting experiments that may place the patient at risk.

Earlier I referred to the conflict of values and obligations in the experimental situation—scientific freedom versus patient inviolability, the moral imperative to provide more effective treatment and the obligation to care for the patient. As delicate as the task of ranking values may be, it appears to be required in the present context. We have drawn attention to pressures to which the patient may be subjected in an experimental context—the exploitation of motives of gratitude, incentives for service, fear, the pressures born of pressures—all of which contribute to a powerfully coercive context for decision making. Given these pressures, as a compensatory move, it is necessary to give greater weight to the patient's rights than to the potential good to be achieved by the research project in which he/she is "invited" to participate. I am claiming with Hans Jonas, that ethically some justification is needed if an infringement of the primary inviolability of the human person is to be permitted. Such justification "must be by values and needs of a dignity commensurate with those sacrificed."[5]

But not only must we rank the individual's rights above the researcher's freedom to seek more effec-

tive remedies, we must also assert the patient's rights against the claims of society on behalf of future sufferers. Since the patient is in the potentially coercive situation outlined earlier it is necessary to give greater weight to his/her rights than to generosity of spirit, compassion for future sufferers, "zeal for humanity, reverence for the Golden Rule, enthusiasm for progress, homage to the call of knowledge...."[6] Only by ranking the patient's rights above the call to sacrifice himself/herself for the common good can we hope to neutralize the combined effect of the convergence of a plurality of powerfully coercive factors in many experimental situations.

It may be objected that the main thrust of this part of the paper has been too negative. The emphasis has been on what is not required of the patient-subject rather than what is required. The subject is not required to act from motives of gratitude, not required to act out of incentives for service, and not to yield to pressures born of pressures. But the question arises: "Is there no positive obligation on the subject's part to participate in experimental procedures?" "If so, in what moral principle or principles is such an obligation grounded?" Two such principles are referred to in the literature—beneficence and justice.

It may be claimed that the patient-subject has a *prima facie* obligation to engage in experimental procedures calculated to benefit others from a motive of beneficence. There are sufferers whose condition may be improved, whether in terms of reduced pain, or by the development of more effective treatment provided that the necessary experimental subjects exhibit a willingness to participate in research. Employed in isolation from other moral principles, however, appeals to beneficence function to predispose the patient to participate in research. Unless moderated by the principle of autonomy, beneficence lacks the necessary checks and balances either to facilitate refusal to participate in, or to withdraw from, an experiment. The respective weighting of beneficence and autonomy depends on an antecedent ranking of our priorities—patient inviolability versus social gain.

Likewise with grounding our obligation to participate in experimental procedures in the principle of justice. It may be claimed with a high degree of plausibility that the burdens as well as the benefits of medical research should be evenly distributed among the members of society. When, however, one recalls Mill's tortuous attempt to harmonize utility and justice, it is clear that justice was invoked to protect minority groups and individuals from undiluted applications of the principle of utility. By contrast, in the present context, the principle of justice is invoked not to moderate but to buttress the principle of utility. We are brought back again in a full circle to the question of weighting the individual against the social components in the context of research projects involving human subjects.

There is yet another constraint on the researcher, one that flows from the nature of the parties to the contract in the research model. The party I refer to is the subject. Herein lies a crucial problem, for human beings in experimental situations are not only subjects but the experimental materials. Because of this dual role it is easy to slip into treating persons as things, and treating ends as means. The difficulty, then, with medical research is that "research" carries overtones of impartiality that are inappropriate to human experimentation. This point may be brought out by contrasting the subject matter of the common-garden variety of scientific research with the subject matter of modern medicine. Originally, experimentation was housed within the domain of natural science, where it deals with inorganic matter. In science, particularly in physics, pure research is both permissible and laudable. A physicist, for example, may push "inert" matter around simply to discover what happens. One may not indulge one's curiosity about human subjects in the same way. The wide discrepancy between "inert" matter and human subjects demands a more conservative approach. "But as soon as animate, feeling beings become the subject of experiment, as they do in the life sciences, and especially in medical research, this innocence of the search for knowledge is lost, and questions of conscience arise."[7] Human subjects have rights which may not be violated simply "to see what happens." In pure science we may indulge ourselves, so far as research funding permits, to pursue knowledge *for its own sake*. Medicine as a profession cannot afford that luxury. Indeed, there are constraints on the pro-

fession of medicine lacking to the field of contemporary philosophical ethics. The professional ethicist may engage in a theoretical inquiry into the meanings of ethical terms, into the validity of ethical arguments, or may try to devise a system for the logic of ethical imperatives, or engage in a comparison of ethical systems noting the analogies and disanalogies between Kantianism and Utilitarianism. And he may do all of these things out of sheer intellectual curiosity.

Medicine as a profession can hardly devote all of its time and energies to such abstract pursuits. As a profession medicine is not concerned with experimental procedures *per se* but with procedures calculated to benefit human beings. There is a built-in practical bent to medicine lacking to pure science.[8] It has a built-in practical bent lacking to both normative and meta-ethics. Another way of putting this is that medicine as a profession is concerned with "the good for *humans*" not with "the good *itself*." If we couple this insight with the uniqueness of the human experimental "material," constraints are imposed upon the medical researcher beyond the ken of the pure physicist or theoretical ethicist. Such constraints impose strict parameters within which guidelines governing human experimentation must be formulated.

In summary, I have no difficulty in acknowledging that experimentation with human subjects results in better medicine provided that the necessary proprieties are observed. As with other human enterprise so with human experimentation, the price of ethically acceptable research is perpetual vigilance. Only when we are sensitive to the implications of the shift in the doctor-patient relationships, alert ourselves to the potentially coercive elements in the experimental situation, and acknowledge the uniqueness of the humane experimental materials can we hope to treat subjects as persons rather than guinea pigs and in Bronowski's phrase, reconcile the welfare of man with the welfare of man.

Acknowledgment

A revised version of a paper presented at the 14th International Conference of Philosophy and Medicine, University of Tel Aviv, September, 1982.

Notes

1 As reported in Jay Katz, *Experimentation with Human Beings* (New York: Russell Sage Foundation, 1972), 64.

2 Hans Jonas, "Philosophical Reflections on Experimenting with Human Subjects," in Tom L. Beauchamp and LeRoy Walters, eds., *Contemporary Issues in Bioethics* (Belmont, CA: Wadsworth, 1982), 2, 531.

3 George H. Kieffer, *Bioethics* (Boston: Addison-Wesley, 1978), 241; Henry K. Beecher, *Research and the Individual* (Boston: Little Brown, 1970), 16.

4 Paul Ramsey, "Consent as a Canon of Loyalty," in Beauchamp and Walters, eds., 534.

5 Jonas, 524.

6 Jonas, 528.

7 Jonas, 524.

8 For a variation on this theme see John E. Thomas, "Medicine and Sociology: A Parting of the Ways," *The Journal of Medicine and Philosophy* 6 (1981): 411-21.

4.
THE NURSE AS PATIENT ADVOCATE

Ellen W. Bernal

SOURCE: *Hastings Center Report* 22.4 (1992): 18-23.

The claim that nurses should be patient advocates is a questionable one, especially when it is mixed in with the professional issue of nurses' freedom to practice. A less combative, more cooperative model of the profession would serve nurses better.

Since the 1970s an extensive discussion in nursing literature has been devoted to the suggestion that nurses be "patient advocates" whose primary responsibility is to protect patient rights and interests in the health care setting.[1] The obligation to patients represents an ideal: in actual practice, institutional and hierarchical constraints often prevent nurses from acting as advocates. Consequently, those espousing patient advocacy argue that unless nurses achieve greater professional autonomy, patients' rights will not be fully protected in hospital settings.[2]

The intertwining of professional and ethical concerns, whereby principles such as patient rights and autonomy are considered in the same context as the professional issue of freedom to practice, is worthy of note. Indeed, such intertwining is a distinguishing feature of nursing ethics in general. While medical ethics rarely needs to address the physician's freedom to establish a professional relationship with patients, nursing ethics has had to deal with ongoing challenges to the freedom to practice, especially in hospital settings.

But even within the context of nursing ethics and its characteristic focus on professional issues, the advocacy literature is distinguished by the frequently explicit claim that patients' rights and interests can only be fully protected in hospital settings if nurses achieve greater professional autonomy. The claim may be misguided. Potential confusions may arise when a call for protection of patient rights is combined with a call for increased political power for nurses.[3]

While the specific features of patient advocacy continue to be debated, it is clear that the central idea—that the primary obligation of nurses is to patients, rather than to physicians or hierarchies within hospitals—has gained wide acceptance within the profession.

Revisions in the American Nurses' Association's Code for Nurses reflect this shift in professional viewpoint. The 1976 code not only omits statements, present in earlier versions, that obliged nurses to maintain confidence in physicians and obey their orders, but also explicitly uses the language of advocacy in its interpretive statements: "In the role of client advocate, the nurse must be alert to and take appropriate action regarding any instances of incompetent, unethical, or illegal practice(s) by any member of the health care team or the health care system itself, or any action on the part of others that is prejudicial to the client's best interests."[4]

The debate over nurses' role as patient advocate affords an opportunity to consider several key issues. First, over the past two decades, nurses' perception of their primary allegiance has shifted from physicians and hospitals to patients. Second, some of the advocacy literature explicitly combines professional aspirations with the expression of obligations to patients. To what extent is this combination of moral and political claims legitimate? Third, patient advocacy assumes that nurses bring a special moral perspective to hospital settings. What is the nature of this moral contribution, and do nurses in fact wish to accept this as a feature of their professional role?

The advocacy literature asserts the moral primacy of autonomy, currently accepted in Western culture, and as a result may risk an impoverished view of illness, suffering, and the obligations of the professional to the patient. Alternative models of the nurse-patient relationship, such as the covenantal models already described in nursing literature, may offer a better construction of the relationship between nursing and the public.

The Advocacy Model

Before the advocacy model gained wide acceptance, nurses believed that their primary obligation was to obey physicians and maintain order within hospitals. This military sense of nursing identity originated in the context of the Crimean war, when Florence Nightingale brought order and greatly improved conditions to military hospitals. Upon her return to England in 1856, Nightingale worked to establish a training school for nurses that would eventually impart the same military discipline to civilian hospitals, through an emphasis on improved education and obedience to institutional hierarchies. Elements of the military ideal included unquestioning loyalty and obedience to the nurse's training school, hospital, and physician's orders; protection of the patient's faith in the physician, even in cases of physician error or incompetence; self-sacrifice under difficult working conditions; and routine indications of discipline such as uniforms and deference to physicians. Despite evidence that some nursing leaders called attention to the conflicts in loyalty that could come about under this model, the military ideal provided an early sense of professional nursing identity. The military language prevalent during the Nightingale era was gradually replaced by the language of advocacy. The primary role of advocacy is defined as the protection of patients' rights and interests. In one of the earliest pieces on the topic, Mary F. Kohnke suggests that advocacy means informing patients about their rights, providing facts about their health care situation, and supporting them in the decisions they make.[5] A more extensive development of this idea is found in a series of articles by George J. Annas, who claims that patients' rights need protection in hospital settings, and that nurses may be able to fill the role of "patient rights advocate."[6]

From the outset, the advocacy literature has frequently associated protection of patient rights with professional development. For example, Annas notes that advocacy will require a level of assertiveness that many nurses may not currently possess. If nurses provided organized support for the idea of patient rights, and taught students the art of advocacy in nursing schools, the position of the patient in the hospital and the public image of the nurse would both be enhanced. "Nurses so trained can act not only as independent practitioners, but can also move into the direct care of patients as partners of doctors rather than servants to them." Similarly, Nancy Quinn and Anne Somers Walsh predict that if nurses support the consumers' movement in health care and become patient advocates, health care and nurses' professional status will improve, while Elsie and Bertram Bandman claim that "patient advocacy is integral with the expanding relationships nurses have in the care of their patients. Models of nurse-patient-physician relationships show that patient advocacy by nurses is essential to patients' health care rights."[7]

The next move in the debate was the claim that hospital power structures prevent nurses from identifying unsafe or unethical practices by instilling a fear of reprisal. That is to say, hospital nurses are limited in their ability to serve as patient advocates because they are unable to protect patients' rights. Unless hospital power structures are changed to permit greater autonomy for nurses, patient rights within hospitals will be compromised. In this view, set forth in an influential article by Roland R. Yarling and Beverly J. McElmurry, optimal protection of patient rights can only be achieved through the development of nurses' professional power:

> unless nursing, through the reform of the institution in which the majority of its members practice, acquires a balance of controlling power in that institution or creates new structures for the organization of practice, it cannot effectively implement standards of care for its own practice. If it cannot realize reform it will compromise the integrity of the nurse-patient relationship, which is the moral foundation of nursing, and it will have lost its status as a profession. Furthermore, the public will have lost its most valuable ally within the health care system. The one action that would most improve the quality of health care in this society is simple and direct: set the nurses free, set the nurses free.[8]

An Ethical Analysis of the Advocacy Argument

The advocacy literature expresses professional identity and aspirations in the context of present nursing practice, displaying a concern for public and interprofessional recognition of nursing's professional status along with the concern to promote patients' rights and best interests. The literature often describes nurses as symbols of moral order within hospitals, and may have captured the imagination of nurses because it seems to offer a constructive way out of current difficult practice conditions, while simultaneously enhancing patients' rights.

The use of autonomy in the arguments for patient advocacy is also worth noting.

The image of the autonomous person is invoked for both the patient whose rights are threatened in the hospital and for the nurse whose moral agency is compromised by institutional power structures. In the most extreme formulation of patient advocacy, the autonomy of the patient is held to be contingent upon the autonomy of the nurse.

The combination of references to actual circumstances, professional frustration and aspiration, and powerful moral ideals tends to promote uncritical assent to the claims for patient advocacy.[9] Criticism of any one of these elements may lead to a defense of advocacy through an appeal to another component. For example, any empirical question raised about nurses' working conditions within hospital settings might be answered by an appeal to nurses' professional aspirations. In a similar fashion, criticism of the search for professional power can be turned aside through a reference to the ideal of autonomy. The complex relationships among the components of the argument may have contributed to the persistence of the advocacy model.

But it is important to distinguish between the interest generated by a model and its adequacy in describing professional realities, values, and ideals. Professional nursing needs to determine whether the current description of patient advocacy actually enhances, or is in fact a detriment to professional development. Toward this end, the elements of the model should be considered separately. For example, the empirical claims and assumptions present in the advocacy literature should be examined. Is the typi-

cal nurse more likely to identify ethical issues than members of other professions, or than the general public? Do nurses currently have adequate freedom to practice? What courses of action are available to nurses when they observe less than optimal care in hospitals or other settings? Do nurses exercise these options, if they are in fact currently available? When nurses hesitate to act because of fear of reprisal, how realistic is this fear? What is the relevance of the advocacy role to situations involving deficiencies in the practice of other nurses? Research in nursing ethics is currently examining related issues that could be extended and brought to bear on the concept of advocacy if the empirical claims used to argue for it could be separated from the accompanying moral principles and professional aspirations.

Professional identity also requires clear conceptual distinctions between intrinsic professional values, the instrumental need for adequate freedom to practice, and the more self-serving goal of increased professional status. Without this differentiation, a key feature of professional identity may be lost: the promise to provide services to the public as an intrinsic value, rather than as a means to achieve professional power. Professional autonomy is not an intrinsic value of nursing and does not constitute part of the services offered to the public.[10] Instead, the ability to take action is a condition for the exercise of other values that are intrinsic to the profession. While freedom to practice is certainly necessary, the advocacy literature repeatedly confuses the distinction between freedom to practice and the less disinterested goal of professional nursing development.

On the Moral Contribution of Nurses to Hospitals

The patient advocacy literature presents symbolic images of the nurse as an individual who identifies ethical concerns, yet because of institutional constraints must either set these concerns aside or take unusually forceful action. If she sets the concerns aside, the nurse compromises personal integrity and the adequacy of patient care; if she takes action, she risks personal and professional harm.

Christine Mitchell's argument for nursing integrity signals the end of the notion that the military model of obedience can provide effective patient care in hospitals, and the beginning of the advocacy literature's claim that the nurse's freedom to act with integrity is essential to the support of patient rights and best interests. In a fictional account, Mitchell describes the moral discord faced by Nurse Andrews, who is caring for two neurologically injured patients, one an alert quadriplegic and the other a comatose individual with a poor prognosis. The two patients are attended by different physicians whose perspectives on cardiopulmonary resuscitation are different. The military model of obedience at the heart of Nurse Andrews's practice leads to inconsistency: she resuscitates the comatose patient several times, but allows the alert quadriplegic to die, despite his interest in recovering. Mitchell comments that "the individual nurse is severely handicapped in acting with integrity. Nurses' interprofessional relationships with physicians come into direct conflict with their relationships with patients. Consequently, the integrity of the whole health care system is threatened."[11] In this story, the nurse is portrayed as central to the protection of moral standards and consistent care within the hospital. When her integrity is compromised, the integrity of the institution is compromised as well.

In other advocacy stories the nurse attempts to champion patient rights and in the process either experiences or narrowly avoids personal harm. Leah Curtin provides a description of an actual situation. Jean S. is a staff nurse who is assigned to care for William R., a recently widowed man in his late sixties who was admitted to the hospital through the emergency room, where he presented with probable bowel obstruction. When the house surgeon operated, he found that Mr. R. had cancer; however, the physician believed that this diagnosis should not be shared with the patient. Jean S. attempted to convince the physician that this lack of disclosure was contrary to the rights of the patient and counterproductive to his well-being, but without success. When the patient continued to ask pointed questions regarding his health, the nurse did inform the patient about his condition. The grateful patient was then able to obtain assistance with home care through a local hospice association and later died peacefully at home. The attending physician was angry with the

nurse and lodged a complaint of insubordination against her, but the director of nursing, social work services, and the chaplain's office supported her decision to share information. In Curtin's commentary upon this case, she observes that "although nurses have a moral duty to be honest in answering patients' questions, ... it is unlikely that nurses will do so (at least in any great numbers) as long as physicians have the professional and institutional power to coerce and punish them."[12]

Whether the nurse in the advocacy stories chooses to act or to remain passive, she brings a moral point of view to patient care. The expectation that nurses are to display a special moral sensitivity, while a key feature of the notion of advocacy, is by no means new. In the culture of ancient Greece and Rome, the perception that women have a natural altruism and an ability to care for others gave a sense of moral obligation to their traditional domestic occupations, such as caring for the sick. But because these occupations were regarded as chores somehow natural to women, and because of women's comparative social invisibility, their work did not appear to merit special notice. Although some of the services performed by women were highly respected, such as preparing the dead for burial and assisting at childbirth, the surrounding culture did not confer professional status on women who performed these activities.[13]

Modern culture persists in the belief that women are naturally altruistic, and altruism is a foundational assumption in the professional development of nursing. The establishment of modern hospitals "played upon the contemporary assumption that there was a necessary and laudable conjunction between nursing and femininity; the trained sensibility of a middle-class woman could alone bring order and morality to the hospital's grim wards."[14] But the view that women are naturally altruistic has restricted the ability of nurses to achieve professional status. Demands for professional autonomy when made by women are taken to be self-interested rather than oriented toward the needs of others, and so are seen as unfeminine.[15]

Patient advocacy appears to offer a way out of this difficulty, as it draws upon the traditional belief that nurses bring a civilizing, altruistic influence to hospitals, but is based on a changed notion of civic virtue. Instead of military obedience, the surrounding culture now values individual rights. Proponents of patient advocacy imply that nurses are the professionals who—given adequate professional freedom—can best ensure the protecting of patient rights within hospitals. Through this maneuver nurses can make a claim for professional power without jeopardizing their traditional image of altruism, self-sacrifice, and high moral ideals.

The advocacy stories, however, contain questionable implications that should be considered carefully by anyone tempted to define nurses as patient advocates. First of all, they suggest that the core values of nursing are ephemeral, and that the profession will take up whatever values are current in the surrounding culture. The stories also contribute to the likelihood that the public will continue to perceive the nursing profession sentimentally, perpetuating longstanding stereotypes of nurses as martyrs or heroes. The martyr, a victim of circumstance, is sacrificed to save others who will not at first honor the sacrifice or recognize its importance. This is the nurse under the military model, who works long hours and sacrifices her own interests to care for the suffering and to save lives. In contrast, the hero, possessing unusual strength and courage, is engaged in a socially visible struggle. This is the nurse under the advocacy model, who both defends patients' rights and seeks to elevate nurses' professional status, in an adversarial struggle against the forces of institutional oppression. Both images are highly unrealistic. Professional authority has legitimate origins in nursing expertise and history, not in romantic images of nurses as guardians of morality. When nurses are portrayed in this fashion, nursing practice is burdened with unrealistic demands and barriers are erected between nurses and the other professionals with whom they cooperate.

The Ideal of Autonomy

Those who promote patient advocacy often confuse the need for an adequate level of professional freedom to practice with an idealized image of autonomy that has attained a privileged moral status in Western culture. In this idealized image, persons select actions from a wide array of choices and are unlimited by situational constraints. Such a vision of autonomy impoverishes our view of social relationships, illness, suffering, and the obligations of the professional to the patient.

On the patient advocate model, social relationships within the hospital are essentially adversarial and manipulative. The rights of the patient are threatened by caregivers and by the institution itself. Nurses' rights too are abridged by physicians, other professionals, and bureaucratic structures. The model assumes that most relationships within hospitals are based on self-preservation and self-interest, rather than on mutual cooperation toward a common end. Within this context, nurses become professionals who assert their own rights and the rights of patients when they are threatened by others. There is a tendency to protest and unmask others' motivations rather than to explore the purposes and ends of social relationships and one's own responsibilities in promoting them.

A misplaced emphasis on autonomy obscures the frequently positive aspects of social relationships within hospitals: the mutually affirmed goals of promoting the patient's best interest in accordance with patient choices and the responsible use of resources in the service of those ends. Although hospitals may sometimes fail in their efforts to achieve their goals, it is not clear that failures are due to a deficit in nursing autonomy. The call for an abstract and unadulterated ideal of autonomy disregards the freedom of action that nurses already have.[16]

It is also not clear that the vision of autonomy invoked by proponents of patient advocacy sufficiently honors the experience of illness for the patient in the hospital. When the patient is suffering and vulnerable, an emphasis on individual rights cannot fully characterize the nurse-client relationship, as Sally Gadow observes when she urges nurses to assist the patient to find meaning in the experience of illness.[17] The interests of third parties and communities are also not encompassed by notions of patient autonomy.

The ascendancy of autonomy in modern culture contributes to the likelihood that the role of nurse as patient advocate will be accepted uncritically, especially by those nurses who actually experience repressive working conditions in hospital settings. Nurses should consider whether a more effective contribution to the growth of professional identity might not be achieved by defining patient advocacy more precisely.

As it now stands, advocacy refers to situations in which the nurse protects the patient from the incompetent or unethical practice of another professional. But other professionals, such as patient representatives, also describe themselves as patient advocates. Are nurses to practice a distinctive, nurse-specific form of advocacy, or is their advocacy to overlap that of other professionals?

Professional nursing might also wish to examine the public's perception of nursing's contributions to health care, and in particular whether the public wishes nurses to assume the role of patient advocate. While public expectations should not define professional identity, extreme disparities between them are an indication that professionals need to examine their assumptions regarding their role.

Nurses should also consider setting aside the idea that they are powerless within hospitals. It would seem to be far more productive to identify and extend currently available resources for action, rather than seeking an idealized version of autonomy that no one working in hospitals actually possesses. If nurses do have restricted autonomy, they are not alone. Increasingly, physicians have their autonomy limited by third-party payers, utilization review, and hospital administration. In any case, what is needed is not greater individuation for nurses but greater cooperation among all professionals who provide health care in a hospital setting.

Professional Virtue
and the Model of a Covenant

With its perplexing claim that patient autonomy is contingent upon nursing autonomy, proponents of patient advocacy tend to disregard crucial empirical questions relating to nursing practice, and to offer an overly romanticized image of the nurse as a moral guardian within the hospital. It would seem important to investigate other descriptions of nursing authority to assess their contribution to the further development of professional identity.

A covenantal model of the professional-public relationship is one alternative that has been suggested. On William May's account, covenantal agreements described in the Bible are based on three elements that provide clues to authentic professional-public relationships: (1) an exchange of gifts, symbolizing mutual indebtedness; (2) an exchange of promises, establishing a set of mutually affirmed intrinsic values; and (3) an ontological change in the persons who create the covenantal agreement. The individual becomes a professional when he or she is given freedom to practice by the public, on the basis of the professional's promise to remain faithful to the ideal of service.[18] These elements, which have their origins in ancient Hebrew thought, afford a different interpretation of issues raised by the proponents of patient advocacy: the relationship between professions and the public, the meaning of personal autonomy and illness, and intrinsic professional values.

A covenantal model calls attention to the reciprocal indebtedness of the public and the profession, suggesting that professional power is a gift from the public to the profession given in exchange for its expertise and orientation toward the service of others. Those who have adopted the notion that nurses should be patient advocates should consider whether the current model of advocacy can fully encompass the extent of services nursing traditionally offers. While protecting patient self-determination is certainly essential, nursing is also, in the language of the American Nurses' Association,

the protection, promotion and restoration of health; the prevention of illness, and the alleviation of suffering in the care of clients, including individuals, family groups, and communities. In the context of these functions, nursing is defined as the diagnosis and treatment of human responses to actual or potential health problems.[19]

Patient advocacy represents only one feature of the range of professional services nursing provides.

Under a covenantal model, gifts are to some degree responsive to the needs and expectations of the recipients. Although the full extent of nursing's gift to the public may not be completely defined by the needs that the public perceives, if patients do not in fact expect or want nurses to be their advocates, the nurse's gift of advocacy may well go unappreciated. Patients presumably regard themselves and their families or other surrogates, rather than nurses, as the primary sources of self-determination, and expect nurses to respond to the wider variety of needs occasioned by illness and health care.

A related concern involves the connection between patient advocacy and professional autonomy. A gift given by the profession to the public should strengthen the covenantal relationship between the nurse and the patient rather than strengthen the profession's independent claim to professional status. A gift with this secondary motivation risks becoming illegitimately self-interested. The risk seems greater when the nurse is presented as the key to moral practice within hospital settings. Surely other professionals within hospitals also provide support for patient self-determination, rights, and interests. Nurses must carefully consider whether they wish to retain this image of moral centrality or whether it is in fact counterproductive to professional development.

A covenantal model describes persons as free to enter into agreements, establish moral principles, and keep promises. This account of practical autonomy, or autonomy within a situation, is an alternative to the more sweeping description of professional autonomy underlying the argument for patient advocacy, which tends to view persons as though they were abstracted from the social obligations, relationships, and contingencies that characterize actual social settings. A covenantal model more clearly engages actual experience, including the need to change institutions that are repressive and inimical to the covenantal relationship.

At present, patient advocacy does not provide a comprehensive description of the role and contributions of nursing. But the question of whether nurses currently possess adequate professional freedom to establish covenantal relationships with patients still remains. It seems clear that professional nursing has an extensive and historically based covenant with the general public. However, especially for nurses who practice in hospitals, the possibility of professional covenants with clients faces several challenges, not only because of the bureaucratic structures of hospitals and the history of the nurse-physician relationship, but also because of the way that nursing services within hospitals are allocated. When patients are admitted to hospitals by physicians, they have little choice regarding which nurses will take care of them. Changes in nursing personnel due to staffing patterns and the frequent lack of primary care nursing also contribute to discontinuity in nurse-patient relationships. These structures place real limitations on hospital nurses' ability to enter into caregiving agreements with individual patients. At the same time, institutions do provide opportunities for cooperative change, which is especially likely to occur if nurses continue to demonstrate the essential contribution that the profession makes to overall patient well-being. The adversarial stance of the advocacy model may not be the best way to achieve needed change.

Professions modify their intrinsic values over time, in response to historical and social conditions. The conditions that prompted the call for patient advocacy should also prompt a consideration of alternative models, given advocacy's theoretical and practical shortcomings. Such consideration will contribute to an expression of professional identity that reflects both the history and traditions of nursing and the challenges of modern practice.

Acknowledgements

This article benefitted greatly from comments received after presentation at the 1991 meeting of the Society for Health and Human Values.

Notes

1   Barbara K. Miller, Thomas J. Mansen, and Helen Lee, "Patient Advocacy: Do Nurses Have the Power and Authority to Act as Patient Advocate?" *Nursing Leadership* 6 (June 1983): 56-60; Gerald R. Winslow, "From Loyalty to Advocacy: A New Metaphor for Nursing," *Hastings Center Report* 14.3 (1984): 32-40; and Terry Pence and Janice Cantrall, eds., *Ethics in Nursing: An Anthology* (New York: National League for Nursing, 1990).

2   George J. Annas, "The Patient Rights Advocate: Can Nurses Fill the Role?" *Supervisor Nurse* 5 (July

1974): 20-23, 25; Mary F. Kohnke, "The Nurse asAdvocate," *American Journal of Nursing* 80 (November 1980): 2038-40; Christine Mitchell, "Integrity in Interprofessional Relationships," in *Responsibility in Health Care*, ed. George J. Agich (Dordrecht: D. Reidel, 1982); Darlene Trandel-Korenchuk and Keith Trandel-Korenchuk, "Nursing Advocacy of Patients' Rights: Myth or Reality?" *Nurse Practitioner* 8 (April 1983): 40-42.

3 See George J. Agich, "Professionalism and Ethics in Health Care," *Journal of Medicine and Philosophy* 5.3 (1980): 186-99.

4 American Nurses' Association, *Code for Nurses with Interpretive Statements* (Kansas City: American Nurses' Association, 1976; 1985).

5 Kohnke, "The Nurse as Advocate."

6 George J. Annas, "Patient Rights: An Agenda for the '80s," *Nursing Law and Ethics* 3 (April 1981), reprinted in *Ethics in Nursing*, ed. Pence and Cantrall, pp. 75-82.

7 Annas, "The Patient Rights Advocate," p. 25; Nancy Quinn and Anne Somers, "The Patient's Bill of Rights: A Significant Aspect of the Consumer Revolution," *Nursing Outlook* 22 (April 1974): 240-44; Elsie L. Bandman and Bertram Bandman, *Nursing Ethics Across the Life Span*, 2nd ed. (Norwalk: Appleton and Lange, 1990), p. 21.

8 Roland R. Yarling and Beverly J. McElmurry, "The Moral Foundation of Nursing," *Advances in Nursing Science* 8.2 (1986): 63-73.

9 Michael Polanyi, *Personal Knowledge: Towards a Post-Critical Philosophy* (New York: Harper Torchbooks, 1964).

10 John S. Packard and Mary Ferrara, "In Search of the Moral Foundation of Nursing," *Advances in Nursing Science* 10.4 (1988): 60-71.

11 Mitchell, "Integrity in Interprofessional Relationships," pp. 163-84.

12 Leah Curtin and Josephine Flaherty, *Nursing Ethics: Theories and Pragmatics* (Bowie, MD: Robert J. Brady Co., 1982), p. 333.

13 Natalie B. Kampen, "Before Florence Nightingale: A Prehistory of Nursing in Painting and Sculpture," in *Images of Nurses: Perspectives from History, Art, and Literature*, ed. Anne Hudson Jones (Philadelphia: University of Pennsylvania Press, 1988), pp. 6-39.

14 Charles E. Rosenberg, *The Care of Strangers: The Rise of America's Hospital System* (New York: Basic Books, 1987), p. 212.

15 Susan Reverby, "A Caring Dilemma: Womanhood and Nursing in Historical Perspective," *Nursing Research* 36.1 (1987): 5-11.

16 Anne H. Bishop and John R. Scudder, Jr., *The Practical, Moral and Personal Sense of Nursing: A Phenomenological Philosophy of Practice* (Albany: State University of New York Press, 1990).

17 Sally Gadow, "Existential Advocacy: Philosophical Foundation of Nursing," in *Nursing Images and Ideals: Opening Dialogue with the Humanities*, ed. Stuart F. Spicker and Sally Gadow (New York: Springer, 1980), pp. 79-101.

18 William F. May, "Code and Covenant or Philanthropy and Contract?" in *Ethics in Medicine: Historical Perspectives and Contemporary Concerns*, ed. Stanley Joel Reiser, Arthur J. Dyck, and William J. Curran (Cambridge, MA: MIT Press, 1977), pp. 65-76; see also Mary Carolyn Cooper, "Covenantal Relationships: Grounding for the Nursing Ethic," *Advances in Nursing Science* 10.4 (1988): 48-59.

19 American Nurses' Association, Code for Nurses, Preamble.

5.
A DEFENSE OF UNQUALIFIED MEDICAL CONFIDENTIALITY[1]

Kenneth Kipnis

SOURCE: *American Journal of Bioethics* 6.2 (2006): 7-18.

It is broadly held that confidentiality may be breached when doing so can avert grave harm to a third party. This essay challenges the conventional wisdom. Neither legal duties, personal morality nor personal values are sufficient to ground professional obligations. A methodology is developed drawing on core professional values, the nature of professions, and the justification for distinct professional obligations. Though doctors have a professional obligation to prevent public peril, they do not honor it by breaching confidentiality. It is shown how the protective purpose to be furthered by reporting is defeated by the practice of reporting. Hence there is no conflict between confidentiality and the professional responsibility to protect endangered third parties.

The Case of the Infected Spouse

The following fictionalized case is based on an actual incident.

1982: After moving to Honolulu, Wilma and Andrew Long visit your office and ask you to be their family physician. They have been your patients ever since.
1988: Six years later the two decide to separate. Wilma leaves for the Mainland, occasionally sending you a postcard. Though you do not see her professionally, you still think of yourself as her doctor.
1990: Andrew comes in and says that he has embarked upon a more sophisticated social life. He has been hearing about some new sexually transmitted diseases and wants to be tested. Testing reveals that he is positive for the AIDS virus, and he receives appropriate counseling.
1991: Visiting your office for a checkup, Andrew tells you Wilma is returning to Hawaii for reconcili-

ation with him. She arrives that afternoon and will be staying at the Moana Hotel. Despite your best efforts to persuade him, Andrew leaves without giving you assurance that he will tell Wilma about his infection or protect her against becoming infected.
Do you take steps to see that Wilma is warned? If you decide to warn Wilma, what do you say to Andrew when, two days later, he shows up at your office asking how you could reveal his confidential test results?
If you decide not to warn Wilma, what do you say to her when, two years later in 1993, she shows up at your office asking how you, her doctor, could possibly stand idly by as her husband infected her with a deadly virus. She now knows she is positive for the virus, that she was infected by her husband, and that you—her doctor—knew, before they reconciled, that her husband would probably infect her.

The ethical challenges here emerge from an apparent head-on collision between medical confidentiality and the duty to protect imperiled third parties. Notwithstanding Andrew's expectation of privacy and the professional duty to remain silent, it can seem unforgivable for anyone to withhold vital assistance in such a crisis, let alone a doctor. The case for breaching confidentiality is supported by at least five considerations: First, the doctor knows, to a medical certainty, that Andrew is both infected with HIV and infectious. Second, knowing Wilma as a patient, let us suppose the doctor reasonably believes that she is not infected. (Wilma cannot be at risk of contracting the disease if she is infected already.) Third, Wilma's vulnerability is both serious and real. HIV infection is both debilitating and, during those years, invariably fatal. The couple's sexuality makes eventual

infection highly likely. Fourth, assuming that preventing Wilma's death is the goal, it is probable that,
were Wilma to be told of Andrew's infection, she
would avoid exposing herself to the risk. This is not
a trivial condition: many people knowingly risk illness and injury out of love and other honorable motivations. Molokai's Father Damien contracted and
died from Hansen's disease while caring for patients
he knew might infect him. Soldiers, police, and firefighters commonly expose themselves to grave risk.
It is not enough that a warning would discharge a
duty to Wilma, merely so she could make an
informed choice. Plainly, the paramount concern has
to be to save Wilma's life. Finally, Wilma is not a
mere stranger. Instead she has an important relationship with you—her doctor—that serves as a basis for
special obligations: You have a special duty to look
out for her health.

In the light of these five considerations, it should
not be a surprise that the conventional wisdom in
medical ethics overwhelmingly supports either an
ethical obligation to breach confidentiality in cases
like this one or, occasionally and less stringently, the
ethical permissibility of doing so (Lo 1995).
Notwithstanding this consensus, it is my intention to
challenge the received view. I will argue in what follows that confidentiality in clinical medicine is far
closer to an absolute obligation than it has generally
been taken to be; doctors should honor confidentiality even in cases like this one. Although the focus
here is on the *Case of the Infected Spouse*, the background idea is that, if it can be demonstrated that
confidentiality should be scrupulously honored in
this one case where so many considerations support
breaching it, the duty of confidentiality should be
taken as unqualified in virtually all other cases as
well (Kottow 1986). I shall not, however, defend that
broader conclusion here.

Although this essay specifically addresses the
obligations of doctors, its approach applies more
broadly to all professions that take seriously the
responsibility to provide distressed practitioners
with authoritative guidance (Kipnis 1986, 63-79;
Wicclair 1986). With its focus narrowly on "professional obligations," the methodology used below
also represents something of a challenge to much of
the conventional thinking in medical ethics.

Clearing the Ground:
What Professional Obligations Are Not

Among philosophers, it is commonplace that if people are not asking the same questions, they are
unlikely to arrive at the same answers. It may be that
the main reason doctors have difficulty reaching
consensus in ethics is that, in general, systematic discussion about professional responsibility is commonly confused with at least three other types of
conversation. When one asks whether one should
call the hotel to warn Wilma, one can be asking: 1)
what the law requires; 2) what one's personal morality requires (e.g., as an Orthodox Jew, a Roman
Catholic, etc.); or 3) what is required by one's most
deeply held personal values (e.g., preventing deaths
or scrupulously honoring other obligations). Discussions can meander mindlessly over all three areas
without attending to boundary crossings. More to the
point, effective deliberation about professional
obligations, as I will try to show, differs importantly
from all three of these discussions. Accordingly, it is
necessary to identify and bracket these other perspectives in order to mark off the intellectual space
within which practitioners can productively reflect
on questions of professional responsibility. Let us
examine these different conversations.

Law

The conventional wisdom on the ethics of medical
confidentiality has been largely shaped by a single
legal case: *Tarasoff v. Regents of the University of
California* (Supreme Court of California; 529 p. 2d
553, Cal. 1974). In 1969, Prosenjit Poddar, a student
at U.C. Berkeley, told a university psychologist he
intended to kill a Ms. Tatiana Tarasoff, a young
woman who had spurned his affections. The psychologist dutifully reported him to the campus
police, who held him briefly and then set him free.
Shortly afterwards, Poddar did as he said he would,
stabbing the young woman to death. The Tarasoff
family sued the University of California for their
daughter's death, finally prevailing in their contention that the psychologist (and, by implication,
the University) had failed in their duty to protect,
since neither Tatiana nor those able to apprise her of

danger were warned. The University was found liable and had to compensate the family for its loss. Today it is hard to find discussions of the ethics of confidentiality that do not appeal to this legal parable and, occasionally, to its California Supreme Court moral: "The protective privilege ends where the public peril begins."

Taking its cue from *Tarasoff*, the prevailing standard in medical ethics now holds that the obligation of confidentiality will give way when a doctor is aware that a patient will seriously injure some identified other person. (One might ask why disclosure is not required when a patient will seriously injure many unidentified persons. Under the narrower standard, there is no duty to alert others about an HIV-infected prostitute who neither informs nor protects a large number of anonymous at-risk clients.) We assume that the physician knows Andrew is seropositive, that Wilma is likely seronegative, that the two will likely engage in activities that transmit the virus, and that breaching confidentiality will probably result in those activities not occurring and Wilma's not becoming infected. Thus, a physician's warning in the *Case of the Infected Spouse* will mean that Wilma is very likely to remain infection-free, and a failure to warn her is very likely to result in her eventual death from AIDS.

Focusing on the legal standard, it is useful to distinguish between "special" and "general" legal duties. Special duties can apply to individuals occupying certain roles. A parent, but not a bystander, has a special duty to rescue a drowning daughter; firefighters and police officers have special duties to take certain occupational risks, and doctors have many special duties toward their patients: confidentiality is a good example. In contrast, virtually everyone has a general duty to be scrupulously careful when handling explosives, to pay taxes on income, to respect others' property, and so on. It is notable that the duty to warn in *Tarasoff* is a special duty, applicable only to those occupying special roles. So if my neighbor casually assures me he is going to kill his girlfriend tomorrow, the *Tarasoff* ruling does not require me to warn her.

It is surprising to many that the default standard in Anglo-American jurisprudence is that there is no general duty to improve the prospects of the precar-

iously placed, no legal obligation to undertake even an easy rescue. As first-year law students discover, one can stand on a pier with a lifeline in hand and, with complete impunity, allow a stranger to drown nearby. Although we will pass over it, it is notable that, in general, the parties who are legally obligated to warn are those who are otherwise ethically obligated not to disclose. One should reflect on the absence of a general duty to warn.

The easy transition from law to ethics reflects a common error. The mistake is to move from the premise that some action is legally required (what the *Tarasoff* opinion establishes in the jurisdictions that have followed it) to the conclusion that the same action is ethically required. But ethical obligations can conflict with legal ones. Journalists, for example, are sometimes ordered by the courts to reveal the identities of their confidential sources. Although law demands disclosure, professional ethics requires silence. Reporters famously go to jail rather than betray sources. Journalists can find themselves in a quandary: while good citizens obey the law and good professionals honor their professional codes, laws requiring journalists to violate their duties to confidential sources force a tragic choice between acting illegally and acting unethically. Conscientious persons should not have to face such decisions.

Similarly in pediatrics, statutes may require doctors to report suspicions of child abuse. But where protective agencies are inept and overworked and foster care is dangerous or unavailable, a doctor's report is more likely to result in termination of therapy and further injury to the child instead of protection and care. To obey the law under these appalling, but too common, circumstances is most likely to abandon and even cause harm to the minor patient, both of which are ethically prohibited in medicine. To assume that legal obligations always trump or settle ethical ones is to blind oneself to the possibility of conflict. Professions have to face these dilemmas head-on instead of masking them with language that conflates legal standards and ethical ones. They must conceive professional ethics as separate from the law's mandate. When law requires what professional responsibility prohibits (or prohibits what professional responsibility requires), professional organizations must press the public, legislatures, and the courts to cease demanding that conscientious practitioners dishonor the duties of their craft. This is an important responsibility of professional organizations. It is a mistake to configure professional obligations merely to mirror the law's requirements. Rather the law's requirements must be configured so that they do not conflict with well-considered professional obligations. Law is a human artifact that can be crafted well or badly. In a well-ordered society no one will have to choose between illegality and immorality. Since the law can require conduct that violates ethical standards (and ethical standards can require conduct that violates the law), it cannot be the case that legal obligations automatically create ethical obligations. As the tradition of civil disobedience shows, it can be ethically permissible or obligatory (though not legal) to violate an unjust law.

Even though laws cannot create ethical obligations by fiat, professions need to distinguish between the state's reasonable interests in the work of doctors (e.g., preventing serious harm to children) and the specific legal mandates a state imposes (e.g., requiring doctors to report suspicion of child abuse to an incompetent state agency). Just as patients can make ill-considered demands that should not be satisfied, so too can the state and its courts.

Accordingly, it is assumed that the state has a legitimate interest in preventing harm to people, and that doctors have an ethical obligation to further that important public objective. The focus in this essay is on the shape of the resulting ethical obligation as it applies narrowly to cases like those involving Wilma Long and Tatiana Tarasoff. Because they introduce complexities that will carry us far afield, we set aside cases involving: (a) children brought in by parents (Kipnis 2004); (b) patients referred for independent medical evaluation; (c) mentally ill or retarded patients in the custody of health care institutions; (d) health care that is the subject of litigation; (e) gunshot, knife wounds, and the like; (f) workers' compensation cases; and a few others. While a much longer discussion could cover these areas, many readers can extend the analysis offered here to discern much of what I would want to say about those other cases.

Though I will not discuss them, institutional policies (hospital rules, for example) function very much like laws. Both involve standards that can be imposed externally upon practitioners. Both can be formulated knowledgeably and wisely or with a disregard for essential professional responsibilities.

Personal Morality

We will understand a "morality" as a set of beliefs about obligations. There are plainly many such sets of beliefs: the morality of Confucius has little in common with the moralities of George W. Bush and Thomas Aquinas. For most of us, morality is uncritically absorbed in childhood, coming to consciousness when we encounter others whose moral beliefs differ.

There are still parts of the world in which virtually all members of a community are participants in a common morality. But moral pluralism now seems a permanent part of the social order. Consider a Jehovah's Witness physician who is opposed, on religious grounds, to administering blood transfusions. If this doctor were the only physician on duty when his patient needed an immediate transfusion, a choice would have to be made between being a good Jehovah's Witness and being a good doctor. The doctor's personal moral convictions are here inconsistent with professional obligations. It follows that clarity about personal morality is not the same as clarity about medical ethics. Professionalism can require that one set aside one's personal morality or carefully limit one's exposure to certain professional responsibilities. Here the rule has to be that doctors will not take on responsibilities that might conflict with their personal morality. Problems could be sidestepped if the Jehovah's Witness doctor specialized in a field that didn't involve transfusion (e.g., dermatology) or always worked with colleagues who could administer them. If I am morally against the death penalty, I shouldn't take on work as an executioner. If I am deeply opposed to the morning-after pill, I shouldn't counsel patients at a rape treatment center. To teach medical ethics in a pluralistic professional community is to try to create an intellectual space within which persons from varied backgrounds can agree upon responsible standards for professional conduct. Participants in such a conversation may have to leave personal morality at the door. For some, it may be a mistake to choose a career in medicine.

If ethics is a critical reflection on our moralities, then the hope implicit in the field of medical ethics is that we might some day reach a responsible consensus on doctors' obligations. While medicine has dozens of codes, it is not hard to observe commonalities: the standards for informed consent, for example. At a deeper level, there can also be consensus on the justifications for those standards. One role for the philosopher is, as in this essay, to assess carefully the soundness of those arguments. A major task for professions is to move beyond the various personal moralities embraced by practitioners and to reach a responsible consensus on common professional standards.

Personal Values

Values are commonly a part of an explanation of personal conduct. It is always reasonable to ask of any rational action: what good was it intended to promote? While some wear shoes to avoid hurting their feet (embracing the value of comfort), others think they look better in shoes (embracing aesthetic values). Where we have to make personal decisions, often we consider how each option can further or frustrate our values, and try to decide among the good and bad consequences.

This strategy can serve when the question is "What should I do?" But the question "What should a good doctor do?" calls for a different type of inquiry. For while I have many personal values, the "good doctor" is an abstraction. She is neither Protestant nor Buddhist, doesn't prefer chocolate to vanilla, and doesn't care about money more than leisure time. Questions about professional ethics cannot be answered in terms of personal values.

A second difficulty appears when we consider that one can give perfect expression to one's most deeply held personal values and still act unethically. Hannibal Lecter in *Silence of the Lambs* and Mozart's Don Giovanni are despicable villains who give vigorous effect to deeply held if contemptible personal values. While personal values can determine action, they do not guarantee that the favored actions are ethical.

Accordingly, we cannot appeal to our personal values to inquire about what physicians in general ought to do. Medicine has no personal values, only individual physicians do. When a physician must decide whether or not to resuscitate a patient, personal values should have nothing to do with the issue. Whether you like the patient or detest him, whether you are an atheist or a fundamentalist believer in a joyous hereafter, should not weigh in the balance. A key part of professionalism involves being able to set personal values aside. While medical students have much to gain by becoming clear about their personal values, that clarity is not the same as responsible certainty about professional obligations.

To summarize the argument so far, discussion about professional obligations in medicine is not the same as discussion about legal and institutional obligations, personal morality or personal values. If a responsible ethical consensus is to be achieved by a profession, it is necessary for physicians to learn to bracket their personal moral and value commitments and to set aside, at least temporarily, their consideration of legal or institutional rules and policies. The practical task is to create an intellectual space within which responsible consensus can be achieved on how physicians, as professionals, ought to act. I will now describe one way in which this might be done.

The Concept of a Professional Obligation

Professional ethics involves disciplined discussion about the obligations of professionals. One place to begin is with a distinction between personal values, already discussed, and what can be called "core professional values." A physician can prefer (1) pistachios to Brazil nuts, and (2) confidentiality to universal candor. While the preference for pistachios is merely personal, the preference for confidentiality is a value all doctors ought to possess. The distinction between personal values and "core professional values" is critical here. There is what this flesh-and-blood doctor happens to care about personally, and what the good doctor ought to care about. This idea of a "good doctor" is a social construction, an aspect of a determinate social role, an integral element of medical professionalism. Our idea of a good doctor includes a certain technical/intellectual mastery coupled with a certain commitment to specific professional values. As with the Jehovah's Witness doctor, personal and professional values may be in conflict. As part of an appreciation of the ethical claims of professionalism, physicians must be prepared to set aside their personal values and morality, to set aside what the legal system and their employers want them to care about, and to take up instead the question of what the responsible physician ought to care about. The profession's core values inform those purposes that each medical professional should have in common with colleagues. In discussing the professionally favored resolution of ethically problematic cases (the *Case of the Infected Spouse*, for example) physicians can ask—together—how medicine's core professional values ought to be respected in those circumstances.

We have alluded to some of these core professional values. Trustworthiness needs to be on the list. Beneficence toward the patient's health needs is essential. Respect for patient autonomy is a third. Others might be collegiality (duties to colleagues), and perhaps a few others: nondiscrimination and a certain deference to families are among the most commonly mentioned candidates. If we were to leave out that doctors should care about the well-being of the public, the argument for confidentiality would be easy. But it too properly goes on the list. Anyone seeing no point in furthering and securing these values would be ill-suited for the practice of medicine.

Each of these professional values has two dimensions. Along one vector, they define the shared aspiration of a profession. At any time, medicine's ability to benefit patients will be limited. But it is a part of the profession's commitment to push its envelope, to enlarge its collective competency and draw upon its knowledge and skill. Those who master and extend the profession's broadest capabilities are exemplary contributors, but practitioners do not discredit themselves by failing to serve in this estimable way.

Along the second vector, values define a bottom line beneath which practitioners shall not sink. Paraphrasing Hippocrates, although you may not always be able to benefit your patients, it is far more important that you take care not to harm them. Knowingly to harm a patient (on balance) is not merely a failure to realize the value of beneficence. It is a culpable betrayal of that value, a far more serious matter.

All the values above can be understood in this second way. Trustworthiness entails that I not lie to patients, or deliberately withhold information they have an interest in knowing. Respect for patient autonomy can require that I not use force or fraud upon them. And the concern for the well-being of the public requires that that interest somehow appear prominently upon every practitioner's radar screen, that doctors not stand idly by in the face of perils the profession can help to avert and, as a lower limit, that they not do anything to increase public peril. Consider that the overutilization of antibiotics, resulting in drug-resistant infectious agents, is professional misconduct that increases public peril.

Ethical problems can arise, first, when core values appear to be in conflict, as with the *Case of the Infected Spouse*. At issue are trustworthiness toward Andrew on one side, and beneficence toward Wilma and a concern for the well-being of the public on the other. If the conflict is real, what is required is a priority rule. For example, the concept of decisional capacity is part of a priority rule resolving the well-studied conflict between beneficence and autonomy: when do physicians have to respect a patient's refusal of life-saving treatment? There is what the patient wants and what the patient needs. But when a patient is decisionally capacitated and informed, his or her refusal trumps the doctor's recommendation.

Second, ethical problems can also arise when it is unclear what some core professional value requires one to do. Though we can all agree that doctors should avoid harming their patients, there is no professional consensus on whether deliberately causing the deaths of certain unfortunate patients—those experiencing irremediable and intense suffering—is always a betrayal of beneficence. Likewise, although doctors may be in a position to prevent harm to third parties, it is not well understood what they must do out of respect for that value. When core values conflict, what is required is a priority rule. When they are unclear, what is required is removal of ambiguity: what philosophers call "disambiguation." These two tasks—prioritizing and disambiguating core professional values—need to be carried out with a high degree of intellectual responsibility.

The above list of medicine's core values is not controversial. Propose a toast to them at an assemblage of physicians and all can likely drink with enthusiasm. What is less clear is why such a consensus should obligate professionals. A criminal organization can celebrate its shared commitment to the oath of silence. But it doesn't follow that those who cooperate with the police are unethical. In addition to organizational "celebratability," three additional elements are required to establish a professional obligation.

The first element is that attention to core values has to be a part of professional education. Most medical education is aimed ·at beneficence. The procedures used in informed consent express a commitment of respect for patient autonomy and trustworthiness. If the profession wholly fails to equip its novices to further its core values, it can be argued that it is not serious about those professed values. Its public commitments will begin to look like they are intended to convey an illusion of concerned attention. In replicating itself, a profession must replicate its commitment. Students of medicine must come to care about the goods that doctors ought to care about. Because justice is rarely explored as a topic in medical education, I do not think it can be counted as a core professional value. However some parts of justice—nondiscrimination, for example—are routinely covered.

The second element is critical. The core values are not just goods that doctors care about and that doctors want other doctors to care about. They are also goods that the rest of us want our doctors to care about. I want my doctor to be trustworthy, to be intent on benefiting my health, to take my informed refusals seriously, and so on. And we want our doctors to look out for the well-being of the public. The core professional values are also social values. (Consider that it is not reasonable to want our mobsters to respect their oaths of silence.)

The third element flows from the second: an exclusive social reliance upon the profession as the means by which certain matters are to receive due attention. We mostly respect medical competence.

But it is precisely because, as a community, we have also come to accept that doctors are reliably committed to their values (our values), that we have, through state legislatures, granted the medical profession an exclusive monopoly on the delivery of medical services. The unauthorized practice of medicine is a punishable crime. If, like the medical profession, one were to make a public claim that, because of unique skills and dedication, some important social concern ought to be exclusively entrusted to you, and the public believes you and entrusts those important matters to you, incidentally prohibiting all others from encroachment upon what is now your privilege, you would have thereby assumed an ethical obligation to give those important matters due attention. Collectively, the medical profession has done exactly this in securing its monopoly on the delivery of certain types of health care. Accordingly the profession has a collective obligation to organize itself so that the shared responsibilities it has assumed in the political process of professionalization are properly discharged by its membership.

A sound code of ethics consists of a set of standards that, if adhered to broadly by the profession's membership, will result in the profession as a whole discharging its responsibilities. Where physician behavior brings about a public loss of that essential trust, society may have to withdraw the monopolistic privilege and seek a better way of organizing health care. Professionalization is but one way of organizing an essential service. There are others.

In summary, the medical profession has ethical obligations toward patients, families, and the community because of its public commitment to secure and further certain critical social values and because of society's exclusive reliance on the profession as its means of delivering certain forms of health care. With the professional privilege comes a reciprocal collective responsibility (Kipnis 1986, 1-14). We can now turn our attention to medicine's responsibility to diminish public perils.

The Duty to Diminish Risks to Third Parties

There is an implication for the way in which we must now understand the problem in the *Case of the*

Infected Spouse. The opening question "Do you take steps to warn Wilma?" has to be understood as a question about medical ethics and not about "you." We want to know what the "good doctor" should do under those circumstance? Each doctor is ethically required to do what a responsible doctor ought to do: in order to properly respect the core values of the profession. To become a doctor without a proper commitment to respect the profession's values is to be unfit for the practice of medicine. So how are trustworthiness and confidentiality to be understood in relationship to medicine's commitment to diminish risks to third parties?

In the *Case of the Infected Spouse* the ethical question is posed in 1991, after the doctor-family relationship has been in place for a decade. The dilemma arises during and immediately after a single office visit, forcing a choice between calling Wilma either you will have to explain to Andrew, in two days, why you disclosed his infection to his wife, or you will have to explain to Wilma, in two years, why you did not disclose his infection to her [sic]. Each option has a bad outcome: the betrayal of Andrew's trust or the fatal infection of Wilma. Either way, you will need to account for yourself.

Infection seems a far worse consequence for Wilma than betrayal is for Andrew. Much of the literature on confidentiality has been shaped by this fact, and perhaps the standard strategy for resolving the problem calls attention to the magnitude and probability of the bad outcomes associated with each option. While predictions of harm can sometimes be wrong, it can be evident that Tatiana Tarasoff and Wilma Long are at grave risk and, accordingly, it can seem honorable to diminish the danger to vulnerable parties like them. Justice Tobriner appeals to a version of this consequentialist argument in *Tarasoff*:

Weighing the uncertain and conjectural character of the alleged damage done the patient by such a warning against the peril to the victim's life, we conclude that professional inaccuracy in predicting violence [or deadly infection] cannot negate the therapist's duty to protect the threatened victim.

Beauchamp and Childress, in their widely read *Principles of Biomedical Ethics* (2001, 309), urge clinicians to take into account "the probability that a harm will materialize and the magnitude of that harm" in any decision to breach confidentiality. (While they also urge that clinicians take into account the potential impact of disclosure on policies and laws regarding confidentiality, they are not very clear about how this assessment is to be carried out.) In brief, the very bad consequences of not disclosing risk to Wilma—disease and death and the betrayal of her trust—outweigh the not-all-that-bad consequence of breached confidentiality to Andrew. Your explanation to Andrew could cover those points.

The preferred argument would go something like this: The state's interest in preventing harm is weighty. Medicine has an obligation to protect the well-being of the community. Because the seriousness of threatened grave injury to another outweighs the damage done to a patient by breaching confidentiality, the obligation of confidentiality must give way to a duty to prevent serious harm to others. Accordingly, despite confidentiality, warning or reporting is obligatory when it will likely avert very bad outcomes in this way. Of course clinicians should try to obtain waivers of confidentiality before disclosure, thereby avoiding the need to breach a duty. But the failure to obtain a waiver does not, on this argument, affect the overriding obligation to report.

A Defense of Unqualified Confidentiality

As powerful as the above justification is, there are problems with it. Go back to 1990, when Andrew comes in to be tested for sexually transmitted diseases. Suppose he asks: "If I am infected, can I trust you not to disclose this to others?" If, following the arguments set out in the previous paragraphs, we are clear that confidentiality must be breached to protect third parties like Wilma, then the only truthful answer to Andrew's question is "No. You can't trust me." If the profession accepts that its broad promise of confidentiality must sometimes be broken, then any unqualified assurances are fraudulent and the profession should stop making them. If there are exceptions, clinicians have a duty to be forthcoming about what they are and how they work. Patients should know up front when they can trust doctors, and when they can't. To withhold this important information is to betray the value of trustworthiness.

Accordingly, the argument for breaching confidentiality has to be modified to support a qualified confidentiality rule, one that carves out an exception from the very beginning, acknowledging an overriding duty to report under defined circumstances. (In contrast, an unqualified confidentiality rule contemplates no exceptions.) Instead of undertaking duties of confidentiality and then violating them, doctors must qualify their expressed obligations so they will be able to honor them. Commentators who have walked through the issues surrounding confidentiality have long understood the ethical necessity of "Miranda warnings" (Bok 1983; Goldman 1980): A clinician would have to say early on, "Certain things that I learn from you may have to be disclosed to ... under the following circumstances ...; and the following things might occur to you as a result of my disclosure: ..." If doctors are ethically obligated to report, they need to say in advance what will be passed along, when, to whom, and what could happen then. They should never encourage or accept trust only to betray their patients afterwards. To do so is to betray the value of trustworthiness.

But now a second problem emerges. If prospective patients must understand in advance that a doctor will report evidence of a threat to others, they will only be willing to disclose such evidence to the doctor if they are willing to accept that those others will come to know. If it is important to them that the evidence not be reported, they will have a weighty reason not to disclose it to those who are obligated to report it.

Some have questioned this proposition, arguing that there is no empirical evidence that prospective patients will avoid or delay seeking medical attention or conceal medically relevant information if confidentiality is qualified in this way. Despite widespread reporting practices, waiting rooms have not emptied and no one really knows if people stop talking openly to their doctors when confidentiality is breached.

Three responses are possible regarding this claim. First, there is a serious difficulty doing empirical research in this area. How, for example, do we determine the number of abusive parents who have not brought their injured children to doctors out of a fear that they will get into trouble with the authorities?

How many HIV+ patients avoid telling their doctors all about their unsafe sexual practices? How many of us would volunteer unflattering truthful answers to direct questions on these and other shameful matters? It is notoriously difficult to gather reliable data on the embarrassing, criminal, irresponsible things people do, and the steps they take to avoid exposure, especially if those are wrongful too. I don't want to suggest that these problems are insurmountable (Reddy et al. 2002), but they are decidedly there and they often make it hard to study the effects of these betrayals.

Second, despite the problems, certain types of indirect evidence can occasionally emerge. Here are two anecdotal examples from Honolulu. There was a time, not long ago, when military enlistees who were troubled by their sexual orientation knew that military doctors and psychologists would report these problems to their officers. Many of these troubled soldiers therefore obtained the services of private psychologists and psychiatrists in Honolulu, despite the fact that free services were available in military clinics. The second example emerged from the failure of the Japanese medical system to keep diagnoses of HIV infection confidential. Many Japanese who could afford it traveled to Honolulu for diagnosis and treatment, avoiding clinics in Japan. At the same time, Japanese data on the prevalence of HIV infection were unrealistically low, especially considering the popularity of Japanese sex tours to the HIV-infected brothels of Thailand. Evidence of this sort can confirm that the failure to respect confidentiality can impair the ability of doctors to do their job.

And third, there is an argument based on the motivational principle that if one strongly desires that event E does not occur, and one knows that doing act A will bring about event E, then one has a weighty reason not to do act A. The criminal justice system is based on this idea. We attach artificial and broadly unwelcome consequences (imprisonment and other forms of punishment) to wrongful, harmful conduct with the expectation that, even if inclined, most people will decide against the conduct in order to avoid the unwelcome consequence. If I don't want to go to prison, and a career in burglary will likely result in my going to prison, then I have a weighty reason to choose a different career. Likewise, if I don't want my marriage to be destroyed by my wife's discovery that I am HIV+, and I know that telling my doctor about reconciliation will result in her discovering just that, then I have a weighty reason not to tell my doctor. The presumption must be in favor of the truth of this seemingly self-evident principle. If critics allege that it is false or otherwise unworthy of endorsement, it seems the burden of disproof belongs to them. It is their responsibility to come up with disconfirming evidence.

It can be argued, in rebuttal, that people still commit burglary and, despite reporting laws, people still go to doctors for HIV testing, even knowing that confidentiality has its limits. But no one would maintain that punishing convicted criminals totally prevents crime and that breaching confidentiality results in all people avoiding or delaying medical treatment, or concealing aspects of their lives. The situation is more complicated.

Consider that Andrew belongs to one of two groups of prospective patients. Members of the first group are willing enough to have reports made to others. Members of the second are deterred from disclosure by the fear of a report. Of course we can't know in advance which type of patient Andrew is, but if both groups are treated alike, uncertainty will not be a problem. (While this division into two groups may be oversimplified, working through the qualifications would take us too far afield.)

Consider the first group: patients who would be willing to have a report made. Recall that the physician in the Case of the Infected Spouse tried to obtain assurance that Wilma would be protected. Under an unqualified confidentiality rule—no exceptions—if the patient were willing to have reports made to others, the doctor should be able to obtain a waiver of confidentiality and Wilma could then be informed. Once permission to report is given, the ethical dilemma disappears. Notice that for this group of patients an exceptionless confidentiality rule works just as well as a rule requiring doctors to override confidentiality when necessary to protect endangered third parties. At-risk parties will be warned just the same, but with appropriate permission from patients. In these cases there is no need to trim back the obligation of confidentiality since patients in this first group are, by definition, willing to have a report made.

Difficulties arise with the second type of patient: those who will not want credible threats reported. Notice that these prospective patients are in control of the evidence doctors need to secure protection for parties at risk. If a patient cannot be drawn into a therapeutic alliance—a relationship of trust and confidence—then doctors will not receive the information they need to protect imperiled third parties (at least so long as patients have options). As a result, doctors will not be able to mobilize protection. When one traces out the implications of a reporting rule on what needs to be said in 1990 (when Andrew asked to be tested and the doctor disclosed the limits to confidentiality), it becomes evident that Wilma will not be protected if Andrew (a) does not want her to know, and (b) understands that disclosure to his doctor will result in her knowing. Depending on his options and the strength of his preferences, he will be careful about what he discloses to his doctor, or will go without medical advice and care, or will find another physician who can be kept in ignorance about his personal life.

We began by characterizing the Case of the Infected Spouse as an apparent head-on collision between the doctor's duty of confidentiality and the duty to protect imperiled third parties. But if the argument above is sound, there is no collision. The obligation to warn third parties does not provide added protection to those at-risk. In particular, a no-exceptions confidentiality rule has a better chance of getting the facts on the table, at least to the extent that honest promises of confidentiality can make it so. To be sure, clinicians would have to set aside the vexing "Should I report?" conundrum and search for creative solutions instead. These strategies will not always prevent harm, but they will sometimes. The nub of the matter is that these strategies can never work if they can't be implemented. And they can't be implemented if the fear of reporting deters patients from disclosure. Accordingly there is no justification for trimming back the obligation of confidentiality since doing so actually reduces protection to endangered third parties, increasing public peril.

The argument advanced here is that—paradoxically—ethical and legal duties to report make it less likely that endangered parties will be protected. Depending on the prospective patient, these duties are either unnecessary (when waivers can be obtained) or counterproductive (when disclosure to the doctor is deterred and interventions other than disclosure are prevented).

In part, the conventional wisdom on confidentiality errs in focusing on the decision of the individual clinician at the point when the choice has to be made to disclose or not. The decision to violate confidentiality reaches backwards to the HIV test administered years earlier and, as we shall see, even before. Perhaps little will be lost if one doctor betrays a single patient one time, or if betrayals are extremely rare. But medical ethics is not about a single decision by an individual clinician. The consequences and implications of a rule governing professional practice may be quite different from those of a single act. Better to ask, what if every doctor did that?

While it is accepted here that doctors have an overriding obligation to prevent public peril, it has been argued that they do not honor that obligation by breaching or chipping away at confidentiality. This is because the protective purpose to be furthered by reporting is defeated by the practice of reporting. The best public protection is achieved where doctors do their best work and, there, trustworthiness is probably the most important prerequisite. Physicians damage both their professional capabilities and their communities when they compromise their trustworthiness.

If the argument above is sound and confidentiality must be respected in this case, we must now return to the question of what the doctor must say to Wilma when, now infected, she returns to the office two years after the reconciliation. Though this question has finally to be faced in 1993, it is on the table before her return to Honolulu. It is there even before Andrew asks to be tested in 1990, and you then have to decide whether to live out the trust he has placed in you or disabuse him of it. In fact, the problem is on the table in 1982, when the couple first enters your office and asks you to be their physician. As a doctor, you have obligations of beneficence and confidentiality and you owe both to each. But now—having read this far—you are aware that something can happen that you cannot control; and, if it does happen, you will face those apparently conflicting

obligations. You can only provide what you owe to one if you betray your obligation to the other. That is the choice you will have to make in 1993, unless you (and the medical profession) contour professional responsibilities now.

If, in choosing a governing ethical principle, the end-in-view is to protect vulnerable third parties; and if this can be done best, as I have tried to show, by honoring confidentiality and doing one's best to protect imperiled third parties within that framework; then what you must say to both Wilma and Andrew, when they enter your office in 1982, should be something like this:

There is an ethical problem physicians sometimes face in taking on a married couple as patients. It can happen that one partner becomes infected with a transmissible disease, potentially endangering the other. If the infected partner won't share information with me because he or she fears I will warn the other, there will be no protection at all for the partner at risk. There may, however, be things I can do if I can talk with the infected partner. What I promise both of you is, if that were to happen, I will do everything I possibly can 'to protect the endangered partner, except for violating confidentiality, which I will not do. You both need to remember that you should not count on me to guarantee the wholesomeness of your spouse, if doing this means betrayal.

It is in these words that the final explanation to Wilma can be found. If Wilma understands from the beginning that medical confidentiality will not be breached; if she (and the public generally) understand that the precariously placed are safer under unqualified confidentiality, she will understand she has final responsibility for her choices. If you are clear enough about it, she will grasp that she can't depend on you to protect her at the cost of betrayal, and that she is better off because of that. Both the doctor and the medical profession collectively need to work through these issues and fully disclose the favored standard to prospective patients before the occasion arises when a doctor must appeal to it. The view defended here is that the profession should continue to make an unqualified pledge of confidentiality, and mean it.

It is also appropriate to consider what should be said to Andrew as he is about to leave your office in

1991 to prepare for a romantic dinner with Wilma. I once spent part of an afternoon with a health care professional who had served in Vietnam. He had counseled married enlistees who had returned from visits with their wives and had been diagnosed with a venereal disease that was probably contracted before they left Vietnam. It is likely that these men may have infected their wives. This clinician had learned how to persuade these men to agree to disclosure. He stressed that their wives would likely find out eventually and that the emotional and medical consequences would be far more severe because of the delay. More importantly—given the soldiers' tentative decisions not to let their at-risk spouses know—he would ask whether this was a marriage they really wanted to preserve? I recall that he claimed a near perfect record in obtaining permission to notify the at-risk spouses. It would be useful if there were skilled allied caregivers, bound by confidentiality, who could routinely conduct these specialized counseling sessions. While this is not the place to set out the full range of options for a profession reliably committed to trustworthiness, it will suffice to point out a direction for professional and institutional development.

Concluding Remarks

Even if the forgoing is accepted, what may trouble doctors still is a fear that they will learn about an endangered person and be barred by this no-exceptions confidentiality rule from doing anything. Actually, there is only one thing they cannot do: disclose. All other paths remain open. Even if a reporting rule keeps many prospective patients out of the office, or silences them while they are there, the rule protects doctors from the moral risk of having to allow injury to third parties when a simple disclosure would prevent it. This distress is significant and has to be faced.

Here we must return to an error discussed earlier: the conflation of personal morality and professional ethics. Like law, personal morality can also conflict with professional responsibility. We considered a Jehovah's Witness surgeon, morally prohibited from administering blood transfusions to patients needing

them. Likewise a Catholic doctor may be unable to discuss certain reproduction-related options. And despite understandable moral misgivings, doctors everywhere must be prepared to administer high-risk treatments they know will cause the deaths of some of their patients. Paradoxically, a personal inability to risk killing patients can disqualify one for the practice of medicine. While personal morality can play a decisive role in career choice, it shouldn't play a decisive role within medical ethics.

Many enter medicine believing that good citizens must prevent serious injury to others, even if that means violating other obligations. But the task of professional ethics in medicine is to set out principles that, if broadly followed, will allow the profession to discharge its collective responsibilities to patients and society. Confidentiality, I have argued, is effective at getting more patients into therapeutic alliances more quickly, it is more effective in bringing about better outcomes for more of them and—counter-intuitively—it is most likely to prevent serious harm to the largest number of at-risk third parties. Now it is ethically praiseworthy for honorable people to belong to a profession that, on balance, diminishes the amount of harm to others, even though these same professionals must sometimes knowingly allow (and sometimes even cause) harm to occur. Although doctors may feel guilty about these foreseeable consequences of their actions and inactions, they are not guilty of anything. They are acting exactly as it is reasonable to want doctors to act.

It is hard enough to create therapeutic alliances that meet patients' needs. But if doctors take on the added duty to mobilize protective responses without waivers of confidentiality, their work may become impossible in too many important cases. And all of us will be the worse for that. The thinking that places the moral comfort of clinicians above the well-being of patients and their victims is in conflict with the requirements of professional responsibility, properly understood. While it will be a challenge for many honorable physicians to measure up to this standard, no one ever said it was easy to be a good doctor.

Note

1 A longer version of this article will appear as "Medical Confidentiality" in *The Blackwell Guide to Bioethics*, ed. R. Rhodes et al. Oxford, UK: Blackwell, 2006. [Editorial note: this article did not appear.]

References

Beauchamp, T.L., and J.F. Childress. 2001. *Principles of Biomedical Ethics*. New York: Oxford University Press.

Bok, S. 1983. *Secrets*. New York: Pantheon Books.

Goldman, A. 1980. *The Philosophical Foundations of Professional Ethics*. Totowa, NJ: Rowman & Littlefield.

Kipnis, K. 1986. *Legal Ethics*. Englewood Cliffs, NJ: Prentice-Hall.

——. 2004. "Gender, sex, and professional ethics in child and adolescent psychiatry." *Child and Adolescent Psychiatric Clinics of North America* 13(3): 695-708.

Kottow, M. 1986. "Medical confidentiality: An intransigent and absolute obligation." *Journal of Medical Ethics* 12: 117-22.

Lo, B. 1995. *Resolving Ethical Dilemmas: A Guide for Clinicians*. Baltimore: Williams and Wilkins.

Reddy, D.M., R. Fleming, and C. Swain. 2002. "Effect of mandatory parental notification on adolescent girls' use of sexual health care services." *Journal of the American Medical Association* 288: 710-14.

Wicclair, M. 1987. "A shield right for reporters vs. the administration of justice and the right to a fair trial: Is there a conflict?" *Business & Professional Ethics Journal* 4(2): 1-14.

6.
SMITH V. JONES [1999] SUPREME COURT OF CANADA

Case Summary by C. Morano

SOURCE: http://scc.lexum.org/en/1999/1999scr1-455/1999scr1-455.html.

[Smith v. Jones is a Supreme Court of Canada decision that focuses on the principle of confidentiality and the public interest. In this case it was determined that the solicitor-client privilege is not absolute but rather subject to exceptions—in this case, the public safety exception.]

Present: Lamer C.J. and L'Heureux-Dubé, Gonthier, Cory, McLachlin, Iacobucci, Major, Bastarache and Binnie JJ.

On appeal from the court of appeal for British Columbia.

Background

Jones was charged with aggravated sexual assault on a prostitute. In the preparation of his client's defence, Jones's lawyer referred him to a psychiatrist, so that even a guilty plea would work in Jones's favour with respect to sentencing. Throughout his sessions with the psychiatrist, Jones described in detail his plan to kidnap, kill, and rape prostitutes. The psychiatrist believed that the accused was dangerous and in need of treatment to prevent him from committing offences of a similar nature in the future. The psychiatrist contacted the defence counsel and found out that his concerns about the accused would not be addressed in the sentencing hearing. As a result, the psychiatrist filed for a declaration that he was entitled to disclose information that was in the interest of public safety.

The trial judge ruled that the public safety exception to the solicitor-client privilege and doctor-patient confidentiality released the psychiatrist from his duties of confidentiality and concluded that the psychiatrist was under a *duty* to disclose to the police

and Crown both the statements made by the accused and the psychiatrist's opinion of them. The Court of Appeal allowed Jones's appeal and changed the order from the psychiatrist being under a *duty* to disclose the statements to one of *permitting* the psychiatrist to disclose the information. Jones appealed the decision of the Court of Appeal.

The Supreme Court of Canada

A majority of the Supreme Court dismissed Jones's appeal and affirmed the order of the Court of Appeal. Speaking on behalf of the majority, Cory J. concluded that "[T]he file will be unsealed and the ban on the publication of the contents of the file is removed, except for those parts of the psychiatrist's affidavit that do not fall within the public safety exception." He said that the solicitor-client privilege is a principle of fundamental importance, but it is not absolute and it is subject to exceptions, including the public safety exception. He continued: "[W]hile only a compelling public interest can justify setting aside solicitor-client privilege, danger to public safety can, in appropriate circumstances, provide such a justification." The majority set out three factors that should be considered when determining whether the solicitor-client privilege should be breached: 1) Is there a clear risk to an identifiable person or group? It is important that such a group or person must always be ascertainable. 2) Is there a risk of serious bodily harm or death? 3) Is the danger imminent? These factors must be defined in the context of each situation and different weights will be given to each, and to the various aspects of each, in any particular case. The Supreme Court's decision did not clarify whether the duty to warn was mandatory or discretionary.

7.
SHOULD JOURNALS PUBLISH
INDUSTRY-FUNDED BIOETHICS ARTICLES?

Carl Elliott

SOURCE: *The Lancet* 366.9483 (2005): 422-24.

North American bioethics has a growing credibility problem. As the influence of bioethics has grown, so has the willingness of bioethicists to seek out funding from the pharmaceutical and biotechnology industries. These industries have begun to fund bioethics centres, lectureships, consultants, advisory panels, conferences, and private regulatory boards.[1-3] The results of this industry-funded work are now making their way into peer-reviewed academic journals. Readers of the medical and bioethics literature have recently seen articles on the ethics of recruiting homeless individuals for research, funded by Eli Lilly;[4] on the ethics of biotechnology and the developing world, funded by Glaxo, Merck, and Pfizer;[5] on the ethics of stem-cell research, funded by Geron;[6] and the ethics of placebo-controlled trials for mood-altering drugs, funded by antidepressant manufacturers.[7] They have also seen pharma-funded university bioethicists collaborating on ethics articles with biotech entrepreneurs[8] and a medical ethics and humanities journal issue funded by a pharmaceutical lobbying organisation.[9] The authors of these articles have disclosed their industry ties, but readers are left to wonder: is an industry-funded bioethicist a bioethicist that we can trust?

Even discussions of conflict of interest have become tainted by questions of conflict of interest— or at least the perception of a potential conflict. The American Journal of Bioethics recently published an article on the ethics of taking gifts from the pharmaceutical industry which was itself funded by Pfizer, while the American Medical Association's Council on Ethics and Judicial Affairs launched an educational project on industry gifts that was funded by a US$675,000 gift from the pharmaceutical industry.[10,11] When the US National Institute of Health (NIH) commissioned a so-called blue-ribbon panel to investigate their conflict-of-interest scandal, in which researchers were found to have undisclosed financial ties to private industry, the blue-ribbon panel included an insurance executive, the vice-president of a for-profit health-care company, the chief executive officer of a leading weapons manufacturer, and the director of the Ethics Resource Center, Washington DC, an ethics institute funded by Merck.[12] One can see the reasoning behind appointing these panellists, but they are hardly likely to inspire trust in observers worried that the NIH has become too close to private industry.

Many North American bioethicists have been reluctant to admit that industry funding is an ethical problem. Three years ago, a task force on bioethics consultation for industry commissioned by the two major US bioethics associations published its recommendations in The Hastings Center Report.[13] The task force found no ethical barrier to industry-funded bioethics consultation, and went on to endorse bioethics advertising (eight of its ten members had done industry-funded work themselves). Similarly, the editors of Theoretical Medicine and Bioethics have argued that financial disclosure in bioethics is positively harmful, because it encourages readers to judge an article by its funding rather than by its merits.[14]

Yet industry funding will surely lead readers to question the impartiality of bioethics as a discipline. And so it should. The pharmaceutical and biotechnology industry has a clear interest in the work that bioethicists do. Bioethicists write scholarly articles about the actions and policies of industry. They lecture on issues of concern to industry at conferences and in university classrooms. They serve on regulatory committees, governmental task forces, and professional bodies. Many offer comments on ethical controversies in the popular press. Bioethicists help write the policies that govern the ethics of medical research, and they sit on the institutional review boards and research ethics committees that decide which research protocols can go forward. It should be no surprise that the pharmaceutical industry is eager to influence them.

Public relations experts clearly understand the advantages of using academic experts to advance a cause. Some companies pay academics to promote their points of view on television, in newspapers and magazines, in academic journals, and in letters to editors.[15] In one case, a Washington speaker's bureau and a public relations firm were found to be recruiting academic experts to attack Eliot Spitzer, the crusading attorney-general for New York who has launched high-profile investigations of the pharmaceutical and insurance industries.[16] In the early 1990s, a tobacco company paid a statistician $10,000 to write one letter to the Journal of the American Medical Association.[17]

Some critics of industry-funded bioethics have argued that the remedy is full disclosure. But disclosure is unlikely to solve the problem. In science, in which far more attention has been paid to issues of conflict of interest, a study[18] found that only 0.5% of over 60,000 published articles included any disclosure of competing financial interests. At the time, it was estimated that about a quarter of researchers actually had industry funding. Those articles were published in science and medical journals with clear guidelines on conflict of interest. Most bioethics journals do not even ask authors to disclose their funding sources. A survey by the Center for Science in the Public Interest in 2002 found that only two of 53 bioethics journals had published guidelines requiring authors to disclose potential conflicts of interest.[19] Even that small number represents an improvement over academic book publishers, who typically have no conflict-of-interest guidelines whatsoever.

Nor have disclosure policies eliminated the problem of bias. In medicine, industry-funded research produces findings that are more favourable to industry than research funded by other sources.[20] Clini-cians who accept gifts and honoraria from industry are more likely to prescribe drugs from that particular industry and more likely to request that those drugs be added to their hospital's formulary, even when they do not themselves believe they have been influenced.[21] It would be very surprising if industry funding, even if disclosed, did not also influence what bioethicists publish.

Disclosure policies raise a red flag and should be retained, but they do nothing to eliminate the real problem of industry funding, which is not secrecy but influence-peddling. The pharmaceutical industry is arguably the most profitable and politically influential industry in the USA.[22] It now funds about 60% of all Americans continuing medical education.[23,24] A large health-care public-relations industry, funded largely by pharmaceutical companies, routinely commissions journalists to cover conferences in which their products are being discussed, distributes copies of favourable journal articles to practitioners and to the press, sponsors disease-awareness campaigns, funds disease-advocacy groups, and commissions key-opinion leaders to present papers at conferences and lectures.[25-27] If bioethics scholarship is to retain any measure of independence and credibility, it will need to take much stronger measures.

Newspapers have understood this for years. Financial columnists are not allowed to accept money from the companies they write about, and film critics are not allowed to accept money from the studios producing the films they review. This standard may well be honoured less in the observation than in the breach, but in principle, it is a standard worth emulating. The Washington Post, for example, states in its ethics code: "We pay our own way. We accept no gifts from news sources. We accept no free trips. We neither seek nor accept preferential treatment that might be rendered because of the positions we hold."[28]

The editors of medical and bioethics journals should adopt a similar policy. If an editorialist writing on ethics or health policy has a financial interest in the topic on which he or she is writing, the journal should not publish the article. Such a policy would prohibit articles on the ethics of antidepressant use funded by antidepressant manufacturers, articles on the ethics of stem-cell research funded by biotechnology companies working on stem cells, and articles on the ethics of genetically modified crops funded by agribusiness. Such a policy would be similar to the one adopted for several years by The New England Journal of Medicine, which stipulated that authors of editorials and review articles (as opposed to scientific reports) "will not have any financial interest in a company (or its competitor) that makes a product discussed in the editorial."[29,30]

The details of such a policy would also need to be worked out carefully. For example, editors would need to decide just how close a tie to industry should be sufficient to trigger the policy. Almost all universities have some ties to industry, but in most cases those ties have little to do with the funding of a bioethics centre or department. These arrangements are clearly not as worrisome as, for example, a bioethics centre directly funded by industry, or one whose faculty members generate their own salaries with grants from industry. Editors would also need to decide what kinds of articles should be prohibited and what kind should merely require disclosure of a financial interest. Journals that are reluctant to prohibit such articles entirely might decide to reserve a special, visibly marked place in the journal for industry viewpoints.

Of course, such a policy would not solve all the problems of industry funding. Bioethicists would still be free to publish their opinions in books, the popular press, and non-peer-reviewed intellectual magazines. But the symbolic effect of such a policy would be very powerful indeed. Bioethicists would be faced with a choice: either forego industry funding, or forego writing scholarly articles about the practices of their funders.

References

1   Elliott C. Pharma buys a conscience. *Am Prospect* 2001; 12: 16.

2   Stolberg S. Bioethicists find themselves the ones being scrutinized. *NY Times* (New York), Aug 2, 2001: A1.

3   Lemmens T, Freedman B. Ethics review for sale? Conflict of interest and commercial research review boards. *Milbank Q* 2000; 78: 547-84.

4   Beauchamp TL, Jennings B, Kinney ED, Levine RJ. Pharmaceutical research involving the homeless. *J Med Philos* 2002; 27: 547-64.

5   Singer PA, Daar AS. Harnessing genomics and biotechnology to improve global health equity. *Science* 2001; 294: 87-89.

6   Mendiola MM, Peters T, Young EW, Zoloth-Dorfman L. Research with human embryonic stem cells: ethical considerations. By Geron Ethics Advisory Board. *Hastings Cent Rep* 1999; 29: 31-36.

7   Charney DS, Nemeroff CB, Lewis L, et al. National Depressive and Manic-Depressive Association consensus statement on the use of placebo in clinical trials of mood disorders. *Arch Gen Psychiatry* 2002; 59: 262-70.

8   Lanza RP, Caplan AL, Silver LM, Cibelli JB, West MD, Green RM. The ethical validity of using nuclear transfer in human transplantation. *JAMA* 2000; 284: 3175-79.

9   *Perspect Biol Med* 2005; 48: (suppl 1).

10   Katz D, Caplan AL, Merz JF. All gifts large and small: toward an understanding of the ethics of pharmaceutical industry gift-giving. *Am J Bioeth* 2003; 3: 39-46.

11   Okie S. AMA criticized for letting drug firms pay for ethics campaign. *Washington Post* (Washington, DC), Aug 30, 2001: A03.

12   Working group of the Advisory Commitee to the Director. Report of the National Institutes of Health Blue Ribbon Panel on Conflict of Interest Policies. http://www.nih.gov/about/ethics_COI_ panelreport.pdf (accessed April 26, 2005). http://www.thelancet.com Published online July 7, 2005 DOI:10.1016/S0140-6736(05)66794-3.

13   Brody B, Dubler N, Blustein J, et al. Bioethics consultation in the private sector. *Hastings Cent Rep* 2002; 32: 14-20.

14   Jansen LA, Sulmasy DP. Bioethics, conflicts of interest and the limits of transparency. *Hastings Cent Rep* 2003; 33: 40-43.

15   Schroeder M. Some professors take payments to express views. *Wall Street Journal* (New York), Dec 10, 2004: B1.

16   Weil J. Insurance hazard: booking agency sought speakers to criticize Spitzer. *Wall Street Journal* (New York), Oct 29, 2004: C3.

17   Hanners D. Documents indicate tobacco industry

paid scientists to write to editors. MN, USA: *St Paul Pioneer Press*, Aug 5, 1998.

18 Krimsky S, Rothenberg LS. Conflict of interest policies in science and medical journals: editorial practices and author disclosures. *Sci Eng Ethics* 2001; 7: 205-18.

19 Center for Science in the Public Interest. CSPI calls for prevention and disclosure of conflicts of interest in bioethics. http://www.cspinet.org/new/bioethics _061102.html (accessed April 26, 2005).

20 Als-Nielsen B, Chen W, Gluud C, Kjaergard LL. Association of funding and conclusions in randomized drug trials: a reflection of treatment effect or adverse events? *JAMA* 2003; 290: 921-28.

21 Chren MM, Landefeld CS. Physicians' behavior and their interactions with drug companies. A controlled study of physicians who requested additions to a hospital drug formulary. *JAMA* 1994; 271: 684-89.

22 Angell M. The truth about the drug companies. New York: Random House, 2004.

23 Hensley S. Drug firms shown classroom door—continuing-ed programs for doctors aim to reduce influence of big companies. *Wall Street Journal* (New York), Jan 14, 2003: D5.

24 Moynihan R. Drug company sponsorship of education could be replaced at a fraction of its cost. *BMJ* 2003; 326: 1163.

25 Burton B, Rowell A. Unhealthy spin. *BMJ* 2003; 326: 1205-07.

26 Payer L. Disease-mongers: how doctors, drug companies, and insurers are making you feel sick. New York: J Wiley, 1992.

27 Relman A. Separating continuing medical education from pharmaceutical marketing. *JAMA* 2001; 285: 2009-12.

28 *The Washington Post*. Washington Post Standards and Ethics. http://www.asne.org/ideas/codes/washington post.htm (accessed April 26, 2005).

29 Drazen J, Curfman G. Financial associations of authors. *N Engl J Med* 2002; 346: 1901-02.

30 Kassirer J. On the take. New York: Oxford University Press, 2004. http://www.thelancet.com Published online July 7, 2005 DOI:10.1016/S0140-6736(05) 66794-3.

CHAPTER TWO

HEALTH CARE
IN CANADA

Web Links

Chapter Two focuses on the social context of health care delivery in Canada, its underlying values, and the challenges to improving Canadian health care. The first two links direct you to the Public Health Agency of Canada website, where you will find a list of the factors that determine health and health care delivery in Canada, some of which are income, social status, gender, education, employment security, and physical environment.

The third link is to the Report authored by Roy Romanow, which focuses on the current challenges to the quality and sustainability of Canadian health care, and how to address those challenges in the future, while considering the values that underlie the system.

(1) Link to the Public Health Agency of Canada, "What Determines Health?"

   http://www.phac-aspc.gc.ca/ph-sp/determinants/index-eng.php

(2) "The Social Determinants of Health: An Overview of the Implications for Policy and the Role of the Health Sector," Public Health Agency of Canada, 22 March 2004.

   http://www.phac-aspc.gc.ca/ph-sp/oi-ar/pdf/01_overview_e.pdf

(3) Link to the Roy Romanow Report, "Building on Values: The Future of Health Care in Canada."

   http://publications.gc.ca/collections/Collection/CP32-85-2002E.pdf

* For an up-to-date list of the web links in this book, please visit:
http://sites.broadviewpress.com/healthcare.

8.
EQUALITY AND EFFICIENCY AS BASIC SOCIAL VALUES

Michael Stingl

SOURCE: Michael Stingl (ed.), *Efficiency versus Equality* (Halifax: Fernwood, 1996).

Social Values and Political Choices

Equality and efficiency are two key terms in the growing national debate over reforming the Canadian health system. Both are widely understood to refer to values basic in the structure and identity of Canadian society. But this is true only on a loose understanding of both terms; in the debate over health reform, both terms mean different things to different people. As long as equality and efficiency remain widely but only loosely understood, the likelihood increases that this debate will become politically intractable and socially divisive.

In this paper, I examine some of the different things that those participating in the debate often mean by equality and efficiency. Taking stock of these different meanings, I distinguish several points of potential reform where we can expect the two values to coincide, as well as several where we can expect them to collide. It is this latter possibility, of course, that is the more ethically interesting and troubling: the fact that in reforming the health system, having more of the one value will sometimes mean having less of the other.

Basic social values guide public policy, and more generally, determine the conditions and limits of social interaction between individuals, groups, and institutions within Canada. They provide the shared social framework within which each of us defines his or her own life. When such values collide, we are individually and collectively faced with a social choice. On the one hand, we might allow our social values to shift in ways that, at least on the surface, avoid conflict; on the other hand, we might simply accept the fact that social values will sometimes collide, and when this happens, face the difficult choice of which value ought to give way to which. In either case, we need to be clear about who the "we" is that is determining the course of social change. Choices regarding basic social values must not be hidden away within governmental bureaucracies, but debated publicly and openly within the larger political context of Canadian society as a whole. In a modern liberal society, determining the basic conditions of our social network with one another is an important right and an important responsibility, for again, basic social values not only determine the structure and identity of Canadian society, but as well, the structure and identity of our lives as individual Canadians.

Determining which basic social value should give way to which is thus a political choice in the broadest sense of the term. What is required to make such choices is public debate and government action. And this is what we are now seeing in varying degrees across Canada: public debate about the importance and possible limits of the Canadian health system and Canadian social services more generally, and government initiatives to make these services more responsive to deficit and debt as well as the needs of all Canadians. To evaluate these initiatives, and to make the social choices they represent wisely, we need a clear public understanding of what the terms equality and efficiency really mean.

Two Different Meanings of Equality

In the debate over health reform it is necessary to distinguish between two very different ways of thinking about human society. On the one hand, we might see society as providing nothing more than the institutional framework necessary for humans to organize the individual pursuit of their own separate ends, as they personally choose to define them. On this picture of society, it is the individual who is of fundamental value; society exists only as a set of formalized arrangements to better enable each individual to pursue his or her own personal good. This is the libertarian view of society.

On the other hand, we might see society as a joint, cooperative venture, participation in which creates the sense of a greater, social good that grounds and gives context to everyone's own personal good. On this second picture of human society individuals will still be fundamentally important, but so too will society. Personal goods may be pursued, but only as part of a larger, cooperative enterprise that works fairly and equally for the good of everyone. This second sort of view might be called liberal egalitarianism, "liberal" because it values the liberty to pursue one's own personal good, but "egalitarian" because it is prepared to limit such liberty for the good of others.[1]

Each of the two different ways of thinking about human society leads to its own idea of what it means to treat persons equally. To understand these two different meanings of equality, we need to examine more fully the views of society on which they are based.[2]

Let us start with what is common between the two views: the value of individual liberty. What makes human beings the interesting, valuable creatures that they are is the fact that they are able to think about and choose the ends towards which they will act. At the most general level, these ends may include such diverse things as material wealth, love and friendship, knowledge, or social power and prestige. Whatever particular mix of such ends a person might choose to pursue, the important thing about people is that they are able to make such choices; they are able, that is, to determine the goals and aims that give structure and meaning to their individual lives.

Acting alone, however, no one individual is likely to get very far towards any of the more interesting or complex ends that make our lives richly or fully human. For the goods that matter most to us, like having children or embarking on a career, we need the help of other people, or at the very least, their non-interference. This, then, is one minimal role that society might play in human life: to insure that no one individual unfairly interferes with the independent choices of another.

This libertarian view of society is developed at length by the philosopher Robert Nozick in his book *Anarchy, State, and Utopia*.[3] According to Nozick, legitimate state authority exists only to enforce rules of non-interference between individual citizens, rules that outlaw things like lying, cheating, stealing, or reneging on promises. Regulating such actions allows a free market to develop between individuals that enables them to trade goods and service in ways that are mutually beneficial. On this free market view of human society, any trade that is consented to is fair, as long as the consent is not the result of coercion; as long, that is, as it is not the result of anything like lying, cheating, or any of the other forms of illicit interference in the life of another. The function of the state is not to create a market of exchanges, but rather to create the social conditions that freely allow such markets to develop and flourish. The markets themselves are nothing more than the separately motivated choices of individuals to enter into trading arrangements with one another.

According to this first view of society, people are ultimately separate from one another, and relationships of interchange and benefit require mutual agreement. Beyond non-interference, no one owes anyone anything. Each may enter into a free market of exchanges to derive whatever goods or services others agree to trade, but no one is obliged to participate in whatever markets might otherwise develop between others, nor to benefit in any way those who are for some reason unable to participate in such markets. Out of charity one might choose to help such a person, but no one is in any way morally obliged to render aid. The motto of this view is that I have my life, and you have yours: and just as I might choose to enter freely into an exchange of goods or services with you, I might just as freely choose not to.

The second way of thinking about human society and human life is not a simple reversal of libertarianism. It does not move to the opposite extreme of declaring that it is society that is of fundamental or primary importance, and individuals of mere derivative value. Liberal egalitarianism, like libertarianism, values individual choice. But unlike libertarianism, it gives independent value to the ongoing social relationships that link the choices of one person to those of the next. It recognizes that although each of us may choose the course of our own life, none of us chooses the background of ongoing social cooperation that makes such a choice possible. Where libertarianism sees society as nothing more than a series of individual agreements, the second conception sees society as having an independent existence and value of its own.

This second view of society is developed at length by the philosopher John Rawls in his book *A Theory of Justice*.[4] According to Rawls, a society is fairly arranged only when it is reasonable for any and all its members to consent to being part of it. Because the rich, full lives that matter most to humans require the shared cooperation of others, some social arrangement will be preferable to no social arrangement in all but the most dire circumstances. The problem is that different arrangements will offer different benefits to different people. A social arrangement that benefits some individuals more will benefit others less, depending on whose natural talents are in greater demand and generate greater social and individual rewards. Moreover, just as some individuals will suffer accidents that diminish whatever opportunities they would have had for developing their talents or lives in ways they might otherwise have chosen, some individuals will be born in ways that similarly limit the range of opportunities available to them.

So the question is, what sort of social arrangement would it be reasonable to enter into, regardless of one's plans, talents, or infirmities? According to Rawls, the only society it would be reasonable for each of us to enter into is one that guarantees every individual the same equal chance to pursue whatever life plan he or she might choose. People being people, such plans will of course vary greatly, some plans requiring more social resources, some fewer. But Rawls' idea is that whatever sort of life we might choose to lead, two basic sorts of goods will be important to us: civil liberties, like freedom of speech, association, and conscience, and material resources, like income and wealth. Since there is no way that those with fewer civil liberties could ever be advantaged by a social system that distributed such liberties unequally, the first principle of a just society is equal liberty for all. But with regard to

material resources, Rawls claims that the situation is markedly different: if more productive individuals are allowed economic incentives, the social pie as a whole will be greater, and so those with lower incomes will have more material resources than they would under a system which distributed income and wealth in a strictly egalitarian fashion. To the extent that those with less material wealth are more advantaged than they otherwise would be, unequal levels of material wealth will be reasonable in a fair and just society.

We will return to Rawls' two principles in the next section, the first governing the fair distribution of basic liberties, and the second governing the fair distribution of material wealth. The question there will be whether health care, or health more generally, is a good more like liberty or more like wealth.

The point here is that just as there are two different ideals of modern society, there are also two different conceptions of equality. For the libertarian, each individual is treated equally by a state that guarantees no more than non-interference between individuals. The state itself treats individuals unequally when it interferes in the lives of its citizens to transfer between them material resources that were initially acquired through free exchange. Enforced charity, by means of a taxation scheme, for example, that transfers resources from those with more to those with less, is not fair or just according to the libertarian view of human life and society. Again, those with more may freely choose to help those with less, but they may just as freely choose not to.

For Rawls, on the other hand, transfers between individuals are required to ensure that each has an equal opportunity to lead whatever life he or she might choose. Since more productive individuals are allowed greater material resources only so far as this is required as an economic incentive to produce more goods and services overall, taxation is just up to the point that the social product as a whole would begin to diminish. Taxation is fair, that is, up to the point that the economic incentives for the better off would cease to motivate them to be more productive.

Something like this second notion of equality is arguably behind the single-tiered structure of the current Canadian health system.[5] The general form of the argument would be that because our health is equally important to all of us regardless of what sort of life we might choose to pursue, taxation schemes that provide equal health benefits to everyone represent a fair and just social arrangement, one that it would be reasonable for all individuals to enter into no matter what their talents or infirmities. Because of the kind of good that health is, each of us is treated as a moral equal only if we are each given an equal amount of health insurance.

In contrast, the current health system of the United States is more nearly libertarian, since individuals are guaranteed only as much health insurance as they are able to purchase in the free market of private insurance plans. This system is not perfectly libertarian, however, because public insurance is provided for people falling below a certain economic baseline or over a certain age limit. Even so, public insurance plans in the U.S. are extremely limited in their coverage, and there are a significant number of Americans above the economic baseline for public insurance who can nevertheless afford little or no private insurance.[6] It is thus unclear to what extent public insurance plans in the U.S. represent charity or justice for those unable to afford adequate private insurance.

More interesting than the U.S. system, and more conceptually problematic, is the sort of hybrid, two-tiered system of health insurance advocated by some Canadian health reformers.[7] Unlike public insurance plans in the United States, all medically necessary services would be covered for all Canadians, but for services deemed not necessary, or for faster or better quality service, access would be available only to people able to afford additional insurance or direct payment. As we shall see in the next section, it is hard to determine whether the idea of equality presupposed by this sort of two-tiered health system is a coherent one.

Health as a Basic Good

Just as there are two importantly different ways in which we might think about society, and hence equality, there are two importantly different ways in which we might think about the value of health services.

On the one hand, we might think of health services as services like any other: just as we might avail ourselves of the services of a travel agent or hair dresser, we might also avail ourselves of the services of a doctor, nurse, or any other health professional. On the other hand we might think of health services as having a direct tie to health, which alongside political liberty and material wealth we might consider a basic social good.[8]

If we follow Rawls in defining basic goods as those things that are likely to matter to us whatever our life plan might be, health seems an obvious addition to the list. Some people, however, seem entirely prepared to trade off at least portions of their health for other goods, such as the pleasures of smoking or high cholesterol diets. Although this does not change the fact that certain levels of health are needed to lead human lives however they might be defined by the individuals leading them, it does raise the possibility of a mixed understanding of the good of health, and hence, of health services. Perhaps only some health services, but not all, need to be understood as integral to the basic good of health. The health services that are not tied directly to the level of health needed to lead a good life, however one might define it, might then be understood as service like any other, commodities to be sought out and paid for by those who desire them.

Let us return here to Rawls' two principles for distributing basic goods. The first principle, the one regarding liberty, is strictly egalitarian. Because of the kind of basic good civil liberties represent, people are treated equally only if they receive equal amounts of this particular good. Here we need to remember the leading idea of Rawls' two principles, that it is equally reasonable for all to participate in a given social arrangement only if that arrangement gives everyone an equal opportunity to pursue their life plans however they might choose to define them. In general, this conception of society requires basic social goods to be distributed equally; the only exception is when distributing a good unequally means more of that same good for all. This is the situation, Rawls says, with material wealth: all do better than they otherwise would if some are given economic incentives to be more productive.

Considered alongside the basic goods of liberty and material wealth, health would seem to be a good more like the former than the latter. Allowing different levels of health does not in any immediate sort of way make those with less health better off than they would otherwise be, and so in this important respect, health seems to have more in common with political liberty than material wealth. If there are no other important differences between them, then it would seem that health ought to be distributed like liberty: in a strictly egalitarian way.

But there are a number of important differences between health services and the sorts of social arrangements needed to guarantee our civil liberties. First, health services can increase in number, kind, and cost. Civil liberties, on the other hand, are limited in number, and tend to be all or nothing. Were a state, for example, to guarantee political but not religious freedom, we would not think it a state that guaranteed freedom of speech, association, and conscience. But it does not seem in principle wrong that a state might provide antibiotics for everyone who needed them but not artificial hearts. Moreover, certain choices of what sort of a life one is going to lead seem legitimately to require or to allow trade-offs involving increased health risks. So while a state can guarantee through its laws and political institutions equal liberty, it cannot through its health services guarantee anything approaching equal health, whatever technologies might be available to it.

Finally, it may be that by allowing a second tier of health services to develop, those with only publicly provided, first-tier services available to them will do better than they otherwise might. There are several ways this might happen, such as less waiting time or innovative treatment options that are developed at and filter down from the more expensive privately purchased second tier of services. But there are also reasons for supposing that things will not be better for those who find themselves limited to first-tier services, as resources, personnel, and finally funding are increasingly drawn away from the first tier to the second. What would in fact happen were the Canadian system to go from one tier to two is far from clear.

Taken together, these differences between liberty and health suggest that health services might be more appropriately distributed in accord with something like Rawls' second principle of justice, the one regarding material wealth. The most straightforward way of doing this would be to incorporate their dis-

tribution directly into the second principle's distribution of material wealth. Assume, that is, that income and wealth were distributed in such a way that whatever inequalities existed made those with less as well off as they could be. To give those with less any more would be to decrease the incentives to the more productive members of society below the level at which they will continue to be as productive as they are.[9] It might then seem to be fair to allow people to purchase as much or as little as they wanted. What rankles about this suggestion given the current free market method of distributing health services in the U.S. is that material wealth is clearly not distributed in accord with Rawls' second principle in either the U.S. or Canada; one result in the U.S., of course, is that a significant number of Americans are unable to purchase health insurance that would be considered in any way adequate or affordable by Canadian standards. But suppose wealth were distributed in a more equal fashion; why not let people spend their money on as much or as little as they wanted?

One practical problem with this market approach to the distribution of health services is that it would seem to require private insurance schemes, which are economically inefficient.[10] A second problem is that preventative services are in some ways more efficient than curative services, and it is not immediately clear how or why people would choose to insure themselves in ways that might allow full realization of the advantages of preventative medicine.[11]

These sorts of practical problems might be resolved with the right sort of public insurance plan, and the right sort of political will to establish and maintain such a plan. But this suggests an even more insurmountable problem for any proposal tying the distribution of health services to a more equal distribution of material wealth: to the extent that the struggle in both Canada and the U.S. for more egalitarian health systems has been uphill, the struggle for greater economic equality has faced a more nearly vertical climb.

This being so, we might wonder whether Rawls' theory of justice has any relevance for the current debate over Canadian health reform. Whatever we might want to say about the overall distribution of material wealth in Canada, all health services are currently available to all Canadians, at least in principle. But this very principle is itself one significant aspect of the Canadian health system that is now being threatened by governmental responses to increasing deficits and debts. Thinking about universality in the context of Rawls' two principles of justice may yet help clarify some of the larger social issues that are at stake in initiatives to trim deficits by trimming health services.

For example, one direct response to the problems involved in tying health services to the principle for distributing material wealth is to insist that health is ultimately more like liberty than not; despite the differences listed above, health services, like liberty, ought to be distributed in a strictly equal fashion. This would respond well to the idea that like liberty, having a certain level of health is central to our having any life plans at all. But we must still recognize at least this one important difference between the two goods: health services can escalate in cost and number in a way that the institutional arrangements guaranteeing equal liberty cannot. This difference could be met, however, by limiting the comprehensiveness of services provided rather than their universal provision. That cost containment should be focused on comprehensiveness rather than universality is suggested by the idea that health is more like liberty than material wealth.

Limiting the comprehensiveness of the public health plan raises a second interesting question regarding current proposals for reforming the health system. Would it be fair to all Canadians to tie basic, medically necessary services to the strictly egalitarian sort of principle appropriate to liberty, and then, in addition, piggyback the accessibility of all other services onto something like Rawls' second principle? This would preserve universal medical coverage for those services determined to be medially necessary, and allow people with more income or wealth to purchase whatever additional services they wanted to. The underlying idea would be that it is only basic health services that are like liberty; whatever life a person might choose to lead, certain basic health services, like liberty, are equally important to everyone. Additional health services, though, are like material wealth: some people will want to pursue more, some people less, depending on the differ-

ent kinds of lives they choose to lead. Unequal access to additional health services, like unequal levels of material wealth, will be a fair social arrangement just so long as those who have less benefit more than they otherwise would have given a completely equal arrangement.

Arguments of precisely this kind were aired at the 1995 annual general meeting of the Canadian Medical Association.[12] Some doctors, agreeing that equality requires all basic health services be provided to all Canadians, suggested that there was nothing wrong with providing additional services to those who were willing to pay for them. They argued that in allowing this second tier of services to develop, the first tier of basic services would in fact be strengthened.

Again, it is an open question whether this last claim is true. But even ignoring the question of how a second tier of health services might in fact impact on the quality of the first tier of publicly funded services, and ignoring, as well, the question of whether material wealth is itself fairly distributed in Canadian society, there is a deeper conceptual problem with this two-tiered sort of approach to reforming the health system. How are we to distinguish between basic and non-basic services? In some few cases, the distinction may appear to be quite clear: face lifts are not a medical necessity, however much one might plan one's life around the availability of such a service. But this is hardly the sort of service that is causing any cost problems for the health system, especially since it is not now included in any public health insurance plan. More relevant in this regard are newly developing life-saving technologies, many of which are costly and publicly available. For the individuals directly affected by them, such technologies will certainly appear to be medically necessary. The problem facing a publicly funded health system, however, is what happens when services of this kind begin to overreach the public's ability to pay for them? What happens when we can't afford to provide life-saving technologies to all those whose lives could thus be saved? Talking about basic versus non-basic services does nothing to resolve this problem.

We might, of course, try to avoid the problem by reinterpreting basic to refer only to those services that could be provided to all who need them, given the limitations of an antecedently determined budget, one that balanced the costs of health against those of other public goods, such as defense, education, social assistance, and economic development. But what this means is that some individuals with life-threatening conditions will be saved, while other individuals, with other life-threatening conditions, will not. Are those who are not saved treated equally to those who are? Even in a single tiered system, one which accepts the economic necessity of limitations on comprehensiveness, this is a question that would have to be faced. But it is an even more difficult question if we allow those who can afford it to purchase life-saving treatments privately. The problem of what it means to call some services but not others part of the basic package of health insurance owed equally to every member of Canadian society is exacerbated by the fact that in a two-tiered system, those who would find themselves unable to purchase the additional treatments available to the economically advantaged would be even more disadvantaged by the advent of their ill health than they already are. Worse yet, those individuals least able to afford to purchase additional services would be the same ones most likely to need to.[13]

It is thus far from clear whether any proposal for two-tiered health reform based on a distinction between basic and non-basic services is workable or coherent. What this suggests, from the perspective of a liberal egalitarian theory of justice, is that the only fair health system is one that is single-tiered.

Conflicts between Equality and Efficiency

Complicating questions about equality is the ambiguity of its companion term in the health reform debate, efficiency. Everyone seems to agree, in a vague, general sort of way, that the health system can and should be more efficiently organized and operated. The differences of opinion are over what exactly this means.

In its simplest use, pursuing greater efficiency means doing what we now do better. Better utilization of the services now available, it is claimed, will cost governments less and at the same time respond more fully to the actual health needs of all Canadians. The argument is that many tests, treatments, and

services are currently being provided to those who do not need them or in ways that have not been proven to be generally effective and that may be even harmful.[14]

Regardless of the extent to which this is in fact true, problems regarding equality arise on even this simplest understanding of efficiency. For example, while the current system overtreats individuals consulting their doctors with nothing more than a common cold, other individuals, such as pregnant women who are economically or otherwise disadvantaged, go without appropriate medical care. Merely eliminating the waste in the health system as it currently exists will do nothing by itself to respond to this second sort of problem, which bears directly on the question of the extent to which the current system is responding equally to the health needs of all Canadians. Achieving better treatment for disadvantaged individuals is, however, one important area of health reform where equality and efficiency might coincide, were the right sorts of reforms to be pursued. Current data suggests that a great many costly medical conditions arise out of early deficiencies in prenatal and childhood nutrition and care. Thus, ensuring that all Canadian fetuses and children receive sufficient nutrition and care is not just a question of greater social equality, but greater economic efficiency as well.

This leads us to a second meaning of efficiency, one that emphasizes preventative over curative health services. The argument here is that it is cheaper to prevent illness rather than to treat it once it has arisen. So far as those who are the most economically disadvantaged are also among the sickest, this is a second important area of health reform where considerations of equality and efficiency might coincide. The extent to which this is so, however, will depend on the extent to which the health statuses of those who are economically less advantaged are tied to social conditions that go beyond the purview of the health system. If a low income job, for example, is bad for your health, it is not clear what the health system can or should do about this fact.

Equality and efficiency are also less clearly connected in a third sense of efficiency, the one at issue in the discussion of the preceding sections. Given the ever expanding horizon of medical possibility, we will soon be at that point, if we are not indeed already there, of not being able to afford to provide every possible medical service to every Canadian who might benefit from it. If we can't provide every service to everyone who might need it, what might it mean to provide as many services to as many people as we can? How are we to measure the efficiency of responding to the health needs of some Canadians, but not others?[15] Even supposing we felt able to answer such questions about efficiency, there is no reason to assume that the most efficient use of services would necessarily be the most equal.

Suppose, for example, that considerations regarding the most efficient use of health services led us to offer hip surgery to those younger than seventy-five but not to those over seventy-five. Would such a policy represent equal treatment for younger and older people, or is it in some sense ageist? Or suppose we were to treat less serious but more prevalent conditions at the expense of more serious but less prevalent conditions; are those affected by the more serious conditions and those affected by the less serious conditions treated as true equals? These sorts of questions are again exacerbated by the data that suggest that those individuals with less advantaged economic backgrounds are likely to experience more, and more serious, medical conditions.

A fourth and final meaning of efficiency involves reforms to the health system that reduce the cost to governments of providing services, but increase the cost to consumers of these services in either time or money. One example of such a reform is shortened hospital stays, which cost the hospital and hence the government less, but cost the consumer more in paying for home care or in relying on the time and energy of family members or friends. Assuming the current tax system to be more or less equal, the question is whether transferring such costs from the citizen as taxpayer to the citizen as consumer of health services introduces more or less equality into Canadian society. Looking back to the discussion of the second section of this paper, we might say, if we were libertarians, that those who are healthy have no social obligation to pay for those who are not. If some people get sick, this is their problem, those of us who are healthy might choose to help those of us who are sick out of charity, but the state should not compel

such help by transferring money from the healthy to the sick through taxation.

On the liberal egalitarian conception of society, however, we must ask ourselves whether it would be reasonable to enter into a society that does not provide equal care for its sick and injured, regardless of their individual ability to pay for health services. For just as any one of us might find ourselves sick or injured, any one of us might experience a dramatic change in our ability to pay for whatever health we might need. This sort of situation is prevalent in the United States, where for many people, losing either their jobs or their health means losing their health insurance.[16]

One way of responding to this problem is the health system adopted by Canada, universally available to all and publicly funded through taxation. Compared to the European Union, taxes in both Canada and the U.S. are low; yet in the U.S., and increasingly in Canada, there is much concern that taxes are too high. There is also concern in the European Union over high taxes, but it exists alongside concern for preserving the basic structure of the egalitarian sort of society that these taxes support. One German, a corporate manager facing a tax rate of nearly 60 percent, put the point this way:

> The European knows that if he gets sick he can go to a good hospital and it won't bankrupt him ... he knows that if his old parents get sick ... they're protected. To Americans, these can be financially disastrous. But we don't fear them. That is why we keep paying. That is why we say we don't like it but the taxes are necessary.[17]

This point returns us the idea that the current health reform debate in Canada is not just about the kind of health system we want for ourselves and our family members. At a deeper and more far-reaching level, it is about the kind of society we want to live in, one that feels an obligation to care for its sick and injured or one that does not. Economic inequalities may be part of a fair and reasonable society, as both libertarians and liberal egalitarians seem to agree. But unless we are willing to adopt the libertarian view of what a modern, liberal society should be, introducing additional inequalities into our health system does not appear to be either reasonable or fair.

Notes

1   This is the term used, for example, by Will Kymlicka in *Contemporary Political Philosophy: An Introduction* (Oxford: Oxford University Press, 1990). Some commentators on the health reform debate call the second view of society communitarianism, but this term has quite a different meaning in contemporary political debate. ...

2   For further discussion of these different approaches to equality, as well as some of their implications for the just distribution of health care services, see Allen Buchanan, "Justice: A Philosophical Review," in *Justice and Health Care*, ed. Earl Shelp (Dordrecht: Reidel, 1981), 3-21.

3   Robert Nozick, *Anarchy, State, and Utopia* (New York: Basic Books, 1974).

4   John Rawls, *A Theory of Justice* (Cambridge, MA: Harvard University Press, 1971).

5   For such an argument see Kai Nielsen, "Autonomy, Equality and a Just Health Care System," *The International Journal of Applied Philosophy* 4 (Spring 1989): 39-44.

6   Robert G. Evans, "Less is More: Contrasting Styles in Health Care," in *Canada and the United States: Differences that Count*, ed. David Thomas (Peterborough, ON: Broadview, 1993), 21-41. For a glimpse into what the statistics mean for the everyday lives of affected Americans, see Eleanor D. Kinney and Suzanne K. Steinmetz, "Note from the Insurance Underground: How the Chronically Ill Cope," *Journal of Health Politics, Policy and Law* 19, 3 (1994): 633-42.

7   Patrick Sullivan, "Private Health Care Dominates Meeting as General Council Calls for National Debate on Issue," *Canadian Medical Association Journal* 153, 6 (1995): 801-03.

8   For a more extended effort to include health in Rawls' theory of justice, see Norman Daniels, *Just Health Care* (Cambridge: Cambridge University Press, 1985). An interesting alternative to Daniels' approach, closer to the one suggested here, is provided in Ronald M. Green, "The Priority of Health Care," *Journal of Medicine and Philosophy* 9 (1983): 373-79. Recent work on the social determinants of health (see note 13) suggests, however, that we might regard health itself, and not just health care services or health more generally, as a primary social good; this is the view I begin to develop here.

9   Again, the idea here is that if the general level of productivity in a society goes down there is less for everybody, those who are less advantaged together with those who are more advantaged. The underlying assumption is that financial incentives, and hence inequalities in the distribution of wealth, are necessary for high levels of productivity in any modern, industrial society. Social programs whose costs cut too deeply into these incentives will thus have less funding available to them than they otherwise might due to a diminished GDP in the society in question. True or not, the underlying assumption of this line of thought is generally accepted among liberal egalitarians.

10 Evans, "Less is More."

11 One important option here is the idea of health maintenance organizations. For the preventative and health promotional potential of this sort of insurance and delivery arrangement, see Michael Rachlis and Carl Kushner, *Strong Medicine: How to Save Canada's Health Care System* (Toronto: Harper Collins, 1994), 248-52, and H.H. Schauffler and T. Rodriguez, "The Availability and Utilization of Health Promotion Programs and Satisfaction with Health Plan," *Medical Care* 32, 12 (1994): 1182-96. But for concomitant problems relating to equal access to all provided services, see H.B. Fox, L.B. Wicks, and P.W. Newacheck, "Health Maintenance Organizations and Children with Special Health Needs: A Suitable Match?" *American Journal of Diseases of Children* 147.5 (1993): 546-52.

12 Sullivan, "Private Health Care."

13 There is a fast-growing literature on the linkages between health and social position. An early work is Michael Marmot and Tores Theorell, "Social Class and Cardiovascular Disease: The Contribution of Work," *International Journal of Health Science* 18.4 (1988): 659-74. Recent collections are Robert G. Evans, M.L. Barer, and T.R. Marmor, eds., *Why are Some People Healthy and Others Not? The Determinants of Health of Populations* (New York: Aldine

de Gruyter, 1994) together with the fall 1994 issue of *Daedalus*. Especially interesting with regard to the version of liberal egalitarianism explored above is Richard G. Wilkinson, "National Mortality Rates: The Impact of Inequality?" *American Journal of Public Health* 82.8 (1992): 1082-84, and Richard G. Wilkinson, "Income Distribution and Life Expectancy," *British Medical Journal* 304.6820 (1992): 165-68.

14   Rachlis and Kushner, *Strong Medicine*.

15   Health economists have, of course, developed an extensive literature devoted to the question of how we might measure the efficiency of different treatment or service options. But whether such precise, technical definitions of efficiency capture what we really ought to mean by the term remains an open question, depending, in part, on how acceptable we find the simplifying assumptions that are necessary to produce precise, technical definitions of such a multifaceted and complex idea. In the debate over health reform, efficiency is in many ways a much more slippery term than equality. For a recent challenge to economic notions of efficiency as they relate to health reform, see Erik Nord, Jeff Richardson, Andrew Street, Helga Kuhse, and Peter Singer, "Who Cares about Cost? Does Economic Analysis Impose or Reflect Social Values?" *Health Policy* 34.2 (1995): 79-94, and Alastair V. Campbell, "Defining Core Health Services: The New Zealand Experience," *Bioethics* 9.3/4 (1995): 252-58.

16   Evans, "Less is More."

17   Nathaniel C. Nash, "Europeans Brace Themselves for Higher Taxes," *Globe and Mail*, 25 February 1995, 4 (D).

9.
CHAOULLI V. THE ATTORNEY GENERAL OF QUEBEC AND THE ATTORNEY GENERAL OF CANADA [2005] SUPREME COURT OF CANADA

Case Summary by C. Morano

SOURCE: http://scc.lexum.org/en/2005/2005scc35/2005scc35.html.

[Chaoulli v. The Attorney General of Quebec and the Attorney General of Canada is a Supreme Court of Canada decision in which a majority ruled that access to private health insurance ought to be permitted when the public system fails to provide health care in a timely manner.]

Present: McLachlin C.J. and Major, Bastarache, Binnie, LeBel, Deschamps and Fish JJ.

On appeal from the Court of Appeal for Quebec.

Background

Z experienced a number of health issues over the years, which motivated him to speak out against wait times in Quebec's health care system. C is a physician, who has tried unsuccessfully to operate an independent private hospital in Quebec. Appellants Z and C contested the validity of a prohibition on private health insurance contained in section 15 of the Health Insurance Act and section 11 of the Hospital Insurance Act. The two argued that the prohibition violates their section 7 and section 1 rights in the Canadian Charter and Quebec Charter respectively. The Superior Court dismissed the motion because although the prohibition did violate section 7 of the Canadian Charter, the infringement was found to be in accordance with the principles of fundamental justice. The Court of Appeal agreed with that decision.

The Supreme Court of Canada

Three out of the four justices held that the appeal should be allowed because the prohibition is incon-sistent with section 1 of the Quebec Charter. They concluded that where a lack of timely health care can result in death, the s. 7 protection of life is engaged; where it can result in serious psychological and physical suffering, the s. 7 protection of security of the person is triggered. In this case, the majority found that the government has prohibited private health insurance that would permit ordinary Quebeckers to access private health care while failing to deliver health care in a reasonable manner, thereby increasing the risk of complication and death. McLachlin C.J. and Major J. held that "the evidence on the experience of other Western democracies with public health care systems that permit access to private health care refutes the government's theory that a prohibition on private health insurance is connected to maintaining quality public health care. It does not appear that private participation leads to the eventual demise of public health care." It follows that s. 15 and s. 11 are arbitrary and the deprivations of the right to life and security of person are not in accordance with the principles of fundamental justice.

All four justices of the majority opinion found that the right to life and to personal inviolability provided for by the Quebec Charter in section 1 is affected by waiting times. Deschamps J. stated that "the evidence shows that, in the case of certain surgical procedures, the delays that are the necessary result of waiting lists increase the patient's risk of mortality or the risk that his or her injuries will become irreparable. The evidence also shows that many patients on non-urgent waiting lists are in pain and cannot fully enjoy any real quality of life." Deschamps J. found that the infringement could not be justified because the purpose of the prohibition on private health insurance is to preserve the integrity of the public health care system, but there is no proportionality between the measure adopted to attain the objective and the objective itself. There are a wide variety of measures that are less drastic and less intrusive in relation to the protected rights and the absolute prohibition on private insurance has not been demonstrated to have met the minimal impairment test.

An interesting component of the Supreme Court's decision is that there were seven justices present and three of the four present in the majority found that the prohibition violated section 7 of the Canadian Charter, so there was no consensus by the majority on whether or not the Canadian Charter was violated.

10.
SUPREME COURT SLAPS FOR-SALE SIGN ON MEDICARE

Lawrie McFarlane

SOURCE: *CMAJ* 173.3 (2005): 269-70.

In 1857 the US Supreme Court issued its now-infamous Dred Scott judgment, decreeing that the constitutional guarantee of equal treatment under the law did not apply to slaves. The decision by Canada's Supreme Court on June 9, 2005, to permit private health insurance in Quebec[1]—and by implication, in the rest of the country—is a moment of comparable judicial folly, for it effectively sets aside a statutory protection of no less significance.

In Canada, every citizen is assured reasonable and equal access to publicly funded health services without regard to class or income. The Canada Health Act permits only one test: medical necessity. The Supreme Court's decision implicitly adds a second, and many fear pre-emptive, test: financial status. As counsel for one of the appellants in the original trial made clear, "I am arguing for the right of more affluent people to have access to parallel health services."[2]

For defenders of universal health care, the court's reasoning is stultifying. The case before the justices amounted to this: a Quebec resident needed orthopedic surgery and was required, because of backlogs in treatment, to wait longer than appropriate. On that basis, he argued he should have access to a separate, private system.

There is no dispute that lengthy wait times cause pain and diminished quality of life. Everyone agrees that delays are unacceptably long in parts of the country. Yet before the court imposed its radical solution, it might have taken more care in its consideration of the nature of the problem.

There are a variety of reasons for lengthening wait lists. Some certainly relate to funding shortfalls or poor management practices. But an equal part of the trend can be linked to excessive compensation demands by various health professions, and to the failure of some medical specialists to practise within appropriate clinical guidelines. Introducing private medicine will not address these problems, and may in fact exacerbate them. More importantly, the waitlist problem is confined mainly to a narrow, albeit essential, area of medical practice. With a few region-specific exceptions, such as radiation therapy in Quebec, most of the concern focuses on elective surgery, and more narrowly still, on orthopedic surgery.

Consider the following growth rates for surgical procedures in British Columbia between 1995 and 2000:

- gynecologic procedures: 4%
- urological surgery: 7.7%
- neurosurgery: 8%
- hip replacement: 42%
- cataract surgery: 66%
- knee replacement: 92%

These figures (and similar rates of increase apply in most of the country) illustrate a critical aspect of the dilemma. Wait times have increased because of an unprecedented surge in procedure volumes. Because this increase exceeds population growth or demographic change by several orders of magnitude, it seems that other causes must be involved. The advent of less invasive surgical procedures, enabling patients to be discharged from hospital more quickly, is likely a critical factor.

Forty years of labour have been cast aside in a spasm of judicial intemperance, and a radical, if not catastrophic, remedy has been imposed to solve a narrow and probably transitory problem.

Given a chance, our health care system will adapt to this changing demand, as it has adapted in the past to other challenges. Six months ago the federal and provincial governments signed a joint Health Accord to attack surgical delay and other related difficulties. One might have hoped the court would allow that initiative time to work before throwing judicial restraint to the wind. At a minimum, whatever remedy was adopted to correct such a narrowly located problem should have been proportionately narrow in its application. Instead, Madame Justice Marie Deschamps, writing for the majority, imposed a sweeping remedy that has the potential to reorder not only orthopedic care but the entire health care spectrum, from family medicine to surgery to acute hospital care.

Critics might wonder why the court doesn't swallow a dose of its own medicine. The problem of trial delay in the judicial field dwarfs whatever difficulties confront our health service. Nation wide, well over half of all criminal cases exceed the guideline, set down by the Supreme Court, of 8 months from arraignment to the start of trial. Many cases take 2 or even 3 times that long. Would the court accept the argument that a parallel judicial system should be created for the well-heeled, to save them the evils of trial delay? Of course not, but it bears thinking why. We have only one court system for the same reason we have only one health care system: the principle of equal treatment demands it. A dual court system would be unthinkable in the same way that two-tier medicine should be unthinkable. (Interestingly, when the issue of trial delay arises, judges apply exactly the same types of remedy as the Supreme Court has now denied the health care system: they ask government for more resources, set guidelines for appropriate wait times and plead for patience when they come up short.)

Madame Justice Ginette Piché of the Quebec Superior Court, whose judgment the Supreme Court overturned, made the link between health care and other basic rights explicit in her decision: "The Court ... considers that if access to the health system is not possible, it is illusory to think that rights to life and security are respected."[3]

In other words, health care is not some commodity to be bartered on the open market. Rather, it is a precondition of the basic rights guaranteed by the Charter. That being so, it should enjoy the same protection, meaning that it must be provided on an equal and indivisible basis.

Had the justices accepted this reasoning, other remedies were at hand. It lay within the court's power to order an improvement in surgical wait lists within the public system, up to some required standard. Perhaps with the imminent threat of a two-tier system to clarify their thinking, the provinces would have made the necessary reforms.

Instead, as the implications sink in, health ministries across the country are aghast. No one has a clue where we go from here. Forty years of labour have been cast aside in a spasm of judicial intemperance, and a radical, if not catastrophic, remedy has been imposed to solve a narrow and probably transitory problem.

The drafters of the Dred Scott judgment thought they had ensured the perpetuation of an underclass in American society, but in fact the opposite came to pass. People were scandalized when they saw such unworthy sentiments dignified in legal reasoning, and in less than a decade, slavery was abolished.

Defenders of medicare can only hope the same thing happens here, and that as people realize the Supreme Court has disfigured a national symbol, they will sweep away two-tier medicine once and for all.

Notes

1   Chaoulli v. Quebec (Attorney General). 2005 SCC 35.
2   Chaoulli v. Quebec (Attorney General) [2000] JQ no 479 at 7.
3   Chaoulli v. Quebec (Attorney General) [2000] JQ no 479 at 138.

11.
PRIVATIZING HEALTH CARE IS NOT THE ANSWER: LESSONS FROM THE UNITED STATES

Marcia Angell

SOURCE: *CMAJ* 179.9 (2008): 916-19.

There are strong moves within Canada to make the Canadian health care system more like the US system by partially privatizing it. Those who favour this approach claim that the US system offers more choice and better quality of care and spares the public purse. Some proponents even go so far as to claim that it is more efficient. My purpose here is to disabuse Canadians of these myths by taking a close look at how the US system works and comparing it with the Canadian system.

In 1972 the Yukon Territory became the last jurisdiction in Canada to adopt the Medical Care Act, which set up a system to provide hospital and physician care to all Canadians.[1] Before then, the Canadian and US health care systems were similar. Both were partly public, partly private, partly for profit and partly nonprofit. Both also left a great many citizens uninsured. The costs were also about the same—a little over $300 per person in 1970—as were outcomes. At that time, life expectancy was about a year longer in the United States.[2]

But with the implementation of Canadian medicare, the two systems rapidly began to diverge in all respects. The US system became more and more costly, leaving increasing numbers of Americans—now about 46 million people—uninsured. In 2005, expenditures were twice as high in the US as in Canada—US$6697 per person v. US$3326 in Canada.[3] And although Canada insures all its population for necessary doctor and hospital care, the US leaves 15% without any insurance whatsoever.[4] Those who are insured often need to pay a substantial fraction of the bill out-of-pocket, and some necessary services may not be covered. In a recent survey, 37% of Americans reported that they went without needed care because of cost, compared with 12% of Canadians.[3]

Outcomes also now favour Canada. Instead of living a year longer, the life expectancy of Americans is now 2.5 years shorter than that of Canadians.[2] Infant mortality rates are higher in the US, as is preventable mortality (death before the age of 75 years from diseases that are amenable to treatment).[5,6] Furthermore, contrary to popular belief, people in the US do not receive more health care services. They visit their doctors much less often and spend less time in hospital than Canadians do (Table 1). Per population, there are also fewer nurses and hospital beds in the US, although there are slightly more doctors and many more magnetic resonance imaging (MRI) units.[5,7]

Why the US Spends More and Gets Less

The only plausible explanation for the US paradox of spending more and getting less is that the US health care system is enormously inefficient compared with the Canadian system. The inefficiency stems from the fact that the US, alone among industrialized countries, relies primarily on private, largely investor-owned corporations to provide health care.[8] It is the only industrialized country that treats health care like a market commodity instead of a social service. Thus, health care is distributed not according to medical need but, rather, according to the ability to pay. There is a great mismatch, however, between medical need and the ability to pay. In fact, those with the greatest need are those least able to pay. Although markets are good for many things, they are not a good way to distribute health care because that is not their primary purpose. Businesses aim to increase revenues and maximize profits. Hospitals in the US, for example, often advertise

---

Key points

- Health care costs per person are twice as high in the United States as in Canada.
- The US health care system has worse outcomes, is less efficient and provides fewer of many basic services than the Canadian system.
- The United States is the only industrialized country that treats health care as a market commodity, not a social service, and leaves uninsured those who cannot pay.
- In the United States, for-profit health care is more expensive and often of lower quality than not-for-profit or government care, with much higher overhead costs.
- The notion that partial privatization in Canada will shorten waiting times for elective procedures is misguided.
- Partial privatization would draw off resources from the public system, increase costs overall and introduce the inequities of the US system.
- The best way to improve the Canadian health care system is to put more resources into it.

---

their services. Like all businesses, they want more, not fewer customers—but only if they can pay. People who are wealthy or well insured may get an MRI they do not need, whereas those without insurance may not get an MRI they do need.

How the US System Works

Most Americans under the age of 65 receive tax-free health benefits from their employers. Employers select the insurance companies and the plans to offer and pay a portion of the premiums—these days, a smaller and smaller portion. There is little choice. But offering benefits is strictly voluntary, and not all employers choose to do so. If offered, the benefits may not be comprehensive. Increasingly, employers cap their contributions, so that the burden of increasing costs falls on the workers.[9] Employees, in turn, often turn down benefits when they are offered, because they cannot afford to pay their growing share of the premiums.

The private insurers with whom employers contract are mostly investor-owned, for-profit businesses. They try to keep premiums down and profits up by stinting on medical services. In fact, the best way for insurers to compete is by not insuring high-risk patients (called "cherry picking" or "cream skimming"), limiting the coverage of those they do insure (e.g., excluding expensive services, such as bone marrow transplantation) and passing costs back to

patients as deductibles, copayments and claim denials. The US is the only country in the world with a health care system based on avoiding sick people. These practices add enormously to overhead costs because they require a great deal of paperwork. They also require creative marketing to attract the affluent and healthy people and to dodge those who are poor or sick. Not surprisingly, the US has by far the highest overhead costs in the world.[5]

It is instructive to follow the health care dollar as it makes its way from employers to the doctors and nurses and hospitals that provide medical services. First, private insurers regularly skim off the top a substantial fraction of the premiums (about 15%-25%) for their administrative costs, marketing and profits.[9] The remainder is passed along a veritable gauntlet of satellite businesses that have sprung up around the health care industry. These include brokers to cut deals, disease-management and utilization review companies, drug-management companies, legal services, marketing consultants, billing agencies and information management firms. They, too, siphon off some of the premiums, including enough for their administrative costs, marketing and profits. It was conservatively estimated that, in 1999, 31.0% of all health care spending in the US was for overhead, nearly twice the estimated 16.7% in Canada. The overhead for Canada's private insurers that year was 13.2%, compared with only 1.3% for its public system.[10]

Table 1: Differences in health care between Canada and the United States

Measure	Canada	United States
Total health care spending per capita (2005)	US$3326	US$6697
Government spending per capita (2005)	US$2322	US$4048
Life expectancy, yr	80.2†	77.8‡
Infant mortality per 1000 births (2004)	5.3	6.8
Amenable mortality* per 100 000 (2002–2003)	77	110
Physician visits per capita	6.1§	3.9¶
Hospital acute care beds per 1000	3.0‡	2.8†
Bed-days per capita	1.0§	0.7‡
Physicians per 1000	2.2‡	2.4†
Nurses per 1000	9.9‡	7.9¶
MRI units per million population	5.5†	26.6‡

Note: MRI = magnetic resonance imaging.
*Deaths before the age of 75 years from diseases amenable to treatment.
†2005 data.
‡2004 data.
§2003 data.
¶2002 data.

The most popular part of the US health care system is the government-administered system for Americans over the age of 65—Medicare. This is a single-payer program embedded within the private, market-based system. It is by far the most efficient part of the US system, with overhead costs to government of about 2%.[11] It covers virtually everyone over the age of 65, not just some of them. It also covers everyone for the full package of benefits, so it cannot be tailored to avoid high-risk or chronically ill patients. But US Medicare is not perfect, and it has been weakened by the Bush administration. Out-of pocket costs for Medicare beneficiaries are substantial and growing. Moreover, because Medicare pays for care in a market-based private system, it experiences many of the same inflationary forces that affect the private insurance system, including profit-maximizing hospitals and physicians' groups. In addition, doctors' fees are skewed to reward highly paid specialists for doing as many expensive procedures as possible. As a result, inflation in the Medicare system is almost as high as inflation in the private sector and is similarly unsustainable.[8]

Attempts to reform the US health care system incrementally have run into the following dilemma. If coverage is expanded, costs rise. If costs are controlled, coverage shrinks. This problem faces the US presidential candidates as they attempt to respond to the increasing calls for reform, and they have embraced opposite horns of the dilemma.[12] Senator John McCain has opted for holding down costs by passing more of the burden to individuals, even though it means reducing coverage. Senator Barack Obama has opted for increasing coverage, even though it means adding to the staggering costs. Neither is a long-term solution. The only way to increase coverage and reduce costs is to change the system entirely.

Polls have shown that about two-thirds of Americans would prefer a Canadian-style system,[13] as would three-fifths of doctors.[14] However, many businesses that profit from the current system, mainly the private insurance industry and for-profit health care facilities, resist any fundamental change. They in turn have inordinate influence over law-makers and many economists and health policy experts, who propagate the myth that a Canadian-style health care system is "unrealistic." In addition, many procedure-oriented specialists are quite happy with the current system. They are generally paid much more than they are in Canada, and that predisposes them to exaggerate the failings of the Canadian system and minimize those of the American system.

Strengths and Failings of the Canadian System

In 1972, after the Yukon Territory signed on to the Medical Care Act, all Canadians were insured for physician and hospital services, but not for other health care needs such as home care, care in long-term facilities and prescription drugs. These and other benefits were left to the individual provinces, if they were covered at all. Moreover, many hospitals added user fees and doctors added extra charges. However, these practices ended with the 1984 Canada Health Act, which required, as a condition of federal contributions to provincial costs, that health care be accessible to everyone, and it essentially abolished user fees and extra charges.[1] The system was able to keep costs in check in part by controlling the supply of certain services—for example, imaging and surgical facilities and the specialist physicians necessary to carry out the procedures. The result was the growth of waiting lists for some procedures. Nevertheless, Canadian medicare remained popular with the public—and still is.

During the 1990s, as Canada went through an economic downturn, Canadian medicare was underfunded. Waiting lists became a political issue, and

public satisfaction with the system, although still high, fell somewhat. Toward the end of the 1990s, as economic conditions improved and the publicity about waiting lists increased, the provinces began to put more money into the health care system.[1] But waiting times are still too long for certain elective procedures, such as hip and knee replacements, and it takes time for increased funding to be translated into more facilities and specialists.

The waiting lists are the ostensible reason for the pressures to partially privatize the Canadian health care system. I say "ostensible" because I believe the main reasons have to do with the desire of businesses and some specialists to profit from the system, just as they do in the US, and the desire of the federal and provincial governments to hold down their costs, even if it means increasing the burden on individuals. Lamenting waiting lists, however, sounds better to the public.

In 2005, the Supreme Court of Canada handed down its decision in Chaoulli v. Quebec.[15] It held that a one-year wait for a hip replacement violated human rights guaranteed by the province of Quebec. Either Quebec would have to shorten waiting times or permit the procedure to be done privately. Although the effect in Quebec itself has been quite limited, the decision added force to a strong move throughout Canada, particularly in British Columbia and Alberta, to permit the marketing of private insurance and the delivery of care in for-profit facilities by doctors working in both the public and private systems. These facilities and doctors would be able to bill medicare and add extra charges.[16]

Why Privatization Is Not the Answer

Whether privatization would shorten waiting lists by creating more facilities is arguable. What it would certainly do is change who would be waiting. In the US, for example, well-insured patients have a very short wait for a hip replacement, but the 46 million Americans without health insurance might wait for the rest of their lives. As in all such parallel systems, privatization would draw off resources—physicians and other assets—from the public system.[17] Waiting lists would be shorter in the private system, but they would almost certainly grow longer in the public system. Access would come to be more about money than medical need, just as it is in the US.

Moreover, it would not be a zero sum game. Money diverted to the private system would not buy the same health care as it would in the public system. There have been many studies comparing for-profit and not-for-profit health care in the US. For-profit care is nearly always more expensive and often of lower quality.[8,18] Indeed, logic and common sense would suggest the same conclusions even without the growing empirical evidence. Unless we believe, without any evidence whatsoever, that for-profit organizations have some secret of efficient operation not known to the not-for-profits, it makes no sense to suppose that, given the same payment system and the same patient population, the for-profit organizations can provide similar services while still extracting their profits and business costs from the system. Neither does it make sense to imagine that investor-owned businesses are charitable organizations that wish to contribute their resources to the community. It is obvious that their responsibilities to their investors require them to take profits from the community. To do this, as many US studies have shown, they skim off the profitable patients and the profitable services, leaving the leftovers to the not-for profits.

I would urge Canadians not to be swayed by the siren song of the privatizers. This is about profiteering as much as it is about health care. The same businesses that have made an exorbitantly expensive and unhealthy mess of the US system stand ready to do the same in Canada. The problem with Canadian medicare is not the system, it is the amount of money put into it. The US problem is exactly the opposite. It is not the money, it is the system. Those wishing to privatize the Canadian system often suggest that waiting times for hip replacements in the US are short because of the market-based system. That is not the case. In the US, most hip replacements are done in the public system for elderly patients. Thus, if we compare waiting times between the two countries, we are not comparing public and private systems. We are comparing two public systems, one of which (in the US) is better funded.

Canada's medicare is one of the best health care systems in the world—far superior to the US system.

I would like to see it broaden its services to include long-term care, home care and prescription drugs. I believe it needs to be better funded from the public purse, although it does not require anywhere near the amount of money Americans put into their system. But it does fulfill its obligations to all Canadians by providing essential health care based on medical need, not on the ability to pay, and it has the great communitarian virtue of requiring everyone to be a part of the system.[19] Thus, it matters to nearly everyone. Privatizing Canada's health care system, even a little, will inevitably cause costs to rise and access to decline. The wisest course for Canada is to expand and reinforce the public system, not undermine it.

Notes

1 Marchildon GP. Health systems in transition: Canada. Toronto: University of Toronto Press; 2005.

2 Organization for Economic Co-operation and Development. OECD health data 2008: statistics and indicators for 30 countries. Paris (France): The Organization; 2008. Available: www.oecd.org/health/healthdata (accessed 2008 Aug 27).

3 Schoen C, Osborn R, Doty MM, et al. Toward higher-performance health systems: adults' health care experiences in seven countries, 2007. *Health Aff* (Millwood) 2007; 26: w717-34.

4 US Bureau of the Census. Income, poverty, and health insurance coverage in the United States. Washington, DC: The Bureau; 2006.

5 American College of Physicians. Achieving a high-performance health care system with universal access: what the United States can learn from other countries. *Ann Intern Med* 2008; 148: 1-21.

6 Nolte E, McKee CM. Measuring the health of nations: updating an earlier analysis. *Health Aff* (Millwood) 2008; 27: 58-71.

7 Anderson GF, Frogner BK, Reinhardt UE. Health spending in OECD countries in 2004: an update. *Health Aff* (Millwood) 2007; 26: 1481-89.

8 Relman AS. A second opinion: rescuing America's health care. New York: Public Affairs; 2007.

9 Geyman J. Do not resuscitate: Why the health insurance industry is dying and how we must replace it. Monroe, ME: Common Courage Press; 2008.

10 Woolhandler S, Campbell T, Himmelstein DU. Costs

of health care administration in the United States and Canada. *N Engl J Med* 2003; 349: 768-75.

11 Potetz L. Financing Medicare: an issue brief. Washington, DC: Kaiser Family Foundation; 2008. Available: www.medicareadvocacy.org/Reform_08_01 .Kaiser BriefReMAFinancing.pdf (accessed 2008 Aug 27).

12 Angell M. Health reform you shouldn't believe in: what the Massachusetts experiment teaches us about incremental efforts to increase coverage by expanding private insurance. *Am Prospect* 2008; May: A15-18.

13 Kuhnhenn J, Thompson T. Election 08 political pulse: the Associated Press/ Yahoo! news poll. The Associated Press; 2008. Available: http://news.yahoo.com /page/election-2008-political-pulse-voter-worries (accessed 2008 Aug 27).

14 Carroll AE, Ackerman RT. Support for national health insurance among US physicians: 5 years later. *Ann Intern Med* 2008; 148: 566-67.

15 Chaoulli v. Quebec (Attorney General), no 29272, Sup Ct of Canada 130 CRR (2d) 99; 2005 CRR LEXIS 76.

16 Steinbrook R. Private health care in Canada. *N Engl J Med* 2006; 354: 1661-64.

17 Flood CM. Chaoulli's legacy for the future of Canadian health care policy. In: Campbell B, Marchildon G, editors. Medicare: facts, myths, problems & promise. Toronto (ON): James Lorimer & Company Ltd.; 2007. p. 156-91.

18 Woolhandler S, Himmelstein DU. Competition in a publicly funded healthcare system. *BMJ* 2007; 335: 1126-29.

19 Romanow R. Commission on the Future of Health Care in Canada. Building on values: the future of health care in Canada—final report. Ottawa: The Commission; 2002. Cat no CP32-85/2002E-IN. Available: www.hc-sc.gc.ca/hcs-sss/alt_formats/hpb-dgps/pdf/ hhr/romanow-eng.pdf (accessed 2008 Sept 22).

CHAPTER THREE

CONSENT

Web Link

(1) Eike-Henner W. Kluge, "After 'Eve': Whither Proxy Decision-Making?"

http://pubmedcentralcanada.ca/articlerender.cgi?accid=PMC1267307&tool=pmcentrez

* For an up-to-date list of the web links in this book, please visit:
http://sites.broadviewpress.com/healthcare.

12.
COMPETENCY TO GIVE AN INFORMED CONSENT: A MODEL FOR MAKING CLINICAL ASSESSMENTS

James F. Drane

SOURCE: *Journal of the American Medical Association* 252.7 (1984): 925-27.

In January 1980, as one more indication of the growing importance of medical ethics, a presidential commission was formed and began work on the moral questions posed by the practice of contemporary medicine. After three years of intense work, the commission published a separate volume on 11 different ethical problems in the hope of stimulating thoughtful discussion. Some broad principles were uncovered that apply to any and every bioethical issue, such as the principle of patient respect and its concrete application in the right of informed consent. But there were also recurring perplexities, one of which was competency or, in the language preferred by the commission, the patient's capacity to choose.[1]

Respect for patients means ensuring their participation in decisions affecting their lives. Such participation is a basic form of freedom and stands at the core of Western values. But freedom, participation, and self-determination suppose a capacity for such acts. No one, for example, assumes that an infant has such a capacity and, time and again, doubts arise about the capacity of some older patients. Not to respect a patient's freedom is undoubtedly wrong. But to respect what may be an expression of freedom only in appearance would be a violation of another basic principle of ethical medicine: promotion of the patient's well-being.

Although the commission's report referred many times to competency or capacity to choose, commissioners and staff members privately expressed frustration and disappointment about their conclusions. The commission reports spelled out what are considered to be the components of competency: the possession of a set of values and goals, the ability to

communicate and understand information, and the ability to reason and deliberate. In addition, the commission criticized some standards for determining competency that either were too lenient and did not protect a patient sufficiently or were too strict and in effect transferred decision making to the physician. But the commission did not come up with its own standard and left unsettled the question of how to decide whether a particular patient's decision should be respected or overridden because of incompetency. Incompetency is not the only reason for overriding a patient's refusal or setting aside a consent, but it is the most common reason for doing so. Defining incompetency or establishing standards of competency is a complex problem because it involves law, ethics, and psychiatry.

Competency Assessment

Competency assessments focus on the patient's mental capacities, specifically, the mental capacities to make an informed medical decision. Does the patient understand what is being proposed? Can the patient come to a decision about treatment based on an adequate understanding? How much understanding and rational decision making capacity are sufficient for this particular patient to be considered competent? Conversely how deficient must this patient's decision-making capacity be before he is declared incompetent? A properly performed competency assessment should eliminate two types of error: (1) preventing a competent person from participating in treatment decisions and (2) failing to protect an incompetent person from the harmful effects of a bad decision.

Model for Making the Assessment

The President's commission did not recommend a single standard for determining competency because any one standard is inappropriate for the many different types of medical decisions that people face. What is proposed here is a sliding standard, i.e., the more dangerous the medical decision, the more stringent the standards of competency. The basic idea, following a suggestion of Mark Siegler,[2] is to connect determination of competency to different medical situations (acute or chronic, critical or noncritical), and next to take this idea a step further by specifying three different standards or definitions of what it means to be competent. These standards are then correlated with three different medical situations, each more dangerous than the other. Finally, the sliding standards and different medical situations are correlated with the types of psychiatric abnormalities that ordinarily undermine competency. The interrelationship of all these entities creates a model that can aid the physician faced with a question about a patient's capacity to choose. This model brings together disparate academic disciplines, but its goal is thoroughly pragmatic: to provide a workable guide for clinical decision making.

Standard 1

The first and least stringent standard of competency to give a valid consent applies to those medical decisions that are not dangerous and objectively are in the patient's best interest. If the patient is critically ill because of an acute illness that is life threatening, if there is an effective treatment available that is low in risk, and if few or no alternatives are available, then consent to the treatment is prima facie rational. Even though patients are seriously ill and thereby impaired in both cognitive and conative functioning, they are usually competent to consent to a needed treatment.

The act of consent to such a treatment is considered to be an informed consent as long as the patient is aware of what is going on. *Awareness* in the sense of orientation or being conscious of the general situation satisfies the cognitive requirement of informed consent. *Assent* alone to what is the rational expecta-

tion in this medical context satisfies the decisional component. When adult patients go along with needed medical treatment, then a legal presumption of competency holds even though the patients are obviously impaired. To insist on higher standards for capacity to give a valid consent in such a medical setting would amount to requiring surplus mental capacities for a simple task and would result in millions of acutely ill patients being considered incompetent. Such an absurd requirement would produce absurd consequences. Altogether rational and appropriate decisions would be set aside as invalid, and surrogate decision makers would have to be selected to make the same decision. For what purpose? To accomplish what objective? To protect what value? None of the values and objectives meant to be safeguarded by the competency requirement is disregarded or set aside by a lenient standard for this type of decision.

Considering as competent seriously ill patients, even the mentally ill, who are aware and assent to treatment, eliminates the ambiguity and confusion associated with terms such as *virtually competent*, *marginally competent*, and *competent for practical purposes* that are used to excuse the commonsense practice of respecting the decisions of patients who would be judged incompetent by a more demanding single standard of decision-making capacity. Refusal by a patient dying of a chronic illness of treatments that are useless and only prolong the dying requires the same modest standard of competency.

Infants, unconscious persons, and the severely retarded would obviously fall short even of this least demanding standard. These persons, and patients who use psychotic defenses that severely compromise reality testing, are the only ones who fail to meet this first definition of decision-making capacity. Children who have reached the age of reason (6 years or older), on the other hand, as well as the senile, the mildly retarded, and the intoxicated, are considered competent.

The law considers 21 and sometimes 18 years to be the age below which persons are presumed incompetent to make binding contracts, including health care decisions. The President's commission, however, endorses a lower age of competency, and so do many authors who write about children and mental retardation. In this model, we are discussing ethical standards, but the physician cannot ignore the law and must obtain consent from the child's legal guardian.

Standard 2

If the illness is chronic rather than acute, or if the treatment is more dangerous or of less definite benefit (or if there are real alternatives to one or another course of action, e.g., death rather than lingering illness), then the risk-benefit balance is tipped differently than in the situation described in the previous section. Consequently, a different standard of competency to consent is required. The patient must be able to *understand* the risks and outcomes of the different options and then be able to *choose* a decision based on this understanding. At this point, competency means capacity to understand the real options and to make an understanding decision, a higher standard than that required for the first type of treatment choice.

Ability to understand is not the same as being able to articulate conceptual or verbal understanding. Some ethicists assume a rationalist epistemology and reduce all understanding to a conceptual or verbal type. Many, in fact, require that patients literally remember what they have been told as a proof of competence. Understanding, however, may be more affective than conceptual. Following an explanation, a patient may grasp what is best for him with strong feelings and convictions, and yet be hard pressed to articulate his understanding/conviction in words.

Competency as capacity for an understanding choice is also reconcilable with a decision to let a trusted physician decide what is the best treatment. Such a choice (waiver) may be made for good reasons and represent a decision in favor of one set of values (safety or anxiety reduction) over another (independence and personal initiative). As such, it can be considered as informed consent and creates no suspicion of incompetency.

Ignorance or inability to understand, however, undermines competency. The same is true of a severe mood disorder or severe shock, which may either impair thought processes or undermine capacity to make an understanding choice. Short-term memory

loss, delusion, dementia, and delirium would also render a patient incompetent. On the other hand, mature adolescents, the mildly retarded, and persons with some personality disorders would be competent to make this type of decision.

Standard 3

The most stringent and demanding standard of competency is reserved for those decisions that are very dangerous and fly in the face of both professional and public rationality. When diagnostic uncertainty is minimal, the available treatment is effective, and death is likely to result from treatment refusal, a presumption is established against refusal of consent to treatment. The medical decision now is not a balancing of what are widely recognized as reasonable alternatives. Any decision other than the one to be treated seems to violate basic reasonableness. A decision to refuse treatment, then, is apparently irrational, besides being harmful. Yet, according to this model, such decisions can be respected as long as the patients satisfy the most demanding standard of competency.

Competency in this context requires a capacity to appreciate the nature and consequences of the decision being made. *Appreciation* is a term used to refer to the highest degree of understanding, one that grasps more than just the medical details of the illness and treatment. To be competent to make apparently irrational and very dangerous choices, the patient must be able to come to a decision based on the medical information and to appreciate the implications of this decision for his life. Competency of this type requires a capacity that is both technical and personal, both cognitive and affective.

Since the patient's decision flies in the face of objective standards of rationality, it must at least be subjectively critical and *rational*. A patient need not conform to what most rational people do to be considered competent, but the competent patient must be able to give reasons for his decision. The patient must be able to show that he has thought through the medical issues and related this information to his personal value system. The patient's personal reasons need not be medically or publicly accepted, but neither can they be purely private, idiosyncratic, or incoherent.

Their intelligibility may derive from a set of religious beliefs or from a philosophical view that is shared by only a small minority. This toughest standard of competency does, however, demand a more rationalistic type understanding: one that includes verbalization, argumentation, and consistency.

The higher-level mental capacities required for competency to make this type of decision are impaired by less severe psychiatric abnormality. In fact, much less serious mental affliction suffices to create an assumption of incompetency to refuse a needed and effective treatment. On the other hand, however, not any mental or emotional disturbance would constitute an impairment of decisional capacity. A certain amount of anxiety, for example, goes with any serious decision and cannot make a patient incompetent. Some mild pain would not impair decisional capacity, but severe pain might do so. Even a slight reactive depression may not render a patient incompetent for this type of decision. But intense anxiety associated with mild or severe shock, and/or a mild endogenous depression, would be considered incapacitating. In fact, any mental or emotional disorder that compromises appreciation and rational decision making would make a patient incompetent. For example, persons who are incapable of making the effort required to control destructive behavior (substance abusers and sociopaths), as well as neurotic persons, hysterical persons, and persons who are ambivalent about their choice, would all be incompetent to refuse life saving treatment. The same standard applies to consent to experiments not related to one's own illness.

Conclusion

Radical advocates of patient rights and doctrinaire libertarians will worry that this model shifts power back toward physicians who make competency determinations and away from patients whose choices ought to be respected. But only in situation 3 does the physician's power increase, and then only for the patient's welfare. Moreover, this loss in the patient's power never reaches the point where patients' self-determination is set aside. Patients can insist on their decision to refuse a treatment even when the physician knows that the outcome will be certain death, as long as every precaution is taken to ensure that such a decision is not the product of a pathological state.

A balancing of values is the cornerstone of a good competency assessment. Rationality is given its place throughout this model. Maximum autonomy is guaranteed for patients because they can choose to do what is not at all beneficial (a non-therapeutic experiment) or refuse to do what is most beneficial. Maximum benefit is also guaranteed because patients are protected against harmful choices that are more the product of abnormality than of their self-determination. All the values, in fact, on which competency requirements were originally based are guaranteed in this model.

No one proposal will settle the question of which standard or standards of competency are appropriate for medical decisions. More empirical research is required on the issue, and more physicians who have valuable practical experience with complex cases need to be heard from. After much more study and discussion, perhaps the medical profession itself, through its ethics committees, will take a stand on the issue. In the meantime, this proposal is meant to be a contribution to the discussion.

Acknowledgment

This investigation was supported in part by grant ED 0652-78 from the National Endowment for the Humanities.

Notes

1   President's Commission for the Study of Ethical Problems in Medicine and Biomedical and Behavioral Research, *Deciding to Forego Life-Sustaining Treatment* (Washington, DC: U.S. Government Printing Office, 1983).

2   M. Siegler and A.D. Goldblatt, "Clinical intuition: A procedure for balancing the rights of patients and the responsibilities of physicians," in S.F. Spicker, J.M. Healey, and H.T. Engelhardt (eds.), *The Law-Medicine Relation: A Philosophical Exploration* (Dordrecht, The Netherlands: D. Reidel Publishing Co., 1981), pp. 5-29; see also A.R. Jonsen, M. Siegler, and W.J. Winslade, *Clinical Ethics* (New York: Macmillan, 1982), pp. 56-85.

13

BIOETHICS FOR CLINICIANS:
INVOLVING CHILDREN IN MEDICAL DECISIONS

Christine Harrison, Nuala P. Kenny, Mona Sidarous, and Mary Rowell

SOURCE: *CMAJ* 156.6 (1997): 825-28.

Eleven-year-old Samantha is a bright, loving child who was treated for osteosarcoma in her left arm. The arm had to be amputated, and Samantha was given a course of chemotherapy. She has been cancer-free for 18 months and is doing well in school. She is self-conscious about her prosthesis and sad because she had to give away her cat, Snowy, to decrease her risk of infection. Recent tests indicate that the cancer has recurred and metastasized to her lungs. Her family is devastated by this news but do not want to give up hope. However, even with aggressive treatment Samantha's chances for recovery are less than 20%.

Samantha adamantly refuses further treatment. On earlier occasions she had acquiesced to treatment only to struggle violently when it was administered. She distrusts her health care providers and is angry with them and her parents. She protests, "You already made me give up Snowy and my arm. What more do you want?" Her parents insist that treatment must continue. At the request of her physician, a psychologist and psychiatrist conduct a capacity assessment. They agree that Samantha is probably incapable of making treatment decisions; her understanding of death is immature and her anxiety level very high. Nursing staff are reluctant to impose treatment; in the past Samantha's struggling and the need to restrain her upset them a great deal.

Why Is It Important to Include Children in Medical Decision-Making?

Ethics

Traditionally, parents and physicians have made all medical decisions on behalf of children. However, just as the concept of informed consent has developed over the last 30 years with respect to competent adult patients, so new ways of thinking about the role of children in medical decision-making have evolved.

Ethical principles that provide guidance in the care of adults are insufficient in the context of caring for children.[1-3] Issues related to the voluntariness of consent, the disclosure of information, capacity assessment, treatment decisions and bereavement are more complex, as is the physician's relationship with the patient and the patient's family.[3,4] Adult models presume that the patient is autonomous and has a stable sense of self, established values and mature cognitive skills; these characteristics are undeveloped or underdeveloped in children.

Although it is important to understand and respect the developing autonomy of a child, and although the duty of beneficence provides a starting point for determining what is in the child's best interest, a family-centred ethic is the best model for understanding the interdependent relationships that bear upon the child's situation.[5] A family-centred approach considers the effects of a decision on all family members, their responsibilities toward one another and the burdens and benefits of a decision for each member, while acknowledging the special vulnerability of the child patient.

A family-centred approach presents special challenges for the health care team, particularly when there is disagreement between parent and child. Such a situation raises profound questions about the nature of the physician-patient relationship in pediatric practice. Integrity in this relationship is fundamental to the achievement of the goal of medicine,[6] which has been defined as "right and good healing action taken in the interest of a particular patient."[7] In the care of adults, the physician's primary relationship is with the particular capable patient. The patient's family may be involved in decision-making, but it is usually the patient who defines the bounds of such involvement.

The care of children, on the other hand, has been described in terms of a "triadic" relationship in which the child, his or her parents and the physician all have a necessary involvement (Dr. Abbyann Lynch, Director, Ethics in Health Care Associates, Toronto: personal communication, 1992). When there is disagreement between parent and child, the physician may experience some moral discomfort in having to deal separately with the child and parent.

The assumption that parents best understand what is in the interest of their child is usually sound. However, situations can arise in which the parents' distress prevents them from attending carefully to the child's concerns and wishes. Simply complying with the parents' wishes in such cases is inadequate. It is more helpful and respectful of the child to affirm the parents' responsibility for the care of their child while allowing the child to exercise choice in a measure appropriate to his or her level of development and experience of illness and treatment. This approach does not discount the parents' concerns and wishes, but recognizes the child as the particular patient to whom the physician has a primary duty of care. This approach seeks to harmonize the values of everyone involved in making the decision.[6,7]

Law

The legal right to refuse medical treatment is related to, but not identical with, the right to consent to treatment. The patient's right to refuse even life-saving medical treatment is recognized in Canadian law[8,9] and is premised on the patient's right to exercise control over his or her own body. Providing treatment despite a patient's valid refusal can constitute battery and, in some circumstances, negligence.

To be legally valid the refusal of medical treatment must be given by a person deemed capable of making health care choices, that is, capable of understanding the nature and consequences of the recommended treatment, alternative treatments and non-treatment. In common law the notion of the "mature minor" recognizes that some children are capable of making their own health care choices despite their age.[10] In common law and under the statutory law of some provinces patients are presumed capable regardless of age unless shown otherwise; in other provinces an age at which patients are presumed capable is specified.[11] When a child's capacity is in doubt an assessment is required.

In the case of children who are incapable of making their own health care decisions, parents or legal guardians generally have the legal authority to act as surrogate decision-makers. The surrogate decision-maker is obliged to make treatment decisions in the best interest of the child. Health care providers who believe that a surrogate's decisions are not in the child's best interest can appeal to provincial child welfare authorities. The courts have the authority to assume a *parens patriae* role in treatment decisions if the child is deemed to be in need of protection. This issue has arisen most commonly with respect to Jehovah's Witnesses who refuse blood transfusions for their children on religious grounds, and courts have authorized treatment in recognition of the state's interest in protecting the health and well-being of children.[12] Every province has child welfare legislation that sets out the general parameters of the "best interest" standard. Courts are reluctant to authorize the withholding or withdrawal of medical treatment, especially in the face of parental support for such treatment.

A special point to consider involves the use of patient restraints. The wrongful or excessive use of restraints could prompt an action of false imprisonment or battery. Restraint can involve the use of force, mechanical means or chemicals. The use of restraint compromises the dignity and liberty of the patient, including the child patient. Restraints should never be used solely to facilitate care but, rather, only when the patient is likely to cause serious bodily harm to himself or herself or to another. If restraint is required, the health care provider should use the least restrictive means possible, and the need for the restraint (as well as its effect on the patient) should be assessed on an ongoing basis.

Policy

The Canadian Paediatric Society has no policy regarding the role of the child patient in medical decision-making. The American Academy of Pediatrics statement on this question articulates the joint responsibility of physicians and parents to make decisions for very young patients in their best interest and states that "[p]arents and physicians should not exclude children and adolescents from decision-making without persuasive reasons."[13]

Empirical Studies

As they grow, children develop decision-making skills, the ability to reason using complex concepts, an understanding of death[14] and the ability to imagine a future for themselves.[15] Children with a chronic or terminal illness may have experiences that endow them with insight and maturity beyond their years. Families often encourage children to participate in decision-making. Allowing even young children to make decisions about simple matters facilitates the development of skills that they will need to make more complex decisions later on.[16-18]

Because tools developed to assess the capacity of adults have not been tested with children, health care professionals working with children should be sensitive to the particular capacity of each child. Children are constantly developing their physical, intellectual, emotional and personal maturity. Although developmental milestones give us a general sense of capacities, two children of the same age will not necessarily have the same ability to make choices. Even when they are deemed capable of making health care choices, children need support for their decisions from family members and the health care team.

How Should I Determine the Appropriate Role of a Child in Medical Decision-Making?

Most children fall into one of three groups with respect to their appropriate involvement in decision-making.[19,20]

Infants and Young Children

Preschool children have no significant decision-making capacity and cannot provide their own consent. As surrogate decision-makers, parents should authorize (or refuse authorization) on their child's behalf, basing their decisions on what they believe to be in the child's best interest.

Primary-School Children

Children of primary-school age may participate in medical decisions but do not have full decision-making capacity. They may indicate their assent or dissent without fully understanding its implications. Nonetheless they should be provided with information appropriate to their level of comprehension. Although the child's parents should authorize or refuse to authorize treatment, the child's assent should be sought and any strong and sustained dissent should be taken seriously.[21]

Adolescents

Many adolescents have the decision-making capacity of an adult.[22,23] This capacity will need to be determined for each patient in light of his or her

- ability to understand and communicate relevant information,
- ability to think and choose with some degree of independence,
- ability to assess the potential for benefit, risks or harms as well as to consider consequences and multiple options, and
- achievement of a fairly stable set of values.[24]

Many children and adolescents, particularly those who have been seriously ill, will need assistance in developing an understanding of the issues and in demonstrating their decision-making capacity. Age-appropriate discussion, perhaps with the assistance of teachers, chaplains, play therapists, nurses, psychologists or others skilled in communicating with children, are helpful. The child's participation may be facilitated by the use of art activities, stories, poems, role-playing and other techniques.[25,26]

Physicians should ensure that good decisions are made on behalf of their child patients. Although the interests of other family members are important and will influence decision-making, the child's interests are most important and are unlikely to be expressed or defended by the child himself or herself. Anxious, stressed or grieving family members may need assistance in focusing on what is best for the child. This may be especially difficult when a cure is no longer possible; in such cases a decision to stop treatment may seem like a decision to cause the child's death.

Whether or not the child participates, the following consideration should bear upon a treatment decision concerning that child:

- The potential benefits to the child
- The potential harmful consequences to the child, including physical suffering, psychological or spiritual distress and death
- The moral, spiritual and cultural values of the child's family

The Case

For Samantha, resuming aggressive treatment will have a serious negative effect on her quality of life. The chances of remission are small, yet a decision to discontinue treatment will likely result in her death. Because death is an irreversible harm, and decisions with serious consequences require a high level of competence in decision-making,[27] the capacity required would be very high. It has been determined that Samantha does not have this capacity.

Nevertheless, Samantha is included in discussions about her treatment options, and her reasons for refusing treatment are explored.[28] Members of the team work hard to re-establish trust. They and Samantha's parents come to agree that refusing treatment is not necessarily unreasonable; a decision by an adult patient in similar circumstances to discontinue treatment would certainly be honoured. Discussions address Samantha's and her parents' hopes and fears, their understanding of the possibility of cure, the meaning for them of the statistics provided by the physicians, Samantha's role in decision-mak-ing and her access to information. They are assisted by nurses, a child psychologist, a psychiatrist, a member of the clergy, a bioethicist, a social worker and a palliative care specialist.

Discussions focus on reaching a common understanding about the goals of treatment for Samantha. Her physician helps her to express her feelings and concerns about the likely effects of continued treatment. Consideration is given to the effects on her physical well-being, quality of life, self-esteem and dignity of imposing treatment against her wishes. Spiritual and psychological support for Samantha and her family is acknowledged to be an essential component of the treatment plan. Opportunities are provided for Samantha and her family to speak to others who have had similar experiences, and staff are given the opportunity to voice their concerns.

Ultimately, a decision is reached to discontinue chemotherapy and the goal of treatment shifts from "cure" to "care." Samantha's caregivers assure her and her family that they are not "giving up" but are directing their efforts toward Samantha's physical comfort and her spiritual and psychological needs. Samantha returns home, supported by a community palliative care program, and is allowed to have a new kitten. She dies peacefully.

Notes

1   Ruddick W. Parents and life prospects. In: O'Neill O., Ruddick W., editors. *Having children: philosophical and legal reflections on parenthood*. New York: Oxford University Press; 1979: 124.

2   Nelson J.L. Taking families seriously. *Hastings Cent Rep* 1992; 22: 6.

3   Hardwig J. What about the family? *Hastings Cent Rep* 1990; 20(2): 5-10.

4   Leikin S. A proposal concerning decisions to forgo life-sustaining treatment for young people. *J Pediatre* 1989; 115: 17-22.

5   Mahowald M. *Women and children in health care*. New York: Oxford University Press; 1993: 187, 189.

6   Hellman J. In pursuit of harmonized values: patient/parent-pediatrician relationships. In: Lynch A, editor. *The "good" pediatrician: an ethics curriculum for use in Canadian pediatrics residency programs*. Toronto: Pediatric Ethics Network; 1996.

7   Pellegrino E.D. Toward a reconstruction of medical morality: the primacy of the act of profession and the fact of illness. *J Med Philos* 1979; 4: 47.

8   *Malett v. Shulman* [1990], 67 DLR (4th) (Ont CA).

9   Art. 11 CCQ.

10   Rozovsky L.E., Rozovsky F.A. *The Canadian law of consent to treatment*. Toronto: Butterworths; 1992: 53-57.

11   Etchells E., Sharpe G., Elliott C., Singer P.A. Bioethics for clinicians 3: Capacity. *Can Med Assoc J* 1996; 155: 657-61.

12   *R.B. v. Children's Aid Society of Metropolitan Toronto*, [1995] 1 SCR 315 (SCC).

13   American Academy of Pediatrics. Informed consent, parental permission and assent in pediatric practice. *Pediatrics* 1995; 95: 314-17.

14   Matthews G.R. Children's conceptions of illness and death. In: Kopelman L.M., Moskop J.C., editors. *Children and health care: moral and social issues*. Dordrecht (Holland): Kluwer Academic Publishers; 1989: 133-46.

15   Koocher G.P., DeMaso D. Children's competence to consent to medical procedures. *Pediatrician* 1990; 17: 68-73.

16   King N.M.P., Cross A.W. Children as decision makers: guidelines for pediatricians. *J Pediatr* 1989; 115: 10-16.

17   Lewis M.A., Lewis C.E. Consequences of empowering children to care for themselves. *Pediatrician* 1990; 17: 63-67.

18   Yoos H.L. Children's illness concepts: old and new paradigms. *Pediatr Nurs* 1994; 20: 134-45.

19   Broome M.E, Stieglitz K.A. The consent process and children. *Res Nurs Health* 1992; 15: 147-52.

20   Erlen J.A. The child's choice: an essential component in treatment decisions. *Child Health Care* 1987; 15: 156-60.

21   Baylis F. The moral weight of a child's dissent. *Ethics Med Pract* 1993; 3(1): 2-3.

22   Weithorn L.A., Campbell S.B. The competency of children and adolescents to make informed treatment decisions. *Child Dev* 1982; 53: 1589-98.

23   Lewis C.C. How adolescents approach decisions; changes over grades seven to twelve and policy implications. *Child Dev* 1981; 52: 538-44.

24   Brock D.W. Children's competence for health care decisionmaking. In: Kopelman L.M., Moskop J.C., editors. *Children and health care: moral and social issues*. Dordrecht (Holland): Kluwer Academic Publishers; 1989: 181-212.

25   Adams P.L., Fras I. *Beginning child psychiatry*. New York: Bruner/Mazel; 1988.

26   Kestenbaum C.J., Williams D., editors. *Handbook of clinical assessment of children and adolescents*. New York: University Press; 1988.

27   Dran J.F. The many faces of competency. *Hastings Cent Rep* 1985; 15(2): 17-21.

28   Freyer D.R. Children with cancer: special considerations in the discontinuation of life-sustaining treatment. *Med Pediatr Oncol* 1992; 20: 136-42.

14.
PROXY CONSENT FOR RESEARCH ON THE INCOMPETENT ELDERLY

Barry F. Brown

SOURCE: James E. Thornton and Earl R. Winkler (eds.), *Ethics & Aging* (Vancouver: UBC Press, 1988).

In the past decade, the ethical issues of research with the elderly have become of increasing interest in gerontology, medicine, law, and biomedical ethics. In particular, the issue has been raised whether the elderly deserve special protection as a dependent group (Ratzan 1980). One of the most profound difficulties in this area of reflection is that of the justification of proxy consent for research on borderline or definitely incompetent patients.

Some diseases of the elderly, such as Alzheimer's disease, cause senile dementia: devastating for the patient and family and, in future, a considerable burden for society. This condition, in turn, renders a patient incapable of giving informed, voluntary consent to research procedures designed to learn about the natural history of the disease, to control it, and to find a cure. The research must be done on human subjects, since there is not as yet a suitable animal model; indeed some feel that there never can be such a model. A protection of the patient, rooted in concern for his best interests, from procedures to which he cannot give consent gives rise to a paradox: "If we can only perform senile dementia research using demented patients, but should not allow them to participate because they are incompetent, then we are left in a quandary. We cannot ethically conduct senile dementia research using demented patients because they are incompetent; but we cannot technically perform it using competent subjects because they are not demented" (Ratzan 1980: 36). Such a position seems to protect demented patients at the expense of their exposure, as a class, to prolonged misery or death.

If the patient cannot give consent, is the proxy consent of relatives ethically valid? That is, do the relatives have the moral right or capacity to give con-

sent for procedures that may not offer much hope for the patient in that they may not offer a direct benefit to him?

Such procedures have by recent convention been called non-therapeutic. They might offer a possible benefit for other sufferers in the future, but little hope of benefit for *this* patient, here and now.

At present, an impasse has developed regarding such research. It appears that such procedures might be illegal under criminal laws on assault. If the research is strictly non-therapeutic, then no benefit is to be found for the patient-subject. If the requirement of therapeutic experimentation is that a direct, or fairly immediate, improvement in the patient's condition is the sole benefit that could count, then it is difficult to see how this could be discovered. For unlike the case of a curable disease or research on preventive measures for childhood diseases, such as polio, the Alzheimer's patients suffer from a presently terminal illness. Studies of the causation of this condition may hold little or no hope of alleviating the condition in them. There appears to be no present or future benefit directly accruing to them. Others may benefit, but they likely will not. Thus, it seems, there is no benefit in view.

If, in fact, such procedures, even relatively innocuous ones, are illegal, then such research cannot go ahead. If so, such persons will remain "therapeutic orphans" just as surely as infants and children unless proxy consent is valid. If proxy consent is also legally invalid, then the legal challenge to this impasse may be either legislative or judicial. In either case, ethical arguments must be offered as justification for the case that proxy consent is or ought to be legally valid. The following explorations are a contribution to that debate.

Can some kind of benefit for the demented be found in research that offers no immediate hope of improvement? I believe that it can, but the nature of that benefit will be unfamiliar or unacceptable to those who are sure that there are only two mutually exclusive alternatives: a utilitarian conception of the social good pitted against a deontological notion of the individual's rights.

Contemporary biomedical ethics routinely employs three principles in its effort to resolve such dilemmas (Reich 1970; Beauchamp & Childress 1983). These are the principle of beneficence, which demands that we do good and prevent harm; the principle of respect for persons (or the principle of autonomy), from which flows the requirement of informed consent; and the principle of justice, which demands the equitable distribution of the benefits and burdens of research. But the first two obviously conflict with each other in human experimentation: the principle of beneficence, which mandates research to save life and restore health, especially if this is seen as directed to the good of society, is in tension with the principle of respect for persons, which requires us to protect the autonomy of subjects. Moreover, the principle of beneficence requires us not only to benefit persons as patients through research, but also to avoid harming them as research subjects in the process. So there is an internal tension between moral demands created by the same principle. Finally, demented patients are no longer fully or sufficiently autonomous. Standard objections to paternalism do not apply. Consequently paternalism of the parental sort is not inappropriate, but rather necessary in order to protect the interest of the patient.

Simple application of these principles, therefore, will not provide a solution. Underlying the manner in which they are applied are radically different conceptions of the relationship of the individual good to the societal or common good.

In the present framework of philosophical opinion, there appear to be two major positions. On the one hand, some consequentialist arguments for non-therapeutic research justify non-consensual research procedures on the grounds that individual needs are subordinate to the general good conceived as an aggregate of individual goods. This good, that of the

society as a whole, can easily be seen to take precedence over that of individuals. This is especially so if the disease being researched is conceptualized as an "enemy" of society. On the other hand, a deontological position argues that the rights of the individual take precedence over any such abstract general good as the advancement of science, the progress of medicine, or the societal good. In this view, to submit an individual incapable of giving or withholding consent to research procedures not for his own direct benefit is to treat him solely as a means, not as an end in himself. In this debate, one side characterizes the general good proposed by the other as much too broad and inimical to human liberty; the other sees the emphasis on individual rights as excessively individualistic or atomistic.

There are strengths and weaknesses in both approaches. The consequentialist rightly insists on a communal good, but justifies too much; the deontologist rightly protects individual interests, but justifies too little. I contend that if we are to resolve the dilemma concerning the incompetent "therapeutic orphan," it is necessary to go between these poles. In order to do so, I wish to draw upon and develop some recent explorations concerning non-therapeutic research with young children. In at least one important respect, that of incompetence, children and the demented are similar. We ought to treat similar cases similarly. I wish also to argue that research ethics requires: (1) a conception of the *common good* that is at once narrower than that of society as a whole and yet transcends immediate benefit to a single individual; and (2) a conception of the common good that sees it not in opposition to the individual good but including it, so that the good is seen as distributed to individuals.

The Lesson of Research with Children

As to the first, we may learn much from the discussions concerning research with children, particularly as they bear upon the distinction between therapeutic and non-therapeutic experimentation. In the 1970s a spirited debate took place between the noted ethicists Paul Ramsey and Richard McCormick on the morality of experimentation with children (Ramsey 1970, 1976, 1977; McCormick 1974, 1976).

Ramsey presented a powerful deontological argument against non-therapeutic experimentation with children. Since infants and young children cannot give consent, an essential requirement of the canon of loyalty between researcher and subject, they cannot be subjected ethically to procedures not intended for their own benefit. To do so, he contended, is to treat children solely as means to an end (medical progress), not as ends in themselves (Ramsey 1970).

McCormick, arguing from a natural law position similar to that developed in the next section, argued that since life and health are fundamental natural goods, even children have an obligation to seek to preserve them. Medical research is a necessary condition of ensuring health, and this is a desirable social goal. Consequently children, as members of society, have a duty in social justice to wish to accept their share of the burdens of participating in research that promise benefit to society and is of minimal or no risk. Thus the parents' proxy consent is a reasonable presumption of the child's wishes if he were able to consent (McCormick 1974).

There are two major puzzles generated by this debate over non-therapeutic research in children. First, Ramsey stressed that the condition to which a child may be at risk need not reside within his skin, but could be an epidemic dread disease. Thus, testing of preventive measures such as polio vaccine on children is justified; indeed it counts for Ramsey as therapeutic. This is interesting for several reasons. First, the therapeutic benefit may be indirect or remote, not necessarily immediate. Second, it embodies the concept of a group or population at risk smaller than society as a whole. Third, it apparently allows for considerable risk. There was a risk of contracting polio from the vaccine. Although the risk might have been slight statistically, the potential damage was grave. By Ramsey's own account, a slight risk of grave damage is a grave risk. Thus, he was prepared to go beyond the limit of minimal or no risk on the grounds that the polio vaccine was *therapeutic*, while McCormick attempted to justify *non-therapeutic* research on children, but confined the risk to minimal or none. It is odd that in the subsequent protracted debate, this difference was not contested.

The second major puzzle arises from McCormick's view that fetuses, infants, and children

ought to participate in low- or no-risk non-therapeutic research in order to share in the burden of social and medical progress in order that all may prosper. Note that only *burdens* are to be shared, not benefits. This is because the topic by definition was non-therapeutic experimentation. By putting it this way he seemed to many to be subordinating the interests of such subjects to a very broadly construed societal good. But let us remember that the argument for such research in the first place was that without it, infants and children would be "therapeutic orphans." That is, without pediatric research, there could be fewer and slower advances in pediatric therapy.

Although not of direct benefit, such research is intended for the long-term benefit of children, and is thus indirectly or remotely therapeutic. It is not conducted for "the benefit of society" or for "the advancement of medical science"; it is for children in the future. Otherwise, it could be carried out on adults. Thus, such research should be construed as done not in view of broad social benefit but for the benefit of children as a group or a sub-set of society. Of course, if advances are made in medicine for the sake of children, society benefits as well, but this is incidental and unnecessary. The sole justification is provided by the benefits now and to come for *children*. At the same time, such benefits set one of the limits for such research: it should be confined to children's conditions, and it should not be directed at conditions for which the research may be done on competent persons.

The Common Good of a Disease Community

Some of the hints arising from the foregoing debate can now be developed. It is indeed wrong to experiment on an incompetent person for "the benefit of society" if the research is unrelated to that person's disease and he is made a subject simply because he is accessible and unresistant. But is it necessarily unethical to conduct experiments on an incompetent person which attempt to discover the cause of the condition which causes the incompetence, and which may cure it or prevent it in others, even if he will not himself be cured?

In a "third way" of conceptualizing the relation between the individual and the group, the good in view is neither that of society as a whole nor that of a single individual. It involves the group of persons with a condition, such as Alzheimer's disease. Here I turn to a conception of the common good articulated by John Finnis of Oxford. Finnis defines the common good not as the "greatest good for the greatest number" but as "a set of conditions which enables the members of a community to attain for themselves reasonable objectives, or to realize reasonably for themselves the value(s) for the sake of which they have reason to collaborate with each other (positively and/or negatively) in a community" (Finnis 1980: 155).

The community may be either the complete community or the political one, or it may be specialized, such as the medical community, the research community, or the community of children with leukemia, and so on. The common good is thus not the sum total of individual interests, but an ensemble of conditions which enable individuals to pursue their objectives or purposes, which enable them to flourish. The purposes are fundamental human goods: life, health, play, esthetic experience, knowledge, and others. Relevant to this discussion are life, health, especially mental integrity, and the consequent capacity for knowledge, all of which are threatened by diseases which cause dementia.

For my purposes, the community should be considered to be, at a minimum, those suffering from Alzheimer's disease. They have, even if they have never explicitly associated with each other, common values and dis-values: their lost health and the remaining health and vitality they possess. It could be said with McCormick that if they could do so, they would reasonably wish the good of preventing the condition in their relatives and friends.

But the community may be rightly construed more broadly than this. It naturally includes families with whom the patients most closely interact and which interact in voluntary agencies devoted to the condition, the physicians who treat them, the nurses, social workers, and occupational therapists who care for them, and the clinical and basic researchers who are working to understand, arrest, cure, and prevent the disease.

The participation of the patient, especially the demented patient, may be somewhat passive. He is a member of the specialized community by accident, not by choice, unless he has indicated his wish to become a research subject while still competent. Efforts to determine what a demented or retarded person would have wished for himself had he been competent have been made in American court decisions involving an incompetent patient's medical care. These "substituted judgment" approaches may have some worth, especially if the patient had expressed and recorded his wishes while still competent.

An individual might execute a document analogous to a human tissue gift—a sort of pre-dementia gift, in which he would officially and legally offer his person to medical research if and when he became demented. This might alleviate the problem of access to some extent, but it has its own difficulties. A pre-dementia volunteer cannot know in advance what types of research procedures will be developed in future, and so cannot give a truly informed consent except to either very specific procedures now known or to virtually anything. Such a pre-commitment may give some support to the decision to allow him to be a subject. But that decision, I contend, is justified by the claim, if valid, that it is for the common good of the dementia-care-research community, of which he is a member and to which, it is presumed, he would commit himself if he were capable of doing so at the time.

It is true, of course, that one might not ever have wished to participate in research procedures. In this case, the individual should be advised to register his or her objection in advance, along the lines that have been suggested for objection to organ donation in those countries that have a system of presumed consent for such donation. This can be achieved by carrying a card on which such an opt-out is recorded, or by placing one's name on a registry which might be maintained by support organizations. I suggest that unless one opts out in this manner, in the early stages of the disease, he or she be considered to have opted-in. That is, there should be a policy of presumed consent. In any event, as experience with organ retrieval has shown, in the final analysis it is the permission of relatives that is decisive in both those cases in which an individual has consented and those in which he or she has not made his or her wishes known.

The other members of the community may not all know each other. They do, however, have common values and, to a considerable degree, common objectives. There can be a high level of deliberate and active interaction, especially if there is close communication between the researchers, family, and volunteers in the voluntary health agencies.

What, then, is the ensemble of conditions which constitute the common good of the Alzheimer's community? Insofar as the purposes of collaboration include the effort to cure or to alleviate the disease, the common good would embrace, in addition to caring health professionals, a policy of promoting research, its ethical review, a sufficient number of committed clinical and scientific researchers, the requisite physical facilities and funding (some or all of which may be within other communities such as hospitals and medical schools), availability of volunteers for research, an atmosphere of mutual trust between research and subject, and finally ongoing research itself. This list is not exhaustive.

If access to the already demented is not allowed, and if this is essential for research on the disease to continue, it may well be impossible to find the answers to key questions about the disease. The common good of the Alzheimer's community would be damaged or insufficiently promoted. Since the goods of life and mental health are fundamental goods, this insufficiency would be profound.

One essential aspect of this common good is distributive justice. Each patient-subject shares not only in the burdens of research in order that all may prosper, but also the benefits. The benefits are not necessarily improved care or cure for the subject, but generally improved conditions for all such patient-subjects: a more aggressive approach to research, improved knowledge of the disease, increased probabilities for a cure, and others. Since the individual participates wholly in that good, he will be deprived of it in its entirety if it is not pursued. The common good is not so much a quantity of benefits as a quality of existence. It can therefore be distributed in its fullness to each member of the community. So, too, each can suffer its diminution.

Richard McCormick (1974) left his description of the common good unnecessarily broad and sweeping. According to some natural law theorists (Mari-

tain 1947) the common good is always a distributed good, not simply the sum of parts. It is construed as flowing back upon the individual members of the community, who are not simply parts of a whole but persons, to whom the common good is distributed in its entirety. Thus, not only can the common good of which McCormick speaks be narrowed to that of children as a group (equivalent to Ramsey's population at risk) but the benefits of such research can be seen as redistributed to the individuals of the group. The benefits are not to be taken in the sense of an immediately available therapy, but in the sense of improved general conditions under which a cure, amelioration, or prevention for all is more likely.

Conclusion

Some of these observations can now be applied to the case of the elderly demented. First, the debate showed the inadequacy of the simple distinction between therapeutic and non-therapeutic experimentation, which has been challenged on several grounds in past years. For example, May (1976: 83) includes diagnostic and preventive types of research under therapeutic experimentation, whereas Reich (1978: 327) observes that the terms "therapeutic" and "non-therapeutic" are inadequate because they do not seem to include research on diagnostic and preventive techniques. In the area of the development of experimental preventive measures such as vaccines for epidemic diseases, and in the area of diseases in which research is carried out on terminal patients with little or no expectation of immediate benefit for these patients, the distinction is somewhat blurred. In each case, there is a defined population at risk: one without the disease but at great risk of contracting it, the other with a disease but with little hope of benefiting from the research.

Such types of research seem to constitute an intermediate category: the "indirectly therapeutic," involving the hope of either prevention or alleviation or cure. This category as applied to dementia shows some characteristics of therapeutic experimentation in the accepted sense, since it is carried out on persons who are ill and it is directed to their own illness. But it also shares some properties of non-therapeutic research, since it is not for their immediate treatment

[handwritten margin note: will be impossible to find a cure for it.]

[handwritten margin note: benefit does not have to be in terms of individual (egoism)]

[handwritten margin note: indirect therapeutic]

and, therefore, benefit. The good to be achieved is more remote, both in time and in application, since it is less sharply located in the individual than is therapy as such.

It must be admitted that there is a difference between the testing of a vaccine for prevention of disease in young, healthy children and research on elderly, seriously ill patients. In the former, the child-subjects will benefit if the vaccine is successful, or at least be protected from harm. In the latter, the subjects will not benefit by way of prevention or cure of their disease, but rather simply by being part of a community in which those goals are being actively pursued. The identification of the demented patient's good with that common good is doubtless less concrete than the identification of the child's good with that of his peers. But it seems to me that underlying both these cases is a notion of the common good required to justify all cases of research that do not promise a hope of direct benefit to a person who is, here and now, ill.

Years ago, Hans Jonas (1969) noted that a physician-researcher might put the following question to a dying patient: "There is nothing more I can do for you. But there is something you can do for me. Speaking no longer as your physician but on behalf of medical science, we could learn a great deal about future cases of this kind if you would permit me to perform certain experiments on you. It is understood that you yourself would not benefit from any knowledge we might gain; but future patients would." Although greatly vulnerable and deserving of maximum protection, such a patient might be ethically approached to be a research subject, because the benefits to future patients are in a way a value to him: "At least that residue of identification is left him that it is his own affliction by which he can contribute to the conquest of that affliction, his own kind of suffering which he helps alleviate in others; and so *in a sense it is his own cause*" (Jonas 1969: 532, emphasis mine).

In this case, the individual apprehends a good greater than his personal good, less than that of society: that of his disease class, which is *his* good. Of course, the identification of which Jonas speaks is psychological; he would likely not agree with the approach herein outlined and might require that such

participation be through a conscious, free choice of the patient. Nevertheless, it is a real, objective good which justifies his choice and prevents us from asking him to participate in research unrelated to his disease. Can a relative, a son or daughter perhaps, ethically make that decision for an incompetent, demented Alzheimer's patient? If so, it is because, in a sense, it is the patient's cause, the patient's good as a member of a community which justifies that choice. It is not a matter of enforcing a social duty or minimal social obligation here, but seeking a good that lies in the relationship one has to others with the same disease. That same good, as noted above, limits the participation of the subject to research related precisely to his disease, not to anything else.

What is the implication of this for risk and the limits of risk? As has been seen, some wish to allow for exposure of subjects to greater than minimal risk provided only that it is classified as "therapeutic" (though the subjects are not ill). Others, in spite of the fact that the research is intended for the benefit of a group at risk, classify it as non-therapeutic and limit the acceptable risk to minimal levels. Are these the only alternatives? One advisory group has allowed, in the case of the mentally incompetent, for a "minor increase over minimal risk" in such circumstances (National Commission for the Protection of Human Subjects 1978: 16). This is presumably permitted because the research is "of vital importance for the understanding or amelioration of the type of disorder or condition of the subjects" or "may reasonably be expected to benefit the subjects in future" (17). But what counts as minor increase in risk? Proposed research into Alzheimer's might involve invasive procedures such as brain biopsies, implantation of electrodes, spinal taps, and injections of experimental drugs. Are these of greater risk than that specified by the National Commission simply because they are invasive of the human brain? Or is there clear statistical risk of serious added damage to the brain? These are matters for empirical study. The invasiveness per se should not rule out a procedure. The major limitations should be whether the procedure is painful, causes anxiety, or adds to the already serious damage to the brain. If research involving procedures of greater risk than "minor increase over minimal" is ever to be justified, it must be so by the intent to avert the proportional evils of death or mental incapacity. If these are insufficient, then I fail to see what grounds might be available upon which to base a case for legislative change.

It is clear, then, that should such research be acceptable it also demands that stringent protective procedures be established in order to ensure that the demented are not drafted into research unrelated to their disease class. This is because the standard, being broader than that of "direct or fairly immediate benefit," is open to an accordion-like expansion, and therefore to abuse. Such safeguards could include: rigorous assurance that the proxy's consent (in reality, simply a permission) is informed and voluntary, the provision of a consent auditor, and various layers of administrative review and monitoring, from a local institutional review board up to a judicial review with a guardian appointed to represent the patient-subject's rights. These procedures may prove to be onerous. But we are on dangerous ground, and as we try to avoid overprotection, which may come at the expense of improved therapy for all, we must also avoid opening up a huge door to exploitation.

References

Beauchamp, T.L., & Childress, J.F. 1983. *Principles of biomedical ethics*. 2nd ed. New York: Oxford University Press.

Finnis, J. 1980. *Natural law and natural rights*. Oxford: Clarendon Press.

Jonas, H. 1969. Philosophical reflections on experimenting with human subjects. In T. Beauchamp and L. Walters (Eds.), *Contemporary issues in bioethics*. 2nd ed. Belmont, CA: Wadsworth.

Maritain, J. 1974. *The person and the common good*. New York: Charles Scribner's Sons.

May, W. 1976. Proxy consent to human experimentation. *Linacre Quarterly* 43: 73-84.

McCormick, R. 1974. Proxy consent in the experimentation situation. *Perspectives in Biology and Medicine* 18: 2-20.

McCormick, R. 1976. "Experimentation in children: sharing in sociality." *Hastings Center Report* 6: 41-46.

National Commission for the Protection of Human Subjects. 1978. *Report and recommendations: Research involving those institutionalized as mentally infirm*. Washington, DC.

Ramsey, P. 1970. *The patient as person*. New Haven: Yale University Press.

Ramsey, P. 1976. The enforcement of morals: Non-therapeutic research on children. *Hastings Center Report* 4: 21-30.

Ramsey, P. 1977. Children as research subjects: a reply. *Hastings Center Report* 2: 40-41.

Ratzan, R. 1980. "Being old makes you different": The ethics of research with elderly subjects. *Hastings Center Report* 5: 32-42.

Reich, W. 1978. Ethical issues related to research involving elderly subjects. *Gerontologist* 18: 326-37.

15.
REIBL V. HUGHES [1980]
SUPREME COURT OF CANADA

Case Summary by C. Morano

SOURCE: http://csc.lexum.org/en/1980/1980scr2-880/1980scr2-880.html.

[Reibl v. Hughes is a Supreme Court of Canada decision that focuses on a physician's duty of care and the factors that are important to informed consent. The court considers three standards of disclosure.]

Present: Laskin C.J. and Martland, Dickson, Beetz, Estey, McIntyre and Chouinard JJ.

On Appeal from the Court of Appeal for Ontario.

Background

The plaintiff appellant 44 underwent serious surgery and following the procedure suffered a massive stroke causing paralysis on the left side of his body as well as impotence. The surgeon did not inform him of the risk of paralysis in having the surgery, but did tell him that the chances of paralysis were greater if he did not have the surgery. The plaintiff recovered damages in both battery and negligence at the trial on the grounds that he had not given informed consent to the procedure, and he was awarded a total sum of $225,000. A majority of the Ontario Court of Appeal ordered a new trial on both liability and damages and ruled out battery as a possible ground of liability based on the facts of the case.

The Supreme Court of Canada

A majority of the Supreme Court agreed with the trial judge's findings, specifically that "the issue of informed consent to treatment is a concomitant of the physician's duty of care. A surgeon's duty to exercise due skill and care in giving his patient reasonable information and advice with respect to the risks specifically attendant on a proposed operative procedure arises out of the special relationship between them.... [T]he scope of this professional duty of care is defined by the evaluation of a variety of inter-related factors which bear uniquely on each case, factors such as the presence of an emergency requiring immediate treatment; the patient's emotional and intellectual make-up, and his ability to appreciate and cope with the relevant facts; the gravity of the known risks, both in terms of their likelihood and the severity of this realization." Therefore, consent is not considered to be informed unless the patient understands the information provided by the doctor. It is the surgeon's duty not only to provide a patient with the information, but to make sure that he or she also understands it. The trial judge concluded that the plaintiff was probably left with the misunderstanding that the operation was being undertaken to alleviate his headaches and hypertension and to permit him to function effectively at his job. "I find that the defendant did not take sufficient care to convey to the plaintiff and assure that the plaintiff understood the gravity, nature and extent of risks specifically attendant on the endarterectomy, in particular the risk that as a result of the operation he could die or suffer a stroke of varying degrees of severity."

The Supreme Court also considered three standards of disclosure and commented on each of them: the professional medical standard, a subjective standard, and an objective standard. The majority found that both the Ontario Court of Appeal and the trial judge had adopted a professional medical standard, not only for determining the material risks that should be disclosed but also, and concurrently, for determining whether there has been a breach of the duty of disclosure. Speaking on behalf of the majority, Laskin C.J. said, "[T]o allow expert medical evidence to determine what risks are material and, hence, should be disclosed and, correlatively, what risks are not material is to hand over to the medical profession the entire question of the scope of the duty of disclosure including the question whether there has been a breach of that duty." As for a subjective test, the court doubted that this kind of test would solve the problem, because it is unlikely that the patient suing would admit that he would have agreed to the surgery if he had been told about all of the risks. The court determined that it is safer on the issue of causation to consider objectively how far the balance in the risks of surgery or no surgery is in favour of undergoing surgery. The adoption of an objective standard does not mean that the issue of causation is completely in the hands of surgeon. The patient's particular situation and the degree to which the risks of surgery or no surgery are balanced would reduce the force of the surgeon's recommendation on an objective evaluation. Laskin concluded that "... the record of evidence amply justifies the trial judge's findings that the plaintiff was told no more or understood no more than that he would be better off to have the operation than not to have it. This was not an adequate, nor a sufficient disclosure of the risk attendant upon the operation itself, a risk well appreciated by the defendant in view of his own experience that of the sixty to seventy such operations that he had previously performed, eight to ten resulted in the death of the patients."

On this issue of causation, the Supreme Court concluded that a reasonable person in the plaintiff's position would have declined surgery at the particular time given the fact that he was within about one and one-half years of earning pension benefits if he continued at his job and there was no neurological deficit then apparent; that there was no immediate emergency making the surgery imperative; that there was a grave risk of a stroke or worse during or as a result of the operation, while the risk of a stroke without it was in the future, with no precise time fixed or which could be fixed except as a guess of three or more years ahead. Since on the trial judge's finding, the plaintiff was under the mistaken impression, as a result of the defendant's breach of the duty of disclosure, that the surgery would relieve his continuing headaches, this would, in the opinion of a reasonable person in the plaintiff's position, also weigh against submitting to the surgery at the particular time. The court restored the judgment at trial and concluded that the plaintiff appellant was entitled to costs throughout.

16.
GAINING FACE OR LOSING FACE? FRAMING THE DEBATE ON FACE TRANSPLANTS

Richard Huxtable and Julie Woodley

SOURCE: *Bioethics* 19.5/6 (2005): 505-22.

I. Introduction

The possibility of transplanting one human face onto another human body was brought to international attention by the British surgeon Dr Peter Butler in 1998.[1] Since then the proposal has attracted much attention in professional, academic and media circles. Professional medical bodies in at least two countries have examined the topic: reports from a British Royal College of Surgeons Working Party and the French National Consultative Ethics Committee for Health and Life Sciences both concluded that the risks currently outweigh any perceived benefits, and have led to a professional moratorium on the procedure.[2] However, a team of surgeons from Louisville, in the United States of America, has recently claimed not only that there is a favourable ethical climate in their institution but also that the risks/benefits ratio is in equipoise, and they therefore wish to proceed.[3]

The Louisville team has, however, invited further discussion of the issues and in this paper we seek to frame that discussion through identifying seven areas of contention and raising a series of questions, albeit without providing answers in all cases. First, we consider what the procedure would and could achieve for the disfigured. That the initial transplants will result in a hybrid appearance and will not improve facial function are important considerations. Equally important, however, is the prospect of the wholesale adoption of another individual's face, which raises concerns that need to be addressed early on. Secondly, we ask why the procedure is being developed, and note that this is a major surgical procedure primarily aimed at addressing psychological difficulties. Thirdly, as the Louisville team

implies, we argue that the procedure is sufficiently novel to warrant thorough analysis and discussion before it is attempted. The British bioethicist Dr Richard Nicholson feels this analysis is premature and unnecessary.[4] We do accept that the technical expertise required and ethical questions posed are certainly familiar, focusing as they do on the autonomy of those involved and the associated risks and benefits. However, the similarities are only skin deep precisely because we are addressing the face, which has considerable importance in terms of identity, self-perception and the way one is perceived by others. The procedure must therefore be considered experimental and analysed accordingly. We then proceed to analyse the issues with particular regard for the recipients of the transplant. Fourthly, then, we ask who are the most likely recipients? Here we identify some difficulties in terms of the autonomy of the recipient, which point to a Catch-22 where those most likely to be able to cope with the transplant and its associated risks ironically appear to be the least 'in need' of receiving it. Fifthly, we consider how receiving a donated face might affect the individual, particularly given the importance of the face in terms of identity and perception. We note, with reference to some analogous scientific developments, that the effects are far from predictable. Our sixth concern is that the patient might be influenced or even coerced by our beauty-fixated society and as such there may be less invasive and certainly less risky means of improving both society's and disfigured individuals' reactions to facial disfigurement. These observations lead us to consider finally whether the question is best posed as 'whether?' or 'when?' facial transplantation should occur. While we have no major problem with the procedure in principle, it seems likely that there will always be a degree of risk, perhaps even a significant degree, for the recipients. Whether autonomy and thus individual choice should govern in this matter is open to debate, and debate is indeed needed in order to establish how far the possibility of gaining face should outweigh the more likely danger of losing face.

II. What Is Envisaged?

As described by the Louisville team, the procedure will involve de-gloving the facial tissue and vasculature from a recently-deceased donor and then attaching it to a recipient. The surgeons claim that this procedure is technically possible as it utilises many established surgical techniques. Indeed, cases of reattachment of an individual's own face and results from animals where the faces of black rats were transplanted onto white ones indicate the feasibility of this procedure.[5]

In terms of the anticipated results, we do not yet appear to be in the realm of the popular John Woo film *Face/Off*, in which a criminal and an FBI agent wholly swap faces. The recipient will be left with a hybrid appearance, since the donor face will be fitted over the tip of their own nose and they will also retain their own lips, eyelids as well as, significantly, their underlying facial skeleton.[6] As the expertise develops, however, there is the possibility that Woo's science fiction will become science fact, since surgeons might also become able to transplant the donor's underlying bone structure, thereby affording the recipient an appearance much closer to the donor's.

III. Why?

Those expected to benefit from the introduction of face transplants include some people born with facial disfigurement and others who have endured, for example, ballistic trauma, severe burns or facial cancers. Whilst skin grafts from the person's own body are already routinely performed, these have their drawbacks, not least in terms of the series of painful operations that are sometimes required. A face transplant would instead mean one operation, which should result in a more continuous visage.

Christine Piff, founder of the support group Let's Face It, has suggested that the procedure might at some point benefit those who cannot eat, drink or speak.[7] That development may be some way away, however. Dr Butler has stated that in the early phase the transplanted face will not function as such; only when extensive nerve regeneration is possible will this occur. The transplanted face may however be more flexible than current skin grafts (using the patient's own non-facial skin),[8] and should provide a better aesthetic appearance, but it may well result in a decrease in function. As such, the recipient would effectively be receiving a 'mask.' If we take the example of an individual with rigid scar tissue resulting from a burn, they would receive a(n allegedly) better aesthetic appearance albeit at the expense of some facial functioning. It is therefore important to note that we are primarily addressing an improvement in appearance.

IV. Where Is the Novelty?

In purely technical terms, it might be argued that a face transplant is merely an extension of techniques already familiar to transplant and plastic surgeons. Transplantation of major organs is regarded as relatively uncontentious in the developed world. Last year, for example, 2,854 organs were transplanted in the United Kingdom alone.[9] Furthermore, surgeons have been performing skin grafts and undertaking reconstructive surgery for years. Of course, neither field is free from ethical controversy, as continuing debates over the sale of human organs and the validity of purely cosmetic surgery demonstrate, but the therapeutic value of such procedures is relatively widely accepted.[10] Equally, the ethicist should be in familiar territory, as the issues pertaining to face transplants are readily articulated in terms of harm, benefit, autonomy, dignity and justice.

However, lest we become too comfortable, we must acknowledge that we are contemplating the transplantation of a face. Certainly, the face, like other currently transplantable body parts, is possessed of blood and nerve supplies. And yet, although we will have more to say on the nature of personal identity, it is undeniable that the face occupies a (loosely drawn) category of organs and tissues that have a special significance to the individual and the wider world within which he or she exists. Hearts, brains and eyes are usually seen as more important and more constitutive of personal identity than organs like, for example, the spleen. In colloquial terms, the heart symbolises our emotional selves (consider terms such as 'heartless,' 'heart-broken' and 'heartfelt'), the brain is connected with our minds and/or souls, and the eyes provide the 'windows of the soul.' This category of 'special' organs may well be relative to time and place: the Ancient Egyptians, for example, believed that the heart was the 'seat of the soul' while the tongue was the 'seat of the mind.' Attitudes do therefore change over time, as has apparently occurred in the case of heart transplants, which were widely condemned when first proposed by Christiaan Barnard in 1967.[11] Nevertheless, we predict that the face will continue to occupy a pivotal perceptual position, important as it is in terms of one's own self-perception and how others perceive one. The very visibility of the face immediately distinguishes it from other, less obviously visible, forms of transplantation that are located beneath the skin. This might go some way to explaining why the recent transplant of a jawbone performed by Professor Giuseppe Spriano did not attract the same degree of attention.[12]

Thus, although it does indeed build upon preexisting knowledge and can indeed be viewed through familiar prisms, there is prima facie good reason for treating facial transplantation as qualitatively different from existing surgical procedures. Furthermore, familiar issues such as the risk of the tissue being rejected assume an even greater significance in this context. For these reasons, this must be viewed as experimental and analysed accordingly. Research ethicists will be used to addressing the risks and benefits of a proposed innovation and in the remainder of this paper we seek to identify the issues relevant to this calculation through consideration of a central question: who are we treating?

V. Who Is the Patient? (Part 1)

The first cluster of issues relates specifically to the recipient of the donor face. Who should be considered for the procedure and according to which criteria? Not infrequently appeals are made to notions of autonomy and beneficence (or non-maleficence), such that the ideal subject (patient?) autonomously decides to submit to the procedure, which it is hoped will provide them with some benefit (or at least be no more harmful than existing options).

Taking the autonomy criterion first, a maximally autonomous agent will make his or her choice while mentally competent, free from outside pressure, and furnished with sufficient information. In terms of information, the consent process will obviously need to be extremely rigorous, especially for those in the first wave of trials, and we will return to this issue below. Momentarily assuming that the subject is appropriately informed (and we note with approval that the Louisville team has considered this in some detail), we then face somewhat thornier dilemmas in the need for competent and voluntary participation.

Dr Butler has indicated that only those demonstrating a high degree of competence, comprehension and the like will be eligible for his study.[13] The potential psychological and physical effects and the likely level of media interest (and even intrusion) certainly suggest that the recipient will need to be a pretty robust character. Yet, if that intuition is correct, will such an individual want (or 'need'?) the procedure, given that, at least at first, there would be no restoration of function? We are reminded here of a barrister, Henry de Lotbiniere, who showed no signs of withdrawal from society or discomfort with his facial disfiguration, as arguably exemplified by his portrait, which was displayed in the Saving Faces exhibition at the National Portrait Gallery, London. Ironically, then, such strong characters appear likely to be the very people reconciled to their disfigurement. Contrary to Butler's view, it is arguable that those most likely to want (or need?) to undergo the procedure will be precisely those who are not so reconciled. These might well be highly vulnerable individuals, whose autonomy could be compromised at least to the extent that their choice is not entirely free. Would it be overly paternalistic or even self-defeating to deny individuals in the latter group the chance to gain face? Furthermore, who would be the judges of—and accordingly gatekeepers to—autonomy? As English law stands, for example, the health care professional offering the relevant treatment, or the researcher conducting the study, assumes this role, and there is no strict requirement to call on assistance from psychiatrists, psychologists and the like.[14] Might the present context not be one in which such additional expertise should be called on, rather than leaving the assessment to the surgeons?

There are also difficulties in terms of the 'harm' to be tackled and the pool of beneficiaries. The Louisville team has already created an online registry in order to identify potential recipients, which it has targeted at those 'suffering from a major facial disfigurement.'[15] This wording, along with the published paper, indicates that the team envisages the application of the procedure to those in perceived medical need. However, this is a notoriously difficult concept to unpack: what is 'medical' and what is 'necessary'? Notably, as the Royal College of Surgeons report recognised, it is not the extent of the disfigurement that determines the individual's reaction thereto.[16] So who then can be said to be in greatest need in this context? Furthermore, can we preclude (as the American team appears to) a move from perceived necessity to choice i.e., facial transplantation as an elective, cosmetic procedure? One could anticipate the desirability of facial transformation for criminals, for example, and the appeal of adopting a popular celebrity's appearance, although such speculation might not be entirely helpful. Nevertheless, we need to think seriously about, and articulate and defend the bases for, distinguishing between the necessary and the elective, before the procedure has begun and certainly before it becomes commonplace.

It is not only the harm associated with the disfigurement that warrants careful consideration, but also the potential harms associated with the procedure. As is the case with other transplantation operations involving foreign tissue, the recipient would need to receive anti-rejection therapy, which can have serious side effects. You will recall that Spriano's jawbone transplant did not attract as much attention as facial transplantation and we suggested that its invisibility could be one reason for this; another reason relevant in the current context relates to the smaller risk of rejection posed by that transplant. The jawbone had been treated with radiotherapy before being inserted into the recipient's face, which less-

ened the need for the immuno-suppressant drugs.[17] This would not be possible for the face transplant. Furthermore, recipients do not always cope well with the side effects of such drugs. The first hand transplant had to be removed after the recipient failed to comply with the regime, after suffering psychological distress and physical symptoms.[18]

Yet even immuno-suppressant drugs cannot guarantee that the body will accept the transplanted tissue. Kidney transplants have the best chances of success, where three-year survival rates are as high as 83%.[19] The face, however, is one of the most antigenic tissues in the body, so the likelihood of comparable success rates is small, particularly in the initial, experimental phases. Even if that rate also obtained for face transplants, this would mean approximately one in five faces rejecting within three years. This prospect rightly troubled the authors of the British and French reports, and the Louisville team also acknowledged the risk, albeit with a rather benign reference to the possible 'loss of the transplanted tissue.'[20] It is better to be frank here: does a recipient literally risk losing face? While a kidney rejecting is of course a major cause for concern, dialysis may still exist as a fall-back; furthermore, the potential for saving life through such transplants means that the benefits more obviously outweigh the risks. What of the face rejecting? Will a skin graft or the like be viable?

To the best of our knowledge a satisfactory fallback position has yet to be published by any of the teams advancing this proposal. Science and society would be all the poorer if scientists lacked the 'courage to fail,' but these risks indicate that we presently need more caution than courage.[21]

In our discussion thus far we have referred to the recipient as both a 'subject' (of research) and a 'patient.' Given the considerations just outlined, however, it could be argued that the recipient only becomes a patient after the procedure has been performed. Guy Foucher, President of the International Federation of Hand Surgeons, opposed hand transplants on this very basis, commenting that the procedure 'transformed a healthy, one-handed man into a sick man with two hands.'[22] Aside from any psychological difficulties that the person might be experiencing, we would assume that the proposed recipient would be otherwise healthy at the time of the face transplant. The healthy person with a facial disfigurement is then transformed into a morbidly ill individual who must endure a toxic regime of drugs for the remainder of their life. At a bare minimum this information would have to be imparted during the consent process.

In terms of the potential recipients there are therefore a host of important questions that demand answers or, perhaps, better answers. The Catch-22 of facial transplantation is especially difficult: if you are robust enough to submit yourself to the procedure and all it might entail, you may be least likely to want it; if, on the other hand, you do desire the new face, you may be less able to cope with the risks posed by this procedure. It is therefore not only the physical effects that matter but also the psychological effects of receiving (or, indeed, not receiving) the face transplant. These effects relate also to questions of principle, primarily concerning personal identity, to which we now turn.

VI. Who's Who?

Some of the risks highlighted in the previous section might be minimised in time, especially if the procedure is allowed to proceed and the science develops accordingly. However, there are other risks that might not be so easily tackled. As Caplan and Katz briefly noted in an early commentary, face transplants 'involve tissues that are associated with each individual's personal identity.'[23] Even in the early stages of the phenomenon we believe there will be threats to individual identity, which would obviously be magnified if the science developed along the *Face/Off* lines. While we do not hold that the recipient would in some way 'become' the donor, we perceive a dynamic relationship between the body and the mind, such that changes in the one will affect the other.

Caplan and Katz rightly talk only of an 'association,' since a popular philosophical account of personal identity actually seems most likely to hold that face transplants present no difficulties in terms of identity. The philosophical literature is replete with attempts to pinpoint the necessary and sufficient conditions for holding that a person is that person; in other words, attempts to answer the related questions, 'who am I?' and 'what makes me me?' These questions are often considered along spatio-temporal lines, in terms of re-identification, where the quest is to discover the conditions that make a person at time T1 the same person as at time T2. Broadly speaking there are two rival criteria, based in physical and psychological attributes, respectively.

The first view essentially holds that sameness of body means sameness of self or person. Supporters of this view of the spatiotemporally-continuous human should readily grasp the significance of face transplants for personal identity. Indeed, if the face is seen as a particularly important identifier, those in the 'body camp' might well ask, who is the donor and who is the recipient? Is my body receiving your face or is your face receiving my body?

There are alternatively those who emphasise the importance of certain psychological properties, such as a functioning brain (or brain stem), personality and memory. Parfit, a leading proponent of this view, suggests that personal identity be characterised by psychological continuity.[24] The essential point of such accounts is that the continuing presence of a particular human body is not sufficiently or even necessarily required for identifying that human body as a particular person. Indeed, on some religious accounts, the 'person' (or soul) is utterly distinct from the body and can therefore exist without a body or after the body's demise. This psychological/spiritual conception has been employed in analyses of for example: the meaning of death; whether the demented patient is continuous with the pre-demented patient; and the validity of advance directives, which are expressed by the competent patient but applicable to the body of that patient when incompetent.[25]

Strict adherents to psychological/spiritual criteria would probably deny that my face is essentially constitutive of who I am. As such, a face transplant appears to pose no problem in principle, even if the science did develop to enable the wholesale adoption of another person's face. Yet while the present authors are most inclined towards the 'mind camp,' we also feel that a face transplant can and will impinge on identity, and accordingly present challenges for both recipients and donors (and their loved ones).

First, we must recall that the face transplant as currently proposed will offer only improvements in aesthetic appearance. In stark contrast to other transplantation procedures, the physical, functional benefits will be absent. Why then would an individual wish to undergo this procedure? Surely the primary motivation must be the psychological benefits offered by the anticipated improvement in appearance. If one's psychological make-up provides the key to identity, it is therefore plausible to hold that a face transplant would indeed have an impact on identity. If this logic succeeds, the question then becomes, is this impact likely to be benign or malign? Unfortunately, this is difficult to predict with certainty before the transplant is attempted, as the following evidence should demonstrate.

Research already suggests that transplanted tissue can feel 'foreign' to the recipient, regardless of the tissue's apparent association (or lack thereof) with personal identity. A Swedish study conducted by Sanner illustrates the differences in opinions expressed over the appropriateness of receiving tissues and organs from other human and non-human sources. Regarding xenotransplantation, one interviewee posed the question, 'Would I become half a pig, if I got an organ from a pig?,' another queried whether he or she 'would start grunting?,' while another opined that 'at least 5% of me would become animal.'[26] Clearly, for these individuals at least, receipt of an animal organ would somehow impinge on their pre-existing notions of personal identity. As Sanner summarised, 'It was less a feeling of influence and more a fear of having the sensation that the body would not be itself, it would be "wrong."'[27] There is equally compelling evidence that some individuals fear the effects on their identity of receiving an organ from another human body. Another of Sanner's interviewees asked, 'If I exchange many parts, I wonder what's left of me as a person?'[28] Such unease has even been cited in evidence before the English High Court. In Re M, reported in 1999, an adolescent was adjudged incompetent and in any case unable to refuse a heart transplant, which she urgently required. Explaining the reasoning behind her initial refusal, M stated:

I don't want to die but I would rather die than have somebody else's heart. I would rather die with fifteen years of my own heart. If I had someone else's heart, I would be different from anyone else—being dead would not make me different from anyone else. I would feel different with someone else's heart, that's a good enough reason not to have a heart transplant, even if it saved my life.[29]

There seem to be two concerns here: one, that she would differ from other people, the other, that she would somehow be a different person, at least in her own perception. However, not everyone shares this unease. Another of Sanner's respondents referred to organs as 'machine parts, in principle nothing strange,' while others commented that 'If you receive a new heart, it will become your own' and 'What is me, is not depending on whose kidney I have received.'[30] Xenotransplantation did not trouble everyone, either: 'My body wouldn't feel different if I get an animal organ. I'm also a kind of animal.'[31] 'Special' tissues can also be accommodated: Lee Brash, who had received a heart and lung transplant as a teenager, understood but did not share M's resistance: 'I used to think that maybe I would be different. With a different heart I might feel different things—even fancy different girls. But I didn't feel any different at all. It doesn't affect the person you are.'[32]

Opinion is therefore divided and, as the Nuffield Council has observed in relation to transplants from animal sources: 'It is difficult to predict what the effects of xenotransplantation might be on individual recipients and, in particular, how people's views of their body and of their identity might be affected by xenotransplantation.'[33]

This is not to deny that some potential recipients can indeed predict the effects for themselves and accordingly stipulate what they are and are not willing to receive. For example, a Jehovah's Witness might oppose a blood transfusion and an Orthodox Jew might object to the use of tissues, valves and organs from pigs.[34] Gillett, albeit writing in a slightly different context, clarifies why such procedures can be seen as threatening. For Gillett, one's personal identity—indeed, one's status as a person—is inextricably connected with one's narrative or life story. As he says,

> A person is largely the cumulative result of a conscious narrative of life ... Once one realises this central role of narrative in human life, the insight soon follows that being a person just is an ongoing process of being inscribed in this way—by the world and the significations impinging on one—and living out the psychic effects of that cumulative inscription under the shaping influence of the values that guide one's self-creation.[35]

If we understand Gillett, he is suggesting that one's identity derives, at least in part, from one's values. Religious faith might occupy a distinctive part of my narrative and hence be to some extent constitutive of my identity. Thus, I might choose to forego a procedure that is contrary to my sincerely and strongly held beliefs on the basis that this would contradict something that defines me; in other words, 'I won't have the blood; it's just not me.' Gillett's observations therefore return us to the suggestion that we should turn the choice over to the recipient, making the conditions for autonomy provide our moral compass. But that will not eradicate the uncertainty: can the individual predict what he or she is getting and whether this will be what he or she wanted? The recipient of the first hand transplant is a case in point as, although he evidently consented to the procedure, he reported feelings of foreignness towards his transplant which, combined with the side effects of the supporting drugs, eventually necessitated its removal.[36] How then could we predict the response of the recipient of a new face?

That a major change in one's appearance can have a significant psychological effect and accordingly impact upon one's self-perception and identity is also poignantly illustrated by the famous situation of 'Dax.' Don Cowart received second and third degree burns over two-thirds of his body in a gas explosion and was consequently hospitalised for 232 days. Despite Don's repeated requests that the painful treatment be discontinued, the health professionals persisted. Prior to the accident, Don had been handsome and athletic; following the accident, he was totally blind, barely able to use his hands, badly scarred, and dependent on others to assist him in performing personal functions. Don then re-named himself 'Dax.' As W.F. May has stated, the bodily changes in turn prompted an 'interior transformation,' in which 'Don Cowart becomes Dax.'[37] Don had worked as a pilot in the Air Force, and was working in real estate at the time of the accident. Dax married and became a lawyer. Evidently Dax felt sufficiently 'other' to re-name himself. His 'old' identity was not completely lost, however, since (for example) his ambition and mental fortitude were just as pronounced after the accident, as evidenced by his subsequent achievements and the fact that, if placed in a similar situation again, he would still decline the burns treatment he endured.[38] But what if Dax was to receive a face transplant? Would he then assume a third identity and third name?

Of course, it is not only one's self-perception that needs to be considered. The human face is, as MacGregor et al. recognised, 'the source of vocal communication, the expression of emotions, and the revealer of personality traits. The face is like the person himself.'[39] This suggests that the defensibility of the procedure cannot be resolved by appealing to the individual and autonomy alone, since the impact on others seems also to matter. These others might comprise the loved ones of the recipient and, importantly, the loved ones of the deceased donor. Potential donors would, we assume, need to be tissue matched and of a similar age and ethnicity to the recipient. Furthermore, because the facial tissue will deteriorate fairly rapidly after death, the recipient and donor will probably need to be geographically proximate as well. There is therefore the prospect of a relative of the deceased being confronted by a familiar face. This might only amount to a recognisable mole or similar feature in the early phase, which might be troubling enough, but could then become an especially significant issue if the science developed to the wholesale assumption of another face.

It therefore appears that not only are we unable to predict the effects on the individual receiving the face transplant but also that the impact on others is somewhat difficult to foresee. Individual choice may be an insufficient solution since the risks and benefits are hard to assess and, as Dax further exemplifies, the aforementioned Catch-22 of receiving the transplant still remains. We therefore need further engagement with the possible effects of receiving the procedure, by scientists, ethicists and, it would appear, society at large. Indeed, the role and influence of society is particularly important here and therefore forms the focus of our penultimate section.

VII. Who Is the Patient? (Part 2)

Having suggested that the effect on identity and self-perception might not be so obviously positive in nature, why offer a face transplant? This leads us to consider again the general question, who are we treating? Another of Sanner's respondents felt that 'It doesn't matter what you have inside your body, it wouldn't be visible from outside.'[40] Visibility and appearance seem to matter, as a respondent to an online BBC poll further suggests:

> There's a lot more to a person than there [sic] face—the person with the transplant will not become you [the donor]. I can see how psychologically it could be very difficult to wake up with someone else's face, but I'd think less difficult than waking up without a face you can show anyone.[41]

Christine Piff, of Let's Face It, acknowledges that facial disfigurement can be a major source of emotional distress and that a transplant could benefit those who have become 'withdrawn.'[42] But this should give us another reason to pause. Such withdrawal is surely due in part to the responses from other members of society. Piff herself has spoken of 'people staring at me' and feeling both 'awful' and in need of 'every bit of courage' she could summon.[43]

In an important sense, one must query whether the 'patient' is actually society, and in particular image-conscious Western society. Macgregor et al. wrote that, 'Every culture has its own standards of attractiveness, and while an infinite number of physical divergences are possible which meet the aesthetic requirements, a certain conformity is demanded.'[44]

This apparent obsession with beauty is probably one of the strongest reasons for permitting this procedure and also ironically one of the main reasons why it gives cause for concern. Ideally, of course,

society would celebrate, rather than alienate, such diversity. There nevertheless lingers the suspicion that the influence of societal norms amounts to a form of coercion, which might again threaten the validity of any consent. Furthermore, we wonder whether alternative responses to disfigurement, such as counselling, would suffer once the transplantation doors are opened. As Strauss has pointed out, 'when something is correctable, our willingness to accept it as untouched is reduced.'[45]

These concerns, particularly when considered alongside the risks of rejection, the risks associated with immuno-suppressants and the uncertain psychological effects of the procedure, combine to suggest that there is more work to do both with those with disfigurements and in this debate specifically. Certainly, the work of charities like the British Changing Faces needs greater recognition, particularly by health care professionals dealing with the disfigured.[46] Although we do not oppose face transplants in principle, more can still be done to respond to the disfigured individual and to facilitate that individual's flourishing in society.

VIII. Conclusion: Whether or When?

We have focused on issues relevant to the recipients of face transplants, which we believe need further analysis and discussion before the procedure is attempted. Other issues that we have not addressed fully include the existence (or otherwise) of a pool of willing donors and the question of cost: would the recipient have to fund the life-long supply of anti-rejection drugs and if so would ability to pay become a criterion for inclusion? Until such questions (and doubtless more) receive defensible answers, we should not be forced into thinking in terms of 'when?' but should instead continue to ask 'whether or not?' In terms of this latter question, it is worth clarifying that (as our discussion of personal identity demonstrated) we have not found a problem with the procedure in principle, but we accept that such opposition may well exist. One might anticipate, for example, appeals to Caplan's 'yuk' factor and charges of meddling with nature. We are not convinced that such arguments will succeed but we are convinced that all such views must be aired at this juncture.

Even if there is no principled objection to the procedure, there is still cause for concern and there remain questions to be answered. Who would be a suitable recipient of the transplant and can the Catch-22 of 'need' and vulnerability be avoided? How can we predict the effects of receiving the donor face on the individual and, indeed, others, such as the loved ones of both the recipient and the donor? While slippery-slope thinking sometimes prompts specious and deliberately extreme metaphors, might this not also be an area in which the potential for future abuse and move to elective transplants are sufficient to prevent the first steps being taken? Is this procedure at least in some sense motivated by society's intolerance of disability? Should not greater efforts be put into other means of addressing the problems associated with facial disfigurement? Finally, and perhaps most importantly, will the anticipated benefits of receiving the transplant ever outweigh the risks? The Working Party of the British Royal College of Surgeons was most influenced by the risk of the face rejecting and the uncertain psychological effects of receiving a donated face.[47] Notably, at a public debate hosted by the Dana Centre at the London Science Museum at least one of the report's authors did not otherwise object in principle to the procedure being undertaken.[48] However, at the same event, the authors appeared to lack a clear view as to when the risks would be sufficiently minimised. We have suggested that this procedure must be viewed as experimental, and research will always carry risks. Should it therefore simply be left to the individual to decide whether or not to run the risks? Whilst mindful of charges of paternalism, we believe autonomy alone cannot govern here. The rights and wrongs of the procedure do not wholly lie in the realm of private morality, since it will surely impact on those close to the recipient and donor and it also involves, and is expressive of the values of, the societies in which the procedure is being contemplated. For these reasons we welcome further analysis and debate not least so that, in the drive to gain face, we do not overlook the risks of losing face.

Notes

1   BBC News Online Network. From Hand to Face. 30 September 1998. Available from: http://news.bbc.co.uk/1/hi/health/183870.stm.

2   The Royal College of Surgeons of England. 2003. Facial Transplantation. Working Party Report. Available from: http://www.rcseng.ac.uk/services/publications/publications/pdf/facial_transplantation.pdf; Comité Consultatif National d'Ethique pour les Sciences de la Vie et de la Santé. 2004. L'allotransplantation de tissu composite (ATC) au niveau de la face (Greffe totale ou partielle d'un visage). *Opinion* 82: 1-20. Available from: http://www.ccne-ethique.fr.

3   O.P. Wiggins et al. On the ethics of facial transplantation research. *Am J Bioeth* 2004; 4(3): 1-12.

4   R. Nicholson. Editorial. *Bull Med Ethics* 2002; 183: 1.

5   D. Concar. The Boldest Cut. *New Sci* 2004; 29 May: 32-37; *Taipei Times* Online. Face Transplants Nearing Reality. 19 November 2003. Available from: http://www.taipeitimes.com/News/taiwan/archives/2003/11/19/2003076393.

6   Royal College of Surgeons, op. cit. note 2.

7   N. McDowell. Surgeons Struggle with Ethical Nightmare of Face Transplants. *Nature* 2002; 420(6915): 449.

8   Ibid.

9   NHS UK Transplant. UK Transplant Activity Report 2003-2004 Summary. 2004. Available from: http://www.uktransplant.org.uk/ukt/statistics/transplant_activity/transplant_activity_uk_2003-2004_summary.jsp.

10 C.A. Erin & J. Harris. An Ethical Market in Human Organs. *J Med Ethics* 2003; 29: 137-38; M.E. Tardy. Ethics and Integrity in Facial Plastic Surgery: Imperatives for the 21st Century. *Facial Plast Surg* 1995; 11(2): 111-15.

11 R. Hoffenberg. Christiaan Barnard: His First Transplants and their Impact on Concepts of Death. *Br Med J* 2001; 323: 1478-80.

12 BBC News Online Network. Doctors Perform Jaw Transplant. 2 February 2003. Available from: http://news.bbc.co.uk/2/hi/health/2712767.stm.

13 P.E. Butler, A. Clarke & R.E. Ashcroft. Face Transplantation: When and for Whom? *Am J Bioeth* 2004; 4(3): 16-17.

14 See Re C (Adult: Refusal of Treatment) [1994] 1 WLR 290. Note, however, that psychiatric assessment is recommended prior to gender reassignment

surgery: K. Wylie. ABC of Sexual Health: Gender Related Disorders. *Br Med J* 2004; 329: 615-17.

15 University of Louisville School of Medicine. Plastic Surgery Research. Information for Potential Face Transplant Patients and Research Subjects. Available from: http://plasticsurgeryresearch.louisville.edu/news.htm#Cleveland.

16 Royal College of Surgeons, op. cit. note 2, p. 10.

17 BBC News Online Network, op. cit. note 12.

18 D. Dickenson & G. Widdershoven. Ethical Issues in Limb Transplants. *Bioethics* 2001; 15(2): 110-24: 116.

19 NHS UK Transplant, op. cit. note 9.

20 Wiggins et al., op. cit. note 4, p. 4.

21 R. Fox & J.P. Swazey. 1979. *The Courage to Fail: A Social View of Organ Transplants and Dialysis.* Chicago. University of Chicago Press.

22 G. Foucher. Commentary: Prospects for Hand Transplantation. *Lancet* 1999; 353: 1286-87.

23 A. Caplan & D. Katz. In Brief: About Face. *Hastings Cent Rep* 2003; 33(1): 8.

24 D. Parfit. 1984. *Reasons and Persons.* New York: Oxford University Press.

25 E.g., M.B. Green & D. Wikler. Brain Death and Personal Identity. *Philos Public Aff* 1980; 9(2): 105-33.

26 M.A. Sanner. People's Feelings and Ideas about Receiving Transplants of Different Origins: Questions of Life and Death, Identity, and Nature's Border. *Clin Transplant* 2001; 15: 19-27: 22.

27 Ibid.

28 Ibid.

29 C. Dyer and S. Boseley. A Matter of Life and Death. *The Guardian* 16 July 1999: 3.

30 Sanner, op. cit. note 26.

31 Ibid. p. 23.

32 G. Davidson. New Life is Heart of the Matter. *Evening News* (Edinburgh) 19 July 1999: 15.

33 Nuffield Council on Bioethics. 1996. Animal-to-Human Transplants: The Ethics of Xenotransplantation: para. 10.45. Available from: http://www.nuffieldbioethics.org/publications/xenotransplantation/rep0000000042.asp.

34 See e.g., http://www.cmf.org.uk/index.htm?nucleus/nucoct93/jehovah.htm; http://www.freeminds.org; http://www.ajwrb.org/index.shtml.

35 G. Gillett. You Always Were a Bastard. *Hastings Cent Rep* 2002; 32: 23-28: 26-27.

36 Dickenson & Widdershoven, op. cit. note 21.

37 W.F. May. 1991. *The Patient's Ordeal.* Indiana. Indiana University Press: 35.

38 See further R. Cavalier, P. Covey & D. Anderson. 1996. A Right to Die? The Dax Cowart Case: An Ethical Case Study on CD-Rom. London. Routledge.

39 F.C. Macgregor et al. 1953. *Facial Deformities and Plastic Surgery: A Psychosocial Study.* Springfield, IL: Charles C. Thomas: 65.

40 Sanner, op. cit. note 26, p. 23.

41 Katie. BBC News Online Network. Talking Point: Face Transplants: Would You Donate Your Face? 29 November 2002. Available from: http://news.bbc.co.uk/1/ hi/talking_point/2518181.stm.

42 McDowell, op. cit. note 7.

43 BBC News Online Network. I Would Consider a Face Transplant. 27 November 2002. Available from: http://news.bbc.co.uk/1/hi/health/2518555.stm.

44 Macgregor et al., op. cit. note 39, p. 65.

45 R.P. Strauss. Ethical and Social Concerns in Facial Surgical Decision Making. *Plast Reconstr Surg* 1983; 72(5): 727.

46 Cf. J. Partridge. Changing Faces: Taking up Macgregor's Challenge. *J Burn Care Rehabil* 1998; 19(2): 174-80.

47 Royal College of Surgeons, op. cit. note 2.

48 See http://www.danacentre.org.uk/.

17.
THE CHALLENGE OF TRANSPLANTS TO AN INTER-SUBJECTIVELY ESTABLISHED SENSE OF PERSONAL IDENTITY

Andrew Edgar

SOURCE: *Health Care Analysis* 17.2 (2009): 123-33.

Introduction

The first face transplant was carried out in France in 2005. The recipient was Isabelle Dinoire, who had been mauled by her dog, losing her nose, lips and chin. The damage was judged to be too severe to be treated through conventional surgical techniques. Most recent reports suggest that problems of rejection of donor tissue have been overcome, that Dinoire has sensation in her new face, and that she has adapted well to her new appearance [9]. What is perhaps most significant about even such a brief summary of Dinoire's case is the emphasis that facial surgery places on the public appearance of the patient, and the need for the patient to become reconciled to a changed appearance. Popular concern over the morality of the face transplant quickly came to focus on the role that one's face plays in one's sense of self or one's personal identity. In order to address these concerns, the current paper will explore the significance of face transplants in the light of a theory of the self that draws on symbolic interactionism, narrative theory, and accounts of embodiment. In the first section of the paper, certain arguments concerning face transplants made by Huxtable and Woodley will be rehearsed. It will be suggested that a significant weakness in their analysis lies in the conception of the self and personal identity that are presumed. In the second section, a theory of the self will be articulated that responds to this concern, by drawing on the work of the phenomenologist Merleau-Ponty on embodiment and the social philosopher G.H. Mead on social interaction. This will allow an account of the nature of the suffering that a face transplant seeks to remedy, and its worth as an operation, and crucially the impact that it may have on the sense of personal identity of the recipient of the transplant. In the conclusion, the treatment will be placed in the context of the prejudices that members of contemporary societies may hold against those with disfigurements.

The Ethics of Face Transplants

Huxtable and Woodley [5] raise a series of questions about the ethical justification of face transplantation, primarily in response to a team of surgeons from Louisville, USA [11]. Around 2005 (and shortly before the Dinoire's transplant) this team proposed that the technological and moral climate was propitious to the operation. Huxtable and Woodley's questions look to the benefits that patients might receive from a face transplant, and in particular the benefits that they may receive over other treatments (be these partial skin grafts or some form of psychological therapy), and the effect that the transplant will have upon the patient. Such questions overtly presuppose that the primary source of distress that the face transplant attempts to overcome is psychological, not physical. The issue at stake is not the physical pain that the original trauma or disease may have caused, but rather the psychological stress that is generated from living with a conspicuous disfigurement in contemporary society [5, p. 506]. Huxtable and Woodley crucially see the effect of the face transplant to be primarily aesthetic, which is to say that it improves the appearance of the face without necessarily improving its functioning (p. 508).

The current paper will put to one side concerns about the technical problems and experimental nature of the operation (see p. 511) (and indeed, due to lack of space, questions about the alternative of psychological therapy), except insofar as they may impact on the social functioning of the post-operative patient, in order to focus on quite specific questions of personal identity that the operation raises. Issues concerning personal identity are addressed by Huxtable and Woodley, and in some detail, while examining the effects that the transplant has upon the patient. Following Caplan and Katz, they accept that the face transplant is distinctive due to the manner in which the face is bound up with personal identity (pp. 513-14). While many forms of transplant can place an emotional burden upon the patient, and the patient can feel alien from the transplanted tissue (pp. 515-16), face transplants serve to intensify that burden, and indeed shift it from being the possibly idiosyncratic reaction of certain individuals or personalities to a more general culturally rooted aversion, precisely because the face plays such a significant role in our self-understanding and in our interaction with others [see 4, p. 1].

Huxtable and Woodley are, therefore, aware that a face transplant, having the potential significantly to transform the most public aspects of one's appearance, may be disruptive at least to one's self-esteem, and in large part the psychological trauma that the transplant seeks to overcome is generated by the antipathy and prejudice that the patient faces, with a resultant inability to function in such a discriminatory society. The face transplant itself may potentially be a further source of disruption to an already fragile sense of self or degree of self-confidence. Indeed, Huxtable and Woodley suggest that the selection of patients for face transplants actually entails a paradoxical form of Catch-22. It is those patients who have the inner strength to cope with disfigurement, and to lead successful social lives, and they alone, who have the strength to handle the further aesthetic changes that the face transplant will bring about. Face transplants are therefore likely to go to those least in (psychological) need of them [5, p. 507].

It may, nonetheless, be suggested that the awareness that Huxtable and Woodley display of the entwining of face transplants with issues of personal identity is only given limited development. This limitation lies in the theory of the self and personal identity that underpins Huxtable and Woodley's arguments. In sketching a theory of personal identity, they outline two opposed camps, the 'mind camp' and the 'body camp.' The former holds that personal identity lies in the continuation of certain psychological or spiritual factors, such as memory, personality or soul. The latter holds that personal identity lies in the continuity of the body. Thus, for the mind camp, facial transformation is largely irrelevant to one's identity, and for the body camp, one potentially acquires the identity of the donor and loses one's own, old, identity (pp. 514-15). Clearly, such accounts are crude, and few theorists would fall dogmatically into either camp. It may nonetheless be suggested, even given this acknowledgement of the failings of the sketch, that setting up an opposition between mind and body camps [with the authors largely situating themselves in the mind camp (p. 515)] tends to reproduce both a mind-body dualism and a highly individualistic view of human being. This is to say that the approach taken by Huxtable and Woodley fails adequately to take account of embodiment, or fully to recognise the social nature of human being.

Huxtable and Woodley do acknowledge that cultural factors may have a significant impact upon the evaluation that the individual has of his or her own facial appearance, and they lament the stress on physical beauty that arises from contemporary 'image conscious Western society' (p. 520). Yet, this amounts to little more than seeing an individual placed within a pre-existing culture. The precise mechanisms through which that culture is reproduced and internalised by the individual are left vague. This may be contrasted with writers such as Hughes [4] or Cole [1], who place emphasis upon the face as a medium of communication with others. The lack of a fully functioning and expressive face serves to exclude the patient from routine social interactions. Prejudiced judgements of the person with a disfigurement, based upon that appearance, or mere embarrassment in their presence, similarly disrupts the possibility of communicating and being understood. More radically, Cole suggests that people with limited facial expression may not just be judged to be boring and uncommunicative, but will begin to behave in a boring and uncommunicative way [see 2, p. 207]. The prejudiced judgement of others thereby becomes a self-understanding and self-enactment.

The objective of the current paper is therefore to offer a richer theory of a social and embodied self than that used by Huxtable and Woodley, and one that may better indicate the risks and benefits of a face transplant, both in terms of the personal identity of the individual patient and the impact upon a society that expresses a high degree of prejudice towards disability and disfigurement. It will be suggested that an adequate understanding of the impact of a face transplant on the patient's sense of self or personal identity requires a narrative account of the self, that again Huxtable and Woodley touch upon, but do not develop (p. 517).

The Self

An alternative account of the self can usefully begin with the question of embodiment, and the distinction between 'being a body' and 'having a body' (that has been articulated by Merleau-Ponty [8], amongst others). A dualism, of the sort implied by Huxtable and Woodley's 'mind camp,' presupposes that the self possesses a body. The body is little more than an instrument or object that the self uses and exploits to its own ends. In contrast, Merleau-Ponty argues that being a body is primary to the human experience. Dualism is rejected, in so far as fundamentally I am my body. I do not experience my body as I experience any other object in the world, for the body is the perspective from which I experience all other objects [see 8, pp. 90-97]. It is through the body that I engage with the world, manipulating it, moving around within it, but also, crucially, by giving it meaning and thus constituting it as more than a mere physical environment. The possibilities that I perceive in that world, and the projects that I can foresee realising in that world, are made possible but also constrained by that body. A different body would open up a different range of possible actions and projects. But further, in being a body I engage in the world in a manner that takes the functioning and co-ordination of the body for granted. Typically I do not have to think about the manipulation and positioning of my body, or the co-ordination of my body with some other instrument or object. My body and the world within which it functions form an integrated and meaningful whole, precisely because my body frames the meaning I can ascribe to the world.

The experience of having a body, where the body is objectified and becomes something problematic upon which the self as a subject reflects, is secondary. The body will become an object when it fails to function in a taken for granted manner. A muscle twinges; my gesturing hand catches painfully against the desk; a fever leaves me weak and shivering. Crucially, the body as the perspective through which one engages with and gives meaning to one's world has changed. The integrity and meaning of that world may break down. Taken-for-granted actions would become problematic, and if possible at all, would require forethought and conscious manipulation of the body. The acquisition of a permanent injury or disability will not merely disrupt the taken-for-granted functioning of the lived body. It will shift the perspective from which the person engages with the world, changing possibilities, projects and meanings. The degree to which a disability, be it acquired or inherited, can become habituated into the lived body of the individual is a complex point, and indeed will depend to some degree upon the psychological resources of the individual involved. Huxtable and Woodley thus cite the example of Henry de Lotbiniere, a London barrister 'who showed no signs of withdrawal from society or discomfort with his facial disfiguration' [5, pp. 510-11]. Yet others, such as Christine Piff, remark on the discomfort they feel enduring the states of others (pp. 519-20).

Piff's experience opens up the second source of objectification, which is, following Sartre, the gaze of others. The body of another person is to me one more object in my world, albeit in many respects a special kind of one. This entails that my body is also an object to others. Being aware of being looked at makes me self-conscious of the objectivity or facticity of my own body [see 10, p. 58]. The crucial point to develop here is that the body is not simply mine, for it is an object that will be interpreted, evaluated and given meaning by others. To a significant degree that meaning may be beyond my control. The body is the medium through which others perceive me, and it is the medium of my communication with them. As Merleau-Ponty puts this: 'It is through my body that I understand other people, just as it is through my body that I perceive "things"' (1962, p. 186). The body is thus the centre of my relations with others, and thus of my intersubjectivity. Others will judge me on the appearance and gesturing of my body just as I judge them. I will strive to offer gestures and an appearance that communicate appropriately. Crucially, again, if my body is damaged or disfigured, then this communication is curtailed.

Merleau-Ponty's phenomenology may begin to indicate the importance of embodiment in understanding the experience of facial disfigurement, and thus the need that face transplants might meet as a therapy. It does not, however, on this account, say much about the self, other than that the self's world and its relationship to that world will depend upon the body. The impact that disfigurement, or more importantly cultural prejudice against disfigurement, may have on one's sense of self, may be further explored in terms of the importance of embodiment to human communication and subjectivity. This entails turning to social interactionist theories [see 7, pp. 15-42], of the sort offered by G.H. Mead.

Mead may be seen to raise issues similar to those of Merleau-Ponty, precisely insofar as he, too, is concerned with the process by which the human being treats herself as an object of reflection. Mead, however, focuses less on the objectification of the body, and more on the objectification of the self as such, and on the manner in which reflection is bound up with being a self and being self-conscious. For Mead, one's sense of self presupposes one's ability to take the attitude or role of the other, which is to say, crudely, that one sees one's own actions, behaviour and, we may add, body, through the eyes of another. This is the Sartrean gaze, although Mead goes further to argue that it is only by internalising this gaze that self-consciousness is developed (and indeed, for Mead, that humanity transcends mere animal existence). Mead's point is that I do not merely become self-conscious by recognising that I am gazed at, but rather that in the recognition of the gaze I internalise a social structure. The other is not simply an everyman, a mere representative of humanity, but is rather the occupant of a quite specific social role. Roles carry with them certain perspectives, evaluations and expectations of behaviour. Thus, in acknowledging the other, I am placing myself in a specific social relationship with them.

Mead develops this observation by suggesting that is it precisely through this social situating that I acquire selfhood. Again, in contrast to the crude Cartesianism of the 'mind camp,' the self is not a given, but rather a condition that is achieved through social interaction. While Mead sees reflection as a crucial human capacity, I am not immediately capable of self-reflection or self-awareness [7, p. 134]. Rather, the mere capacity for reflexivity that I have is given substance precisely insofar as I reflect and judge upon myself from the position of the other. Such reflection will begin for the child by internalising the judgements of the mother. The child's most basic perspectives, values (and thus, in Merleau-Ponty's phenomenological terminology, 'world') is developed by seeing the world and him or herself from the mother's perspective. For the competent adult, internalisation is of the 'generalised other' [7, pp. 154-56] of the immediate society in which they live and function. The generalised other is a system of roles, and Mead finds an important model of such systems is team sports, where each player understands their own position in the team by understanding the positions of the other players (pp. 151-63). Thus, for example, to occupy the role of patient entails that I understand, internalise and judge myself in terms of the roles of doctor, nurse, surgeon, and so on.

Any individual within a complex society will occupy multiple social roles, either sequentially or simultaneously, as she moves for example between parenthood, work and leisure, or sees herself in terms of the family, the local community, the business and so on. The possibility is thereby opened up that a person has multiple selves, or more precisely in Mead's terminology, there is more than one possible 'me.' This is to suggest that, according to the role one is occupying, one will perceive the world differently (or more radically, actually live in a distinct world, for one will ascribe different meanings and possibilities to one's environment), and will adopt different attitudes and judgements to others and to oneself. For Mead, the 'me' is thus the objectified self. The 'me' is the self under reflection, and will shift, according to the social context of the person.

The 'I,' conversely, is the self as subject. It is the self that reflects upon the 'me.' Understood negatively, it is the self when not determined by a social role. Positively, it is the capacity to respond to new situations and challenges, and thus to distance itself from the restrictions of any given social role [7, p. 199].

Drawing a further parallel between Mead and Merleau-Ponty, it may be suggested that typically the role one occupies is performed habitually. The expectations of the role fall into a taken for granted background. Critical objectification, exploiting the tension between the 'I' and the 'me,' occurs either as one is learning the role or when performance of the role encounters unforeseen problems. Disease and injury may thus be triggers to objectification. Many roles will become harder to perform due to physical impairment. However, the Meadian analysis goes beyond that offered above via Merleau-Ponty, precisely insofar as it suggests that the gaze that falls on the body is always part of system of roles. This is indeed to follow the phenomenologist in order to suggest that the body is not a mere object in a physical environment, but always already something interpreted in a (cultural and meaningful) world. Yet in Mead's terms, it is to argue that the evaluation given to the body, by either the I or the other, depends upon the role in which the body is part of the performance. The evaluation of a disfigured body will thus be relative to the perspective of a particular system of roles. Within the intimacy of the family, the disfigurement may be irrelevant. In the fleeting and impersonal interactions of public spaces, it may be highly significant, not least if the generalised other of this public space expresses a prejudice towards disfigurement. The experience of Christine Piff noted above may thereby be understood as reflection on one's self (or 'me') from the perspective of a highly critical and uncomprehending generalised other. One becomes self-conscious, objectifying oneself and thus 'having' rather than 'being' a body, precisely because the internalisation of the attitudes and roles of the other make problematic one's routine performance of almost any public role.

More radically, it may be suggested that disfigurement and other forms of visible impairment disrupt the possibility of communication. On one level, this occurs through the importance of the face and body within communication. The inability to move one's face may hamper the expression of emotion, or even the articulation of one's voice. Here, Cole's example of Mary is illustrative. Mary gradually lost facial mobility. Her family did not notice the loss (which at once highlights how role performance may be better enabled in the intimacy of the family than in public). The loss of facial mobility had led others to assume that she was suffering from dementia, confusing the inability to express emotion with an actual lack of emotional and intellectual activity. In addition, Mary found herself isolated as friends ceased to visit her, conceivably because the taken for granted performance of conversational roles had become impossible for Mary, and her friends lacked any resources to compensate or indeed understand the breakdown of the taken for granted world [2, pp. 189-90].

Following this example, it may be suggested that, on a deeper level, communication breaks down not simply due to physical impediments, but to prejudice and misunderstanding within the generalised other. Appropriate forms of communication may not exist that could embrace those with disabilities and disfigurements. At the extreme, this is to suggest that disfigurement becomes itself a role, and crucially a deviant role, falling outside the normal communication and interaction of society. This is part of Goffman's analysis of stigma (which include physical deformities), whereby the body of the person is so categorised by a prejudiced society as to spoil that person's 'social identity.' That is to say, the prior expectations of the generalised other confine the role that the stigmatised person can perform, effectively excluding them from full participation in society [see 4, pp. 19-21].

Crucially, if one's self-understanding is dependent upon the internalisation of the attitudes of the other, the implication of any analysis deriving from Mead (and Goffman) is to suggest that disfigurement, if marked and stigmatised by the generalised other, impacts upon the self and personal identity. Stigmatisation affects not just one's ability to perform a public role, but also one's personal perspective and self-evaluation. A case offered by Huxtable and Woodley is significant here [5, p. 518]. Don Cowart received severe burns over two-thirds of his body. While he had been handsome and athletic prior to the accident, after treatment he was blind and badly and visibly scarred. Don renamed himself 'Dax,' thereby marking the fundamental change in personal identity that the accident and treatment brought about. Huxtable and Woodley ask, a little disingenuously, if Dax would assume a third identity and a third name if he were to receive a face transplant. A Meadian analysis would answer 'yes,' or at least, 'in all likelihood.' It is this line of inquiry, which is to say, the impact that a face transplant might have on the socially constituted identity of the patient, that the remainder of this paper will pursue.

Face Transplants, Appearance and Personal Identity

Disfigurement, it has been suggested, serves to alienate a person from their body. The body becomes something one has, rather than something one is. The body ceases to fall into the taken for granted background of the patient's life, either because it ceases to function effectively (and thus, for example, inhibits the usual processes of communication), or because it becomes the focus of the disapproving and disempowering gaze of others. A face transplant attempts to remedy this, allowing the patient once more to be her body, by transforming and 'normalising' her appearance. However, if the body is as intimately bound up with personal identity as has been suggested above, the face transplant, precisely because it will not restore the patient's original appearance, may present the patient with a further perspective through which her world is shaped, and an appearance that will stimulate new and different responses (albeit hopefully less critical ones) from others. The result of a face transplant may thus be a new self, at the very least in Mead's sense, of facilitating a new cluster of 'me's.'

This issue may be analysed by considering the nature of the face transplant as an operation. A face transplant may appear to be a radical form of cosmetic surgery. It touches only the appearance of the patient, while possibly leaving the functioning of the face further impaired [5, p. 508]. In effect, the operation may leave the patient with a mere mask, that they have but, precisely because of its lack of function and alien appearance, he cannot be. As such, its

worth as a medical procedure may be questioned. In the light of this, an argument may be borrowed from Habermas. In the context of concerns about the therapeutic legitimacy of genetic engineering, Habermas has suggested what he calls a 'categorical' distinction between the 'grown' and the 'made.' In effect, these terms represent two different attitudes that the agent can take to the transformation of their environment, and thus to the transformation of their bodies. The former is the attitude inherent to cultivation, medical and other therapy, and to the selective breeding of plant or animal species. It is the approach of the agriculturist, the doctor and the animal or plant breeder, and crucially entails that they work with 'the inherent dynamics of auto-regulated nature' [3, p. 45]. That is to say, that they respect the dynamics in the material with which they work. In contrast, the technician or engineer treats their material as dead matter, upon which they can freely exercise their will.

In the context of a face transplant, it may be suggested that if the treatment is merely a radical form of cosmetic surgery, then it is concerned merely to engineer (rather than cultivate) a new appearance for the patient. The patient's body, crucially, is treated as something he or she merely has. It is a possession, that is to be shaped so as to facilitate the person's competent functioning in society. The disfigured face and body elicit disapproval and perhaps disgust from the other. The post-operative body will remove or at least reduce and possibly remove this disapproval. The recipient of the new face might then be seen to be manipulating people around her, perhaps even a little cynically, presenting a face that she knows will elicit a specific (sympathetic) response, and behind which she hides. In the light of Mead's arguments, it may be acknowledged that the lack of disapproval will feedback positively on the patient's self-esteem, and the range of roles that she can occupy successfully and competently will be greatly expanded. But, crucially, any socially acceptable appearance will suffice. There need be no continuity with the patient's appearance prior to the disfiguring trauma. The face transplant patient therefore seems to be radically alienated from her body, and presupposes in line with the 'mind camp' that she will have a continuity of personality and thus selfhood despite changes in bodily appearance. The intuition of the problematic nature of this belief, grounding above in the analysis of Mead and Merleau-Ponty, may be suggested to underpin popular concerns about face transplants as a procedure.

It may, nonetheless, be suggested that a face transplant can never be pure making. An example much used in the literature is that of the film *Face-Off*, where plastic surgery is used to exchange, perfectly, the faces of characters played by Nicolas Cage and John Travolta [5, p. 507]. Amongst many other fictional examples, Fay Weldon imagines a similar surgical transformation of a woman's appearance, into that of another, in *The Life and Loves of a She Devil*. In practice, a face transplant cannot so radically change the recipient's appearance. The bone structure of the face remains untouched, and the surgeons must work, in a manner that is suggestive of cultivation rather than making, with the existing face, its bone structure and tissue type. The resultant postoperative face is thus neither that of the donor, as the *Face-Off* scenario suggests, nor yet a restoration of the recipient's pre-trauma appearance. It is rather a new face, albeit one that has an important degree of continuity with the recipient's previous appearance. It may be suggested that it is this somewhat fractured continuity that is fundamental to the success of the face transplant, and in effect makes the new face expressive of the complex self that has been through trauma and therapy. Such a face is not a cynically worn mask. It has been argued above that, following Mead, the self should not be understood as necessarily unified. The self is composed of multiple 'me's,' through the performance of diverse social roles. MacIntyre [6] responds to precisely this characterisation of modernity, where the self is fragmented between different social roles, in his defence of virtue ethics. The challenge for MacIntyre, to which virtue ethics responds, is to find unity in that fragmentation, and importantly to do so through the quest for an overriding narrative of self-identity. The victim of trauma has additionally to struggle to incorporate that trauma in his or her biography, constructing some sense of unity and coherence out of the fragmentation. The body is necessarily part of that story, because, following Merleau-Ponty, the narrator should strive once more to be that body, and

not merely to have it. The narrative is not to be of a mere manipulator, who has retreated behind the mask of her body. Without developing the role that a narrative ethics might play here in any great depth, it may nonetheless be suggested that face transplants, as currently conceived and practised, respect the historical and narrative nature of the self. That is to say that some traces of the transplant will remain visible, however successful the operation may have been. The new face will thus acquire the status of a transplanted face, rather than a 'natural' face. The new face may therefore be understood as an expression, not of the pre-accident self, but of a self that has experienced both the accident and the therapy. The traces of surgery become acceptable, expressive, marks of their complex and painful biography, and thus the embodiment of any story that he could tell about himself. The patient thereby once again becomes his body, not by restoring a pre-trauma appearance, for that appearance is as alien to his present self as is the appearance of another person, but by learning to live in a body that is his history.

Conclusion

The foregoing analysis has suggested that the recipient of a face transplant must be understood as an embodied and social self. Only then can the nature of the face transplant as a therapy, as well as the nature of the suffering it seeks to remedy, be understood. It has been suggested above that the suffering that face transplants are designed to remedy is a social-psychological suffering. Huxtable and Woodley, in contrast, see the treatment as dealing with 'psychological difficulties' [5, p. 506]. The arguments derived from Merleau-Ponty and especially from Mead emphasise the importance of qualifying this suffering as resulting from society. This, however, highlights a further important question posed by Huxtable and Woodley, who ask if the patient should be society, not the disfigured individual (p. 520). The above arguments have stressed the role that prejudice within the ambient culture, and the internalisation of that prejudice in the disfigured person's self-understanding, play in the suffering involved. The transformation of attitudes within society is indeed to be urgently encouraged (and organisations such as the charity Changing Faces play a vital role here). However, social change is slow, and more pessimistically it may be suggested that all societies mark some boundary between acceptable and unacceptable appearance [see 4, p. 17]. Appeals to the current obsession with beauty in contemporary society may, in practise, be naive in the light of a more thorough understanding of human cultural history. Further, it is also unclear why certain individuals, who could be aided by surgery, should be expected to spearhead challenges to widespread prejudice through the public display of their appearance. Finally, if the face transplant is understood as growth, and not making, as the acceptance of being a body rather than having a body, then it may be seen, not to be a capitulation to an obsession with beauty, but rather an expression of, and bearing witness to, the complexity of physical appearance and the biographical entwining of the social self and the body. This itself may serve to challenge superficial and prejudiced evaluations of physical appearance in contemporary society.

References

1. Cole, J. (1998). *About face*. Cambridge MA: MIT.
2. Cole, J. (2000). Relations between the face and the self as revealed by neurological loss: The subjective experience of facial difference. *Social Research* 67(1): 187-218.
3. Habermas, J. (2003). *The future of human nature*. Cambridge: Polity.
4. Hughes, M.J. (1998). *The social consequences of facial disfigurement*. Aldershot: Ashgate.
5. Huxtable, R., & Woodley, J. (2005). Gaining face or losing face? Framing the debate on face transplants. *Bioethics* 19(5-6): 505-22.
6. MacIntyre, A. (2007). *After virtue: A study in moral theory*. 3rd ed. London: Duckworth.
7. Mead, G.H. (1934). *Mind, self and society: From the standpoint of a social behaviorist*. Chicago: University of Chicago Press.
8. Merleau-Ponty, M. (1962). *Phenomenology of perception*. Trans. C. Smith. London: Routledge.
9. Murphy, C. (2008). 'Facing up to face transplants.' BBC News website, http://news.bbc.co.uk/2/hi/health/7277582.stm. Accessed 1 March 2009.
10. Toombs, S.K. (1992). *The meaning as illness: A phenomenological account of the different perspectives of physician and patient*. London: Kluwer.
11. Wiggins, O.P., et al. (2004). On the ethics of facial transplantation research. *The American Journal of Bioethics* 4(3): 1-12. doi:10.1080/15265160490496507. 123

CHAPTER FOUR

REPRODUCTION

Web Link

(1) Link to Canada's Assisted Human Reproduction Act 2004.

http://laws-lois.justice.gc.ca/eng/acts/A-13.4/

Canada's Assisted Human Reproduction Act is a comprehensive piece of legislation developed by Health Canada regarding reproductive technologies and related research. Although it may overlap with ethics, it is not considered to be an ethical code; it is law.

* For an up-to-date list of the web links in this book, please visit: http://sites.broadviewpress.com/healthcare.

18.
REFLECTIONS ON REPRODUCTIVE RIGHTS IN CANADA

Christine Overall

SOURCE: *Human Reproduction: Principles, Practices, Policies* (Toronto: Oxford University Press, 1993).

The concept of "reproductive rights" plays a central role in discussions of issues relating to women's reproductive health. While the concept of rights in general does not by any means constitute all that is important in ethical discourse, and the concept of reproductive rights in particular does not exhaust all that is significant in the moral evaluation of reproductive issues, the idea of reproductive rights is, at this point at least, indispensable to a complete discussion of reproductive ethics and social policy.

Barbara Katz Rothman has expressed reservations about the use of the term "reproduction," arguing that we do not literally produce babies or reproduce ourselves.[1] While I agree with this observation, I shall continue to use the phrase "reproductive right" because I specifically want to explore the strengths and the ambiguities of that phrase. In particular, this chapter will analyse and evaluate the ways in which this notion of reproductive right has been given a unique legal and moral expression within Canadian society during the last two decades, manifesting itself within the struggle for abortion, the debates about midwifery and the place of birth, and the introduction of social practices relating to new reproductive technologies such as *in vitro* fertilization.

Originally, the concept of reproductive rights seemed to find a natural home within the abortion debate, but it is now being extended to discussions of new reproductive technologies. What is extraordinary is that the idea of reproductive rights is used not only by feminists concerned with promoting women's well-being and ending oppression, but also by non-feminists, whose agenda usually includes preservation of the traditional family, extension of male sexual and reproductive entitlements, and enforcement of a "pro-life" morality that sees women's bodies as instruments for the production of babies. In other words, while the idea of reproductive rights is both useful and central to the advancement of women's reproductive freedom, there are also ways in which it can be and is being used against women's best interests. For this reason feminists need to think carefully about what they mean when making claims for reproductive rights.

The Right Not to Reproduce

The term "reproductive right" has more than one meaning.[2] It is necessary, first, to distinguish between the right to reproduce and the right *not* to reproduce. The two are sometimes mistakenly conflated as, for example, when Justice Bertha Wilson referred in her Supreme Court decision on the Morgentaler case to "[t]he right to reproduce or not to reproduce which is in issue in this case."[3] The right not to reproduce is the entitlement not to be compelled to beget or bear children against one's will: the entitlement not to have to engage in forced reproductive labour. To say that women have a right not to reproduce implies that they have no obligation to reproduce. In its weak (liberty) sense it is the entitlement not to be compelled to donate gametes (eggs or sperm) or embryos against one's will. The right not to reproduce in the strong (welfare) sense is the right of access to services like abortion and contraception that enable women to avoid procreation. Women do not owe their reproductive products or labour to any person or institution, including male partners or the state.

Recognition of the right not to reproduce has been slower to develop in Canada than in the United States. Full exercise of such a right requires, among other protections, access to safe and effective contraception and abortion services. In other words, the moral entitlement to abortion access follows from the broader right not to reproduce. In 1969, stipulations were introduced into the Criminal Code that provided for the possibility, under certain carefully specified conditions, of therapeutic exceptions to the general law that using any means or permitting any means to be used for the purpose of procuring a miscarriage on a female person was an indictable offence. According to the then new Section 251 of the Code, such a therapeutic abortion had to be performed by a qualified medical practitioner who was not a member of a therapeutic abortion committee; in an accredited or approved hospital; and only after a decision by the hospital's therapeutic abortion committee, consisting of at least three members, each of them a qualified medical practitioner, that the continuation of the pregnancy would, or would be likely to, endanger the life or health of the pregnant woman.

In the ensuing years, variations in interpretation of and conformity to Section 251 gave rise in many cases to outright injustice. In some areas hospitals could not obtain accreditation or approval; in some hospitals there were not sufficient doctors to constitute a therapeutic abortion committee. Hospitals had no legal obligation to set up such a committee; and those committees that did exist had no obligation to meet. Some hospitals imposed quotas on the numbers of abortions performed, or limitations on patient eligibility based on place of residence. Women had no right to appear before the committees to present their case, and interpretation of the phrase "life or health" of the pregnant woman was left entirely to committee members. Interpretations varied enormously from one committee to another, and some even introduced extraneous considerations such as marital status of the applicant, consent of her spouse, or number of previous abortions.[4]

Section 251 of the Criminal Code placed severe constraints on Canadian women's right not to reproduce. In effect, it said that some women—directly, those whose abortion requests were rejected by therapeutic abortion committees, and indirectly, those who had no opportunity to bring their request to such a committee—had a legal obligation to procreate; it sentenced them to forced reproductive labour. This surely was a major violation of what the Charter of Rights and Freedoms now refers to as "security of the person." In the words of Supreme Court Judge Jean Beetz in the Morgentaler decision, "A pregnant woman's person cannot be said to be secure if, when her life or health is in danger, she is faced with a rule of criminal law which precludes her from obtaining effective and timely medical treatment."[5]

The so-called "pro-life" movement in North America places heavy emphasis upon what is alleged to be the foetus's right to life. Even without specifically recognizing such a right, however—indeed, without making any direct references at all to the foetus or its physical condition—Section 251 implicitly attributed to the foetus a right to the use and occupancy of the woman's uterus. In effect, the woman's body was regarded simply as a container, with various utilities, that the foetus happened to need for nine months. Indeed, foetuses are the only group of entities that have been given entitlement under Canadian law to the medical use of the bodies of adult persons.

Section 251 also helped to perpetuate a right of access to women's reproductive labour that potentially benefited both individual men and the state. In the words of Justice Bertha Wilson, Section 251 of the Criminal Code "assert[ed] that the woman's capacity to reproduce is not to be subject to her own control. It is to be subject to the control of the state.... She is truly being treated as a means—a means to an end which she does not desire but over which she has no control."[6]

Fortunately, in January 1988 the Supreme Court removed these Criminal Code impediments to women's access to abortion.[7] No longer is a woman seeking an abortion required to obtain the approval of a therapeutic abortion committee. According to the judicial decision, "Forcing a woman, by threat of criminal sanction, to carry a foetus to term unless she meets certain criteria unrelated to her own priorities and aspirations, is a profound interference with a woman's body and thus a violation of security of the person."[8]

But this decision has by no means permanently removed a significant danger to women's right not to reproduce. Like women in the United States,[9] Canadian women cannot assume that access to abortion will remain indefinitely protected. Potential threats to abortion access can be found in at least three areas.

First, there is a danger that the recent expression of concerns about the reasons for abortion and abortion-related procedures may lead to renewed limitations on access to abortion. One example is the growing media discussion of abortion for the purpose of sex selection.[10] Another is the demand for regulation of and limitations on so-called selective termination in pregnancy (discussed in detail in Chapter 3 below [*Human Reproduction*]). This procedure, performed in cases of multiple pregnancy in order to reduce the number of foetuses in the uterus, usually involves the injection of potassium chloride into the thorax of one or more of the foetuses to stop the heart. The "terminated" foetus is reabsorbed into the woman's body, without further need for surgery.[11] Recent media news reports have quoted Canadian ethicists and physicians as challenging the justification of the procedure and calling for limitations on the number of foetuses to be terminated.[12]

A second reason for concern about potential threats to the right not to reproduce is the persistence of the claim that there is a need for protection of foetal life and alleged foetal rights. In March 1989 the Supreme Court of Canada dismissed Joseph Borowski's argument that Section 251 of the Criminal Code contravened the life, security, and equality rights of the foetus, as a "person" protected by sections 7 and 15 of the Canadian Charter of Rights and Freedoms. In the absence of a law governing abortion, the Court found the appeal to be moot, and stated that the appellant no longer had standing to pursue the appeal. It added:

> In a legislative context any rights of the foetus could be considered or at least balanced against the rights of women guaranteed by s. 7.... A pronouncement in favour of the appellant's position that a foetus is protected by s. 7 from the date of conception would decide the issue out of its proper context. Doctors and hospitals would be left to speculate as to how to apply such a ruling consistently with a woman's rights under s. 7.[13]

Nevertheless, it is not impossible that a future government could use the decision in the Borowski case as part of the rationale for reintroducing a law to recriminalize some abortions. Indeed, even the 1988 decision striking down the existing abortion law left open the very real possibility that legal steps might be taken to protect so-called foetal rights. For example, Justice Wilson stated that "Section 1 of the Charter authorizes reasonable limits to be put upon the woman's right having regard to the fact of the developing foetus within her body." She added:

> A developmental view of the foetus ... supports a permissive approach to abortion in the early stages of pregnancy and a restrictive approach in the later stages.... [The woman's] reasons for having an abortion would ... be the proper subject of inquiry at the later stages of her pregnancy when the state's compelling interest in the protection of the foetus would justify it in prescribing conditions. The precise point in the development of the foetus at which the state's interest in its protection becomes "compelling" I leave to the informed judgment of the legislature which is in a position to receive guidance on the subject from all the relevant disciplines. It seems to me, however, that it might fall somewhere in the second trimester.[14]

Similarly, Chief Justice Brian Dickson said, "State protection of foetal interests may well be deserving of constitutional recognition under s. 1."[15] And Justice Beetz stated:

> [A] rule that would require a higher degree of danger to health in the latter months of pregnancy, as opposed to the early months, for an abortion to be lawful, could possibly achieve a proportionality which would be acceptable under s. 1 of the Charter.... Parliament is justified in requiring a reliable, independent and medically sound opinion in order to protect the state interest in the foetus.... [T]here would be a point in time at which the state interest in the foetus would become compelling. From this point in time, Parliament would be entitled to limit abortions to those required by therapeutic reasons and therefore require an independent opinion as to the health exception.... I am of the

view that the protection of the foetus is and ... always has been, a valid objective in Canadian criminal law.... I think s. 1 of the Charter authorizes reasonable limits to be put on a woman's right having regard to the state interest in the protection of the foetus.[16]

More recently it has been claimed that without protection of foetal rights there is nothing to prevent abortion for purposes of sex selection, harm to foetuses by the use of dangerous drugs and by third-party attacks, and the buying and selling of foetuses and foetal parts.[17] The Law Reform Commission of Canada's Working Paper entitled "Crimes Against the Foetus" expresses serious concern about dangers to the foetus, and proposes a new category of criminal offence, "Foetal Destruction or Harm."[18] Thus the stage is set for a potential continuation of major conflict between women's right not to reproduce and the alleged rights of the foetus. Unfortunately, as the Working Paper makes clear, recognition of foetal rights would almost inevitably mean the judicial recognition, via the recriminalization of abortion,[19] of the foetus's alleged right to occupancy and use of a woman's body, and concomitant limitations on women's autonomy and self-determination.

A third reason for concern about threats to Canadian women's right not to reproduce is the growing use by anti-abortion groups of not only non-violent civil disobedience but also active interference in the operations of abortion clinics.[20] In addition, "pro-life" leaders such as Joseph Borowski have threatened the use of violence in defence of their cause:

The war goes on. There is no end to this fight, and certainly no compromise. They [pro-choice] are the enemy. It's a war. Our side has one advantage. We pray. They don't.... I'm glad I did not come to Ottawa for the [Morgentaler Supreme Court] decision. I probably would have gone into the court and punched the judges in the nose.... I'm a non-violent man, and I don't believe in violence but if the seven judges or whoever were here right now, I would have great difficulty restraining myself from punching them in the mouth.[21]

In the face of these potential threats to the right not to reproduce, feminist research and activism must insist that there is no need for the recriminalization of abortion, including late abortion. No woman deliberately sets out to kill a highly developed foetus, and abortion is not sought by women for its own sake. Rather, in the words of philosopher Caroline Whitbeck, it is often a "grim option."[22] While abortions late in pregnancy may seem particularly problematic, they are usually requested for one of the following reasons. In some instances it was impossible for the woman to obtain the abortion earlier, because convoluted legal procedures delayed its approval. Cases such as these can be avoided by making very early abortions easily available and accessible. In other instances, a late abortion is sought either because prenatal testing reveals a foetal condition that is or is perceived as being severely disabling or even life-threatening, or because the woman's own life or health is endangered.[23] There is, therefore, insufficient justification for the introduction of legislation to protect the late-term foetus from the pregnant woman, or indeed for any new Criminal Code limitations on abortion.

Moreover, the entitlement to choose how many foetuses to gestate, and of what sort, should be seen as a part of the right not to reproduce. The protection of this choice is essential within a cultural context where mothering receives little social support, people with disabilities are subject to bias and stigmatization, and raising several infants simultaneously represents a personal and financial challenge of heroic dimensions. (It is also significant that the upsurge in the incidence of multiple pregnancies has been generated by the administration of fertility drugs and by the use of *in vitro* fertilization and the technology of gamete intrafallopian transfer, or GIFT.) There is no more reason to demand that a woman gestate a certain number of foetuses or type of foetus than there is to demand that she gestate a given foetus or foetuses. To set such requirements is to accord those foetuses an unjustified right of occupancy of the woman's uterus.

If protection of the foetus seems to be a worthwhile and neglected social goal, then what is needed is greater protection of the pregnant woman herself.

Even, surely, on the basis of the non-feminist and implausible assumption of an adversarial relationship between pregnant woman and foetus, the reinstallation of physicians as "body police" enforcing foetal rights[24] is unlikely to improve the behaviour of pregnant women towards their foetuses. Furthermore, in order to prevent the commodification of foetuses and foetal parts, and other undesirable uses of the foetus, there is no more need to assign personhood or rights to the foetus than there is to assign personhood or rights to blood or body parts. Instead of using that blunt instrument the criminal law in *post hoc* fashion to attempt to manage undesirable reproductive practices, use can be made of existing regulations governing health care and the utilization of human tissues. Ultimately, of course, it will be necessary to minimize and finally eliminate the powerful underlying conditions of oppression that generate such practices as foetal commodification and sex selection.

The Right to Reproduce

The right not to reproduce is distinct from the right to reproduce. In other words, it is independent, neither implying a right to reproduce nor following from such a right.

The right to reproduce has two senses, which may be called the weak (or liberty) sense and the strong (or welfare) sense. The weak sense of the right to reproduce is the entitlement not to be interfered with in reproduction, or prevented from reproducing. It would imply an obligation on the part of the state not to inhibit or limit reproductive liberty through, for example, racist marriage laws, forced sterilization,[25] or coercive birth-control programs.

In this weak sense, the right to reproduce is also compromised by restrictions on the place of birth and on birth attendants, and by court-ordered Caesarean sections for competent but unwilling pregnant women. Like the United States, Canada has a history of the gradual medicalization of birth. Midwives have been replaced by physicians, from general practitioners to obstetricians; hospitals have replaced the home; and medical innovations from foetal monitoring, amniotomy (the premature puncturing of the amniotic sac), and forceps deliveries to anaesthesia and Caesarean sections have made birthing into a health crisis. Without the genuine freedom to choose home birth, to be attended by midwives, and to avoid obstetrical technology, women's right to reproduce in the weak sense is seriously compromised.

In its strong sense, the right to reproduce would be the right to receive all necessary assistance to reproduce. It would imply entitlement to access to any and all available forms of reproductive products, technologies, and labour, including the gametes of other women and men, the gestational services of women, and the full range of procreative techniques including *in vitro* fertilization, gamete intrafallopian transfer, uterine lavage (a process in which one woman is inseminated with sperm, her uterus is flushed with fluid, and the embryo is retrieved for implantation in another woman's uterus), embryo freezing, and sex preselection.

Non-feminist writers such as American legal theorist John A. Robertson defend the right to reproduce in the strong sense by claiming that it is simply an extension of the right to reproduce in the weak sense. As he puts it, "the right of the married couple to reproduce noncoitally" and "the right to reproduce noncoitally with the assistance of donors and surrogates" both follow from "constitutional acceptance of a married couple's right to reproduce coitally."[26] (Robertson's heterosexist bias is not much mitigated by his later concession that there is "a very strong argument for unmarried persons, either single or as couples, also having a positive right to reproduce.")[27] Robertson believes that these rights entitle married couples certainly, and perhaps single persons, to "create, store, transfer, donate and possibly even manipulate extra-corporeal embryos"; and "to contract for eggs, sperm, embryos, or surrogates." They would also, he thinks, justify compelling a contract mother to hand over a child to its purchasers, even against her will.[28]

In addition, American attorney Lori B. Andrews argues that the right to reproduce in the strong sense is probably founded upon the right to marital privacy, which, she claims, protects the full range of married people's choices about both sexual and reproductive behaviour.[29] Hence some feminists may want to claim the right to reproduce in the strong sense both because of arguments such as those of Robertson and Andrews, and because of a fear that otherwise access to reproductive technologies such as IVF may be treated by the state as a privilege—one to be gained only through possession of the requisite social criteria, such as being heterosexual and married.

Nevertheless, the legitimacy and justification of this right to reproduce are questionable. To recognize it would be to shift the burden of proof onto those who have doubts about the morality of technologies such as IVF and practices such as contract motherhood. For it suggests that a child is somehow owed to each of us, as individuals or as members of a couple, and that it is indefensible for society to fail to provide all possible means for obtaining one. Thus it might be used, as Robertson advocates, to imply an entitlement to hire contract mothers, to obtain other women's eggs, and to make use of donor insemination and uterine lavage of another woman, all in order to maximize the chances of reproducing.[30] In other words, recognition of the right to reproduce in the strong sense would create an active right of access to women's bodies and in particular to our reproductive labour and products. For example, it would condone the hiring of contract mothers, and force the latter to surrender their infants after birth. And it might be used to found a claim to certain kinds of children—for example, children of a desired sex, appearance, or intelligence.

Exercise of the alleged right to reproduce in this strong sense could potentially require violation of some women's right not to reproduce. There is already good evidence, in both the United States and Great Britain, that eggs and ovarian tissue have been taken from some women without their knowledge or informed consent.[31] It is not difficult to imagine that recognizing a strong right to reproduce could require either a similar theft of eggs or embryos from some women, if none can be found to offer them willingly, or a commercial inducement to sell these products. Such a right could be used as a basis for requiring fertile people to "donate" gametes and embryos. Even if some people would willingly donate gametes, there is no *right* on the part of the infertile that would entitle them to demand such donations.

The feminist language of reproductive rights is illegitimately co-opted when it is used to defend an alleged right to become or to hire a contract mother, to buy or to sell eggs, embryos, or babies, or to select or preselect the sex of one's offspring. There can be no genuine entitlement to women's reproductive labour, nor to buying or otherwise obtaining human infants. Contract motherhood entails a type of slave trade in infants, and it commits women to a modern form of indentured servitude.

It is to be hoped that Canada will choose neither the legalization of contract motherhood nor the criminalization of contract mothers. We should opt instead to reduce the potential motivation for such contracts by making them unenforceable and by rendering criminal both the operation of contract motherhood agencies and the actions of professionals who participate in such arrangements. It is important for Canadian social policy to resist the incursion of US-style commercialization of reproduction and reproductive entrepreneurialism, the most likely victims of which would be poor women and women of colour [...].

At the same time, there is no need to treat procedures like *in vitro* fertilization as privileges to which access may be limited on arbitrary and unfair grounds—grounds such as marital status, sexual orientation, putative stability or parenting potential, or economic level. While I cannot wholeheartedly support and endorse highly ineffective, costly, and painful procedures such as IVF, I also cannot endorse the call by some feminists for a total ban on the procedure. State provision and financing of IVF is different from state provision of contract motherhood. Many compelling reasons—primary among them being the sale of babies and the exploitation of women's reproductive labour—militate against state recognition of contract motherhood through legalization or financial support. These two reasons are not present, or not inevitably present, in the case of IVF.

Rather, without asserting a strong right to all possible reproductive assistance, we can critically examine the artificial barriers, such as marital status, sexual orientation, and ability to pay, that get in the way of women's fair access to reproductive technologies. We can also provide protections for women entering and participating in infertility treatment programs. This would require ensuring that applicants make a genuinely informed choice, in full knowledge of the short- and long-term risks, possible benefits, chances of success and failure, alternative approaches and treatments, and perhaps even the pronatalist social pressures to procreate. *If* IVF seems to be a valuable medical service (and that view is still debatable) then it deserves to be made available, like other medical services, through medicare, as is now the case in Ontario. It would also be important to ensure thorough screening of egg and sperm donors; to maintain adequate records that will make it possible to track the long-term effects of IVF on women and their offspring; and to ensure that any women who provide eggs for the program have genuinely chosen to do so. Finally, in the long run, feminists should be thinking about whether it is possible to incorporate high-tech infertility treatments such as IVF into women-centred and women-controlled reproductive health centres.

The approach sketched here avoids two tendencies that I believe are undesirable: on the one hand, treating access to reproductive technology as a privilege to be earned through the possession of certain personal, social, sexual, and/or financial characteristics; and on the other hand, a kind of feminist maternalism that seeks, in the best interests of women, to terminate IVF research and treatment.[32] While many feminists have stressed both the social construction of the desire for motherhood and the dangers and ineffectiveness of *in vitro* fertilization,[33] it is surely dangerous for feminists to claim to understand better than infertile women themselves the origins and significance of their desire for children. It is not the role of feminist research and action to protect women from what is interpreted as their own "false consciousness." Instead, we should assume that when women are provided with full information about the possibilities they will be empowered to make reproductive decisions that will genuinely benefit themselves and their children.[34]

Conclusion

The two themes that have structured the struggle over reproductive rights in Canada appear to have little in common: on the one hand, access to various reproductive services and technologies; on the other, the use and exploitation of women's bodies for reproductive purposes.

Nevertheless, the goals of access to reproductive technologies and access to women's bodies come together within conservative discourse on reproduction. Pronatalist, pro-family, and in favour of traditional roles for women, this discourse is also classist, racist, ableist, and heterosexist. The oppressive nature of this discourse is often disguised by the co-optation of feminist language and concepts. In recent lectures and papers, for example, members of the anti-abortion movement have claimed that there is "sexism" in the pro-choice movement,[35] which is alleged to favour the sexual agenda of men over the reproductive needs of women, and have depicted the foetus as a member of a maligned minority group. The same voices that want to ban abortion because women engage in sexual intercourse "by choice" also want to compel contract mothers to sell their babies because they enter the contracts "by choice." Meanwhile, nonfeminists are proclaiming that new reproductive technologies actually promote women's autonomy and reproductive choice.[36]

Paradoxically, however, both the non-existence and the existence of certain reproductive "choices" or alternatives can be coercive. While lack of access to contraception or abortion clearly violates reproductive choice by failing to respect the right not to reproduce, conversely practices such as contract motherhood and the sale of gametes and embryos have the potential to violate reproductive choice. In other words, respecting a right to reproduce in the strong sense for some may violate the right not to reproduce of others.

Feminists want to preserve and enhance access to the reproductive services and technologies that benefit women while preventing further encroachments on access to women's bodies, whether by the state or by individuals. The way to do this is by insisting upon both women's right not to reproduce and our right to reproduce in the weak sense, and also by developing a critical analysis of the ways in which the right to reproduce in the strong sense is now being exercised.

Notes

1 Barbara Katz Rothman, remarks at a conference on "Legal and Ethical Aspects of Human Reproduction," Canadian Institute of Law and Medicine, Toronto, Dec. 1989.

2 Christine Overall, *Ethics and Human Reproduction: A Feminist Analysis* (Boston: Allen and Unwin, 1987), Chapter 8.

3 R v. Morgentaler [1988] 1 SCR 30, 172.

4 Ibid., 56-61, 64-73.

5 Ibid., 90.

6 Ibid., 173.

7 Ignoring the Criminal Code provisions on abortion, community health clinics in Quebec had already been providing abortions for more than a decade before the Supreme Court decision.

8 R v. Morgentaler [1988] 1 SCR 32.

9 See George J. Annas, "Webster and the Politics of Abortion," *Hastings Center Report* 19 (March/April 1989): 36-38. In July 1989 the United States Supreme Court ruled that the state of Missouri had the right to ban the performance of abortions by public hospitals and public employees. It is anticipated that the court may in future uphold additional state-imposed restrictions on abortion services, seriously limiting access to abortion, particularly for poor women. See *Webster v. Reproductive Health Services*, 109 S. Ct. 3040 (1989).

10 For example, Brenda Large's editorial "If Sex-Based Abortions Are Wrong, So Are All," *Kingston Whig-Standard* (11 Feb. 1989).

11 Mark I. Evans, John C. Fletcher, Evan E. Zador, Burritt W. Newton, Mary Helen Quigg, and Curtis D. Struyk, "Selective First-Trimester Termination in Octuplet and Quadruplet Pregnancies: Clinical and Ethical Issues," *Obstetrics and Gynecology* 71, 3, pt. 1 (March 1988): 291.

12 Dorothy Lipovenko, "Infertility Technology Forces People to Make Life and Death Choices," *The Globe and Mail* (21 Jan. 1989): A4; "Multiple Pregnancies Create Moral Dilemma," *Kingston Whig-Standard* (21 Jan. 1989): 3.

13 Borowski v. Canada (Attorney General) [1989] 1 SCR 342.

14 R. v. Morgentaler, 181, 183.

15 Ibid., 76.

16 Ibid., 82-83, 110, 113, 124.

17 Neil Reynolds, "Fetal Status Cannot Depend on Momentary Opinion," *Kingston Whig-Standard* (16 March 1989): 6.

18 Law Reform Commission of Canada, Working Paper 58, "Crimes Against the Foetus" (Ottawa, 1989), 64.

19 Ibid., 42, 56, and 64.

20 A. Johnson, "Clinic Fights to Survive in B.C.," *Rites* (March 1989): 4; and Helen Armstrong, Debi Brock and Jennifer Stephen, "'Operation Rescue' Turns Into Fiasco," *Rites* (March 1989): 5.

21 Joseph Borowski, quoted in *The Toronto Star* and *The Globe and Mail*, 10 March 1989.

22 Caroline Whitbeck, "The Moral Implications of Regarding Women as People: New Perspectives on Pregnancy and Personhood," in William B. Bondeson, H. Tristram Engelhardt, Jr, Stuart F. Spicker, and Daniel H. Winship, eds., *Abortion and the Status of the Fetus* (Boston: Reidel, 1984), 251.

23 This is argued by Sanda Rodgers in "The Future of Abortion in Canada," in Christine Overall, ed., *The Future of Human Reproduction* (Toronto: Women's Press, 1989). This argument in no way endorses the use of abortion for supposed eugenic purposes. As disabled women and their allies have pointed out, feminists should be highly critical of the use of reproductive technologies to discriminate among human beings on the basis of their physical or mental condition, or to promote the notion of human perfectibility. See Marcia Saxton, "Prenatal Screening and Discriminatory Attitudes About Disability," in Elaine Hoffman Baruch, Amadeo F. D'Adamo, Jr, and Joni Seager, eds., *Embryos, Ethics, and Women's Rights: Exploring the New Reproductive Technologies* (New York: Haworth Press, 1988), 217-24, and Ruth Hubbard, "Eugenics: New Tools, Old Ideas," in ibid., 225-35.

24 In my view, this is the effect of the proposal of the Law Reform Commission of Canada's "Crimes Against the Foetus," which would require "medical authorization" of an abortion by one "qualified medical practitioner" before foetal viability, and by two such practitioners after the foetus is capable of independent survival (64).

25 In North America there is a long history of the forced sterilization of native women and women of colour.

26 John A. Robertson, "Procreative Liberty, Embryos, and Collaborative Reproduction: A Legal Perspec-

tive," in Baruch et al., eds., *Embryos, Ethics and Women's Rights*, 180. Cf. Lori B. Andrews, "Alternative Modes of Reproduction," in Sherrill Cohen and Nadine Taub, eds., *Reproductive Laws for the 1990s* (Clifton, N.J.: Humana Press, 1989), 364.

27 Robertson, "Procreative Liberty," 181.

28 Ibid., 180, 186, and 190.

29 Lori B. Andrews, *New Conceptions: A Consumer's Guide to the Newest Infertility Treatments* (New York: Ballantyne Books, 1985), 138.

30 From this point of view, then, IVF with donor gametes is more problematic than IVF in which a woman and a man make use of their own eggs and sperm.

31 Genoveffa Corea, "Egg Snatchers," in Rita Arditti, Renate Duelli Klein, and Shelley Minden, eds., *Test-Tube Women: What Future for Motherhood* (London: Pandora Press, 1984), 37-51.

32 Renate Duelli Klein, quoted in Christine St. Peters, "Feminist Discourse, Infertility, and the New Reproductive Technologies," *National Women's Studies Association Journal* 1, 3 (Spring 1989): 358.

33 See, for example, Susan Sherwin, "Feminist Ethics and In Vitro Fertilization," in Marsha Hanen and Kai Nielsen, eds., *Science, Morality and Feminist Theory* (Calgary: University of Calgary Press, 1987), 265-84.

34 For a more detailed discussion of the fair provision of IVF, see "Access to *In Vitro* Fertilization: Costs, Care, and Consent," Chapter 8 [in *Human Reproduction*, Oxford University Press, 1993].

35 See, for example, Diane Marshall and Martha Crean, "The Human Face of a Woman's Agony," in Ian Gentles, ed., *A Time to Choose Life: Women, Abortion and Human Rights* (Toronto: Stoddart, 1990), 134-42, and Janet Ajzenstat, "The Sexism of Pro-Choice," Queen's University, Kingston, Ont., 14 March 1989. Ajzenstat is a member of the Department of Political Science, McMaster University.

36 John Robertson ("Procreative Liberty") claims that "[e]xtra-corporeal conception seems to promote choice, to promote the autonomy of women (and men) in helping them overcome infertility, which for many women (and men) is a very serious problem" (192). It "makes possible new, partial reproductive roles for women" as "egg and embryo donors and surrogates" (193).

19.
CLASS, FEMINIST, AND COMMUNITARIAN CRITIQUES OF PROCREATIVE LIBERTY

John A. Robertson

SOURCE: *Children of Choice: Freedom and the New Reproductive Technologies*
(Princeton: Princeton University Press, 1994).

With procreative liberty as a beacon, this book[1] has visited the ethical, legal, and social conflicts presented by new reproductive technology. The journey has fleshed out the meaning of procreative liberty by arguing for presumptive moral and legal protection for reproductive technologies that expand procreative options. Those technologies that are not centrally connected to the values that underlie procreative liberty deserve less respect. The resulting picture is a growing array of sophisticated technologies that can help individuals achieve their reproductive goals. As with many technologies, a bright, hopeful side coexists with dismay and distrust over how reproductive technologies might be used. For many people the technical ability to prevent or end pregnancy, to relieve infertility, to increase the chance of healthy offspring, or to obtain tissue for research and therapy is a great boon, and confirms one's faith in scientific progress.

Yet others feel profound discomfort with reproductive manipulations, and urge strict regulation or even prohibition. The source of their disquiet may be traced back to fears of manipulating nature and interfering with God's plans that have plagued science since its inception. Here the danger is even more ominous, because reproductive technologies manipulate the earliest stages of human life and potentially harm prenatal life, offspring, women, and the family.

In responding to this technology, individuals and society are both caught between autonomy and ambivalence—between the demands of personal choice and the disquiet that uses of autonomy causes them and society. One is damned either way—either overly technologizing the intimate, or losing the very real benefits that this technology provides.

The burden of this book has been to show the importance of procreative liberty in resolving these controversies. The lens of procreative liberty is essential because reproductive technologies are necessarily bound up with procreative choice. They are means to achieve or avoid the reproductive experiences that are central to personal conceptions of meaning and identity. To deny procreative choice is to deny or impose an all-encompassing reproductive experience on persons without their consent, thus denying them respect and dignity at the most basic level.

Although procreative liberty is a deeply held value, its scope and contours have never previously been fully elaborated. Past controversies have concerned contraception and abortion, and rarely, with the exception of eugenic sterilization and overpopulation in the Third World, dealt with limitations on procreation itself. The advent of new reproductive technologies has changed the landscape of conflict, and forced us to inquire into the meaning and scope of procreative liberty.

This book's discussion of seven controversial reproductive technologies has shown the intimate connection between procreative liberty and technology. Once this connection is made, the choice of individuals to use or not use these technologies should be presumptively respected because of the privileged position that procreative liberty occupies as a moral and legal right. Where only peripheral aspects of procreation are involved, the right to use those techniques must rest on some basis other than procreative liberty.

The invocation of procreative liberty as a dominant value is not intended to demolish opposition or end discussion. It is offered as a template to guide inquiry and evaluation, and to assure that moral inquiry and public policy do not ignore the importance of personal choice in these matters. No right is absolute. Even procreative liberty can be limited or restricted when adequate cause can be shown. Procreative choices that clearly harm the tangible interest of others are subject to regulation or even prohibition. Even if they cannot be prohibited, their use can be condemned as irresponsible or ill-advised, or not encouraged.

With this approach, however, we have seen that there are few instances in which the feared harms of the new technology are compelling enough to justify restrictive legal intervention (though the need for responsible use remains). Again and again the dire warnings of harm turn out to be baseless or speculative fears, or to reflect highly contested positions about fetal or embryo status, gestational motherhood, and the nature of families—positions that are usually insufficient to justify interference with procreation. In nearly every instance, public policy should keep the gateway to technology open, allowing individuals the freedom to enter as they will.

In the few instances in which choice could be limited, the core values of procreative liberty do not appear to be directly implicated, as with restrictions on pregnant women using drugs, Norplant for the retarded, and nontherapeutic genetic engineering. Even when a good case for restricting reproductive choice exists, the regulatory emphasis should be on counseling, education, notice, and noncoercive incentives, though criminal penalties or injunctions may in some cases be justified.

Some people, of course, will disagree with this analysis, either because they dispute the privileged position accorded procreative liberty or the assessment of harms from individual choice. For example, they may think that I have underestimated the impact of these technologies on women, children, and the family, or undervalued the moral status of embryos and fetuses. Or they may simply be more cautious. With technologies that have not yet been widely used, much less assimilated into the social fabric, it may be premature to pronounce them socially acceptable or even essential to procreative choice.

Yet even if one differs with the book's position in particular instances, the importance of procreative liberty in assessing other applications of technology should remain. For example, persons holding pro-life views will disagree with a biologically based, symbolic analysis of abortion and other prenatal conflicts. But this disagreement should affect only those situations in which embryos or fetuses are directly threatened, and not all other instances of procreative choice.

Even persons with pro-life beliefs might grant the importance of procreative liberty in deciding whether persons may or may not use technologies that do not destroy prenatal life. They may still recognize the right of infertile couples to use IVF, at least within certain limits, and may favor prenatal screening where therapeutic interventions are possible. They may also support uses of Norplant and other technologies when people are not equipped to raise children, as long as embryos and fetuses are not destroyed. Despite differences in some areas, considerable room remains for respecting procreative choice.

An additional advantage of a procreative liberty framework for assessing reproductive technology is the guidance that this approach provides in evaluating future innovations. The development of IVF, prenatal screening, contragestion, and other techniques marks a watershed in human reproduction from which there is no turning back. Future developments will push the envelope of technological control even further, as extracorporeal gestation, cloning, embryo splitting, genetic engineering, embryo tissue farms, posthumous birthing, and other variations come on line. Each of them will present the same dilemmas of individual choice and public policy that we now face.

Procreative liberty should provide a useful framework for evaluating those future developments as well. The effect of each new technology on procreative choice will have to be assessed. If procreative interests are centrally implicated, then only strong countervailing interests will justify limitation. As illustrated repeatedly throughout this book, many of the concerns and fears will, upon closer analysis, turn out to be speculative fears or symbolic perceptions that do not justify infringing core procreative interests. If we accept a strong version of procreative liberty, then public policy for those technologies, as for most of those surveyed in this book, may have to rely on education and persuasion rather than coercion.

The Problems of a Rights-Based Approach

The approach of this book has been explicitly and unswervingly rights based. Taking procreative liberty as a fundamental moral and legal right, it has assumed that the individual's procreative liberty should rule unless there are compelling reasons to the contrary.

While such an approach characterizes many social issues in the United States, a right-based approach has been strongly criticized in recent years as overly individualistic and insufficiently sensitive to the needs of the community. In a recent book, for example, Professor Mary Ann Glendon has argued that rights talk is limiting because it is absolutist, individualist, and inimical to a sense of social responsibility.[2] Others have argued that rights talk is too private and individualistic, ignoring how public claims interpenetrate the private sphere.[3] It also exposes a social blindness to the claims of interdependence and mutual responsibility that are at the heart of social living.[4]

These criticisms of rights talk are especially applicable to reproduction. A rights-based perspective tends to view reproduction as an isolated, individual act without effects on others. The determinative consideration is whether an individual thinks that a particular technology will serve his or her personal reproductive goals. Except for the rare case of compelling harm, the effects of reproductive choices on offspring, on women, on family, on society and on the general tone and fabric of life are treated as irrelevant to moral analysis or public policy.[5]

Yet reproduction is the act that most clearly implicates community and other persons. Reproduction is never solipsistic. It always occurs with a partner, even if that partner is an anonymous egg or sperm donor, and usually requires the collaboration of physicians and nurses. Its occurrence also directly affects others by creating a new person who in turn affects them

and society in various ways. Reproduction is never exclusively a private matter and cannot be completely accounted for in the language of individual rights. Emphasizing procreative rights thus risks denying the central, social dimensions of reproduction.

Critics of rights talk point particularly to the abortion debate, where the pro-choice claim ignores both the interests of fetuses and the interests of fathers and potential grandparents.[6] This criticism might also be leveled against other reproductive technologies, from IVF and collaborative reproduction to genetic screening and fetal tissue transplants. Emphasizing procreative rights necessarily deemphasizes the effects of these technologies on prenatal life, offspring, handicapped children, the family, women, and collaborators.

Although powerful and important, however, this critique of rights does not defeat the priority assigned to procreative rights anymore than it defeats the priority of free speech, due process, travel, and other important rights. To begin with, the critique does not always prove the ill effects that it claims. Glendon, for example, overlooks the fact that many rights "encourage precisely the form of deliberation and communal interaction" that Glendon herself favors.[7] This is true of political and social rights, which make communal deliberation and democracy possible.[8] It is also true of rights to use procreative technologies. Thus IVF encourages the formation of families and the cooperative, dependent relationships that inhere therein. The use of donors and surrogates requires a special kind of cooperation, often among strangers, that leads to new forms of community. Even aborting to get fetal tissue for a loved one can be a sacrifice that binds rather than divides.

Second, rights-based approaches to reproduction or other issues do not ignore other interests so much as judge them, after careful scrutiny, as inadequate to sustain interference with individual choice. If harmful effects are clearly established or the action in question does not implicate central features of fundamental liberty, public concerns may take priority over private choice. In many cases, however, the state is relegated to exhortation and noncoercive sanctions to protect communal interest because it cannot satisfy the burden of serious harm necessary to justify overriding fundamental rights.

A third problem with the critique of rights is that the alternative it offers is weak and thin, even less desirable than whatever excesses rights might breed. Without the protection of rights, important aspects of individual dignity and integrity have no protection from legislative majorities or policymakers. Elizabeth Kingdom's hope that getting beyond rights will enable public policy to make "a wider calculation of the proper distribution of social benefits" overlooks the need for rights to protect us from the policy calculations of zealous administrators.[9] Indeed, the emergence of rights is due to the failure of the community and public officials to give due regard to the needs of affected individuals.

This is especially clear in the case of abortion, which Glendon and Elizabeth Fox-Genovese claim shows the divisive, individualistic vices of a rights approach. The claim for a right to abortions comes out of a failed collective responsibility toward motherhood, which makes abortion an essential option. If pro-life groups were truly concerned with the weak and vulnerable, as their concern with the fetus claims, they would make greater efforts to rectify the social and economic conditions that make abortion a necessary option for women. Their failure in this regard suggests rather an interest in controlling "women's reproductive capacities ... (in order) ... to continue a system of discrimination that is based on sex."[10] Rights are essential precisely to guard against discriminatory agendas that deny dignity and integrity to women and men. They are responses to failures of social responsibility, not the causes of them.[11]

To be convincing, however, a right-based approach must acknowledge its defects even while proclaiming its strengths. It cannot ignore the social dimension, even if social claims are seldom sufficient to limit procreative choice. To assure that full credence is given to these dimensions, three specific criticisms of a rights-based approach are discussed. In each case we will see that procreative liberty, despite some qualifications, emerges alive and well.

Money and Class

A major problem with a rights-based approach is that it ignores the social and economic context in which exercise of rights is embedded. Procreative rights are negative in protecting against private or state interference, but they give no positive assistance to someone who lacks the resources essential to exercise the right. A rights-based approach to reproductive choice thus has no way to take the effects of money and class into account. As Rhonda Copeland has noted:

The negative theory of privacy is ... profoundly inadequate as a basis for reproductive and sexual freedom because it perpetuates the myth that the ability to effectuate one's choices rests exclusively on the individual, rather than acknowledging that choices are facilitated, hindered or entirely frustrated by social conditions. In doing so negative privacy theory exempts the state from responsibility for contributing to the material conditions and social relations that impede, and conversely, could encourage autonomous decision-making.[12]

The truth of this statement is evident in how the distribution of wealth operates as a prime determinant of who exercises reproductive rights. The most obvious wealth effect concerns access to reproductive technology. For example, women who lack the money to pay for Norplant or abortions are much less able to avoid reproduction than those who can pay. Yet the Supreme Court has held that the state's failure to fund abortions for indigent women does not violate their right to terminate pregnancy because it places no obstacle in their path that was not already there.[13] It is also the poor who feel the brunt of 24-hour waiting periods for abortions, and who would be most acutely affected if *Roe v. Wade* were ever reversed.

Lack of resources also affect one's ability to undergo IVF and related assisted reproductive techniques. At a cost of $7,000 per cycle, only middle- and upper-class couples can afford this treatment. Since several cycles may be needed to establish pregnancy, this is a technique that will clearly be wealth-based. Similarly, egg donation and surrogacy, which have equivalent or higher costs, will also be distributed according to wealth. Nor will prenatal screening and genetic manipulation be widely available to those who cannot pay for them.

There is irony in the financial disparities that determine differential access here. Poor and minorities have greater rates of infertility than middle and upper classes, yet only the latter can afford the high costs of IVF and other assisted reproductive treatment. Given the current crisis of access to health care for poor people, the idea of Medicaid payments for infertility treatments is politically unlikely, so these disparities are likely to continue.

Allocating reproductive technologies and other essential goods and services according to ability to pay raises profound questions of social justice. Because infertility impairs a basic aspect of species-typical functioning, a strong argument for including it in any basic health-care package can be made.[14] Yet it does not follow that society's failure to assure access to reproductive technologies for all who would benefit justifies denying access to those who have the means to pay. Such a principle has not been followed with other medical procedures, even life-saving procedures such as heart transplants. As troubled as we might be by differential access, the demands of equality should not bar access for those fortunate enough to have the means.

Class and money may also influence the roles individuals play in the collaborative reproductive process. Under the theory of procreative liberty proposed in this book, individuals have the right to hire or engage donors and surrogates, or to serve as donors and surrogates themselves.[15] Since donors and surrogates are usually paid for their contribution, the danger is that only the middle class and wealthy will have the resources to hire them, while only the lower classes will be inclined to assume these roles. If this is so, money and class will greatly skew the distribution of roles and services in collaborative reproduction.

The latter concern, however, may be most acute for surrogacy. Although lack of funds may prevent poor people from obtaining gamete donations, poverty has not been a determinant of who provides sperm and egg donations. Proximity, reliability, health, and fertility have been the main factors physicians have sought in gamete donors. While egg donations are paid as much as $1,500 to $2,000 per cycle, it is unlikely that only poor women in need of money will choose to be donors.

Class, however, may be a stronger factor in the selection of surrogate mothers. Again, poor people will not usually be able to buy surrogate services, if a willing family member is not available. However, they are more likely to be recruited as surrogates because of the $10,000 or more that they will be paid. It is not surprising that Mary Beth Whitehead, the surrogate in the *Baby M* case, was of a lower social class and less educated then the recipient couple. Similarly, in the *Anna C. v. Mark J.* gestational surrogate case, the surrogate was black, while the hiring couple was white/Asian.[16] Although many surrogates have gone to high school or college, there is a danger that class bias and financial need will determine the supply of surrogates. Carried to extremes, a breeder class of poor, minority women whose reproductive capacity is exploited by wealthier people could emerge.

But what is to be done about this practice? Denying poorer women that opportunity by prohibiting payment or by allowing payment only to middle-class surrogates denies them a reproductive role which they find meaningful. Given that poorer women serve as nannies, babysitters, housekeepers, and factory workers, gestational services might also be sold, even though it will offend the respect that some persons have for maternal gestation. Should couples be denied access to surrogacy because of the risk of class bias, when the surrogate is freely and intelligently choosing that role? Whatever our qualms about such a practice, it may have to be tolerated because the procreative liberty of all the parties is so intimately involved.

A final area in which class and money will make itself felt is in state interventions to protect offspring from harmful prenatal conduct or to limit irresponsible reproduction by compulsory contraception. Punishing women for prenatal child abuse or ordering cesarean sections against their will appears to have a disproportionate racial and class impact. For example, a Florida study showed that while the same percentage of white and black women have signs of illegal drugs in their blood at birth, the state refers black women disproportionately to the criminal justice system or to child welfare agencies.[17] Other studies have shown that mandatory cesarean sections are most commonly sought for black and poor women, not for whites who also refuse the operation.[18] Similarly, compulsory contraception for child abusers or HIV women seems to target the poor and minorities more than other groups. Although an invidious discriminatory purpose has not been shown to underlie these disparities, the danger that wealth, class, and race will be factors in the state's coercive use of reproductive technology cannot be ignored.

These points about the role of money and class in distributing reproductive technologies and procreative choice show the limits of a negative rights-based approach to procreative liberty. It is another example of the disparities that differential distribution of wealth in a liberal society inevitably brings. One can decry the disparities that exist and urge that society correct distributive inequities, however, without denying all persons the right to make these choices. In the end, the need for social justice is not a compelling reason for limiting the procreative choice of those who can pay.

The Feminist Critique

A strong emphasis on procreative liberty has also been questioned by feminists who fear that technology will lessen women's control over reproduction and further oppression of women. Feminist critics have usually focused on the dangers to women in surrogate motherhood or objected to prenatal interventions for the sake of offspring. However, the feminist critique goes deeper than a challenge to these techniques, and calls into question all reproductive technologies that redound to the benefit of a male-dominated society at the expense of women.[19]

The feminist critique of a rights-based approach to reproductive technology has several strands. Sometimes the objections go to the very idea of subjecting the natural reproductive process to technological control, because such control is viewed as a male-driven violation of the natural order. The more central fear, however, is that because of men's greater access to wealth and power, they will use reproductive technologies to control and oppress women. Indeed, some feminists assert that men devised these techniques in order to control female reproduction just when women began gaining social and economic power. They fear that a rights-based approach to

reproductive technology will further patriarchal domination of women by reinforcing the traditional identification of women with childbearing and child rearing. At the very least, it will result in women taking on additional reproductive burdens to serve male procreative agendas.

Given the long history of sexism in medicine, the feminist critique must be taken seriously. A long tradition exists of men controlling female reproduction. Male doctors wrested control of the birth process from female midwives in the eighteenth and nineteenth centuries. In the early twentieth century they developed techniques of twilight sleep and anesthesia to further that control, which the natural childbirth movement of the 1960s and 1970s fought hard to overcome.[20] Hysterectomy, involuntary sterilization, and mastectomy reflect further assaults on female sexuality and reproduction. Electronic fetal monitoring and high rates for cesarean births may also be seen as further examples of male control.[21]

Some developments in reproductive technology seem to be cut from the same cloth. Forced cesarean section or jail for drug use discovered by doctors during pregnancy strikes some people as a form of medical violence against women. Forced contraception to limit "irresponsible reproduction" could be viewed as a way to bring untrammeled female sexuality under control. Restrictions on abortion often seem more concerned with imposing sexual and reproductive orthodoxy than on protecting fetuses.

Noncoital treatments of infertility can also be seen in this light. Women undergo the burdensome roller-coaster ride of IVF treatment to please their husbands. IVF technologies assault the woman's body with powerful hormones to coax out eggs and make the uterus receptive to embryos. Women may also feel compelled to screen out defective embryos and fetuses to make sure that they deliver a "good baby."

Because women bear the brunt of reproductive work, injustice in the distribution of reproductive burdens and benefits is inescapable. However, the view that a rights-based view of reproductive technology places power increasingly in the hands of men to the detriment of women overlooks the many ways in which technology offers options that expand the freedom of women. It also overlooks how a rights-based approach, despite its contextual limitations, assures women a large measure of control over their reproductive lives.

Consider how several technologies discussed in this book help women to avoid unwanted pregnancy or to have healthy offspring. Norplant is a safe, effective, and reversible long-lasting contraception that many women will welcome. When RU486 becomes available in the United States, it will allow unwanted pregnancies to be terminated at early stages without surgery, and thus increase access to abortion. IVF and the other assisted reproductive techniques enable women to rear offspring when they previously would have had to remain childless or adopt. Earlier and less invasive prenatal diagnosis allows a woman to avoid giving birth to handicapped children. Tissue production techniques may eventually allow a woman to save the life of a child, a parent, or even herself. Given these possibilities, reproductive technologies would appear to advance the interests of women.

Although a rights-based approach to reproduction cannot eliminate the inherent inequalities in male and female procreation, it can provide substantial protection for women. It is the best guarantee of a woman's control over the options these technologies offer. Legal recognition of procreative liberty will protect women from public sector impositions on their procreative choice. Respecting this liberty will stop the state from outlawing early abortion. Respect of this right will also protect women against forced sterilization, forced abortion, or forced contraception to prevent harm to offspring or taxpayers. Some limits on reproductively related conduct, such as drug use during pregnancy, might still be possible, but the threat here is not procreative liberty and neither men nor women have the right to harm offspring by egregious or irresponsible prenatal conduct. When everything is considered, a strong commitment to procreative liberty will protect more than it will harm the interests of women.

Of course this is not to deny the ways in which technology can be used to harm women, or the barriers that stand in the way of women having the means and the situational power to exercise free choice in decisions about technology. However, the most common target of feminist attacks is the argument that procreative liberty leads to the enforce-ment of surrogate mother contracts against the wishes of the gestational mother. Although much less common than other assisted reproductive techniques, surrogacy has come to symbolize the struggle of women to gain control of pregnancy and reproduction.[22]

Many feminists always favor the gestational mother in these disputes, as do most of the courts and legislatures that have addressed the issue.[23] Yet which solution is most protective of women is debatable—the woman who provides the egg for gestational surrogacy also has important reproductive interests at stake as do women who wish to serve as surrogates who are denied the opportunity because of the legal unenforceability of their preconception promise. Many liberal feminists now argue that the intentions of the contracting parties should control rearing.[24] In their view, such a solution puts women in ultimate control, even though it requires that they be bound by surrogacy contracts just as they are by their contracts in other settings. It also undercuts traditional notions of reproductive orthodoxy that identify women with gestation and child rearing.

In the private sphere, the main issue for women will be whether they will be free to use—to have access to—the technologies they desire. Pro-creative liberty will protect them against state restrictions that are based on speculative harms or particular moral views of proper reproductive behavior, a major threat in this area. They will thus be free to use or not use IVF, egg and embryo donation, gestational surrogacy, genetic screening, embryo biopsy, and fetal therapy to treat infertility or to have healthy children.

Of course, a right against the state to use these techniques will not overcome contextual constraints on a women's freedom. It does not help her if she lacks the funds to purchase the services in question. Nor will it remove the financial pressures that might lead her to choose to be an egg donor or a surrogate. It also does not protect her from her partner's, her family's, or her own internally generated demands—the product of socialization in a patriarchal society—to have children, despite the physical, social, or psychological burdens to her of doing so. Yet these limitations do not diminish the importance of the negative protections that a recognition of procreative liberty establishes, even if women do end up carrying a heavier reproductive load than men.

Some philosophers argue that more reproductive choices are not always better for women because new options do not always leave all of a woman's previous alternatives unchanged.[25] As evidence they cite how the development of IVF led to pressure on women to undergo several burdensome cycles of treatment, and how prenatal sex determination might lead to pressure to abort. They also point to how prenatal genetic testing now makes a woman responsible for having handicapped offspring if she rejects amniocentesis, when previously she would have been seen as a victim of the natural lottery.[26]

One cannot deny that reproductive choices will not increase self-determination for all women, because some will be pressured to make choices that they previously would not have had to face, or will lack the resources to take advantage of the opportunities presented. On balance, however, there is no reason to think that women do not end up with more rather than less reproductive freedom as a result of technological innovations. If so, procreative liberty is an important bulwark that helps women achieve the greater freedom that reproductive advances make possible. The more important lesson for social policy is the need to protect women from new forms of private sector coercion that arise because of these techniques, and to support their efforts to exercise procreative autonomy.

One need only imagine a world without procreative liberty to appreciate its contribution to the well-being of women. Although procreative liberty gives little protection from family or internal pressures to procreate or from lack of resources, it does prevent arbitrary, moralistic, or speculative governmental impositions on a woman's procreative choice. Even in a world without the technological options now available, recognition of negative procreative liberty would be an important achievement.

The Communitarian Critique: Rights and Responsibility

Rights-based approaches are also criticized for their disregard of the needs of community. An emphasis on rights is necessarily individualist. It reflects a "do your own thing" mentality that ignores the impact of exercising rights on the shape, the tone, and the overall well-being of communities, and may obstruct the resolution of pressing economic and social problems.[27] Responsibility in the exercise of rights is essential if communities are to survive and be vital, yet rights talk invariably slights one's responsibility to the community.

This criticism is especially applicable to reproductive rights. Procreative liberty emphasizes individual satisfaction and deemphasizes the social consequences of procreative choice. It respects individual desire but denigrates duty and responsibility in how desire is fulfilled. Yet responsibility in procreation is essential because of its effects on resulting offspring. Indeed, many persons would argue that no one should reproduce unless they are able and willing to care and nurture the children they produce. Yet this book ... largely rejects that conception of procreative liberty, as do feminists and others who want strict walls against any governmental intervention in reproductive choice.

Procreative liberty arguments for use of new reproductive technologies are vulnerable to the communitarian critique on several grounds. Many consumers of these techniques—and professionals who profit from offering them—rush to use them with little thought of their impact on offspring, family, and society. One may ask whether it is socially responsible to spend a billion dollars a year on assisted reproduction when so many other health needs are unmet, and when so many children await in foster homes for adoption.[28] Couples who spend thousands of dollars on such treatments may be less concerned about their child's welfare than their own selfish desires. Cumulatively, such practices could undermine the bonds on which the welfare of children and the community depend.

The community also suffers from routinization of prenatal screening practices. Embryos and fetuses become objects to be discarded or destroyed if they do not meet standards of quality or convenience, thus diminishing respect for the first stages of human life and the well-being of children who are born simply ordinary or with minor handicaps. The willingness to employ gamete donors and surrogates as reproductive collaborators also undermines community.

Infertile couples might view donors and surrogates not as equals in a mutually collaborative enterprise, but as depersonalized cogs in the production of children. Written contracts distance the infertile couple and surrogate from the emotional reality of their joint endeavor.[29] Disaggregation and recombination of reproductive components also undermine the traditional importance of genetic and gestation bonds in defining families, and may leave children and parents confused about their lineage and social responsibilities. Finally, couples who harvest the uterus for transplant and research material contribute, like slash-and burn farmers in the rain forest, to the increasing erosion of community conceptions of the sanctity of human life.

These concerns should be taken seriously, but the assumption that a rights-based approach to reproductive technology will inevitably diminish community greatly overstates the case. Procreative liberty does entitle women on welfare, convicted child abusers, and those with HIV to procreate, but as we saw in chapter 4 [all chapter references from *Children of Choice*], it is not clear that such reproduction is always irresponsible. We have also seen, in chapter 8, that procreative liberty does not give women or men the right to engage in prenatal conduct that will harm offspring. The expense and burdens of assisted reproduction is as likely to make the child loved and cherished as it is to commodify it as a product to satisfy parental selfishness. Prenatal genetic interventions to enhance the health of offspring may be more rooted in love than in narcissism.

Nor will the use of surrogates and donors necessarily be depersonalized and adversarial. Couples usually meet the surrogate, have frequent contact during pregnancy, and may correspond or meet in later years. Often egg donors are friends or family, and are increasingly sought out even when they are strangers. Written contracts; by providing certainty and understanding of mutual obligations, bring parties together more often than they divide. Contrary to rights critics, the use of donors and surrogates is as likely to be truly collaborative and cooperative as it is to be adversarial and antagonistic. Rather than undermine family, these practices present new variations of family and community that could help fill the void left by flux in the shape of the American family.

If this is so, an emphasis on reproductive rights is not inconsistent with reproductive responsibility and the needs of community, and is unlikely to damage individuals, families or larger social concerns more than it benefits them. The fears raised, however, do remind us of the possible reverberations of reproductive decisions on individuals and the community and thus the need for sensitivity and respect for others in their use.

Efforts to assure responsible use of reproductive technologies could take several forms. One is for both providers and consumers to resist the seductive urge to use a technology because it is there and might work. A technological solution of infertility is a powerful temptation, as the readiness of couples to try IVF and related procedures shows. Because the technology may be more onerous and less effective than at first appears, couples should be accurately informed of their prospects and counseled about the complications that could arise.[30]

A second approach is to ask potential users to think carefully about the social and psychological ramifications of collaborative reproduction for themselves, the children, and the donors and surrogates who assist them. Infertile couples, donors, and surrogates should explore the social and emotional uncertainties they face before embarking on such a weighty venture. They should be especially careful before undertaking truly novel procedures, such as splitting embryos to create twins born years apart, using related or intergenerational surrogates, creating embryos for tissue, and the like.[31]

A third approach is to develop guidelines or canons of ethical behavior. A legal right to use reproductive technologies does not necessarily entitle one to private-sector access. Health professionals are gatekeepers who ultimately determine who will use these technologies. They should use discretion in accepting patients and in acceding to their demands for technological help, yet not exclude persons on the basis of sexual preference, disability, or life-style alone. Above all, they should treat their patients with dignity and respect, and not mislead or exploit their desire to reproduce merely to make a profit. Regulatory measures to protect consumers from provider overreaching, as discussed in chapter 5, are clearly justified.

Finally, a rights approach to reproductive technology is not an imprimatur on all uses of the technology. It does not require that the state subsidize or otherwise encourage the use of all reproductive techniques, and provides no immunity from moral condemnation, persuasion, or noncoercive instruction in how that technology should be used. Thus not all forms of collaborative reproduction need be subsidized, even if health insurance should or does cover some infertility treatment. States may also refuse to enact laws that facilitate collaborative reproduction, though that approach might cause more problems than it presents.[32] In short, there is ample room for protecting the community while also respecting individual choice. How to encourage responsible use without infringing procreative liberty will remain a major challenge for public policy.

Conclusion: Autonomy and Ambivalence

Resort to technology is a powerful temptation to persons who wish to have or to avoid having offspring. Reliance on technology, however, has both a bright and a dark side. It can be used in a caring, supportive, and communal way, or it can be used to oppress, dominate, and alienate. The ultimate challenge is to use it well.

Despite the problems of a rights-based approach, I have argued that procreative liberty should be presumptively protected in moral analysis and in public policy determinations about new reproductive technology. Procreation is central to individual meaning and dignity, and respect for procreative liberty best resolves the many controversies surveyed. A commitment to autonomy, however, does not eliminate the ambivalence that use of these techniques creates at both the individual and societal level.

At the individual level, persons may be ambivalent about the manipulations and social uncertainties that technologized means of reproduction entail, yet feel that they have few alternatives if they are to overcome infertility, avoid handicapped children, or save a loved one. At the societal level, ambivalence arises from the unknown social effects of permitting individuals to engineer offspring and to alter traditional understandings of family. Yet restricting individual efforts to find reproductive meaning through technology engenders further ambivalence, for it violates procreative freedom and implicates the state in intimate decisions best left to personal choice.

As science produces more technologies to control reproduction, public response will oscillate between attraction and repulsion, between respect for autonomy and concern for how that freedom is used. In the end, the reception of individual reproductive technologies will depend on their efficacy, the goals they serve, and their real and symbolic effects. Ambivalence will dissipate only when a clear verdict on the desirability or undesirability of a particular technology is possible. Given normative differences and uncertain empirical effects, that will not quickly occur.

There is no stopping the desire for greater control of the reproductive process. Since this is so value-laden an area, ethical, legal, and social conflicts over reproductive technology are likely to continue for many years. In confronting those conflicts, we must not deny the importance of procreative liberty just to escape the discomfort that its use often engenders. There is no better alternative than leaving procreative decisions to the individuals whose procreative desires are most directly involved.

Notes

1 [John A. Robertson, *Children of Choice: Freedom and the New Reproductive Technologies* (Princeton University Press, 1994)—Ed.]

2 *Rights Talk: The Impoverishment of Political Discourse* (New York: Free Press, 1991).

3 Elizabeth Fox-Genovese, "Society's Child" (Review of *Life Itself: Abortion in the American Mind* by Roger Rosenblatt), *The New Republic*, 18 May 1992, 40-41.

4 This is one of Elizabeth Kingdom's criticisms of rights in *What's Wrong with Rights: Problems for Feminist Politics of Law* (Edinburgh U.K.: Edinburgh University Press 1991), 79-84.

5 I am grateful to Daniel and Sidney Callahan for first making me aware of this aspect of reproductive rights.

6 See Fox-Genovese, "Society's Child"; Daniel Callahan, "Bioethics and Fatherhood," *Utah Law Review* 1992 (3): 735.

7   Cass Sunstein, "Right talk," *The New Republic*, 2 September 1991, 34.

8   As Sunstein notes, rights of speech and association, jury trial and antidiscrimination, are basic preconditions for social involvement, thus enhancing rather than dividing community. In addition, rights and duties are correlative, thereby creating an implicit sense of social responsibility. Id. At 35.

9   Kingdom, *What's Wrong with Rights*, 83.

10 Sunstein, "Right talk," 36. Sunstein further notes: "If one looks at the context in which restrictions on abortion take place, at their real purposes and real effects, then the abortion right is most plausibly rooted not in privacy but in the right to equality on the basis of sex. Current law nowhere compels men to devote their bodies to the protection of other people, even if life is at stake, and even if men are responsible for the very existence of those people.... Such restrictions are an important means of reasserting traditional gender roles." Id. See also chapter 3 [of *Children of Choice*—Ed.].

11 If the social vision of reproduction is to claim our allegiance, then society's commitment to the sanctity of life must be reflected in a social commitment to support it at all stages, including in those pregnant women who desire an abortion because they lack the resources to care for a child.

12 "Losing the Negative Right of Privacy: Building Sexual and Reproductive Freedom," *New York University Review of Law and Social Change* 18 (1991): 46.

13 Maher v. Roe, 432 U.S. 464 (1977); Harris v. McCrae, 448 U.S. 297 (1980).

14 Norman Daniels, *Just Health Care* (New York: Cambridge University Press, 1985), 26-28.

15 Either directly or as a derivative right of the recipient. See chapters 2 and 6 [of *Children of Choice*—Ed.].

16 822 p. 2d 1317, 4 Cal. Rptr. 2nd 170 (1992).

17 Ira J. Chasnoff, "The Prevalence of Illicit Drug Use during Pregnancy and Discrepancies in Mandatory Reporting in Pinellas County, Florida," *New England Journal of Medicine* 322 (1990): 1202. However, the differential treatment could be explained by the fact that the white women were more likely to have evidence of marijuana in their blood, while the black women had evidence of cocaine.

18 V.E. Kolder, J. Gallagher, and M.T. Parsons, "Court-Ordered Obstetrical Interventions," *New England Journal of Medicine* 316 (1987): 1192-1196.

19 Almost any issue of "Issues in Reproductive and Genetic Engineering": *Journal of International Feminist Analysis* contains criticism of the dangers of new reproductive technologies, including IVF. See, for example, Bette Vanderwater, "Meanings and Strategies of Reproductive Control: Current Feminist Approaches to Reproductive technology," 5 (1992): 215.

Part of the feminist objection to the medicalization of pregnancy through ultrasound, amniocentesis, cesarean sections, and IVF, to name but a few examples, is that women lose control over their own pregnancies and childbirths. Martha Field, "Surrogacy Contracts—Gestational and Traditional: The Argument for Nonenforcement," *Washburn Law Journal* 31 (1991): 1, 16. It is usually men who then control the process.

20 Judith Leavitt, "Birthing and Anesthesia: The Debate Over Twilight Sleep," *Signs* 6 (1980): 147.

21 Adrienne Rich, *Of Woman Born: Motherhood as Experience and Institution* (New York: W.W. Norton, 1976). 117-148; Bottoms, Rosen, and Sokol, "The Increase in the Cesarean Birth Rate," *New England Journal of Medicine* 302 (1980): 559; Banta, "Benefits and Risks of Electronic Fetal Monitoring," in *Birth Control and Controlling Birth*, ed., H. Holmes, B. Hoskins, and M. Gross (Atlantic Highlands, NJ: Humanities Press, 1980), 147.

22 Martha Field notes: "A final thing about surrogacy is allocation of power between the sexes. Seen through one lens surrogacy concerns who will control pregnancy and reproduction. Surrogacy is one way for men to take control of reproduction, to have babies without being dependent upon women, or at least to be dependent only upon those women who are under contract.... The surrogacy debate is part of a range of hard-fought issues over who is going to make the greater part of the decision in this important facet of life." Field, *Surrogacy Contracts*, 31.

23 See chapter 6 [of *Children of Choice*—Ed.].

24 M. Shultz, "Reproductive Technology and Intent-Based Patenthood: An Opportunity for Gender Neutrality," *Wisconsin Law Review* (1990): 298; L. Andrews, *New Conceptions* (New York: St. Martin's Press, 1984); L. Andrews, *Between Strangers: Surrogate Mothers, Expectant Fathers, and Brave New Babies* (New York: Harper and Row, 1989).

25 I am indebted to Dan Brock's "Reproductive Freedom: Its Nature, Bases, and Limits" (unpublished paper, 1992) for this particular formulation of the problem.

26 Barbara Katz Rothman, *The Tentative Pregnancy* (New York: Viking Press, 1986).

27 Sunstein notes that rights talk can sometimes "stop discussion in its tracks," leaving the impression that much more needs to be said but making it difficult to say it. Rights talk can also lead to "conclusions that masquerade as reasons." "Right talk," 34. Ideally, the claim of a right should not cut off the detailed argument about social consequences that recognition of rights often encapsulates.

28 Most of the money comes from persons buying reproductive services with their own funds, and thus would not be available to satisfy other health needs of the community. For a discussion of IVF, surrogacy, and adoption, see Field, *Surrogacy Contracts*, and Elizabeth Bartholet, *Family Bonds: Adoption and the Politics of Parenting* (Boston: Houghton Mifflin, 1993). Field and Bartholet never state why infertile couples alone and not all persons who reproduce have the obligation to adopt kids in need of parents.

29 See Maura Ryan, "The Argument for Unlimited Procreative Liberty: A Feminist Critique," *Hastings Center Report*, July/August 1990, 6.

30 See chapter 5 [of *Children of Choice*—Ed.].

31 Knowing when to proceed and when to stop is difficult precisely because so little is known about so many procedures.

32 See chapter 6 [of *Children of Choice*—Ed.] for elaboration of this point.

20.
CHOOSING SURGICAL BIRTH:
DESIRE AND THE NATURE OF BIOETHICAL ADVICE[1]

Raymond G. De Vries, Lisa Kane Low, and Elizabeth (Libby) Bogdan-Lovis

SOURCE: Hilde Lindemann, Marian Ververk, and Margaret Urban Walker (eds.), *Naturalized Bioethics* (Cambridge: Cambridge University Press, 2009), 42-64.

All is clouded by desire: as fire by smoke, as a mirror by dust.... Wisdom is clouded by desire, the ever present enemy of the wise.
—Krishna to Arjuna, Bhagavadgita, book 3

Most of us, academics or laypersons, accept the straightforward and simple syllogism: scientific discovery → change or improvement in medical practices → new ethical problems → bioethical advice or solutions. While there are some cynics among us,[2] the progression from science to practice to ethical adjustment seems logical, if not natural. But the real world, alas, is not a clean and logical place. Our tidy idea of a natural progression conceals a messy process where competing information, demands, pressures, values, and emotions interact to produce scientific discovery, new medical practices, and bioethical advice. We may prefer to see bioethics as part of a well-organized division of labor, but it is, in fact, one part of the complex world of science, medicine, and health care.

Called upon to provide reasoned and defensible advice on the ethical quandaries that emerge from this jumble, bioethicists must find a way to collect information, strip away confounding factors, and zero in on the essential dilemma. Clearing away the clutter provides clarity for bioethics, but it also obscures the social origins of the facts that are brought to bear in bioethical deliberation. When consultant bioethicists consider ethical problems associated with genetic therapy, for example, they ask about risks and benefits of the procedure, scrutinize the informed-consent process, question the effects of altered genes on the population, and consider who will and will not have access to new treatments.

They do *not* ask about the more foundational issues: How did this medical practice and the science that supports it come to be (i.e., what are the social and cultural forces that produced genetic therapies as opposed to other approaches to disease)? What influences the desires and demands for these therapies by patients and their families? How does this approach to disease reflect the desires and anxieties of caregivers? And last but decidedly not least: How does the social location of bioethics—in the worlds of medicine, science, and in the larger culture—influence bioethical judgment? In distilling the "facts of the case" of genetic therapy—about risk and benefit, personal autonomy, and justice—consultant bioethicists ignore the way these facts are produced by cultural ideas, social structures, organizational constraints, group norms, and social relationships.

Academic bioethicists may protest that the principlism implicit in our description of the bioethical approach to genetic therapy is passé. They will point to far more nuanced and elegant approaches to ethical quandaries, including casuistry, narrative ethics, and care ethics. Yet nearly all bioethical deliberations that occur in hospital ethics committees, in committees that advise professional bodies, and in research ethics committees invoke the four principles of autonomy, beneficence, nonmaleficence, and justice. This is no surprise. Principlism provides an easily understood and easy-to-apply template for recognizing and resolving ethical dilemmas. Such routinization of bioethical deliberation makes organizational sense. After all, do we really want bioethical advice at the end of life to include reflection on the science that brought us life-prolonging technologies, the culture that shapes the wishes of family members and the anxieties of caregivers, and the place of bioethics in hospital organizations? Well, yes and no. We social scientists are convinced that these issues *should* be part of the conversation, but we also recognize the social conditions that make this kind of broader conversation impractical and thus unlikely. Our goal here is to show what is lost when bioethicists fail to attend to these larger questions. We are convinced that inattention to the social facts of bioethical quandaries diminishes the possibility of achieving the goals of bioethics, whether those goals are described modestly (helping those in the life sciences to see the moral implications of their actions) or immodestly (assuring that medicine and medical science are done ethically).

We make our case by taking a close look at the issue of cesarean delivery on maternal request (CDMR).[3] Unlike areas of medical practice where the presence of bioethicists has become routine and almost taken for granted, this relatively new and still controversial procedure gives us the opportunity to see how social and cultural forces shape bioethical advice. Providers of maternity care have reported a recent—and, by their reckoning, dramatic—increase in women with uncomplicated pregnancies asking to have their babies delivered surgically. The central question engendered by these requests—should elective surgery be used to intervene in what is essentially a natural and healthy process?—has led to lively discussions among professionals and the public. Pregnant women want to know about the risks and benefits to their babies, themselves, their partners, and their families. Physicians want to see the evidence and understand how CDMR affects the health of their patients, the use of their skills, and the management of their practices. Bioethicists want to understand the moral dimensions of choosing more and less technological approaches to care at birth.

Because we are at a remove from the clinic, the questions we ask of CDMR have a more "meta" feel. We start by asking: Why now? How did CDMR become a medical and bioethical issue? What roles have been played by professions, professionals, clients, medical institutions, and third-party payers in the emergence of this issue? How has the evidence brought to bear on CDMR been created and used? How—from what materials and toward what ends—

are bioethical arguments about CDMR fashioned? These questions situate medical and bioethical practice in personal, social, and political space, offering a naturalistic account of the way bioethics (and in particular the principle of autonomy) is engaged in the everyday work of medicine. Rather than extracting the moral questions from the environment in which they arise (as is common in bioethics), we examine this bioethical issue as it is found in the social and cultural situation of health care.

Surgical Birth on Demand

In the late 1990s studies investigating a possible link between vaginal delivery and pelvic floor damage began to populate the medical literature, expanding along with the rise of urogynecology, a medical specialty that focuses on the integrity and function of a woman's pelvic floor. Case studies suggesting a correlation between vaginal delivery and pelvic floor damage were cited as a rationale for introducing informed consent for elective cesarean delivery. This consideration in turn raised a related question of whether informed consent should be provided for vaginal delivery. Obstetric and urogynecological specialists cautiously surmised that harm to the pelvic floor might be averted with surgical delivery. It followed (in a self-fulfilling fashion) that "preserving the pelvic floor" could then be a medically indicated rationale for choosing a surgical instead of a vaginal birth (O'Boyle et al. 2002; Sultan and Stanton 1996; Handa et al. 1996; Devine et al. 1999; DeLancey 2000).

The United States is experiencing a rapid rise in surgical births—in 2005, 30.2 percent of U.S. births were accomplished surgically (Hamilton et al. 2007)—but it is difficult to distinguish between elective and medically indicated cesarean births, and there are no credible data on the extent of CDMR. In spite of this, the program of a 2006 National Institutes of Health (NIH) "State of the Science" conference on the procedure asserted that CDMRs make up 2.5 percent of all surgical births.[4] To support this assertion, those convinced of an attention-worthy rise in the CDMR rate used a statistical sleight of hand: they introduced graphics that showed the number of primary (first-time) cesarean sections rising, even though maternal risk profiles remained unchanged. Their conclusion? The "unexplained" rise in the rate of primary cesarean deliveries must be the result of maternal request. Disregard for other sources of the rise in surgical births, including, for example, changed professional practice patterns, allowed conference organizers to frame the question in terms of women's choices. The evidence brought to bear focused on balancing respect for women's autonomy with the benefits and risks of surgical birth. By posing CDMR as an ethical dilemma, the NIH conference created space to consider CDMR in terms of women's desires.[5]

The autonomy principle figured prominently in conference discussions. In the absence of direct and convincing evidence of increased risk, how could a physician deny the desire of a woman giving birth? Following the conference, NIH conveners issued a press release with the headline, "Panel Finds Insufficient Evidence to Recommend for or against Maternal Request Caesarean Delivery." A tagline recommended that those women requesting a cesarean delivery should be thoroughly counseled on potential risks and benefits. Neither the press release nor subsequent media coverage mentioned that the evidence supporting the claim that vaginal birth damages the pelvic floor was very weak; this oversight is interesting because concern with pelvic floor damage is a primary rationale for choosing elective surgery. Thus, the practical result of the conference was to conclude that there can be *no* ethical objection when the desire of an "informed" woman for a surgical birth meets the desire of a physician to apply the "best" of medical technology to the natural process of birth.

Desire and Surgical Birth

How did we get to this point? A lot of time, energy, and money are being spent on a situation that, in statistical terms, is vanishingly small. In a recent nationally representative survey of mothers in the United States, "just one mother among the 252 survey participants with an initial (primary) cesarean reported having had a planned cesarean at her own request with no medical reason" (Declercq et al. 2006). That is 0.4 percent of the women with a pri-

mary cesarean and 0.2 percent of first time mothers. What is at stake here? In order to understand what seems to be disproportionate attention being paid to CDMR, we must look at the way desire influences medicine and bioethics.

We use the term "desire" to replace the more often invoked "interests." It is commonplace for social scientists to describe how interests shape knowledge and practice. Although it is clear that interests *do* shape the generation of knowledge, patterns of practice, and the development of technologies, the connotations of interest often are limited to *material* interests. Desire expands and more accurately describes the interests that inform decision making in health care.

In the case of surgical birth, for example, it often is claimed that obstetricians prefer surgical birth because it is in their (material) interest. In some places, so the argument goes, the remuneration is higher for surgical birth, and even if it is not, the time demands of surgery are comparatively less because an elective procedure can be scheduled, and surgery is more "efficient" than waiting for labor. These arguments may be true, but there are at least two problems with this analysis of the link between interest and practice. First, more than material interests are involved in a preference for surgical birth. It is a rare obstetrician that would choose surgery simply for his or her convenience and pecuniary gain; it is far more likely that a physician, after years of education and the socialization experience of residency, sees surgery as the *best* way to promote the health of a mother and her child. The second problem follows from the first: physicians do not recognize themselves in descriptions of the interest-practice link and thus see little reason to reflect on the non-medical influences on their practice.

Replacing *interests* with *desire* broadens our understanding of professional knowledge and practice. Desire stresses the depth and strength of feeling and implies strong intention or aim. Desire begins with the assumption that medical professionals want to do their best for their clients, but it allows analytic room to explore the genesis of desires, how they represent a mix of material, psychological, social, political, and cultural motivations. Desire has the added advantage of bringing in other actors whose interests are less easily described as "material." In our case, it allows us to explore how CDMR is produced by the desires of women, medical institutions, *and* bioethicists.

Our first glimpse of the role of desire comes in the name used to describe the use of surgery to assist in a birth absent a medical indication. While it may seem simply descriptive, the term CDMR imports professional attitudes and desires. Notice that the active agent is defined as the mother: it is she who is setting the surgical wheels in motion and she whose wishes must be honored. Notice, too, how "cesarean delivery" masks the fact that this procedure involves major surgery.[6] Many women whose babies are delivered surgically are subsequently surprised by the attendant postoperative pain and lengthy period of recovery.[7]

In an effort to be more neutral, to remove assumptions about agency, and to make clear that "cesarean birth" is indeed a *surgical* procedure, from here on we refer to this phenomenon as "non-medically indicated surgical birth" (NMISB).

Professional Desire

Professional desires, acquired in the long process of becoming a doctor, influence the creation and use of medical science, define professional fears, and influence the organization of health care delivery. When we look at NMISB through the lens of professional desire, we gain a clearer picture of the forces at work in medical decisions, a necessary but often ignored first step in bioethical deliberation.

Desire Diminishes Science

No one knows what the best cesarean delivery rate should be—or even what is a good range. Obstetricians are obliged to recommend cesarean delivery in any given case based on the best available evidence of the balance of risks and benefits for mother and child. If the mother agrees, a cesarean is performed. *The statistics shouldn't matter.* (W.B. Harer Jr., past president of the American College of Obstetricians and Gynecologists, 2000, 13, emphasis added)

What role does science play in the decision of an obstetrician to intervene in birth? Harer's statement is revealing: he acknowledges that a doctor's judgment should be informed by the "best available evidence," but in the end he stakes his claim for physician autonomy, asserting that "statistics shouldn't matter." He recognizes that the credibility of medicine rests on science, but he preserves a place for the "art" of medicine, that is, the freedom of doctors to practice as they see best. Science becomes secondary to the wisdom of the physician.

This same attitude is found in the work of Mary Hannah, a physician-researcher widely known for her study that concluded surgery was safer than vaginal birth for babies in the breech position at term (Hannah et al. 2000).[8] Writing about "planned elective cesarean section" with no medical indication, Hannah (2004) concludes that it is a reasonable choice for some women. But she makes her case in a rather odd way. She first describes the *known* risks of cesarean delivery, which include higher maternal mortality, longer recovery time, major bleeding, subsequent placenta previa, neonatal respiratory distress, and unexplained stillbirth in a second pregnancy. She then shifts to a more tentative voice to list the benefits that *may* be associated with surgical birth, including reducing the risk of urinary incontinence, fecal incontinence, unexplained or unexpected stillbirth, and certain complications of labor. Hannah (2004, 814) uses this inconclusive and disputed evidence to advise her fellow obstetricians:

If a woman without an accepted medical indication requests delivery by elective cesarean section and, after a thorough discussion about the risks and benefits, continues to perceive that the benefits to her and her child of a planned elective cesarean outweigh the risks, then most likely the overall health and welfare of the woman will be promoted by supporting her request.

Although she qualifies her position ("most likely"), Hannah, like Harer, defends professional autonomy in the face of evidence. Verified and unverified facts have equal weight; statistics do not matter.

There is another interesting commonality in the reasoning used by Hannah and Harer. In both we see how their desire to help women is limited by what they know about birth. Because vaginal birth is already beset by so much intervention, the surgical option seems appropriate to Hannah (2004, 813). "Labour and vaginal birth, complete with hospital stay, continuous electronic fetal heart rate monitoring, induction or augmentation of labor, epidural anesthesia, forceps delivery, episiotomy, and multiple caregivers, may also not be considered 'natural' or 'normal.'" For Harer (2000, 13), surgical birth is a *remedy* for (poorly managed) vaginal births: he points out that incontinence is associated with "episiotomy and sphincter damage" and "use of forceps" and that "cesarean delivery [is] protective against these risks." Both seem unaware of the possibility that birth can be attended in less invasive and disruptive ways and that well-managed vaginal births with minimal interventions are the more appropriate comparison group for studies of surgical birth.

Desire Determines Science

Not only does professional desire give preference to professional autonomy over science; it also *determines* science by dictating research questions and the interpretation of results. This becomes clear when looking at cross-societal variation in medical science: the design, results, and use of scientific studies are products of professional desires forged by cultural ideas and the organization of health care systems and medical research.

The universalizing nature of science obscures this variation. In spite of Payer's (1988) now twenty-year-old observations about culture and medicine, it can be difficult to find differences between, for example, British and Finnish nephrology. A kidney is a kidney, after all. Interestingly, one place where we *do* find variation in medical science is in maternity care, an area of medicine where cultural ideas about women, family, the body, pain, and the efficacy of medical intervention shape both science and policy (De Vries et al. 2001).

Most striking in this regard is maternity care policy and obstetric science in the Netherlands, where nearly one-third of the births take place at home. In no other country with a modern health system do more than 3 percent of births occur at home. Mid-

wives are primary attendants at 71 percent of Dutch home births (general practitioners attend the other 29 percent); midwives are the primary caregiver at 48 percent of all of that nation's births. It is a system that works quite well in terms of cost-efficiency and quality; the high rate of midwife-attended home birth is coupled with the world's lowest rates of surgical intervention in birth and very low rates of infant mortality.

The peculiarity of birth in the Netherlands creates a special problem for Dutch gynecologists and obstetrical researchers. In light of the uniformity of obstetrics outside the Netherlands, and in light of the need to scientifically support health care practices, how do the Dutch defend what seems an old-fashioned way of birth?[9] In fact, some researchers in the Netherlands are committed to the Dutch view of birth, whereas others, whose allegiance lies with the larger world of obstetric medicine, are skeptical of (and slightly embarrassed by) Dutch birth practices. Not surprisingly, those in the first camp do scientific research that supports the maternity policy of the Netherlands, whereas the skeptics do scientific research that exposes the Dutch way of birth as dangerous.

All those who would do research on the mode and place of birth face the same inherent difficulties. First, it is impossible to do randomized clinical trials on this topic. Assigning a woman to give birth in a setting she would not ordinarily choose not only would be unethical but also would create a confounding variable: the emotional state of a woman birthing in an environment she finds unfriendly would influence the outcome of birth. Second, extremely large samples are required to find significant differences in the outcomes of healthy women having their babies at home or in the hospital. Given this reality, researchers have three choices: they can use existing statistics, do "prospective studies" that analyze outcomes based on an "intention to treat" design,[10] or devise new measures capable of discovering small differences in outcomes. Dutch researchers have used all three methods, but the best illustration of the way desire shapes obstetric science comes from research using new types of measurement.

The desire to find a better, more scientific way of comparing the outcomes of home and hospital birth led several researchers to develop a research design based on objective measures of umbilical cord blood pH and neonatal behavior. The researchers surmised—not unreasonably—that, in spite of favorable outcomes shown in prospective studies, midwife-assisted birth at home was unsafe. Women who give birth at home in the Netherlands must be healthy, as defined by a set of guidelines published by the Ministry of Health, and thus will have excellent outcomes, regardless of where they give birth. In order to get around this problem, the team devised a research strategy that would allow comparisons to be made even when there was no *overt* morbidity and mortality. Researchers would look for small but significant differences in the pH of blood taken from the umbilical cord. Lower pH values are suggestive of oxygen deprivation (acidosis), which is associated with growth retardation and damage to the central nervous system, and hence less than optimal outcomes for the neonatal brain. In conjunction with measures of cord blood pH, researchers also assessed outcomes using a scale that measured the neurological condition of the newborn.

In a series of articles and papers these researchers proposed, tested, and defended their use of measures of umbilical cord blood pH and neurological scores as a fitting way to examine more closely the outcomes of home and hospital births (see Stolte et al. 1979; Van den Berg-Helder 1980). Throughout the 1980s, several studies were done using these outcome measures, the most prominent of which, published in *American Journal of Obstetrics and Gynecology*, showed care in hospitals to be superior to birth at home with midwives: on average, babies born at home or under midwife care were more acidotic and had poorer neurological scores (Lievaart and De Jong 1982).

This widely read study presented a clear challenge to the Dutch way of birth. Pieter Treffers (a champion of home birth and then chair of obstetrics at the University of Amsterdam) and his colleagues replicated the research, paying careful attention to the collection and storage of cord blood. When researchers took pains to assure that cord blood samples from the clients of midwives and gynecologists were treated in an identical manner, the results were opposite to those reported by Lievaart and De Jong:

women attended by midwives had significantly *higher* cord blood pH values. The researchers concluded that there was no cause for concern about the use of midwives.

Eager to get these results to the readers of *American Journal of Obstetrics and Gynecology*, Treffers and his colleagues submitted this research to the journal in two studies, but neither study was accepted for publication. Instead, the first was published in the *Journal of Perinatal Medicine* (Pel and Treffers, 1983), an English-language journal published in Germany, and the second was accepted by the *Nederlands Tijdschrift voor Geneeskunde* (*Dutch Journal of Medicine*) (Knuist et al. 1987).

This case study from the Netherlands reveals that accepted definitions of what is "normal" in pregnancy determine what is accepted by journal editors as good science.[11] Editors of the *American Journal of Obstetrics and Gynecology*, most of whom do *not* share the cultural assumptions of the Dutch, accepted the work of Lievaart and De Jong and rejected the work of Treffers because of what they "know" to be true about birth. They are unwilling to let research evidence influence their belief that "birth is normal only in retrospect."[12]

The "Dutch difference" illustrated here also shows up in the science that directs the use of surgery to birth babies in the breech position at the onset of labor. The often-cited "term breech trial" done by Hannah (a Canadian) and her colleagues (2000, 1375) concluded: "Planned caesarean section is better than planned vaginal birth for the term fetus in the breech presentation; serious maternal complications are similar between the groups." But in their analysis, Leeuw and Verhoeven (2006), two physicians whose desires are shaped in the Dutch maternity care system, conclude that the data from the term breech trial are "very controversial" and, looking at data from the Netherlands, argue for an increase in *vaginal* delivery of breech babies.

Here we see how ideology about the "best" way to give birth affects both the generation and interpretation of the scientific facts about birth. Desires, shaped by training and practice, influence science. The assumed relation between science and practice is turned on its head: practice is not based on science; rather, science is based on practice.

Desire Varies by Professional Specialty

The desires of medical professionals vary by specialty. While the first years of medical school are quite
similar for all physicians-in-training, the later years
and the years of residency expose students to different
experiences, different regimes of socialization, and
different bodies of knowledge. Specialties also differ
in typical demands of energy and time, types of clients
and complaints, types and rates of remuneration, and
nature and amount of interaction with clients.

Urogynecology is a relatively new profession: the
United States specialty group, the American Urogy-
necologic Society, was founded in 1979, and the first
issue of the professional journal of this specialty, the
International Urogynecology Journal, was published
in 1989. The specialty grew in response to a particular set of clinical problems, as the society explains
on its Web site:

> A Urogynecologist is an Obstetrician/ Gynecolo-
> gist who has specialized in the care of women
> with Pelvic Floor Dysfunction. The Pelvic Floor is
> the muscles, ligaments, connective tissue, and
> nerves that help support and control the rectum,
> uterus, vagina, and bladder. The pelvic floor can
> be damaged by childbirth, repeated heavy lifting,
> chronic disease or surgery. (http://www.augs.org/
> 14a/pages/index.cfm?pageid=210, last accessed
> October 5, 2007)

The Web site goes on to list "some problems due to
Pelvic Floor Dysfunction," the first of which is
"Incontinence: Loss of bladder or bowel control,
leakage of urine or feces."

Not all physicians deal with pelvic floor dysfunction on a daily basis, and this difference in ailments
seen and treated leads to a different set of desires.
Doctors in family practice, for example, have a view
of women that is less specialized and that encompasses many more aspects of their lives. Writing in
their specialty journal, *Annals of Family Medicine*,
Leeman and Plante (2006, 265) respond to the move
toward NMISB:

> Patient-choice cesarean delivery may become
> widely disseminated before the potential risks to

women and their children have been well analyzed. The growing pressure for cesarean delivery
in the absence of a medical indication may ultimately result in a decrease of women's childbirth
options. Advocacy of patient-choice requires preserving vaginal birth options as well as cesarean
delivery.

Because they are not driven by daily encounters with
the heartbreak of incontinence, family practice
physicians emphasize the need to preserve choice in
mode of childbirth, even in cases where women
desire a vaginal birth for a breech presentation or
after a previous surgical birth.

Fear Replaces Confidence

Desire often operates as a pull factor—a yearning to
possess a wished-for goal or object. But the pull
toward a goal or object can include a desire to avoid
other outcomes. In the case of birth and surgical
birth, fear is an important source of action. It is
worth noting that *all* published studies of fear of
childbirth are studies of birthing women: it is simply
assumed that "fear of childbirth" means a *woman's*
fear of childbirth. No consideration is given to the
caregivers' fears and how these fears may influence
the way babies get born.[13] Before we discuss the
fears of women, we mention two ways that fear
shapes the desires of physicians: fear of natural
processes and fear of legal action.

Technology, broadly defined, has always been
present at birth. In premodern times, midwives did
not often use instruments to assist at birth, but they
had a variety of techniques, including positioning,
movement, and hands-on maneuvers, to help a
woman give birth to her child. During the twentieth
century, the technologies of birth became more
mechanical and more automated, moving from a
simple fetoscope to the electronic fetal monitor,
from forceps to vacuum extraction, from simple
blood and urine tests to amniocentesis and chorionic
villus sampling. While advances in technology offer
much, they also move the caregiver away from the
natural process of birth and low-technology solutions to the problems of labor. Technology replaces
traditional knowledge. With the rise in popularity of

the "doptone" (a device that uses sonar to locate and modify the heart tones of the fetus), caregivers have forgotten how to use a fetoscope. This may seem a small loss, but the fetoscope is capable of giving a wealth of important information about mother and baby. The doptone can pick up a heart tone from nearly anywhere on the mother's belly; the fetoscope requires careful placement and registers the strength of the heartbeat. The latter procedure allows the caregiver to assess the position of the baby and puts the caregiver close to mother, where touch and smell provide measures of wellness. Similarly, the resort to surgery for all babies in the breech position has all but eliminated the knowledge of how to manage a breech birth vaginally. Doctors no longer trust themselves to guide a natural process without technology.

There is also the very real fear of being sued. This fear drives beliefs, actions, and advice to mothers. Stories abound about obstetricians leaving their practices because of fear of lawsuits and the high costs of malpractice insurance (Xu et al. 2007). Silverman (2004, 1) reports that "one in seven fellows with the American College of Obstetricians and Gynecologists has stopped practicing obstetrics because of the risk of medical liability claims." In their study of "cesarean on request" in eight European countries, Habiba et al. (2006, 651) discovered "a consistent, statistically significant trend emerged between obstetricians' self-reported feeling that their medical practice was influenced, occasionally or often, by fear of litigation and the willingness to perform a caesarean delivery at the client's request."

The Influence of Physician Desire

With the rise of for-profit hospitals and the push for greater efficiency in the nonprofit sector,[14] a business model is replacing a care model. Cost recovery is increasingly important. Speaking about the cost of cancer treatments, Dr. Robert Geller, an oncologist who worked in private practice from 1996 to 2005 before leaving to join a biotechnology company, points out that cancer doctors know that certain drug regimens are more profitable than others: "It's clear that physicians stopped making decisions based on what made scientific or clinical sense in lieu of what made better business sense" (quoted in Berenson,

2007). The same is true for hospitals and surgical birth. While physicians are often paid the same for vaginal and surgical births, hospitals can bill for far more services for surgical births. In 2003 the average cost of surgical birth was $12,468, compared to $6,240 for a vaginal birth (Baicker et al. 2006).

The desires of nurses also are shaped by physician desire and organizational needs. In their innovative research, Regan and Liaschenko (2007) discovered three discrete orientations toward birth among labor and delivery nurses. Shown a drawing of a woman in labor and asked to describe what was occurring, the nurses went on to characterize birth as a "natural process," a "lurking risk," or a "risky process." These attitudes were correlated with the environments in which the nurses worked: nurses working in a unit that employed midwives (whose desires are less oriented toward medical intervention) were less likely to see birth as a lurking risk or a risky process. According to Regan and Liaschenko (2007, 623), "Nurses' beliefs about the risks of childbirth focus nursing care along a specified trajectory of nursing action whereby the use of childbirth technologies and their associated physiological response might influence the use of CS [cesarean section]."

Women's Desires

How does professional desire shape what women want? The desires of women are heavily influenced by their perception of birth, the importance of choice, concerns about sexuality, and the demands of work and career. We examine the first three of these influences through the lens of a discussion that occurred on the Web site of a popular media outlet. In September 2006, MSNBC put the issue of elective surgical birth to the public in an e-discussion, inviting readers to respond to the following query in its online health section: "A study shows that the infant death rate for babies born via C-section is three times higher than those born vaginally. Some C-sections are medically necessary, but others are not. What are your views on elective C-sections?"

The subsequent interactive e-discussion generated a rich and telling discourse, touching on the themes most commonly mentioned in NMISB debates. We use selected responses (posted between September

14 and September 20, 2006) to explore what these themes reveal about women's desires.[15] As with professional desires, individual desires do not emerge spontaneously: the desires of childbearing women are threads within a complex tapestry of cultural and social forces.

While a few e-respondents described childbirth as an inherently healthy process, a majority of discussants accepted the prevailing medical perception of birth as fraught with risk. "Caring Mom"[16] claimed: "If C-sections weren't here most of us women couldn't have kids." And "cuddliemamma" pondered: "How many infant/mother fatalities have resulted from c-sections being avoided or delayed?" "SamsMom" tells others that she received *authoritative* reassurance from her doctors that, "when performed in a sterile OR, the risks from a C-section are the same as risks of a vaginal birth." In this pathological view, surgical delivery is a welcome antidote to the "predictable dangers" of birth, supporting the conventional wisdom that birth simply will not work in the absence of medical intervention.

Another prominent theme in the e-discussion was *choice*, calling on a presumed liberal entitlement *to* choose. Notice how the notion of autonomous choice, so important in reproductive health advocacy efforts, is (mis)appropriated here. "Animalover" had an elective cesarean: "I was glad that I had the choice to decide what was best for me and my child. I wish every woman would become more aware of her options." "Haveaniceday" is "VERY pro-c section! And I believe it is up to the mom to decide what she wants, and for what reason." "ProfessorMD" suggests: "The mother must have total and unlimited choice."

The long-term negative effects of childbirth in terms of incontinence and sexuality were on the mind of several e-discussants. "Lonnie" says:

> Celebrities get c-sections because it preserves the elasticity of their vagina. My obgyn said that no amount of kegel exercises can bring it back to what it was before a natural delivery.... The new term according to my obgyn for having an elective c-section is "perineum preservation." Would you rather have stitches on your abdomen or on your vagina if you tear?

"SamsMom," who chose a cesarean delivery, notes that during vaginal birth "severe tearing can occur on the mother." She goes on to defend her choice with doctor-supplied "facts" such as "the incontinence rate in Argentina. Women [there] ... have one of the lowest incontinence rates in the world [and] one of the highest C-section [rates]."

The notion that bypassing the vagina for birth is desirable to preserve future perineal, urinary, and anal sphincter function (see Nygaard and Cruikshank 2003) is a curious perversion of the precautionary principle, where wisdom dictates that one should take action proactively to forestall imminent disaster. In this case, the risks and harms of the intervention—major abdominal surgery—are ignored. Many comments by participants repeat the same suspect information (about pelvic floor damage) that influences providers, exemplifying a "medical false consciousness." In turn, this false consciousness presses providers of obstetrical care to support women's autonomous choice of NMISB.

Bioethics' patient-choice literature presumes a rational actor capable of evaluating available options and considering their consequences to ultimately achieve ends that will increase the individual's overall happiness (Jaeger et al. 2001, 246). Critics of mandatory informed consent point to weaknesses in the rational-actor paradigm, noting the many systematic errors of reasoning that occur in estimating probabilities. These critics tell us that overestimates of injury are especially likely for events prone to excessive vividness (Schneider 2006, 57). The e-discussants offer a case in point: they frame NMISB as an action that selects among expected "risk" options of uncertain labor and birth trajectories. The "childbirth is always risky" frame amplifies the likelihood of bad outcomes (Jaeger et al. 2001), and, seen in that light, the responses to MSNBC's question are both reasonable and rational.

Surgical birth also can be regarded as a rational choice when seen in the context of women's work. One's location in the world of employment is an important influence on one's desires in choices about birth. The number of births to women aged thirty and older has increased markedly in the past thirty years (Hamilton et al. 2007). These women are more likely to be established in their careers, and thus must organize their childbearing around the demands of work. A scheduled birth fits more easily with the needs of employers and has the added advantage of allowing family members who live at a distance to organize their travel efficiently and economically.

But Is It Ethical? Moralizing Obstetric Desire

There was a time when professional desire was sufficient justification for treatment decisions. In the "golden age of doctoring" (McKinley and Marceau, 2002), the considered decision of a medical professional about proper treatment went largely unchallenged by patients, hospitals, and third-party payers. We now live in a society where professional desire is constrained by insurance companies, risk managers, drug formularies, and yes, bioethicists. Although there is some dispute as to the power of bioethics committees and bioethicists, it is commonplace for professional associations and hospitals to have ethics committees at the ready to review controversial clinical decisions and medical practices.

NMISB is a procedure that begs for ethical advice. The use of an expensive, highly technological, and risky procedure to assist at a birth that everyone agrees could occur without intervention pushes all the buttons of contemporary clinical ethics. As we noted, the opinion of academic ethicists about principlism—that it is simplistic and passé—has little influence on clinical ethics, where autonomy, beneficence, nonmaleficence, and justice continue to be used to make decisions and generate advice. In deciding if NMISB can be justified ethically, ethicists and ethics committees must strike a balance between autonomy (the right of a woman to determine her own care), beneficence (promoting the welfare of the woman and her baby), nonmaleficence (avoiding unnecessary harm to the woman and her baby), and justice (seeking the proper and fair use of health care resources).

One reason the principlist approach has remained popular is that abstract principles can float above, and yet account for, the peculiarities of culture. Regardless of our cultural differences, we can all agree that nonmaleficence is a good thing; but we must hasten to add that what you and I *call* harm may vary. The same can be said of autonomy: in the

United States autonomy is conceived in a radically individualist manner, but in other cultures we can adjust the idea to incorporate more familial and communal ideas of autonomy. In the atomistic United States, a free and independent individual should (must?) determine her care, whereas in more communal societies autonomous decisions occur in consultation with, or by decision of, recognized authorities. Pushed too far in this direction, of course, the principles become meaningless. Can we really speak of autonomy if a treatment decision for an adult woman is made by others?

Bioethical advice about NMISB reflects the variation in desires we described previously. This is clearly seen in looking at the responses to NMISB offered by two professional associations of obstetricians, one based in the United States and the other being an international organization: the American College of Obstetricians and Gynecologists (ACOG), and the International Federation of Gynecologists and Obstetricians (FIGO). Interestingly, both organizations base their advice on the same principles, but different desires result in different advice.

In 1998 FIGO's Committee for the Ethical Aspects of Reproduction and Women's Health published its position on NMISB in a document titled *Ethical Aspects of Caesarean Delivery for Non-Medical Reasons*. Its opinion, reaffirmed in 2003, was based on the principles of nonmaleficence and justice. The committee starts with two observations: "Cesarean section is a surgical intervention with potential hazards for both mother and child"; and "[Cesarean section] uses more resources than normal vaginal delivery." Given that FIGO members "have a professional duty to do nothing that may harm their patients" and "an ethical duty to society to allocate health care resources wisely," the committee concludes: "At present, because hard evidence of net benefit does not exist, performing cesarean section for non-medical reasons is not justified" (http://www.figo.org/docs/Ethics%20Guidelines.pdf).

ACOG's position on NMISB is found in an opinion from its Committee on Ethics, "Surgery and Patient Choice," dated 2007 (www.acog.org/from _home/publications/ethics/co395.pdf). The ACOG committee considers how each of the four principles of bioethics may be applied to the request of healthy women for a surgical birth. The principle of autonomy lends support for the "permissibility of elective cesarean delivery in a normal pregnancy (after adequate informed consent)." The principle of justice "regarding the allocation of medical resources must be considered" in the debate over NMISB, but (unlike FIGO), the committee adds, "It is not clear whether widespread implementation of elective cesarean birth would increase or decrease the resources required to provide delivery services." With regard to the other principles, the committee notes that "the application of the principles of beneficence and nonmaleficence ... is made problematic by the limitations of the scientific data. Different interpretations of the risks and benefits are the basis for reasonable differences among obstetricians regarding this challenging issue." The committee then concludes: "If the physician believes that cesarean delivery promotes the overall health and welfare of the woman and her fetus more than vaginal birth, he or she is ethically justified in performing a cesarean delivery."

Autonomy and Desire

The story of NMISB demonstrates how medical science, medical practice, and bioethics are shaped by the desires of professionals, organizations, and patients. Our analysis offers four lessons for bioethicists.

First, like medicine, bioethics is shaped by desire. This occurs in at least two ways: the need to survive professionally and the desire to frame an issue in ways that are familiar. With regard to survival: unlike other professions in medicine, clinical bioethics has no visible means of support. Clinicians fund themselves by seeing patients, and those who teach in medical schools are funded by tuition dollars, but who will fund bioethics consultations? Bioethical advice has no billing code and no RVU (relative value unit).[17] Given this situation, bioethicists must be keenly attentive to the needs of their colleagues in the clinic. Saying no too often will not help secure bioethicists a place. Thus, bioethics is likely to go along with the reigning clinical mentality.

Second, bioethical advice must cast a wider net when looking for facts relevant to the dilemma in

question. Because of its roots in philosophy and the humanities, bioethics tends to ignore social context. In a recent listserv discussion that offers an apt illustration, bioethicists weighed in on a case of a woman who refused an "emergency" cesarean section. The facts of the case are these: after twelve hours of labor and more than two hours of pushing, an obstetrician informed his patient that it was time for either a vacuum extraction or a cesarean section. The woman agreed to the vacuum but would not sign a consent that also allowed a cesarean. While the obstetrician was out of the room, deciding how to handle the refusal (what if surgery became necessary during the extraction procedure?), the woman spontaneously delivered a healthy child. The listserv discussion ignored the healthy, spontaneous birth and instead centered on the fine points of law, ethics, autonomy, paternalism, and the duty to rescue. Uninteresting to the bioethicists was the fact that the professional judgment of the physician was wrong. The desires of bioethicists, shaped in the crucible of philosophical debate, center on intellectual puzzles and elegant arguments.

When bioethicists are called on for advice, it is their habit to wade through a sea of facts to find the key issue(s) in question. This important and useful skill serves the needs of clinicians well. In the midst of a heated and emotionally charged family debate about what to do with a laboring woman or a dying parent, bioethical parsimony is useful. But the clean cut of Occam's razor excises facts that are essential to good bioethical advice. The "stuff" of bioethical advice—the data from which one assembles a judgment—must include all the social and cultural forces at play in the dilemma in question. In the case of NMISB, to ignore the many ways that desire shapes and constrains the choices of women and caregivers is to concede the power to define the situation to one institution: medicine. When bioethical advice fails to account for the social and cultural contexts of bioethical dilemmas, it is all too easy for critics to label bioethicists as apologists for medicine and science (Elliott 2001).

Third, NMISB and the ethical advice it generates call into question the way autonomy gets used by bioethics in the United States. ACOG's opinion, that there is no ethical reason to deny the request of an informed, healthy woman for a surgical birth, rests on a socially and culturally limited idea of "informed consent." Missing in the information given to a woman choosing surgical birth is discussion of the way in which professional desires shape medical science and medical practice and thus bias the information she receives. Absent also is comment on the way a woman's desires are produced by culture. Like Odysseus—who, in his cautious approach to the songs of the Sirens, recognized that desires could be bent and misdirected in ways that caused harm—bioethicists must be aware that unreflective obeisance to autonomy is dangerous.

The fourth and final lesson of NMISB is that the distinction between autonomy and paternalism can no longer be maintained. We see here (and it is true elsewhere) that informed consent imports paternalism. Concealed in the information given to a woman to obtain her consent is the paternalism of medical science and clinical practice that generate facts in line with professional desire. It is time to rethink paternalism. "False" paternalism—the self-interested assertion of one's will upon another—is clearly objectionable. But "true" paternalism, defined as the selfless love of a parent for a child, recognizes the corrupting influence of professional desire and looks for ways to respect persons—to serve the interests of patients—that go beyond the formula of informed consent.

Notes

1 A grant from the National Institutes of Health (U.S.) National Library of Medicine (1G13LM008781-01) supported De Vries's work on this chapter.

2 Stevens (2000), for example, posits that bioethical solutions *preceded*, and indeed made possible, the development of new medical practices. She describes how the work of bioethicists helped to change the definition of death in a way that allowed physicians to move ahead with organ transplantation.

3 CDMR is among the most popular of the many terms used to describe the phenomenon of healthy women submitting to a surgical birth in the absence of a medical indication for the intervention.

4 See http://consensus.nih.gov/2006/2006Cesarean SOS027main.htm.

5 The significance of the "problem" of CDMR was repeatedly challenged by skeptical members of the audience during the program. The proceedings of the conference can be watched in the NIH videocast Web site (http://videocast.nih.gov/).

6 The term "cesarean section" had this same masking effect: most women are unaware that "section" implies "cutting or separating by cutting." Replacing "section" with "delivery" further obscures the fact this procedure is major abdominal surgery.

7 Compared to women who give birth vaginally, women who have their babies surgically are far more likely to report pain that interferes with their daily activities in the first two months after birth (Declercq et al. 2006, 91).

8 Several more recent studies have challenged Hannah's findings. See http://www.lamaze.org/Research/WhenResearchisFlawed/VaginalBreechBirth/tabid/167/Default.aspx.

9 This review of the scientific debate over Dutch maternity care is based on several years of research in the Netherlands by De Vries (2005).

10 This design, where analyses are based on *planned*, rather than the *actual*, place of birth, is necessary because of the simple fact that most complicated births end up in the hospital; to simply compare home and hospital births builds in a negative bias toward the hospital and a positive bias toward home birth.

11 Two researchers whose work challenged the status quo in obstetrics—Tew, whose epidemiological work in Britain suggested home birth was safe, and Klein, whose research suggested that routine episiotomies were unnecessary—faced great difficulties in getting their research published in British and American journals. See Tew 1995 and Klein 1995.

12 One interviewee reported that the *American Journal of Obstetrics and Gynecology* refused to publish an article by Berghs and Spanjaards based on their research that showed extremely low interobserver agreement about the interpretation of electronic fetal monitoring recordings taken during the second stage of labor (see Berghs and Spanjaards 1988, 129-40). The letter of refusal stated that it would be "immoral" to publish these results (De Vries, 2005, 207).

13 In their innovative work with labor and delivery nurses, Regan and Liaschenko (2007) have identified a range of attitudes toward birth (from normal, to lurk-

ing risk, to risky), and they are at work studying how these influence the course of labor. So far, there is no similar work with physicians.

14 With the rise of diagnosis-related groups (DRGs) and managed care, nonprofit hospitals have been forced to find ways to be efficient.

15 Unfortunately, the Web site with these comments has been taken down.

16 All e-discussion names have been changed.

17 Schneiderman and his colleagues (2003, 1166) have suggested a creative solution: they studied the effect of bioethics consultations on the "use of life-sustaining treatments delivered to [intensive care] patients who ultimately did not survive to hospital discharge." Using a randomized controlled trial where patients were randomly assigned to consultation or standard care (i.e., no consultation), they discovered that ethics consultation significantly reduced the use of life-sustaining treatments *and* was regarded as helpful by a majority of nurses, patients or surrogates, and physicians. In other words, bioethicists are paying for themselves by reducing futile care at the end of life.

References

1. Berghs, G. and E. Spanjaards (1988). De normale zwangerschap: Bevalling en beleid (The normal pregnancy: Birth and policy). PhD dissertation, Catholic University, Nijmegen.

2. Declercq, E.R.C., Sakala, M.P. Corry, and S. Applebaum (2006). *Listening to mothers 2: Report of the second national survey of women's childbearing experiences.* New York: Childbirth connection.

3. De Vries, Raymond G. (2005). *A pleasing birth: Midwifery and maternity care in the Netherlands.* Philadelphia: Temple University Press.

4. Klein, M. (1995). Studying episiotomy: When beliefs conflict with science. *Journal of Family Practice* 41 (5): 483-88.

5. Regan, M. and J. Liaschenko (2007). In the mind of the beholder: Hypothesized effect of intrapartum nurses' cognitive frames of childbirth cesarean section rates. *Qualitative Health Research* 17 (5): 612-24.

6. Schneiderman, L., et al. (2003). Effects of ethics consultations on non-beneficial life-sustaining treatments in the intensive care setting: A randomized controlled trial. *Journal of the American Medical Association* 290: 1166-72.

7. Stevens, M.L.T. (2000). *Bioethics in America: Origins and cultural politics.* Baltimore: Johns Hopkins University Press.

8. Tew, M. (1995). *Safer childbirth? A critical history of maternity care.* London: Chapman & Hall.

21.
ASSISTED REPRODUCTIVE TECHNOLOGIES AND EQUITY OF ACCESS ISSUES

M.M. Peterson

SOURCE: *Journal of Medical Ethics* 31.5 (2005): 280-85.

[Note: Since this article was written, changes have taken place in the regulation of assisted reproduction services in Australia. All Assisted Reproduction Technology units must comply with the Reproductive Technology Accreditation Committee Code of Practice and the National Health and Medical Research Council Ethical Guidelines on the Use of ART in Clinical Practice and Research. However, law and policy on access to services are governed and set by each state and territory. At the time of publication of the current volume, each state and territory except South Australia had passed legislation providing lesbians access to reproductive services. In May 2011, the South Australia Social Development Committee tabled a Report to the South Australia Parliament in which it recommended changes to the law to allow increased access by same sex couples. Ethical challenges relating to equity, age, and disability persist.]

In Australia and other countries, certain groups of women have traditionally been denied access to assisted reproductive technologies (ARTs). These typically are single heterosexual women, lesbians, poor women, and those whose ability to rear children is questioned, particularly women with certain disabilities or who are older. The arguments used to justify selection of women for ARTs are most often based on issues such as scarcity of resources, and absence of infertility (in lesbians and single women), or on social concerns: that it "goes against nature"; particular women might not make good mothers; unconventional families are not socially acceptable; or that children of older mothers might be orphaned at an early age. The social, medical, legal, and ethical reasoning that has traditionally promoted this lack of equity in access to ARTs, and whether the criteria used for client deselection are ethically appropriate in any particular case, are explored by this review. In addition, the issues of distribution and just "gatekeeping" practices associated with these sensitive medical services are examined.

Although many think of assisted reproduction as a recent development, the first recorded case of medical assistance, in the normally private act of procreation, occurred nearly one hundred and twenty years ago in Philadelphia when a doctor used sperm, donated by a medical student, to inseminate a woman whose husband was sterile. When the successful case was published in a medical journal, the public was outraged.[1] Today, as well as artificial insemination by donor (AID), there are numerous other artificial reproductive technology (ART) procedures available and it has been estimated that around 300 000 babies have been born worldwide as a result of ARTs.[1,2] Many of the initial objections to in vitro fertilisation (IVF) technology were based on fears and assumptions that the physical and/or psychosocial development of children born as a result of these technologies would be impaired by the artificial way in which they had been conceived. There was a perceived anticipation of increase in potential for aberrant parental bonding as well as an expectation of probable social stigmatisation of IVF offspring. The vast majority of studies undertaken to investigate these concerns have, however, found very little, if any, significant difference in physical development or psychological wellbeing in IVF children as compared to non-IVF children.[3-6]

The symbiotic relationship between medical advances and social values is well established. Technologies such as IVF and other ARTs inevitably provide normative challenges as they widen the scope of reproductive options and contest the traditional notions of motherhood, pregnancy, and childbirth. Inevitably, new technologies and capabilities prompt medical and legal discourses, usually representative of the dominant power groups within society, which may act to either encourage or discourage consequential social adjustment. Throughout history there have been numerous examples of initial intense public resistance to new medical treatments and procedures that later become commonplace and manifestly socially acceptable. The introduction of the IVF procedure for heterosexual, infertile couples is a modern example of this type of initial resistance, prompted by fear of the unknown, followed by relatively swift social adaptation.[1,7]

An appreciation of the relationship between procreative freedom and professional agency is necessary to understand why and how women make their particular reproductive choices. The options made available to, or withheld from, women are determined centrally by the medical profession with reference to legal issues and social values.

The fact that the vast majority of IVF services are private can sometimes allow the operators to use their own paternalistic forms of discretion in patient selection and, in effect, in the USA at least, legally allows them to set their own criteria for client selection or deselection.[8] In Australia, access to ART programmes may be restricted by legislation or specific codes of practice in some states, which, in turn, may be inconsistent with the Commonwealth Sex Discrimination Act (CSDA). In such cases of legal conflict, state law prevails and ART programmes may seek exemption from the CSDA by application to the Human Rights and Equal Opportunity Commission.[9]

Indeed, it is only in recent times that the provision of established common medical services, public or private, has appreciably diverged from a paternalistic delivery model to one that respects the client as an autonomous agent capable of making medical decisions (if provided with appropriate information) based on personal values and beliefs. Autonomy has been defined as "freedom from external constraint and the presence of critical mental capacities such as understanding, intending, and voluntary decision

making capacity."[10] The concept of respect for autonomy is based on the Kantian notion of humans as "ends in themselves" capable of the determination of their own destinies. This, in turn, implies that each individual has autonomy based rights that require a morally appropriate response from others. In medical service provision, however, exceptions to the demand for respect for autonomy are deemed acceptable when "an individual's choices endanger the public health, potentially harm another party, or involve a scarce resource for which a patient cannot pay."[10]

The predominance of white, middle class, able bodied women living as heterosexual couples is evident across private IVF clientele. This is, in part, due to the "out of pocket" costs to the client associated with the procedure, which in Australia is between AUD$1200 and AUD$2800 (depending on level of private health insurance) for one basic IVF cycle; pregnancy success may require several cycles.[11,12] In the USA, non-Hispanic white women are twice as likely as Hispanic women, and four times as likely as black women, to have used ARTs. Age, income, and education level are also positively correlated with use of infertility services.[13] Some might interpret this to suggest that ART services are increasingly used by older, professional women because they more often choose to delay childbearing to benefit their own professional advancement. It is known, however, that those in the lowest socioeconomic groups actually have higher infertility rates because of poverty, poor nutrition, and increased rates of infectious diseases and sexually transmitted diseases such as chlamydia.[8]

The cost of ongoing research and development associated with artificial reproductive technologies is significant and it has often been noted that funds are allocated to this lucrative field of medical treatment to the detriment of less financially profitable projects such as screening and treatment for sexually transmitted diseases that could effectively reduce the rising rate of infertility. Thus, a majority of poorer, less educated women suffer a double loss with respect to reproductive medical services as their health needs are ignored because of preferential attention to consumer demand from a selected minority of advantaged women.[14]

"Procreative liberty," as defined by Robertson,[8] is the widely accepted fundamental individual right to either have or avoid having children. This entails reproductive freedom as a negative personal right, meaning that the person "violates no moral duty in making a procreative choice and other persons have a duty not to interfere with that choice."[8] Thus, the ideal of "procreative liberty" for some women often cannot be realised unless they "qualify" or have the necessary means to access all available treatments for infertility. It is a valid interpretation to suggest that denial of procreative choice equates to denial of basic personal respect and dignity. Individuals or couples that experience infertility often experience guilt, low self esteem, disappointment, depression, increased rates of relationship conflict, and sexual dysfunction.[8] When the 1948 Charter of the United Nations endorsed the democratic ideal that "men and women of full age, without any limitation due to race, nationality or religion, have the right to marry and to found a family" and that "the family is the natural and fundamental group unit of society and is entitled to protection by society and the state" in Article 16 of the Universal Declaration of Human Rights, it signified the wide acceptance that the family unit is central to human existence and dignity.[15]

The Report of the Committee of Enquiry into Human Fertilisation and Embryology (known as the Warnock Report) in the UK acknowledged the stress suffered by those who are childless, even if they have intentionally chosen this state, because of the importance that society places on the family unit as a valued institution. The report concluded that whether child bearing is considered a "wish" or a "need" is irrelevant, as medicine no longer only deals with preservation of life but addresses any bodily malfunction.[16] Thus, it is not unreasonable to acknowledge that it is the state of childlessness that is of grave concern for many women and men as opposed to merely the actual cause of infertility.

The Warnock report concluded with a recommendation that a statutory licensing authority be established to regulate reproductive technologies and licence ART service providers. As a result, the UK Human Fertilisation and Embryology Act 1990 code of practice clearly states that licensed centres providing ART services "must also take into account the welfare of any child who may be born ... as a result of treatment (including the need of that child for a father)" before providing a woman with such treatment. The act also notes that "centres should avoid adopting any policy or criteria which may appear arbitrary or discriminatory."[17,18] There is no recommendation or reference, however, to an appropriate agent or the necessary standardised methods of assessment required to facilitate this process. By default, ART medical professionals have accepted this role but whether this is an acceptable situation is a debatable issue. There has been little, if any, open resistance by doctors to assuming this extraordinary role of social and psychological evaluator.

"Welfare" is a broad notion comprising both material and psychosocial wellbeing; however, it is widely accepted that the most important aspects of a child's welfare are those that pertain to "stability and security, the loving and understanding care and guidance, the warmth and compassionate relationships that are the essential for the full development of the child's own character, personality and talents."[18]

In Australia, the individual states control ART services, with three states having enacted legislation (Victoria 1995, West Australia 1991, and South Australia 1988) to control the procedures involved, while the remaining states and territories have traditionally adhered to the NHMRC (National Health and Medical Research Council) guidelines supplementary note 4.[19] The latter guidelines, for many years, referred to the fact that "IVF should only be available to people within an accepted family relationship" but failed to provide a definition of this concept. In 1996, the NHMRC replaced supplementary note 4 (SN4) with a revised version, entitled "Ethical guidelines on assisted reproductive technology," which omits reference to "accepted family relationships" but effectively ignores access issues by failing to address them at all, recommending that they be addressed by complementary ART legislation in all states and territories. Over eight years later, however, none of the remaining four Australian states and territories has enacted legislation and thus, by default, their ART services still refer to the 1996 NHMRC guidelines, which are currently under review.[20] In addition, the introduction to the guidelines includes a reference to the impact of social values, citing the need for "a serious regard for the long term welfare" of any children who may be born as a result of ARTs. As opposed to advocating equity of access this manoeuvre can be interpreted as tacit endorsement of the status quo effectively promoted by the initial guidelines.[2]

Hitherto, legal regulation of reproductive technologies has occurred belatedly in response to the challenges to social and cultural norms that these new capabilities instigate.[21] Thus far, the most common initial legal response has been to form regulations that reinforce and protect the traditional patterns of procreation, thereby promoting the very narrow opinion of the "appropriate" family unit as being composed of children with heterosexual parents who are married or have been in a stable de facto cohabiting relationship for at least five years. A recent legal decision in Queensland upheld the right of a fertility service doctor to refuse AID unless the requesting woman could provide written consent to the procedure from her male partner. Stuhmcke notes that, in this way, the law acts to limit the possibility of social change by controlling the medical advances that may enable such change.[2,22]

Steinberg's study of attitudes held by ART medical staff found that there was a common belief that, inherent in their medical responsibilities, IVF professionals were obliged to use their "common sense" about facilitation of "appropriate" reproduction and in the judgement of parenting ability. The vast majority of respondents admitted that they would refuse to treat women who were neither married nor living in a long term heterosexual relationship out of concern for the potential child's need to have an appropriate family unit that included both male and female parents.[14] This provides confirmation that many ART medical professionals feel entitled to exercise power over the reproductive autonomy of their referred potential clients, denying some women freedom of procreative choice by electing to reinforce entrenched ideologies about the family unit and sexuality.[2,23]

Social learning theory views human development in terms of the child's tuition experiences based on their prime models within family, peer, gender, and culture groups. There is much evidence that psychosocial influences of families and peers affect children's self-esteem, beliefs, aspirations, and levels of self regulation, which, in turn, causally affect their emotional, moral, and academic development.[24] It has traditionally been assumed that it is important for children to have both male and female role models, within the primary family unit, for healthy psychosocial development. Psychological studies of children raised in family units with homosexual parents have, however, found no significant negative impact on cognitive development and function, emotional adjustment, gender identity or behaviour when compared with children of heterosexual couples or single mothers.[2,5,22,25]

With the failure rate of modern marriages approaching 40-50% in many countries which also have the highest number of ART services, a significant number of families have minimal or no contact with a father figure and there are obviously no guarantees that heterosexual couples will remain married or as a couple throughout their offspring's childhood.[2,5,18,26] Thus, it would constitute an inappropriate discrimination to exclude lesbian, single heterosexual, or postmenopausal women from access to ARTs because of concern for the welfare of their potential offspring.

Around twenty five per cent of children in Western societies are currently being raised in homes that do not include both a mother and a father for a variety of reasons. Today, the definition of family is often not restricted to a biological characterisation but may be broadened to encompass those committed relationships between individuals that fulfil the functions of a family. Apart from law and custom, subjective intention can also define family and, using this method of determination, a homosexual couple, in a stable relationship, caring for a child or children, functions as a family.[26,27] The clinical importance of embracing a wider definition of family has also been recognised as crucial for good medical practice by family physicians.[28]

At present, homosexual couples who seek the assistance of ART services necessarily request the use of donor gametes. Thus the question of whether offspring are psychologically harmed by collaborative reproduction or by lack of knowledge or contact with a genetic parent might be considered. Concerns raised about the lack of knowledge of, and contact with, a genetic parent have been well debated and studied with respect to artificial insemination by donor (AID), but have not proven to be a deterrent to the provision of this service to heterosexual couples. Ethically, there should be no difference in consideration of this issue in the case of homosexual couples.

The claim of non-qualification due to absence of medical infertility is routinely used as a reason to deny ART services to lesbian women. Yet, fertile heterosexual couples who are at high risk for having a child with some specific genetic disorders are currently not only able, but encouraged, to access IVF services to increase, as far as possible, their likelihood of a producing a healthy baby by using preimplantation genetic diagnosis to select embryos without the condition. Some ART units have specifically annotated this latter category of client as an exception to the requirement for infertility and it is sometimes claimed that these fertile couples have a "legitimate" medical need for ART services.[29] On the other hand, as Pearn highlighted, because neither member of a lesbian couple can produce sperm, they could be considered to be technically infertile and thus qualify to access donor sperm in the same manner as a heterosexual couple in which the male partner is unable to produce enough healthy sperm to achieve conception naturally.[25] Although it is feasible for lesbians to obtain private sperm donation and selfinseminate, the potential health risks combined with the possibility of future demands for paternal involvement in child rearing decisions or access make anonymous donation via ART services preferable.[2]

In 1997, the Queensland Anti-Discrimination Tribunal found that a lesbian who was refused access to donor sperm insemination by a clinic had been treated as "less than the equal of a heterosexual woman."[30] Also, more recently, the decision of the Court of Appeal of the Supreme Court of Queensland, in JM v QFG (Queensland Fertility Group), helped to maintain limitation of access to ART through the legal sanctioning of a restricted medical definition of infertility. The decision was based on the finding that "the refusal was not due to her lesbianism but rather due to her not complying with the definition of 'infertility' stated by the clinic."[22,31] The 1996 Supreme Court of South Australia deci-

sion, in Pearce v South Australian Health Commission, held that the Reproductive Technology Act's limitation of access to ART services to married couples is inconsistent with the provisions of the Sex Discrimination Act, making this limitation constitutionally invalid.[32] Although single women are now able to access ART in South Australia, the Sex Discrimination Act does not protect women from discrimination associated with sexual preference. It does, however, signify the beginning of hope for further legal sanction of "alternative" family units.[2]

As a result of a legal challenge in 2000, an amendment was made to the Infertility Treatment Act 1997, which directed that women who were not married or in a heterosexual de facto relationship should not be treated unless they were medically assessed as "clinically infertile." Thus, this medical diagnosis, in its narrowest form, has become the basic test for eligibility, with non-clinical or "social" factors theoretically excluded from the process, for a subset of potential recipients of ART services, whereas the wider application of "otherwise being unlikely to become pregnant" applies to women who are married or in a de facto relationship.[33,34] In 2001, an Australian Government social policy research paper examined, in detail, the main arguments, based on the issue of medical legitimacy, which have been routinely used against extending ART services to lesbians and single women and were able to "with some degree of confidence, conclude that these leading reasons for denying socially infertile women access to ART on medical grounds have not sufficiently made their case."[29]

As Pearn notes, it is unreasonable to expect doctors to be "mechanistic agents of State policy" and conscientious objectors who have sound personal or religious convictions must be allowed to refrain from the provision of ethically sensitive services such as abortion and some ART practices.[25] This needs to be balanced, however, by restraint from judgmental or negative behaviour toward the client seeking these services. Although the suggestion that homosexual doctors should develop specialised "alternative" ART services to provide lesbians with access to reproductive procedures denied elsewhere might appear to be supportive, it simply promotes further marginalisation of this minority group and, therefore, is inappropriate. A recent position statement launched by the Australian Medical Association (AMA) notes the high social status held by doctors in this culture and indicates that, therefore, they "have a role to play in promoting acceptance of sexual and gender diversity."[35]

It is interesting to note that much resistance to provision of ART services to lesbians focuses on concern for just distribution of scarce resources. International estimates identify lesbian sexual identity in around 0.8% of women, although estimates as high as 4 to 10% have also been suggested. However, these higher estimates usually include women who identify themselves as bisexual or merely report same sex attraction or sexual experience.[36] A recent epidemiological study specifically designed to estimate the incidence of lesbian identity in a single county in the USA determined an incidence of 1.87% of the adult female population.[37] As only a proportion of individuals who identify themselves as lesbians are anticipated to request access to ART services, this indicates that the actual impact on resource utilisation is unlikely to be significant enough to warrant such vehement resistance and suggests that the actual motivation for prohibition is more likely to be discriminatory homophobia or heterosexism.

Postmenopausal women require donated ova to achieve IVF pregnancies. In the past, excess ova harvested after hormonal stimulation of young women undergoing IVF were donated in significant numbers. Improved techniques, including embryo freezing, have, however, reduced the number of excess ova available for donation.[38] Recent legislation in Victoria, which is likely to be repeated in other Australian states, has given offspring of donor gametes the right to request identifying information about their donor biological parent once they reach 18 years of age.[39] This change is expected to impact negatively on the number of anonymous sperm donors and suggests that donated gametes will become an increasingly scarce resource.

The allocation of scarce medical resources is often an ethically contentious problem. The scarcity argument is applied to a number of varied services in medicine today and different units devise their own methods of assessment of potential recipients to determine the allocation of their particular scarce resource. Transplant units routinely allocate scarce donor organs to waiting recipients who will be the lucky few among many on a long waiting list. Many potential recipients die waiting. In part, the transplant coordinators' decisions are determined by the imperative to closely match donor and recipient tissue by immune system compatibility; however, some ethical guidelines are still necessary.

Considerations of medical and social utility are often appealed to as part of the decision making process. It is accepted within the discipline of transplant medicine that psychosocial and lifestyle criteria should be considered by coordinators for patient selection or rejection for organ transplant. Order of priority is usually based on a perception of how deserving potential recipients are, informed by their demonstrated compliance with general health advice. Higher level compliance is assumed to be an indicator of potential to care appropriately for the transplanted organ and, therefore, predictive of a more successful long term outcome.[40,41] In parallel terms of medical utility in the case of ART services, lesbian women are expected to achieve the same rate of pregnancy success from AID and general childrearing success as heterosexual women. In terms of social utility, it is impossible to make generalised claims about discernible difference between the contributions to society's welfare of lesbians and heterosexual women or that of either's offspring.

On consideration of medical utility, it would be unjust to assess recipient priority based on age alone because the medical fact remains that pregnancy success rate is most strongly correlated with the age of ova, donated or otherwise. Also, it is doubtful that large numbers of postmenopausal women are likely to inundate IVF services.[42] If older women are discriminated against, the remaining option of negotiation with private donors, who are known or related to the recipient, would circumvent competition for anonymously donated ova but may provoke regrettable familial or interpersonal stresses. A desire for just process must be counterbalanced against the concern that consumer demand for the right to procreative choice via new technologies might create pressures for young and underprivileged women to undergo invasive procedures associated with some long term health risks in order to sell gametes or act as surrogate mothers.

Another point of resistance to allowing post-menopausal women access to ART services is the claim that older women might not have the energy and patience to cope with babies when they are in their fifties and teenagers when they are in mid to late sixties. It is salient to note that older women have, since time immemorial, played an important role in child rearing, including being the sole carer for their grandchildren if they become orphaned or the children's parents are physically or mentally incapacitated or otherwise rendered incapable of parenting. Nor has there ever been any strong condemnation of men aged fifty or older becoming fathers, which is a regular event. A study of assisted reproductive technology clinics in the USA determined that although most clinics set age limits for women, most do not do so for men.[43] Additionally, although the average age of menopause remains around 52, life expectancy has increased dramatically over the twentieth century, more so for women than for men. It is also true that some women have borne babies naturally in their mid to late fifties prior to the advent of ART services. These facts indicate that expressed concerns about whether older women will survive long enough to properly care for their children are logically tenuous.[44]

The argument against postmenopausal childbearing based on the belief that this state in older women goes "against nature" is contrived, as it conveniently ignores the fact that, at present, it is socially and medically perfectly acceptable to create a temporary or permanent "against nature" infertile state in young women with the use of contraceptives or surgery. It is also considered appropriate for older women to "defy nature" by using hormone replacement therapy to postpone the untoward effects of menopause.[45] As Singer also notes, if the descriptive view of what is natural (nature untouched by human intervention) is employed, then all of medicine goes against nature. Alternatively, the ideological view (that human nature involves exercising human capacities) also indicates that pregnancy resulting from ART technology is natural because it is a result of the exercise of current human capacity.[46]

Very much in the realm of non-natural, researchers at the University of Pennsylvania have now created artificial ova from mouse embryonic stem cells and believe that the process will be just as simple using human stem cells. Obviously, this will force society to further rethink philosophical ideas of parenthood but could negate some of the current ethical and legal dilemmas associated with the use of donor gametes. This technology would, theoretically, make it easier for postmenopausal women to access IVF services and could enable homosexual couples to have offspring genetically related to both same sex parents.[47] Similarly, although researchers claim to be developing the artificial uterus specifically to improve survival chances for premature new born infants, this technology may, in the future, provide a reproductive option to couples or individuals that will be equally feasible for postmenopausal women, women who have undergone hysterectomy, and male homosexual couples.[48]

Even though there is occasional evidence of incremental adjustment in medical and legal discourse towards accommodation of non-traditional concepts of the family unit and parenting, much resistance still persists. One only needs to be reminded of the fear of stigmatisation that accompanied the advent of the first births of "test tube babies," which failed to materialise, to hope that equity of access to ARTs can and will exist in the future and also that non-standard families become a welcomed and accepted part of the social, medical, and legal fabric of life.

On the other hand, issues raised in the debate about access to ARTs are inextricably entwined with other debates, such as those to do with feminist issues, reproductive politics, public health policy and funding as well as the ethics of future human reproductive potentials such as cloning, artificial ova, and artificial wombs. As Van Dyck notes, the public debate of ARTs is often restricted to doctors, scientists, religious groups, politicians, and a few feminists who have strong cultural authority in Western societies. Many groups, however, such as the poor, the elderly, the uneducated, and ethnic minorities, have an equal right to participate in the debate but have neither opportunity nor appropriate skills to effectively present their views.[45] It is noteworthy that these latter groups are the same ones who are commonly barred access to ARTs by the more powerful parties.

In the absence of universally accepted psychological or other criteria for adequate parenting, medical ART gatekeepers often fall back on traditional unfounded beliefs and socially accepted biases to justify deselection of particular individuals. There is a great deal of variability in the processing of perceived ethical challenges and most ART services have no openly available information or written policy regarding their exclusion criteria. Some IVF units request the support of staff psychologists or psychiatrists in decisions to exclude applicants for treatment on the basis of sexual orientation, marital status, or personal beliefs. Increasingly, these professionals are refusing to allow an inappropriate inference of assumed mental health problems related to personal, innocuous lifestyle preferences and are reminding IVF practitioners that these are, instead, ethical and moral questions.[49]

According to Stern's study of ART services in the US, many use various professionals, including nurses, mental health providers, and laboratory staff to make access decisions but only 31% of the clinics use ethics committees and there is no requirement for such committees to include individuals who hold formal qualifications in ethics. As Seal notes: "Social and 'ethical' decisions about the suitability of the individual to be treated based on class, race or lifestyle are unacceptable."[50] To ensure equity of access to reproductive services and just distribution of medical resources, it is imperative that ART clinics should provide valid, defensible policies that encourage deliberation of ethically contentious cases with consistency and fairness.[43] Such policies must be determined, with reference to law, by ethics committees, which include members who represent the underserved and minority groups whose needs otherwise remain unrecognised.

Notes

1   Rigby M. In vitro fertilisation. *The Courier Mail* 1984 Sept 11:33.

2   Stuhmcke A. Lesbian access to in vitro fertilisation. *Australas Gay Les Law J* 1997;7:15-40.

3   Colpin H. Parenting and psychosocial development of IVF children: review of the research literature. *Dev Rev* 2002;22:644-73.

4   Golombok S, MacCallum F, Goodman E. The "test-tube" generation: parent child relationships and the psychological wellbeing of in vitro fertilisation children at adolescence. *Child Dev* 2001;72:599-608.

5   Anderssen N, Amlie C, Ytteroy E. Outcomes for children with lesbian or gay parents: a review of studies from 1978 to 2000. *Scand J Psychol* 2002;43:335-51.

6   Kovacs G. Assisted reproduction: a reassuring picture. *Med J Aust* 1996;164:628-30.

7   Morgan J. Ethics and in vitro fertilisation. *The Courier Mail* 1984 Sept 11:33.

8   Robertson JA. *Children of choice: freedom and the new reproductive technologies*. Princeton NJ: Princeton University Press, 1994.

9   NHMRC. Ethical guidelines on assisted reproductive technology. *Canberra: Australian Government Publishing Service*, 1996:22.

10 Beauchamp TL. Ethical theory and bioethics. In: Beauchamp TL, Walters L, eds. *Contemporary issues in bioethics* [5th ed]. Belmont, CA: Wadsworth, 1999:1-32.

11 About infertility: costs, http://ivf.wesley.com.au/index.cfm?MenuID = 268&TopMenuID = 234 {accessed 19 Oct 2003).

12 IVF Australia. IVF Australia: costs, http://www.ivf.com.au/htmlpages/costs.html (accessed 19 Oct 2003).

13 Beauchamp TL, Walters L, eds. *Contemporary issues in bioethics* [5th ed]. Belmont, CA: Wadsworth, 1998:622-26.

14 Steinberg DL. A most selective practice: the eugenic logic of IVF. *Women's Studies International Forum* 1997;20:33-48.

15 United Nations. Charter of the United Nations: universal declaration of human rights http://www.un.org/aboutun/charter/index.html (accessed 19 Oct 2003).

16 Warnock M. Infertility. In: Beauchamp TL, Walters L, eds. *Contemporary issues in bioethics* [5th ed]. Belmont, CA: Wadsworth, 1984:626-27.

17 The Human Fertilisation and Embryology Act. http://www.hmso.gov.uk/acts/acts!990/ukpga_1990 0037_en_l .htm (accessed 5 Oct 2004).

18 Lee RG, Morgan D. *Human fertilisation and embryology: regulating the reproductive revolution*. London: Blackstones Press, 2001.

19 South Australian Council on Reproductive Technology. Reproductive technology: legislation around Aus-

tralia, http://www.dhs.sa.gov.au/reproductive_tech nology/other.asp (accessed 21 Mar 2004).

20 NHMRC. Notice under section 13: review of NHMRC ethical guidelines on assisted reproductive technology (1996). http://www.health.gov.au/nhmrc/ issues/reptech.htm (accessed 21 Mar 2004).

21 Law Reform Commission. Artificial conception: in vitro fertilisation 1987 19/10/03. http://www.lawlink .nsw.gov.au/lrc.nsf/pages/dpl 5chp6 (accessed 19 Oct 2003).

22 Stuhmcke A. Limiting access to assisted reproduction: JM v QFG. *Aus J Fam Law* 2002;16:245-52.

23 Corea G. *The mother machine: reproductive technologies from artificial insemination to artificial wombs.* New York: Harper & Row, 1985.

24 Zimmerman BJ. Social learning, cognition and personality development. http://www.sciencedirect.com /science/referenceworks/0080430767 (accessed 18 Oct 2003).

25 Pearn JH. Gatekeeping and assisted reproductive technologies: the rights and responsibilities of doctors. *Med J Aust* 1997;167:318-20.

26 Fasouliotis S, Sehenker JG. Social aspects in assisted reproduction. *Hum Reprod Update* 1999;5:26-39.

27 Macklin R, Delaney SR. Artificial means of reproduction and our understanding of the family. *Hastings Cent Re*p 1991;21:5-1 1.

28 Medalie JH, Cole-Kelly K. The clinical importance of defining family. Am Fam *Physician* 2002;65:1277-79.

29 Rickard M. Is it medically legitimate to provide assisted reproductive treatments to fertile lesbians and single women? Canberra: Parliament of Australia, 2001. Report no 23 2000-01.

30 JM v QFG and GK and State of Queensland [1997] QADT 5 31 Jan 1997.

31 Queensland State Government. Supreme Court of Queensland Court of Appeal: JM v QFG & GK[1998] QCA 228 (18 Aug 1998). http://www.austlii.edu.au /cgi-bin/disp.pl/au/cases/qld/QCA/1998/ 228.html?query=title+%28+%22?m+v+qfg%22+ %29 (accessed 21 Mar 2004).

32 South Australian State Government. South Australian Supreme Court decisions. Gail Deborah Dorothy Pearce v South Australian Health Commission, North-Western Adelaide Health Service, Gregory John Russell, Repromed Ply Ltd and Roger John Sta-

bles no SCGRG 96/1114 judgment no 5801. http://www.austlii.edu.au/cgi-bin/disp.pl/au/cases /sa/SASC/1996/5801.html?query=title+%28+%22 pearce+%22+%29 (accessed 21 Mar 2004).

33 Infertility Treatment Act 1995. http://www.dms.dpc .vic.gov.au/Domino/Web_Notes/LDMS/PubLaw Today.nsf?OpenDatabase (accessed 30 Aug 2004).

34 Victorian Law Reform Commission. Assisted reproduction & adoption: should the current eligibility criteria in Victoria be changed? Melbourne: Victorian State Government, 2003:162.

35 Australian Medical Association. Position statement: sexual diversity and gender identity. Chicago, IL: AMA, 2002. http://www.ama.com.au/web.nsf/doc /WEEN-5GA2YX (accessed 14 Oct 2003).

36 McNair R. Lesbian health inequalities: a cultural minority issue for health professionals. *Med J Aust* 2003;178:643-45.

37 Aaron DJ, Chang YF, Markovic N, et al. Estimating the lesbian population: a capture-recapture approach. *J Epidemiol Community Health* 2003;57:207-09.

38 Monash IVF. IVF factsheet: donor egg program, http://www.monashivf.edu.au/library/factsheets /donor_egg.html (accessed 19 Oct 2003).

39 Monash IVF. IVF factsheet: donor insemination. http://www.monashivf.edu.au/library/factsheets /donor_insemination.html (accessed 19 Oct 2003).

40 Corley MC, Westerberg N, Elswick RK Jr, et al. Rationing organs using psychological and lifestyle criteria. *Res Nurs Health* 1998;21:327-37.

41 The CARI guidelines: recipient suitability, http://www.kidney.org.au/cari/drafts/new/recipient .html (accessed 14 Oct 2003).

42 Monash IVF. IVF factsheet: age and fertility, http://www.monashivf.edu.au/library/factsheets/age _and_infertility.html (accessed 19 Oct 2003).

43 Stem JE. Access to services at assisted reproductive technology clinics? a survey of policies and practices. *Am J Obstet Gynecol* 2001;184(4):591-97.

44 Fisher F, Sommerville A. To everything there is a season? Are there medical grounds for refusing fertility treatment to older women. In: Harris J, Holm S, eds. *The future of human reproduction.* Oxford: Oxford University Press, 1998:203-20.

45 Van Dyck J. *Manufacturing babies and public consent: debating the new reproductive technologies.* New York: New York University Press, 1995.

46   Singer P, Wells D. In vitro fertilisation: the major issues. *J Med Ethics* 1983;9:192-95.

47   Newson AJ. Artificial egg creation: new paths to parenthood, http://jme.bmjjournals.com/misc/ecurrent .shtml#now (accessed 16 Sept 2003).

48   Knight J. Artificial wombs: an out of body experience. *Nature* 2002;419:106-07.

49   Stotiand NL. Women's mental health: psychiatric issues related to infertility, reproductive technologies, and abortion. *Prim Care* 2002;29:13-26.

50   Seal V. *Whose choice? Working class women and the control of fertility.* London: Fortress, 1990.

22.
DONATING FRESH VERSUS FROZEN EMBRYOS
TO STEM CELL RESEARCH: IN WHOSE INTERESTS?

Carolyn McLeod and Françoise Baylis

Source: *Bioethics* 21.9 (2007): 465-77.

In countries that limit human embryo research to embryos in excess of clinical need,[1] there is considerable controversy about the use of fresh versus frozen-thawed embryos for the derivation of embryonic stem cell lines.[2] On the one hand, there are those who insist that all embryos deemed suitable for transfer to a woman's uterus should be transferred or frozen for later transfer. On the other hand, there are those who want women to donate (some of) their fresh embryos for stem cell research instead of freezing them or discarding them. Among the latter are stem cell scientists who have tried to persuade (and some have succeeded in persuading) in vitro fertilization (IVF) physicians to have their patients donate to research fresh embryos in excess of the maximum recommended for transfer in a single IVF cycle.[3]

People who want women in fertility treatment to donate their fresh embryos to stem cell research tend to be unclear, however, about what kinds of fresh embryos they have in mind. They could mean fresh embryos deemed unsuitable for transfer for morphological, biological or genetic reasons,[4] which would certainly be consistent with statements offered in defense of fresh embryo donation: 'Those embryos which have been tested positive for illness will never be used for reproductive purposes, nor will they be frozen.... They are, however, very valuable for research';[5] and '[t]here are embryos going down the drain all the time. It's a biological waste.'[6] But in terms of the value for research of fresh embryos unsuitable for transfer (for morphological reasons, at least), available evidence suggests that these embryos are less efficient than frozen-thawed embryos in deriving embryonic stem cell lines.[7] Research by Sjögren and colleagues involving women in IVF who donated fresh and frozen embryos to stem cell research found that it was better to use frozen-thawed rather than fresh embryos. Those who favour fresh embryo donation tend to ignore or dismiss this finding, however and, without supporting evidence, insist that it is better to derive human embryonic stem cell lines from fresh embryos.[8] Their insistence leads us to believe that by 'fresh embryos,' they actually mean to include both embryos deemed suitable for transfer as well as embryos deemed unsuitable for transfer (which would be consistent with policy statements permitting embryonic stem cell research involving fresh embryos of either type).[9]

But if fresh embryos suitable for transfer are what advocates of fresh embryo donation have in mind, then they equivocate on the use of the term 'fresh embryos' (since these are not the embryos that are going down the drain), and more importantly, their proposals are immensely worrisome, ethically speaking, because donating fresh embryos suitable for transfer is contrary to the interests of female IVF patients.

In this paper, we explain why donating fresh embryos suitable for transfer to stem cell research specifically, and to embryo research more generally, is not in the self-interests of female IVF patients.[10] Next, we consider the other-regarding interests of these patients and conclude that while fresh embryo donation may serve those interests, it does so at unnecessary cost to patients' self-interests. Lastly, we review some of the potential barriers to the autonomous donation of fresh embryos to research and highlight the risk that female IVF patients invited to donate their excess fresh embryos to research will misunderstand key aspects of the donation decision, be coerced to donate, or be exploited in the consent process. For the purposes of this discussion, we focus on female IVF patients (hereafter patients), because the implications of fresh embryo donation are more serious for them than for male IVF patients.

On the basis of our analysis, we conclude that patients should not be asked to donate fresh embryos suitable for transfer to stem cell research, even if (at some future date) there was overwhelming evidence that such embryos were highly efficient in establishing stem cell lines. In our view, such donation should be prohibited as a matter of sound public policy because allowing it would ultimately contribute to women's continued oppression. Thus, social justice demands no less than a total ban on the research use of fresh embryos from IVF patients, when these embryos have been deemed suitable for transfer (hereafter 'fresh embryos,' unless otherwise noted).[11]

Relevant Interests of Women Undergoing IVF

It is important for the physical and psychological health of women undergoing IVF to avoid ovarian stimulation and egg retrieval, where possible. Doing so is not possible in the first cycle of IVF, but it may be possible thereafter if there are excess embryos and if these embryos are frozen for later possible use. Hence, most IVF clinics recommend freezing excess embryos. But now, in Canada—where the law prohibits creating 'an in vitro embryo for any purpose other than creating a human being or improving or providing instruction in assisted reproduction procedures'[12]—stem cell researchers are asking IVF physicians to invite their patients to donate their fresh embryos to research, instead of freezing them for later reproductive use.[13] Some IVF physicians have acquiesced. Others have declined: 'It's so controversial. I'm not going to touch it.'[14] We think that IVF physicians should decline such requests, because accepting them would require that they act in a manner inconsistent with their obligation to protect and promote patients' interests.

Self-Interests

Current live birth rates with IVF are such that any one IVF cycle probably will not result in a live birth

(as live birth rates per cycle are less than 50%, and often substantially less than 50%). Thus, patients determined to reproduce using IVF likely will need a subsequent cycle, and it is common practice for this cycle to involve the transfer of frozen-thawed embryos from a prior cycle.

Donating fresh embryos to research, instead of freezing them for use in a future IVF cycle, is contrary to the self-interests of most patients for at least five reasons: first, donating fresh embryos can decrease the chance of pregnancy and childbearing; second, it can increase the number of risky or painful procedures that women must undergo; third, it can increase the psychological stress experienced by women as a result of IVF; fourth, it can increase the social disruption that IVF causes; and fifth, it can increase the financial burden of fertility treatment.

First, donating fresh embryos to research can decrease women's chances of pregnancy and childbearing,[15] especially for women who become unwilling or unable to consent to further ovarian stimulation and egg retrieval and who have no (more) frozen embryos available for thawing and transfer because of a prior decision to donate fresh embryos to research. Any woman could develop an unwillingness or inability to do further ovarian stimulation and egg retrieval, because of how burdensome—physically, psychologically, and socially—these processes tend to be for women (as we explain below). Also, any woman could become unwilling or unable to do more ovarian stimulation and egg retrieval because of financial or other (e.g., health) reasons. Since these are possibilities for all women, all women who give away fresh embryos that they could freeze for later reproductive use lessen their chances of reproducing and thereby possibly thwart their goal of childbearing.

Second, donating fresh embryos to research means that women who undertake another IVF cycle may again have to accept the physical risks and pain involved in ovarian stimulation and egg retrieval, which could be avoided with an IVF cycle using frozen-thawed embryos. There are significant physical risks associated with ovarian stimulation. The short-term health risk is that of ovarian hyperstimulation syndrome (OHSS). Mild forms of OHSS involve 'transient lower abdominal discomfort, mild nausea, vomiting, diarrhea, and abdominal distention (observed in up to a third of superovulation cycles).'[16] More serious forms of OHSS entail 'rapid weight gain, tense ascites, hemodynamic instability (orthostatic hypotension, tachycardia), respiratory difficulty, progressive oliguria and laboratory abnormalities. Life-threatening complications of OHSS include renal failure, adult respiratory distress syndrome (ARDS), hemorrhage from ovarian rupture, and thromboembolism.'[17] It was reported at the 2006 meeting of the European Society for Human Reproduction and Embryology that six women had died of OHSS.[18] The long-term risks of ovarian stimulation are less well documented. Two studies, however, suggest a link between ovarian stimulation and ovarian cancer.[19] In addition, egg retrieval can be very painful and is therefore feared by many women.[20] The short- and long-term risks of ovarian stimulation as well as the pain and fear of egg retrieval can all be avoided by transferring frozen-thawed embryos.

Third, donating fresh embryos to research could mean more psychological stress for patients than they would otherwise experience. Women in general report higher levels of psychological stress from IVF than men, presumably because they have more invested in the outcome (including their self-image, their time, and their physical well-being).[21] Arguably, an IVF cycle that includes ovarian stimulation and egg retrieval is more stressful psychologically for women than a cycle using frozen-thawed embryos. The added effort and risk involved in a cycle using fresh embryos can make it all the more difficult for women to await the outcome of treatment, knowing that if it doesn't work, they will have done it all for nothing.

A fourth reason why fresh embryo donation can violate women's interests is that typically an IVF cycle that involves ovarian stimulation and egg retrieval is more socially disruptive than a cycle using frozen-thawed embryos because of the daily blood tests and routine ultrasounds involved. The blood tests typically occur in the early morning (around 7am) and if the women also need an ultrasound that day, then they may have to wait around or make a return visit. For women who work outside of the home or who have children at home to care for, frequent early morning blood tests and ultrasounds

are difficult to schedule, especially for those women who have to travel great distances to get to these appointments.

Lastly, donating fresh embryos to research is problematic insofar as it is contrary to the financial interests of many patients. An IVF cycle that involves ovarian stimulation and egg retrieval is more expensive than an IVF cycle using frozen-thawed embryos, even when the additional cost of embryo freezing is taken into account. With a frozen-thawed embryo cycle, one typically avoids the expense of sperm collection, sperm-washing, ovarian stimulation, and egg retrieval, as well as associated clinic and physician charges. One study estimates the cost saving with frozen-thawed embryo transfer at between 55-75% as compared with other assisted reproductive procedures.[22]

Thus, for many patients, donating fresh embryos to research is not in their self-interests. It is not in their reproductive self-interest; not in their interest in maintaining their overall physical and mental health; not in their career or family interests; and likely also not in their financial interests. Overall, for their own sakes, patients are better off freezing their excess fresh embryos, rather than donating them to research. The overwhelming majority of women seem to recognize this fact; rates of embryo freezing are as high as 99%.[23]

The only possible caveat here is that donating excess fresh embryos to stem cell research may be in patients' self-interests if they are (or believe themselves to be) at risk for one of the medical problems for which stem cell research may lead to effective treatment. We do not explore this possible future self-interest in this section of the paper, not because it is unimportant, but because at best it would be secondary to the primary self-interest in initiating a pregnancy. Our analysis of this secondary self-interest parallels our analysis below of other-regarding interests (which we also consider secondary to the primary self-interest in initiating a pregnancy).

Since fresh embryo donation to research goes against the self-interests of most women undergoing IVF, it is worth asking why stem cell researchers would expect patients to donate fresh embryos in sufficient numbers to allow them to undertake the research they are interested in. Perhaps they do not (or choose not to) accept that these embryos have reproductive potential. Or, they expect that fresh embryo donation will cohere with patients' other-regarding interests, and that patients will allow these interests to outweigh or supersede their self-interests. In other words, perhaps stem cell researchers (and IVF physicians) assume that women undergoing IVF will be altruistic and sacrifice their self-interest(s) to help others. But why make this assumption?

Other-Regarding Interests

Usually, when people make big sacrifices, they do so for people with whom they have some affinity. In the context of health care that affinity might be shared membership in a 'disease' group. Thus, infertile IVF patients might be willing to make big sacrifices in support of embryo research to treat infertility. But is there any reason why they might be willing to make big sacrifices to support embryonic stem cell research, where the sacrifice would not be for the sake of people who are like them in being infertile, but for the sake of people with any number of medical problems? One possible answer is that some infertile IVF patients have intimate relations with people who have one or more of the medical problems for which stem cell research may lead to effective treatment (e.g., a parent with Parkinson's disease); and these patients might be willing to promote this secondary interest at some cost to their primary interest in achieving a pregnancy. As Harvard stem cell scientist, Kevin Eggan, puts it, 'women who have families that are afflicted with diseases that we study might step forward.'[24] For it to be reasonable for them to step forward, however, it would have to be true that they could not achieve their secondary interest without cost to their primary interest. And available scientific data does not support this assumption. To be clear on this last point, researchers could develop stem cell therapies using frozen-thawed rather than fresh embryos. There is evidence that human embryonic stem cell lines can be derived from frozen-thawed embryos,[25] but as yet, there is no evidence that using fresh embryos would be better than using frozen-thawed embryos. Alternatively, researchers could use somatic tissues

instead of embryos. In short, available data does not show that diverting the use of fresh embryos created for reproductive purposes to stem cell research is necessary for the eventual (possible) development of stem cell therapies. It follows that women do not have to risk undermining their primary interest in pregnancy for a secondary interest in promoting embryonic stem cell research.

The upshot of this discussion about women's interests—self- and other-regarding—is that it is perfectly reasonable for women to be self-interested when faced with the option of donating their fresh embryos to stem cell research (where their self-interest demands that they not take this option). Moreover, it is unreasonable for others to expect women to act any differently. Our view is not that altruism in this domain is impossible, or would always be morally unacceptable, but simply that researchers (and IVF physicians) should not expect women to have such other-regarding interests. Nor should they invite them to act against their self-interests.

Possible Barriers to Autonomous Donation

In response to our claim that fresh embryo donation is contrary to the self- and other-regarding interests of women, some stem cell researchers and IVF physicians might insist that there are patients ready and willing to donate their fresh embryos to stem cell research. For these donations to be fully autonomous, however, they would have to be made with full understanding and without coercion or exploitation. Below, we dispute each of these possibilities.

Misunderstanding

Misunderstanding that results in mistaken beliefs can thwart autonomous decision making, as happens with: i) patients who mistakenly believe that fresh embryo donation is in their reproductive interests; ii) patients who understand that fresh embryo donation generally is not in the reproductive interests of women in an IVF program, but who mistakenly believe that they are not to be counted among these women because they are in their 'last' cycle of IVF; and iii) patients who mistakenly believe that they are obligated to be altruistic and donate their excess fresh embryos to research.

First, consider the group of patients who mistakenly believe that fresh embryo donation serves their reproductive interests, which it does not. Are patients truly at risk of developing such a wildly mistaken belief? We think so, especially since the persons requesting that patients donate fresh embryos to research, or the persons offering patients the opportunity to do so, are physicians or other care providers. (While in some jurisdictions, researchers are responsible for getting consent to donate embryos to specific research projects, typically physicians, or other care providers, make the initial inquiry into whether patients are willing to donate embryos to research.) Patients might believe that physicians would only suggest interventions that would further their reproductive interests, since their purpose in being at the clinic is to promote these interests and the stated goal of the clinic is to help patients succeed in having children. In addition, physicians might be unclear about how different fresh embryo donation is from other options in fertility treatment, insofar as fresh embryo donation does not improve one's chances of reproducing. (Such lack of clarity is possible given how short appointments with physicians can be.[26]) Alternatively, patients might have stopped listening to details about 'options' presented by physicians, because of how complex the information often is, and simply decided to accept what their physicians recommend/offer, on the grounds, again, that physicians would only recommend/offer to them whatever could further their reproductive goals. The problems alluded to here are of informational complexity and of undue deference to physicians by patients.

To be sure, the same problem of confusing embryo donation with a choice that furthers one's reproductive interests can occur with frozen as well as fresh embryo donation. But the donation of frozen embryos usually takes place once the women are no longer patients (and may never again be patients), and for this reason the women are less likely to see donation as a positive step toward reproducing. Also, at the time of frozen embryo donation the women are likely at a distance, both physically and psychologically, from their physicians and so they are less likely to be influenced by what their physicians want (or by what they perceive them to want).[27] Notably, many IVF patients who consent to the future donation of excess frozen embryos to research at the outset of treatment change their mind once they are no longer in active treatment and no longer potentially influenced by what their physicians might want.[28]

Second, consider the group of patients who mistakenly believe that they do not need to freeze excess fresh embryos for later reproductive use because they are done with IVF. This mistaken belief could be the result of them misunderstanding their chances of success with IVF, misunderstanding how psychologically prepared they are or will be for future IVF cycles, or misunderstanding their financial ability to continue with IVF. We address each of these possibilities in turn.

Perhaps the most common reason why a very few patients do not freeze excess fresh embryos for use in subsequent IVF cycles is that they are very confident that IVF will work for them the first time (i.e., result in a pregnancy and a healthy live birth), so they will not need further IVF cycles.[29] Being overconfident about the success of IVF is common among patients, especially those who are in their first cycle.[30] Such optimism can function as a kind of coping mechanism. ('I need to believe it is going to work; otherwise why would I be putting myself through all of this?') But IVF does not always (often) work. Failure in a first cycle can make obvious what may not have been obvious before: that IVF is not foolproof or that one may have a serious fertility problem.

Extreme optimism (especially in one's first IVF cycle) could stem from various sources. One source of optimism is clinic staff members, who sometimes express more optimism about treatment than they ought to.[31] Another source is family members or friends, especially those for whom reproduction was easy and who simply do not understand how the treatment could not work given that everything is timed so perfectly. A third source of optimism is society, which teaches us, especially through secondary school, that the chances of getting pregnant are about as high as the chances of it raining in June.[32] Society—more specifically the media—also tells us repeatedly of the miracles that reproductive technologies create, thereby distorting the success rates of these technologies. A fourth source of optimism is the women themselves who probably have internalized these social messages, along with other messages that connect womanhood with pregnancy and motherhood. The latter could make it impossible for women even to recognize themselves as women if they were to accept that they had a serious fertility problem. As a consequence, they may not accept this fact and may be overly optimistic about IVF.

No patient can be fully informed about whether her current IVF cycle will be successful and about what her preferences will be in terms of doing another cycle if the current one is unsuccessful. Thus, it is in women's interests to freeze all embryos suitable for transfer for possible future use in a later cycle.

Another reason why some IVF patients may say they are finished with IVF is that they do not feel that they have it in them to do more cycles. (In all likelihood, these are patients who have been through several IVF cycles.) But, of course, these patients could be wrong in thinking that they are done with IVF. Patients can and do change their minds about continuing with IVF, especially if their most recent cycle was 'unexpectedly' unsuccessful. For many patients, giving up on IVF is very difficult. It requires of women that they accept their infertility (which some deny, unjustifiably, even while they are in treatment),[33] and perhaps their childlessness as well. For some women, accepting either or both of these things is tantamount to admitting that they will never attain true womanhood and will never have good lives.

A further reason why some women may believe they are finished with IVF is that they no longer have the money to pursue their reproductive dream. IVF is costly. For some patients one IVF cycle will represent their entire life savings. Other patients may have more disposable income, yet have reached the limit of what they are prepared to invest in their reproductive project. In either case, financial circumstances or beliefs could change, making it possible to proceed with one or more future IVF cycles (each of which would be less costly if there were frozen embryos available for thawing and transfer).

In summary, women could want to donate fresh embryos to research because, for any number of reasons, they mistakenly believe that they are done with IVF and so will not need frozen embryos for future reproductive purposes.

Lastly, patients willing to donate fresh embryos to research could be mistaken in their belief that they are morally obligated to donate. Patients might assume that they ought to donate their excess fresh embryos because doing so would benefit humanity and they are morally obligated to act so as to benefit humanity, even at some risk to themselves. But we know from our previous discussion about altruism that donations of fresh embryos to stem cell research by patients is not the only (or perhaps even the best) way to proceed with this research and patients would be wrong to assume otherwise. Moral philosophy also tells us that whether people are morally required to help others while putting their own well-being at risk is complicated. It is certainly not obvious in the case of IVF treatment that women are obligated to donate fresh embryos that could, if the embryos implanted, put an end to their struggle with infertility, even if the relevant research would inevitably create a breakthrough in stem cell therapy.

Thus, various factors (psychological, social, and financial) can interfere with patients' understanding key aspects of the decision of whether to donate their fresh embryos to research. Failing to see that donation is not connected with reproduction, believing in error that one is truly done with IVF, or wrongly assuming that one is morally required to donate fresh embryos to research can prevent patients from truly knowing whether donation fits with their autonomous desires.

Coercion

Patients may fully understand everything that is relevant to a decision to donate fresh embryos to stem cell research, and still not choose autonomously because they are coerced. The coercion may be the result of a coercive offer, or of a threat of harm.[34]

To be coerced is to be compelled to accept and possibly act upon a proposal (e.g., to donate fresh embryos to stem cell research) on the grounds that failure to do so would worsen one's situation relative to the pre-proposal situation (a non-normative baseline of comparison) or to a situation that is fair (a normative baseline). The proposal—whether intentional or unintentional—alters or influences the will of the person coerced, making her choose differently than she otherwise would, it being rational or necessary for her to do what the coercer wants her to do.

In practice, the coercer can be an institution or an institutionalized set of social norms rather than an actual person.[35] Following Ann Cudd, we call such coercion simply, 'institutional coercion.' Sometimes people have trouble identifying institutional coercion because they take the relevant institutions or norms for granted (i.e., as simply the way things are), as many people do, for example, with the institutions of motherhood and heterosexuality. Widespread acceptance of institutionalized norms in no way diminishes their coercive effect, however.

Further, for there to be coercion, the offer or threat need not be real in the sense that the person's circumstances really would improve if she responded to the offer, or worsen if she failed to respond to the threat. The offer or threat need only be credible and compelling to the person for there to be coercion. For example, an offer or threat could be a bluff, yet still have a coercive effect.

Finally, coercion is prima facie wrong because it violates autonomy. People who are coerced do not choose freely, although they may make choices (e.g., the choice to save their skins by complying with a particular threat).[36]

In this paper, we focus on threats of abandonment (i.e., by one's physician or other care providers) and threats of stereotyping, both of which could coerce women to donate fresh embryos for research. These threats most likely stem from social norms and structures, although they could also issue from individuals, most notably physicians (and other care providers) or researchers. Moreover, the threat of being abandoned is perhaps most common, or most severe, when the person who asks whether the patient wants to donate her fresh embryos to stem cell research is her physician as opposed to a stem cell researcher. But a threat of abandonment could also exist when the request/offer comes from a researcher, because a physician ultimately directs the patient to the researcher, thus indicating to the patient that s/he, the physician, supports what the researcher is doing.

No matter who asks the patient about fresh embryo donation, therefore, the patient might reason that if she does not consent to the donation, then her physician will abandon her as a patient or treat her less well than s/he otherwise would. But why might a patient think she will be abandoned? First, she might assume that her physician would not ask her about fresh embryo donation, or direct her to a researcher who would ask her to consent to embryonic stem cell research (or have a nurse or other care provider direct her to such a researcher), if the physician did not believe that donating was a reasonable (possibly even good) thing to do. This assumption would flow from the commonly held view that physicians only have their patients' best interests in mind and at heart. Second, patients might know that the treatment they are receiving is elective, which suggests that they do not have the same right to it as they do to medically necessary therapies and that their physicians are not under the same obligation to provide it. Also, many patients may not have other physicians to turn to, especially if there is only one fertility clinic in their area. Taken together these thoughts could help to form a strong desire in patients to be compliant with what they take to be the physician's own view, namely, that fresh embryo donation is a reasonable (possibly even good) thing to do. These thoughts also make a threat of abandonment credible, although the threat may not be real. Patients who respond to this perceived threat in deciding to donate their fresh embryos to research are coerced.

The threat of abandonment, as we have described it, arises out of social norms and structures. But the behaviour of physicians and other care providers could also enhance (or diminish) this threat. For example, it matters how a physician or other care provider presents a proposal for donating fresh embryos to research, or presents a proposal for the patient to talk with a stem cell researcher who wants to obtain fresh embryos. Does s/he make it sound as though fresh embryo donation is something that patients ought to accept? Further, does the culture of the clinic bolster the perceived threat? For example, if physicians, nurses and other clinic staff tend to expect compliance (and label patients 'noncompliant' or 'problem patients' if they are demanding or questioning), then the perceived (or real) threat of abandonment for refusing a certain option or recommendation may be quite high.

Stereotyping by physicians or researchers is another potential threat that might compel patients to donate fresh embryos to research.[37] Like the threat of abandonment, the perception of a stereotype threat here begins with the assumption that the physician, or in this case perhaps the researcher, favours donation because it is a rational, praiseworthy thing to do. On this assumption, women who do not donate are at risk of being labeled 'hormonal,' that is, irrational or overly emotional. The threat of this stereotype is unusually high in fertility treatment because of the hormone medication(s) that women take. In an effort to avoid this stereotype, patients may respond positively to the 'rational' proposal that they donate their fresh embryos to research. Another stereotype that might compel patients to donate fresh embryos to research is that of the selfless woman, dedicated to caring for others. Here, the goal is not to avoid the stereotype, but rather to satisfy it. Patients can achieve this by donating their fresh embryos to research, which shows substantial concern for others.

But why assume that many patients in fertility treatment would perceive themselves to be at serious risk of animating stereotypes, especially with their physician, with whom they presumably have a meaningful relationship, at least compared to what they have with a researcher? Stereotypes prevail more easily in the absence of meaningful relationships. (To illustrate, we often stereotype strangers and cease to do so only once they cease to be strangers to us.) Unfortunately, however, one cannot assume that patients undergoing fertility treatment usually have meaningful relationships with their physician; in fact, there is good reason to believe that in general, these relationships are quite poor. One study in Finland shows that for women who are dissatisfied with fertility treatment, the greatest source of dissatisfaction is their relationship with their physician: s/he did not spend enough time with them, was not empathetic enough, did not understand their particular worries and concerns, etc.[38] In some cases, the dissatisfaction came from the team approach to fertility treatment, in which patients

receive care most of the time from a team of physicians and nurses rather than from one particular physician or nurse. With this approach, patients often do not know who will provide what care when: they may get a different physician every day or every other day that they go in for an ultrasound to monitor their follicle production; and they may get a different nurse every day calling them to tell them their blood test results. The team approach, which is common in fertility clinics, can benefit patients to be sure (e.g., by allowing them to get treatment quicker than they otherwise would); but it also denies patients the ability to have a relationship, of any meaningful sort, with their care providers. Consequently, it enhances the risk for patients of experiencing stereotype threats.

Thus, various social norms (e.g., stereotypes) and social structures (e.g., the team approach) are in place that can coerce patients to donate fresh embryos to stem cell research. We accept that these norms and structures can compromise consent not only for fresh embryo donation, but for other options as well. Yet their coercive force is particularly worrisome in the context of fresh embryo donation, because of how much worse off patients can be as a result of making such a donation.

Exploitation and Coercion

Agreements that IVF patients make to donate fresh embryos to stem cell research can be purely coercive. But they can also be exploitative and coercive. With the latter, we have in mind agreements that take unfair advantage of how beholden some patients feel to their IVF physicians and who donate their fresh embryos as a way of giving back to their physicians. These patients may have a strong desire to donate; yet their desire may originate or be influenced by coercive forces in our society (as illustrated below). Coercion can make us go against our immediate desires, as it does in the case of patients who would rather not donate their fresh embryos to research, but who do so anyway to avoid abandonment or stereotyping. Or, coercion can explain, in part or in whole, why we have some of the immediate desires that we do: we were coerced into having them, even though we may not now recognize this fact. The latter sort of coercion, combined with exploitation, is a further potential barrier to women autonomously donating their fresh embryos to stem cell research.

Assuming we understand coercion, let us explore the nature of exploitation briefly. Exploitation involves taking unfair advantage of someone. If you are taking unfair advantage, then you, the exploiter, must benefit. By contrast, the person you exploit either receives no (net) benefit or some benefit but not what she deserves. In the former case, the exploitation is harmful and in the latter, it is mutually advantageous, that is, relative to a baseline of non-cooperation.[39] Exploitation that is mutually advantageous is not advantageous to both parties in a way that is fair, as happens, for example, when the person exploited was in a vulnerable position to begin with (e.g., she was oppressed or impoverished), did not deserve to be in this position, and her vulnerability explains why she agrees to cooperate in the first place. While relative to her initial circumstances, she benefits from cooperating with the person who ultimately exploits her, relative to circumstances that are fair, she does not benefit to the degree that she ought to. (Here, the baseline of comparison is a normative baseline.) Rather than getting what she deserves, she gets the scraps offered to her by the person who takes advantage of her vulnerable state.

One further point about exploitation: like coercion, exploitation can be intentional or non-intentional. Out of charity, we assume that exploitation of patients in the context of fresh embryo donation for stem cell research is non-intentional: researchers or physicians who exploit the donors do not intend to take unfair advantage of them, but do so as a result of their interactions. For example, stem cell researchers and some physicians may take unfair advantage of the fact that some patients feel beholden to physicians for treating their infertility (and thus are in a state of moral vulnerability) and see fresh embryo donation as a way to relieve their (sense of) indebtedness. The researchers could be the exploiters—taking unfair advantage of patients who feel beholden—even though the physicians are the ones to whom patients feel beholden.

Why might some patients feel so beholden to IVF physicians that they would be willing to donate fresh embryos to research, and possibly compromise their reproductive future in order to repay the debt that they feel they owe? For some patients, physicians manage to get them government subsidies for their care, or, in rare cases, they pay for the treatment, as one physician did on Mother's Day 2006 for a woman who 'desperately' needed IVF but could not afford it.[40] Intense feelings of gratitude would be common in these cases. But such feelings could also arise among patients who have to pay for the treatment themselves. They might feel beholden because of a deep desire to get pregnant and a perception of their physician as a saviour to them—that is, someone who will rescue them from an 'empty, childless life.' Some physicians encourage this perception of themselves when they are optimistic with patients about being able to 'cure' them.

Patients who donate fresh embryos out of a sense of indebtedness benefit in being relieved of their perceived debt. But this benefit may not outweigh the harm that they experience (i.e., to their reproductive goals and to their overall physical and mental health), in which case, the agreement to donate would be harmful to them. Alternatively, the agreement could be mutually advantageous, as it is when the benefit of expressing their gratitude outweighs the harm that may ensue as a result of the decision to donate.

Why assume that patients who benefit from donating fresh embryos to research to relieve their feelings of indebtedness are exploited in the process? Surely, not all agreements that are born out of indebtedness are exploitative. We agree. But when feelings of indebtedness are morally inappropriate or unjust (as with patients who do not deserve to feel indebted), people who take advantage of these feelings to secure an agreement take unfair advantage of another's vulnerabilities. Some women may feel beholden enough to be willing to donate fresh embryos to research only because of an intense desire to reproduce that comes from an oppressed and coerced self-image. They were coerced into believing that they are not real women if they cannot reproduce. So a desire that is a product of coercion fuels their sense of indebtedness and explains why they donate. Here, they are taken advantage of in their vulnerable state of having internalized a social mandate of reproduction for women. They are exploited because the advantage taken is unfair. The only potential benefit they receive is relief from a sense of indebtedness that is not authentic to them anyway. As such, one could argue that the women receive no real benefit, while the researchers clearly benefit; and therefore, the agreements that the women make with them must be exploitative.

Donations of fresh embryos by women who are vulnerable in the above way are also not purely consensual. A coercive social structure that makes some women desperate when they discover that they are infertile or cannot reproduce with their partners is what ultimately explains why these women donate their fresh embryos to research. In accepting their donation, physicians and, in turn, researchers not only take unfair advantage of them in their vulnerable state, but also compromise their freedom.

Thus, exploitation combined with a certain form of coercion is a possible barrier to women autonomously donating their fresh embryos to research. This barrier adds another layer—on top of misunderstanding and other forms of coercion—to the difficulty involved in having women make informed, autonomous choices about donating excess fresh embryos to stem cell research.

The Possibility of Autonomous Donation of Excess Fresh Embryos

According to the Ethics Committee of the American Society for Reproductive Medicine, '[w]ithout evidence that fresh embryos are significantly preferable to frozen embryos for ES [embryonic stem] cell use, it is appropriate to use only spare embryos that have been frozen.'[41] At the present time, such evidence is definitely lacking; we do not know whether fresh embryos in general are better than frozen-thawed embryos for this purpose, although we do know that fresh embryos deemed unsuitable for transfer are worse than frozen-thawed embryos in this regard.[42] From the perspective of evidence-based research therefore, only frozen-thawed embryos ought to be used for stem cell research. We have reached the same conclusion from an ethics perspective, and more particularly, from the perspective of patients. We have focused on donating fresh embryos suitable for transfer to stem cell research, and argued that

such donations violate women's self-and other-regarding interests, and that profound barriers exist to women making these donations in an autonomous fashion.

One might object to our claims about autonomy and insist that some patients will not misunderstand, be coerced or be exploited and that these patients ought to have the opportunity to donate their fresh embryos to stem cell research (whether suitable or unsuitable for transfer), provided that they perceive donation to be in their interests. Our response to this objection is twofold. First, the prospects of being able to identify the few patients who either are not subject to the above barriers to autonomy or could overcome them are dim. Second, the objection assumes that patients expressly prefer to donate fresh rather than frozen embryos; yet there are no grounds for this assumption. In fact, it would be most unusual for women who are fully informed to have this preference, even if they were staunch supporters of embryonic stem cell research, given that the goals of stem cell research could be achieved without their fresh embryos and thus without them having to incur the possible additional harms associated with fresh embryo donation. Importantly, the claim that research goals could be achieved without using fresh embryos would continue to be true if it were shown that human embryonic stem cell derivation was more efficient when using fresh embryos. Sometimes the most efficient option is not the most ethically sound option.

In closing, others have acknowledged that the consent process for the donation of fresh embryos to research is complicated;[43] but we go further in this paper and argue that the process is so fraught with difficulties that it simply ought not to take place. As we have shown, the barriers to autonomous decision-making are too severe; and, perhaps more importantly, fresh embryo donation is contrary to the interests of female infertility patients and furthers their oppression. Women's interests are best served and their autonomy best promoted if they have the time and distance from their IVF treatment that would allow them to reflect carefully on whether they want to donate excess embryos to research (as happens with the usual delay when patients donate frozen embryos to research). Studies show that with time and distance, women often withdraw prior consent to donating frozen embryos to research or simply do not give final consent to donation. This pattern creates an incentive for researchers to get access to fresh embryos before women can reflect and change their mind. But this pattern also speaks loudly against allowing or, worse, endorsing such a practice. We join others in insisting that final consent for donation to embryo research ought to be delayed 'until a significant time after IVF treatment,' which would definitely preclude the donation of fresh embryos.[44]

Notes

1   These countries include Canada, China, Germany, Iceland, and Italy. See Canada. Assisted Human Reproduction Act, S.C. 2004, c. 2; China, Hong Kong, The Human Reproductive Technology Ordinance, An Ordinance no. 47, Available at: http://www.hklii.org.hk/hk/legis/ord/561 [Accessed on 10 Aug 2007]; Germany. Act Ensuring Protection of Embryos in Connection with the Importation and Utilization of Human Embryonic Stem Cells—Stem Cell Act—of 28 June 2002. Available at: http://www.bmj.bund.de/files/-/1146/Stammzellgesetz%20englisch.pdf [Accessed on 13 Aug 2007]; Iceland. Regulation No. 568/1997 on Artificial Fertilization, Available at: http://eng.heilbrigdisra duneyti.is/lawsand-regulations/nr/686 [Accessed on 10 Aug 2007]; and G. Benagiano & L. Gianaroli. The New Italian IVF Legislation. *Repro BioMed Online* 2004; 9, 2: 117-125. Available at: http://www .rbmonline.com/4DCGI/ Article/Detail?38%091%09 =%201376%09 [Accessed on 13 Aug 2007].

2   On the controversy, see for example, Canada. The Standing Senate Committee on Social Affairs, Science and Technology. 2007. Ninth Report of the Committee. Available at: http://www.parl.gc.ca/39 /1/parlbus/commbus/senate/com-e/soci-e/rep-e/rep09 feb07-e.htm [Accessed on 10 Aug 2007]; and Canadian Institutes of Health Research. 2007. 11th Meeting of the Stem Cell Oversight Committee (SCOC). Available at: http://www.cihr-irsc.gc.ca/e/33704.html [Accessed on 10 Aug 2007].

3   In practice, the maximum varies from country to country, from clinic to clinic, and from patient to patient (based on age, reason for treatment, number of previous cycles, etc.). See for example, Joint SOGCCFAS (Society for Obstetricians and Gynaecologists of Canadian Fertility and Andrology Society) Guideline. Guidelines for the Number of Embryos to Transfer Following In Vitro Fertilization. *J Obstet Gynaecol Can*, 2006; 28, 9: 803-804.

4   F. Baylis. Embryological Viability. *AmJBio* 2005; 5, 6: 17-18; K. Elder. 2005. Routine Gamete Handling: Oocyte Collection and Embryo Culture. In *In Vitro Fertilization and Assisted Reproduction*. P.R. Brinsden, ed. London, UK: Taylor & Francis. ch. 15: 287-307; L. Scott. 2003. *Classification of Pronuclei and Polarity of the Zygote: Correlations with Outcome. In A Color Atlas for Human Assisted Reproduction: Laboratory and Clinical Insights*. P. Patrizio, M. Tucker, V. Guelman, eds. Lippincott Williams & Wilkins. ch. 5: 71-88.

5   Andras Nagy, first Canadian stem cell scientist to derive human embryonic stem cell lines from fresh embryos, quoted in Flawed Embryos Sought for Research, Vancouver Sun, cited in: 2005. *University of Toronto News Digest* 6 Oct. Available at: http://www.news.utoronto.ca/inthenews/archive/2005 _10_06.html [Accessed on 10 Aug 2007].

6   A. Nagy, quoted in M. Munro. 2006. Controversial Stem Cell Project Gets Green Light: Canadian Agency Authorizes use of 'Fresh' Embryos for First Time. *The Ottawa Citizen*. 27 June. Available at: http://www.canada.com/ottawacitizen/story.html?id= b46a30c6-c67e-4c14ace3-fd8f269e548b&k=86316 &p=2 [Accessed on 10 Aug 2007].

7   A. Sjögren et al. Human Blastocysts for the Development of Embryonic Stem Cells. Reprod *Biomed Online* 2004; 9: 326-29. This is the only study we know of that compares the efficiency of fresh versus frozen-thawed embryos for stem cell derivation.

8   H. Greely. Moving Human Embryonic Stem Cells from Legislature to Lab: Remaining Legal and Ethical Questions. *PLoS Med* 2006; 3, 5, e143: 0571-0575, at 0572; K. Rook. 2005. Canadian Stem-Cell Research Wins Approval. *The Globe and Mail* 9 June: A13. Available at: http://www.utoronto.ca/health studies/newsitems/06.09.05canadianstemcell.html [Accessed on 10 Aug 2007]; M. Munro. 2006. 'Fresh' Embryos OK for Research. *National Post* 27 June. Available at: http://www.canada.com/nationalpost

/news/story.html?id=0c72d357-626d-4fac9446-6b8d62e4d054&k=59768&p=2 [Accessed on 10 Aug 2007]; M. Munro. 2006. Ban Fresh Embryo Donations, Ethics Adviser Insists. *Vancouver Sun* 28 June. Available at: http://www.canada.com/vancouver sun/news/story.html?id=47687071-4a17-4e10-b708-820e6dbdf81a&k=82919 [Accessed on 10 Aug 2007].

9   See for example, Canadian Institutes of Health Research. 2007. Updated Guidelines for Human Pluripotent Stem Cell Research. 29 June. Available at: http://www.irsc.gc.ca/e/34460.html [Accessed on 10 Aug 2007]. Permitted research includes: 'Research to derive and study human embryonic stem (ES) cell lines or other cell lines of a pluripotent nature from human embryos, provided that: The embryos used, *whether fresh or frozen*, were originally created for reproductive purposes and are no longer required for such purposes' (emphasis added).

10 J. Nisker & A. White. The CMA Code of Ethics and the Donation of Fresh Embryos for Stem Cell Research. *Can Med Assoc J* 2005; 173, 6: 621-622, at 621; F. Baylis & N. Ram. Eligibility of Cryopreserved Human Embryos for Research in Canada. *J Obstet Gynaecol Can* 2005; 27, 10: 949-955, at 950; F. Baylis & C. McInnes. Women at risk: Embryonic and fetal stem cell research in Canada. *McGill Health Law Publication* 2007; 1: 53-67 [Online]. Available: http://mhlp.mcgill.ca/pdfs/baylis-mcinnes.pdf [Accessed on 10 Aug 2007]; and F. Baylis et al. 2007. Nothing Extreme about Protecting Fresh Embryos. *The Globe and Mail* 16 Jan: A15.

11 Notice that our objection is not to all human embryo research involving embryos in excess of clinical need. We have no principled objection to the research use of either frozen embryos or fresh embryos deemed unsuitable for transfer.

12 Assisted Human Reproduction Act, S.C. 2004, c.2. s.5 (1)(b). Available at: http://www.canlii.org/ca/sta/a-13.4/ [Accessed on 10 Aug 2007].

13 Rook, op. cit. note 8; H. Branswell. 2005. Toronto Institute Develops Canada's First Two Embryonic Stem Cell Lines. *Canadian Press* 8 June; Munro, op. cit. note 6. Controversial Stem Cell Project; Munro, op. cit. note 8. 'Fresh' Embryos OK.

14 Dr. Cal Greene of the Calgary-based Regional Fertility Program quoted in P.J. Smith. 2006. Alberta Scientist begins Stem-Cell Extraction on Human Embryos. LifeSiteNews.com: 10 August. Available at: http://www.lifesite.net/ldn/2006/aug/06080902.html [Accessed on 10 Aug 2007]. Similar comments were made to us by clinicians at the 52nd annual meeting of the Canadian Fertility and Andrology Society (CFAS) in Ottawa, Canada (Nov 2006), where we presented the poster, 'The Ethics of Inviting Female IVF Patients to Donate Fresh Embryos to Stem Cell Research.' Available at http://www.novel techethics.ca/site_genetic.php?page=209 [Accessed on 10 Aug 2007].

15 Nisker & White, op. cit. note 10, p. 621.

16 Ovarian Hyperstimulation Syndrome, National Guidelines Clearinghouse (a comprehensive database of evidence-based clinical practice guidelines and related documents). Available at: http://www.guide-line.gov/summary/summary.aspx?doc_id=4845 [Accessed on 10 Aug 2007]. Information based on: Practice Committee of the American Society of Reproductive Medicine. Ovarian Hyperstimulation Syndrome. *Fertil Steril* 2003; 80, 5: 1309. See also A. Delvigne & S. Rozenberg. Epidemiology and Prevention of Ovarian Hyperstimulation Syndrome (OHSS): a review. *Hum Reprod Update* 2002; 8: 559-577.

17 Ibid. 18 H. Pearson. Health Effects of Egg Donation may take Decades to Emerge. News@Nature.com 9 August 2006, available at: http:// www.nature.com/news/2006/060807/full/442607a.html [Accessed on 10 Aug 2007].

18 H. Pearson. Health Effects of Egg Donation may take Decades to Emerge. News@Nature.com 9 August 2006, available at: http://www.nature.com/news /2006/060807/full/442607a.html [Accessed on 10 Aug 2007].

19 A.S. Whittemore et al. Characteristics Relating to Ovarian Cancer Risk: Collaborative Analysis of 12 US Case-control Studies. II Invasive Epithelial Ovarian Cancers in White Women. *Am J Epidemiol* 1996; 136, 10: 1184; and M.A. Rossing et al. Ovarian Tumors in a Cohort of Infertile Women. *NEJM* 1994; 331, 12: 771; L.A. Brinton et al. Ovarian Cancer Risk After the Use of Ovulation-Stimulating Drugs. *Obstet Gynecol* 2004; 103: 1194-1203.

20 A. Eugster & A.J.J.M. Vingerhoets. Psychological Aspects of In vitro Fertilization: A Review. *Soc Sci Med* 1999; 48: 575-589.

21 A.L. Greil. Infertility and Psychological Distress: A Critical Review of the Literature. *Soc Sci Med* 1997; 45: 1697-1704.

22 B.J. Van Voorhis et al. The Efficacy and Cost Effectiveness of Embryo Cryopreservation Compared with Other Assisted Reproductive Techniques. *Fertil Steril* 1995; 64, 3: 647-650.

23 L. Lornage et al. Six Year Follow-up of Cryopreserved Embryos. *Hum Reprod* 1995; 10: 2610-2616.

24 R. Waters & J. Lauerman. Harvard Scientists Try Cloning to Create Stem Cells (Update2). 2006. Bloomberg.com 6 June. Available at: http://www.bloomberg.com/apps/news?pid=newsarchive&sid=a9obSc92m0Zk [Accessed on 10 Aug 2007].

25 S.P. Park et al. Establishment of Human Embryonic Stem Cell Lines from Frozen-Thawed Blastocysts using STO Cell Feeder Layers. *Human Reprod* 2004; 19: 676-684.

26 M. Malin et al. What Do Women Want? Women's Experiences of Infertility Treatment. *Soc Sci Med* 2001; 53: 123-133.

27 For this reason, among others, the Ethics Committee of the American Society for Reproductive Medicine (ASRM) recommends that only frozen embryos be used for research. Ethics Committee of the ASRM. Donating Spare Embryos for Embryonic Stem-Cell Research. *Fertil Steril* 2004; 82, *Suppl* 1: S224-27 at S226.

28 S.C. Klock, S. Sheinin & R.R. Kazer. The Disposition of Unused Frozen Embryos [letter]. *NEJM* 2001; 345, 1: 69-70; J. Nisker et al. Development and Investigation of a Free and Informed Choice Process for Embryo Donation to Stem Cell Research in Canada. *J Obstet Gynaecol Can* 2006; 28, 10: 903-908.

29 Personal communication between Angela White (research assistant to C. McLeod) and Dr. Valter Feyles, reproductive endocrinologist, London Health Sciences Centre.

30 V.L. Peddie, E. van Teijlingen & S. Bhattacharya. A Qualitative Study of Women's Decision-making at the End of IVF Treatment. *Hum Reprod* 2005; 20, 7: 1944-1951.

31 Ibid.

32 The comparison with rain in June comes from V. Hey et al. 1996. *Hidden Loss: Miscarriage and Ectopic Pregnancy*, 2nd ed. London, UK: Women's Press. They say that society leads us to believe the chances of having a child after getting pregnant are as high as rain in June.

33 Y. Benjamini, M. Gozlan & E. Kokia. On the Self-regulation of a Health Threat: Cognitions, Coping, and Emotions among Women undergoing Treatment for Infertility. *Cognit Ther Res* 2004; 28, 5: 577-592; O.B.A. van den Akker. Coping, Quality of Life and Psychological Symptoms in Three Groups of Sub-fertile Women. *Patient Educ Couns* 2005; 57: 183-189.

34 Not everyone agrees that coercion can be the result of an offer rather than a threat, but we find this view persuasive. (See S. Anderson. 2006. Coercion. *Stanford Encyclopedia of Philosophy online*. E.N. Zalta, ed. Available at http://plato.stanford.edu/entries/coercion/#CoeOff [Accessed on 10 Aug 2007], section 2.4 'Coercive offers?.')

35 A. Cudd. Oppression by Choice. *J Soc Philos* 1994; 25th Anniversary Special Issue: 22-44, at 29.

36 Ibid.

37 On stereotype threats, see C. Steele. A Threat in the Air: How Stereotypes Shape Intellectual Identity and Performance. *Am Psychol* 1997; 52, 6: 613-629.

38 Malin et al., op. cit. note 26.

39 A. Wertheimer. 2001. Exploitation. *Stanford Encyclopedia of Philosophy online*. E.N. Zalta, ed. Available at: http://plato.stanford.edu/entries/exploitation [Accessed on 10 Aug 2007]. On exploitation, see also R.J. Sample. 2003. *Exploitation: What It Is and Why It's Wrong*. Lanham: Rowman & Littlefield.

40 Canadian Television Network (CTV) Local News, 13 May 2006.

41 Ethics Committee of the ASRM, op. cit. note 27.

42 Sjögren et al., op. cit. note 7.

43 Greely, op. cit. note 8.

44 Nisker et al., op. cit. note 28, p. 907.

23.
REPRODUCTIVE CLONING AND A (KIND OF) GENETIC FALLACY

Neil Levy and Mianna Lotz

Source: *Bioethics* 19.3 (2005): 232-49.

Whatever credibility we attach to the recent announcement, by the leader of the Raelian cult, of the birth of the first cloned human being, the prospect of human reproductive cloning appears imminent. Should we be alarmed, morally, by this prospect? Our purpose is to examine the claim, gaining in popularity, that we ought, on the contrary, to welcome it. Proponents argue that there are circumstances in which cloning ought to be permitted: at the very least, they say, once it has become safe, and can be used to allow the otherwise infertile to have children of their own, cloning should take its place as just one additional means of assisting reproduction.

The claim that cloning is morally supportable on the grounds that it would allow the otherwise infertile to have genetically related children, is, we believe, the strongest argument in its favour. Moreover, permitting cloning for this reason alone would render many of the arguments commonly advanced against it irrelevant. Thus, the genetic argument for reproductive cloning (as we shall call it) deserves centre stage in our ethical deliberations. Cloning should be permitted if and only if the fact that it offers a kind of 'cure' for infertility constitutes a morally significant argument in its favour.

Yet the genetic argument for cloning is not sound. It rests upon assumptions and beliefs, concerning the importance of a genetic connection to our children, which are false. Moreover, these false beliefs have undesirable consequences, consequences which would be magnified if we allowed human cloning. Accordingly, consideration of the genetic argument gives us reason to prohibit cloning, not to welcome it.

The Genetic Argument

Proponents of human reproductive cloning offer several reasons why it ought to be permitted. However, the most weighty are variations on a single theme: cloning ought to be permitted when it is the only, or the only practicable, way in which people can have healthy children who are closely related to them biologically. Consider the following cases:

- Liz and Sean are married and wish to start a family, but Sean is infertile. Liz could have a child using donor sperm. However, both prefer that their child be the physical product of their loving union, and therefore theirs, and theirs alone, biologically speaking.
- Robyn and her partner are lesbians. They, too, wish to start a family. In the jurisdiction in which they live, they might be permitted to adopt a child; failing that, either partner could use donor sperm. Once again, however, the resulting child would not be the embodiment of their love for one another.
- Matthew and Lynn are a married couple who wish to have a child. Unfortunately, Lynn is a carrier for a rare and serious genetic illness, and there is a high probability that any biological child of hers will develop this disease.

In these cases cloning opens up a possibility for the couples that is entirely new. It would allow them to have a child that is theirs, biologically. Liz could bear a child who is the genetic clone of Sean. In that case, they would both be the biological parents of the child. If her own, denucleated, egg is used, then they will both be the genetic parents as well, since in that case she supplies the mitochondrial DNA.[1] Similar techniques would permit Robyn and her partner, and Matthew and his, to have children who are their genetic offspring. Even in surrogacy cases, in which the mitochondrial DNA is supplied by the surrogate mother, the resulting child will share well over 90% of its DNA with one of its 'parents.' Thus, even male homosexuals could have children who were their genetic offspring.

These cases share one interesting feature. In them, the motivation to clone stems not from desires that might seem pernicious, but from the (supposedly) natural desire many of us have to bring children into the world who are closely related to us, genetically speaking. In these cases, cloning could cure infertility, a condition which causes many people great distress.[2] This is the genetic argument for human reproductive cloning.

Notice that cloning utilized solely for the purpose of allowing the otherwise infertile to have biological children is cloning which raises few of the spectres that commonly haunt the cloning debate. Few people will see in such cloning the prospect of armies of obedient replicants, for instance.[3] More seriously, the genetic argument helps to allay fears that those who might employ cloning must be motivated by the narcissistic desire to create duplicates of themselves.[4] Moreover, cloning in these cases is not driven by a desire to produce the perfect child, or to replicate a desirable genome, which, given fears that the search for perfection will make us less tolerant of imperfection, is also widely regarded as a suspect motivation.[5] To be sure, some objections to cloning retain their original force even in cases in which it is permitted solely as a 'treatment' for infertility. The objection that cloning represents a threat to the child's supposed 'right to an open future,' or her closely related 'right to ignorance,' would still need to be confronted.[6] So, too, will the contention that cloning represents a (further) commodification of human life, the hubristic extension of human powers beyond the limits that give meaning and value to human life.[7] However, if the contention that people should be given every opportunity to have biological children is as morally weighty as many believe, it will almost certainly outweigh these considerations. If there really is a strong, morally decisive, interest in having biologically related children, then irrespective of the cogency of the above arguments, we shall have to permit human reproductive cloning.

As noted, cloning would not permit the otherwise infertile to be parents in the (usual) genetic sense. We can, however, ignore this complication. If the genetic connection matters as much as commonly thought, then the fact that the child will be rather more closely related to one of its social parents than is usual, ought to strengthen the case for allowing cloning for the otherwise infertile. If it is true that parents care for and protect their children in part because of the genetic connection they have to them, how much more will this be the case when the child is the clone of one of them?

How Important Is Genetics?

These days, most people take the importance of genetics for granted. The genome, we are frequently told, is the key to life; it is what makes us what we are, individually and as a species. It explains intelligence, propensities, and sexual orientation. No wonder, then, that in assessments of the relative importance of the genetic and the social (and indeed, the gestational) in accounting for the parent-child relationship, the genetic is a clear winner. In fact, however, there are strong reasons to doubt the cogency of all of these claims for the importance of the genetic.[8] Supposed claims for the supremacy of the genetic stand in need of justification, and it is to that analysis that we now turn.

Carson Strong, in the most sustained consideration of this question in the context of cloning, identifies six reasons why people might be thought to have a legitimate interest in having a biological child:

1) It involves participation in the creation of a person;
2) It can be an affirmation of a couple's mutual love and acceptance of each other;
3) It can contribute to sexual intimacy;
4) It provides a link to future persons;
5) It involves experiences of pregnancy and childbirth; and
6) It leads to experiences associated with child rearing.[9] To these six reasons, we can add three more:

7) Genetic parents will provide better care for children than will non-genetic parents;

8) Genetic relatedness is more natural than other means of assuming responsibility for children;

9) A genetic connection will best ensure that the child shares the significant interests and outlook of her parents, thus making for more satisfying parenting and allowing greater intimacy between parents and child.[10]

Not all of these considerations are of relevance to cloning. For obvious reasons, allowing cloning for the otherwise infertile would on its own do nothing to enhance their sexual intimacy. Moreover, (6) is not specifically relevant to biological children; an adopted child will allow for parenting experience just as well. The same might be said regarding (4), though as we shall see, this can be disputed. Nevertheless, this still leaves a formidable list of apparently weighty considerations.

Let us, then, assess the items on the list, taking them in reverse order. Is it, first of all, true that a genetic connection will better ensure that the child shares significant characteristics with its parents, especially with that parent with whom it shares most of its DNA? Gregory Pence is among those who believe that it is, and that allowing parents to clone will reduce the chances that they will be disappointed in the child:

> One reason why some parents are disappointed stems from the random pattern of gene assortment. It is true that two parent-musicians would certainly be disappointed if their child was tone-deaf, but how likely is that if the ancestor has perfect pitch?[11]

Others share his view. Michael Tooley holds that allowing cloning would have benefits for the child, because at least one of her parents would be better able to appreciate her point of view, due to their great psychological similarity.[12] Brenda Almond goes further, suggesting that the biological relation is the bearer of 'what might be called psychic similarity':

> Shared attitudes, appraisals, interests, tendencies, common qualities of character, a common Weltan-

schauung—a characteristic way of looking at the world.[13]

Unfortunately for these philosophers, there is very little evidence that genetics is anywhere near as important as they suggest. It is extremely unlikely that a child's genes determine its fundamental outlook, its Weltanschauung. This is mere superstition, in the guise of modern science. There is no gene for conservatism, nor for Catholicism.[14] Of course, our genetic make-up contributes something to our characteristics; but the extent to which this is so is very far from clear, and is certainly very much less than is commonly suggested. Evidence for the (often touted) heritability of intelligence, for instance, is flawed at best.[15] A corollary of the exaggerated attention paid to the genetic, of course, is a significant disregard of the social: of the ways in which parents form their children by educating and nurturing them. Yet the evidence suggests that social factors are at least as important in making us who we are. In this context, Pence's example is well chosen. Parents do not best ensure that their child will have perfect pitch by paying attention to its genetic makeup. Perfect pitch is an ability that all, or very nearly all, children can acquire, if they need it. Speakers of tonal languages—in which pitch is grammatically significant—require much greater sensitivity to it than do speakers of non-tonal languages such as English or French. Thus, whereas the incidence of perfect pitch amongst speakers of European languages is about 1 in 10,000, it seems to be near universal among speakers of Chinese and Vietnamese.[16] We suggest that this case is typical: our most important individual characteristics are acquired, not innate. This is most obviously the case for those traits that constitute what Almond calls our Weltanschauung: our political and world-views, our religion, our sense of what is important and what trivial.[17]

We turn, then, to (8), the claim that the genetic connection is natural, and ought to be strengthened and protected for this reason. At least in its crudest form, this claim can be dispensed with relatively quickly. It is simply false to believe that the (supposed) fact that something is natural supplies any normative reasons. In spite of its temptations, the argument from the naturalness of something to its desirability is open to decisive counterexamples. For instance, it is true that one of this article's authors is naturally short-sighted. That is to say, unless he 'interferes' with his physiological processes, he will not see clearly. Yet it does not follow that it is inadvisable to so interfere. Indeed, it is more plausible to believe that he is better off for having interfered: for having had a pair of glasses made for him. Thus the mere fact that something is natural does not suffice to show that it is normative for us, in any sense. It does not set standards by which we ought to live.[18]

However, there is perhaps another sense in which the genetic connection to children is natural, and for that reason ought to be preferred to other ways of becoming a parent. We have a sociobiological argument in mind: perhaps parents are (unconsciously?) motivated to have children by the urgings of their 'selfish genes.' If this is the case, then perhaps parents will care more deeply for a child who is a close relative of theirs. In other words, perhaps (8) provides the explanation for why (7) is true: for why parents can be expected to care better for biological children than for adopted ones.

Brenda Almond is the most forceful advocate of this position. She invokes the wisdom of Solomon here. His famous judgment was predicated on the recognition that: The true—that is, the biological—mother would prefer even to sacrifice her own rights and her relationship with the child if that was necessary to preserve the child's life, and that it was for this very reason that her rights and relationship should be preserved.[19]

In contrast, the quality of care when 'purely social connections are involved' is questionable. When one considers 'recent abuse cases connected with children's homes' and sexual abuse of children by stepparents, one realizes that biology remains the best guarantee that children will be cared for, today as in Solomon's day. Human beings, like other animals, have 'natural tendencies and inclinations' to care for their biological offspring, and we disrupt these at our peril.[20] Or so it might be claimed.

Unfortunately, this is complete fantasy, just as it was in Solomon's day. Neither the sociobiological underpinnings nor the supposed cross-cultural consensus to which Almond appeals hold water. It is simplistic, from an evolutionary biological point of

view, to think that the characteristic of caring for one's own children, or at least for those who share a large proportion of our genes, will automatically be selected for. It is certainly possible that selective pressures would increase the proportion of genes for this kind of behaviour in a given population (assuming for the moment, and very simplistically, that it even makes sense to talk about genes for a complex behaviour of this kind). But it is equally possible that selective pressures might favour other sorts of behaviour, such as the tendency to care for those who are physically proximate.[21]

As for the cross-cultural consensus Almond cites, it too is nonexistent. As remarked earlier, an emphasis on the biological often correlates with a disregard of the social and historical. Almond does not need to check the facts concerning attitudes to children in other times and places, since she knows that the dispositions to care for biological offspring are innate, and therefore cannot be subject to change. If she had checked, she might have been surprised. It is neither true that all cultures value blood ties to children more than social ones, nor that blood ties are always valued at all. Richard Lewontin, for instance, notes that some cultures do not appear to value the blood connection at all:

> The cultural pressure to preserve a biological continuity as the form of immortality and family identity is certainly not a human universal. For the Romans, as for the Japanese, the preservation of family interest was the preeminent value, and adoption was a satisfactory substitute for reproduction. Indeed, in Rome the foster child (alumnus) was the object of special affection by virtue of having been adopted, i.e., acquired by an act of choice.[22]

Thus, not all cultures care more for the genetic than for the social. Indeed, not all cultures care very much for either—including our own, until fairly recently. In 1960 Philippe Ariès controversially argued that maternal relationships to children in the Middle Ages were characterized by indifference.[23] More recent evidence indicates that Ariès actually underestimated the extent of that indifference. According to him, attitudes to children began to alter in the sixteenth and seventeenth centuries. However, he drew his evidence too narrowly from the upper classes, and failed to notice that among the poverty stricken relative indifference persisted well into the eighteenth century and probably later.[24] It simply is not true that a biological connection itself ensures that children will be well treated. It is neither necessary nor sufficient for good childcare.

We can, then, discount the proposed biological justifications for the claim that genetic parents can be expected to provide better care for children than non-genetic parents. It is true that studies into the patterns of child abuse appear to show that the incidence of abuse is higher amongst children living with step parents than amongst those living with parents with whom they have a genetic relationship.[25] This suggests, prima facie, some causal connection between biological relatedness and childcare quality. However, that causal connection may be socially rather than biologically constituted. That is, its existence may be explained solely by reference to prevailing social attitudes about the importance of genetic relatedness and the degree of responsibility that flows from it. In a culture that venerates genetic relationships, we might expect neglect of or harm to biological offspring to be especially taboo. Thus, not only is there no sound evidence to support the existence of a biological basis for better parental care for biological offspring, there is no need even to look for biological explanations. The social explanation offers both a sufficient and sound causal account, should there be a phenomenon to be accounted for.

Since we are here concerned with whether there is good reason to have a biological child, and not with whether there is good reason to have a child at all, we ignore the question of whether child-rearing is a valuable experience. An adopted child provides for this interest, if indeed it is significant. We also ignore the question of whether the experience of pregnancy is valuable. It may be that it is, but this is somewhat tangential to our concerns. If a woman is otherwise infertile, but capable of bearing a child, and if the experience of doing so is valuable, then it is an experience that is available to her independently of cloning. A donated egg, fertilized with sperm from her partner or from someone else, could be implanted in her uterus. On the other hand, if the genetic

connection is itself valuable, the question of gestation ought to be irrelevant. (5) therefore has no bearing on our discussion.

We turn now to (4). The notion that the biological connection provides a link to future persons is of course true, but it is a confusion to think that this justifies the biological. The person or couple who adopts, or the woman who gestates an embryo to which she has no genetic connection, assumes a connection to future persons just as surely as does the genetic parent. It might be argued, however, that the nature of this connection is different in these cases, and that this difference is crucially important. However, there seems to us to be no version of such an argument that does not beg the question of the value of the genetic. Some philosophers have urged an 'immortality' argument in favor of the genetic: courtesy of the genetic connection, they argue, our genes will survive our death; if we are lucky, they will continue to do so for centuries or even millennia.[26] We can discount this argument, for two reasons. Firstly, such a form of immortality, in which copies of our genes persist whilst our psychological continuity— that all-important signifier of identity—is lost, is surely a very poor sort indeed, and barely worth its name. Secondly, a brief consideration of the facts casts doubt on the value of and need for this kind of genetic 'immortality.' In the normal case, our children share 50% of our genes.[27] Thus, our grandchildren will each have 25% of our genes, and so on. In just a few generations, the genetic proportion for which we are causally responsible will be very low. Unless we advocate its repeated and widespread use, cloning is a poor way to ensure even an ersatz kind of immortality. In any case, if we are concerned that our genes survive our deaths, there are alternatives to having biological children. Our efforts could be expended on caring for nephews and nieces instead, for instance—each of them carries 25% of our genes.

There are, moreover, different ways of 'surviving' one's death. One is genetic; another is social. Children can inherit not only genes but also ideas and interests, political views and religious commitments, and the like. We have a tendency to assume that genetic 'survival' is superior, but we have no non-question-begging arguments that support that assumption.

We turn, then, to the final two arguments in favour of a genetic relationship to one's children: (1) that it involves participation in the creation of a person; and (2) that it is an expression of a couple's love for one another. These, we think, are prima facie the most weighty moral considerations in favour of the biological. It is a fact that many couples view the creation of a child, brought forth out of both of their bodies, as the physical manifestation of a union that is otherwise 'merely' symbolic. It makes real and concrete their love for one another.[28] The belief that it does so is solidly based upon the biological fact that their sexual love has begun the process of creating a new life. Through this expression of love we 'participate in the mystery of the creation of self-consciousness.'[29] Thus, we might think, the biological child as an affirmation of love has a metaphysical and spiritual significance for which there is no social substitute.

While the two arguments appear closely bound—at least in the above formulation—they are in fact not necessarily so. As will become clear, there is no reason to think that biological children embody their parents' love in a way that social children do not and cannot. The linking of these two arguments is a symptom of precisely that which we seek to overturn: namely, an unwarranted emphasis on the importance of biological as opposed to social connectedness. Furthermore, the two arguments raise distinct issues and are therefore best treated separately.

Let us start with the argument that biological parenting involves participation in the 'creation of a person.' Strong's reference to the activity of 'person creation' is, of course, ambiguous in the light of philosophical notions of 'personhood.' If by 'creation' Strong simply has in mind 'conception,' then there is no sense in which people who decide to have a biological child are—by dint of bringing about conception—engaged in the creation of a 'person.' If, on the other hand, Strong's intended emphasis is on the parents' participation in the (gradual) development of a person, then non-biological parents of adopted children engage as surely in the 'creation of a person' as do biological parents. Many of the preconditions for personhood—such as a sense of a distinct self and identity, a Theory of Mind, and the like—do not begin to emerge until the second year of life.[30] It is the social parents, and the social family more generally, who have the most direct participation in, and make the greatest contribution to, the development of the child's self concept; and this is true irrespective of whether the social parents are also the biological parents.

Taken in the second sense, then, the desire to participate in the creation of a person cannot count as a reason specifically and exclusively in favour of biological parenting (by means of cloning or otherwise).[31]

Consider, then, the second argument, viz. that biological parenting is the expression and affirmation of a couple's love for one another. It is worth testing our intuitions here against a range of cases, real and imagined, in order to see whether the biological connection continues to have this significance across a range of situations. Consider, first, an actual case, that of Kimberly Mays:

In 1978, two baby girls were born within hours of each other at a Florida hospital, the children of Robert and Barbara Mays and Ernest and Regina Twiggs. At the age of nine, the Twiggs' daughter died of a congenital heart defect. However, blood tests revealed that she wasn't their biological daughter. The Twiggs' realized that the children must have been swapped in the hospital, and sued for custody of Kimberly.[32]

Now, according to the biological story just considered, it is Kimberly Mays who is the living symbol of the Twiggs' love for one another. They were making a mistake when they lavished affection on Arlena Twiggs. But surely this is implausible. Surely a decade of raising a child has forged bonds more significant than the mere biological, bonds that are more potent in their capacity to affirm the Twiggs' love for one another than is the fact of biological relatedness. To be sure, perhaps the strength and depth of those bonds owe something to each party's belief that there is a strong genetic connection. But the fact that it is belief in, and not actual existence of, a genetic connection that secures the salient bonds, only serve to emphasize that it is not biology that underlies our personal ties, but (at best) beliefs about biology. Such beliefs are social, and amenable to alteration.

Consider now a thought experiment, one well beyond our current technological means, but in principle possible—the baby-making machine:

> The machine allows its operator to construct a viable embryo, which is then implanted into a uterus (natural or artificial) and brought to term. The operator can select the genotype of the embryo, gene for gene. Thus she can build the baby from the ground up. She can even, if she likes, make a genetic copy of herself.

Notice that the operator of our machine is participating—very directly—in the creation of new life. She is causally responsible for the creation of a future person, who will be self-conscious. Yet it is hard to endow her work with great spiritual significance. Notice, too, that many of our common intuitions, which normally strengthen our conviction that the genetic is important, are confused by this thought experiment. One frequently cited piece of alleged evidence for the importance of the genetic is the wish commonly expressed by the adopted to meet their biological parents.[33] Now, even if it was granted that, given the current climate of interest in the genetic, we all have a degree of curiosity and desire to know the people responsible for our genotype, is there any reason to think that such a desire would survive the baby-making machine? Would the child want to meet the machine's operator? The only case in which she would, we suspect, would be when her genotype is identical to that of the operator, and then it would be out of mere curiosity rather than any natural desire (and even this curiosity would be the expression of an inadequate understanding of genetics). Consideration of these cases ought to help us shake off the overemphasis on biology that too often structures our thinking. There are actual and possible cases in which sharing a genotype is of little significance. At the same time, there is no reason to believe that other methods of entering into relationship with a child cannot be imbued with all of the significance normally attributed to the biological. There is no reason why an adopted child cannot be considered the physical expression of a couple's love for one another, in a sense that is just as real as that invoked by Lauritzen and Strong. The adopted child is the physical result and embodiment of a joint decision of the couple to commit, together, to the project of rearing and nurturing another human being. It is the decision to parent together that expresses the mutual love, trust, and commitment of partners in a relationship; and it does so irrespective of whether the resulting child is the biological product of the parents or not.

There are, then, no sound arguments for cloning that do not rest upon a mistaken view of the significance of a genetic connection of parents to their children. Why would anyone go to all the expense and trouble of cloning, either themselves or another person, unless they thought that genotype really mattered?[34] If they simply wanted a child, they could adopt; if they believed that a biological (though not genetic) connection was important, and they were capable of bearing a child, they could have an embryo implanted. Perhaps the biological connection matters, to some extent; perhaps, that is, the experience of pregnancy and childbirth forms bonds that are significant and valuable. But that is irrelevant to the topic of cloning. Such experiences are available to those physically capable of them, whether cloning is permitted or not. It is simply a modern form of superstition that leads us to attribute such importance to the genetic.

So far, however, we have at best shown that the strongest argument for cloning—the genetic argument—is in fact rather weak. Undermining this argument for cloning is therefore undermining the argument for cloning. But undermining an argument for a policy or action is not the same thing as showing that the policy or action is impermissible. We turn now to a consideration of why cloning ought not to be permitted.

Reinforcing the Genetic

We have shown that the grounds most commonly cited for pursuing cloning do not withstand critical scrutiny. But there are independent reasons for opposing cloning, which are broadly consequentialist in nature. The core of the argument we have in mind is that cloning should be opposed because permitting it will reinforce an over-emphasis on the genetic that is both unwarranted and unfortunate. Permitting cloning will allow people to give free reign to their biologistic fantasies; it will strengthen the impression that biology is destiny, or at least a significant constraint upon destiny. And there are strong consequentialist reasons for preventing such views from becoming further entrenched.

Whatever benefits we might still think cloning could provide, permitting cloning would bring certain harms that, we believe, outweigh the potential benefits. One class of potential harms is of particular concern: namely those harms that will be incurred as a result of the impact of cloning upon the practice of adoption. If cloning were to become widely available, the primary motive for adoption would be removed. It may be that some people adopt children primarily out of altruistic motives; that is, they recognise that there are children with significant needs that they are in a position to satisfy, and they decide to adopt a child (or more than one) in order to fulfil those needs. However, if they exist at all, purely altruistic adopters of this kind are almost certainly in a small minority. The majority of those who adopt children do so because they desire to have a child, and adoption offers them the (only) opportunity to do so.

What, then, will be the likely impact of cloning upon current adoption practices? In a climate in which genetic connection is so highly (yet unwarrantedly) esteemed, it is reasonable to think that widespread access to cloning will result in (i) more unwanted children languishing in institutional care (while people who could have provided them with good homes, and have a desire to have a child, choose to clone themselves instead of adopting someone else's biological offspring); and (ii) those parents who are averse to the likelihood of (i), will opt to keep their children rather than offering them for adoption, a 'choice' that is both not fully free and potentially counterproductive for parent(s) and child(ren).

The result is an overall diminution in the satisfaction of needs (or desires or preferences).[35] This can be seen from a comparison of need-satisfaction in the adoption scenario and need-satisfaction in the cloning scenario. In the case of adoption, need fulfilment is symmetrical: an existing child's need for a parent is fulfilled by an adoptive parent whose own need (or preference/desire) for a child is, in turn, satisfied. By contrast, cloning involves unilateral and asymmetrical need-satisfaction: of the parents for a (biological) child. Cloning fulfils no need on the part of the future clone-child (who does not yet exist, and would not otherwise have existed). What is more, not only does cloning not fulfil any needs of the clone-child, it involves the avoidable neglect of the significant needs of existing children. Where cloning is unavailable (and unnecessary institutional barriers to adoption are removed) some people will be forced to satisfy their own needs (or preferences/desires) in a way that simultaneously satisfies other significant existing needs. Thus need satisfaction is maximised in a world in which cloning is unavailable; and on such consequentialist grounds cloning should be opposed.

There is a second consequentialist consideration worth noting. It might be suggested that the genetic bias is based on, or at least heavily influenced by, a proprietarian conception of the relationship of children to parents. One reason given for the preference for genetic connectedness is that the genetically related child is, in some sense, 'more my own' than the child who is purely socially connected to me.[36] According to one version of the proprietarian view, whatever we produce, we justifiably own. Parental ownership rights are sometimes grounded in Lockean labour theories of ownership; or they may be based on the principle of self-ownership, according to which '… genetic parents maintain a defeasible right over the child, since they provide the constitutive genetic material.'[37] Proponents of this view argue that ownership and property rights over the child are based upon the parents' ownership over their own genetic material, a proposition that is itself open to serious question.[38]

Whatever the precise intentions of those who express the view that biological children are more 'their own' than non-biological children, genuinely proprietarian views of children have been discredited, and for good reason. The rights and obligations of parents with respect to children cannot be rendered analogous to the rights and obligations of private ownership. Theorists point out that the rights of parenthood are: contingent on the fulfilment of certain social obligations; regulated by the wellbeing of the thing that is 'owned' (the child, in this case); not based on any notion of the owned object's scarcity; not readily distributable between mother and father; subject to legitimate claims by the 'owned' (the child); and wane over time in a way that private property ownership in the main does not.[39] In addition, modern conceptions of the moral status of human beings—even minors—preclude them from being justifiably regarded as the sorts of things that can be owned as private property. To most, the idea that parents own their children in much the same way as they might own their cars, is 'deeply and rightly, repugnant.'[40] Yet we might plausibly think that permitting cloning in a context in which the genetic is over-valued will give proprietarian attitudes more 'leash' than is desirable.

Finally, we believe that permitting cloning would tend to encourage the current over-valuation of the importance of genetics in general, not just in relation to children. In the midst of a resurgence of interest in innateness and biology, a corresponding reduction in the importance accorded to the social and the political is conceivable and worth resisting. There is a danger that what are in fact false genetic determinist views will be used to buttress opposition to, or at least a reduction in, the use of public funds to improve the life prospects of the disadvantaged. We believe that the genetic arguments for disadvantage are confused, and that a great deal can be accomplished through properly designed and targeted social programs. We therefore oppose cloning, because we believe that permitting it would encourage the kind of social and political climate in which these social programs are threatened.

By contrast, opposing cloning can play a part in the wider project of shifting perceptions about the genetic. The vast resources that would otherwise be expended on cloning can be used on encouraging adoption,[41] and on educating the public on the real (limited) importance of the role of genes in forming the traits we come to possess. Most importantly, this money could be spent on the social programs that the emphasis on genetics would otherwise lead us to downplay: programs aimed at poverty alleviation, at education, and at improving the life prospects of those born into the under-classes. The belief, all too frequently expressed, that the problems of these people are genetic in origin, is pernicious and false; permitting cloning would tend only to reinforce it.

Notes

1 Neither Liz nor Sean would be biological parents in the usual genetic sense. Liz would bear the child, and give birth to it, but it would not carry her genetic material (other than her mitochondrial DNA). Sean would have an offspring that bore a genetic relationship to him closer to that borne by a (near identical) sibling, than to a genetic child. The child's social grandparents will also be her genetic parents. Notwithstanding this, cloning offers Sean a degree of genetic relatedness to the resultant child that sperm donorship would not.

2 D.B. Hershenov. An Argument for Limited Human Cloning. *Public Affairs Quarterly* 2000; 14: 245-258; P. Kitcher. 2000. There Will Never Be Another You. In *Human Cloning*. B. MacKinnon, ed. Urbana. University of Illinois Press: 53-67.

3 22% of respondents in a February 2001 Time/CNN poll gave this fear as their reason for opposing reproductive cloning.

4 L. Kass. 1998. The Wisdom of Repugnance. In *Flesh of My Flesh: The Ethics of Human Cloning*. G.E. Pence, ed. Lanham. Rowman and Littlefield: 13-37.

5 B. Appleyard. 1999. Would We Let It Live? In *Goodbye Normal Gene: Confronting the Genetic Revolution*. G. O'Sullivan, E. Sharman & S. Short, eds. Sydney. Pluto Press: 157-168.

6 Defenders of such rights argue that the child's knowledge of her future—the illnesses from which she is likely to suffer, the abilities and weaknesses she will possess, how she will look as she ages—represent a serious limit to her sense of individuality and ability to make free choices. For consideration of these objections, see B. Steinbock. 2000. *Cloning Human Beings: Sorting through the Ethical Issues*. In MacKinnon, op. cit. note 2, pp. 68-84, and National Bioethics Advisory Commission. 1998. *Cloning Human Beings*. In Pence, op. cit. note 4, pp. 45-65. M. Tooley. The Moral Status of the Cloning of Humans. *Monash Bioethics Review* 1999; 18: 27-49, provides plausible considerations against the 'open future' argument.

7 Kass, op. cit. note 4; J. Haldane. 2000. Being Human: Science, Knowledge and Virtue. In *Philosophy and Public Affairs*. J. Haldane, ed. Cambridge. Cambridge University Press: 189-202.

8   J.M. Kaplan. 2000. *The Limits and Lies of Human Genetic Research: Dangers for Social Policy.* New York. Routledge; R.C. Lewontin, R. Rose & L.J. Kamin. 1984. *Not in Our Genes: Biology, Ideology, and Human Nature.* New York. Pantheon Books.

9   C. Strong. 2000. Cloning and Infertility. In *The Human Cloning Debate* (2nd ed.). G. McGee, ed. Berkeley. Berkeley Hills Books: 184-215; at 188.

10 Reasons seven to nine are advanced forcefully in B. Almond. 1999. Family Relationships and Reproductive Technology. *In Having and Raising Children: Unconventional Families, Hard Choices, and the Social Good.* U. Narayan & J.J. Bartkowiak, eds. University Park, Penn. The Pennsylvania State University Press: 103-118.

11 G.E. Pence. 1998. *Who's Afraid of Human Cloning?* Lanham. Rowman & Littlefield: 137.

12 Tooley, op. cit. note 6, p. 42.

13 Almond, op. cit. note 10, p. 104.

14 Kaplan, op. cit. note 8, p. 162, notes that an attorney specializing in contract pregnancies in the United States allows his clients to select their 'surrogate mother' on the basis, inter alia, of religion. Genetic determinism has become so entrenched that people now attribute quasi-magical powers to genes.

15 Lewontin, et al., op. cit. note 8.

16 Scientific American Online. Perfect Pitch. (http://www.sciam.com/exhibit/1999/110199pitch). Of course, Asians typically differ genetically from Europeans in many—rather superficial—ways, but these genetic differences do not correlate with ability to learn a tonal language as a first language. Indeed, the genetic differences across 'races' are tiny and insignificant. For an overview, see H. Kassim. 2002. 'Race,' Genetics, and Human Difference. In *A Companion to Genethics.* J. Burley & J. Harris, eds. Oxford. Blackwell 2002: 302-316.

17 In stressing the importance of a genetic connection to children, proponents of cloning find themselves in a bind that they appear not to have noticed. To the extent that phenotypic traits are genetically determined, the Weltanschauung argument is strengthened, but so is the 'open future' objection. Typically, they have tried to circumvent this objection by arguing against genetic determinism (Pence, op. cit. note 11; Tooley, op. cit. note 6, pp. 38-39). But to the extent that they succeed, they undercut the Weltanschauung argument.

18 L.M. Antony. Nature and Norms. *Ethics* 2000; 111: 8-36. In any case, there is no definition of 'natural' that would permit cloning to count as securing a natural connection between people (unless one illegitimately substitutes the term 'natural' for 'genetic'). Offspring that are the near-identical genetic siblings of their parents do not occur 'naturally,' but instead require a great deal of technological intervention.

19 Almond, op. cit. note 10, pp. 109-110.

20 Ibid., p. 108.

21 E. Sober. 1994. Did evolution make us psychological egoists? In his *From a Biological Point of View: Essays in Evolutionary Philosophy.* Cambridge. Cambridge University Press: 8-27.

22 R.C. Lewontin. 1998. The Confusion over Cloning. In Pence, op. cit. note 4, pp. 129-139; at 134. Kaplan (op. cit. note 8, p. 167) notes that the Trobriand Islander (social) fathers do not distinguish between their (biological) children and those born to the same mother but a different father.

23 P. Ariès. 1960. *L'enfant et la vie familale sous l'ancien regime.* Paris. Plon.

24 E. Stocker. 1976. *The Making of the Modern Family.* London. Collins.

25 M. Daly and M. Wilson. Evolutionary social psychology and family homicide. *Science* 1988; 242: 519-524.

26 Pence, op. cit. note 11, p. 110.

27 More precisely, a child receives 50% of the small number of genes that vary between human beings, from each of her parents. She shares the overwhelming majority of her genes with all human beings; indeed, with other primates as well.

28 P. Lauritzen. 1993. *Pursuing Parenthood: Ethical Issues in Assisted Reproduction.* Bloomington. Indiana University Press: 72-76.

29 Strong, op. cit. note 9, p. 188.

30 See, for example, L.E. Berk. 1991. *Child Development,* 2nd edition. Boston. Allyn and Bacon: 434-437.

31 Of course, it is true that people who engage in procreation are causally responsible for the existence of beings who—all things going well—will become persons. But since personhood develops gradually, after birth, this causal role does not have the moral significance Strong imputes to it.

32 This case is discussed in Lauritzen, op. cit. note 28,

pp. 76-78. He differs from us in continuing to hold that Kimberly is the embodiment of the Twiggs' love. More recent cases that test our intuitions about the significance of genetic relatedness arise out of bungled IVF procedures. The *Journal of Medical Ethics* recently reported on a case—whose broad type is not unique—in which a white couple gave birth to black twins (M. Sprigge. IVF Mix-up: White Couple have Black Babies. *JME* Data Supplement: eCurrent Controversies, at www.jme.bmjjournals.com/cgi/content/full/27/6/DC1. We note that in such cases as these, in which the unintended absence of genetic relationship becomes clear before the social process of parenting has really commenced (i.e., at birth), our moral intuitions are likely to be less clear than in the Kimberly Mays case, where we might feel that there has been ample opportunity for the Mays couple to have the love-affirming quality of their (albeit non-genetic) offspring manifested.

33 Pence, op. cit. note 11, p. 110.

34 Current estimates of the cost of a single live birth of a human clone are about $150 million; the process would require approximately fifty surrogate mothers. See P. Singer. The Year of the Clone? *Free Inquiry* 2001; 21: 13.

35 Needs are more appropriately attributed to infant human beings than are preferences. However, in respect of would-be parents, it may be more appropriate and less controversial to speak of preferences or desires for children, rather than of needs. Importantly, the consequentialist calculation is not adversely affected by this slippage between terms. Indeed, one avenue open to the consequentialist is to compare the moral significance of need satisfaction with the moral significance of (mere) preference satisfaction, finding that adoption is morally desirable on the grounds that needs as opposed to (mere) preferences are fulfilled.

36 Strong does not explicitly refer to this reason, but it is not rare, and indeed may accompany (9), that is, the view that a genetic connection best ensures that children share the significant interests and outlook of their parents, thus making for more satisfying parenting and allowing for greater parent-child intimacy.

37 See, for example, B. Hall. The Origin of Parental Rights. *Public Affairs Quarterly* 1999; 13: 73-82.

38 See A. Kolers & T. Bayne. 'Are You My Mommy?': On the Genetic Basis of Parenthood. *Journal of Applied Philosophy* 2001; 18: 273-286.

39 Ibid; D. Archard. Child Abuse: Parental Rights and the Interests of the Child. *Journal of Applied Philosophy* 1990; 7: 183-194, especially 186-187.

40 Ibid.

41 Lauritzen (op. cit. note 28, p. 126) points out that mothers who give up their children for adoption almost invariably so do because of poverty. This is not, however, a reason to discourage adoption, as he seems to think, at least not under current conditions. If we limit the number of adoptions, whilst leaving the causes of poverty unaltered, we worsen the situation of these mothers and their children.

24

THE WISDOM OF REPUGNANCE

Leon R. Kass

SOURCE: *The New Republic* 216.22 (1997): 17-26.

Our habit of delighting in news of scientific and technological breakthroughs has been sorely challenged by the birth announcement of a sheep named Dolly. Though Dolly shares with previous sheep the "softest clothing, woolly, bright," William Blake's question, "Little Lamb, who made thee?" has for her a radically different answer: Dolly was, quite literally, made. She is the work not of nature or nature's God but of man, an Englishman, Ian Wilmut, and his fellow scientists. What's more, Dolly came into being not only asexually—ironically, just like "He who calls Himself a Lamb"—but also as the genetically identical copy (and the perfect incarnation of the form or blueprint) of a mature ewe, of whom she is a clone. This long-awaited yet not quite expected success in cloning a mammal raised immediately the prospect—and the specter—of cloning human beings: "I a child and Thou a lamb," despite our differences, have always been equal candidates for creative making, only now, by means of cloning, we may both spring from the hand of man playing at being God.

After an initial flurry of expert comment and public consternation, with opinion polls showing overwhelming opposition to cloning human beings, President Clinton ordered a ban on all federal support for human cloning research (even though none was being supported) and charged the National Bioethics Advisory Commission to report in ninety days on the ethics of human cloning research. The commission (an eighteen-member panel, evenly balanced between scientists and nonscientists, appointed by the president and reporting to the National Science and Technology Council) invited testimony from scientists, religious thinkers and bioethicists, as well as from the general public. It is now deliberating about what it should recommend, both as a matter of ethics and as a matter of public policy.

Congress is awaiting the commission's report, and is poised to act. Bills to prohibit the use of federal funds for human cloning research have been introduced in the House of Representatives and the Senate; and another bill, in the House, would make it illegal "for any person to use a human somatic cell for the process of producing a human clone." A fateful decision is at hand. To clone or not to clone a human being is no longer an academic question.

Taking Cloning Seriously, Then and Now

Cloning first came to public attention roughly thirty years ago, following the successful asexual production, in England, of a clutch of tadpole clones by the technique of nuclear transplantation. The individual largely responsible for bringing the prospect and promise of human cloning to public notice was Joshua Lederberg, a Nobel Laureate geneticist and a man of large vision. In 1966, Lederberg wrote a remarkable article in *The American Naturalist* detailing the eugenic advantages of human cloning and other forms of genetic engineering, and the following year he devoted a column in *The Washington Post*, where he wrote regularly on science and society, to the prospect of human cloning. He suggested that cloning could help us overcome the unpredictable variety that still rules human reproduction, and allow us to benefit from perpetuating superior genetic endowments. These writings sparked a small public debate in which I became a participant. At the time a young researcher in molecular biology at the National Institutes of Health (NIH), I wrote a reply to the Post, arguing against Lederberg's amoral treat-

Kass views

ment of this morally weighty subject and insisting on the urgency of confronting a series of questions and objections, culminating in the suggestion that "the programmed reproduction of man will, in fact, dehumanize him."

Much has happened in the intervening years. It has become harder, not easier, to discern the true meaning of human cloning. We have in some sense been softened up to the idea—through movies, cartoons, jokes and intermittent commentary in the mass media, some serious, most lighthearted. We have become accustomed to new practices in human reproduction: not just in vitro fertilization, but also embryo manipulation, embryo donation and surrogate pregnancy. Animal biotechnology has yielded transgenic animals and a burgeoning science of genetic engineering, easily and soon to be transferable to humans.

accustomed to new practices

Even more important, changes in the broader culture make it now vastly more difficult to express a common and respectful understanding of sexuality, procreation, nascent life, family, and the meaning of motherhood, fatherhood and the links between the generations. Twenty-five years ago, abortion was still largely illegal and thought to be immoral, the sexual revolution (made possible by the extramarital use of the pill) was still in its infancy, and few had yet heard about the reproductive rights of single women, homosexual men and lesbians. (Never mind shameless memoirs about one's own incest!) Then one could argue, without embarrassment, that the new technologies of human reproduction—babies without sex—and their confounding of normal kin relations—who's the mother: the egg donor, the surrogate who carries and delivers, or the one who rears?—would "undermine the justification and support that biological parenthood gives to the monogamous marriage." Today, defenders of stable, monogamous marriage risk charges of giving offense to those adults who are living in "new family forms" or to those children who, even without the benefit of assisted reproduction, have acquired either three or four parents or one or none at all. Today, one must even apologize for voicing opinions that twenty-five years ago were nearly universally regarded as the core of our culture's wisdom on these matters. In a world whose once-given natural boundaries are

Parenthood

blurred by technological change and whose moral boundaries are seemingly up for grabs, it is much more difficult to make persuasive the still compelling case against cloning human beings. As Rsonikov put it, "man gets used to everything—the beast!"

Indeed, perhaps the most depressing feature of the discussions that immediately followed the news about Dolly was their ironical tone, their genial cynicism, their moral fatigue: "an udder way of making lambs" (*Nature*), "who will cash in on breakthrough in cloning?" (*The Wall Street Journal*), "is cloning baaaaaaaad?" (*The Chicago Tribune*). Gone from the scene are the wise and courageous voices of Theodosius Dobzhansky (genetics), Hans Jonas (philosophy) and Paul Ramsey (theology) who, only twenty-five years ago, all made powerful moral arguments against ever cloning a human being. We are now too sophisticated for such argumentation; we wouldn't be caught in public with a strong moral stance, never mind an absolutist one. We are all, or almost all, post-modernists now.

people

Cloning turns out to be the perfect embodiment of the ruling opinions of our new age. Thanks to the sexual revolution, we are able to deny in practice, and increasingly in thought, the inherent procreative teleology of sexuality itself. But, if sex has no intrinsic connection to generating babies, babies need have no necessary connection to sex. Thanks to feminism and the gay rights movement, we are increasingly encouraged to treat the natural heterosexual difference and its preeminence as a matter of "cultural construction." But if male and female are not normatively complementary and generatively significant, babies need not come from male and female complementarity. Thanks to the prominence and the acceptability of divorce and out-of-wedlock births, stable, monogamous marriage as the ideal home for procreation is no longer the agreed-upon cultural norm. For this new dispensation, the clone is the ideal emblem: the ultimate "single-parent child."

Thanks to our belief that all children should be wanted children (the more high-minded principle we use to justify contraception and abortion), sooner or later only those children who fulfill our wants will be fully acceptable. Through cloning, we can work our wants and wills on the very identity of our children,

picking and choosing — *we would only want those who have our wants & wills. Those are the ones who we will accept*

exercising control as never before. Thanks to modern notions of individualism and the rate of cultural change, we see ourselves not as linked to ancestors and defined by traditions, but as projects for our own self-creation, not only as self-made men but also man-made selves; and self-cloning is simply an extension of such rootless and narcissistic self-re-creation.

Unwilling to acknowledge our debt to the past and unwilling to embrace the uncertainties and the limitations of the future, we have a false relation to both: cloning personifies our desire fully to control the future, while being subject to no controls ourselves. Enchanted and enslaved by the glamour of technology, we have lost our awe and wonder before the deep mysteries of nature and of life. We cheerfully take our own beginnings in our hands and, like the last man, we blink.

Part of the blame for our complacency lies, sadly, with the field of bioethics itself, and its claim to expertise in these moral matters. Bioethics was founded by people who understood that the new biology touched and threatened the deepest matters of our humanity: bodily integrity, identity and individuality, lineage and kinship, freedom and self-command, eros and aspiration, and the relations and strivings of body and soul. With its capture by analytic philosophy, however, and its inevitable routinization and professionalization, the field has by and large come to content itself with analyzing moral arguments, reacting to new technological developments and taking on emerging issues of public policy, all performed with a naive faith that the evils we fear can all be avoided by compassion, regulation and a respect for autonomy. Bioethics has made some major contributions in the protection of human subjects and in other areas where personal freedom is threatened; but its practitioners, with few exceptions, have turned the big human questions into pretty thin gruel.

One reason for this is that the piecemeal formation of public policy tends to grind down large questions of morals into small questions of procedure. Many of the country's leading bioethicists have served on national commissions or state task forces and advisory boards, where, understandably, they have found utilitarianism to be the only ethical vocabulary acceptable to all participants in discussing issues of law, regulation and public policy. As many of these commissions have been either officially under the aegis of NIH or the Health and Human Services Department, or otherwise dominated by powerful voices for scientific progress, the ethicists have for the most part been content, after some "values clarification" and wringing of hands, to pronounce their blessings upon the inevitable. Indeed, it is the bioethicists, not the scientists, who are now the most articulate defenders of human cloning: the two witnesses testifying before the National Bioethics Advisory Commission in favor of cloning human beings were bioethicists, eager to rebut what they regard as the irrational concerns of those of us in opposition. One wonders whether this commission, constituted like the previous commissions, can tear itself sufficiently free from the accommodationist pattern of rubber-stamping all technical innovation, in the mistaken belief that all other goods must bow down before the gods of better health and scientific advance.

If it is to do so, the commission must first persuade itself, as we all should persuade ourselves, not to be complacent about what is at issue here. Human cloning, though it is in some respects continuous with previous reproductive technologies, also represents something radically new, in itself and in its easily foreseeable consequences. The stakes are very high indeed. I exaggerate, but in the direction of the truth, when I insist that we are faced with having to decide nothing less than whether human procreation is going to remain human, whether children are going to be made rather than begotten, whether it is a good thing, humanly speaking, to say yes in principle to the road which leads (at best) to the dehumanized rationality of Brave New World. This is not business as usual, to be fretted about for a while but finally to be given our seal of approval. We must rise to the occasion and make our judgments as if the future of our humanity hangs in the balance. For so it does.

The State of the Art

If we should not underestimate the significance of human cloning, neither should we exaggerate its imminence or misunderstand just what is involved. The procedure is conceptually simple. The nucleus of a mature but unfertilized egg is removed and replaced with a nucleus obtained from a specialized cell of an adult (or fetal) organism (in Dolly's case, the donor nucleus came from mammary gland epithelium). Since almost all the hereditary material of a cell is contained within its nucleus, the renucleated egg and the individual into which this egg develops are genetically identical to the organism that was the source of the transferred nucleus. An unlimited number of genetically identical individuals—clones—could be produced by nuclear transfer. In principle, any person, male or female, newborn or adult, could be cloned, and in any quantity. With laboratory cultivation and storage of tissues, cells outliving their sources make it possible even to clone the dead.

The technical stumbling block, overcome by Wilmut and his colleagues, was to find a means of reprogramming the state of the DNA in the donor cells, reversing its differentiated expression and restoring its full totipotency, so that it could again direct the entire process of producing a mature organism. Now that this problem has been solved, we should expect a rush to develop cloning for other animals, especially livestock, in order to propagate in perpetuity the champion meat or milk producers. Though exactly how soon someone will succeed in cloning a human being is anybody's guess, Wilmut's technique, almost certainly applicable to humans, makes attempting the feat an imminent possibility.

Yet some cautions are in order and some possible misconceptions need correcting. For a start, cloning is not Xeroxing. As has been reassuringly reiterated, the clone of Mel Gibson, though his genetic double, would enter the world hairless, toothless and peeing in his diapers, just like any other human infant. Moreover, the success rate, at least at first, will probably not be very high: the British transferred 277 adult nuclei into enucleated sheep eggs, and implanted twenty-nine clonal embryos, but they achieved the birth of only one live lamb clone. For this reason, among others, it is unlikely that, at least for now, the practice would be very popular, and there is no immediate worry of mass-scale production of multicopies. The need of repeated surgery to obtain eggs

and, more crucially, of numerous borrowed wombs for implantation will surely limit use, as will the expense; besides, almost everyone who is able will doubtless prefer nature's sexier way of conceiving.

Still, for the tens of thousands of people already sustaining over 200 assisted-reproduction clinics in the United States and already availing themselves of in vitro fertilization, intracytoplasmic sperm injection and other techniques of assisted reproduction, cloning would be an option with virtually no added fuss (especially when the success rate improves). Should commercial interests develop in "nucleus-banking," as they have in sperm-banking; should famous athletes or other celebrities decide to market their DNA the way they now market their autographs and just about everything else; should techniques of embryo and germline genetic testing and manipulation arrive as anticipated, increasing the use of laboratory assistance in order to obtain "better" babies—should all this come to pass, then cloning, if it is permitted, could become more than a marginal practice simply on the basis of free reproductive choice, even without any social encouragement to upgrade the gene pool or to replicate superior types. Moreover, if laboratory research on human cloning proceeds, even without any intention to produce cloned humans, the existence of cloned human embryos in the laboratory, created to begin with only for research purposes, would surely pave the way for later baby-making implantations.

In anticipation of human cloning, apologists and proponents have already made clear possible uses of the perfected technology, ranging from the sentimental and compassionate to the grandiose. They include: providing a child for an infertile couple; "replacing" a beloved spouse or child who is dying or has died; avoiding the risk of genetic disease; permitting reproduction for homosexual men and lesbians who want nothing sexual to do with the opposite sex; securing a genetically identical source of organs or tissues perfectly suitable for transplantation; getting a child with a genotype of one's own choosing, not excluding oneself; replicating individuals of great genius, talent or beauty—having a child who really could "be like Mike"; and creating large sets of genetically identical humans suitable for research on, for instance, the question of nature versus nurture, or for special missions in peace and war (not excluding espionage), in which using identical humans would be an advantage. Most people who envision the cloning of human beings, of course, want none of these scenarios. That they cannot say why is not surprising. What is surprising, and welcome, is that, in our cynical age, they are saying anything at all.

The Wisdom of Repugnance

"Offensive." "Grotesque." "Revolting." "Repugnant." "Repulsive." These are the words most commonly heard regarding the prospect of human cloning. Such reactions come both from the man or woman in the street and from the intellectuals, from believers and atheists, from humanists and scientists. Even Dolly's creator has said he "would find it offensive" to clone a human being.

People are repelled by many aspects of human cloning. They recoil from the prospect of mass production of human beings, with large clones of look-alikes, compromised in their individuality; the idea of father-son or mother-daughter twins; the bizarre prospects of a woman giving birth to and rearing a genetic copy of herself, her spouse or even her deceased father or mother; the grotesqueness of conceiving a child as an exact replacement for another who has died; the utilitarian creation of embryonic genetic duplicates of oneself, to be frozen away or created when necessary, in case of need for homologous tissues or organs for transplantation; the narcissism of those who would clone themselves and the arrogance of others who think they know who deserves to be cloned or which genotype any child-to-be should be thrilled to receive; the Frankensteinian hubris to create human life and increasingly to control its destiny; man playing God. Almost no one finds any of the suggested reasons for human cloning compelling; almost everyone anticipates its possible misuses and abuses. Moreover, many people feel oppressed by the sense that there is probably nothing we can do to prevent it from happening. This makes the prospect all the more revolting.

Revulsion is not an argument; and some of yesterday's repugnances are today calmly accepted—though, one must add, not always for the better. In crucial cases, however, repugnance is the emotional expression of deep wisdom, beyond reason's power fully to articulate it. Can anyone really give an argument fully adequate to the horror which is father-daughter incest (even with consent), or having sex with animals, or mutilating a corpse, or eating human flesh, or even just (just!) raping or murdering another human being? Would anybody's failure to give full rational justification for his or her revulsion at these practices make that revulsion ethically suspect? Not at all. On the contrary, we are suspicious of those who think that they can rationalize away our horror, say, by trying to explain the enormity of incest with arguments only about the genetic risks of inbreeding.

The repugnance at human cloning belongs in this category. We are repelled by the prospect of cloning human beings not because of the strangeness or novelty of the undertaking, but because we intuit and feel, immediately and without argument, the violation of things that we rightfully hold dear. Repugnance, here as elsewhere, revolts against the excesses of human willfulness, warning us not to transgress what is unspeakably profound. Indeed, in this age in which everything is held to be permissible so long as it is freely done, in which our given human nature no longer commands respect, in which our bodies are regarded as mere instruments of our autonomous rational wills, repugnance may be the only voice left that speaks up to defend the central core of our humanity. Shallow are the souls that have forgotten how to shudder.

The goods protected by repugnance are generally overlooked by our customary ways of approaching all new biomedical technologies. The way we evaluate cloning ethically will in fact be shaped by how we characterize it descriptively, by the context into which we place it, and by the perspective from which we view it. The first task for ethics is proper description. And here is where our failure begins.

Typically, cloning is discussed in one or more of three familiar contexts, which one might call the technological, the liberal and the meliorist. Under the first, cloning will be seen as an extension of existing techniques for assisting reproduction and determining the genetic makeup of children. Like them, cloning is to be regarded as a neutral techhnique, with no inherent meaning or goodness, but subject to multiple uses, some good, some bad. The morality of cloning thus depends absolutely on the goodness or badness of the motives and intentions of the cloners: as one bioethicist defender of cloning puts it, "the ethics must be judged only by the way the parents nurture and rear their resulting child and whether they bestow the same love and affection on a child brought into existence by a technique of assisted reproduction as they would on a child born in the usual way."

The liberal (or libertarian or liberationist) perspective sets cloning in the context of rights, freedoms and personal empowerment. Cloning is just a new option for exercising an individual's right to reproduce or to have the kind of child that he or she wants. Alternatively, cloning enhances our liberation (especially women's liberation) from the confines of nature, the vagaries of chance, or the necessity for sexual mating. Indeed, it liberates women from the need for men altogether, for the process requires only eggs, nuclei and (for the time being) uteri— plus, of course, a healthy dose of our (allegedly "masculine") manipulative science that likes to do all these things to mother nature and nature's mothers. For those who hold this outlook, the only moral restraints on cloning are adequately informed consent and the avoidance of bodily harm. If no one is cloned without her consent, and if the clonant is not physically damaged, then the liberal conditions for licit, hence moral, conduct are met. Worries that go beyond violating the will or maiming the body are dismissed as "symbolic"—which is to say, unreal.

The meliorist perspective embraces valetudinarians and also eugenicists. The latter were formerly more vocal in these discussions, but they are now generally happy to see their goals advanced under the less threatening banners of freedom and technological growth. These people see in cloning a new prospect for improving human beings—minimally, by ensuring the perpetuation of healthy individuals by avoiding the risks of genetic disease inherent in the lottery of sex, and maximally, by producing "optimum babies," preserving outstanding genetic material, and (with the help of soon-to-come techniques for precise genetic engineering) enhancing inborn human capacities on many fronts. Here the

morality of cloning as a means is justified solely by the excellence of the end, that is, by the outstanding traits or individuals cloned—beauty, or brawn, or brains.

These three approaches, all quintessentially American and all perfectly fine in their places, are sorely wanting as approaches to human procreation. It is, to say the least, grossly distorting to view the wondrous mysteries of birth, renewal and individuality, and the deep meaning of parent-child relations, largely through the lens of our reductive science and its potent technologies. Similarly, considering reproduction (and the intimate relations of family life!) primarily under the political-legal, adversarial and individualistic notion of rights can only undermine the private yet fundamentally social, cooperative and duty-laden character of child-bearing, child-rearing and their bond to the covenant of marriage. Seeking to escape entirely from nature (in order to satisfy a natural desire or a natural right to reproduce!) is self-contradictory in theory and self-alienating in practice. For we are erotic beings only because we are embodied beings, and not merely intellects and wills unfortunately imprisoned in our bodies. And, though health and fitness are clearly great goods, there is something deeply disquieting in looking on our prospective children as artful products perfectible by genetic engineering, increasingly held to our willfully imposed designs, specifications and margins of tolerable error.

The technical, liberal and meliorist approaches all ignore the deeper anthropological, social and, indeed, ontological meanings of bringing forth new life. To this more fitting and profound point of view, cloning shows itself to be a major alteration, indeed, a major violation, of our given nature as embodied, gendered and engendering beings—and of the social relations built on this natural ground. Once this perspective is recognized, the ethical judgment on cloning can no longer be reduced to a matter of motives and intentions, rights and freedoms, benefits and harms, or even means and ends. It must be regarded primarily as a matter of meaning: Is cloning a fulfillment of human begetting and belonging? Or is cloning rather, as I contend, their pollution and perversion? To pollution and perversion, the fitting response can only be horror and revulsion; and conversely, generalized horror and revulsion are prima facie evidence of foulness and violation. The burden of moral argument must fall entirely on those who want to declare the widespread repugnances of humankind to be mere timidity or superstition.

Yet repugnance need not stand naked before the bar of reason. The wisdom of our horror at human cloning can be partially articulated, even if this is finally one of those instances about which the heart has its reasons that reason cannot entirely know.

The Profundity of Sex

To see cloning in its proper context, we must begin not, as I did before, with laboratory technique, but with the anthropology—natural and social—of sexual reproduction.

Sexual reproduction—by which I mean the generation of new life from (exactly) two complementary elements, one female, one male, (usually) through coitus—is established (if that is the right term) not by human decision, culture or tradition, but by nature; it is the natural way of all mammalian reproduction. By nature, each child has two complementary biological progenitors. Each child thus stems from and unites exactly two lineages. In natural generation, moreover, the precise genetic constitution of the resulting offspring is determined by a combination of nature and chance, not by human design: each human child shares the common natural human species genotype, each child is genetically (equally) kin to each (both) parent(s), yet each child is also genetically unique.

These biological truths about our origins foretell deep truths about our identity and about our human condition altogether. Every one of us is at once equally human, equally enmeshed in a particular familial nexus of origin, and equally individuated in our trajectory from birth to death—and, if all goes well, equally capable (despite our mortality) of participating, with a complementary other, in the very same renewal of such human possibility through procreation. Though less momentous than our common humanity, our genetic individuality is not humanly trivial. It shows itself forth in our distinctive appearance through which we are everywhere recognized; it is revealed in our "signature" marks of fingerprints and our self-recognizing immune system; it symbolizes and foreshadows exactly the unique, never-to-be-repeated character of each human life.

Human societies virtually everywhere have structured child-rearing responsibilities and systems of identity and relationship on the bases of these deep natural facts of begetting. The mysterious yet ubiquitous "love of one's own" is everywhere culturally exploited, to make sure that children are not just produced but well cared for and to create for everyone clear ties of meaning, belonging and obligation. But it is wrong to treat such naturally rooted social practices as mere cultural constructs (like left- or right-driving, or like burying or cremating the dead) that we can alter with little human cost. What would kinship be without its clear natural grounding? And what would identity be without kinship? We must resist those who have begun to refer to sexual reproduction as the "traditional method of reproduction," who would have us regard as merely traditional, and by implication arbitrary, what is in truth not only natural but most certainly profound.

Asexual reproduction, which produces "single-parent" offspring, is a radical departure from the natural human way, confounding all normal understandings of father, mother, sibling, grandparent, etc., and all moral relations tied thereto. It becomes even more of a radical departure when the resulting offspring is a clone derived not from an embryo, but from a mature adult to whom the clone would be an identical twin; and when the process occurs not by natural accident (as in natural twinning), but by deliberate human design and manipulation; and when the child's (or children's) genetic constitution is pre-selected by the parent(s) (or scientists). Accordingly, as we will see, cloning is vulnerable to three kinds of concerns and objections, related to these three points: cloning threatens confusion of identity and individuality, even in small-scale cloning; cloning represents a giant step (though not the first one) toward transforming procreation into manufacture, that is, toward the increasing depersonalization of the process of generation and, increasingly, toward the "production" of human children as artifacts, products of human will and design (what others have called the problem of "commodifica-

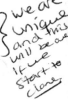
[margin note] We are unique and this will be loss if we start to clone

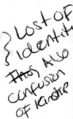
[margin note] Lost of identity & also confusion of kinship

[margin note] embryo derive from adult : Both parent & child would be identical twins

[margin note] Kass 3 points against cloning

[margin note, bottom] ★ such biological truths tells us about our identity & our origins

tion" of new life); and cloning—like other forms of eugenic engineering of the next generation—represents a form of despotism of the cloners over the cloned, and thus (even in benevolent cases) represents a blatant violation of the inner meaning of parent-child relations, of what it means to have a child, of what it means to say "yes" to our own demise and "replacement."

Before turning to these specific ethical objections, let me test my claim of the profundity of the natural way by taking up a challenge recently posed by a friend. What if the given natural human way of reproduction were asexual, and we now had to deal with a new technological innovation—artificially induced sexual dimorphism and the fusing of complementary gametes—whose inventors argued that sexual reproduction promised all sorts of advantages, including hybrid vigor and the creation of greatly increased individuality? Would one then be forced to defend natural asexuality because it was natural? Could one claim that it carried deep human meaning?

The response to this challenge broaches the ontological meaning of sexual reproduction. For it is impossible, I submit, for there to have been human life—or even higher forms of animal life—in the absence of sexuality and sexual reproduction. We find asexual reproduction only in the lowest forms of life: bacteria, algae, fungi, some lower invertebrates. Sexuality brings with it a new and enriched relationship to the world. Only sexual animals can seek and find complementary others with whom to pursue a goal that transcends their own existence. For a sexual being, the world is no longer an indifferent and largely homogeneous otherness, in part edible, in part dangerous. It also contains some very special and related and complementary beings, of the same kind but of opposite sex, toward whom one reaches out with special interest and intensity. In higher birds and mammals, the outward gaze keeps a lookout not only for food and predators, but also for prospective mates; the beholding of the many splendored world is suffused with desire for union, the animal antecedent of human eros and the germ of sociality. Not by accident is the human animal both the sexiest animal—whose females do not go into heat but are receptive throughout the estrous cycle and whose

males must therefore have greater sexual appetite and energy in order to reproduce successfully—and also the most aspiring, the most social, the most open and the most intelligent animal.

The soul-elevating power of sexuality is, at bottom, rooted in its strange connection to mortality, which it simultaneously accepts and tries to overcome. Asexual reproduction may be seen as a continuation of the activity of self-preservation. When one organism buds or divides to become two, the original being is (doubly) preserved, and nothing dies. Sexuality, by contrast, means perishability and serves replacement; the two that come together to generate one soon will die. Sexual desire, in human beings as in animals, thus serves an end that is partly hidden from, and finally at odds with, the self-serving individual. Whether we know it or not, when we are sexually active we are voting with our genitalia for our own demise. The salmon swimming upstream to spawn and die tell the universal story: sex is bound up with death, to which it holds a partial answer in procreation.

The salmon and the other animals evince this truth blindly. Only the human being can understand what it means. As we learn so powerfully from the story of the Garden of Eden, our humanization is coincident with sexual self-consciousness, with the recognition of our sexual nakedness and all that it implies: shame at our needy incompleteness, unruly self-division and finitude; awe before the eternal; hope in the self-transcending possibilities of children and a relationship to the divine. In the sexually self-conscious animal, sexual desire can become eros, lust can become love. Sexual desire humanly regarded is thus sublimated into erotic longing for wholeness, completion and immortality, which drives us knowingly into the embrace and its generative fruit—as well as into all the higher human possibilities of deed, speech and song.

Through children, a good common to both husband and wife, male and female achieve some genuine unification (beyond the mere sexual "union," which fails to do so). The two become one through sharing generous (not needy) love for this third being as good. Flesh of their flesh, the child is the parents' own commingled being externalized, and given a separate and persisting existence. Unification is enhanced also by their commingled work of rearing. Providing an opening to the future beyond the grave, carrying not only our seed but also our names, our ways and our hopes that they will surpass us in goodness and happiness, children are a testament to the possibility of transcendence. Gender duality and sexual desire, which first draws our love upward and outside of ourselves, finally provide for the partial overcoming of the confinement and limitation of perishable embodiment altogether.

Human procreation, in sum, is not simply an activity of our rational wills. It is a more complete activity precisely because it engages us bodily, erotically and spiritually, as well as rationally. There is wisdom in the mystery of nature that has joined the pleasure of sex, the inarticulate longing for union, the communication of the loving embrace and the deep-seated and only partly articulate desire for children in the very activity by which we continue the chain of human existence and participate in the renewal of human possibility. Whether or not we know it, the severing of procreation from sex, love and intimacy is inherently dehumanizing, no matter how good the product. We are now ready for the more specific objections to cloning.

The Perversities of Cloning

First, an important if formal objection: any attempt to clone a human being would constitute an unethical experiment upon the resulting child-to-be. As the animal experiments (frog and sheep) indicate, there are grave risks of mishaps and deformities. Moreover, because of what cloning means, one cannot presume a future cloned child's consent to be a clone, even a healthy one. Thus, ethically speaking, we cannot even get to know whether or not human cloning is feasible.

I understand, of course, the philosophical difficulty of trying to compare a life with defects against nonexistence. Several bioethicists, proud of their philosophical cleverness, use this conundrum to embarrass claims that one can injure a child in its conception, precisely because it is only thanks to that complained-of conception that the child is alive to complain. But common sense tells us that we have no reason to fear such philosophisms. For we surely know that people can harm and even maim children in the very act of conceiving them, say, by paternal transmission of the aids virus, maternal transmission of heroin dependence or, arguably, even by bringing them into being as bastards or with no capacity or willingness to look after them properly. And we believe that to do this intentionally, or even negligently, is inexcusable and clearly unethical.

The objection about the impossibility of presuming consent may even go beyond the obvious and sufficient point that a clonant, were he subsequently to be asked, could rightly resent having been made a clone. At issue are not just benefits and harms, but doubts about the very independence needed to give proper (even retroactive) consent, that is, not just the capacity to choose but the disposition and ability to choose freely and well. It is not at all clear to what extent a clone will truly be a moral agent. For, as we shall see, in the very fact of cloning, and of rearing him as a clone, his makers subvert the cloned child's independence, beginning with that aspect that comes from knowing that one was an unbidden surprise, a gift, to the world, rather than the designed result of someone's artful project.

Cloning creates serious issues of identity and individuality. The cloned person may experience concerns about his distinctive identity not only because he will be in genotype and appearance identical to another human being, but, in this case, because he may also be twin to the person who is his "father" or "mother"—if one can still call them that. What would be the psychic burdens of being the "child" or "parent" of your twin? The cloned individual, moreover, will be saddled with a genotype that has already lived. He will not be fully a surprise to the world. People are likely always to compare his performances in life with that of his alter ego. True, his nurture and his circumstance in life will be different; genotype is not exactly destiny. Still, one must also expect parental and other efforts to shape this new life after the original—or at least to view the child with the original version always firmly in mind. Why else did they clone from the star basketball player, mathematician and beauty queen—or even dear old dad—in the first place?

Since the birth of Dolly, there has been a fair amount of doublespeak on this matter of genetic identity. Experts have rushed in to reassure the public that the clone would in no way be the same person, or have any confusions about his or her identity: as previously noted, they are pleased to point out that the clone of Mel Gibson would not be Mel Gibson. Fair enough. But one is shortchanging the truth by emphasizing the additional importance of the intrauterine environment, rearing and social setting: genotype obviously matters plenty. That, after all, is the only reason to clone, whether human beings or sheep. The odds that clones of Wilt Chamberlain will play in the NBA are, I submit, infinitely greater than they are for clones of Robert Reich.

Curiously, this conclusion is supported, inadvertently, by the one ethical sticking point insisted on by friends of cloning: no cloning without the donor's consent. Though an orthodox liberal objection, it is in fact quite puzzling when it comes from people (such as Ruth Macklin) who also insist that genotype is not identity or individuality, and who deny that a child could reasonably complain about being made a genetic copy. If the clone of Mel Gibson would not be Mel Gibson, why should Mel Gibson have grounds to object that someone had been made his clone? We already allow researchers to use blood and tissue samples for research purposes of no benefit to their sources: my falling hair, my expectorations, my urine and even my biopsied tissues are "not me" and not mine. Courts have held that the profit gained from uses to which scientists put my discarded tissues do not legally belong to me. Why, then, no cloning without consent—including, I assume, no cloning from the body of someone who just died? What harm is done the donor, if the genotype is "not me"? Truth to tell, the only powerful justification for objecting is that genotype really does have something to do with identity, and everybody knows it. If not, on what basis could Michael Jordan object that someone cloned "him," say, from cells taken from a "lost" scraped-off piece of his skin? The insistence on donor consent unwittingly reveals the problem of identity in all cloning.

Genetic distinctiveness not only symbolizes the uniqueness of each human life and the independence of its parents that each human child rightfully attains. It can also be an important support for living a worthy and dignified life. Such arguments apply

with great force to any large-scale replication of human individuals. But they are sufficient, in my view, to rebut even the first attempts to clone a human being. One must never forget that these are human beings upon whom our eugenic or merely playful fantasies are to be enacted.

Troubled psychic identity (distinctiveness), based on all-too-evident genetic identity (sameness), will be made much worse by the utter confusion of social identity and kinship ties. For, as already noted, cloning radically confounds lineage and social relations, for "offspring" as for "parents." As bioethicist James Nelson has pointed out, a female child cloned from her "mother" might develop a desire for a relationship to her "father," and might understandably seek out the father of her "mother," who is after all also her biological twin sister. Would "grandpa," who thought his paternal duties concluded, be pleased to discover that the clonant looked to him for paternal attention and support?

Social identity and social ties of relationship and responsibility are widely connected to, and supported by, biological kinship. Social taboos on incest (and adultery) everywhere serve to keep clear who is related to whom (and especially which child belongs to which parents), as well as to avoid confounding the social identity of parent-and-child (or brother-and-sister) with the social identity of lovers, spouses and co-parents. True, social identity is altered by adoption (but as a matter of the best interest of already living children: we do not deliberately produce children for adoption). True, artificial insemination and in vitro fertilization with donor sperm, or whole embryo donation, are in some way forms of "prenatal adoption"—a not altogether unproblematic practice. Even here, though, there is in each case (as in all sexual reproduction) a known male source of sperm and a known single female source of egg— a genetic father and a genetic mother—should anyone care to know (as adopted children often do) who is genetically related to whom.

In the case of cloning, however, there is but one "parent." The usually sad situation of the "single-parent child" is here deliberately planned, and with a vengeance. In the case of self-cloning, the "offspring" is, in addition, one's twin; and so the dreaded result of incest—to be parent to one's sibling—is here brought about deliberately, albeit without any act of coitus. Moreover, all other relationships will be confounded. What will father, grandfather, aunt, cousin, sister mean? Who will bear what ties and what burdens? What sort of social identity will someone have with one whole side—"father's" or "mother's"—necessarily excluded? It is no answer to say that our society, with its high incidence of divorce, remarriage, adoption, extramarital child-bearing and the rest, already confounds lineage and confuses kinship and responsibility for children (and everyone else), unless one also wants to argue that this is, for children, a preferable state of affairs.

Human cloning would also represent a giant step toward turning begetting into making, procreation into manufacture (literally, something "handmade"), a process already begun with in vitro fertilization and genetic testing of embryos. With cloning, not only is the process in hand, but the total genetic blue-print of the cloned individual is selected and deter-mined by the human artisans. To be sure, subsequent development will take place according to natural processes; and the resulting children will still be rec-ognizably human. But we here would be taking a major step into making man himself simply another one of the man-made things. Human nature becomes merely the last part of nature to succumb to the tech-nological project, which turns all of nature into raw material at human disposal, to be homogenized by our rationalized technique according to the subjec-tive prejudices of the day.

How does begetting differ from making? In natur-al procreation, human beings come together, com-plementarily male and female, to give existence to another being who is formed, exactly as we were, by what we are: living, hence perishable, hence aspir-ingly erotic, human beings. In clonal reproduction, by contrast, and in the more advanced forms of man-ufacture to which it leads, we give existence to a being not by what we are but by what we intend and design. As with any product of our making, no mat-ter how excellent, the artificer stands above it, not as an equal but as a superior, transcending it by his will and creative prowess. Scientists who clone animals make it perfectly clear that they are engaged in instrumental making; the animals are, from the start, designed as means to serve rational human purposes.

In human cloning, scientists and prospective "par-ents" would be adopting the same technocratic men-tality to human children: human children would be their artifacts.

Such an arrangement is profoundly dehumaniz-ing, no matter how good the product. Mass-scale cloning of the same individual makes the point vividly; but the violation of human equality, freedom and dignity are present even in a single planned clone. And procreation dehumanized into manufac-ture is further degraded by commodification, a virtu-ally inescapable result of allowing babymaking to proceed under the banner of commerce. Genetic and reproductive biotechnology companies are already growth industries, but they will go into commercial orbit once the Human Genome Project nears com-pletion. Supply will create enormous demand. Even before the capacity for human cloning arrives, estab-lished companies will have invested in the harvesting of eggs from ovaries obtained at autopsy or through ovarian surgery, practiced embryonic genetic alter-ation, and initiated the stockpiling of prospective donor tissues. Through the rental of surrogate-womb services, and through the buying and selling of tis-sues and embryos, priced according to the merit of the donor, the commodification of nascent human life will be unstoppable.

Finally, and perhaps most important, the practice of human cloning by nuclear transfer—like other anticipated forms of genetic engineering of the next generation—would enshrine and aggravate a pro-found and mischievous misunderstanding of the meaning of having children and of the parent-child relationship. When a couple now chooses to procre-ate, the partners are saying yes to the emergence of new life in its novelty, saying yes not only to having a child but also, tacitly, to having whatever child this child turns out to be. In accepting our finitude and opening ourselves to our replacement, we are tacitly confessing the limits of our control. In this ubiqui-tous way of nature, embracing the future by procre-ating means precisely that we are relinquishing our grip, in the very activity of taking up our own share in what we hope will be the immortality of human life and the human species. This means that our chil-dren are not our children: they are not our property, not our possessions. Neither are they supposed to live our lives for us, or anyone else's life but their own. To be sure, we seek to guide them on their way, imparting to them not just life but nurturing, love, and a way of life; to be sure, they bear our hopes that they will live fine and flourishing lives, enabling us in small measure to transcend our own limitations. Still, their genetic distinctiveness and independence are the natural foreshadowing of the deep truth that they have their own and never-before-enacted life to live. They are sprung from a past, but they take an uncharted course into the future.

Much harm is already done by parents who try to live vicariously through their children. Children are sometimes compelled to fulfill the broken dreams of unhappy parents; John Doe Jr. or the III is under the burden of having to live up to his forebear's name. Still, if most parents have hopes for their children, cloning parents will have expectations. In cloning, such overbearing parents take at the start a decisive step which contradicts the entire meaning of the open and forward-looking nature of parent-child relations. The child is given a genotype that has already lived, with full expectation that this blueprint of a past life ought to be controlling of the life that is to come. Cloning is inherently despotic, for it seeks to make one's children (or someone else's children) after one's own image (or an image of one's choosing) and their future according to one's will. In some cases, the despotism may be mild and benevolent. In other cases, it will be mischievous and downright tyrannical. But despotism—the control of another through one's will—it inevitably will be.

Meeting Some Objections

The defenders of cloning, of course, are not wittingly friends of despotism. Indeed, they regard themselves mainly as friends of freedom: the freedom of individuals to reproduce, the freedom of scientists and inventors to discover and devise and to foster "progress" in genetic knowledge and technique. They want large-scale cloning only for animals, but they wish to preserve cloning as a human option for exercising our "right to reproduce"—our right to have children, and children with "desirable genes." As law professor John Robertson points out, under our "right to reproduce" we already practice early forms of unnatural, artificial and extramarital reproduction, and we already practice early forms of eugenic choice. For this reason, he argues, cloning is no big deal.

We have here a perfect example of the logic of the slippery slope, and the slippery way in which it already works in this area. Only a few years ago, slippery slope arguments were used to oppose artificial insemination and in vitro fertilization using unrelated sperm donors. Principles used to justify these practices, it was said, will be used to justify more artificial and more eugenic practices, including cloning. Not so, the defenders retorted, since we can make the necessary distinctions. And now, without even a gesture at making the necessary distinctions, the continuity of practice is held by itself to be justificatory.

The principle of reproductive freedom as currently enunciated by the proponents of cloning logically embraces the ethical acceptability of sliding down the entire rest of the slope—to producing children ectogenetically from sperm to term (should it become feasible) and to producing children whose entire genetic makeup will be the product of parental eugenic planning and choice. If reproductive freedom means the right to have a child of one's own choosing, by whatever means, it knows and accepts no limits.

But, far from being legitimated by a "right to reproduce," the emergence of techniques of assisted reproduction and genetic engineering should compel us to reconsider the meaning and limits of such a putative right. In truth, a "right to reproduce" has always been a peculiar and problematic notion. Rights generally belong to individuals, but this is a right which (before cloning) no one can exercise alone. Does the right then inhere only in couples? Only in married couples? Is it a (woman's) right to carry or deliver or a right (of one or more parents) to nurture and rear? Is it a right to have your own biological child? Is it a right only to attempt reproduction, or a right also to succeed? Is it a right to acquire the baby of one's choice?

The assertion of a negative "right to reproduce" certainly makes sense when it claims protection against state interference with procreative liberty, say, through a program of compulsory sterilization.

But surely it cannot be the basis of a tort claim against nature, to be made good by technology, should free efforts at natural procreation fail. Some insist that the right to reproduce embraces also the right against state interference with the free use of all technological means to obtain a child. Yet such a position cannot be sustained: for reasons having to do with the means employed, any community may rightfully prohibit surrogate pregnancy, or polygamy, or the sale of babies to infertile couples, without violating anyone's basic human "right to reproduce." When the exercise of a previously innocuous freedom now involves or impinges on troublesome practices that the original freedom never was intended to reach, the general presumption of liberty needs to be reconsidered.

We do indeed already practice negative eugenic selection, through genetic screening and prenatal diagnosis. Yet our practices are governed by a norm of health. We seek to prevent the birth of children who suffer from known (serious) genetic diseases. When and if gene therapy becomes possible, such diseases could then be treated, in utero or even before implantation—I have no ethical objection in principle to such a practice (though I have some practical worries), precisely because it serves the medical goal of <u>healing existing individuals</u>. But therapy, to be therapy, implies not only an existing "patient." It also implies a norm of health. In this respect, even germline gene "therapy," though practiced not on a human being but on egg and sperm, is less radical than cloning, which is in no way therapeutic. But once one blurs the distinction between health promotion and genetic enhancement, between so-called negative and positive eugenics, one opens the door to all future eugenic designs. "To make sure that a child will be healthy and have good chances in life": this is Robertson's principle, and owing to its latter clause it is an utterly elastic principle, with no boundaries. Being over eight feet tall will likely produce some very good chances in life, and so will having the looks of Marilyn Monroe, and so will a genius-level intelligence.

Proponents want us to believe that there are legitimate uses of cloning that can be distinguished from illegitimate uses, but by their own principles no such limits can be found. (Nor could any such limits be enforced in practice.) Reproductive freedom, as they understand it, is governed solely by the subjective wishes of the parents-to-be (plus the avoidance of bodily harm to the child). The sentimentally appealing case of the childless married couple is, on these grounds, indistinguishable from the case of an individual (married or not) who would like to clone someone famous or talented, living or dead. Further, the principle here endorsed justifies not only cloning but, indeed, all future artificial attempts to create (manufacture) "perfect" babies.

A concrete example will show how, in practice no less than in principle, the so-called innocent case will merge with, or even turn into, the more troubling ones. In practice, the eager parents-to-be will necessarily be subject to the tyranny of expertise. Consider an infertile married couple, she lacking eggs or he lacking sperm, that wants a child of their (genetic) own, and propose to clone either husband or wife. The scientist-physician (who is also co-owner of the cloning company) points out the likely difficulties—a cloned child is not really their (genetic) child, but the child of only one of them; this imbalance may produce strains on the marriage; the child might suffer identity confusion; there is a risk of perpetuating the cause of sterility; and so on—and he also points out the advantages of choosing a donor nucleus. Far better than a child of their own would be a child of their own choosing. Touting his own expertise in selecting healthy and talented donors, the doctor presents the couple with his latest catalog containing the pictures, the health records and the accomplishments of his stable of cloning donors, samples of whose tissues are in his deep freeze. Why not, dearly beloved, a more perfect baby?

The "perfect baby," of course, is the project not of the infertility doctors, but of the eugenic scientists and their supporters. For them, the paramount right is not the so-called right to reproduce but what biologist Bentley Glass called, a quarter of a century ago, "the right of every child to be born with a sound physical and mental constitution, based on a sound genotype ... the inalienable right to a sound heritage." But to secure this right, and to achieve the requisite quality control over new human life, human conception and gestation will need to be brought *packaging process of "the perfect baby"*

fully into the bright light of the laboratory, beneath which it can be fertilized, nourished, pruned, weeded, watched, inspected, prodded, pinched, cajoled, injected, tested, rated, graded, approved, stamped, wrapped, sealed and delivered. There is no other way to produce the perfect baby.

Yet we are urged by proponents of cloning to forget about the science fiction scenarios of laboratory manufacture and multiple-copied clones, and to focus only on the homely cases of infertile couples exercising their reproductive rights. But why, if the single cases are so innocent, should multiplying their performance be so off-putting? (Similarly, why do others object to people making money off this practice, if the practice itself is perfectly acceptable?) When we follow the sound ethical principle of universalizing our choice—"would it be right if everyone cloned a Wilt Chamberlain (with his consent, of course)? Would it be right if everyone decided to practice asexual reproduction?"—we discover what is wrong with these seemingly innocent cases. The so-called science fiction cases make vivid the meaning of what looks to us, mistakenly, to be benign.

Though I recognize certain continuities between cloning and, say, in vitro fertilization, I believe that cloning differs in essential and important ways. Yet those who disagree should be reminded that the "continuity" argument cuts both ways. Sometimes we establish bad precedents, and discover that they were bad only when we follow their inexorable logic to places we never meant to go. Can the defenders of cloning show us today how, on their principles, we will be able to see producing babies ("perfect babies") entirely in the laboratory or exercising full control over their genotypes (including so-called enhancement) as ethically different, in any essential way, from present forms of assisted reproduction? Or are they willing to admit, despite their attachment to the principle of continuity, that the complete obliteration of "mother" or "father," the complete depersonalization of procreation, the complete manufacture of human beings and the complete genetic control of one generation over the next would be ethically problematic and essentially different from current forms of assisted reproduction? If so, where and how will they draw the line, and why? I draw it at cloning, for all the reasons given.

Ban the Cloning of Humans

What, then, should we do? We should declare that human cloning is unethical in itself and dangerous in its likely consequences. In so doing, we shall have the backing of the overwhelming majority of our fellow Americans, and of the human race, and (I believe) of most practicing scientists. Next, we should do all that we can to prevent the cloning of human beings. We should do this by means of an international legal ban if possible, and by a unilateral national ban, at a minimum. Scientists may secretly undertake to violate such a law, but they will be deterred by not being able to stand up proudly to claim the credit for their technological bravado and success. Such a ban on clonal baby-making, moreover, will not harm the progress of basic genetic science and technology. On the contrary, it will reassure the public that scientists are happy to proceed without violating the deep ethical norms and intuitions of the human community.

This still leaves the vexed question about laboratory research using early embryonic human clones, specially created only for such research purposes, with no intention to implant them into a uterus. There is no question that such research holds great promise for gaining fundamental knowledge about normal (and abnormal) differentiation, and for developing tissue lines for transplantation that might be used, say, in treating leukemia or in repairing brain or spinal cord injuries—to mention just a few of the conceivable benefits. Still, unrestricted clonal embryo research will surely make the production of living human clones much more likely. Once the genies put the cloned embryos into the bottles, who can strictly control where they go (especially in the absence of legal prohibitions against implanting them to produce a child)?

I appreciate the potentially great gains in scientific knowledge and medical treatment available from embryo research, especially with cloned embryos. At the same time, I have serious reservations about creating human embryos for the sole purpose of experimentation. There is something deeply repugnant and fundamentally transgressive about such a utilitarian treatment of prospective human life. This total, shameless exploitation is worse, in my opinion, than the "mere" destruction of nascent life. But I see no added objections, as a matter of principle, to creating and using cloned early embryos for research purposes, beyond the objections that I might raise to doing so with embryos produced sexually.

And yet, as a matter of policy and prudence, any opponent of the manufacture of cloned humans must, I think, in the end oppose also the creating of cloned human embryos. Frozen embryonic clones (belonging to whom?) can be shuttled around without detection. Commercial ventures in human cloning will be developed without adequate oversight. In order to build a fence around the law, prudence dictates that one oppose—for this reason alone—all production of cloned human embryos, even for research purposes. We should allow all cloning research on animals to go forward, but the only safe trench that we can dig across the slippery slope, I suspect, is to insist on the inviolable distinction between animal and human cloning.

Some readers, and certainly most scientists, will not accept such prudent restraints, since they desire the benefits of research. They will prefer, even in fear and trembling, to allow human embryo cloning research to go forward.

Very well. Let us test them. If the scientists want to be taken seriously on ethical grounds, they must at the very least agree that embryonic research may proceed if and only if it is preceded by an absolute and effective ban on all attempts to implant into a uterus a cloned human embryo (cloned from an adult) to produce a living child. Absolutely no permission for the former without the latter.

The National Bioethics Advisory Commission's recommendations regarding this matter should be watched with the greatest care. Yielding to the wishes of the scientists, the commission will almost surely recommend that cloning human embryos for research be permitted. To allay public concern, it will likely also call for a temporary moratorium—not a legislative ban—on implanting cloned embryos to make a child, at least until such time as cloning techniques will have been perfected and rendered "safe" (precisely through the permitted research with cloned embryos). But the call for a moratorium rather than a legal ban would be a moral and a practical failure. Morally, this ethics commission would

(at best) be waffling on the main ethical question, by refusing to declare the production of human clones unethical (or ethical). Practically, a moratorium on implantation cannot provide even the minimum protection needed to prevent the production of cloned humans.

Opponents of cloning need therefore to be vigilant. Indeed, no one should be willing even to consider a recommendation to allow the embryo research to proceed unless it is accompanied by a call for prohibiting implantation and until steps are taken to make such a prohibition effective.

Technically, the National Bioethics Advisory Commission can advise the president only on federal policy, especially federal funding policy. But given the seriousness of the matter at hand, and the grave public concern that goes beyond federal funding, the commission should take a broader view. (If it doesn't, Congress surely will.) Given that most assisted reproduction occurs in the private sector, it would be cowardly and insufficient for the commission to say, simply, "no federal funding" for such practices. It would be disinguous to argue that we should allow federal funding so that we would then be able to regulate the practice; the private sector will not be bound by such regulations. Far better, for virtually everyone concerned, would be to distinguish between research on embryos and baby-making, and to call for a complete national and international ban (effected by legislation and treaty) of the latter, while allowing the former to proceed (at least in private laboratories).

The proposal for such a legislative ban is without American precedent, at least in technological matters, though the British and others have banned cloning of human beings, and we ourselves ban incest, polygamy and other forms of "reproductive freedom." Needless to say, working out the details of such a ban, especially a global one, would be tricky, what with the need to develop appropriate sanctions for violators. Perhaps such a ban will prove ineffective; perhaps it will eventually be shown to have been a mistake. But it would at least place the burden of practical proof where it belongs: on the proponents of this horror, requiring them to show very clearly what great social or medical good can be had only by the cloning of human beings.

We Americans have lived by, and prospered under, a rosy optimism about scientific and technological progress. The technological imperative—if it can be done, it must be done—has probably served us well, though we should admit that there is no accurate method for weighing benefits and harms. Even when, as in the cases of environmental pollution, urban decay or the lingering deaths that are the unintended by-products of medical success, we recognize the unwelcome outcomes of technological advance, we remain confident in our ability to fix all the "bad" consequences—usually by means of still newer and better technologies. How successful we can continue to be in such post hoc repairing is at least an open question. But there is very good reason for shifting the paradigm around, at least regarding those technological interventions into the human body and mind that will surely effect fundamental (and likely irreversible) changes in human nature, basic human relationships, and what it means to be a human being. Here we surely should not be willing to risk everything in the naive hope that, should things go wrong, we can later set them right.

The president's call for a moratorium on human cloning has given us an important opportunity. In a truly unprecedented way, we can strike a blow for the human control of the technological project, for wisdom, prudence and human dignity. The prospect of human cloning, so repulsive to contemplate, is the occasion for deciding whether we shall be slaves of unregulated progress, and ultimately its artifacts, or whether we shall remain free human beings who guide our technique toward the enhancement of human dignity. If we are to seize the occasion, we must, as the late Paul Ramsey wrote, "raise the ethical questions with a serious and not a frivolous conscience. A man of frivolous conscience announces that there are ethical quandaries ahead that we must urgently consider before the future catches up with us." By this he often means that we need to devise a new ethics that will provide the rationalization for doing in the future what men are bound to do because of new actions and interventions science will have made possible. In contrast a man of serious conscience means to say in raising urgent ethical questions that there may be some things that men should never do. The good things that men do can be made complete only by the things they refuse to do.

CHAPTER FIVE

FETUSES AND NEWBORNS

25.
WHY ABORTION IS IMMORAL

Don Marquis

SOURCE: *Journal of Philosophy* 86.4 (April 1989): 182-202.

The view that abortion is, with rare exceptions, seriously immoral has received little support in the recent philosophical literature. No doubt most philosophers affiliated with secular institutions of higher education believe that the anti-abortion position is either a symptom of irrational religious dogma or a conclusion generated by seriously confused philosophical argument. The purpose of this essay is to undermine this general belief. The essay sets out an argument that purports to show, as well as any argument in ethics can show, that abortion is, except possibly in rare cases, seriously immoral, that it is in the same moral category as killing an innocent adult human being.

The argument is based on a major assumption. Many of the most insightful and careful writers on the ethics of abortion—such as Joel Feinberg, Michael Tooley, Mary Anne Warren, H. Tristram Engelhardt, Jr., L.W. Sumner, John T. Noonan, Jr., and Philip Devine[1]—believe that whether or not abortion is morally permissible stands or falls on whether or not a fetus is the sort of being whose life it is seriously wrong to end. The argument of this essay will assume, but not argue, that they are correct.

Also, this essay will neglect issues of great importance to a complete ethics of abortion. Some anti-abortionists will allow that certain abortions, such as abortion before implantation or abortion when the life of a woman is threatened by a pregnancy or abortion after rape, may be morally permissible. This essay will not explore the casuistry of these hard cases. The purpose of this essay is to develop a general argument for the claim that the overwhelming majority of deliberate abortions are seriously immoral.

I

A sketch of standard anti-abortion and pro-choice arguments exhibits how those arguments possess certain symmetries that explain why partisans of those positions are so convinced of the correctness of their own positions, why they are not successful in convincing their opponents, and why, to others, this issue seems to be unresolvable. An analysis of the nature of this standoff suggests a strategy for surmounting it.

Consider the way a typical anti-abortionist argues. She will argue or assert that life is present from the moment of conception or that fetuses look like babies or that fetuses possess a characteristic such as a genetic code that is both necessary and sufficient for being human. Anti-abortionists seem to believe that (1) the truth of all of these claims is quite obvious, and (2) establishing any of these claims is sufficient to show that abortion is morally akin to murder.

A standard pro-choice strategy exhibits similarities. The pro-choicer will argue or assert that fetuses are not persons or that fetuses are not rational agents or that fetuses are not social beings. Pro-choicers seem to believe that (1) the truth of any of these claims is quite obvious, and (2) establishing any of these claims is sufficient to show that an abortion is not a wrongful killing.

In fact, both the pro-choice and the anti-abortion claims do seem to be true, although the "it looks like a baby" claim is more difficult to establish the earlier the pregnancy. We seem to have a standoff. How can it be resolved?

As everyone who has taken a bit of logic knows, if any of these arguments concerning abortion is a good argument, it requires not only some claim characterizing fetuses, but also some general moral principle that ties a characteristic of fetuses to having or not having the right to life or to some other moral characteristic that will generate the obligation or the lack of obligation not to end the life of a fetus. Accordingly, the arguments of the anti-abortionist and the pro-choicer need a bit of filling in to be regarded as adequate.

Note what each partisan will say. The anti-abortionist will claim that her position is supported by such generally accepted moral principles as "It is always prima facie seriously wrong to end the life of a baby." Since these are generally accepted moral principles her position is certainly not obviously wrong. The pro-choicer will claim that her position is supported by such plausible moral principles as "Being a person is what gives an individual intrinsic moral worth" or "It is only seriously prima facie wrong to take the life of a member of the human community." Since these are generally accepted moral principles, the pro-choice position is certainly not obviously wrong. Unfortunately, we have again arrived at a standoff.

Now, how might one deal with this standoff? The standard approach is to try to show how the moral principles of one's opponent lose their plausibility under analysis. It is easy to see how this is possible. On the one hand, the anti-abortionist will defend a moral principle concerning the wrongness of killing which tends to be broad in scope in order that even fetuses at an early stage of pregnancy will fall under it. The problem with broad principles is that they often embrace too much. In this particular instance, the principle "It is always prima facie wrong to take a human life" seems to entail that it is wrong to end the existence of a living human cancer-cell culture, on the grounds that the culture is both living and human. Therefore, it seems that the anti-abortionist's favored principle is too broad.

On the other hand, the pro-choicer wants to find a moral principle concerning the wrongness of killing which tends to be narrow in scope in order that fetuses will *not* fall under it. The problem with narrow principles is that they often do not embrace enough. Hence, the needed principles such as "It is prima facie seriously wrong to kill only persons" or "It is prima facie wrong to kill only rational agents" do not

explain why it is wrong to kill infants or young children or the severely retarded or even perhaps the severely mentally ill. Therefore, we seem again to have a standoff. The anti-abortionist charges, not unreasonably, that pro-choice principles concerning killing are too narrow to be acceptable; the pro-choicer charges, not unreasonably, that anti-abortionist principles concerning killing are too broad to be acceptable.

Attempts by both sides to patch up the difficulties in their positions run into further difficulties. The anti-abortionist will try to remove that problem in her position by reformulating her principle concerning killing in terms of human beings. Now we end up with: "It is always prima facie seriously wrong to end the life of a human being." This principle has the advantage of avoiding the problem of the human cancer-cell culture counterexample. But this advantage is purchased at a high price. For although it is clear that a fetus is both human and alive, it is not at all clear that a fetus is a human *being*. There is at least something to be said for the view that something becomes a human being only after a process of development, and that therefore first trimester fetuses and perhaps all fetuses are not yet human beings. Hence, the anti-abortionist, by this move has merely exchanged one problem for another.[2]

The pro-choicer fares no better. She may attempt to find reasons why killing infants, young children, and the severely retarded is wrong which are independent of her major principle that is supposed to explain the wrongness of taking human life, but which will not also make abortion immoral. This is no easy task. Appeals to social utility will seem satisfactory only to those who resolve not to think of the enormous difficulties with a utilitarian account of the wrongness of killing and the significant social costs of preserving the lives of the unproductive.[3] A pro-choice strategy that extends the definition of "person" to infants or even to young children seems just as arbitrary as an anti-abortion strategy that extends the definition of "human being" to fetuses. Again, we find symmetries in the two positions and we arrive at a standoff.

There are even further problems that reflect symmetries in the two positions. In addition to counterexample problems, or the arbitrary application problems that can be exchanged for them, the standard anti-abortionist principle "It is prima facie seriously wrong to kill a human being," or one of its variants, can be objected to on the grounds of ambiguity. If "human being" is taken to be a *biological* category, the anti-abortionist is left with the problem of explaining why a merely biological category should make a moral difference. Why, it is asked, is it any more reasonable to base a moral conclusion on the number of chromosomes in one's cells than on the color of one's skin?[4] If "human being," on the other hand, is taken to be a *moral* category, then the claim that a fetus is a human being cannot be taken to be a premise in the anti-abortion argument, for it is precisely what needs to be established. Hence, either the anti-abortionist's main category is a morally irrelevant, merely biological category, or it is of no use to the anti-abortionist in establishing (noncircularly, of course) that abortion is wrong.

Although this problem with the anti-abortionist position is often noticed, it is less often noticed that the pro-choice position suffers from an analogous problem. The principle "Only persons have the right to life" also suffers from an ambiguity. The term "person" is typically defined in terms of psychological characteristics, although there will certainly be disagreement concerning which characteristics are most important. Supposing that this matter can be settled, the pro-choicer is left with the problem of explaining why *psychological* characteristics should make a *moral* difference. If the pro-choicer should attempt to deal with this problem by claiming that an explanation is not necessary, that in fact we do treat such a cluster of psychological properties as having moral significance, the sharp-witted anti-abortionist should have a ready response. We do treat being both living and human as having moral significance. If it is legitimate for the pro-choicer to demand that the anti-abortionist provide an explanation of the connection between the biological character of being a human being and the wrongness of being killed (even though people accept this connection), then it is legitimate for the anti-abortionist to demand that the pro-choicer provide an explanation of the connection between psychological criteria for being a person and the wrongness of being killed (even though that connection is accepted).[5]

Feinberg has attempted to meet this objection (he calls psychological personhood "commonsense personhood"):

> The characteristics that confer commonsense personhood are not arbitrary bases for rights and duties, such as race, sex or species membership; rather they are traits that make sense out of rights and duties and without which those moral attributes would have no point or function. It is because people are conscious; have a sense out of their personal identities; have plans, goals, and projects; experience emotions; are liable to pains, anxieties, and frustrations; can reason and bargain, and so on—it is because of these attributes that people have values and interests, desires and expectations of their own, including a stake in their own futures. And a personal well-being of a sort we cannot ascribe to unconscious or nonrational beings. Because of their developed capacities they can assume duties and responsibilities and can have and make claims on one another. Only because of their sense of self, their life plans, their value hierarchies, and their stakes in their own futures can they be ascribed fundamental rights. There is nothing arbitrary about these linkages.[6]

The plausible aspects of this attempt should not be taken to obscure its implausible features. There is a great deal to be said for the view that being a psychological person under some description is a necessary condition for having duties. One cannot have a duty unless one is capable of behaving morally, and a being's capability of behaving morally will require having a certain psychology. It is far from obvious, however, that having rights entails consciousness or rationality as Feinberg suggests. We speak of the rights of the severely retarded or the severely mentally ill, yet some of these persons are not rational. We speak of the rights of the temporarily unconscious. The New Jersey Supreme Court based their decision in the Quinlan case on Karen Ann Quinlan's right to privacy, and she was known to be permanently unconscious at that time. Hence, Feinberg's claim that having rights entails being conscious is, on its face, obviously false.

legitimacy?s

Of course, it might not make sense to attribute rights to a being that would never in its natural history have certain psychological traits. This modest connection between psychological personhood and moral personhood will create a place for Karen Ann Quinlan and the temporarily unconscious. But then it makes a place for fetuses also. Hence, it does not serve Feinberg's pro-choice purposes. Accordingly, it seems that the pro-choicer will have as much difficulty bridging the gap between psychological personhood and personhood in the moral sense as the anti-abortionist has bridging the gap between being a biological human being and being a human being in the moral sense.

Furthermore, the pro-choicer cannot any more escape her problem by making person a purely moral category that the anti-abortionist could escape by the analogous move. For if person is a moral category, the pro-choicer is left without the resources for establishing (noncircularly, of course) the claim that a fetus is not a person, which is an essential premise in her argument. Again, we have both a symmetry and a standoff between pro-choice and anti-abortion views.

Passions in the abortion debate run high. There are both plausibilities and difficulties with the standard positions. Accordingly, it is hardly surprising that partisans of either side embrace with fervor the moral generalizations that support the conclusions they preanalytically favor, and reject with disdain the moral generalizations of their opponents as being subject to inescapable difficulties. It is easy to believe that the counterexamples to one's own moral principles are merely temporary difficulties that will dissolve in the wake of further philosophical research, and that the counterexamples to the principles of one's opponents are as straightforward as the contradiction between A and O propositions in traditional logic. This might suggest to an impartial observer (if there are any) that the abortion issue is unresolvable.

There is a way out of this apparent dialectible quandary. The moral generalizations of both sides are not quite correct. The generalizations hold for the most part, for the usual cases. This suggests that they are all *accidental* generalizations, that the moral claims made by those on both sides of the dispute do not touch on the *essence* of the matter.

This use of the distinction between essence and accident is not meant to invoke obscure metaphysical categories. Rather, it is intended to reflect the rather atheoretical nature of the abortion discussion. If the generalization a partisan in the abortion dispute adopts were derived from the reason why ending the life of a human being is wrong, then there could not be exceptions to that generalization unless some special case obtains in which there are even more powerful countervailing reasons. Such generalizations would not be merely accidental generalizations; they would point to, or be based upon, the essence of the wrongness of killing, what it is that makes killing wrong. All this suggests that a necessary condition of resolving the abortion controversy is a more theoretical account of the wrongness of killing. After all, if we merely believe, but do not understand, why killing adult human beings such as ourselves is wrong how could we conceivably show that abortion is either immoral or permissible?

II

In order to develop such an account, we can start from the following unproblematic assumption concerning our own case: it is wrong to kill *us*. Why is it wrong? Some answers can be easily eliminated. It might be said that what makes killing us wrong is that a killing brutalizes the one who kills. But the brutalization consists of being inured to the performance of an act that is hideously immoral; hence, the brutalization does not explain the immorality. It might be said that what makes killing us wrong is the great loss others would experience due to our absence. Although such hubris is understandable, such an explanation does not account for the wrongness of killing hermits, or those whose lives are relatively independent and whose friends find it easy to make new friends.

A more obvious answer is better. What primarily makes killing wrong is neither its effect on the murderer nor its effect on the victim's friends and relative, but its effect on the victim. The loss of one's life is one of the greatest losses one can suffer. The loss of one's life deprives one of all the experiences, activities, projects, and enjoyments that would otherwise have constituted one's future. Therefore, killing someone is wrong, primarily because the killing inflicts (one of) the greatest possible losses on the victim. To describe this as the loss of life can be misleading, however. The change in my biological state does not by itself make killing me wrong. The effect of the loss of my biological life is the loss to me of all those activities, projects, experiences, and enjoyments which would otherwise have constituted my future personal life. These activities, projects, experiences, and enjoyments are either valuable for their own sakes or are means to something else that is valuable for its own sake. Some parts of my future are not valued by me now, but will come to be valued by me as I grow older and as my values and capacities change. When I am killed, I am deprived both of what I now value which would have been part of my future personal life, but also what I would come to value. Therefore, when I die, I am deprived of all of the value of my future. Inflicting this loss on me is ultimately what makes killing me wrong. This being the case, it would seem that what makes killing *any* adult human being prima facie seriously wrong is the loss of his or her future.[7]

How should this rudimentary theory of the wrongness of killing be evaluated? It cannot be faulted for deriving an "ought" from an "is" for it does not. The analysis assumes that killing me (or you, reader) is prima facie seriously wrong. The point of the analysis is to establish which natural property ultimately explains the wrongness of the killing, given that it is wrong. The point of the analysis is to establish which natural property ultimately explains the wrongness of the killing, given that it is wrong. A natural property will ultimately explain the wrongness of killing, only if (1) the explanation fits with our intuitions about the matter and (2) there is no other natural property that provides the basis for a better explanation of the wrongness of killing. This analysis rests on the intuition that what makes killing a particular human or animal wrong is what it does to that particular human or animal. What makes killing wrong is some natural effect or other of the killing. Some would deny this. For instance, a divine-command theorist in ethics would deny it. Surely this denial is, however, one of those features of divine-command theory which renders it so implausible.

The claim that what makes killing wrong loss of the victim's future is directly suppor~~~ two considerations. In the first place this theory explains why we regard killing as one of the worst of crimes. Killing is especially wrong, because it deprives the victim of more than perhaps any other crime. In the second place, people with AIDS or cancer who know they are dying believe, of course, that dying is a very bad thing for them. They believe that the loss of a future to them that they would otherwise have experienced is what makes their premature death a very bad thing for them. A better theory of the wrongness of killing would require a different natural property associated with killing which better fits with the attitudes of the dying. What could it be?

The view that what makes killing wrong is the loss to the victim of the value of the victim's future gains additional support when some of its implications are examined. In the first place, it is incompatible with the view that it is wrong to kill only beings who are biologically human. It is possible that there exists a different species from another planet whose members have a future like ours. Since having a future like that is what makes killing someone wrong, this theory entails that it would be wrong to kill members of such a species. Hence, this theory is opposed to the claim that only life that is biologically human has great moral worth, a claim which many anti-abortionists have seemed to adopt. This opposition, which this theory has in common with personhood theories, seems to be a merit of the theory.

In the second place, the claim that the loss of one's future is the wrong-making feature of one's being killed entails the possibility that the futures of some actual nonhuman mammals on our own planet are sufficiently like ours that it is seriously wrong to kill them also. Whether some animals do have the same right to life as human beings depends on adding to the account of the wrongness of killing some additional account of just what it is about my future or the futures of other adult human beings which makes it wrong to kill us. No such additional account will be offered in this essay. Undoubtedly, the provision of such an account would be a very difficult matter. Undoubtedly, any such account would be quite controversial. Hence, it surely should not reflect badly on this sketch of an elementary theory of the wrongness of killing that it is indeterminate with respect to some very difficult issues regarding animal rights.

In the third place, the claim that the loss of one's future is the wrong-making feature of one's being killed does not entail, as sanctity of human life theories do, that active euthanasia is wrong. Persons who are severely and incurably ill, who face a future of pain and despair, and who wish to die will not have suffered a loss if they are killed. It is, strictly speaking, the value of a human's future which makes killing wrong in this theory. This being so, killing does not necessarily wrong some persons who are sick and dying. Of course there may be other reasons for a prohibition of active euthanasia, but this is another matter. Sanctity-of-human-life theories seem to hold that active euthanasia is seriously wrong even in an individual case where there seems to be good reason for it independently of public policy considerations. This consequence is most implausible, and it is a plus for the claim that the loss of a future of value is what makes killing wrong that it does not share this consequence.

In the fourth place, the account of the wrongness of killing defended in this essay does straightforwardly entail that it is prima facie seriously wrong to kill children and infants, for we do presume that they have futures of value. Since we do believe that it is wrong to kill defenseless little babies, it is important that a theory of the wrongness of killing easily account for this. Personhood theories of the wrongness of killing, on the other hand, cannot straightforwardly account for the wrongness of killing infants and young children.[8] Hence, such theories must add special ad hoc accounts of the wrongness of killing the young. The plausibility of such ad hoc theories seems to be a function of how desperately one wants such theories to work. The claim that the primary wrong-making feature of a killing is the loss to the victim of the value of its future accounts for the wrongness of killing young children and infants directly; it makes the wrongness of such acts as obvious as we actually think it is. This is a further merit of this theory. Accordingly, it seems that this value of a future-like-ours theory of the wrongness of killing shares strengths of both sanctity-of-life and personhood accounts while avoiding weaknesses of both.

In addition, it meshes with a central intuition concerning what makes killing wrong.

The claim that the primary wrong-making feature of a killing is the loss to the victim of the value of its future has obvious consequences for the ethics of abortion. The future of a standard fetus includes a set of experiences, projects, activities, and such which are identical with the futures of adult human beings and are identical with the futures of young children. Since the reason that is sufficient to explain why it is wrong to kill human beings after the time of birth is a reason that also applies to fetuses, it follows that abortion is prima facie seriously morally wrong.

This argument does not rely on the invalid inference that, since it is wrong to kill persons, it is wrong to kill potential persons also. The category that is morally central to this analysis is the category of having a valuable future like ours; it is not the category of personhood. The argument to the conclusion that abortion is prima facie seriously morally wrong proceeded independently of the notion of person or potential person or any equivalent. Someone may wish to start with this analysis in terms of the value of a human future, conclude that abortion is, except perhaps in rare circumstances, seriously morally wrong, infer that fetuses have the right to life, and then call fetuses "persons" as a result of their having the right to life. Clearly, in this case, the category of person is being used to state the *conclusion* of the analysis rather than to generate the *argument* of the analysis.

The structure of this anti-abortion argument can be both illuminated and defended by comparing it to what appears to be the best argument for the wrongness of the wanton infliction of pain on animals. This latter argument is based on the assumption that it is prima facie wrong to inflict pain on me (or you, reader). What is the natural property associated with the infliction of pain which makes such infliction wrong? The obvious answer seems to be that the infliction of pain causes suffering and that suffering is a misfortune. The wanton infliction of pain on other adult humans causes suffering. The wanton infliction of pain on animals causes suffering. Since causing suffering is what makes the wanton infliction of pain wrong and since the wanton infliction of pain on animals causes suffering, it follows that the wanton infliction of pain on animals is wrong.

This argument for the wrongness of the wanton infliction of pain on animals shares a number of structural features with the argument for the serious prima facie wrongness of abortion. Both arguments start with an obvious assumption concerning what it is wrong to do to me (or you, reader). Both then look for the characteristic or the consequence of the wrong action which makes the action wrong. Both recognize that the wrong-making feature of these immoral actions is a property of actions sometimes directed at individuals other than postnatal human beings. If the structure of the argument for the wrongness of the wanton infliction of pain on animals is sound, then the structure of the argument for the prima facie serious wrongness of abortion is also sound, for the structure of the two arguments is the same. The structure common to both is the key to the explanation of how the wrongness of abortion can be demonstrated without recourse to the category of person. In neither argument is that category crucial.

This defense of an argument for the wrongness of abortion in terms of a structurally similar argument for the wrongness of the wanton infliction of pain on animals succeeds only if the account regarding animals is the correct account. Is it? In the first place, it seems plausible. In the second place, its major competition is Kant's account. Kant believed that we do not have direct duties to animals at all, because they are not persons. Hence, Kant had to explain and justify the wrongness of inflicting pain on animals on the grounds that "he who is hard in his dealings with animals becomes hard also in his dealing with men."[9] The problem with Kant's account is that there seems to be no reason for accepting this latter claim unless Kant's account is rejected. If the alternative to Kant's account is accepted, then it is easy to understand why someone who is indifferent to inflicting pain on animals is also indifferent to inflicting pain on humans, for one is indifferent to what makes inflicting pain wrong in both cases. But, if Kant's account is accepted, there is not intelligible reason why one who is hard in his dealings with animals (or crabgrass or stones) should also be hard in his dealings with men. After all, men are persons: animals

are no more persons than crabgrass or stones. Persons are Kant's crucial moral category. Why, in short, should a Kantian accept the basic claim in Kant's argument?

Hence, Kant's argument for the wrongness of inflicting pain on animals rests on a claim that, in a world of Kantian moral agents, is demonstrably false. Therefore, the alternative analysis, being more plausible anyway, should be accepted. Since this alternative analysis has the same structure as the anti-abortion argument being defended here, we have further support for the argument for the immorality of abortion being defended in this essay.

Of course, this value of a future-like-ours argument, if sound, shows only that abortion is prima facie wrong, not that it is wrong in any and all circumstances. Since the loss of the future to a standard fetus, if killed, is, however, at least as great a loss as the loss of the future to a standard adult human being who is killed, abortion, like ordinary killing, could be justified only by the most compelling reasons. The loss of one's life is almost the greatest misfortune that can happen to one. Presumably abortion could be justified in some circumstances, only if the loss consequent on failing to abort would be at least as great. Accordingly, morally permissible abortions will be rare indeed unless, perhaps, they occur so early in pregnancy that a fetus is not yet definitely an individual. Hence, this argument should be taken as showing that abortion is presumptively very seriously wrong, where the presumption is very strong—as strong as the presumption that killing another adult human being is wrong.

III

How complete an account of the wrongness of killing does the value of a future-like-ours account have to be in order that the wrongness of abortion is a consequence? This account does not have to be an account of the necessary conditions for the wrongness of killing. Some persons in nursing homes may lack valuable human futures, yet it may be wrong to kill them for other reasons. Furthermore, this account does not obviously have to be the sole reason killing is wrong where the victim did have a valuable future. This analysis claims only that, for any killing where the victim did have a valuable future like ours, having that future by itself is sufficient to create the strong presumption that the killing is seriously wrong.

One way to overturn the value of a future-like-ours argument would be to find some account of the wrongness of killing which is at least as intelligible and which has different implications for the ethics of abortion. Two rival accounts possess at least some degree of plausibility. One account is based on the obvious fact that people value the experience of living and wish for the valuable experience to continue. Therefore, it might be said, what makes killing wrong is the discontinuation of that experience for the victim. Let us call this the *discontinuation account*.[10] Another rival account is based upon the obvious fact that people strongly desire to continue to live. This suggests that what makes killing us so wrong is that it interferes with the fulfillment of a strong and fundamental desire, the fulfillment of which is necessary for the fulfillment of any other desires we might have. Let us call this the *desire account*.[11]

Consider first the desire account as a rival account of the ethics of killing which would provide the basis for rejecting the anti-abortion position. Such an account will have to be stronger than the value of a future-like-ours account of the wrongness of abortion if it is to do the job expected of it. To entail the wrongness of abortion, the value of a future-like-ours account has only to provide a sufficient, but not a necessary condition for the wrongness of killing. The desire account, on the other hand, must provide us also with a necessary condition for the wrongness of killing in order to generate a pro-choice conclusion on abortion. The reason for this is that presumably the argument from the desire account moves from the claim that what makes killing wrong is interference with a very strong desire to the claim that abortion is not wrong because the fetus lacks a strong desire to live. Obviously, this inference fails if someone's having the desire to live is not a necessary condition of its being wrong to kill that individual.

One problem with the desire account is that we do regard it as seriously wrong to kill persons who have little desire to live or who have no desire to live or, indeed, have a desire not to live. We believe it is seri-

ously wrong to kill the unconscious, the sleeping, those who are tired of life, and those who are suicidal. The value-of-a-human-future account renders standard morality intelligible in these cases; these cases appear to be incompatible with the desire account.

The desire account is subject to a deeper difficulty. We desire life, because we value the goods of this life. The goodness of life is not secondary to our desire for it. If this were not so, the pain of one's own premature death could be done away with merely by an appropriate alteration in the configuration of one's desires. This is absurd. Hence, it would seem that it is the loss of the goods of one's future, not the interference with the fulfillment of a strong desire to life, which accounts ultimately for the wrongness of killing.

It is worth noting that, if the desire account is modified so that it does not provide a necessary, but only a sufficient, condition for the wrongness of killing, the desire account is compatible with the value of a future-like-ours account. The combined accounts will yield an anti-abortion ethic. This suggests that one can retain what is intuitively plausible about the desire account without a challenge to the basic argument of this essay.

It is also worth noting that, if future desires have moral force in a modified desire account of the wrongness of killing, one can find support for an anti-abortion ethic even in the absence of a value of a future-like-ours account. If one decides that a morally relevant property, the possession of which is sufficient to make it wrong to kill some individual, is the desire at some future time to live—one might decide to justify one's refusal to kill suicidal teenagers on these grounds, for example—then, since typical fetuses will have the desire in the future to live, it is wrong to kill typical fetuses. Accordingly, it does not seem that a desire account of the wrongness of killing can provide a justification of a pro-choice ethic of abortion which is nearly as adequate as the value of a human-future justification of an anti-abortion ethic.

The discontinuation account looks more promising as an account of the wrongness of killing. It seems just as intelligible as the value of a future-like-ours account, but it does not justify an anti-abortion position. Obviously, if it is the continuation of one's activities, experiences, and projects, the loss of which makes killing wrong, then it is not wrong to kill fetuses for that reason, for fetuses do not have experiences, activities, and projects to be continued or discontinued. Accordingly, the discontinuation account does not have the anti-abortion consequences that the value of a future-like-ours account has. Yet it seems as intelligible as the value of a future-like-ours account, for when we think of what would be wrong with our being killed, it does seem as if it is the discontinuation of what makes our lives worthwhile which makes killing us wrong.

Is the discontinuation account just as good an account as the value of a future-like-ours account? The discontinuation account will not be adequate at all, if it does not refer to the *value* of the experience that may be discontinued. One does not want the discontinuation account to make it wrong to kill a patient who begs for death and who is in severe pain that cannot be relieved short of killing. (I leave open the question of whether it is wrong for other reasons.) Accordingly, the discontinuation account must be more than a bare discontinuation account. It must make some reference to the positive value of the patient's experiences. But, by the same token, the value of a future-like-ours account cannot be a bare future account either. Just having a future surely does not itself rule out killing the above patient. This account must make some reference to the value of the patient's future experiences and projects also. Hence, both accounts involve the value of experiences, projects, and activities. So far we still have symmetry between the accounts.

The symmetry fades, however, when we focus on the time period of the value of experiences, etc., which has moral consequences. Although both accounts leave open the possibility that the patient in our example may be killed, this possibility is left open only in virtue of the utterly bleak future for the patient. It makes no difference whether the patient's immediate past contains intolerable pain, or consists in being in a coma (which we can imagine is a situation of indifference), or consists in a life of value. If the patient's future is a future of value, we want our account to make it wrong to kill the patient. If the patient's future is intolerable, whatever his or her

immediate past, we want our account to allow killing the patient. Obviously, then, it is the value of the patient's future which is doing the work in rendering the morality of killing the patient intelligible.

This being the case, it seems clear that whether one has immediate past experiences or not does no work in the explanation of what makes killing wrong. The addition the discontinuation account makes to the value of a human future account is otiose. Its addition to the value-of-a-future account plays no role at all in rendering intelligible the wrongness of killing. Therefore, it can be discarded with the discontinuation account of which it is a part.

IV

The analysis of the previous section suggests that alternative general accounts of the wrongness of killing are either inadequate or unsuccessful in getting around the anti-abortion consequences of the value of a future-like-ours argument. A different strategy for avoiding the anti-abortion consequences involves limiting the scope of the value of a future argument. More precisely, the strategy involves arguing that fetuses lack a property that is essential for the value-of-a-future argument (or for any anti-abortion argument) to apply to them.

One move of this sort is based upon the claim that a necessary condition of one's future being valuable is that one values it. Value implies a valuer. Given this one might argue that, since fetuses cannot value their futures, their futures are not valuable to them. Hence, it does not seriously wrong them deliberately to end their lives.

This move fails, however, because of some ambiguities. Let us assume that something cannot be of value unless it is valued by someone. This does not entail that my life is of no value unless it is valued by me. I may think, in a period of despair, that my future is of no worth whatsoever, but I may be wrong because others rightly see value—even great value—in it. Furthermore, my future can be valuable to me even if I do not value it. This is the case when a young person attempts suicide, but is rescued and goes on to significant human achievements. Such young people's futures are ultimately valuable to them, even though such futures do not seem to be valuable to them at the moment of attempted suicide. A fetus' future can be valuable to it in the same way. Accordingly, this attempt to limit the anti-abortion argument fails.

Another similar attempt to reject the anti-abortion position is based on Tooley's claim that an entity cannot possess the right to life unless it has the capacity to desire its continued existence. It follows that, since fetuses lack the conceptual capacity to desire to continue to live, they lack the right to life. Accordingly, Tooley concludes that abortion cannot be seriously prima facie wrong.[12]

What could be the evidence for Tooley's claim? Tooley once argued that individuals have a prima facie right to what they desire and that the lack of the capacity to desire something undercuts the basis of one's right to it.[13] This argument plainly will not succeed in the context of the analysis of this essay, however, since the point here is to establish the fetus' right to life on other grounds. Tooley's argument assumes that the right to life cannot be established in general on some basis other than the desire for life. This position was considered and rejected in the preceding section.

One might attempt to defend Tooley's basic claim on the grounds that, because a fetus cannot apprehend continued life as a benefit, its continued life cannot be a benefit or cannot be something it has a right to or cannot be something that is in its interest. This might be defended in terms of the general proposition that, if an individual is literally incapable of caring about or taking an interest in some X, then one does not have a right to X or X is not a benefit or X is not something that is in one's interest.[14]

Each member of this family of claims seems to be open to objections. As John C. Stevens has pointed out, one may have a right to be treated with a certain medical procedure (because of a health insurance policy one has purchased), even though one cannot conceive of the nature of the procedure.[15] And, as Tooley himself has pointed out, persons who have been indoctrinated, or drugged, or rendered temporarily unconscious may be literally incapable of caring about or taking an interest in something that is in their interest or is something to which they have a right, or is something that benefits them. Hence, the Tooley claim that would restrict the scope of the

value of a future-like-ours argument is undermined by counterexamples.[16]

Finally, Paul Bassen[17] has argued that, even though the prospects of an embryo might seem to be a basis for the wrongness of abortion, an embryo cannot be a victim and therefore cannot be wronged. An embryo cannot be a victim, he says, because it lacks sentience. His central argument for this seems to be that, even though plants and the permanently unconscious are alive, they clearly cannot be victims. What is the explanation of this? Bassen claims that the explanation is that their lives consist of mere metabolism and mere metabolism is not enough to ground victimizability. Mentation is required.

The problem with this attempt to establish the absence of victimizability is that both plants and the permanently unconscious clearly lack what Bassen calls "prospects" or what I have called "a future life like ours." Hence, it is surely open to one to argue that the real reason we believe plants and the permanently unconscious cannot be victims is that killing them cannot deprive them of a future life like ours; the real reason is not their absence of present mentation.

Bassen recognizes that his view is subject to this difficulty, and he recognizes that the case of children seems to support this difficulty, for "much of what we do for children is based on prospects." He argues, however, that, in the case of children and in other such cases, "potentiality comes into play only where victimizability has been secured on other grounds."[18]

Bassen's defense of this view is patently question-begging, since what is adequate to secure victimizability is exactly what is at issue. His examples do not support his own view against the thesis of this essay. Of course, embryos can be victims: when their lives are deliberately terminated, they are deprived of their futures of value, their prospects. This makes them victims, for it directly wrongs them.

The seeming plausibility of Bassen's view stems from the fact that paradigmatic cases of imagining someone as a victim involve empathy, and empathy requires mentation of the victim. The victims of flood, famine, rape, or child abuse are all persons with whom we can empathize. That empathy seems to be part of seeing them as victims.[19]

In spite of the strength of these examples, the attractive intuition that a situation in which there is victimization requires the possibility of empathy is subject to counterexamples. Consider a case that Bassen himself offers: "Posthumous obliteration of an author's work constitutes a misfortune for him only if he had wished his work to endure."[20] The conditions Bassen wishes to impose upon the possibility of being victimized here seem far too strong. Perhaps this author, due to his unrealistic standards of excellence and his low self-esteem, regarded his work as unworthy of survival, even though it possessed genuine literary merit. Destruction of such work would surely victimize its author. In such a case, empathy with the victim concerning the loss is clearly impossible.

Of course, Bassen does not make the possibility of empathy a necessary condition of victimizability; he requires only mentation. Hence, on Bassen's actual view, this author, as I have described him, can be a victim. The problem is that the basic intuition that renders Bassen's view plausible is missing in the author's case. In order to attempt to avoid counterexamples, Bassen has made his thesis too weak to be supported by the intuitions that suggested it.

Even so, the mentation requirement on victimizability is still subject to counterexamples. Suppose a severe accident renders me totally unconscious for a month, after which I recover. Surely killing me while I am unconscious victimizes me, even though I am incapable of mentation during that time. It follows that Bassen's thesis fails. Apparently, attempts to restrict the value of a future-like-ours argument so that fetuses do not fall within its scope do not succeed.

V

In this essay, it has been argued that the correct ethic of the wrongness of killing can be extended to fetal life and used to show that there is a strong presumption that any abortion is morally impermissible. If the ethic of killing adopted here entails, however, that contraception is also seriously immoral, then there would appear to be a difficulty with the analysis of this essay.

But this analysis does not entail that contraception is wrong. Of course, contraception prevents the actualization of a possible future of value. Hence, it follows from the claim that futures of value should be maximized that contraception is prima facie immoral. This obligation to maximize does not exist, however; furthermore, nothing in the ethics of killing in this paper entails that it does. The ethics of killing in this essay would entail that contraception is wrong only if something were denied a human future of value by contraception. Nothing at all is denied such a future by contraception, however.

Candidates for a subject of harm by contraception fall into four categories: (1) some sperm or other, (2) some ovum or other, (3) a sperm and an ovum separately, and (4) a sperm and an ovum together. Assigning the harm to some sperm is utterly arbitrary, for no reason can be given for making a sperm the subject of harm rather than an ovum. Assigning the harm to some ovum is utterly arbitrary, for no reason can be given for making an ovum the subject of harm rather than a sperm. One might attempt to avoid these problems by insisting that contraception deprives both the sperm and the ovum separately of a valuable future like ours. On this alternative, too many futures are lost. Contraception was supposed to be wrong, because it deprived us of one future of value, not two. One might attempt to avoid this problem by holding that contraception deprives the combination of sperm and ovum of a valuable future like ours. But here the definite article misleads. At the time of contraception, there are hundreds of millions of sperm, one (released) ovum and millions of possible combinations of all of these. There is not actual combination at all. Is the subject of the loss to be a merely possible combination? Which one? This alternative does not yield an actual subject of harm either. Accordingly, the immorality of contraception is not entailed by the loss of a future-like-ours argument simply because there is no nonarbitrarily identifiable subject of the loss in the case of contraception.

VI

The purpose of this essay has been to set out an argument for the serious presumptive wrongness of abortion subject to the assumption that the moral permissibility of abortion stands or falls on the moral status of the fetus. Since a fetus possesses a property, the possession of which in adult human beings is sufficient to make killing an adult human being wrong, abortion is wrong. This way of dealing with the problem of abortion seems superior to other approaches to the ethics of abortion, because it rests on an ethics of killing which is close to self-evident, because the crucial morally relevant property clearly applies to fetuses, and because the argument avoids the usual equivocations on "human life," "human being," or "person." The argument rests neither on religious claims nor on Papal dogma. It is not subject to the objection of "speciesism." Its soundness is compatible with the moral permissibility of euthanasia and contraception. It deals with our intuitions concerning young children.

Finally, this analysis can be viewed as resolving a standard problem—indeed, *the* standard problem—concerning the ethics of abortion. Clearly, it is wrong to kill adult human beings. Clearly, it is not wrong to end the life of some arbitrarily chosen single human cell. Fetuses seem to be like arbitrarily chosen human cells in some respects and like adult humans in other respects. The problem of the ethics of abortion is the problem of determining the fetal property that settles this moral controversy. The thesis of this essay is that the problem of the ethics of abortion, so understood, is solvable.

Notes

1 Joel Feinberg, "Abortion," in *Matters of Life and Death: New Introductory Essays in Moral Philosophy*, ed. Tom Regan (New York: Random House, 1986), pp. 256-93; Michael Tooley, "Abortion and Infanticide," *Philosophy and Public Affairs*, II, no. 1 (1972), pp. 37-65; idem, *Abortion and Infanticide* (New York: Oxford, 1984); Mary Anne Warren, "On the Moral and Legal Status of Abortion," *The Monist* 57, no. 1 (1973), pp. 43-61; Tristram Engelhardt Jr., "The Ontology of Abortion," *Ethics* 84, no. 3 (1974), pp. 217-34; L.W. Sumner, *Abortion and Moral Theory* (Princeton: University Press, 1981); John T. Noonan Jr., "Almost Absolute Value in History," in *The Morality of Abortion: Legal and Historical Perspective*, ed. Noonan (Cambridge: Harvard, 1970); and Philip Devine, *The Ethics of Homicide* (Ithaca: Cornell University Press, 1978).

2 For interesting discussions of this issue, see Warren Quinn, "Abortion: Identity and Loss," *Philosophy and Public Affairs* 13, no. 1 (1984), pp. 24-54; and Lawrence C. Becker, "Human Being: the Boundaries of the Concept," *Philosophy and Public Affairs* 4, no. 4 (1975), pp. 334-59.

3 See, e.g., Don Marquis, "Ethics and the Elderly: Some Problems," in *Aging and the Elderly: Humanistic Perspectives in Gerontology*, ed. Stuart Spicker, Kathleen Woodwark, and David Van Tassel (Atlantic Highlands, NJ: Humanities Press, 1978), pp. 341-55.

4 See Warren, "Moral and Legal Status"; and Tooley, "Abortion and Infanticide."

5 This seems to be the fatal flaw in Warren's treatment of this issue.

6 Feinberg, "Abortion," p. 270.

7 I have been most influenced on this matter by Jonathan Glover, *Causing Death and Saving Lives* (New York: Penguin, 1977), chap. 3; and Robert Young, "What is So Wrong with Killing People?" *Philosophy* 54, no. 210 (1979), pp. 515-28.

8 Feinberg, Tooley, Warren, and Engelhardt have all dealt with this problem.

9 Immanuel Kant, "Duties to Animals and Spirits," in *Lectures on Ethics*, trans. Louis Infeld (New York: Harper, 1963), p. 239.

10 I am indebted to Jack Bricke for raising this objection.

11 Presumably a preference utilitarian would press such an objection. Tooley once suggested that his account has such a theoretical underpinning; "Abortion and Infanticide," pp. 46-47.

12 Tooley, "Abortion and Infanticide," pp. 46-47.

13 Ibid., pp. 44-45.

14 Donald VanDeVeer seems to think this is self-evident; see his "Whither Baby Doe?" in Regan, *Matters of Life and Death*, p. 233.

15 John C. Stevens, "Must the Bearer of a Right Have the Concept of That to Which He Has a Right?" *Ethics* 95, no. 1 (1984), pp. 68-74.

16 See Tooley, "Abortion and Infanticide," pp. 47-49.

17 Paul Bassen, "Present Sakes and Future Prospects: The Status of Early Abortion," *Philosophy and Public Affairs* 11, no. 4 (1982), pp. 322-26.

18 Ibid., p. 333.

19 Note carefully the reasons he gives on the bottom of ibid., p. 316.

20 Ibid., p. 318.

26.
THE MORAL SIGNIFICANCE OF BIRTH

Mary Anne Warren

SOURCE: *Hypatia* 4.3 (1989): 46-65.

English common law treats the moment of live birth as the point at which a legal person comes into existence. Although abortion has often been prohibited, it has almost never been classified as homicide. In contrast, infanticide generally is classified as a form of homicide, even where (as in England) there are statutes designed to mitigate the severity of the crime in certain cases. But many people—including some feminists—now favor the extension of equal legal rights to some or all fetuses (S. Callahan 1984, 1986). The extension of legal personhood to fetuses would not only threaten women's right to choose abortion, but also undermine other fundamental rights. I will argue that because of these dangers, birth remains the most appropriate place to mark the existence of a new legal person.

Speaking of Rights

In making this case, I find it useful to speak of moral as well as legal rights. Although not all legal rights can be grounded in moral rights, the right to life can plausibly be so construed. This approach is controversial. Some feminist philosophers have been critical of moral analyses based upon rights. Carol Gilligan (1982), Nel Noddings (1984), and others have argued that women tend to take a different approach to morality, one that emphasizes care and responsibility in interpersonal relationships rather than abstract rules, principles, or conflicts of rights. I would argue, however, that moral rights are complementary to a feminist ethics of care and responsibility, not inconsistent or competitive with it. Whereas caring relationships can provide a moral ideal, respect for rights provides a moral floor—a minimum protection for individuals which remains morally binding even where appropriate caring rela-

tionships are absent or have broken down (Manning 1988). Furthermore, as I shall argue, social relationships are part of the foundation of moral rights.

Some feminist philosophers have suggested that the very concept of a moral right may be inconsistent with the social nature of persons. Elizabeth Wolgast (1987, 41-42) argues convincingly that this concept has developed within an atomistic model of the social world, in which persons are depicted as self-sufficient and exclusively self-interested individuals whose relationships with one another are essentially competitive. As Wolgast notes, such an atomistic model is particularly inappropriate in the context of pregnancy, birth, and parental responsibility. Moreover, recent feminist research has greatly expanded our awareness of the historical, religious, sociological, and political forces that shape contemporary struggles over reproductive rights, further underscoring the need for approaches to moral theory that can take account of such social realities (Harrison 1983; Luker 1984; Petchesky 1984).

But is the concept of a moral right necessarily incompatible with the social nature of human beings? Rights are indeed individualistic, in that they can be ascribed to individuals, as well as to groups. But respect for moral rights need not be based upon an excessively individualistic view of human nature. A more socially perceptive account of moral rights is possible, provided that we reject two common assumptions about the theoretical foundations of moral rights. These assumptions are widely accepted by mainstream philosophers, but rarely stated and still more rarely defended.

The first is what I shall call the intrinsic-properties assumption. This is the view that the only facts that can justify the ascription of basic moral rights[1] or moral standing[2] to individuals are facts about *the intrinsic properties of those individuals.* Philosophers who accept this view disagree about which of the intrinsic properties of individuals are relevant to the ascription of rights. They agree, however, that relational properties—such as being loved, or being part of a social community or biological ecosystem—cannot be relevant.

The second is what I shall call the single-criterion assumption. This is the view that there is some single property, the presence or absence of which divides the world into those things which have moral rights or moral standing, and those things which do not. Christopher Stone (1987) locates this assumption within a more general theoretical approach, which he calls "moral monism." Moral monists believe that the goal of moral philosophy is the production of a coherent set of principles, sufficient to provide definitive answers to all possible moral dilemmas. Among these principles, the monist typically assumes, will be one that identifies some key property which is such that, "Those beings that possess the key property count morally ... [while those] things that lack it are all utterly irrelevant, except as resources for the benefit of those things that do count" (1987, 13).

Together, the intrinsic-properties and single-criterion assumptions preclude any adequate account of the social foundations of moral rights. The intrinsic-properties assumption requires us to regard all personal or other relationships among individuals or groups as wholly irrelevant to basic moral rights. The single-criterion assumption requires us to deny that there can be a variety of sound reasons for ascribing moral rights, and a variety of things and beings to which some rights may appropriately be ascribed. Both assumptions are inimical to a feminist approach to moral theory, as well as to approaches that are less anthropocentric and more environmentally adequate. The prevalence of these assumptions helps to explain why few mainstream philosophers believe that birth can in any way alter the infant's moral rights.

The Denial of the Moral Significance of Birth

The view that birth is irrelevant to moral rights is shared by philosophers on all points of the spectrum of moral views about abortion. For the most conservative, birth adds nothing to the infant's moral rights, since all of those rights have been present since conception. Moderates hold that the fetus acquires an equal right to life at some point after conception but before birth. The most popular candidates for this point of moral demarcation are (1) the stage at which the fetus becomes viable (i.e., capable of surviving outside the womb, with or without medical assistance), and (2) the stage at which it becomes sentient (i.e., capable of having experiences, including that of pain). For those who hold a view of this sort, both infanticide and abortion at any time past the critical stage are forms of homicide, and there is little reason to distinguish between them either morally or legally.

Finally, liberals hold that even relatively late abortion is sometimes morally acceptable, and that at no time is abortion the moral equivalent of homicide. However, few liberals wish to hold that infanticide is not—at least sometimes—morally comparable to homicide. Consequently, the presumption that being born makes no difference to one's moral rights creates problems for the liberal view of abortion. Unless the liberal can establish some grounds for a general moral distinction between late abortion and early infanticide, she must either retreat to a moderate position on abortion, or else conclude that infanticide is not so bad after all.

To those who accept the intrinsic-properties assumption, birth can make little difference to the moral standing of the fetus/infant. For birth does not seem to alter any intrinsic property that could reasonably be linked to the possession of a strong right to life. Newborn infants have very nearly the same intrinsic properties as do fetuses shortly before birth. They have, as L.W. Sumner (1983, 53) says, "the same size, shape, internal constitution, species membership, capacities, level of consciousness, and so forth."[3] Consequently, Sumner says, infanticide cannot be morally very different from late abortion. In his words, "Birth is a shallow and arbitrary criterion of moral standing, and there appears to be no way of connecting it to a deeper account" (52).

Sumner holds that the only valid criterion of moral standing is the capacity for sentience (136). Prenatal neurophysiology and behavior suggest that human fetuses begin to have rudimentary sensory experiences at some time during the second trimester of pregnancy. Thus, Sumner concludes that abortion should be permitted during the first trimester but not thereafter, except in special circumstances (152).[4]

Michael Tooley (1983) agrees that birth can make no difference to moral standing. However, rather than rejecting the liberal view of abortion, Tooley boldly claims that neither late abortion nor early infanticide is seriously wrong. He argues that an entity cannot have a strong right to life unless it is capable of desiring its own continued existence. To be capable of such a desire, he argues, a being must have a concept of itself as a continuing subject of conscious experience. Having such a concept is a central part of what it is to be a person, and thus the kind of being that has strong moral rights (41). Fetuses certainly lack such a concept, as do infants during the first few months of their lives. Thus, Tooley concludes, neither fetuses nor newborn infants have a strong right to life, and neither abortion nor infanticide is an intrinsic moral wrong.

These two theories are worth examining, not only because they illustrate the difficulties generated by the intrinsic-properties and single-criterion assumptions, but also because each includes valid insights that need to be integrated into a more comprehensive account. Both Sumner and Tooley are partially right. Unlike "genetic humanity"—a property possessed by fertilized human ova—sentience and self-awareness are properties that have some general relevance to what we may owe another being in the way of respect and protection. However, neither the sentience criterion nor the self-awareness criterion can explain the moral significance of birth.

The Sentience Criterion

Both newborn infants and late-term fetuses show clear signs of sentience. For instance, they are apparently capable of having visual experiences. Infants will often turn away from bright lights, and those who have done intrauterine photography have sometimes observed a similar reaction in the late-term fetus when bright lights are introduced in its vicinity. Both may respond to loud noises, voices, or other sounds, so both can probably have auditory experiences. They are evidently also responsive to touch, taste, motion, and other kinds of sensory stimulation.

The sentience of infants and late-term fetuses makes a difference to how they should be treated, by contrast with fertilized ova or first-trimester fetuses. Sentient beings are usually capable of experiencing painful as well as pleasurable or affectively neutral sensations.[5] While the capacity to experience pain is valuable to an organism, pain is by definition an intrinsically unpleasant experience. Thus, sentient beings may plausibly be said to have a moral right not to be deliberately subjected to pain in the absence of any compelling reason. For those who prefer not to speak of rights, it is still plausible that a capacity for sentience gives an entity some moral standing. It may, for instance, require that its interests be given some consideration in utilitarian calculations, or that it be treated as an end and never merely as a means.

But it is not clear that sentience is a sufficient condition for moral equality, since there are many clearly-sentient creatures (e.g., mice) to which most of us would not be prepared to ascribe equal moral standing. Sumner examines the implications of the sentience criterion primarily in the context of abortion. Given his belief that some compromise is essential between the conservative and liberal viewpoints on abortion, the sentience criterion recommends itself as a means of drawing a moral distinction between early abortion and late abortion. It is, in some ways, a more defensible criterion than fetal viability.

The 1973 *Roe v. Wade* decision treats the presumed viability of third-trimester fetuses as a basis for permitting states to restrict abortion rights in order to protect fetal life in the third trimester, but not earlier. Yet viability is relative, among other things, to the medical care available to the pregnant woman and her infant. Increasingly sophisticated neonatal intensive care has made it possible to save many more premature infants than before, thus altering the average age of viability. Someday it may be possible to keep even first-trimester fetuses alive and developing normally outside the womb. The viability criterion seems to imply that the advent of total ectogenesis (artificial gestation from conception to birth) would automatically eliminate women's right to abortion, even in the earliest stages of pregnancy.

At the very least, it must imply that as many aborted fetuses as possible should be kept alive through artificial gestation. But the mere technological possibility of providing artificial wombs for huge numbers of human fetuses could not establish such a moral obligation. A massive commitment to ectogenesis would probably be ruinously expensive, and might prove contrary to the interests of parents and children. The viability criterion forces us to make a hazardous leap from the technologically possible to the morally mandatory.

The sentience criterion at first appears more promising as a means of defending a moderate view of abortion. It provides an intuitively plausible distinction between early and late abortion. Unlike the viability criterion, it is unlikely to be undermined by new biomedical technologies. Further investigation of fetal neurophysiology and behavior might refute the presumption that fetuses begin to be capable of sentience *at some point in the second trimester*. Perhaps this development occurs slightly earlier or slightly later than present evidence suggests. (It is unlikely to be much earlier or much later.) However, that is a consequence that those who hold a moderate position on abortion could live with; so long as the line could still be drawn with some degree of confidence, they need not insist that it be drawn exactly where Sumner suggests.

But closer inspection reveals that the sentience criterion will not yield the result that Sumner wants. His position vacillates between two versions of the sentience criterion, neither of which can adequately support his moderate view of abortion. The strong version of the sentience criterion treats sentience as a sufficient condition for having full and equal moral standing. The weak version treats sentience as sufficient for having some moral standing, but not necessarily full and equal moral standing.

Sumner's claim that sentient fetuses have the same moral standing as older human beings clearly requires the strong version of the sentience criterion. On this theory, any being which has even minimal capacities for sensory experience is the moral equal of any person. If we accept this theory, then we must conclude that not only is late abortion the moral equivalent of homicide, but so is the killing of such sentient nonhuman beings as mice. Sumner evident-

ly does not wish to accept this further conclusion, for he also says that "sentience admits of degrees ... [a fact that] enables us to employ it both as an inclusion criterion and as a comparison criterion of moral standing" (144). In other words, all sentient beings have some moral standing, but beings that are more highly sentient have greater moral standing than do less highly sentient beings. This weaker version of the sentience criterion leaves room for a distinction between the moral standing of mice and that of sentient humans—provided, that is, that mice can be shown to be less highly sentient. However, it will not support the moral equality of late-term fetuses, since the relatively undeveloped condition of fetal brains almost certainly means that fetuses are less highly sentient than older human beings.

A similar dilemma haunts those who use the sentience criterion to argue for the moral equality of nonhuman animals. Some animal liberationists hold that all sentient beings are morally equal, regardless of species. For instance, Peter Singer (1981, 111) maintains that all sentient beings are entitled to equal consideration for their comparably important interests. Animal liberationists are primarily concerned to argue for the moral equality of vertebrate animals, such as mammals, birds, reptiles and fish. In this project, the sentience criterion serves them less well than they may suppose. On the one hand, if they use the weak version of the sentience criterion then they cannot sustain the claim that all nonhuman vertebrates are our moral equals—unless they can demonstrate that they are all sentient *to the same degree* that we are. It is unclear how such a demonstration would proceed, or what would count as success. On the other hand, if they use the strong version of the sentience criterion, then they are committed to the conclusion that if flies and mosquitos are even minimally sentient then they too are our moral equals. Not even the most radical animal liberationists have endorsed the moral equality of such invertebrate animals,[6] yet it is quite likely that these creatures enjoy some form of sentience.

We do not really know whether complex invertebrate animals such as spiders and insects have sensory experiences, but the evidence suggests that they may. They have both sense organs and central nervous systems, and they often act as if they could see, hear, and feel very well. Sumner says that all invertebrates are probably nonsentient, because they lack certain brain structures—notably forebrains—that appear to be essential to the processing of pain in vertebrate animals (143). But might not some invertebrate animals have neurological devices for the processing of pain that are different from those of vertebrates, just as some have very different organs for the detection of light, sound, or odor? The capacity to feel pain is important to highly mobile organisms which guide their behavior through perceptual data, since it often enables them to avoid damage or destruction. Without that capacity, such organisms would be less likely to survive long enough to reproduce. Thus, if insects, spiders, crayfish, or octopi can see, hear, or smell, then it is quite likely that they can also feel pain. If sentience is the sole criterion for moral equality, then such probably sentient entities deserve the benefit of the doubt.

But it is difficult to believe that killing invertebrate animals is as morally objectionable as homicide. That an entity is probably sentient provides a reason for avoiding actions that may cause it pain. It may also provide a reason for respecting its life, a life which it may enjoy. But it is not a sufficient reason for regarding it as a moral equal. Perhaps an ideally moral person would try to avoid killing any sentient being, even a fly. Yet it is impossible in practice to treat the killing of persons and the killing of sentient invertebrates with the same severity.

Even the simplest activities essential to human survival (such as agriculture, or gathering wild foods) generally entail some loss of invertebrate lives. If the strong version of the sentience criterion is correct, then all such activities are morally problematic. And if it is not, then the probable sentience of late-term fetuses and newborn infants is not enough to demonstrate that either late abortion or infanticide is the moral equivalent of homicide. Some additional argument is needed to show that either late abortion or early infanticide is seriously immoral.

The Self-Awareness Criterion

Although newborn infants are regarded as persons in both law and common moral conviction, they lack certain mental capacities that are typical of persons. They have sensory experiences, but, as Tooley points out, they probably do not yet think, or have a sense of who they are, or a desire to continue to exist. It is not unreasonable to suppose that these facts make some difference to their moral standing. Other things being equal, it is surely worse to kill a self-aware being that wants to go on living than one that has never been self-aware and that has no such preference. If this is true, then it is hard to avoid the conclusion that neither abortion nor infanticide is quite as bad as the killing of older human beings. And indeed many human societies seem to have accepted that conclusion.

Tooley notes that the abhorrence of infanticide which is characteristic of cultures influenced by Christianity has not been shared by most cultures outside that influence (315-322). Prior to the present century, most societies—from the gatherer-hunter societies of Australia, Africa, North and South America, and elsewhere, to the high civilizations of China, India, Greece, Rome, and Egypt—have not only tolerated occasional instances of infanticide but have regarded it as sometimes the wisest course of action. Even in Christian Europe there was often a de facto toleration of infanticide—so long as the mother was married and the killing discreet. Throughout much of the second millennium in Europe, single women whose infants failed to survive were often executed in sadistic ways, yet married women whose infants died under equally suspicious circumstances generally escaped legal penalty (Piers 1978, 45-46). Evidently, the sanctions against infanticide had more to do with the desire to punish female sexual transgressions than with a consistently held belief that infanticide is morally comparable to homicide.

If infanticide has been less universally regarded as wrong than most people today believe, then the self-awareness criterion is more consistent with common moral convictions than it at first appears. Nevertheless, it conflicts with some convictions that are almost universal, even in cultures that tolerate infanticide. Tooley argues that infants probably begin to think and to become self-aware at about three months of age, and that this is therefore the stage at which they begin to have a strong right to life (405-406). Perhaps this is true. However the customs of most cultures seem to have required that a decision about the life of an infant be made within, at most, a few days of birth. Often, there was some special gesture or ceremony—such as washing the infant, feeding it, or giving it a name—to mark the fact that it would thenceforth be regarded as a member of the community. From that point on, infanticide would not be considered, except perhaps under unusual circumstances. For instance, Margaret Mead gives this account of birth and infanticide among the Arapesh people of Papua New Guinea:

> While the child is being delivered, the father waits within ear-shot until its sex is determined, when the midwives call out to him. To this information he answers laconically, "Wash it," or "Do not wash it." If the command is "Wash it," the child is to be brought up. In a few cases when the child is a girl and there are already several girl-children in the family, the child will not be saved, but left, unwashed, with the cord uncut, in the bark basin on which the delivery takes place. (Mead [1935] 1963, 32-33)

Mead's account shows that among the Arapesh infanticide is at least to some degree a function of patriarchal power. In this, they are not unusual. In almost every society in which infanticide has been tolerated, female infants have been the most frequent victims. In patriarchal, patrilineal and patrilocal societies, daughters are usually valued less than sons, e.g., because they will leave the family at marriage, and will probably be unable to contribute as much as sons to the parents' economic support later. Female infanticide probably reinforces male domination by reducing the relative number of women and dramatically reinforcing the social devaluation of females.[7] Often it is the father who decides which infants will be reared. Dianne Romaine has pointed out to me that this practice may be due to a reluctance to force women, the primary caregivers, to decide when care should not be given. However, it also suggests that infanticide often served the interests of individual men more than those of women, the family, or the community as a whole.

Nevertheless, infanticide must sometimes have been the most humane resolution of a tragic dilem-

ma. In the absence of effective contraception or abortion, abandoning a newborn can sometimes be the only alternative to the infant's later death from starvation. Women of nomadic gatherer-hunter societies, for instance, are sometimes unable to raise an infant born too soon after the last one, because they can neither nurse nor carry two small children.

But if infanticide is to be considered, it is better that it be done immediately after birth, before the bonds of love and care between the infant and the mother (and other persons) have grown any stronger than they may already be. Postponing the question of the infant's acceptance for weeks or months would be cruel to all concerned. Although an infant may be little more sentient or self-aware at two weeks of age than at birth, its death is apt to be a greater tragedy—not for it, but for those who have come to love it. I suspect that this is why, where infanticide is tolerated, the decision to kill or abandon an infant must usually be made rather quickly. If this consideration is morally relevant—and I think it is—then the self-awareness criterion fails to illuminate some of the morally salient aspects of infanticide.

Protecting Nonpersons

If we are to justify a general moral distinction between abortion and infanticide, we must answer two questions. First, why should infanticide be discouraged, rather than treated as a matter for individual decision? And second, why should sentient fetuses not be given the same protections that law and common sense morality accord to infants? But before turning to these two questions, it is necessary to make a more general point.

Persons have sound reasons for treating one another as moral equals. These reasons derive from both self-interest and altruistic concern for others—which, because of our social nature, are often very difficult to distinguish. Human persons—and perhaps all persons—normally come into existence only in and through social relationships. Sentience may begin to emerge without much direct social interaction, but it is doubtful that a child reared in total isolation from human or other sentient (or apparently sentient) beings could develop the capacities for self-awareness and social interaction that are essential to personhood. The recognition of the fundamentally social nature of persons can only strengthen the case for moral equality, since social relationships are undermined and distorted by inequalities that are perceived as unjust. There may be many nonhuman animals who have enough capacity for self awareness and social interaction to be regarded as persons, with equal basic moral rights. But, whether or not this is true, it is certainly true that if any things have full and equal basic moral rights then persons do.

However we cannot conclude that, because all persons have equal basic moral rights, it is always wrong to extend strong moral protections to beings that are not persons. Those who accept the single-criterion assumption may find that a plausible inference. By now, however, most thoughtful people recognize the need to protect vulnerable elements of the natural world—such as endangered plant and animal species, rainforests, and rivers—from further destruction at human hands. Some argue that it is appropriate, as a way of protecting these things, to ascribe to them legal if not moral rights (Stone 1974). These things should be protected not because they are sentient or self-aware, but for other good reasons. They are irreplaceable parts of the terrestrial biosphere, and as such they have incalculable value to human beings. Their long-term instrumental value is often a fully sufficient reason for protecting them. However, they may also be held to have inherent value, i.e., value that is independent of the uses we might wish to make of them (Taylor 1986). Although destroying them is not murder, it is an act of vandalism which later generations will mourn.

It is probably not crucial whether or not we say that endangered species and natural habitats have a moral right to our protection. What is crucial is that we recognize and act upon the need to protect them. Yet certain contemporary realities argue for an increased willingness to ascribe rights to impersonal elements of the natural world. Americans, at least, are likely to be more sensitive to appeals and demands couched in terms of rights than those that appeal to less familiar concepts, such as inherent value. So central are rights to our common moral idiom, that to deny that trees have rights is to risk being thought to condone the reckless destruction of rainforests and redwood groves. If we want to communicate effectively about the need to protect the natural world—and to protect it for its own sake as well as our own—then we may be wise to develop theories that permit us to ascribe at least some moral rights to some things that are clearly not persons.

Parallel issues arise with respect to the moral status of the newborn infant. As Wolgast (1987, 38) argues, it is much more important to understand our responsibilities to protect and care for infants than to insist that they have exactly the same moral rights as older human beings. Yet to deny that infants have equal basic moral rights is to risk being thought to condone infanticide and the neglect and abuse of infants. Here too, effective communication about human moral responsibilities seems to demand the ascription of rights to beings that lack certain properties that are typical of persons. But, of course, that does not explain why we have these responsibilities towards infants in the first place.

Why Protect Infants?

I have already mentioned some of the reasons for protecting human infants more carefully than we protect most comparably-sentient nonhuman beings. Most people care deeply about infants, particularly—but not exclusively—their own. Normal human adults (and children) are probably "programmed" by their biological nature to respond to human infants with care and concern. For the mother, in particular, that response is apt to begin well before the infant is born. But even for her it is likely to become more intense after the infant's birth. The infant at birth enters the human social world, where, if it lives, it becomes involved in social relationships with others, of kinds that can only be dimly foreshadowed before birth. It begins to be known and cared for, not just as a potential member of the family or community, but as a socially present and responsive individual. In the words of Loren Lomasky (1984, 172), "birth constitutes a quantum leap forward in the process of establishing ... social bonds." The newborn is not yet self-aware, but it is already (rapidly becoming) a social being.

Thus, although the human newborn may have no intrinsic properties that can ground a moral right to life stronger than that of a fetus just before birth, its emergence into the social world makes it appropriate to treat it as if it had such a stronger right. This, in effect, is what the law has done, through the doctrine that a person begins to exist at birth. Those who accept the intrinsic-properties as assumption can only regard this doctrine as a legal fiction. However, it is a fiction that we would have difficulty doing without. If the line were not drawn at birth, then I think we would have to draw it at some point rather soon thereafter, as many other societies have done.

Another reason for condemning infanticide is that, at least in relatively privileged nations like our own, infants whose parents cannot raise them can usually be placed with people who will love them and take good care of them. This means that infanticide is rarely in the infant's own best interests, and would often deprive some potential adoptive individual or family of a great benefit. It also means that the prohibition of infanticide need not impose intolerable burdens upon parents (especially women). A rare parent might think it best to kill a healthy[8] infant rather than permitting it to be reared by others, but a persuasive defense of that claim would require special circumstances. For instance, when abortion is unavailable and women face savage abuses for supposed sexual transgressions, those who resort to infanticide to conceal an "illegitimate" birth may be doing only what they must. But where enforcement of the sexual double standard is less brutal, abortion and adoption can provide alternatives that most women would prefer to infanticide.

Some might wonder whether adoption is really preferable to infanticide, at least from the parent's point of view. Judith Thomson (1971, 66) notes that "a woman may be utterly devastated by the thought of a child, a bit of herself, put out for adoption and never seen or heard of again." From the standpoint of narrow self-interest, it might not be irrational to prefer the death of the child to such a future. Yet few would wish to resolve this problem by legalizing infanticide. The evolution of more open adoption procedures which permit more contact between the adopted child and the biological parent(s) might lessen the psychological pain often associated with adoption. But that would be at best a partial solution. More basic is the provision of better social support for child-rearers, so that parents are not forced by

economic necessity to surrender their children for adoption.

These are just some of the arguments for treating infants as legal persons, with an equal right to life. A more complete account might deal with the effects of the toleration of infanticide upon other moral norms. But the existence of such effects is unclear. Despite a tradition of occasional infanticide, the Arapesh appear in Mead's descriptions as gentle people who treat their children with great kindness and affection. The case against infanticide need not rest upon the questionable claim that the toleration of infanticide inevitably leads to the erosion of other moral norms. It is enough that most people today strongly desire that the lives of infants be protected, and that this can now be done without imposing intolerable burdens upon individuals or communities.

But have I not left the door open to the claim that infanticide may still be justified in some places, e.g., where there is severe poverty and a lack of accessible adoption agencies or where women face exceptionally harsh penalties for "illegitimate" births? I have, and deliberately. The moral case against the toleration of infanticide is contingent upon the existence of morally preferable options. Where economic hardship, the lack of contraception and abortion, and other forms of sexual and political oppression have eliminated all such options, there will be instances in which infanticide is the least tragic of a tragic set of choices. In such circumstances, the enforcement of extreme sanctions against infanticide can constitute an additional injustice.

Why Birth Matters

I have defended what most regard as needing no defense, i.e., the ascription of an equal right to life to human infants. Under reasonably favorable conditions that policy can protect the rights and interests of all concerned, including infants, biological parents, and potential adoptive parents.

But if protecting infants is such a good idea, then why is it not a good idea to extend the same strong protections to sentient fetuses? The question is not whether sentient fetuses ought to be protected: of course they should. Most women readily accept the responsibility for doing whatever they can to ensure that their (voluntarily continued) pregnancies are successful, and that no avoidable harm comes to the fetus. Negligent or malevolent actions by third parties which result in death or injury to pregnant women or their potential children should be subject to moral censure and legal prosecution. A just and caring society would do much more than ours does to protect the health of all its members, including pregnant women. The question is whether the law should accord to late-term fetuses *exactly the same* protections as are accorded to infants and older human beings.

The case for doing so might seem quite strong. We normally regard not only infants, but all other post-natal human beings as entitled to strong legal protections *so long as they are either sentient or capable of an eventual return to sentience*. We do not also require that they demonstrate a capacity for thought, self-awareness, or social relationships before we conclude that they have an equal right to life. Such restrictive criteria would leave too much room for invidious discrimination. The eternal propensity of powerful groups to rationalize sexual, racial, and class oppression by claiming that members of the oppressed group are mentally or otherwise "inferior" leaves little hope that such restrictive criteria could be applied without bias. Thus, for human beings past the prenatal stage, the capacity for sentience—or for a return to sentience—may be the only pragmatically defensible criterion for the ascription of full and equal basic rights. If so, then both theoretical simplicity and moral consistency may seem to require that we extend the same protections to sentient human beings that have not yet been born as to those that have.

But there is one crucial consideration which this argument leaves out. It is impossible to treat fetuses *in utero* as if they were persons without treating women as if they were something less than persons. The extension of equal rights to sentient fetuses would inevitably license severe violations of women's basic rights to personal autonomy and physical security. In the first place, it would rule out most second-trimester abortions performed to protect the woman's life or health. Such abortions might sometimes be construed as a form of self-defense. But the right to self-defense is not usually taken to

mean that one may kill innocent persons just because their continued existence poses some threat to one's own life or health. If abortion must be justified as self-defense, then it will rarely be performed until the woman is already in extreme danger, and perhaps not even then. Such a policy would cost some women their lives, while others would be subjected to needless suffering and permanent physical harm.

Other alarming consequences of the drive to extend more equal rights to fetuses are already apparent in the United States. In the past decade it has become increasingly common for hospitals or physicians to obtain court orders requiring women in labor to undergo cesarean sections, against their will, for what is thought to be the good of the fetus. Such an extreme infringement of the woman's right to security against physical assault would be almost unthinkable once the infant has been born. No parent or relative can legally be forced to undergo any surgical procedure, even possibly to save the life of a child, once it is born. But pregnant women can sometimes be forced to undergo major surgery, for the supposed benefit of the fetus. As George Annas (1982, 16) points out, forced cesareans threaten to reduce women to the status of inanimate objects—containers which may be opened at the will of others in order to get at their contents.

Perhaps the most troubling illustration of this trend is the case of Angela Carder, who died at George Washington University Medical Center in June 1987, two days after a court-ordered cesarean section. Ms. Carder had suffered a recurrence of an earlier cancer, and was not expected to live much longer. Her physicians agreed that the fetus was too undeveloped to be viable, and that Carder herself was probably too weak to survive the surgery. Although she, her family, and the physicians were all opposed to a cesarean delivery, the hospital administration—evidently believing it had a legal obligation to try to save the fetus—sought and obtained a court order to have it done. As predicted, both Carder and her infant died soon after the operation.[9] This woman's rights to autonomy, physical integrity, and life itself were forfeit—not just because of her illness, but because of her pregnancy.

Such precedents are doubly alarming in the light of the development of new techniques of fetal therapy. As fetuses come to be regarded as patients, with rights that may be in direct conflict with those of their mothers, and as the *in utero* treatment of fetuses becomes more feasible, more and more pregnant women may be subjected against their will to dangerous and invasive medical interventions. If so, then we may be sure that there will be other Angela Carders.

Another danger in extending equal legal protections to sentient fetuses is that women will increasingly be blamed, and sometimes legally prosecuted, when they miscarry or give birth to premature, sick, or abnormal infants. It is reasonable to hold the caretakers of infants legally responsible if their charges are harmed because of their avoidable negligence. But when a woman miscarries or gives birth to an abnormal infant, the cause of the harm might be traced to any of an enormous number of actions or circumstances which would not normally constitute any legal offense. She might have gotten too much exercise or too little, eaten the wrong foods or the wrong quantity of the right ones, or taken or failed to take certain drugs. She might have smoked, consumed alcohol, or gotten too little sleep. She might have "permitted" her health to be damaged by hard work, by unsafe employment conditions, by the lack of affordable medical care, by living near a source of industrial pollution, by a physically or mentally abusive partner, or in any number of other ways.

Are such supposed failures on the part of pregnant women potentially to be construed as child abuse or negligent homicide? If sentient fetuses are entitled to the same legal protections as infants, then it would seem so. The danger is not a merely theoretical one. Two years ago in San Diego, a woman whose son was born with brain damage and died several weeks later was charged with felony child neglect. It was said that she had been advised by her physician to avoid sex and illicit drugs, and to go to the hospital immediately if she noticed any bleeding. Instead, she had allegedly had sex with her husband, taken some inappropriate drug, and delayed getting to the hospital for what might have been several hours after the onset of bleeding.

In this case, the charges were eventually dismissed on the grounds that the child protection law invoked had not been intended to apply to cases of this kind. But the multiplication of such cases is inevitable if the strong legal protections accorded to infants are extended to sentient fetuses. A bill recently introduced in the Australian state of New South Wales would make women liable to criminal prosecution if they are found to have smoked during pregnancy, eaten unhealthful foods, or taken any other action which can be shown to have adversely affected the development of the fetus (*The Australian*, July 5, 1988, 5). Such an approach to the protection of fetuses authorizes the legal regulation of virtually every aspect of women's public and private lives, and thus is incompatible with even the most minimal right to autonomy. Moreover, such laws are apt to prove counterproductive, since the fear of prosecution may deter poor or otherwise vulnerable women from seeking needed medical care during pregnancy. I am not suggesting that women whose apparent negligence causes prenatal harm to their infants should always be immune from criticism. However, if we want to improve the health of infants we would do better to provide the services women need to protect their health, rather than seeking to use the law to punish those whose prenatal care has been less than ideal.

There is yet another problem, which may prove temporary but which remains significant at this time. The extension of legal personhood to sentient fetuses would rule out most abortions performed because of severe fetal abnormalities, such as Down syndrome or spina bifida. Abortions performed following amniocentesis are usually done in the latter part of the second trimester, since it is usually not possible to obtain test results earlier. Methods of detecting fetal abnormalities at earlier stages, such as chorion biopsy, may eventually make late abortion for reasons of fetal abnormality unnecessary; but these methods are not yet widely available.

The elimination of most such abortions might be a consequence that could be accepted, were the society willing to provide adequate support for the handicapped children and adults who would come into being as a result of this policy. However, our society is not prepared to do this. In the absence of adequate communally-funded care for the handicapped, the prohibition of such abortions is exploitative of women. Of course, the male relatives of severely handicapped persons may also bear heavy burdens. Yet the heaviest portion of the daily responsibility generally falls upon mothers and other female relatives. If fetuses are not yet persons (and women are), then a respect for the equality of persons should lead to support for the availability of abortion in cases of severe fetal abnormality.[10]

Such arguments will not persuade those who deeply believe that fetuses are already persons, with equal moral rights. How, they will ask, is denying legal equality to sentient fetuses different from denying it to any other powerless group of human beings? If some human beings are more equal than others, then how can any of us feel safe? The answer is twofold.

First, pregnancy is a relationship different from any other, including that between parents and already-born children. It is not just one of innumerable situations in which the rights of one individual may come into conflict with those of another; it is probably the *only* case in which the legal personhood of one human being is necessarily incompatible with that of another. Only in pregnancy is the organic functioning of one human individual biologically inseparable from that of another. This organic unity makes it impossible for others to provide the fetus with medical care or any other presumed benefit, except by doing something to or for the woman. To try to "protect" the fetus other than through her cooperation and consent is effectively to nullify her right to autonomy, and potentially to expose her to violent physical assaults such as would not be legally condoned in any other type of case. The uniqueness of pregnancy helps to explain why the toleration of abortion does not lead to the disenfranchisement of other groups of human beings, as opponents of abortion often claim. For biological as well as psychological reasons, "It is all but impossible to extrapolate from attitudes towards fetal life attitudes toward [other] existing human life" (D. Callahan 1970, 474).

But, granting the uniqueness of pregnancy, why is it *women's* rights that should be privileged? If women and fetuses cannot both be legal persons then why not favor fetuses, e.g., on the grounds that they are more helpless, or more innocent, or have a longer life expectancy? It is difficult to justify this apparent bias towards women without appealing to the empirical fact that women are already persons in the usual, nonlegal sense—already thinking, self-aware, fully social beings—and fetuses are not. Regardless of whether we stress the intrinsic properties of persons, or the social and relational dimensions of personhood, this distinction remains. Even sentient fetuses do not yet have either the cognitive capacities or the richly interactive social involvements typical of persons.

This "not yet" is morally decisive. It is wrong to treat persons as if they do not have equal basic rights. Other things being equal, it is worse to deprive persons of their most basic moral and legal rights than to refrain from extending such rights to beings that are not persons. This is one important element of truth in the self-awareness criterion. If fetuses were already thinking, self-aware, socially responsive members of communities, then nothing could justify refusing them the equal protection of the law. In that case, we would sometimes be forced to balance the rights of the fetus against those of the woman, and sometimes the scales might be almost equally weighted. However, if women are persons and fetuses are not, then the balance must swing towards women's rights.

Conclusion

Birth is morally significant because it marks the end of one relationship and the beginning of others. It marks the end of pregnancy, a relationship so intimate that it is impossible to extend the equal protection of the law to fetuses without severely infringing women's most basic rights. Birth also marks the beginning of the infant's existence as a socially responsive member of a human community. Although the infant is not instantly transformed into a person at the moment of birth, it does become a biologically separate human being. As such, it can be known and cared for as a particular individual. It can also be vigorously protected without negating the basic rights of women. There are circumstances in which infanticide may be the best of a bad set of options. But our own society has both the ability and the desire to protect infants, and there is no reason why we should not do so.

We should not, however, seek to extend the same degree of protection to fetuses. Both late-term fetuses and newborn infants are probably capable of sentience. Both are precious to those who want children; and both need to be protected from a variety of possible harms. All of these factors contribute to the moral standing of the late-term fetus, which is substantial. However, to extend equal legal rights to fetuses is necessarily to deprive pregnant women of the rights to personal autonomy, physical integrity, and sometimes life itself. *There is room for only one person with full and equal rights inside a single human skin.* That is why it is birth, rather than sentience, viability, or some other prenatal milestone that must mark the beginning of legal personhood.

Notes

My thanks to Helen Heise, Dianne Romaine, Peter Singer, and Michael Scriven for their helpful comments on earlier versions of this paper.

1   Basic moral rights are those that are possessed equally by all persons, and that are essential to the moral equality of persons. The intended contrast is to those rights which arise from certain special circumstances—for instance, the right of a person to whom a promise has been made that that promise be kept. (Whether there are beings that are not persons but that have similar basic moral rights is one of the questions to be addressed here.)

2   "Moral standing," like "moral status" is a term that can be used to refer to the moral considerability of individuals, without being committed to the existence of moral rights. For instance, Sumner (1983) and Singer (1981) prefer these terms because, as utilitarians, they are unconvinced of the need for moral rights.

3   It is not obvious that a newborn infant's "level of consciousness" is similar to that of a fetus shortly before birth. Perhaps birth is analogous to an awakening, in that the infant has many experiences that were previously precluded by its prenatal brain chemistry or by its relative insulation within the womb. This speculation is plausible in evolutionary terms, since a rich subjective mental life might have little survival value for the fetus, but might be highly valuable for the newborn, e.g., in enabling it to recognize its mother and signal its hunger, discomfort, etc. However, for the sake of the argument I will assume that the newborn's capacity for sentience is generally not very different from that of the fetus shortly before birth.

4   It is interesting that Sumner regards fetal abnormality and the protection of the woman's health as sufficient justifications for late abortion. In this, he evidently departs from his own theory by effectively differentiating between the moral status of sentient fetuses and that of older humans—who presumably may not be killed just because they are abnormal or because their existence (through no fault of their own) poses a threat to someone else's health.

5   There are evidently some people who, though otherwise sentient, cannot experience physical pain. However, the survival value of the capacity to experience pain makes it probable that such individuals are the exception rather than the rule among mature members of sentient species.

6   There is at least one religion, that of the Jains, in which the killing of any living thing—even an insect—is regarded as morally wrong. But even the Jains do not regard the killing of insects as morally equivalent to the killing of persons. Laypersons (unlike mendicants) are permitted some unintentional killing of insects—though not of vertebrate animals or persons—when this is unavoidable to the pursuit of their profession (See Jaini 1979, 171-73).

7   Marcia Guttentag and Paul Secord (1983) argue that a shortage of women benefits at least some women, by increasing their "value" in the marriage market. However, they also argue that this increased value does not lead to greater freedom for women; on the contrary, it tends to coincide with an exceptionally severe sexual double standard, the exclusion of women from public life, and their confinement to domestic roles.

8   The extension of equal basic rights to infants need not imply the absolute rejection of euthanasia for infant patients. There are instances in which artificially extending the life of a severely compromised infant is contrary to the infant's own best interests. Competent adults or older children who are terminally ill sometimes rightly judge that further prolongation of their lives would not be a benefit to them. While infants cannot make that judgment for themselves, it is some-

times the right judgment for others to make on their behalf.

9 See *Civil Liberties* 363 (Winter 1988), 12, and Lawrence Lader, "Regulating Birth: Is the State Going Too Far?" *Conscience* IX: 5 (September/October, 1988), 5-6.

10 It is sometimes argued that using abortion to prevent the birth of severely handicapped infants will inevitably lead to a loss of concern for handicapped persons. I doubt that this is true. There is no need to confuse the question of whether it is good that persons be born handicapped with the very different question of whether handicapped persons are entitled to respect, support, and care.

References

Annas, George. 1982. "Forced Cesareans: The Most Unkindest Cut of All," *Hastings Center Report* 12, 3: 16-17, 45.

The Australian, Tuesday, July 5, 1988, 5.

Callahan, Daniel. 1970. *Abortion: Law, Choice and Morality*. New York: Macmillan.

Callahan, Sydney. 1984. "Value choices in abortion," in Sydney Callahan and Daniel Callahan, eds., *Abortion: Understanding Differences*. New York and London: Plenum Press.

Callahan, Sydney. 1986. "Abortion and the Sexual Agenda," *Commonweal*, April 25: 232-38.

Gilligan, Carol. 1981. *In a Different Voice: Psychological Theory and Women's Development*. Cambridge, MA: Harvard University Press.

Guttentag, Marcia, and Paul Secord. 1983. *Too Many Women: The Sex Ratio Question*. Beverly Hills: Sage Publications.

Harrison, Beverly Wildung. 1983. *Our Right to Choose: Toward a New Ethic of Abortion*. Boston: Beacon Press.

Jaini, Padmanab S. 1979. *The Jaina Path of Purification*. Berkeley, Los Angeles, London: University of California Press.

Lomasky, Loren. 1984. "Being a Person—Does It Matter?" in Joel Feinberg, ed., *The Problem of Abortion*. Belmont, California.

Luker, Kristen. 1984. *Abortion and the Politics of Motherhood*. Berkeley, Los Angeles and London: University of California Press.

Manning, Rita. 1988. *Caring For and Caring About*. Paper presented at conference entitled *Explorations in Feminist Ethics*, Duluth, Minnesota. October 8.

Mead, Margaret. [1935] 1963. *Sex and Temperament in Three Primitive Societies*. New York: Morrow Quill Paperbacks.

Noddings, Nel. 1984. *Caring: A Feminine Approach to Ethics and Moral Education*. Berkeley, Los Angeles and London: University of California Press.

Petchesky, Rosalind Pollack. 1984. *Abortion and Women's Choice*. New York, London: Longman.

Piers, Maria W. 1978. *Infanticide*. New York: W.W. Norton and Company.

Singer, Peter. 1981. *The Expanding Circle: Ethics and Sociobiology*. New York: Farrar, Straus and Giroux.

Stone, Christopher. 1974. *Should Trees Have Standing: Towards Legal Rights for Natural Objects*. Los Altos: William Kaufman.

Stone, Christopher. 1987. *Earth and Other Ethics*. New York: Harper & Row.

Sumner, L.W. 1983. *Abortion and Moral Theory*. Princeton, NJ: Princeton University Press.

Taylor, Paul W. 1986. *Respect for Nature: A Theory of Environmental Ethics*. Princeton, NJ: Princeton University Press.

Thomson, Judith Jarvis. 1971. "A Defense of Abortion," *Philosophy and Public Affairs* 1, 1: 47-66.

Tooley, Michael. 1983. *Abortion and Infanticide*. Oxford: Oxford University Press.

Wolgast, Elizabeth. 1987. *The Grammar of Justice*. Ithaca and London: Cornell University Press.

27.
ABORTION THROUGH A FEMINIST ETHICS LENS

Susan Sherwin

SOURCE: *Dialogue* 30.3 (1991): 327-42.

Abortion has long been a central issue in the arena of applied ethics, but, the distinctive analysis of feminist ethics is generally overlooked in most philosophic discussions. Authors and readers commonly presume a familiarity with the feminist position and equate it with liberal defences of women's right to choose abortion, but, in fact, feminist ethics yields a different analysis of the moral questions surrounding abortion than that usually offered by the more familiar liberal defenders of abortion rights. Most feminists can agree with some of the conclusions that arise from certain non-feminist arguments on abortion, but they often disagree about the way the issues are formulated and the sorts of reasons that are invoked in the mainstream literature.

Among the many differences found between feminist and non-feminist arguments about abortion, is the fact that most non-feminist discussions of abortion consider the questions of the moral or legal permissibility of abortion in isolation from other questions, ignoring (and thereby obscuring) relevant connections to other social practices that oppress women. They are generally grounded in masculinist conceptions of freedom (e.g., privacy, individual choice, individuals' property rights in their own bodies) that do not meet the needs, interests, and intuitions of many of the women concerned. In contrast, feminists seek to couch their arguments in moral concepts that support their general campaign of overcoming injustice in all its dimensions, including those inherent in moral theory itself.[1] There is even disagreement about how best to understand the moral question at issue: non-feminist arguments focus exclusively on the morality and/or legality of performing abortions, whereas feminists insist that other questions, including ones about accessibility and delivery of abortion services must also be addressed.

Although feminists welcome the support of non-feminists in pursuing policies that will grant women control over abortion decisions, they generally envision very different sorts of policies for this purpose than those considered by non-feminist sympathizers. For example, Kathleen McDonnell. (1984) urges feminists to develop an explicitly "'feminist morality' of abortion.... At its root it would be characterized by the deep appreciations of the complexities of life, the refusal to polarize and adopt simplistic formulas" (p. 52). Here, I propose one conception of the shape such an analysis should take.

Women and Abortion

The most obvious difference between feminist and non-feminist approaches to abortion can be seen in the relative attention each gives to the interests and experiences of women in its analysis. Feminists consider it self-evident that the pregnant woman is a subject of principal concern in abortion decisions. In most non-feminist accounts, however, not only is she not perceived as central, she is rendered virtually invisible. Non-feminist theorists, whether they support or oppose women's right to choose abortion, focus almost all their attention on the moral status of the developing embryo or the fetus.

In pursuing a distinctively feminist ethics, it is appropriate to begin with a look at the role of abortion in women's lives. Clearly, the need for abortion can be very intense; women have pursued abortions under appalling and dangerous conditions, across widely diverse cultures and historical periods. No one denies that if abortion is not made legal, safe, and accessible, women will seek out illegal and life-threatening abortions to terminate pregnancies they cannot accept. Anti-abortion activists seem willing to accept this price, but feminists judge the inevitable loss of women's lives associated with restrictive abortion policies to be a matter of fundamental concern.

Although anti-abortion campaigners imagine that women often make frivolous and irresponsible decisions about abortion, feminists recognize that women have abortions for a wide variety of reasons. Some women, for instance, find themselves seriously ill and incapacitated throughout pregnancy; they cannot continue in their jobs and may face enormous difficulties in fulfilling their responsibilities at home. Many employers and schools will not tolerate pregnancy in their employees or students, and not every woman is able to put her job, career, or studies on hold. Women of limited means may be unable to take adequate care of children they have already borne and they may know that another mouth to feed will reduce their ability to provide for their existing children. Women who suffer from chronic disease, or who feel too young, or too old, or who are unable to maintain lasting relationships may recognize that they will not be able to care properly for a child at this time. Some who are homeless, or addicted to drugs, or who are diagnosed as carrying the AIDS virus may be unwilling to allow a child to enter the world under such circumstances. If the pregnancy is a result of rape or incest, the psychological pain of carrying it to term may be unbearable, and the woman may recognize that her attitude to the child after birth will always be tinged with bitterness. Some women have learned that the fetuses they carry have serious chromosomal anomalies and consider it best to prevent them from being born with a condition bound to cause suffering. Others, knowing the fathers to be brutal and violent, may be unwilling to subject a child to the beatings or incestuous attacks they anticipate; some may have no other realistic way to remove the child (or themselves) from the relationship.

Or a woman may simply believe that bearing a child is incompatible with her life plans at this time, since continuing a pregnancy is likely to have profound repercussions throughout a woman's entire life. If the woman is young, a pregnancy will very likely reduce her chances of education and hence limit her career and life opportunities: "The earlier a woman has a baby, it seems, the more likely she is to drop out of school; the less education she gets, the more likely she is to remain poorly paid, peripheral to the labour market, or unemployed, and the more children she will have—between one and three more than her working childless counterpart" (Petchesky 1984, p. 150). In many circumstances, having a child will exacerbate the social and economic forces already stacked against her by virtue of her sex (and her race, class, age, sexual orientation, or the effects of some disability, etc.). Access to abortion is a necessary option for many women if they are to escape the oppressive conditions of poverty.

Whatever the reason, most feminists believe that a pregnant woman is in the best position to judge whether abortion is the appropriate response to her circumstances. Since she is usually the only one able to weigh all the relevant factors, most feminists reject attempts to offer any general abstract rules for determining when abortion is morally justified. Women's personal deliberations about abortion include contextually defined considerations reflecting her commitment to the needs and interests of everyone concerned—including herself, the fetus she carries, other members of her household, etc. Because there is no single formula available for balancing these complex factors through all possible cases, it is vital that feminists insist on protecting each woman's right to come to her own conclusions. Abortion decisions are, by their very nature, dependent on specific features of each woman's experience; theoretically dispassionate philosophers and other moralists should not expect to set the agenda for these considerations in any universal way. Women must be acknowledged as full moral agents with the responsibility for making moral decisions about their own pregnancies.[2] Although I think that it is possible for a woman to make a mistake in her moral judgment on this matter (i.e., it is possible that a woman may come to believe that she was wrong about her decision to continue or terminate a pregnancy), the intimate nature of this sort of decision makes it unlikely that anyone else is in a position to arrive at a more reliable conclusion; it is, therefore, improper to grant others the authority to interfere in women's decisions to seek abortions.

Feminist analysis regards the effects of unwanted pregnancies on the lives of women individually and collectively as a central element in the moral evaluation of abortion. Even without patriarchy, bearing a child would be a very important event in a woman's life. It involves significant physical, emotional, social, and (usually) economic changes for her. The ability to exert control over the incidence, timing, and frequency of child-bearing is often tied to her ability to control most other things she values. Since we live in a patriarchal society, it is especially important to ensure that women have the authority to control their own reproduction.[3] Despite the diversity of opinion among feminists on most other matters, virtually all feminists seem to agree that women must gain full control over their own reproductive lives if they are to free themselves from male dominance.[4] Many perceive the commitment of the political right wing to opposing abortion as part of a general strategy to reassert patriarchal control over women in the face of significant feminist influence (Petchesky 1980, p. 112).

Women's freedom to choose abortion is also linked with their ability to control their own sexuality. Women's subordinate status often prevents them from refusing men sexual access to their bodies. If women cannot end the unwanted pregnancies that result from male sexual dominance, their sexual vulnerability to particular men can increase, because caring for an(other) infant involves greater financial needs and reduced economic opportunities for women.[5] As a result, pregnancy often forces women to become dependent on men. Since a woman's dependence on a man is assumed to entail that she will remain sexually loyal to him, restriction of abortion serves to channel women's sexuality and further perpetuates the cycle of oppression.

In contrast to most non-feminist accounts, feminist analyses of abortion direct attention to the question of how women get pregnant. Those who reject abortion seem to believe that women can avoid unwanted pregnancies by avoiding sexual intercourse. Such views show little appreciation for the power of sexual politics in a culture that oppresses women. Existing patterns of sexual dominance mean that women often have little control over their sexual lives. They may be subject to rape by strangers, or

by their husbands, boyfriends, colleagues, employers, customers, fathers, brothers, uncles, and dates. Often, the sexual coercion is not even recognized as such by the participants, but is the price of continued "good will"—popularity, economic survival, peace, or simple acceptance. Few women have not found themselves in circumstances where they do not feel free to refuse a man's demands for intercourse, either because he is holding a gun to her head or because he threatens to be emotionally hurt if she refuses (or both). Women are socialized to be compliant and accommodating, sensitive to the feelings of others, and frightened of physical power; men are socialized to take advantage of every opportunity to engage in sexual intercourse and to use sex to express dominance and power. Under such circumstances, it is difficult to argue that women could simply "choose" to avoid heterosexual activity if they wish to avoid pregnancy. Catherine MacKinnon neatly sums it up: "the logic by which women are supposed to consent to sex [is]: preclude the alternatives, then call the remaining option 'her choice'" (MacKinnon 1989, p. 192).

Nor can women rely on birth control alone to avoid pregnancy. There simply is no form of reversible contraception available that is fully safe and reliable. The pill and the IUD are the most effective means offered, but both involve significant health hazards to women and are quite dangerous for some. No woman should spend the 30 to 40 years of her reproductive life on either form of birth control. Further, both have been associated with subsequent problems of involuntary infertility, so they are far from optimum for women who seek to control the timing of their pregnancies.

The safest form of birth control involves the use of barrier methods (condoms or diaphragms) in combination with spermicidal foams or jelly. But these methods also pose difficulties for women. They may be socially awkward to use: young women are discouraged from preparing for sexual activity that might never happen and are offered instead romantic models of spontaneous passion. (Few films or novels interrupt scenes of seduction for the fetching of contraceptives.) Many women find their male partners unwilling to use barrier methods of contraception and they do not have the power to insist. Further, cost is a limiting factor for many women. Condoms and spermicides are expensive and are not covered under most health care plans. There is only one contraceptive option which offers women safe and fully effective birth control: barrier methods with the back-up option of abortion.[6]

From a feminist perspective, a central moral feature of pregnancy is that it takes place in *women's bodies* and has profound effects on *women's* lives. Gender-neutral accounts of pregnancy are not available; pregnancy is explicitly a condition associated with the female body.[7] Because the need for abortion is experienced only by women, policies about abortion affect women uniquely. Thus, it is important to consider how proposed policies on abortion fit into general patterns of oppression for women. Unlike non-feminist accounts, feminist ethics demands that the effects on the oppression of women be a principal consideration when evaluating abortion policies.

The Fetus

In contrast, most non-feminist analysts believe that the moral acceptability of abortion turns on the question of the moral status of the fetus. Even those who support women's right to choose abortion tend to accept the central premise of the anti-abortion proponents that abortion can only be tolerated if it can be proved that the fetus is lacking some criterion of full personhood.[8] Opponents of abortion have structured the debate so that it is necessary to define the status of the fetus as either valued the same as other humans (and hence entitled not to be killed) or as lacking in all value. Rather than challenging the logic of this formulation, many defenders of abortion have concentrated on showing that the fetus is indeed without significant value (Tooley 1972, Warren 1973); others, such as Wayne Sumner (1981), offer a more subtle account that reflects the gradual development of fetuses whereby there is some specific criterion that determines the degree of protection to be afforded them which is lacking in the early stages of pregnancy but present in the later stages. Thus, the debate often rages between abortion opponents who describe the fetus as an "innocent," vulnerable, morally important, separate being whose life is threatened and who must be protected

at all costs, and abortion supporters who try to establish some sort of deficiency inherent to fetuses which removes them from the scope of the moral community.

The woman on whom the fetus depends for survival is considered as secondary (if she is considered at all) in these debates. The actual experiences and responsibilities of real women are not perceived as morally relevant (unless they, too, can be proved innocent by establishing that their pregnancies are a result of rape or incest). It is a common assumption of both defenders and opponents of women's right to choose abortion that many women will be irresponsible in their choices. The important question, though, is whether fetuses have the sort of status that justifies interfering in women's choices at all. In some contexts, women's role in gestation is literally reduced to that of "fetal containers"; the individual women disappear or are perceived simply as mechanical life-support systems.[9]

The current rhetoric against abortion stresses the fact that the genetic make-up of the fetus is determined at conception and the genetic code is incontestably human. Lest there be any doubt about the humanity of the fetus, we are assailed with photographs of fetuses at various stages of development demonstrating the early appearance of recognizably human characteristics, e.g., eyes, fingers, and toes. The fact that the fetus in its early stages is microscopic, virtually indistinguishable from other primate fetuses to the untrained eye, and lacking in the capacities that make human life meaningful and valuable is not deemed relevant by the self-appointed defenders of fetuses. The anti-abortion campaign is directed at evoking sympathetic attitudes towards this tiny, helpless being whose life is threatened by its own mother; it urges us to see the fetus as entangled in an adversarial relationship with the (presumably irresponsible) woman who carries it. We are encouraged to identify with the "unborn child" and not with the (selfish) woman whose life is also at issue.

Within the non-feminist literature, both defenders and opponents of women's right to choose abortion agree that the difference between a late-term fetus and a newborn infant is "merely geographical" and cannot be considered morally significant. But a fetus

[handwritten margin note: Sympath with fetus & not with mother]

inhabits a woman's body and is wholly dependent on her unique contribution to its maintenance while a newborn is physically separate though still in need of a lot of care. One can only view the distinction between being in or out of a woman's womb as morally irrelevant if one discounts the perspective of the pregnant woman; feminists seem to be alone in recognizing her perspective as morally important.[10]

Within anti-abortion arguments, fetuses are identified as individuals; in our culture which views the (abstract) individual as sacred, fetuses *qua* individuals should be honoured and preserved. Extraordinary claims are made to try to establish the individuality and moral agency of fetuses. At the same time, the women who carry these fetal individuals are viewed as passive hosts whose only significant role is to refrain from aborting or harming their fetuses. Since it is widely believed that the woman does not actually have to *do* anything to protect the life of the fetus, pregnancy is often considered (abstractly) to be a tolerable burden to protect the life of an individual so like us.[11]

Medicine has played its part in supporting these sorts of attitudes. Fetal medicine is a rapidly expanding specialty, and it is commonplace in professional medical journals to find references to pregnant women as "fetal environments." Fetal surgeons now have at their disposal a repertory of sophisticated technology that can save the lives of dangerously ill fetuses; in light of such heroic successes, it is perhaps understandable that women have disappeared from their view. These specialists see fetuses as their patients, not the women who nurture them. Doctors perceive themselves as the *active* agents in saving fetal lives and, hence, believe that they are the ones in direct relationship with the fetuses they treat.

Perhaps even more distressing than the tendency to ignore the woman's agency altogether and view her as a purely passive participant in the medically controlled events of pregnancy and childbirth is the growing practice of viewing women as genuine threats to the well-being of the fetus. Increasingly, women are viewed as irresponsible or hostile towards their fetuses, and the relationship between them is characterized as adversarial (Overall 1987, p. 60). Concern for the well-being of the fetus is taken as licence for doctors to intervene to ensure

that women comply with medical "advice." Courts are called upon to enforce the doctors' orders when moral pressure alone proves inadequate, and women are being coerced into undergoing unwanted Caesarean deliveries and technologically monitored hospital births. Some states have begun to imprison women for endangering their fetuses through drug abuse and other socially unacceptable behaviours. An Australian state recently introduced a bill that makes women liable to criminal prosecution "if they are found to have smoked during pregnancy, eaten unhealthful foods, or taken any other action which can be shown to have adversely affected the development of the fetus" (Warren 1989, p. 60).

In other words, physicians have joined with anti-abortionist activists in fostering a cultural acceptance of the view that fetuses are distinct individuals, who are physically, ontologically, and socially separate from the women whose bodies they inhabit, and who have their own distinct interests. In this picture, pregnant women are either ignored altogether or are viewed as deficient in some crucial respect and hence subject to coercion for the sake of their fetuses. In the former case, the interests of the women concerned are assumed to be identical with those of the fetus; in the latter, the women's interests are irrelevant because they are perceived as immoral, unimportant, or unnatural. Focus on the fetus as an independent entity has led to presumptions which deny pregnant women their roles as active, independent, moral agents with a primary interest in what becomes of the fetuses they carry. Emphasis on the fetus's status has led to an assumed licence to interfere with women's reproductive freedom.

A Feminist View of the Fetus

Because the public debate has been set up as a competition between the rights of women and those of fetuses, feminists have often felt pushed to reject claims of fetal value in order to protect women's claims. Yet, as Addelson (1987) has argued, viewing abortion in this way "tears [it] out of the context of women's lives" (p. 107). There are other accounts of fetal value that are more plausible and less oppressive to women.

On a feminist account, fetal development is examined in the context in which it occurs, within women's bodies rather than in the imagined isolation implicit in many theoretical accounts. Fetuses develop in specific pregnancies which occur in the lives of particular women. They are not individuals housed in generic female wombs, nor are they full persons at risk only because they are small and subject to the whims of women. Their very existence is relational, developing as they do within particular women's bodies, and their principal relationship is to the women who carry them.

On this view, fetuses are morally significant, but their status is relational rather than absolute. Unlike other human beings, fetuses do not have any independent existence; their existence is uniquely tied to the support of a specific other. Most non-feminist commentators have ignored the relational dimension of fetal development and have presumed that the moral status of fetuses could be resolved solely in terms of abstract metaphysical criteria of personhood. They imagine that there is some set of properties (such as genetic heritage, moral agency, self-consciousness, language use, or self-determination) which will entitle all who possess them to be granted the moral status of persons (Warren 1973, Tooley 1972). They seek some particular feature by which we can neatly divide the world into the dichotomy of moral persons (who are to be valued and protected) and others (who are not entitled to the same group privileges); it follows that it is a merely empirical question whether or not fetuses possess the relevant properties.

But this vision misinterprets what is involved in personhood and what it is that is especially valued about persons. Personhood is a social category, not an isolated state. Persons are members of a community; they develop as concrete, discrete, and specific individuals. To be a morally significant category, personhood must involve personality as well as biological integrity.[12] It is not sufficient to consider persons simply as Kantian atoms of rationality; persons are all embodied, conscious beings with particular social histories. Annette Baier (1985) has developed a concept of persons as "second persons" which helps explain the sort of social dimension that seems fundamental to any moral notion of personhood:

A person, perhaps, is best seen as one who was long enough dependent upon other persons to acquire the essential arts of personhood. Persons essentially are *second* persons, who grow up with other persons.... The fact that a person has a life *history*, and that a people collectively have a history depends upon the humbler fact that each person has a childhood in which a cultural heritage is transmitted, ready for adolescent rejection and adult discriminating selection and contribution. Persons come after and before other persons. (p. 84-85; her emphasis)

Persons, in other words, are members of a social community which shapes and values them, and personhood is a relational concept that must be defined in terms of interactions and relationships with others.

A fetus is a unique sort of being in that it cannot form relationships freely with others, nor can others readily form relationships with it. A fetus has a primary and particularly intimate relationship with the woman in whose womb it develops; any other relationship it may have is indirect, and must be mediated through the pregnant woman. The relationship that exists between a woman and her fetus is clearly asymmetrical, since she is the only party to the relationship who is capable of making a decision about whether the interaction should continue and since the fetus is wholly dependent on the woman who sustains it while she is quite capable of surviving without it.

However much some might prefer it to be otherwise, no one else can do anything to support or harm a fetus without doing something to the woman who nurtures it. Because of this inexorable biological reality, she bears a unique responsibility and privilege in determining her fetus's place in the social scheme of things. Clearly, many pregnancies occur to women who place very high value on the lives of the particular fetuses they carry, and choose to see their pregnancies through to term despite the possible risks and costs involved; hence, it would be wrong of anyone to force such a woman to terminate her pregnancy under these circumstances. Other women, or some of these same women at other times, value other things more highly (e.g., their freedom, their health, or previous responsibilities which conflict with those generated by the pregnancies), and choose not to continue their pregnancies. The value that women ascribe to individual fetuses varies dramatically from case to case, and may well change over the course of any particular pregnancy. There is no absolute value that attaches to fetuses apart from their relational status determined in the context of their particular development.

Since human beings are fundamentally relational beings, it is important to remember that fetuses are characteristically limited in the relationships in which they can participate; within those relationships, they can make only the most restricted "contributions."[13] After birth, human beings are capable of a much wider range of roles in relationships with an infinite variety of partners; it is that very diversity of possibility and experience that leads us to focus on the abstraction of the individual as a constant through all her/his relationships. But until birth, no such variety is possible, and the fetus is defined as an entity within a woman who will almost certainly be principally responsible for it for many years to come.

No human, and especially no fetus, can exist apart from relationships; feminist views of what is valuable about persons must reflect the social nature of their existence. Fetal lives can neither be sustained nor destroyed without affecting the women who support them. Because of a fetus's unique physical status—*within* and dependent on a particular woman—the responsibility and privilege of determining its specific social status and value must rest with the woman carrying it. Fetuses are not persons because they have not developed sufficiently in social relationships to be persons in any morally significant sense (i.e., they are not yet second persons). Newborns, although just beginning their development into persons, are immediately subject to social relationships, for they are capable of communication and response in interaction with a variety of other persons. Thus, feminist accounts of abortion stress the importance of protecting women's right to continue as well as to terminate pregnancies as each sees fit.

Feminist Politics and Abortion

Feminist ethics directs us to look at abortion in the context of other issues of power and not to limit dis-

cussion to the standard questions about its moral and legal acceptability. Because coerced pregnancy has repercussions for women's oppressed status generally, it is important to ensure that abortion not only be made legal but that adequate services be made accessible to all women who seek them. This means that within Canada, where medically approved abortion is technically recognized as legal (at least for the moment), we must protest the fact that it is not made available to many of the women who have the greatest need for abortions: vast geographical areas offer no abortion services at all, but unless the women of those regions can afford to travel to urban clinics, they have no meaningful right to abortion. Because women depend on access to abortion in their pursuit of social equality, it is a matter of moral as well as political responsibility that provincial health plans should cover the cost of transport and service in the abortion facilities women choose. Ethical study of abortion involves understanding and critiquing the economic, age, and social barriers that currently restrict access to medically acceptable abortion services.[14]

Moreover, it is also important that abortion services be provided in an atmosphere that fosters women's health and well-being; hence, the care offered should be in a context that is supportive of the choices women make. Abortions should be seen as part of women's overall reproductive health and could be included within centres that deal with all matters of reproductive health in an open, patient-centred manner where effective counselling is offered for a wide range of reproductive decisions.[15] Providers need to recognize that abortion is a legitimate option so that services will be delivered with respect and concern for the physical, psychological, and emotional effects on a patient. All too frequently, hospital-based abortions are provided by practitioners who are uneasy about their role and treat the women involved with hostility and resentment. Increasingly, many anti-abortion activists have personalized their attacks and focussed their attention on harassing the women who enter and leave abortion clinics. Surely requiring a woman to pass a gauntlet of hostile protesters on her way to and from an abortion is not conducive to effective health care. Ethical exploration of abortion raises questions about how women are treated when they seek abortions;[16] achieving legal permission for women to dispose of their fetuses if they are determined enough to manage the struggle should not be accepted as the sole moral consideration.

Nonetheless, feminists must formulate their distinctive response to legislative initiatives on abortion. The tendency of Canadian politicians confronted by vocal activists on both sides of the abortion issue has been to seek "compromises" that seem to give something to each (and, thereby, also deprives each of important features sought in policy formation). Thus, the House of Commons recently passed a law (Bill C-43) that allows a woman to have an abortion only if a doctor certifies that her physical, mental, or emotional health will be otherwise threatened. Many non-feminist supporters of women's right to choose consider this a victory and urge feminists to be satisfied with it, but feminists have good reason to object. Besides their obvious objection to having abortion returned to the Criminal Code, feminists also object that this policy considers doctors and not women the best judges of a woman's need for abortion; feminists have little reason to trust doctors to appreciate the political dimension of abortion or to respond adequately to women's needs. Abortion must be a woman's decision, and not one controlled by her doctor. Further, experience shows that doctors are already reluctant to provide abortions to women; the opportunity this law presents for criminal persecution of doctors by anti-abortion campaigners is a sufficient worry to inhibit their participation.[17] Feminists want women's decision-making to be recognized as legitimate, and cannot be satisfied with a law that makes abortion a medical choice.

Feminists support abortion on demand because they know that women must have control over their reproduction. For the same reason, they actively oppose forced abortion and coerced sterilization, practices that are sometimes inflicted on the most powerless women, especially those in the Third World. Feminist ethics demands that access to voluntary, safe, effective birth control be part of any abortion discussion, so that women have access to other means of avoiding pregnancy.[18]

Feminist analysis addresses the context as well as the practice of abortion decisions. Thus, feminists also object to the conditions which lead women to abort wanted fetuses because there are not adequate financial and social supports available to care for a child. Because feminist accounts value fetuses that are wanted by the women who carry them, they oppose practices which force women to abort because of poverty or intimidation. Yet, the sorts of social changes necessary if we are to free women from having abortions out of economic necessity are vast; they include changes not only in legal and health-care policy, but also in housing, child care, employment, etc. (Petchesky 1980, p. 112). Nonetheless, feminist ethics defines reproductive freedom as the condition under which women are able to make truly voluntary choices about their reproductive lives, and these many dimensions are implicit in the ideal.

Clearly, feminists are not "pro-abortion," for they are concerned to ensure the safety of each pregnancy to the greatest degree possible; wanted fetuses should not be harmed or lost. Therefore, adequate pre- and post-natal care and nutrition are also important elements of any feminist position on reproductive freedom. Where anti-abortionists direct their energies to trying to prevent women from obtaining abortions, feminists seek to protect the health of wanted fetuses. They recognize that far more could be done to protect and care for fetuses if the state directed its resources at supporting women who continue their pregnancies, rather than draining away resources in order to police women who find that they must interrupt their pregnancies. Caring for the women who carry fetuses is not only a more legitimate policy than is regulating them; it is probably also more effective at ensuring the health and well-being of more fetuses.

Feminist ethics also explores how abortion policies fit within the politics of sexual domination. Most feminists are sensitive to the fact that many men support women's right to abortion out of the belief that women will be more willing sexual partners if they believe that they can readily terminate an unwanted pregnancy. Some men coerce their partners into obtaining abortions the women may not want.[19] Feminists understand that many women oppose abortion for this very reason, being unwilling to support a practice that increases women's sexual vulnerability (Luker 1984, p. 209-15). Thus, it is important that feminists develop a coherent analysis of reproductive freedom that includes sexual freedom (as women choose to define it). That requires an analysis of sexual freedom that includes women's right to refuse sex; such a right can only be assured if women have equal power to men and are not subject to domination by virtue of their sex.[20]

In sum, then, feminist ethics demands that moral discussions of abortion be more broadly defined than they have been in most philosophic discussions. Only by reflecting on the meaning of ethical pronouncements on actual women's lives and the connections between judgments on abortion and the conditions of domination and subordination can we come to an adequate understanding of the moral status of abortion in our society. As Rosalind Petchesky (1980) argues, feminist discussion of abortion "must be moved beyond the framework of a 'woman's right to choose' and connected to a much broader revolutionary movement that addresses all of the conditions of women's liberation" (p. 113).

Notes

* Earlier versions of this paper were read to the Department of Philosophy, Dalhousie University and to the Canadian Society for Women in Philosophy in Kingston. I am very grateful for the comments received from colleagues in both forums; particular thanks go to Lorraine Code, David Braybrooke, Richmond Campbell, Sandra Taylor, Terry Tomkow and Kadri Vihvelin for their patience and advice.

1   For some idea of the ways in which traditional moral theory oppresses women, see Morgan (1987) and Hoagland (1988).

2   Critics continue to want to structure the debate around the *possibility* of women making frivolous abortion decisions and hence want feminists to agree to setting boundaries on acceptable grounds for choosing abortion. Feminists ought to resist this injunction, though. There is no practical way of drawing a line fairly in the abstract; cases that may appear "frivolous" at a distance, often turn out to be substantive when the details are revealed, i.e., frivolity is in the eyes of the beholder. There is no evidence to sug-

gest that women actually make the sorts of choices worried critics hypothesize about: e.g., a woman eight months pregnant who chooses to abort because she wants to take a trip or gets in "a tiff" with her partner. These sorts of fantasies, on which demands to distinguish between legitimate and illegitimate personal reasons for choosing abortion chiefly rest, reflect an offensive conception of women as irresponsible; they ought not to be perpetuated. Women, seeking moral guidance in their own deliberations about choosing abortion, do not find such hypothetical discussions of much use.

3   In her monumental historical analysis of the early roots of Western patriarchy, Gerda Lerner (1986) determined that patriarchy began in the period from 3100 to 600 BCE when men appropriated women's sexual and reproductive capacity; the earliest states entrenched patriarchy by institutionalizing the sexual and procreative subordination of women to men.

4   There are some women who claim to be feminists against choice in abortion. See, for instance, Callahan (1987), though few spell out their full feminist program. For reasons I develop in this paper, I do not think this is a consistent position.

5   There is a lot the state could do to ameliorate this condition. If it provided women with adequate financial support, removed the inequities in the labour market, and provided affordable and reliable childcare, pregnancy need not so often lead to a woman's dependence on a particular man. The fact that it does not do so is evidence of the state's complicity in maintaining women's subordinate position with respect to men.

6   See Petchesky (1984), especially Chapter 5, "Considering the Alternatives: The Problems of Contraception," where she documents the risks and discomforts associated with pill use and IUD's and the increasing rate at which women are choosing the option of diaphragm or condom with the option of early legal abortions as backup.

7   See Zillah Eisenstein (1988) for a comprehensive theory of the role of the pregnant body as the central element in the cultural subordination of women.

8   Thomson (1971) is a notable exception to this trend.

9   This seems reminiscent of Aristotle's view of women as "flower pots" where men implant the seed with all the important genetic information and the movement necessary for development and women's job is that of

passive gestation, like the flower pot. For exploration of the flower pot picture of pregnancy, see Whitbeck (1973) and Lange (1983).

10 Contrast Warren (1989) with Tooley (1972).

11 The definition of pregnancy as a purely passive activity reaches its ghoulish conclusion in the increasing acceptability of sustaining brain-dead women on life support systems to continue their functions as incubators until the fetus can be safely delivered. For a discussion of this new trend, see Murphy (1989).

12 This apt phrasing is taken from Petchesky (1986), p. 342.

13 Fetuses are almost wholly individuated by the women who bear them. The fetal "contributions" to the relationship are defined by the projections and interpretations of the pregnant woman in the latter stages of pregnancy if she chooses to perceive fetal movements in purposeful ways (e.g., "it likes classical music, wine, exercise").

14 Some feminists suggest we seek recognition of the legitimacy of non-medical abortion services. This would reduce costs and increase access dramatically, with no apparent increase in risk, provided that services were offered by trained, responsible practitioners concerned with the well-being of their clients. It would also allow the possibility of increasing women's control over abortion. See, for example McDonnell (1984), chap. 8.

15 For a useful model of such a centre, see Wagner and Lee (1989).

16 See CARAL/Halifax (1990) for women's stories about their experiences with hospitals and free-standing abortion clinics.

17 The Canadian Medical Association has confirmed those fears. In testimony before the House of Commons committee reviewing the bill, the CMA reported that over half the doctors surveyed who now perform abortions expect to stop offering them if the legislation goes through. Since the Commons passed the bill, the threats of withdrawal of service have increased. Many doctors plan to abandon their abortion service once the law is introduced, because they are unwilling to accept the harassment they anticipate from anti-abortion zealots. Even those who believe that they will eventually win any court case that arises, fear the expense and anxiety involved as the case plays itself out.

18 Therefore, the Soviet model, where women have access to multiple abortions but where there is no other birth control available, must also be opposed.

19 See CARAL/Halifax (1990), p. 20-21, for examples of this sort of abuse.

20 It also requires that discussions of reproductive and sexual freedom not be confined to "the language of control and sexuality characteristic of a technology of sex" (Diamond and Quinby 1988, p. 197), for such language is alienating and constrains women's experiences of their own sexuality.

References

Addelson, Kathryn Pyne. 1987. "Moral Passages," in Eva Feder Kittay and Diana T. Meyers, eds., *Women and Moral Theory*. Totowa, N.J.: Rowman & Littlefield.

Baier, Annette. 1985. *Postures of the Mind: Essays on Mind and Morals*. Minneapolis: University of Minnesota Press.

Callahan, Sidney. 1987. "A Pro-life Feminist Makes Her Case," *Utne Reader* (March/April): 104-14.

CARAL/Halifax. 1990. *Telling Our Stories: Abortion Stories from Nova Scotia*. Halifax: CARAL/Halifax (Canadian Abortion Rights Action League).

Daly, Mary. 1973. *Beyond God the Father: Toward a Philosophy of Women's Liberation*. Boston: Beacon Press.

Diamond, Irene, and Lee Quinby. 1988. "American Feminism and the Language of Control," in Irene Diamond and Lee Quinby, eds., *Feminism and Foucault: Reflections on Resistance*. Boston: Northeastern University Press.

Eisenstein, Zillah R. 1988. *The Female Body and the Law*. Berkeley: University of California Press.

Hoagland, Sara Lucia. 1988. *Lesbian Ethics: Toward New Value*. Palo Alto, CA: Institute of Lesbian Studies.

Lange, Lynda. 1983. "Woman is Not a Rational Animal: On Aristotle's Biology of Reproduction," in Sandra Harding and Merill B. Hintickka, eds., *Discovering Reality: Feminist Perspectives on Epistemology, Metaphysics, Methodology, and Philosophy of Science*. Dordrecht, Holland: D. Reidel.

Lerner, Gerda. 1986. *The Creation of Patriarchy*. New York: Oxford.

Luker, Kristin. 1984. *Abortion and the Politics of Motherhood*. Berkeley: University of California Press.

MacKinnon, Catherine. 1989. *Toward a Feminist Theory*

of the State. Cambridge, MA: Harvard University Press.

McDonnell, Kathleen. 1984. *Not an Easy Choice: A Feminist Re-examines Abortion*. Toronto: The Women's Press.

McLaren, Angus, and Arlene Tigar McLaren. 1986. *The Bedroom and the State: The Changing Practices and Politics of Contraception and Abortion in Canada, 1880-1980*. Toronto: McClelland and Stewart.

Morgan, Kathryn Pauly. 1987. "Women and Moral Madness," in Marsha Hanen and Kai Nielsen, eds., *Science, Morality and Feminist Theory. Canadian Journal of Philosophy*, Supplementary Volume 13: 201-26.

Murphy, Julien S. 1989. "Should Pregnancies Be Sustained in Brain-dead Women?: A Philosophical Discussion of Postmortem Pregnancy," in Kathryn Strother Ratcliff et al., eds., *Healing Technology: Feminist Perspectives*. Ann Arbor: The University of Michigan Press.

Overall, Christine. 1987. *Ethics and Human Reproduction: A Feminist Analysis* Winchester, MA: Allen & Unwin.

Petchesky, Rosalind Pollack. 1980. "Reproductive Freedom: Beyond 'A Woman's Right to Choose,'" in

Catharine R. Stimpson and Ethel Spector Person, eds., *Women: Sex and Sexuality*. Chicago: University of Chicago Press.

——. 1984. *Abortion and Woman's Choice: The State, Sexuality, and Reproductive Freedom*. Boston: Northeastern University Press.

Sumner, L.W. 1981. *Abortion and Moral Theory*. Princeton: Princeton University Press.

Thomson, Judith Jarvis. 1971. "A Defense of Abortion," *Philosophy and Public Affairs*, 1: 47-66.

Tooley, Michael. 1972. "Abortion and Infanticide," *Philosophy and Public Affairs*, 2, 1 (Fall): 37-65.

Van Wagner, Vicki, and Bob Lee. 1989. "Principles into Practice: An Activist Vision of Feminist Reproductive Health Care," in Christine Overall, ed., *The Future of Human Reproduction*. Toronto: The Women's Press.

Warren, Mary Anne. 1973. "On the Moral and Legal Status of Abortion," *The Monist*, 57: 43-61.

——. 1989. "The Moral Significance of Birth," *Hypatia*, 4, 2 (Summer): 46-65.

Whitbeck, Carolyn. 1973. "Theories of Sex Difference," *The Philosophic Forum*, 5, 1-2 (Fall/Winter 1973-74): 54-80.

28.
WINNIPEG CHILD AND FAMILY SERVICES (NORTHWEST AREA) V. G. (D.F.) [1997] SUPREME COURT OF CANADA

Case Summary by C. Morano

SOURCE: http://scc.lexum.org/en/1997/1997scr3-925/1997scr3-925.html.

[This case focuses on the rights of the mother as an autonomous decision maker and on the legal status of the fetus until birth. The court determined that any right or interest of the fetus remains incomplete until after birth.]

Present: Lamer C.J. and La Forest, L'Heureux-Dubé, Sopinka, Gonthier, Cory, McLachlin, Iacobucci and Major JJ.

Background

The respondent was five months pregnant with her fourth child and she was addicted to glue sniffing, which could damage the nervous system of the fetus. As a result of her addiction, two of her previous children are permanently disabled and are permanent wards of the state. On a motion by the appellant, a superior court judge ordered that the respondent be placed in the custody of the director of child and family services and detained in a health centre for treatment until the birth of the child. The Court of Appeal held that the law of *parens patriae*, which is the power of the court to act in the best interests of a child, did not support the order. Given the complexity of extending the law to permit such an order, the court of appeal concluded that this was more of a task for the legislature, rather than the courts to carry out. The defendant remained voluntarily at the health centre until she was discharged in August and stopped sniffing glue. In December she gave birth to an apparently normal child that is she is now raising.

The Supreme Court of Canada

A majority of the Supreme Court concluded that the appeal should be dismissed. Speaking on behalf of the Majority, McLachlin J. pointed out that the appeal raises two legal issues: first, "Does tort law as it exists or may properly be extended by the court, permit an order detaining a pregnant woman against her will in order to protect her unborn child from conduct that may harm the child?"; the second is whether or not the court's *parens patriae* jurisdiction as it exists or may properly be extended by the court to permit such an order? With respect to the first legal issue, McLachlin stated, "the law of Canada does not recognize the unborn child as a legal or juridical person. Once a child is born, alive and viable, the law may recognize that its existence began before birth for certain limited purposes. But the only right recognized is that of the born person. This is a general proposition, applicable to all aspects of the law, including the law of torts." McLachlin referred to the case of *Tremblay v. Daigle*, where it was established that any right or interest that the fetus may have remains inchoate and incomplete until the child's birth. In terms of whether or not the law of tort should be extended to permit such an order, McLachlin held that such a change was too drastic to be left up to the common law: "To permit intervention prior to birth in recognition of a duty of care owed to the fetus in utero would constitute a major departure from the common law as it has stood for decades." Recognizing a duty of care owed by a mother to her child for negligent prenatal behavior may create a conflict between the pregnant woman as an autonomous decision maker and her fetus. It would increase the level of outside scrutiny that she would be subjected to. Partners, parents, friends, and neighbours are among the potential classes of people who might monitor the pregnant woman's actions to ensure that they remain within the legal parameters. Difficulty in determining what conduct is and is not permissible might be expected to give rise to conflicts between the interested persons and the pregnant woman.

The second issue raised by this case is whether *parens patriae* can be extended to permit the order of detention in this particular case. McLachlin found that the *parens patriae* power of the courts over born children permits the courts to override the liberty of the parents to make decisions on behalf of their children where a parental choice may result in harm to the child, but extending *parens patriae* to unborn children would affect a much broader range of interests. Not only would the parent's power to make decisions for his or her child be affected, but the court would end up making decisions for the mother herself. It would seriously intrude on the rights of the woman. Therefore, *parens patriae* does not support the order for the detention of the respondent. This would not be an incremental change, but a drastic one that the legislature is in a much better position to decide.

29.
IGNORANCE, INDETERMINACY, AND ABORTION POLICY

Peter Alward

SOURCE: *The Journal of Value Inquiry* 41.2-4 (2007): 183-200.

It is commonly assumed in discussions of abortion that the moral question and the policy question coincide, that a legal prohibition of abortion is justified if and only if abortion is morally wrong. It should be noted, however, that even if this bi-conditional holds in the special case of abortion, moral questions and policy questions do not generally coincide. Lying and promise-breaking, for example, are morally wrong, but a legal prohibition of these activities is unlikely to be justified. More controversially, Sunday shopping prohibitions might be justified by appeal to the detrimental effects on families that ensue when parents are forced to work on the days their children are home from school. It would be difficult, however, to establish that buying and selling goods on Sundays, as opposed to Saturdays or Mondays, is morally suspect.

The lesson that can be drawn here is that the connection between moral questions and policy questions is loose enough that they can at least in principle be answered independently. This is important because abortion policies have serious consequences for women and yet the moral question increasingly appears to be intractable. We will consider the extent to which justification can be found for policies governing abortion in the absence of any definitive answer to question of the morality of abortion.

The Moral Question

The most prominent approach to the moral question centers on the notion of moral personhood. According to advocates of this approach, the moral question reduces to the question of whether or not the biologically human organism, which comes into existence at conception, acquires the status of moral personhood before birth. If an unborn human being is, at some time, a person with a right to life, then, ceteris paribus, abortion is seriously morally wrong at that time, and if an unborn human being is not a person, at some time, then abortion is more or less morally unproblematic at that time. Broadly speaking, there are three positions someone can take vis-à-vis personhood: the conservative position, the liberal position, and the moderate position. According to conservatives, unborn human beings acquire personhood at or soon after conception. According to liberals, human beings become persons only at or after birth. According to moderates, unborn human beings acquire personhood gradually, starting out as nonpersons at conception and ending up as persons by the time they are born.

The conservative position on personhood faces two serious difficulties. It is far too inclusive; and it leaves open an insurmountable explanatory gap between the physical or biological properties of the entities to which personhood is attributed and the moral properties that come with having this status. The first difficulty is that if human beings at or near conception are persons, then all relevantly similar entities are persons as well. But since human beings at this stage are merely integrated clusters of cells, the conservative position seems to imply that all relevantly similar integrated cell clusters are persons. Moreover, the only available strategies to restrict personhood are either unjustifiably chauvinistic or empirically suspect. The second difficulty is that an explanation is required as to why entities of this kind are persons with a right to life and other moral entitlements, and no such explanation is forthcoming. What we find in the literature are equivocations between biological humanity and moral personhood and obscurities, as well as various theological appeals.[1] This paucity of plausible explanation is not surprising. There is simply no reason to believe that anything about a small cluster of cells entitles it to the protection that comes with personhood.

The liberal position runs into related difficulties. It is too exclusive; and although plausible explanations of the possession of moral properties are given in core cases, an explanatory gap emerges in important residual cases. Liberals normally take the mark of personhood to be the possession of certain higher-order cognitive capacities which can be roughly characterized as rational self-consciousness. The trouble is some human beings that are normally thought of as entitled to the moral protection which comes with personhood, such as infants and small children, the severely developmentally challenged, and human beings suffering from extreme senility, lack these capacities. The standard liberal strategy for handling such cases is to take the moral protection to which such human beings are entitled to stem from the value placed upon them by other persons.[2] But not only does this render these otherwise vulnerable human beings morally vulnerable to the vicissitudes of the human heart, it also yields moral protection for at least some unborn human beings. Moreover, any attempt to exclude unborn human beings from such protection will likely prove ad hoc.

In addition, liberals typically analyze personhood in terms of the possession of a desire or interest in continued existence, or in terms of actual or hypothetical contractual agreements into which persons have entered to refrain from killing each other.[3] Both approaches require higher order cognitive capacities including, among other things, the possession of a self-concept and the concept of this self existing in the future. But there are human beings who possess the relevant capacities who do not desire continued existence or have not, and would not, entered into contractual agreements of that kind. This includes not only those who are depressed, unconscious, or indoctrinated, but also people who just happen to be dark or angry or uncooperative.[4] Moreover, liberal attempts to explain why such human beings are nevertheless persons remain unpersuasive.[5]

The moderate position on personhood does better than both liberals and the conservatives on the extension of the concept of a person, excluding many of the entities conservatives include and including many which liberals exclude. Typically, moderates identify personhood with sentience, which consists in being conscious and having the capacities to feel pleasure and pain and to perceive.[6] They also take the moral protection afforded by personhood to come in degrees: unborn human beings acquire minimal protection at the onset of sentience and come to have quite strong protection as a result of their rather more complex conscious states at the time of birth. As a result, most simple cell-clusters turn out not to be persons, and infants and the senile turn out to possess personhood. Nevertheless, the moderate position does run afoul of the explanatory gap problem. It is plausible that an entity with even minimal sentience has interests which entitle to it to some kind of moral protection. An entity with the capacity for pleasure and pain, for example, has an interest in not suffering pain, and this may well obligate others to refrain from engaging in any course of action that would cause it pain. But the issue here is with abortion, which kills unborn human beings. The fact that an entity has an interest in not undergoing pain does not entail that it has an interest in continued existence. Hence any moral protection to which it is entitled as a result of this former interest does not protect it from being killed, as long as it is killed painlessly. More generally, it is far from clear how a moderate could explain why an entity which is sentient but lacking higher order cognitive capacities could have the kind of interests that would ground a right to continued existence, regardless of what other interests it might have.

There have been a number of solutions offered to the moral question of abortion which do not strictly speaking hang on the issue of personhood. Proponents of one prominent approach appeal to the potential properties of unborn human beings rather than their currently actualized properties. Underlying such appeals to potentiality is a basic strategy shared by valuable-future accounts of the wrongness of killing, latent-capacity accounts of unborn persons, and some conservative, and even some liberal, accounts of personhood.[7] Proponents of the strategy proceed by first identifying a diachronic relation of some kind, and then claiming that whenever a non-person stands in this relation to a future person, the non-person inherits the moral protection to which the future person is entitled. The diachronic relation can be taken to be either an identity relation or a continuity relation. Moreover, since the future is uncertain, the non-person is typically required only to likely stand in this relation to a future person in order to inherit the desired moral protection.

This diachronic strategy, however, runs into the same sorts of difficulties that infected the various positions on personhood. There is reason to believe that at least some diachronic relations are too inclusive, yielding moral protection to the material precursors to conception and other entities subjected to currently hypothetical technological interventions.[8] Attempts to exclude such entities by appeal to substantial change or the absence of a subject of harm, while not entirely implausible, nevertheless do have an air of ad hoc-ness to them.[9] In addition, an analogue of the explanatory gap problem arises for the diachronic strategy. Just as an explanation is needed from advocates of various positions regarding personhood as to why their favored entities are entitled to the moral protection that comes with this status, an explanation is needed from advocates of the diachronic strategy as to why standing in some such diachronic relationship to a person enables an entity to inherit the moral protection due a person. No such explanation, however, is forthcoming. There is simply no reason to think that non-persons who happen to stand in such diachronic relations to future persons thereby acquire interests that can be frustrated by being killed or otherwise treated as a non-person. Without the acquisition of such interests, the inheritance of moral protection is simply mysterious.

Finally, Judith Jarvis Thomson has attempted to avoid the personhood argument by arguing that abortion is permissible in most cases, even if the unborn human being is a person.[10] According to Thomson, a right to life does not entitle a person to the bare minimum needed to survive. In depriving someone of what she needs to survive, a person does not thereby violate her right to life. Since what abortion does is merely deprive an unborn human being of what it needs to survive, continued use of the pregnant woman's body, abortion does not violate its right to life, although in some circumstances it may nevertheless be morally indecent. The trouble with Thom-

son's argument is that many abortion techniques involve killing the unborn rather than merely removing it from the woman's body. Hence, by Thomson's own lights, many abortions violate the unborn human being's right to life.[11] More to the point, Thomson attaches far too much moral significance to the distinction between killing and letting die. Someone could, for example, imagine circumstances in which the bare minimum someone needs to survive is continued use of a ledge high up on a skyscraper. Thomson's view seems to imply that someone with proprietary rights over this ledge could permissibly push the interloper off to her death if there was no other available exit, but it would be a serious rights violation to stab her to death. The distinction between killing and letting die may not be as morally flimsy as James Rachels would have us believe, but it could not be as load-bearing as all that.[12] Finally, since Thomson's argument entails that a pregnant woman has the right to remove the unborn human being from her body but not to secure its death, it does not fully address the moral question of abortion. The point of having an abortion is not merely to terminate a continued state of pregnancy, or even to avoid a life path encumbered by the responsibilities of parenthood. It is to prevent the existence of a person to whom the woman stands in a special biological relationship. Only given the contingencies of current fetal-removal techniques and incubator technology does Thomson's argument secure rights for pregnant women that will satisfy most abortion rights advocates.

The lesson of this discussion is that the moral problem of abortion increasingly appears to be intractable. The fact that there is no currently adequate solution to it does not by itself show this problem to be intractable. After all, advocates of the various views considered here might eventually be able to solve the difficulties they face, or some other less problematic solution might be developed. But there are few grounds for optimism on this count. Not only is it far from clear how someone might go about solving these difficulties, or what shape a novel solution might take, the fact that the vast amount of intellectual labor that has thus far been spent on the moral problem has yielded so little progress suggests that further attempts to solve it may prove futile.

Even if the considerations raised here fall short of establishing the intractability of the moral problem, they do suffice to show that we currently lack knowledge concerning the morality of abortion. In particular, they show that we currently lack sufficient justification for our moral beliefs about abortion for moral knowledge, even if these beliefs are true. Nevertheless there still might be some evidence that counts more weakly in favor of one or more views concerning the status of unborn human beings or the morality of abortion. Someone might, for example, point to the putative fact that one of the views considered here coheres better with our background moral knowledge than the alternatives as evidence for the view. Whether or not there is any weak evidence of this kind regarding the morality of abortion will not be adjudicated here. Instead, a preliminary assumption will be made to the effect that we are in a state of complete ignorance, and an account of what kind of abortion policy would be appropriate under such conditions will be developed. Subsequently, the issue of what difference it makes if we have some such weak evidence will be considered.

Justifying Policy

Before going on to consider the justification of abortion policy under conditions of ignorance, it is worth pausing to say a few things about the justification of policy more generally. The kinds of policies at issue are policies which prohibit or place restrictions on classes of behavior, which are normally backed by the threat of legal sanction for failure to comply. What is important to note about such policies is that they restrict the liberty of people to engage in behavior in which they otherwise might be inclined to engage. For present purposes it will simply be assumed that ceteris paribus restricting liberty in this way is seriously wrong and, hence, that justifying such policies is a matter of justifying the restrictions on liberty that they require.[13]

There are three central kinds of arguments used to justify policies which restrict liberty: harm arguments, paternalistic arguments, and utilitarian arguments. Advocates of harm arguments attempt to justify restrictions on behavior by appeal to the

detrimental effects of such behavior on people other than the agents who engage in it.[14] Harm arguments are clearly relevant to abortion policy. Since abortion kills the unborn human being, if the entity is a person, then this behavior causes serious harm to a moral person. As a result, if the unborn human being is a person, policies prohibiting or severely restricting abortion are presumably justified, even though they place significant restrictions on the liberty of pregnant or, more generally, fertile women.

Paternalistic and utilitarian arguments are, however, less relevant to abortion policy. Advocates of paternalistic arguments attempt to justify restrictions on behavior by appeal to the detrimental effects of the behavior on the agents who engage in it.[15] Normally paternalistic considerations are persuasive only when the restrictions on liberty are minimal and the harm risked by the restricted behavior is severe, or when the policy in question applies only to agents who are not competent to make decisions regarding the behavior in question. Legislation requiring seat belt use, or prohibiting underage drinking, for example, might be justified on paternalistic grounds. In the case of abortion, such considerations might justify requiring that abortions be done by licensed practitioners, or requiring that legal proxies make abortion decisions on behalf of those deemed incompetent. But given the significant effect on women's life paths that carrying a child to term can have, as well as the increased health risks, paternalistic considerations are unlikely to justify substantial restrictions on abortion.

Advocates of utilitarian arguments attempt to justify restrictions on behavior by appeal to the societal benefits that will likely ensue, rather than by appeal to the effects of such behavior on those directly involved in it. As with paternalism, utilitarian considerations are persuasive only when the restrictions on liberty in question are quite minimal and the societal benefits are significant. For example, given that being prohibited from shopping is for most of us merely a minor inconvenience, a Sunday shopping ban might be justified on utilitarian grounds. But, as above, prohibitions of abortion place a significant restriction on the freedom of women, and it remains unclear what sort of societal benefit such a restriction would accrue.

Given their importance to the justification of abortion policy, it is worth pausing to look at harm arguments in more detail. The question that needs to be addressed is what kinds of behavior-restricting policies can be justified by appeal to such arguments. In general, this is a function of three factors: the nature and severity of the harm caused by the behavior; the intimacy of the connection between the behavior and the harm; and the extent to which the behavior-restricting policy would interfere with the pursuit by people of their central goals and life paths.

The kinds of behavioral effects that count as harms include both physical damage and psychological damage to an organism, as well as interference with autonomy and the deprivation of property. Because these sorts of behavioral consequences come in degrees, the harmfulness of a species of behavior can be loosely measured in terms of the severity of its effect upon its victim, where ceteris paribus the limiting case is causing death. What is important to note, however, is that, for the purpose of harm arguments, such effects count as harms only if the victim is entitled to moral protection from that sort of treatment. If, for example, rats are not entitled to moral protection from psychological damage, then a policy prohibiting the use of rodent repellents that emit high frequency screeching noises cannot be justified on harm grounds, even if the noises do severe damage to rat minds.

The behavior a legislator might want to restrict or prohibit can be more or less intimately connected to the harm which justifies restricting or prohibiting it. The most intimate connection is a definitional connection. In such cases, the criteria for successfully engaging in the behavior are such that an agent cannot do so without causing the harm. For example, a person cannot commit homicide without causing someone's death. A strong but less intimate connection exists in cases in which the behavior in question generates a high risk of harm. A person can, for example, successfully perform the act of driving drunk without harming anyone, but in so doing generates an unacceptably high risk of harm to others, at least under normal circumstances.[16] The connection between the behavior and the risk of harm might be thought of as more or less direct if little can feasibly be done to reduce the risk to acceptable levels short

of prohibiting the behavior altogether. There are, however, cases in which the connection between some species of behavior and the risk it generates is more or less indirect. In such cases, the risk of harm is somewhat causally downstream of the behavior which generates it. For example, alcohol consumption generates a risk of harm to others; people under the influence of alcohol are much more likely to commit assaults of various kinds, as well as being more dangerous when operating heavy machinery. But while the risks generated by drunk driving cannot be alleviated without prohibiting it, the risks generated by alcohol consumption can arguably be adequately reduced without prohibiting drinking, by instead prohibiting public drinking and drunkenness.

The final factor in harm arguments for behavior-restricting policies is the significance of the behavior at issue to individuals who engage in it. Although no precise measure of behavioral significance can be made, there are a few general things that can be said. We can distinguish between behavior which is an end in itself and behavior which is engaged in as a means to some further end. Normally, behavior whose value is instrumental is less significant than behavior whose value is intrinsic. After all, any other behavior which yielded the ultimately desired outcome would serve as well. Shopping on Sunday, for example, is a means of acquiring goods whose use may be intrinsically valuable; but Saturday or Monday shopping would serve just as well. The main exception occurs when the behavior in question is the only readily available means to achieve the end at which it is directed. In such circumstances, the significance of the behavior approaches the significance of the end at issue. In addition, we can distinguish between intrinsically valuable behaviors which correspond to central ends and behaviors which correspond to peripheral ends. Even if, for example, many people value driving without wearing a seatbelt as an end in itself, for most of them this is a much more peripheral end than ends connected with their personal relationships, their careers, and their hobbies. Finally, we can distinguish between discrete ends, such as having a vacation in Cuba, and valued life paths, such as being a philosopher. In general, policies which prevent someone from pursuing a valued life path place a more significant restriction on freedom than do policies which prevent the satisfaction of more discrete ends.

In order to justify behavior-restricting policies by appeal to harm arguments it has to be established that the expected harm of the behavior in question sufficiently outweighs its typical significance. The expected harm of species of behavior is, roughly, the product of the severity of harm the behavior could cause and the likelihood it will cause such harm. Given that a number of different harms of varying likelihoods might ensue from any given type of behavior, a more accurate formula for expected harm is the sum of the products of the severity and likelihood of each possible harm. By itself, however, that the expected harm of some behavior is high does not justify a policy prohibiting it. For example, the expected psychological harm of breaking off romantic relationships is reasonably high, but a policy prohibiting break-ups would nevertheless remain unjustified. Whether or not some such policy is justified depends also on the significance of the behavior to individuals who would otherwise engage in it. Most behavior varies in its significance to members of a population. As a result, the justification of policy prohibiting the behavior will have to be framed in terms of its significance to the average or typical member of that population. Only when the expected harm of a species of behavior sufficiently outweighs its significance to the typical member of a population is a policy prohibiting or restricting that behavior by members of the population justified. If the behavior is more or less directly connected to the harm, a policy prohibiting it would be justified. If the behavior is more or less indirectly connected to the harm, only a policy regulating it is likely to be justified.

Let us consider, by way of comparison, drunk driving and breaking off romantic entanglements. The expected harm of both sorts of behavior is relatively high: the potential harm of the former is very severe, but its occurrence is only somewhat likely; the potential harm of the latter is somewhat less severe but a lot more certain. Nevertheless prohibitions of drunk driving are justified on harm grounds whereas prohibitions against ending romantic relationships on the same basis would not be. The central difference is that ending romantic relationships is of far

greater significance to typical members of society than is driving drunk.

Driving drunk is for most people merely a means of returning home or to some other desirable location after a bout of drinking. Not only are there normally other available means to this end, such as taxis, the end itself can hardly be counted among the most important ends for typical people, although it is not entirely insignificant. In contrast, romantic relationships are among the most important aspects of the lives of typical people, and being able to break off relationships is essential to their ability to shape and nurture this central facet of their lives. Given this difference in significance, a much higher expectation of harm would be required to justify prohibiting break ups than is required to prohibit drunk driving.

Ignorance and the Policy Question

Let us consider harm arguments for the prohibition of abortion. The first thing to note is that the significance of this activity is very high. It is the only effective means available to a pregnant woman of avoiding the disruptions to her life that may occur during the nine month period of pregnancy, disruptions which may interfere with valued relationships, her chosen career, and other things of importance to her. Moreover, it is the most effective means of avoiding the whole scale usurpation of a valued life path by the responsibilities of parenthood that could ensue were the pregnancy carried to term. This could also be avoided by putting the child up for adoption. But it can be very difficult for a woman to bring herself to give away a child to which she has given birth, and in so doing she risks feelings of guilt and remorse, as well as other more serious psychological problems. In addition, adoption yields the existence of a person to whom the woman stands in a unique biological relationship; thus a woman who chooses the adoption route thereby risks future interference in her chosen life path as a result of demands for a personal relationship or claims made on her resources, for example, which the existence of such a person might yield.

Given that abortion is a species of behavior with a high degree of significance, the expected harm of this behavior would have to be very high in order for it to be justifiably prohibited on harm grounds. The outcome of abortion which might count as a harm is the death of the unborn human being, which is a near certainty. But whether or not this yields a high enough expectation of harm to justify an anti-abortion policy depends on the moral status of unborn human beings. If it is a moral person with a full right to life then expected harm of abortion is certainly high enough to justify a policy prohibiting it. If it is not a person, then there is no expected harm at all; hence a policy prohibiting abortion could not be justified. The problem is that, as argued above, we simply do not know whether or not the unborn human being is a person.

Nevertheless an abortion policy must be adopted, even if it is a policy of refraining from placing any restrictions on access to abortion. Given the effect of abortion policy on the interests of women and its possible effect on the interests of unborn human beings, inaction is not morally neutral. Moreover, policy is regularly formed under conditions of at least partial ignorance. The standard against which such policy is appropriately evaluated is not the judgment of a transcendent omniscient legislator of some kind. Instead, it should be evaluated by the standard of some similarly situated, epistemically responsible legislator. In what follows, a number of cases in which policy might be required under conditions of ignorance will be considered. From these cases a number of general principles will be derived which can then be applied to the case of abortion policy. For present purposes, it will be assumed that newborn babies are persons with a full right to life and that the precursors to conception are morally insignificant. Initially, it will also be assumed that we are completely ignorant of the moral status of the unborn human being throughout the whole period from conception to birth, that at no point during gestation do we have any evidence one way or the other as to whether the entity is a person. Subsequently, we will consider the difference it makes if at various points during this period, if we take ourselves to have some reason to believe the unborn human being is or is not a person.

Let us consider first the following case which is modeled on the market in artworks in Europe after World War II, many of whose exchanges involved works plundered from museums and private collections during the war. Let us suppose that a couple of generations after a major conflict, a large body of artworks produced prior to the conflict are in the possession of a number of museums, private collectors and art dealers. Moreover, let us suppose that there are few if any records establishing ownership of the works immediately prior to or during the conflict and, hence, that there is no evidence that some, all, or none of the artworks came into the possession of their current possessors by means of theft or plunder. Finally, let us suppose that as a matter of law, any artworks that were plundered during the conflict are the property of the legal heirs of those from who they were taken, rather than their current possessors.

The question to be raised here is whether or not a policy prohibiting the buying and selling of the artworks would be justified under such circumstances. The first thing to note is that if the artworks were known, as a matter of fact, to belong to their current possessors, such a policy would not be justified. People are, after all, entitled to buy and sell their property more or less as they choose. If the artworks were known not to belong to their current possessors, this prohibition would be justified. It would, in effect, simply be a prohibition against buying and selling a class of stolen goods. But in the case at hand, the artworks are neither known to belong to their possessors nor known not to belong to their possessors. There is simply no evidence one way or the other. Given the epistemological situation in which legislators in the hypothetical society find themselves, a prohibition of market transactions involving the artworks in question cannot be justified. A policy prohibiting the behavior would involve a restriction of people's freedom to engage in a species of behavior without any evidence that the behavior harms the interests of anyone else. There is not any evidence that it does not harm the interests of third parties. But, on the view being defended here, this is not relevant. What is, in effect, being suggested is that there is an epistemic presumption in favor of freedom: behavior-restricting policies are justified only if there is evidence that the behavior is harmful.

If this presumption is applied to the case of abortion policy and, as we have been assuming, we are completely ignorant of the status of the unborn human being from conception to birth, then it follows that any policy prohibiting abortion is unjustified. There are, however, at least three ways someone might go about resisting this conclusion. She might deny that there is any presumption in favor of freedom, even in the hypothetical artwork case. Alternatively, she might appeal to dissimilarities between the artwork example and the case of abortion and argue that they show that the presumption does not apply to the case of abortion, or is overridden by other considerations. Finally, she could argue that, despite the arguments presented above, we have at least some evidence concerning the status of the unborn human being and that this evidence suffices for at least some restrictions to abortion. The first strategy is a non-starter. To say that the freedom to engage in a species of behavior can be justifiably restricted in the absence of any evidence of harm is incompatible with any claim of the substantive value of freedom. The other two strategies are more promising.

One disanalogy between the artwork example and abortion is that even if it turns out that the possessor of a work is not its real owner, by selling the work the possessor does not undermine the owner's interests in any substantial way. After all, the legitimate owner is not any worse off when her artwork comes to be newly in the possession of a buyer than she was when it was previously in the possession of the seller. But if it turns out that an unborn human being is a person, an abortion seriously undermines that person's interests. It might be argued on this basis that the possibility of genuine harm to the interests of affected parties by a species of behavior overrides any epistemic presumption there might be in favor of the freedom to engage in that behavior.

This sort of concern can be addressed by changing our hypothetical case as follows. Instead of artworks, let us suppose that a couple of generations after the conflict a large quantity of fine wine of a pre-conflict vintage is in the possession of a number of high end retailers, fancy restaurants, and individual wine connoisseurs. Let us assume again that few if any records establishing ownership of the works immediately prior to or during the conflict exist and, hence, that there is no evidence that some, all, or none of the wine came to be possessed by their current possessors as a result of the wartime plunder of wine cellars. Moreover, let us suppose that the behavior we might want to prohibit is not buying and selling the wine, but rather consuming it.

It is clear that even a prohibition of the consumption of the wine in question would be unjustified in these circumstances. Prohibiting individuals, who for all anyone knows are the legitimate possessors of some good, from enjoying the benefits of the good without any evidence that in so doing they are harming others is simply unjustifiable. Someone might urge a course of caution and defend a prohibition of consuming the wine until such a time as all the evidence comes in. But a policy of this kind risks overgeneralization. For example, from time to time people come home with extra bags of groceries belonging to other customers. A similar course of caution might count in favor of holding off eating any groceries, even when there is no reason to suppose they have been misdirected, until clear title has been established. Moreover, in the case at hand, there is no reason to suppose that any new evidence is forthcoming. Under such circumstances, waiting for the evidence to come in might require waiting indefinitely, in effect depriving the possessors of the wine of its central benefit. Finally, if the goods in question are perishable merely temporarily delaying consumption can deprive their possessors of their benefits. It is worth reiterating that the policy of caution at issue has this effect in the absence of any evidence that the goods do not belong to their possessors.

Another disanalogy between the hypothetical cases discussed thus far and abortion is that even if the possessor of an artwork or some wine is not its owner, the behavior at issue only has the effect of depriving the real owner of some property. But if an unborn human being is a person, an abortion severely harms the person herself. Someone might argue that the possibility of serious harm to a person overrides any epistemic presumption in favor of freedom, even if the possibility of harm to a person's property does not.

There is, however, another kind of case which may shed some light here. Let us suppose that there is a tissue transplant technique which can be used not only to cure conditions which risk harm to a patient's life or health, but also to rectify defects of various kinds which impede her pursuit of valued life paths. Let us suppose also that living donors could not survive the tissue-extraction process. Hence, ignoring the possibility of volunteers, the only sources of the tissue are cadavers and people killed for the purpose. Finally, let us suppose that, for whatever reason, there are no records or any other evidence of the origin of the tissue in any given case, or evidence of other facts that would indicate the general likelihood of one or the other source of tissue. There is simply no reason to believe that some, all, or none of the tissue used in the various instances of the procedure was procured from people murdered for this purpose.

The question is whether or not a policy of prohibiting this tissue transplant technique would be justified under these circumstances. Again, a policy of this sort would involve restricting the freedom of people to engage in a species of behavior without any evidence that it is harmful. As a result, such a policy would be suspect for the reasons advanced above. It might be objected that because the possible harm of the procedure is so severe and because typical patients value undergoing the procedure only as a means to achieve some further end, it is reasonable to permit people to use only alternate means to the same end. But appeals to possible harm cannot reasonably be used as a basis for justifying behavior-restricting policies. If a person is unlucky enough, practically any course of action could cause severe harm to others. This is why the likelihood of harm has to be sufficiently high before a policy restricting the behavior is appropriate. Moreover, while it could be conceded that an unknown expectation of harm suffices to justify prohibiting behavior with mere instrumental value as long there are there are equally effective and accessible alternatives available, if there are no effective or accessible alternative procedures it certainly does not do so. It would, in effect, amount to requiring people to forgo the benefits of a procedure which, for all anyone knows, is entirely harmless; and this is especially unpalatable when the benefits in question, such as prolonged life, improved health, and unimpeded pursuit of a chosen life path, are highly significant to the typical patient.

Finally, it might be objected that, unlike the hypothetical cases we have been considering, we are not in a state of complete ignorance regarding the moral status of unborn human beings. Someone might, for example, present an argument along the following lines. We know that normal newborn human beings are persons, even if we do not know why they are persons. It is unlikely that birth marks a morally significant transition in the life of a human organism. After all, there are no typical differences between human beings just before birth and just after birth that are likely to support the difference in moral status that exists between persons and non-persons. Hence, it is reasonably likely that unborn human beings near the point of birth are persons. An analogous argument which appealed to the similarity between unborns immediately after conception and either the precursors of conception or non-human cell-clusters could be taken to establish the unlikelihood that early-term unborns are persons as well.

This is not an implausible argument, although some might balk at the suggestion that we know newborn human beings are persons. After all, if we do not know what features make newborns persons, whatever reasons we have for thinking they nonetheless are persons likely do not provide sufficient justification to yield knowledge. Nevertheless if we do assume that newborns are persons with a full right to life, the high degree of similarity between newborns and unborn human beings immediately prior to birth and the near certainty that an abortion procedure will result in the death of an unborn human being together render the expected harm of late-term abortions high. Behavior that, for example, has an even chance of killing what is definitely a person has the same expected harm as behavior that will certainly kill what has an even chance of being a person. But even given this assumption, the radical dissimilarity between newborns and newly conceived human beings renders this argument impotent to establish that earlier term abortions have any expected harm. Similarity considerations presumably establish that at some point midterm abortions begin having increasing degrees of expected harm, again given our assumption about the moral status of newborns.

In absence of any other putative evidence for or against the personhood of unborn human beings, these sorts of considerations have the following implications for the justification of abortion policy. Since no reason has been provided for thinking newly conceived human beings are persons, there is no more justification for prohibiting early-term abortions than there is for prohibiting the behavior discussed in the hypothetical cases above. In addition, given the typical significance of abortion to pregnant women, relatively high levels of expected harm must be tolerated before a policy prohibiting it would be justified. As a result, any prohibition of mid-term abortions is unlikely to be justified. Finally, given the higher degree of expected harm from late term abortions, a policy placing broad restrictions on it would likely be justified. But it is worth emphasizing that this is all premised on the assumption that newborn human beings are persons. If reasonable grounds can be found to deny personhood to newborns, all bets are off.

From Ignorance to Indeterminacy

It may prove fruitful to conclude with a discussion of the possibility that it is simply indeterminate whether or not unborn human beings are persons. Not only is indeterminacy the metaphysical analogue of that epistemic vice ignorance, one tempting explanation of our failure to determine the moral status of unborn human beings is because their moral status is indeterminate. Since the jury is out on the inference from ignorance to indeterminacy, this suggestion does not yet provide any grounds for rethinking the conclusions drawn above regarding abortion policy. But there are some interesting parallels between the effect of ignorance on the policy question and the effect of indeterminacy on the moral question.

To say that the moral status of unborn human beings is indeterminate is to say that neither the criteria for being a person nor the criteria for being a non-person apply to unborn human beings. It is useful to distinguish between what might be called complete and graduated indeterminacy. If the indeterminacy is complete, then no sense can be attached to the idea that some unborn human beings are more or less person-like and others are more or less non-person-like, or even that they are all equally person-like

and non-person-like. The idea here is that to have any degree of personhood an entity must meet all of the personhood criteria and to have any degree of non-personhood an entity must meet all of the non-personhood criteria, but unborn human beings meet neither set of criteria. If the indeterminacy is graduated, then an unborn human being can fail to be either a person or non-person, but nevertheless can have a high degree of personhood by meeting a large number of the personhood criteria or a high degree of non-personhood by meeting a large number of the non-personhood criteria.

If the status of the unborn human being is completely indeterminate, the morality of abortion, arguably at least, is indeterminate as well. After all, abortion is morally permissible if and only if the reproductive rights of the pregnant woman outweigh the putative right to life of the unborn human being, assuming the life or health of the woman is not at risk. If the unborn is a person, then its right to life outweighs reproductive rights, and if it is not a person, it does not have a right to life and reproductive rights trump. But if there is no fact of the matter as to whether the unborn is a person with a right to life, then there is no fact of the matter whether reproductive rights are outweighed by a right to life. Someone might appeal to a moral analogue of the epistemic presumption invoked above and argue that exercising reproductive rights is impermissible only if in so doing a woman violates the determinate moral entitlements of other parties. For present purpose, the defensibility of some such argument will not be addressed. If, however, the indeterminacy in the status of the unborn human being is graduated, then there is, at least in principle, a determinate answer to the moral question of abortion. Because recently conceived unborn human beings presumably have a low degree of personhood, if any, reproductive rights of women are trumping; hence early-term abortions are morally unproblematic. Moreover, because unborn human beings just prior to birth presumably have a high degree of personhood, late-term abortions are impermissible except to preserve the woman's life or health. Finally, although unborn human beings come to have a non-negligible degree of personhood by the mid-point of pregnancy, given the importance of reproductive rights, they presumably outweigh the relatively weak right to life that comes with low to medium degrees of personhood.

This is, in effect, the solution to the moral question endorsed by advocates of the moderate position on personhood, and it coheres nicely with the solution to the policy question defended on epistemic grounds above. There is a reasonably broad consensus that there ought to be few or no restrictions on early-term abortions and fairly serious restrictions on late-term abortions. As a result, many people find the moderate position intuitively very appealing. But as we have seen, this view, along with its competitors, runs into serious difficulties. The advantage of the approach defended here is that it retains the intuitive appeal of the moderate position but provides these intuitions with a firmer theoretical basis.

Notes

1 See John Noonan, "The Morality of Abortion: Legal and Historical Approaches," in Louis Pojman and Francis Beckwith, eds., *The Abortion Controversy: 25 Years After Roe v. Wade* 2nd Edition (Toronto: Wadsworth, 1998), p. 207, and John Finnis, "Abortion and Health Care Ethics," in Helga Kuhse and Peter Singer, eds., *Bioethics: An Anthology* 2nd Edition (Oxford: Blackwell, 2006), pp. 17-24.

2 See Louis Pojman, "Abortion: A Defense of the Personhood Argument," in Louis Pojman and Francis Beckwith, eds., op. cit., p. 286.

3 See Michael Tooley, "Abortion and Infanticide," in Helga Kuhse and Peter Singer, eds., op. cit., pp. 25-39.

4 Ibid, pp. 29-30.

5 See Michael Tooley, "In Defense of Abortion and Infanticide," in Louis Pojman and Francis Beckwith, eds., op. cit., p. 217.

6 See Wayne Sumner, *Abortion and Moral Theory* (Princeton, NJ: Princeton University Press, 1981).

7 See Don Marquis, "Why Abortion is Immoral," in Helga Kuhse and Peter Singer, eds., op. cit., pp. 51-62, Stephen Schwarz, *The Moral Question of Abortion* (Chicago: Loyola University Press, 1990), Finnis, op. cit., and Michael Tooley, "In Defense of Abortion and Infanticide," in Louis Pojman and Francis Beckwith, eds., op. cit., pp. 209-33.

8 See Michael Tooley, "Abortion and Infanticide," in Helga Kuhse and Peter Singer, eds., op. cit., p. 36.

9 See Finnis, op. cit., p. 19, and Marquis, op. cit., p. 61.

10 See Judith Jarvis Thomson, "A Defense of Abortion," *Philosophy and Public Affairs* 1 (1971).

11 See Peter Alward, "Thomson, the Right to Life, and Partial Birth Abortion," *Journal of Medical Ethics*, 28 (2002).

12 See James Rachels, "Active and Passive Euthanasia," *New England Journal of Medicine* 9 (1975).

13 See John Stuart Mill, *On Liberty* (London: Longman, Roberts & Green, 1869).

14 Ibid.

15 See Gerald Dworkin, "Paternalism," *The Monist* 56 (1972).

16 See Richard Parker, "Blame, Punishment, and the Role of Result," *American Philosophical Quarterly* 21 (1984).

30.
HOW IS THE ETHICS OF STEM CELL RESEARCH DIFFERENT FROM THE ETHICS OF ABORTION?

Elizabeth Harman

Source: *Metaphilosophy* 38.2-3 (2007): 207-24.

Destroying Leftover Embryos

While my central conclusions will concern the practice of creating and then destroying embryos to make stem cells, I will draw a conclusion about that practice by contrasting it with another method of using embryos to make stem cells: using embryos left over from fertility treatments. In order to do embryonic stem cell research, researchers need to extract the inner cell mass from early human embryos. The embryos are destroyed in the process.[1] Some stem cell researchers have extracted cells from frozen embryos that are left over from fertility treatments. The leftover embryos stand no practical chance of developing into persons; their fate has been sealed before the researchers have anything to do with them. This suggests the following argument: because the researchers do not themselves deprive the embryos of lives as persons, the researchers do not harm the embryos, and so there can be no objection on behalf of the embryos to the researchers' actions. One might point out that the researchers do destroy the embryos. But it does not seem to be better for the embryos to live on as frozen embryos than to be destroyed; what's bad for them is not getting to develop.

This argument is too quick as it stands. First, the mere fact that a bad outcome was going to befall someone anyway does not always make it permissible to ensure that outcome. If two assassins both independently target one victim, the one who gets there first is not off the hook because the other assassin was about to act (even if he knew that). Nevertheless, the fact that an outcome was going to happen anyway does often mitigate causing or ensuring that

outcome. A second way in which the argument is too quick is that it's not certain that any particular leftover embryo won't get to develop into a person. While this might seem inevitable, it's possible that the relevant people will decide to have this embryo implanted into a woman's womb: the embryo's parents might suddenly decide to donate it to aid an infertile couple. Because this small chance exists, the researchers do lower the probability that the embryo will get to develop into a person—they lower it from very low to zero—and so they do deprive the embryo of a chance (a small chance) of getting to live life as a person.

Thus, destroying a leftover embryo does harm the embryo by depriving it of the chance to live life as a person. This harm is not very serious, however, due to the fact that the embryo was very unlikely to get to live life as a person anyway.[2]

Now let's suppose that the destroyed embryo has the full moral status of a person. Because the harm to the embryo of being destroyed is not very serious, it seems the harm can be justified by consideration of the incredible benefits that may be gained from stem cell research. Thus, I conclude that extracting cells from leftover embryos is permissible, even on the assumption that these embryos have the full moral status of persons.

Harm and Moral Status

Note that my discussion above kept two questions separate: Does this action harm this thing? and Does this thing have moral status? These two questions are often not separated. Indeed, some philosophers have the substantive view that the things that have moral status are exactly the things that can be harmed. Thus, in the literature on the ethics of abortion there is a substantial tradition of arguing that fetuses are not harmed by abortions, because the deprivation of their futures is not bad for them, or because they are not really deprived of any futures. Yet it would clearly be very good for a fetus if it got to live on and have all the benefits involved in getting to be a person. Abortion thwarts a fetus's natural development and keeps it from getting these benefits. Thus, it is clear that fetuses are harmed by being aborted. But that does not settle whether there is thereby any moral reason against abortion; whether there is, depends on whether the harm to the fetus is a morally significant harm—it depends on whether the fetus has moral status.

To see that something can be susceptible to harm while lacking moral status, consider the example of a dandelion growing in my backyard. If I put a picnic table in my backyard, I deprive the dandelion of light. Clearly, this harms it. However, equally clearly, there is no moral reason at all against my putting the table there in virtue of the harm to the dandelion. The dandelion lacks moral status; harms to it simply do not provide reasons. Nevertheless, the dandelion can be harmed.

In the next section, I argue that if a researcher creates an embryo and then destroys the embryo to make stem cells, the researcher has significantly harmed the embryo. It is important that nothing follows about whether there are thereby any moral reasons against this practice. If the embryos in question lack moral status, then there are no moral reasons against the practice in virtue of the harms to the embryos. While the practice is very bad for them, there is no moral badness to it. However, if the embryos in question have moral status, then there is a moral reason against the practice due to the harm to the embryos.

Creating Embryos to Make Stem Cells

Suppose that a researcher creates an embryo and then destroys the embryo to make stem cells. Does the researcher do anything that significantly harms the embryo?

Here is an argument that she does not. The researcher performs two relevant actions: first, the creation of the embryo; second, the destruction of the embryo. Surely creating the embryo does not harm it. And once the embryo is created, its fate is pretty much sealed. It is never going to be implanted into a womb; it is never going to get to develop into a person. No one wants it. Those who may have a right to decide what becomes of it (its genetic parents, let's assume) do not want it implanted into a womb. If the researcher never destroyed the embryo, it would not get to develop into a person. Thus, destroying it does not harm it; its fate was sealed before it was destroyed.

This argument makes two crucial claims: creating the embryo does not significantly harm it, and destroying the embryo does not significantly harm it. I think the second of these claims is true: once an embryo has been created for the purposes of extracting cells, the destruction of this embryo is no worse for it than the destruction of embryos left over from fertility treatments. However, I think the first claim is false: creating the embryo does significantly harm it. Let's suppose that the stem cell research lab is up and running. This makes the following counterfactual true and knowable: "If the researcher creates an embryo, the embryo will fail to get to live life as a person." What will happen is this. The embryo will be created, and it will need a great deal of help and aid to develop normally. This help and aid, in the form of a woman willing to nurture it in her womb, will not be forthcoming. No one will owe it this aid, so no one will be mistreating it in not providing the aid. Nevertheless, it will fail to get the aid it needs, and it will not be able to develop normally. It will not get to live life as a person. It will lose out on all the tremendous benefits involved in getting to live life as a person. Its whole existence will be as a mere embryo, compared to a much more meaningful life it could have had as a person. From the embryo's perspective, this is a tragedy. Of course, the embryo does not literally have a perspective, in that it does not have any experiences. But things can be better or worse for the embryo, and this is a tragedy for it. Not getting to live life as a person is a huge loss. It is very bad for the embryo that it does not get to live life as a person.

The researchers know that if they create the embryo, it will fail to get to live life as a person. They knowingly do something that leads to the embryo's suffering this fate, which I have argued is very bad for it. Thus, they harm the embryo.

Just how bad is it to be deprived of the chance to live life as a person? I think that few harms are worse. Perhaps some are worse: perhaps having a rich life cut off abruptly in the middle is worse; perhaps suffering extreme torture is worse. But this is certainly one of the worst things that can happen to something.[3]

I claim that it is very bad for an embryo if it comes to exist and is then destroyed. What follows about the ethics of stem cell research? Nothing. It depends on whether what is bad for the embryo matters morally—on whether the embryo has moral status.

If the embryo has the full moral status of a person, then there is a very significant moral reason against this form of stem cell research, due to the harm to the embryo. But even on the assumption that the embryo has the full moral status of a person, this does not settle whether this form of stem cell research is wrong.

Perhaps this case is like abortion. Thomson has argued that even if the fetus has the full moral status of a person, abortion is permissible because a pregnant woman has the right to refuse to suffer significant hardships in order to provide aid to the fetus, and if the only way to avoid providing this aid to the fetus is to kill it, she may do so.

However, nothing like that is going on when we are considering creating embryos that would be destroyed to make stem cells. There is no existing being we are refusing to aid. Rather, we are bringing a being into existence, knowing it will need aid that it will not receive. (Note that Thomson's arguments do not show that, even if a fetus has the full moral status of a person, it is permissible to bring a fetus into existence in order to abort it.[4]) Furthermore, if we fail to engage in this practice—if we fail to create embryos that would be destroyed to make stem cells—it is not the case that anyone will find himself providing aid to something against his will, as a pregnant woman will find herself if she does not abort.

Given that there is a strong reason against this form of stem cell research, due to the badness [sic] to the embryos of this practice, how might the practice be justified? We may think that the practice is justified because although it is bad for the embryos, it is very good for many people, future people who will be saved by the therapies that stem cell research will provide. However, this is the wrong kind of consideration to justify severely harming something—if that thing has the full moral status of a person. For example, it is impermissible to cut up one healthy person and use his or her organs to save five patients with organ failure.[5] The cases appear to be parallel. The embryos we would create, if they have the full moral status of persons, would be severely harmed in order to save many other, unconnected people.

If we assume that human embryos and fetuses have the full moral status of persons from the moment of conception, then any tragedy for one of them is a morally significant tragedy that provides a compelling moral reason. Abortion is a tragedy for the fetus in question. Thomson argues that abortion is permissible even given the assumption that the fetus has the full moral status of a person. But that's because the only way to prevent the tragedy for the fetus is for a woman to undergo significant hardship to provide aid; because the woman doesn't owe this sacrifice to the fetus, she may abort it in order to avoid aiding it. Similarly, if we create an embryo that will be destroyed to make stem cells, the embryo will suffer a tragedy. However, this practice cannot be justified in a parallel way, if we assume that the embryo has the full moral status of a person. Failing to create the embryo does not force anyone to suffer burdens in order to aid the embryo in the way that failing to abort a pregnancy imposes burdens on a pregnant woman in forcing her to aid the fetus.[6]

Objections

In this section, I discuss five objections to the argument of my previous section. In that section, I argued that creating an embryo that will be destroyed to extract stem cells significantly harms the embryo. I furthermore argued that if the embryo has the full moral status of a person, this practice is impermissible. The first two objections that I will consider maintain that this practice is not bad for the embryo. The third objection maintains that, although the practice is bad for the embryo, the practice is not wrong—even on the assumption that the embryo has the full moral status of a person. The fourth and fifth objections maintain that the picture I am presenting has implausible further implications. Each objection could be discussed at great length; I will confine myself to articulating each objection and then very briefly arguing that it fails.

The first objector maintains that the embryo is not harmed by coming to exist and then failing to get to live life as a person. The objector asserts that an embryo (or fetus) that dies is not deprived of a future as a person because if it had developed into a person, the embryo would not have been identical to the person.

In my discussion, I have assumed the relevant identity claim: when an embryo does develop into a person, there is a single thing that is first an embryo and then later a person. Some philosophers deny the identity claim because they are convinced of a psychological criterion of identity for persons. However, Derek Parfit (1984) has shown that what matters in survival does not coincide with identity; and in the face of his arguments, we should see that a psychological criterion is merely a good guide to what matters in survival, not to identity. Some philosophers hold that certain early embryos are not identical to any later-existing persons: these are embryos that are early enough to be capable of twinning. I do not understand why the mere possibility of twinning should be enough to undermine identity in a case where twinning did not actually occur. Had the embryo twinned, though it would have developed into two different persons, it would have been identical to neither. Nevertheless, if the embryo did actually develop without twinning, it is identical to the person it developed into. (Compare: an amoeba today is identical to itself yesterday, although it could have divided yesterday into two amoebas, in

which case it would not have been identical to either one.)

The second objector makes the following argument for the permissibility of creating an embryo in a circumstance in which the embryo will be destroyed. "It's better to exist and have a small chance of getting to live life as a person, and then be destroyed, than never to exist at all. An action cannot be wrong in virtue of its effects on something, if it makes that thing better off than it would otherwise have been. Therefore, creating an embryo in a situation in which the embryo will be destroyed is permissible."

This argument fails because it can be impermissible to create something although that thing has a life that is better than nonexistence. For example, it's impermissible to conceive while one has a temporary condition that will cause one's conceived child to be deaf; one should wait until the temporary condition ends and then conceive. But an argument parallel to the objector's argument would license this action. The objector's argument raises a problem known as "the non-identity problem." In my 2004 paper, I discuss the non-identity problem in detail and argue that we can impermissibly harm someone by creating her even if she has a life worth living (and so, even if her existence is better than not existing at all).

The third objector argues that I have misdescribed the way in which an embryo's not getting to live life as a person is bad for it. I have suggested that an embryo's not getting to live life as a person is bad for it in the way that being in pain, losing a limb, or losing one of his five senses would be bad for a person—that the event is in itself bad, not merely bad because the alternative would be better. The objector points out that events that are in themselves bad for a person provide much stronger reasons than events that are merely failures to receive benefits. While we have some reasons to avoid causing persons to fail to receive benefits, these reasons are much weaker than our reasons against causing events that are in themselves bad for persons. Suppose I have been planning to give Anne a million dollars but then decide not to. This decision is very bad for Anne.

But there is no strong moral reason against my deciding this way, and part of the explanation is that while the decision is very bad for Anne, it merely results in Anne's failing to get a benefit. It does not cause anything that is in itself bad for Anne. The objector suggests that the embryo's failing to get to live life as a person is like Anne's failing to get a million dollars: it would have been wonderful for the embryo to get to become a person, but not getting to become a person does not involve suffering a fate that is in itself bad. My response to this objection is that it's certainly true that we have much weaker reasons against failing to provide certain positive benefits than we do against causing events that are in themselves bad for a person. I agree with the objector that if the badness for the embryo is merely like the failure to get some spectacular benefit, then—on the assumption that the embryo has the full moral status of a person—creating the embryo and destroying it to get cells can be justified by the benefits that will come from stem cell research. But the badness for the embryo of failing to get to live life as a person is not like failing to get a million dollars, for two reasons. First, it's a tricky business to draw the line between the things that are in themselves bad for something and the things that provide weaker reasons because they are mere failures to receive a certain kind of benefit; as I suggested above, becoming blind and losing a limb fall in the first category, although the explanation of what is bad about these crucially involves the benefits of having what is lost. Second, the death of a person is clearly in itself bad, not merely like failing to receive a great benefit. But the right story about the badness of death for a person crucially involves the deprivation of future life (though that is not the whole story). Given these considerations, it seems clear that the embryo's failing to get to live life as a person falls in the first category: it is like becoming blind, losing a limb, or a person's death; it is not like failing to get a million dollars.

The fourth objector claims that my embracing the argument of Thomson's paper is in tension with my claim that, on the assumption that the embryo has the full moral status of a person, it is wrong to create the embryo in a circumstance in which it will be destroyed. In her paper, Thomson clearly advocates the view that it is permissible to abort a fetus that was the result of voluntary sex—at least if contraception was used, and the pregnancy was a result of failure of the contraception. And (though this is even less explicit in the paper) Thomson also seems to advocate the view that it is permissible to engage in sex with contraception even if one knows that there is a small chance that one will create a fetus and then destroy it by aborting it. The objector maintains that I should claim that this behavior is wrong—on the assumption that the fetus has the full moral status of a person. But I need not say this. What's crucial for my purposes here is that there is a big moral difference between doing something that might create a being that would then need aid and would not get it, while minimizing the likelihood of this creation, and on the other hand doing something that is very likely to create a being that will then need aid and will not get it. I am arguing that the latter action harms the created being. (I can embrace Thomson's defense of a woman who aborts a fetus after contraception fails. Thomson argues that a woman is not obligated to refrain from a basic life activity such as sex in order to avoid pregnancy due to contraception failure—and if she does get pregnant as a result of contraception failure, she is not obligated to aid the fetus whose existence was a foreseeable but unlikely result of her behavior, even on the assumption that the fetus has the full moral status of a person.)

A further question is whether it is permissible to use fertility treatments that are very likely (indeed, nearly certain) to result in the creation of "extra" embryos that will not get to develop into persons. For reasons parallel to those I have given about creating embryos for stem cell research, I claim that such a practice is not permissible, on the assumption that the created embryos have the full moral status of persons. (I believe this assumption is false, however, and that such fertility treatments are permissible.)

(I won't go into the question of whether, if the created embryos have the full moral status of persons, then after having created them—with the goal of destroying them—stem cell researchers in fact owe them aid. That is a hard question. But I think it is not a pressing question, because I think the assumption that the created embryos have the full moral status of persons is false.)

The fifth objector points out that, on the view I am advocating, if embryos have moral status, then there is much more morally significant harm in the world than we generally realize or worry about. Many embryos fail to implant and thus suffer the fate of being created but not getting to live life as a person. The objector maintains that it's just not plausible that these events are morally significant. My response is that because I do not claim that these embryos have moral status, I am not committed to the view that their failure to implant is morally significant. But I am committed to the claim that those who think these embryos have moral status should think these are morally significant events. Are they also committed to the claim that we should try to prevent these events? That is a hard question, and it depends on how we could prevent these failures of implantation.

A Low Level of Moral Status?

Now that we've seen what follows from the embryo's having the full moral status of a person, let's consider a different claim: the claim that the embryo has some moral status. Suppose this claim is true. What follows?

In short, I think the same reasoning applies and the same conclusion follows. Creating an embryo and then destroying it significantly harms the embryo, and there is a strong moral reason against doing so, if the embryo has any moral status at all. An objector will say this does not take seriously the possibility that the embryo may have a low level of moral status.

There do seem to be different levels of moral status: for example, gnats have a lower level of moral status than fish, which have a lower level of moral status than rabbits, which have a lower level of moral status than persons. Gnats never give us strong reasons at all. Fish may give us some reasons, but these reasons aren't as strong as the reasons that rabbits give us; and persons give us yet much stronger reasons.

Here's a first reason to think that levels of moral status don't help much in this case. Even though we think that rabbits have lower moral status than persons, we still acknowledge that in a particular case, a reason given by harm to a rabbit may be stronger than a reason given by harm to a person. For example, suppose that I see that a rabbit is about to fall from such a great height that it will be killed; the only way to stop it from falling is to rush past a person, Jim, causing Jim to fall over and very likely get a bruise or two. In this case, it seems that I should save the rabbit, causing Jim his bruises: the harm to the rabbit would be so serious that it outweighs the harm to Jim. This shows that reasons to do with persons don't always win out over reasons to do with lesser beings—but also that reasons against harming things with lower levels of moral status can be very weighty reasons.

When it comes to an embryo not getting to live life as a person, this harm is so serious that it seems it must provide a very strong reason indeed.

At this point, an objector might say that a low level of moral status greatly diminishes the significance of any particular harm: something's having a low level of moral status is just the thing's being such that there isn't ever a very strong reason against harming it. Even if a harm to it would be very much worse than some other harm to a person, the harm to the person may provide a stronger reason because its victim is a person.

Many people do think that there are levels of moral status that work like this; but there are reasons to think otherwise. We tend to think that fish have much lower moral status than persons. Does this mean we think that some harm which is very bad for a fish matters less than a harm that is much less bad for a person? It's not clear we do think this. It's true we don't treat the deaths of fish as seriously as we treat the deaths of humans; but this can be explained by the fact that fish are less harmed by death than humans are. When fish die, they are deprived of their future lives as fish; by contrast, when a person dies, he is deprived of something much better—life as a person. (And death harms a person in other ways as well.)

Consider gnats. Gnats have very uneventful mental lives.[7] Nothing is ever very pleasurable for a gnat. Nothing is ever very painful for a gnat. Gnats give us only very weak moral reasons because they are susceptible to only very minor benefits and harms. Similarly, fish give us reasons that do not go beyond a certain strength because they are not susceptible to harms and benefits of a certain degree. Rabbits are susceptible to greater harms and benefits than fish are; for example, their pain may be more involved or acute, and they can enjoy loving relationships and mourn the death of a loved one. Thus, we have stronger reasons to avoid harming rabbits and to benefit them. Finally, persons are susceptible to yet greater harms and benefits. Thus we have stronger reasons to treat them in particular ways.

I do not deny that there are levels of moral status. There are levels of moral status in the following sense. Some things are susceptible to less significant harms and benefits than other things. The former things are thus typically the source of less strong moral reasons, and it is in this sense that they have a lower level of moral status.

But I deny that there are levels of moral status in another sense. I deny that there is a status that makes a harm of a particular degree matter more because it happened to a thing with high moral status; and I deny that there is such a thing as a status that makes a harm matter less because it happened to a thing with low moral status.[8] Rather, there are systematic differences in the types of harms and benefits that different kinds of things can suffer. So some kinds of things, such as persons, systematically give us stronger reasons than are given by other kinds of things, such as fish. The low moral status of fish is not a function of their suffering terribly bad things that matter little—it is a function of their not suffering anything that is very bad at all.

I think people are misled by the existence of things like gnats and fish that never provide really strong moral reasons. They think that embryos could be like those things in not providing really strong moral reasons. But the explanation for the lack of really strong moral reasons to treat gnats and fish in a certain way is that they are not susceptible to very severe harms, or to very great benefits. Embryos are not like that: they can suffer a truly terrible harm, the loss of the chance to live life as a person.

A View of Moral Status

I have focused on a particular form of stem cell research: the practice of creating embryos and then destroying them to make stem cells. I have argued that this practice significantly harms the embryos, and that if the embryos have moral status, this practice is wrong. Many people think this practice is permissible even though they also think that the embryos have at least some moral status. My arguments are meant to show that if these people are to maintain their view that the practice is permissible, they must come around to the view that the embryos in question lack moral status.

In this section, I articulate a view of which things have moral status that has the result that the created and destroyed embryos lack moral status. I argue that the particular view I am proposing is more plausible than other views on which the created and destroyed embryos lack moral status. Furthermore, I respond to some objections to the particular view I am proposing.

Here is the view of moral status that I propose:

The Ever Conscious View: A being has moral status at a time just in case it is alive at that time and there is a time in its life at which it is conscious.[9]

What does this view say? Consider plants. There is no time in their lives that they are conscious; so, on the Ever Conscious View, they lack moral status. Nevertheless, the Ever Conscious View is compatible with strong environmentalist ethical obligations; humans and other animals provide adequate reasons to protect the environment.

Consider you and me. We are conscious now, so there is a time in our lives at which we are conscious, so, on the Ever Conscious View, we have moral status at every time during our lives: from the moment we came to exist until the last moment before our deaths. Consider the dead human bodies we will become; they are not alive, so they do not have moral status. Nevertheless, the Ever Conscious View is compatible with the view that we have obligations to people after they die, and that we can wrong people after they die. But it implies that these obligations are not obligations to the presently existing dead bodies; they are obligations to the past living persons. On the Ever Conscious View, if something is ever conscious during its life, either in the past, present, or future, then it has moral status at all times throughout its life. This has the result that temporarily unconscious persons have moral status, and that permanently unconscious though still living human beings have moral status. Nevertheless, the Ever Conscious View is compatible with the view that it is permissible to kill permanently unconscious living humans—indeed, it is compatible with the view that we may owe it to them to kill them. (But it is incompatible with the view that the reason we may kill them is that they lack moral status.)

For our purposes, what's most important about the view is what it says about embryos and fetuses. The Ever Conscious View holds that some early embryos have moral status and some lack moral status—even two intrinsically identical early embryos, with intrinsically identical pasts, may differ in moral status due to their differing actual futures. One embryo is in fact going to be destroyed before it is ever conscious; thus, on the Ever Conscious View, it now lacks moral status. An intrinsically identical embryo is in fact going to develop into a conscious being; thus, on the Ever Conscious View, it now has moral status. It's natural to think that these two fetuses must have the same moral status; that is, it's natural to overlook a view on which actual future determines current moral status.

If we assume that pre-conscious fetuses and embryos must either all have moral status or all lack moral status, then it becomes quite plausible that they all have some moral status. Two facts in particular suggest that they must have some moral status. First, consider a woman who becomes pregnant. Suppose she and her partner decide to continue the pregnancy and to raise the child. They know that

there is a living being in her womb who is the beginning stage of their child. They have attitudes toward that very being, the fetus—indeed, they love it. Plausibly, it is inappropriate to love something that lacks moral status, that is in itself morally irrelevant. But the woman and her partner are not making any kind of mistake in already loving the fetus.[10] This suggests that the fetus has moral status. Second, consider another woman who becomes pregnant and plans to continue her pregnancy. Suppose that she smokes and drinks while the fetus is not yet conscious, even though she knows this will damage the fetus and interfere with its development. This woman's behavior is wrong. It seems that we miss what is wrong with the behavior if we say merely that while the fetus now lacks moral status, her behavior is wrong because she is causing there to be, in the future, something with moral status that is harmed by her current behavior. Rather, it seems that she owes it to the fetus not to smoke and drink, and that this is best explained by the fetus's already having moral status. Thus, if we focus our attention on fetuses and embryos that are going to continue to develop, it appears that pre-conscious fetuses and embryos do have moral status.

However, if we focus our attention on fetuses and embryos that will die before ever becoming conscious, we are led toward a very different conclusion. These fetuses and embryos are living beings, but they are much more similar to plants than to persons or animals, considering the properties that seem relevant to having moral status. These beings go through their whole lives without ever being conscious. They never have a bad experience, or a good one. When considering the death of a pre-conscious embryo or fetus, many people are tempted to think that this death is morally irrelevant. I think that many people give up this belief in the face of considerations to do with embryos and fetuses that do have futures as conscious beings—it seems that these pre-conscious embryos and fetuses must have moral status, so it seems that all pre-conscious embryos and fetuses must have moral status.

The Ever Conscious View provides a way to hold on to both natural views: the view that some pre-conscious embryos and fetuses lack moral status—

those that die before becoming conscious—and the view that some pre-conscious embryos and fetuses have moral status—those that will ever become conscious.

The Ever Conscious View is more plausible than the view that all preconscious fetuses and embryos lack moral status, because unlike that view, the Ever Conscious View does not dictate a cold attitude toward all pre-conscious fetuses: it allows that some already have moral status. I have not provided a substantial argument for the Ever Conscious View here; but I have shown that the view accommodates all of a number of common and natural views, some of which otherwise must be given up. These views are: the view that it is appropriate to love a pre-conscious fetus; the view that our reasons not to smoke and drink during a pregnancy that will be carried to term are due to the moral status of the fetus; and the view that the death of a pre-conscious fetus in an abortion, or of an embryo to extract cells, is morally insignificant. I will turn now to considering two objections to the Ever Conscious View.

The first objection is that the Ever Conscious View must be false because whether something has moral status must be a matter of the thing's nature and facts about a fetus's actual future are not facts about its nature. According to the objector, we could differentiate fetuses in all sorts of different ways and say that some fetuses have moral status and some lack moral status—but drawing a line between two intrinsically identical fetuses is arbitrary; and the moral-status facts couldn't possibly be arbitrary.

I agree with the objector that something's moral status must be determined by its nature. Some properties of a thing are not part of its nature and thus could not possibly determine whether it has moral status: what the woman who carries it intends for it (that is, whether she intends to abort it), what part of the world it is located in, whether those around it believe that pre-conscious embryos and fetuses have moral status—all of these factors are far too extrinsic to be relevant to whether an embryo or a fetus has moral status. However, the Ever Conscious View does not allow any similarly extrinsic factors to enter into whether something has moral status. On the Ever Conscious View, only a thing's intrinsic prop-

erties are relevant to whether it has moral status; but future and past intrinsic properties count too.[11] Thus, I think that something's nature is a matter of the intrinsic properties the thing has throughout its life. On this understanding of a thing's nature, its nature does determine its moral status, according to the Ever Conscious View.

The second objection is that the Ever Conscious View makes it contingent whether some activities, such as abortion, are permissible. The objector says: "You and I have moral status—and did, according to the Ever Conscious View, back when we were pre-conscious fetuses. So it would have been wrong to abort us! But then actual abortions of preconscious fetuses are permissible, because those fetuses lack moral status, whereas merely possible abortions are all impermissible—it would have been wrong to perform them. But that's just crazy."

The objector assumes that whether a fetus has moral status is a necessary feature of that fetus. But on the Ever Conscious View, that's not true. On the Ever Conscious View, pre-conscious fetuses and embryos that lack moral status are such that they would have had moral status if they had had futures in which they were conscious. And, on the Ever Conscious View, pre-conscious fetuses and embryos that actually have moral status—like the embryos that you and I once were—would have lacked moral status if we had died before ever becoming conscious. Suppose we ask whether it would have been permissible to abort the preconscious fetus that developed into me. If it had been aborted, that preconscious fetus would have lacked moral status. So killing it would have been killing something that lacked moral status; killing it would have been permissible. Thus, the view does not make it contingent whether abortion of a pre-conscious fetus is permissible: actual abortions are permissible, and merely possible abortions are permissible as well.

Conclusion

While it is natural to think that embryonic stem cell research is easier to justify than abortion, I have argued that in one important respect the opposite is true. On the assumption that human embryos and fetuses have the full moral status of persons from the moment of conception, abortion is easier to justify than one method of obtaining embryonic stem cells. Abortion can be justified as the only way of protecting a woman from suffering burdens in order to aid the fetus. But no corresponding justification is available for creating an embryo and then destroying it to extract cells: while lives may be saved and improved by this process, we are not in general entitled to impose great harm on one person—or a being with the moral status of a person—in order to save the lives of people who are otherwise unconnected to that person. The difference between the two cases is that the permissibility of abortion—on the assumption the fetus has the full moral status of a person—stems from the fact that the very burdens to the woman which would be prevented by killing the fetus are caused by the fetus's getting the woman's aid. Abortion is permissible because a pregnant woman's only way of withdrawing aid from the fetus, to spare herself the burdens of providing this aid, is to kill the fetus; no parallel claims can be made to justify stem cell research.

I have argued that this surprising conclusion holds even on the weaker assumption that human embryos and fetuses have some moral status from the moment of conception. This part of my argument relied on my claim that to have low moral status is to be susceptible to only minor harms and benefits—it is for this reason, and only for this reason, that things with low moral status do not provide strong reasons. Embryos are not like that, so they do not have low moral status. On the assumption that an embryo has any moral status at all, a significant harm to it provides a significant moral reason.

From my two conclusions, it follows that it is permissible to create embryos and then destroy them to extract cells only if the destroyed embryos lack moral status. While the view that all pre-conscious fetuses and embryos lack moral status is implausible, because it dictates a cold attitude toward those embryos and fetuses that are the early stages of persons, the Ever Conscious View is a more plausible alternative. On this view, pre-conscious embryos that will die without ever being conscious lack moral status; but pre-conscious embryos that will become conscious already have moral status.

Acknowledgments

For helpful comments on drafts of this essay, I thank Stephanie Beard-man, Macalester Bell, Matt Evans, Laura Grabel, Peter Graham, Lori Gruen, Alex Guerrero, Sarah McGrath, Nishi Shah, Peter Singer, Sharon Street, and the Lawrence S. Rockefeller Visiting Fellows at the Princeton University Center for Human Values (in 2006 and 2007).

Notes

1 See my footnote 9 for a discussion of how the ethics of the situation would be different if the cells could be extracted without destroying the embryo.

2 Although I claim that the harm to the embryo is not very serious, considerable argument is needed to establish this claim in the face of the objection from the case of the two assassins. That is work for another occasion, but I will briefly suggest how the argument might be made. One could begin by denying that the case of destroying the leftover embryo is really analogous to the case of the two assassins. One could then propose a case that provides a better analogy, such as the following. Suppose that we are in a remote area and we have a hospital, but it is not well equipped. We have lost power and are running a life-support machine on a generator, which is going to give out in two hours. We have sent someone to report our power problems and to bring in more doctors, but she is not due to reach anyone for several hours, and it should take several more hours before anyone can reach us with more generators. The life-support machine is keeping a man in a coma alive; we know that if we could keep him on life support until help arrives, he could be fully revived and would end up perfectly healthy. But we also know that help is not due to arrive until long after the generator has given out. Another man has just stumbled into the clinic, having a heart attack, and slumped onto the ground. We have very good reason to think that if we detach the generator from the man in a coma, we will be able to use it to power a defibrillator to save the life of the

man who has just stumbled in—but then the man in a coma will die. This, I claim, is a case in which we may detach the generator from the man in a coma, even though we would be killing him—and in this case, causing his death is mitigated by the fact that he is overwhelmingly likely to die soon anyway. Indeed, it is a practical certainty that he will die; the only way he would not die would be if by some bizarre and happy accident someone happened to decide to bring us a generator and set out toward us many hours ago, so as to reach us before we even lose power. If destroying a leftover embryo is analogous to detaching the man in a coma from the generator, it is plausible that the harm to the embryo is not very serious.

3 In unusual cases, the deprivation of the chance to live life as a person may be good for an embryo. For example, if an embryo is such that if it gets to live life as a person this life will involve utter misery, then the deprivation of the chance to have this life is good for it.

4 See the fourth objection discussed in the section below entitled "Objections" for further discussion of this point.

5 A consequentialist would disagree with my claims here. These claims are assumptions of this essay.

6 Recently, news stories have reported that it may be possible to extract cells from an embryo, in order to make stem cells, without damaging or destroying the embryo. How would this change the moral picture I am laying out? If this new technology reduces the need to create any embryos for the sole purpose of stem cell research, it may mean that the practice this essay focuses on will rarely (or never) occur. But if a researcher creates an embryo knowing that this new technology will be used to extract cells and that the undamaged embryo will then continue to exist without ever developing, this practice is on a moral par with creating an embryo knowing it will be destroyed. In either case, the created embryo will not get to live life as a person, which is a tragedy for it. In either case, on the assumption that the embryo has the full moral status of a person, the practice is impermissible.

7 I am assuming that gnats do have some conscious experiences, though minimal ones. If they don't, what I say about gnats can be taken to apply to whatever beings do have some conscious experiences, though minimal ones.

8 In this essay, I have only given a sketch of an argument for my view about levels of moral status. My 2003 paper argues that there are no levels of moral status of the second kind I describe in the text above: there is no status that makes severe harms provide weak moral reasons. In that paper, I discuss and respond to a number of objections, including objections to do with the greater significance of human pain over animal pain, and the difficulty of drawing interspecies comparisons of harm. Peter Singer (1993; chap. 3) argues that there are no levels of moral status, merely differences in the degree of harm and benefit a being tends to undergo. (I do not think Singer would agree with my extension of his view to the case of embryos and fetuses.)

9 In my 1999 paper, I argue that pre-conscious fetuses that will actually become persons have moral status, and that pre-conscious fetuses that will die before becoming persons lack moral status. The Ever Conscious View is a more general version of this view. I previously stated the Ever Conscious View in my 2003 paper; I showed that the view helped to solve a problem, but I did not provide further argument for it (I did not, for example, argue that it was the only view that could solve that problem).

10 If the pregnant woman who loves her fetus suffers an early miscarriage, we need not say she was making a mistake in loving her fetus—although on the Ever Conscious View it turns out that her fetus is not the kind of thing it is appropriate to love. She had a reasonable belief that the fetus was the beginning stage of a person, and was the kind of thing that is the appropriate object of love.

11 I am assuming that whether something is conscious is an intrinsic matter. This is compatible with externalism about mental content: it may be an intrinsic matter whether something has any conscious states at all, while it is not an intrinsic matter what the content of those mental states is.

References

Harman, Elizabeth. 1999. "Creation Ethics: The Moral Status of Early Fetuses and the Ethics of Abortion." *Philosophy and Public Affairs* 28, no. 4 (Fall): 310-324.

———. 2003. "The Potentiality Problem." *Philosophical Studies* 114, nos. 1-2 (May): 173-98. FFF.

———. "Can We Harm and Benefit in Creating?" *Philosophical Perspectives* 18:89-113.

Parfit, Derek. 1984. *Reasons and Persons*. Oxford: Clarendon Press.

Singer, Peter. 1993. *Practical Ethics*. Cambridge: Cambridge University Press.

Thomson, Judith Jarvis. 1971. "A Defense of Abortion." *Philosophy and Public Affairs* 1 (Fall): 47-66.

31.
SHOULD SELECTING SAVIOUR SIBLINGS BE BANNED?

S. Sheldon and S. Wilkinson

SOURCE: *Journal of Medical Ethics* 30.6 (2004): 533-37.

Recent high profile cases in Australia,[1] the UK,[2] and the USA[3] have brought to the public's attention a new kind of embryo selection. By using HLA (human leucocyte antigen) typing, popularly known as "tissue typing," in conjunction with preimplantation genetic diagnosis (PGD), doctors are now able to pick an embryo for implantation which, if all goes well, will become a "saviour sibling,"[4] a brother or sister capable of donating life-saving tissue to an existing child. In the UK, the most recent case to reach the courts and the newspapers is that of the Hashmis.[5] Their son, Zain, has thalassaemia, a blood disorder which could be cured using tissue from the umbilical cord of a sibling, but only if the sibling is a tissue match. The Human Fertilisation and Embryology Authority gave permission for the Hashmis to select a saviour sibling for Zain. This decision was swiftly challenged in the courts, with the UK High Court finding that the selection of a saviour sibling was unlawful.[6] In May 2003, the Court of Appeal overturned this decision, declaring that tissue typing can be authorised under current legislation.[7]

Prior to the recent Court of Appeal ruling, it looked as if this form of preimplantation selection might be prohibited in the UK and our aim in this paper is to assess whether this and similar bans are defensible. Our focus throughout is on cases where doctors plan just to use umbilical cord tissue, as opposed to those in which the use of non-renewable solid organs (such as kidneys) is intended, and we concede from the outset that the latter raise additional objections that (for reasons of space) we do not consider here. We will concentrate on critically assessing the arguments for prohibition (rather than, for example, positive arguments for reproductive liberty). This is because banning the use of PGD to create saviour siblings will lead to the death of a number of children who could have been saved by sibling donation. And given that a ban will be fatal for a section of the population, the onus of proof rests clearly with the prohibitionists who must demonstrate that these children's deaths are less terrible than the consequences of allowing this particular use of PGD. As Glover puts it:[8] "You have got to have a very powerful reason to resist the means by which a child's life can be saved."

In what follows, we divide the prohibitionist arguments into three categories. First, there is the idea that saviour siblings would be wrongfully instrumentalised, treated as mere means rather than ends-in-themselves, or treated as commodities. Secondly, there are arguments according to which the creation of saviour siblings would either cause or constitute a move towards the creation of "designer babies." Finally, there are arguments which focus on the welfare of saviour siblings.

Means, Ends, and Commodification

The idea of deliberately creating a saviour sibling often provokes comments like these:

> It is totally unethical. You are not creating a child for itself.[9]

> We would have very serious concerns that he is a commodity rather than a person.[10]

> The trouble really is that this child as it grows up has been brought into the world because it is a commodity.[11]

Such comments run together two distinct worries: concerns about people having children for the wrong reasons, on the one hand, and concerns about the way in which the child will be treated by his or her parents, on the other. Thoughts of the second kind are really concerns about the welfare of the resultant child and so we will discuss these in a later section, focusing for the time being on the idea that deliberately conceiving a child is wrong if done for certain kinds of reason. Clearly, conceiving can be wrong if done for the wrong reasons. Conceiving a child in order later to eat it or torture it would be uncontentious, if extreme, supporting examples for this principle. The real question then is: Which reasons are the wrong reasons? One answer is that a child should be wanted for his or her own sake and not for some other purpose:[12]

> The commonest objection to this procedure is that it is wrong to bring children into existence "conditionally." This objection finds its philosophical foundation in Immanuel Kant's famous dictum, "Never use people as a means but always treat them as an end."

As an argument against selecting saviour siblings, though, this is defective in at least two ways (as Boyle and Savulescu, quoted above, go on to point out). First, it relies on a misreading of Kant's "famous dictum." This does not prohibit treating people as means, but rather prohibits treating them merely or solely as means. As Harris notes:[13] "We all ... [treat people as means] perfectly innocuously much of the time. In medical contexts, anyone who receives a blood transfusion has used the blood donor as a means to their own ends...." So there is nothing objectionable about creating a baby as a "means to an end" provided that it is also viewed and treated as a human being.

A second more practical objection to this argument is that it does not adequately distinguish between creating a child as a saviour sibling and creating a child for some other "instrumental" purpose for example, "completing a family," being a playmate for an existing child, saving a marriage, delighting prospective grandparents, or providing an heir. Perhaps these things are different from creating a saviour sibling but, if they are, the difference isn't

that they are any less "instrumental" for in all these cases, the child is used as a means.

The concern then cannot really be about having a child as a means since people frequently do this and it is not in itself objectionable. What might be objectionable, from the Kantian view, is creating a child solely to advance some further end. For example, it would obviously be wrong to create a saviour sibling and then just to discard him or her once it had "served the purpose." But this is clearly not what is proposed and so, overall, this argument fails, as a purely ethical argument and a fortiori as a case for legal prohibition.

Designer Babies and Slippery Slopes

A second argument against permitting the deliberate creation of saviour siblings is that to do so would be to step onto a slippery slope towards allowing "designer babies."[5] This argument combines two distinct objections. The general form of the first is that if we allow something to happen which, considered in itself, is either acceptable or only slightly bad, it will later cause something else to happen which is very bad or clearly wrong (this being what is at the bottom of the proverbial slope).

So applied to saviour siblings, it says that if we allow the creation of saviour siblings (which is only slightly bad) this will lead to something much worse: the creation of fully-fledged designer babies. As Quintavalle puts it "the new technique is a dangerous first step towards allowing parents to use embryo testing to choose other characteristics of the baby, such as eye colour and sex".[14] So the claim is that we will start off by allowing the deliberate creation of saviour siblings and "slide down the slope" towards permitting the selection of embryos on wholly frivolous grounds.

The second version of the slippery slope argument is either a point about consistency or a reductio ad absurdum that is, an attempt to refute a position by showing that it has absurd implications. Lying behind it is the following argument:

1) Allowing the selection of saviour siblings isn't morally different from allowing people to choose "designer" characteristics (for example, hair colour).

2) Therefore: (from (1)) if we ban one, we should ban the other. Conversely, if we allow one, we should allow the other.

3) Allowing people to choose designer characteristics is wrong and should be banned.

4) Therefore: (from (2) and (3)) allowing the selection of saviour siblings is wrong and should be banned.

This kind of argument can be used in two closely related ways. First, it is asserted that people who oppose designer babies but not saviour siblings are inconsistent and should really oppose both. Secondly, there is an attempted reductio of the view that selecting saviour siblings should be permitted: the idea being that this has the (supposedly absurd, or at least unpalatable) implication that selecting embryos with designer characteristics should also be permitted.

The objections to these "slope" arguments fall into three main categories. First, one could reject the premise (shared by both arguments) that allowing people to choose embryos with designer characteristics is wrong. Secondly (specifically in relation to the consequence based argument), one could argue that allowing the selection of saviour siblings won't, or needn't, cause us to become "permissive" about designer babies. Finally (specifically in relation to the consistency or reductio argument), one could argue that saviour siblings and designer babies are relevantly different and therefore one can oppose the latter and not the former without inconsistency.

Purely for the sake of argument, we will grant that allowing people to choose embryos with designer characteristics is wrong and should be prohibited and move straight onto the second objection.[15] This says that allowing the selection of saviour siblings won't, or needn't, cause us to become permissive about designer babies. There are at least three reasons for supporting this objection. The first is that those who propound the empirical slippery slope argument rarely, if ever, support it with any hard evidence. Merely asserting that saviour siblings are the "first step towards allowing parents to use embryo testing to choose other characteristics" is inadequate. The second is that it is very easy to envisage how,

through careful regulation, a "slide down the slope" might be averted. In particular, there is no reason why selection can't be allowed for some purposes but not others. Indeed, that is the present position and there is no reason to believe that such a position couldn't be maintained, if Parliament (or a regulatory body such as the UK's Human Fertilisation and Embryology Authority) decided that that is what it wanted. So a slide is not inevitable. Thirdly, and finally, there is the fact that to get a fully-fledged designer baby—that is, one in whom numerous traits were selected for—a very large pool of preimplantation embryos would be required from which to select, thus imposing considerable extra cost, discomfort, and inconvenience on women.

The third objection to the slippery slope argument is that saviour siblings and designer babies are morally different, and therefore there is nothing inconsistent about opposing one but not the other. Obviously there is a preliminary complication about what exactly counts as a "designer baby" but, for the sake of argument, let us just stipulate that a designer baby is one selected for his or her superficial characteristics (for example brown eyes, black hair, or tallness). Given this definition, is selecting a saviour sibling relevantly different from selecting a designer baby?

One reason for answering "yes" is the following. In the saviour sibling case, but not in designer babies case, there is a very weighty reason for using PGD saving an existing child's life. But the same cannot be said of designer babies because the reasons for choosing a designer baby (insofar as there are reasons at all) are generally trivial such as a mere fondness for particular hair colour. So the prima facie case for permitting saviour sibling selection is much stronger than that for permitting designer baby selection because there are important reasons for the first but not the second. This constitutes a relevant difference between them and explains why one could without inconsistency oppose the latter but not the former. There is of course much more to be said about how we might in general distinguish important from trivial reasons and we do not claim that this will always be a straightforward matter. But at least in this case the distinction seems relatively clear and unproblematic, for it is hard to deny that saving a child's life is a much more weighty consideration than getting a child with one's preferred hair colour.

We conclude therefore that the slippery slope or designer babies objection fails to justify a ban on the creation on saviour siblings because: (a) even if there is a "slope" there is no reason to believe that a "slide" down it is inevitable and (b) there are important differences between saviour siblings and designer babies which the slippery slope argument overlooks.

The Welfare of the Child

Finally, those who oppose the deliberate creation of saviour siblings often make claims about the welfare of those children who will be thus created. These claims are based on a widely held moral belief (one enshrined in English Law) that, when making decisions about the use of reproductive technologies, we are under an obligation to take into account the welfare of any child created.[16]

The fundamental empirical premise of the child welfare argument is that saviour siblings will, on average, have worse lives than either (a) children conceived "naturally" or (b) other children created using PGD. The second comparator, (b), is of particular relevance if what is argued is that there is nothing wrong with PGD per se but that its use in this context is wrong. Given that the use of PGD for other purposes (that is, screening for a variety of genetic disorders) has been widely accepted, it seems appropriate to take the latter as our main focus.

Two types of damage are suggested by the proponents of the child welfare objection: harm to physical health caused directly by the PGD process and psychological harm. Let's start with physical health. Given that we are considering only the use of umbilical cord stem cells, any physical health problems for the saviour sibling must be caused by the PGD process itself (since no postnatal intervention using the child is envisaged). Is PGD physically harmful to the child thus selected? A recent editorial in The Lancet suggests that "embryo biopsy for PGD does not seem to produce adverse physical effects in the short term, but it is too early to exclude the possibility of later effects."[17] What we can say though is that,

as far as direct effects on physical health are concerned, there is no reason to think that saviour siblings will be any worse off than other children created using PGD. So a child welfare argument based on physical health considerations will either simply fail (because the evidence of harm is inadequate) or will prove too much, counting not only against the creation of saviour siblings but against all uses of PGD. Either way, the argument doesn't successfully single out saviour sibling selection for especially restrictive treatment.

An obvious response to this is to claim that a future child should be exposed to the risks of PGD only if she will probably derive enough benefits to outweigh those risks a view that we will call the net benefit principle. On this view, the potential person is rather like an existing patient and doctors should expose her to risk only if, on the balance of probabilities, she will be a net beneficiary. If this principle is accepted, then (it is argued) there is an important difference between using PGD to select a saviour sibling and using it to screen for a serious genetic disorder since only the latter procedure benefits the child created, and so only the latter can be ethically acceptable.

However, this net benefit argument relies on some confused thinking about what it means to "benefit an embryo." It appears to depend on something like the following model. When we screen for a disorder, an embryo (D) is subjected to an intervention (T) which has the following effects:

1) T prevents D from having a serious genetic disorder.
2) T involves as yet unknown long term health risks for D.

So subjecting D to T can (according to this model) be justified solely by reference to D's interests because the benefit of (1) outweighs the harm or risk involved in (2). In saviour sibling cases, however, things seem importantly different. For an embryo (S) is subjected to an intervention (T*) with the following effects:

1) T* will make S (more likely to be) a donor for an existing child.

2) T* involves as yet unknown long term health risks for S.

T* cannot be justified by reference to S's interests since there is no benefit for S and some risk and so, if we accept the net benefit principle, inflicting T* on S is wrong. This then provides the (supposed) ethical basis for allowing preimplantation screening for genetic disorders, while not allowing saviour sibling selection namely, that only the former conforms to the net benefit principle.

What's wrong with this model? The main difficulty is that it is not the case that T (PGD) prevents D from having a serious genetic disorder. Rather, D was selected because it did not have the genetic disorder in question (and so had D been naturally implanted, rather than implanted as a result of T, D still would not have had the disorder). So we cannot think of T as benefiting D in a straightforwardly causal way, because T has not cured D or removed a disorder. Rather, T involved choosing D on the grounds that it was already a "healthy" embryo.

Given this, what can it mean to say that D has been benefited by T? The only way to make sense of this claim is to say that D derives benefit because T causes D to be implanted, and being implanted is better for D than not being implanted (assuming that, if implanted, D will go on to have a "life worth living" and that the alternative to implantation is destruction). So, if there is any benefit at all for D, it is not "being healthy rather than having a genetic disorder." Rather, the benefit is "existing rather than not existing."

This style of argument raises a number of thorny philosophical problems which we cannot explore in any depth here. One obvious difficulty, for example, is the question of whether it really makes sense to say of an individual that they were benefited by events that caused them to exist. But there are more practical and more decisive objections too. The most relevant for our purposes is that the argument just outlined applies equally to screening for genetic disorders and saviour sibling selection. For if the relevant benefit is being caused to exist (rather than being cured of a genetic disorder) then clearly both D and S stand to gain more or less equally in this respect since both are caused to exist by the selection

process and probably would not have existed without it. And furthermore this will apply (again, more or less equally) to all selected embryos, except in those few cases where the life in question is so bad that it is "not worth living." So the net benefit principle (even if true) fails to justify drawing a moral distinction between screening for genetic disorders and saviour sibling selection.

We turn now to the idea that saviour siblings will be psychologically scarred. There seem to be two linked analytically separate concerns here: first, that a future child may suffer psychological harm if she finds out that she was wanted not for herself, but as a means to save the life of a sibling; and second, that a child conceived for this reason is likely to enjoy a less close and loving relationship with its parents who are less likely to value and nurture the child given that they wanted it primarily to save the life of the sibling.[18] However, even if we concede for the sake of argument that it would be hurtful or upsetting for a specially selected sibling (A) to discover that she had been conceived for the primary purpose of saving the life of an existing child (B), it seems unlikely that A would be less happy than another, randomly selected sibling (C) who was unable to act as a tissue donor. For it could surely be argued here that A would benefit from B's company and may well derive pleasure from knowing that[19] he has saved B's life. Furthermore, as Robertson et al point out:

> the fact that the parents are willing to conceive another child to protect the first suggests that they are highly committed to the well-being of their children, and that they will value the second child for its own sake as well.

In contrast, imagine the psychological impact on C, born into a bereaved family and later to discover that she was a huge disappointment to her parents because of her inability to save B's life. Of course, a full consideration of the issue of psychological harm would involve marshalling substantial bodies of empirical evidence (not something that we can do here). But while this discussion remains entirely speculative, we can at least say that it is far from obvious that considerations of child welfare should count against, rather than for, the practice of saviour sibling selection.

Next, we want to look at a more philosophical response to the child welfare argument and ask: If it were established that saviour siblings were (on average) less happy than other children, would this fact be sufficient to justify banning the selection of saviour siblings?

We need to start by making a general distinction between two kinds of policy. First, there are "make people happier" policies; these aim to make actual (present or future) people happier than they otherwise would be.[20] Secondly, there are "prevent unhappy people" policies, which aim to prevent unhappy people from coming into existence. Make people happier policies are ubiquitous. Prevent unhappy people policies, on the other hand, are much rarer and often highly controversial because they are seen as "eugenic." An example of a prevent unhappy people policy would be encouraging the termination of fetuses with severe physical impairments (or at least this is one possible rationale for such a policy).[21]

Within this category (prevent unhappy people policies) a further distinction can be drawn. First, there are policies that aim to prevent the creation of A so that B (who will be more happy than A would have been) can be created instead. B, in a manner of speaking, takes A's place. Kuhse and Singer provide what seems to be a clear example of this way of thinking (emphasis added):[22]

> If the test shows that the foetus does have Down's syndrome, the woman is able to have an abortion. The same happens with women who are shown to be carriers of the gene for haemophilia: the foetus can be checked to see if it has the disease. If it does, the woman can have an abortion, and then try again, so that she can have a normal baby. Why do we regard this as a reasonable thing to do, even when the handicap is one like haemophilia, which is quite compatible with a worthwhile life? ... *[Because] we are offsetting the loss of one possible life against the creation of another life with better prospects.*

Secondly, there are policies that simply aim to prevent the creation of A (without any appeal to

"substitution") the thought being that, if A were to be born, she'd have a not merely low, but a negative quality of life, one such that she'd be "better off dead". As Glover puts it:[23]

> some kinds of life are perhaps worse than not being alive at all ... if it makes sense for people to see death as in their interests, there seems a parallel possibility of parents or doctors thinking that not being born may be in the interests of a potential child.

Many regulations governing reproduction are of the "make people happier" kind. Other legislation, though, is not about making actual children happier but is, rather, about reducing the number of "disadvantaged" children born either directly, through prohibition, or indirectly, through measures which are calculated to discourage. Such legislation clearly falls into the "prevent unhappy people" category. But can child welfare considerations justify such restrictions?

These restrictions could be defended in one (or both) of two ways. The first justification is that they lead to the "replacement" of less happy future people with more happy ones. The second is that they prevent misery and suffering by stopping the births of people with "negative quality lives." Let's take the second justification first. This is extremely unlikely to work against saviour sibling selection, even if any children created face very severe psychological problems. For, in the absence of other unconnected problems (for example severe painful illness) the chances of saviour siblings having negative quality lives are remote. Are we really expected to believe that these children will live lives that are worse than not being alive at all? Also relevant here are thoughts about how our attitudes to saviour siblings cohere with our attitudes to children with disabilities. For in the debate about prenatal screening, selective termination, eugenics and suchlike, the thought that people with severe and painful disabilities are "glad to be alive" is (rightly) taken seriously. If we allow (as we should) that these people, faced with extraordinarily unfavourable circumstances, have lives worth living, then surely we must also allow that most saviour siblings will have lives worth living too.

So proponents of restrictive regulation are forced to fall back on the first justification: selecting saviour siblings should be banned because this will lead to the children who would otherwise have been created in this way being "replaced" by a roughly equal number of other "happier" children (children who would not have existed at all if saviour sibling selection had been allowed). This, though, is problematic because there are general theoretical reasons for not allowing any arguments of this sort (replacement arguments) to influence the regulation of reproduction. The main one is that if arguments of this type are acceptable, then there seems no reason to restrict their application to particular practices like saviour sibling selection. Once we start thinking in this way, it is hard to limit the scope of such arguments because, as Glover suggests:[24]

If someone with a handicap is conceived instead of a normal person, things turn out less well than they might have done. It would have been better if the normal person had been conceived. But things of this sort can be said about almost any of us. If my own conception was an alternative to the conception of someone just like me except more intelligent, or more athletic or more musical, it would have been better if that person had been conceived.

This has troubling implications. The main one is that if a replacement argument is deemed sufficient to justify prohibiting saviour sibling selection then (other things being equal) parallel arguments should, for reasons of consistency, be deemed sufficient to justify (amongst other things) making compulsory the use of prenatal screening or PGD so as to reduce the amount of disease in the world, and making women impregnate themselves with enhanced donor sperm rather than the "normal" sperm of their partners. The replacement justification of these coercive state actions would be fundamentally the same as the one lying behind the prohibition of saviour sibling selection that is, people's procreative autonomy would be restricted on the grounds that it would be better if a "happier" group of future persons came into existence instead of a "less happy" group.[25]

Our contention is not that all of these practices are exactly the same; they are not. But we would argue that there is something troubling about allowing this style of reasoning to underpin restrictions on procreative liberty. We would be the first to admit that this argument needs much more fleshing out (not something there is space to do here). However, what is clear, even from this short version is that there is something problematic about using replacement arguments to justify coercive state action. Hence, this justificatory strategy is not one on which prohibitionists should rely.

Conclusion

In this paper, we have critically assessed the three main arguments for prohibiting the use of PGD and tissue typing to select saviour siblings. These arguments are (a) that saviour siblings would be wrongfully treated as means rather than ends, (b) that they would cause or constitute a slide towards designer babies, and (c) that they would suffer physically and/or emotionally. We have found each of these arguments to be flawed and therefore conclude that the selection of saviour siblings should be permitted, especially given that prohibiting it would result in the preventable deaths of a number of existing children.

Notes

1 Spriggs M, Savulescu J. "Saviour siblings." *J Med Ethics* 2002,28:289. Davies J-A, "'Designer' baby goes ahead." *The Age* 12 March 2003, www.theage.com.au/articles/2003/03/!1/l 047144972401.html.

2 BBC News. Hashmi decision sparks ethics row, 22 February 2002, http://news.bbc.co.uk/1/hi/health/1836827.stm.

3 BBC News. Genetics storm girl "responding well," 19 October 2002, http://news.bbc.co.uk/1/hi/health/979884.stm.

4 This term is taken from Spriggs M, Savulescu J. "Saviour siblings." *J Med Ethics* 2002,28:289.

5 Robertson JA, Kahn JP, Wagner JE. Conception to obtain hematopoietic stem cells. *Hastings Cent Rep* 2002;32:34-40.

6 R (Quintavalle) v Human Fertilisation and Embryology Authority [2003] EWHC 2785 (Admin).

7   R (Quintavalle) v Human Fertilisation and Embryology Authority [2003] EWCA Civ 667.

8   Glover J. Quoted in: BBC News. Doctor plans "designer baby" clinic. 11 December 2001, http://news.bbc.co.Uk/l/hi/health/1702854.stm.

9   Quintavalle J. Quoted in: BBC News. Doctor plans "designer baby" clinic. 11 December 2001, http://news.bbc.co.Uk/l/hi/health/1702854.stm. Quintavelle is a leading, member of the group, Comment on Reproductive Ethics, which brought me judicial review action described in reference 5 above.

10 Nathanson V. Quoted in: BBC News. Baby created to save older sister. 4 October 2000, http://news.bbc.co.Uk/l/hi/health/1702854.stm.

11 Winston R. Quoted in: BBC News. Go-ahead for "designer babies." 13 December 2001, http://news.bbc.co.Uk/l/hi/health/1706926.stm.

12 Boyle R, Savulescu J. Ethics of using preimplantation genetic diagnosis to select a stem cell donor for an existing person. *BMJ* 2001;323:1240-43, 1241.

13 Harris J. *The Value of Life.* London: Routledge, 1985:143.

14 Attributed to Josephine Quintavalle by BBC News. Pro-life challenge to embryo testing, 12 July 2002, http://news.bbc.co.uk/!/hi/health/ 2125482.stm.

15 This is partly because contesting this would take us too far from the issue at hand and into very complex territory, and partly because we don't need to contest it to undermine the slippery slope argument.

16 Under s. 13, Human Fertilisation and Embryology Act 1990, we are directed that: "A woman shall not be provided with treatment services unless account has been taken of the welfare of any child who may be born as a result of the treatment (including the need of that child for a father), and of any other child who may be affected by the birth." It should be noted here that this section also explicitly invites us to consider the welfare of existing children. Whilst it is probable that the architects of the 1990 Act were thinking here of the prevention of harm rather than the according of benefits to existing children, the wording of the law is clearly broad enough also to include the latter. This was recognised by the Court of Appeal in its consideration of the Hashmi case, see the judgment of Manee U at 133.

17 Preimplantation donor selection [editorial]. *Lancet* 2001,358:1195.

18 This possibility was specifically denied by both the Hashmis and the Whitakers, who claimed that they wanted another child in any case.

19 These kinds of arguments are routinely advanced by the courts in allowing parents to consent to allow one sibling to act as a donor to another. Such donation is held to be in the donor's best interests, notwithstanding the pain and physical risks associated with the procedure, because of the donor's interest in a continued relationship with his or her sibling. Strunk v Strunk (1969)445SW2dl45(KyCA).

20 We use terms like "happy" and "unhappy" here as a shorthand for quality of life (as perceived from the perspective of the person living that life).

21 Sheldon S, Wilkinson S. Termination of pregnancy for reason of foetal disability: are there grounds for a special exception in law? *Med Law Rev* 2001;9:85-109.

22 Kuhse H, Singer P. *Should the Baby Live?* Oxford: Oxford University Press, 1985:158.

23 Glover J. *Fertility and the Family: the Glover Report on reproductive technologies to the European Commission.* London: Fourth Estate, 1989, 129. See also reference 27.

24 Glover J. *Causing Death and Saving Lives.* Harmondsworth: Penguin, 1977:148.

25 Sheldon S, Wilkinson S. Termination of pregnancy for reason of foetal disability: are there grounds for a special exception in law? *Med Law Rev* 2001;9:85-109.

32.
CHALLENGING THE RHETORIC OF CHOICE IN PRENATAL SCREENING

Victoria Seavilleklein

SOURCE: *Bioethics* 23.1 (2009): 68-77.

Introduction

Prenatal screening in Canada is on the verge of expanding in multiple different directions. This screening, consisting of maternal serum screening and nuchal translucency screening, is designed to identify pregnant women likely to have fetuses with chromosomal anomalies and open neural tube defects; once identified, these women can be offered further diagnostic testing with the option of abortion if test results are positive. While prenatal screening has traditionally been limited to pregnant women considered to be 'high-risk,' the Society of Obstetricians and Gynaecologists of Canada (SOGC) has recently recommended that it be offered to all pregnant women regardless of age, disease history or risk status.[1] Similar recommendations have been made by the American College of Obstetricians and Gynecologists (ACOG).[2] In addition to broadening the target population of screening, the number of conditions being screened for is likely to increase. For decades, prenatal screening has been used to screen for Down syndrome, open neural tube defects, and Trisomy18. Current studies, however, show that prenatal screens might also be used to detect conditions such as Smith-Lemli-Opitz syndrome,[3] Trisomy13, Turner's syndrome,[4] and cystic fibrosis.[5] Hence, this particular juncture is an ideal moment to pause and reflect on the reasons for this proliferation of screening and the values that it is deemed to support.

One of the principal values that is offered in support of prenatal screening is autonomy. The value of autonomy, often framed in terms of women's choice, is widely recognized by those who fund, research, develop, and implement prenatal screening[6] and is central in obstetrics and genetics departments and public information pamphlets.[7] Even those who object to some or many aspects of prenatal screening, such as disability rights activists, prioritize autonomy when they state that decisions about the kind of children one will raise—if such decisions must be made at all—are better left to individual women than to society or the medical profession.[8] In this paper, I critically examine the value of autonomy in the context of prenatal screening to determine whether it justifies the expansion of prenatal screening to all pregnant women. I argue that current screening practice does not protect or promote women's autonomy in the vast majority of cases, either on a narrow analysis of choice reflecting individual autonomy or on a broad analysis of choice reflecting relational autonomy. Consequently, we should hesitate before expanding screening to more pregnant women.

Autonomy and Informed Consent

The value of autonomy is deeply entrenched in contemporary society. It is a reflection of broad social-political change brought about in the second half of the 20th century by second-wave feminism, the civil rights movement in the US, and the development of the Charter of Rights and Freedoms in the new Canadian Constitution. It also represents efforts to distance current genetics practices from the coercive and discriminatory practices of past eugenics movements and from other abuses in human experimentation and clinical medicine.

Despite its importance in society and particularly in genetics, there is incontrovertible evidence that women are not making free informed choices about prenatal screening. Autonomy is protected in health care by the theory and practice of informed consent, the most authoritative and widely disseminated theory of which is described by Tom Beauchamp and James Childress.[9] In a specific decision-making context, informed consent is deemed to be reached if the person is competent, if adequate standards of disclosure and understanding about the intervention are attained, and if consent (i.e., authorization) is given voluntarily. According to studies conducted in North America and in the Western world, informed consent is not being met in the vast majority of cases in prenatal screening.[10] In particular, a recent Health Technology Assessment, conducted by Green at al. for the UK's National Health Service, identified and surveyed 78 studies that have been conducted internationally about the psychosocial implications of prenatal screening. Most of these studies were conducted in the US and the UK, although several are from Canada and other European countries. The overwhelming conclusion drawn from all of this research concerned 'the inadequacy of current procedures for achieving informed consent.'[11]

There is no one element of informed consent that consistently fails to achieve an adequate threshold level in prenatal screening. Rather, any of disclosure, understanding, voluntariness and consent[12] can be challenged as inadequate in light of the empirical evidence of current practice. I will give some examples of each. First of all, while some pregnant women may not be competent to give informed consent, the vast majority of women are and so this precondition for decision-making is not a central concern in most analyses.

Disclosure is important because its quality determines women's ability to understand the test. The SOGC recommends that the following information be provided to pregnant women prior to a screening test: details about the conditions being screened, the likelihood of detection, the method of screening, the meaning of a screen-positive result and a screen-negative result, the choices following a screen-positive result (amniotic fluid alpha fetoprotein, acetylcholinesterase and fetal karyotype, detailed ultrasound for fetal anomaly), the choices following a positive diagnosis (abortion or continuation of the pregnancy) and details as to how further information can be obtained.[13]

While full counselling is not recommended, this still encompasses a great deal of information to disclose in a short clinical encounter. Describing the details of the conditions screened for alone will take several minutes.[14] Nevertheless, a 1993 report of the Royal Commission on New Reproductive Technologies revealed that physicians spent less than five minutes on average discussing maternal serum screening.[15] A US study reported a discussion time of approximately two minutes.[16] This is a very limited period of time in which to disclose all the relevant material listed by the SOGC. In practice, relevant details are often disclosed incorrectly to pregnant women,[17] not disclosed at all (such as the possibility of abortion if consequent tests are positive), or a discussion does not even take place.[18]

In health care, patients must not only be given information relevant to their decision-making, they must also understand the information that they have been given. Full understanding is not required for informed consent but patients should understand the salient aspects of the proposed procedure and the consequences of proceeding with the intervention or not.[19] Studies evaluating women's knowledge and understanding of prenatal screening overwhelmingly show that women do not understand the testing, including basic facts such as why the test is being done, what conditions are being looked for, what the results mean, and what will (or may) follow after testing.[20] These findings are the same both for women who choose to have testing and for those who decline.[21] Researchers of one of the most comprehensive studies done on this topic in Canada concluded that despite the high educational level of their study cohort and the existence of a well-organized provincial screening program, there were 'information gaps overall and in all domains.'[22]

A contributing factor to this difficulty in comprehension may be that probabilities are very difficult for people to understand. For example, when women are told that they have an increased risk of having a fetus with Down syndrome, some women think this means a) that they have a fetus with Down syndrome[23] or b) that their chance of having a child with Down syndrome is 50-50.[24] This reaction reflects the difficulty in applying a population statistic at an individual level; after all, a chance of 1 in 250 of having a child with a certain condition is meaningful when considering a group of 250 women, but it does not say anything specific about the child of any particular woman in that group.

Once the relevant information has been disclosed and understood, a decision must be made voluntarily, or in the absence of a substantially controlling influence.[25] Whether an act is controlled, non-controlled, or somewhere in between depends on the degree to which a patient acts on the basis of her own will. The most obvious cases where voluntariness is undermined are when women are not asked for their authorization at all or when they believe that testing is mandatory. Screening was originally performed frequently without giving women the ability to consent or decline. For example, in the first Canadian prenatal screening program, established in Manitoba in 1985, only 38% of clinicians asked for women's express consent for maternal serum alphafetoprotein (AFP) screening while more than 40% incorporated the test into routine blood work without asking for consent.[26] A more recent prospective study performed in Ontario in 1996 found that 360 out of 941 respondents reported that they had not been given a choice about having maternal serum screening.[27] Their belief that they did not have a choice about testing is sufficient to undermine voluntariness.

The influence that a health-care provider has on a woman's decision-making is widely recorded in the literature on prenatal diagnosis,[28] with decision-making correlating with factors such as the provider's approach, gender, and specialty (i.e., obstetrician versus general practitioner).[29] This same trend has been observed in prenatal screening. Nancy Press and Carole Browner found that the very diverse group of women in their study—who almost unanimously accepted screening—were influenced primarily by the way in which the screening was described to them by their health-care provider and in patient information pamphlets (both of which were biased in favour of screening).[30] Diane Paul goes so far as to say that the strongest determining factor in whether women choose to have screening is not in the attitudes of the women but in the approach taken by their health-care provider.[31] Whether this influence is sufficient to undermine voluntariness may be debated. However,

in some cases, health-care providers may use their influence to more directly determine the choices of pregnant women. For instance, concerns about litigation, if women do not have screening and end up having a child with a disability, may cause some physicians to err on the 'safe' side and convince women to have screening in a way that may be regarded as substantially controlling.[32]

Consent, the final element, refers to the authorization given for a specific procedure or intervention to be performed. It can be express, tacit (given through silence or by omission), implicit or implied (when consent is interpreted by certain actions), or presumed (based on assumptions of what a person will or should do).[33] It is clear from documents on prenatal screening that the form of consent considered to be appropriate is express consent. For example, the SOGC Practice Guidelines for maternal serum screening state that 'The decision whether or not to have testing may be verbally communicated between the woman and her health care provider but, ideally, should be recorded.'[34] The empirical evidence discussed above shows that express consent for prenatal screening is not always asked for or given by women undergoing the testing.

Hence, while some health-care providers may be very skilled at clearly disclosing the relevant information and some pregnant women may understand the test sufficiently to provide express voluntary consent (or refusal), in the majority of cases adequate levels of informed consent are not being achieved. Given the importance of autonomy in our society and in genetics in particular, it is essential that efforts be made to improve the process of informed consent in order to protect free informed choice for pregnant women. The fact that reproductive autonomy is not being well protected in current prenatal screening practice should also make us wary about expanding the scope of screening to pregnant women population-wide.

A Relational Approach

Even if the process of informed consent were improved, however, this theory reflects a very narrow conception of choice; it reflects a bias in the literature about choice traditionally understood as individual choice, or individual autonomy, in a specific decision-making context. An analysis of women's choice is thereby restricted to their ability to accept or decline a particular option that is offered to them. It allows no room for reflection on the practice that is making those particular choices available or on other contextual influences outside the clinic that may not qualify as coercive or substantially controlling but may nevertheless have a significant impact on women's decision-making. If prenatal screening is intended to represent something more than an additional consumer choice for women, then a broader conception of choice is required.

A broader conception of choice requires a different kind of theory. In traditional theories of autonomy, persons are characterized as independent, self-sufficient, rational decision-makers who can receive information and make decisions by weighing the costs and benefits of various options. By contrast, in theories of relational autonomy, persons are viewed as relational beings embedded within and shaped by a web of interconnected relationship.[35] As a result of this conception of selves, persons, and their values, desires, etc. are seen as constructed in part by their social environment.[36] Relational autonomy (understood in a broad sense) has a much larger scope than informed consent, or individual autonomy. It explicitly includes consideration not only of women's decision-making in the clinic, but also of the social and political context in which practices develop and choices are offered;[37] it is not just the quality of the information disclosed to pregnant women that matters but the kinds of choices that are available, how these choices are framed, and what opportunities or pressures women experience as a result. These contextual features, illuminated by a relational approach, provide additional reason to challenge the claim that prenatal screening should be promoted and expanded on the basis of autonomy.

Contextual factors, such as the research agenda, political and economic interests, and historical circumstance, are worth exploring because they provide insight into the practice of prenatal screening and determine the choices that women will face in the clinic.[38] Carine Vassy argues that in the UK prenatal screening was not developed in response to the demands of women, as is often claimed, but that pro-

grams were initiated by government organizations, interested sectors of the medical profession, and the medical supply industry for their own purposes.[39] In France, she notes the role of biomedical researchers in implementing and expanding screening services. While there were undoubtedly numerous factors and actors influencing the initial developments and implementations of screening programs, Vassy claims that testing is established to suit particular interests in society—but not directly those of pregnant women—and that women are then screened without much attention to informed consent. Citing various studies, she argues that most women in France simply followed along with offers of testing and did not make engaged, informed decisions to be tested.[40] As we have seen, there was a similar lack of express consent sought by health-care providers in Canada in the early years of screening.[41] Since the number of women being screened increases when informed consent is not a priority, Vassy argues that institutions and organizations involved in the screening receive the false impression that women want the testing and therefore invest more resources into expanding the services. Expanded services result in more women being tested, and so the cycle continues. At some point during this feedback loop, however, the testing becomes normalized as part of routine prenatal care, such that women come to expect it; stopping the programs then becomes perceived as removing choice even though women's wishes about screening may never have been established.

Similarly, despite the rhetoric of choice in screening programs and the conviction of clinicians that 'women want this testing' and that 'we are just offering women what they want,' there is little support in the literature for women driving the initiative to develop and implement prenatal screens; this creative impetus seems to have come from elsewhere. There is some information collected on the wishes of couples regarding future use of prenatal genetic testing when they have already had a child with a particular condition,[42] but there is not much evidence available regarding the wishes of low-risk populations for screening services. Some of the evidence that does exist does not provide much clarity. For example, the health technology assessment by Green et al. reports that most women seem to have favourable attitudes towards the screening although they have 'ambiguous or conflicting evaluations of the role of screening and the information it provides to the individual and society.'[43] Moreover, the authors found that efforts to study the desires of women were inconsistent, that some perspectives were likely misrepresented in the data, and that others were affected by 'cognitive readjustment' or post-choice bias.[44] Another complicating factor was that women's choices were not fully informed and relied mostly on wishes for reassurances and/or on the recommendations of their health-care provider.[45]

Once prenatal screening is established, its implementation and uptake may be propelled by cultural attitudes about the value of information and of science. 'Information is power,' 'more information is better than less,' and 'information increases choice' are all familiar mantras. The emphasis on informed choice that is pervasive in prenatal screening seems to reinforce this view. For example, in a study conducted by Press and Browner of Catholic pregnant women, the participants thought it was better to have the information about a positive screen result despite the fact that nothing could be done about it (or would be done about it, since most did not want to abort).[46] Moreover, the belief appeared to be unanimous that scientific information 'could not, or should not, be refused.'[47] Similarly, a study conducted for the late onset condition of Alzheimer's found that, despite most participants remembering almost nothing about their genotype or risk factors for the condition, they all stated that they would recommend testing to their friends and relatives partly because they thought it would 'provide useful information.'[48] Hence, whether women want genetic or biological information is debatable. For those who do come to value it, it is not clear why they value it; in the latter case, for instance, the information was prized even though it was not fully understood or needed for decision-making.

Whether more information, obtained via new screening options, will increase choice is also unclear. Barbara Katz Rothman explains that sometimes new options quietly foreclose on old possibilities.[49] She gives the example of contraception. When it was first introduced, it was hailed as a tool of liberation—especially for the middle classes—

because women were able to control the size of their families and have fewer children. A consequence of this choice, especially when it came to be made by more and more women, was that it became socially difficult to have large families. She notes the difficulty of finding apartments and even vehicles large enough to accommodate a family with more than two or three children, not to mention the wealth that is necessary to make large families feasible.[50] Women on welfare who have 'too many children' have been threatened at various times in the past with a loss of welfare payments if they have any more.[51] This example demonstrates a 'narrowing and structuring of choices.'[52] According to Ruth Hubbard, '[a]s choices become available, they all too rapidly become compulsions to "choose" the socially endorsed alternative.'[53]

When the focus of society is on a new option, such as prenatal screening, other possibilities might become harder to choose or may silently disappear. In other words, once women exercise their ability to make the choice to use prenatal screening, they might lose their ability not to choose it. For instance, increased use of maternal serum screening enabled the SOGC to recommend that amniocentesis only be routinely offered to pregnant women over the age of 40; this strategy assumes that all women aged 35 to 39 who are interested in amniocentesis will make use of maternal serum screening, as indeed they must in order to have access to amniocentesis. The testing pathway that older pregnant women can take has been re-shaped by these new recommendations and their option to choose amniocentesis directly (or at all, if they receive a negative screen result) has disappeared.[54]

Social-political forces and entrenched cultural assumptions can also affect how choices are framed and how free women may feel to make certain decisions. For instance, recommendations for the widespread offering of amniocentesis were instigated by two major lawsuits filed (and won) by women who had not been offered testing and had given birth to children with disabilities.[55] Because of the fear that any problems with a newborn must be assigned a culprit, clinicians may be worried that even if a woman does not wish for screening now, in retrospect, she might have wanted it, in which case clinicians may be liable.[56] As a result, health-care providers may be more persuasive when offering a test than strict standards of disclosure would allow[57] and make it hard for women to decline screening.[58]

The language used to describe the screening may also affect choice. For example, disability rights activists have challenged the use of language such as 'abnormalities,' 'defects,' and 'risks' because they are normative and have built-in negative connotations.[59] Women's decisions may be subtly influenced by how they interpret these terms. Language may also mislead when comments referring to screening as a way to 'make sure your baby is healthy' imply that testing is meant to ensure health rather than to detect certain conditions.[60] Also, any comments that suggest directiveness are influential to some degree. Statements like 'when a screening test is positive, further investigation is *usually recommended*' and 'if the test shows a higher risk, it can also cause a lot of worry until *we can find out for sure* if there really is a problem'[61] imply that further testing should or will normally follow after a positive screen result instead of emphasizing that it is up to the woman whether she chooses to pursue the results further.

Entrenched cultural assumptions about the roles and responsibilities of women and mothers may increase the difficulty women face in refusing screening. Abby Lippman argues that claims that women themselves need or choose prenatal screening is something constructed by the context of testing.[62] The fact that women are generally responsible for the health of the family and that screening is often portrayed as part of routine prenatal care makes screening seem like the responsible course to take.[63] The commonly expressed belief that testing is reassuring goes hand-in-hand with this assumption, since it builds on the belief held by some women that testing will somehow promote the birth of a healthy child, such that a caring woman is not doing her motherly duty if she foregoes this testing. The framing of screening in this way makes the refusal of screening seem irresponsible or irrational.

The labelling of pregnant women as 'at-risk' is also likely to construct a perceived need for testing according to Lippman. A woman labelled 'high-risk' may feel that she requires testing in order to reduce her risk, whatever her actual risk figure.[64] Indeed, in pregnancy, everyone is categorized as 'at-risk'; they are either low or high risk, at least until all the results are in. No one is 'no-risk'[65] despite the fact that the vast majority of children are born healthy and at term.[66] Because of the negative and fearful connotations of risk, the label of risk may make women feel more dependent on technology for their pregnancies to reduce this risk and to provide reassurance that their pregnancy is progressing normally.[67] The impact of risk labels can be demonstrated by looking at the uptake of prenatal screening in the Netherlands where pregnancy is considered natural and not medicalized to anywhere near the degree that it is in North America.[68] In a study of 1400 pregnant women who received the offer of screening along with detailed information about the advantages and disadvantages of screening, the 35% who declined screening did so on the basis of the fact that they believed testing to be unnecessary; one of the primary reasons given for this judgment was that they were not categorized as belonging to a risk group.[69] In North America, every pregnant woman is categorized as belonging to a risk group, thereby eliminating the reasonableness of declining screening based on lack of need.

The very offer of screening, however it is framed, may create a perceived need for testing, especially when screens have been selected and implemented by the medical system; this decision establishes screening as a legitimate use of scarce medical resources and thereby surreptitiously underlines its importance. The offer of screening is widely recognized to raise anxiety levels in pregnant women, in addition to positive screen results.[70] Susan Sherwin argues that the medicalization of pregnancy elevates the importance of medical interventions and distances women from their own pregnancies; this distance increases their anxiety and causes women to rely even more on medical expertise to assure them that everything is progressing normally, thus reinforcing the cycle of dependence.[71] Indeed, reassurance is one of the primary reasons for which women pursue prenatal screening.[72] In the same Dutch study described above, where pregnancy is not medicalized and prenatal screening is not routine, pregnant women do not feel these levels of anxiety about their pregnancies. Of the 1400 pregnant women offered prenatal screening in the study, 'reassurance' was almost insignificant (8%) as a contributing factor for accepting testing.[73]

Hence, the existence of the technology and the way it is portrayed creates the perception that it is a necessary part of prenatal care, not merely an optional one. Once screening becomes even more normalized, it may not even be reassuring to be in a low risk bracket or to have one's risk reduced; the impetus for testing may remain due to the fact that fears over the conditions being screened for may become enhanced due to the constant public focus created by prenatal screening and diagnosis.[74] Also, as tests become more normalized, they become harder to question or decline and they become part of the care that is desired by women and expected of women.[75]

Ultrasonography is a classic example of a technology that was adapted for pregnancy and increasingly became offered to assess gestational age, detect fetal anomalies and monitor fetal development.[76] This technology is now entrenched in prenatal care and has come to play an important social and emotional role in pregnancy because of its ability to visualize the fetus.[77] This role has been fulfilled despite a continued lack of evidence as to its clinical efficacy.[78] Regardless of its clinical import, ultrasound is so central to the pregnancy experience and so widely valued that most women who are offered it have difficulty refusing it at the risk of being judged to be irrational or irresponsible.[79] In prenatal interventions that are as normalized as ultrasound, to decline their use poses an 'enormous burden of proof' on those who might want to challenge the norm.[80]

Ultrasonography also presents an example of how familiarity with a technology and its routinization or normalization in prenatal care can reduce the impact of choice and even the perceived need to ask for authorization. Informed consent in relation to ultrasonography as a screening test is significantly below any reasonable threshold[81] and counselling women prior to screening is no longer even a standard of practice.[82] A study conducted in Canada in 2002 found that out of 113 women surveyed before undergoing their 18 week ultrasound, 55% had not received any information about ultrasound screening from their health-care provider, 46% did not understand the ultrasound to be a screen for anomalies,

and 26% were unclear about its diagnostic capabilities.[83] Hence, the widespread desire for and use of ultrasound screening is not accompanied by any significant level of understanding about the meaning or implications of the screen, at least relative to the purpose for which the technology has been medically justified.[84] Since pre-test counselling for ultrasound is no longer a standard of practice, it is naïve to suppose that informed consent will increase with more widespread use of prenatal screening if it is not even being satisfied now. In fact, as a practice becomes more accepted, it often ceases to become a focus of critical attention.[85]

A framework of relational autonomy also allows us to look beyond the available choices to consider other possibilities. The choice that is being offered with prenatal screening is not the choice to have a blood test but the choice to avoid having a child with a certain condition, primarily one that could result in a disability. Prenatal screening is the first step in offering women this choice. Why is this choice being supported and not others? For example, women can choose to abort a fetus with Down syndrome or spina bifida at 20 weeks gestation but they cannot choose to abort a fetus at 20 weeks based on fetal sex (in the absence of a sex-linked disorder). Abortions on the basis of fetal sex are considered to be morally objectionable because of entrenched sex discrimination against female fetuses; hence, abortions based on this trait are not supported by the medical profession. Nor is it widely supported for women to choose to give birth under water or using a birthing stool, to give birth at home,[86] or to stay several days in the hospital after labour in order to have time to rest and adjust to being a mother. In other words, it is only possible to make choices about a narrow range of options that are defined by the medical system. Whether certain options will be available to pregnant women depends on the eligibility criteria set by the medical system, and these occasionally shift in light of professional practice guidelines as is the case with prenatal screening. Likewise, prenatal technologies are not freely available for women to choose but can only be accessed through the medical system acting as gatekeeper.

Interestingly, part of the emphasis on prenatal screening over the last several years has been due to the fact that women are having children later in life. Since the risk of chromosomal anomalies increases with age, the incidence of Down syndrome is suspected to have increased dramatically in correlation.[87] This suspicion has been used in part to justify widescale implementation of prenatal screening and to motivate the case to secure provincial funding for these programs.[88] While prenatal screening, diagnosis, and abortion have been targeted as a means by which to counter this increasing incidence, alternatives such as creating more possibilities for women to have children earlier have not been sufficiently promoted or endorsed. While women may delay childbirth for many reasons, the fact that having a child early in a woman's career may be damaging to her chances of success is a significant reason to postpone pregnancy. Increased acceptance in the workplace of child care demands and maternity leaves might remove some of the social pressure that encourages some women to put their childbearing plans on hold until their career paths are secure.

A societal commitment to support children with disabilities is another option that is often not given as much attention as prenatal screening, diagnosis and abortion options. For instance, it is hard to make a free choice about pursuing prenatal screening options when there are not adequate socially-supported alternatives, such as social supports, that would make the decision to raise a child with disabilities easier and/or when the availability of these services is not known to women during pregnancy. Social and economic pressures (in addition to pervasive discrimination) may make a woman feel that she is not able to care for a child with disabilities and turn to screening options as a result.[89] Hence, improved social supports and the communication of these supports to pregnant women may have an impact on some women's reproductive decisions.[90] While many pregnant women may still choose to pursue screening, diagnosis, and abortion even when social supports are very good and known to them during pregnancy (or before), knowing that there are adequate supports available may enhance the ability of some women to make the choice to continue a pregnancy if the choice to do so might otherwise have been restrained by a concern about resources.

In summary, there are a multitude of factors in society that might influence women's choices in the clinical context; while these factors might not be characterized as coercive or substantially controlling, as described in the theory of informed consent, they may nevertheless restrict the ability of women to make a free choice in the face of screening options. These forces include the normalization of technology combined with a cultural desire for information, cultural assumptions about women and mothers being responsible for health combined with the misperception of medical technology as promoting the birth of a healthy child, the categorization of pregnant women into risk categories with technology offering risk reduction and reassurance, and medical and societal values that determine which choices will be supported and made available to pregnant women. Hence, a broader conception of choice using a relational framework reveals additional reasons to worry that the expansion of prenatal screening may undermine women's autonomy.

To be clear, I am not advocating that prenatal screening be withheld from pregnant women. Reproductive autonomy is highly valued in our society and is important because of past coercive practices in reproduction and continued gender oppression. Because having a child with a disability may have a significant impact on a woman's life (depending on the severity) and because she is more likely to be responsible for the care work, she is in the best position to judge whether having a child with a disability is something that she could manage. However, it is not clear that women are being given the opportunity to make informed choices about screening. Some women are being subtly directed down a path that, given greater understanding, they might not have chosen. Increased normalization through the continued expansion of prenatal screening will extend these concerns to all pregnant women. In order to promote reproductive autonomy for women who want testing while protecting the autonomy of women who may not, alternative means of implementing prenatal screening should be pursued. One possibility that I explore elsewhere is to make screening available to all women who want it without routinely offering it as part of standard prenatal care.[91]

Conclusion

In short, whether choice is interpreted narrowly as informed consent or broadly as relational, there are reasons to worry that women's autonomy is not being protected or promoted by the routine offer of screening. At minimum, efforts must be made to improve the process of informed consent, which is no easy task. Steps should also be taken to address some of the contextual factors that restrain choice. In the meantime, however, incorporating the offer of prenatal screening into routine prenatal care for all pregnant women is not supported by the value of autonomy and ought to be reconsidered.

Notes

1   A. Summers et al. Prenatal Screening for Fetal Aneuploidy—SOGC Clinical Practice Guidelines. *J Soc Obstet Gynaecol Can*. 2007; 29: 146-161.

2   American College of Obstetricians and Gynecologists. ACOG Practice Bulletin no. 77: Screening for Fetal Chromosomal Abnormalities. *Obstet Gynecol*. 2007; 109: 217-228.

3   Smith-Lemli-Opitz syndrome is already being screened for in some health districts, e.g., Nova Scotia.

4   Summers et al., op. cit. note 1.

5   The SOGC does not currently recommend prenatal screening for cystic fibrosis (R.D. Wilson. Cystic Fibrosis Carrier Testing in Pregnancy in Canada—SOGC Committee Opinion. *J Obstet Gynaecol Can*. 2002; 24: 644-647). However, it may soon be offered as part of routine screening in the US (CBC Radio One. August 15, 2007. Preparing Parents for the News: Interview with Dr. David Young. Information Mornings. Available at: http://www.cbc.ca/informationmorningns/interviews.html [Accessed 1 Nov 2007].

6   For example, see E.M. Hutton et al. Practice Guidelines for Health Care Providers Involved in Prenatal Screening and Diagnosis. SOGC Clinical Practice Guidelines. 1998: 1-5.

7   For example, see Ontario Maternal Serum Screening Steering Committee. 2004. Integrated Prenatal Screening (IPS): It's Your Choice. Available at: http://www.lhsc.on.ca/programs/rmgc/mss/pamphlet.

htm [Accessed 1 Nov 2007]; Women's and Children's Health Programs: Obstetrics/Gynaecology. Maternal Serum Testing: A Pamphlet for Women who are Pregnant, or Planning Pregnancy. Available at: http://www.ahsc.health.nb.ca/prenatalscreening/PrintableMaterials6.htm [Accessed 1 Nov 2007].

8   E. Parens & A. Asch. 2000. *The Disability Rights Critique of Prenatal Genetic Testing: Reflections and Recommendations. In Prenatal Testing and Disability Rights*. E. Parens & A. Asch, eds. Washington, D.C.: Georgetown University Press: 3-43.

9   T. Beauchamp & J. Childress. 2001. *Principles of Biomedical Ethics*. 5th ed. New York: Oxford University Press. For a thorough exploration of an earlier account, see R. Faden, T. Beauchamp & N. King. 1986. *A History and Theory of Informed Consent*. New York: Oxford University Press.

10 J.M. Green et al. Psychosocial Aspects of Genetic Screening of Pregnant Women and Newborns: A Systematic Review. *Health Technol Assess*. 2004; 8: iii, ix-x, 1-109; V. Goel et al. Evaluating Patient's Knowledge of Maternal Serum Screening. *Prenat Diagn*. 1996; 16: 425-430; A.M. Jaques, L.J. Sheffield & J.L. Halliday. Informed Choice in Women Attending Private Clinics to Undergo First-Trimester Screening for Down Syndrome. *Prenat Diagn*. 2005; 25: 656-664; J. Gekas et al. Informed Consent to Serum Screening for Down Syndrome: Are Women Given Adequate Information? *Prenat Diagn*. 1999; 19: 1-7.

11 Green et al., op. cit. note 10, p. 76.

12 'Consent' should not be confused with 'informed consent.' Consent is one of the elements of informed consent, and simply refers to the decision that is made to accept or decline a medical intervention. For example, agreeing to a procedure without proper discussion or understanding would satisfy the criterion of consent, but informed consent would not be achieved because adequate threshold levels of the other three elements would not also have been met.

13 J. Johnson & A. Summers. Prenatal Genetic Screening for Down Syndrome and Open Neural Tube Defects Using Maternal Serum Marker Screening. *SOGC Clinical Practice Guidelines: Committee Opinion*. 1999: 4.

14 For example, Down syndrome, Trisomy 18, and open neural tube defects are all known by other names

(Trisomy 21, Edwards' syndrome, spina bifida, myelomeningocele) and each is distinct and variable in terms of clinical outcomes and clinical expression. It is also important to clarify the non-medical aspects of the conditions.

15 B.N. Chodirker & J.A. Evans. 1993. *Maternal Serum AFP Screening: The Manitoba Experience. In Current Practice of Prenatal Diagnosis in Canada: Research Studies of the Royal Commission on New Reproductive Technologies*, Vol. 13. Royal Commission on New Reproductive Technologies, ed. Ottawa: Canada Communications Group: 535-610.

16 N. Press & C. Browner. 1994. Collective Silences, Collective Fictions: How Prenatal Diagnostic Testing Became Part of Routine Prenatal Care. In *Women and Prenatal Testing: Facing the Challenges of Genetic Technology*. K.H. Rothenberg & E.J. Thomson, eds. Columbus: Ohio State University Press: 201-218.

17 Chodirker & Evans, op. cit. note 15, pp. 577-582; J.C. Carroll et al. Ontario Maternal Serum Screening Program: Practices, Knowledge and Opinions of Health Care Providers. *Can Med Assoc J.* 1997; 156: 775-784.

18 Of almost a thousand women surveyed in Ontario just before many of them were about to undergo maternal serum screening, almost half (48%) reported that they had not discussed the screen with their health care provider (Goel et al., op. cit. note 10).

19 Beauchamp & Childress, op. cit. note 9; Faden & Beauchamp, op. cit. note 9.

20 Green et al., op. cit. note 10; Goel et al., op. cit. note 10; Jaques et al., op. cit. note 10; Gekas et al., op. cit. note 10; Press & Browner, op. cit. note 16.

21 Goel et al., op. cit. note 10; Press & Browner, op. cit. note 16.

22 Goel et al., op. cit. note 10, p. 428.

23 M. Garel et al. Ethical Decision-Making in Prenatal Diagnosis and Termination of Pregnancy: A Qualitative Survey Among Physicians and Midwives. *Prenat Diagn.* 2002; 22: 811-817.

24 Gekas et al., op. cit. note 10.

25 Beauchamp & Childress, op. cit. note 9; Faden et al, op. cit. note 9.

26 Chodirker & Evans, op. cit. note 15.

27 Goel et al., op. cit. note 10.

28 R. Rapp. 1994. Women's Responses to Prenatal Diagnosis: A Sociocultural Perspective on Diversity. In *Women and Prenatal Testing: Facing the Challenges of Genetic Technology*. K.H. Rothenberg, E.J. Thomson, eds. Columbus: Ohio State University Press: 219-233.

29 L. Stranc. 2000. Patterns of Referral and Invasive Prenatal Diagnosis in Women of Advanced Maternal Age: Manitoba 1990-1995. Doctoral Dissertation. University of Manitoba, Winnipeg, Manitoba; J. Rothschild. 2005. *The Dream of the Perfect Child.* Bloomington, IN: Indiana University Press.

30 Press & Browner, op. cit. note 16.

31 D.B. Paul. 1998. *The Politics of Heredity: Essays on Eugenics, Biomedicine, and the Nature-Nurture Debate.* Albany: State University of New York Press.

32 Press & Browner, op. cit. note 16.

33 Beauchamp & Childress, op. cit. note 9.

34 Johnson & Summers, op. cit. note 13, p. 4.

35 S. Sherwin. 1998. A Relational Approach to Autonomy in Health Care. In *The Politics of Women's Health: Exploring Agency and Autonomy*. S. Sherwin, ed. Philadelphia: Temple University Press: 19-47.

36 Ibid.

37 For a thorough exploration of theories of relational autonomy, see C. Mackenzie & N. Stoljar, eds. 2000. *Relational Autonomy: Feminist Perspectives on Autonomy, Agency, and the Social Self.* Oxford: Oxford University Press. For an example of relational autonomy applied to the health care context, see Sherwin, op. cit. note 35.

38 For an exploration of the contextual factors influencing the development of prenatal diagnostic technologies, see R. Rapp. 1999. *Testing Women, Testing the Fetus: The Social Impact of Amniocentesis in America.* New York: Routledge.

39 C. Vassy. From a Genetic Innovation to Mass Health Programmes: The Diffusion of Down's Syndrome Prenatal Screening and Diagnostic Techniques in France. *Soc Sci Med.* 2006; 63: 2041-2051. These purposes include the costs that would be saved by having fewer children with Down syndrome and spina bifida to care for and the money that could be made from the sale of obstetric ultrasound equipment and the testing kits for the screens.

40 Ibid.

41 Chodirker & Evans, op. cit. note 15.

42 For example, see T. Dudding et al. Reproductive

Decisions after Neonatal Screening Identifies Cystic Fibrosis. Arch Dis Child—*Fetal Neonatal Ed.* 2000; 82: F124-F127.

43   Green et al., op. cit. note 10, p. 55.

44   Ibid.

45   Ibid.

46   Press & Browner, op. cit. note 16. Advance knowledge of a child with disabilities can allow women the opportunity to prepare for this outcome. However, this knowledge can only be achieved through the pursuit of an additional, diagnostic, test such as amniocentesis. Because of the risk of miscarriage associated with this procedure, some women who would not consider an abortion may not pursue this option and be left instead with the uncertain probability assessment from a prenatal screen result.

47   Ibid: 213.

48   M. Lock. 2006. Grappling with a Shape Shifter: Social Repercussions of Genetic Testing for the APOE Gene. Public Lecture. Dalhousie University, Halifax, Nova Scotia.

49   B.K. Rothman. 1986. *The Tentative Pregnancy: Prenatal Diagnosis and the Future of Motherhood.* New York: Viking Penguin, Inc.; D. Davis. 2001. *Genetic Dilemmas: Reproductive Technologies, Parental Choices, and Children's Futures.* New York: Routledge.

50   Rothman, op. cit. note 49.

51   Ibid. Having too few children can also be a problem, however, as developed countries with falling birth rates have begun to discover, or in populations that feel culturally threatened, such as Quebec. In these social and/or political circumstances, some countries may offer incentives for having more children.

52   Ibid: 13.

53   Ibid: 12.

54   In many cases, the option of maternal serum screening will be a benefit because it may avoid the need for invasive testing. However, for some women who are particularly anxious about their fetus, not having direct (or possibly any) access to amniocentesis may be considered an unwelcome restriction of autonomy.

55   R.S. Cowan. 2001. Medicine, Technology, and Gender in the History of Prenatal Diagnosis. In *Feminism in Twentieth-Century Science, Technology, and Medicine.* A. Creager, E. Lunbeck & L. Schiebinger, eds. Chicago: The University of Chicago Press: 186-196.

56   For example, health-care providers interviewed in the US when maternal serum AFP screening was first offered reported feeling required to test all their patients because of liability concerns (Press & Browner, op. cit. note 16).

57   D.B. Paul. 1994. *Eugenic Anxieties, Social Realities, and Political Choices. In Are Genes Us?: The Social Consequences of the New Genetics.* C. Cranor, ed. New Brunswick, NJ: Rutgers University Press: 142-154.

58   Press & Browner, op. cit. note 16.

59   E. Parens & A. Asch, eds. 2000. *Prenatal Testing and Disability Rights.* Washington, DC: Georgetown University Press; R. Grant & K. Flint. Prenatal Screening for Fetal Aneuploidy: A Commentary by the Canadian Down Syndrome Society. *J Obstet Gynaecol Can.* 2007; 29: 580-582.

60   Press & Browner, op. cit. note 16; E. Gates. 1994. Prenatal Genetic Testing: Does it Benefit Pregnant Women? In *Women and Prenatal Testing: Facing the Challenges of Genetic Technology.* K.H. Rothenberg & E.J. Thomson, eds. Columbus: Ohio State University Press: 183-200.

61   Women's and Children's Health Programs: Obstetrics/Gynaecology. Prenatal Screening & Prenatal Diagnosis: Basic Information; my emphasis. Available at: http://www.ahsc.health.nb.ca/prenatalscreening/index.htm [Accessed 1 Nov 2007]. Interestingly, this site was developed by Maritime women, their partners, and health-care providers so this phrasing might reflect the perception of pregnant women of their experiences.

62   A. Lippman. Prenatal Genetic Testing and Screening: Constructing Needs and Reinforcing Inequalities. *Am J Law Med.* 1991; 17: 15-50.

63   Gates, op. cit. note 60; S. Sherwin. 2001. Normalizing Reproductive Technologies and the Implications for Autonomy. In *Globalizing Feminist Bioethics: Crosscultural Perspectives.* R. Tong, with G. Anderson & A. Santos, eds. Boulder, CO: Westview Press: 96-113.

64   Lippman, op. cit. note 62.

65   Ibid.

66   R. Kohut & I.D. Rusen. 2002. Congenital Anomalies in Canada—A Perinatal Health Report, 2002. Ottawa, Canada: Minister of Public Works and Government Services Canada.

67 Lippman, op. cit. note 62; T. Pearce. July 10, 2007. 40 is the New 35 When it Comes to[sic] High-Risk Pregnancy. *Globe and Mail*. Available at: http://www.the globeandmail.com/servlet/story/RTGAM. 20070710.wlamnio10/BNStory/lifeFamily/home [Accessed 1 Nov 2007].

68 For instance, midwives perform most of the prenatal care, there are high rates of home births and low rates of epidurals (M. van den Berg et al. Accepting or Declining the Offer of Prenatal Screening for Congenital Defects: Test Uptake and Women's Reasons. *Prenat Diagn*. 2005; 25: 84-90).

69 Ibid.

70 Green et al., op. cit. note 10; Carroll et al., op. cit. note 17; J.M. Green. Serum Screening for Down's Syndrome: Experiences of Obstetricians in England and Wales. *BMJ*. 1994; 309: 769-772. In the event of a negative screen result, anxiety levels either return to their pre-test level or continue to stay at a residual, elevated level throughout the pregnancy and even after birth.

71 Sherwin, op. cit. note 63.

72 Green et al., op. cit. note 10.

73 van den Berg et al., op. cit. note 68.

74 Lippman, op. cit. note 62.

75 Sherwin, op. cit. note 63.

76 R. Kohut, D. Dewey & E.J. Love. Women's Knowledge of Prenatal Ultrasound and Informed Choice. *J Genet Couns*. 2002; 11: 265-276.

77 As an example, in some baby books the spot for 'baby's first picture' is designated as the place to put the fetus' ultrasound photo (Anna Sheridan-Jonah, personal communication).

78 B.G. Ewigman et al. Effect of Prenatal Ultrasound Screening on Perinatal Outcome. *N Engl J Med*. 1993; 329: 821.

79 Sherwin, op. cit. note 63.

80 Ibid: 104.

81 Kohut et al., op. cit. note 76.

82 Garel et al., op. cit. note 23; R. Kohut. 2000. Prenatal Services Report, 2000: National Survey. Personal Communication: 1-22.

83 Kohut et al., op. cit. note 76.

84 Pregnant women may, of course, understand it perfectly well in terms of the ability of ultrasound to provide her with a visual of her fetus and a picture to take home.

85 Green et al., op. cit. note 10.

86 Some of these possibilities may be options for women who are able to access the services of a midwife in provinces where midwifery is accepted and available.

87 Kohut & Rusen, op. cit. note 66. This statement cannot be confirmed, however, since abortion rates for fetuses with Down syndrome is also suspected to have increased, thereby keeping the live birth rate of children with Down syndrome approximately the same.

88 For example, see Alberta Public Health Association. 2004. Support for a Provincially Funded and Centrally Organized Maternal Serum Screening Program. Available at: http://www.apha.ab.ca/Resolutions/ 2004res01.html [Accessed 11 Apr 2006].

89 Philip Ferguson, Alan Gartner, and Dorothy Lipsky propose that many of the difficulties reported from raising a child with disabilities in the 1950s and 1960s may have had more to do with the complete lack of social supports available to families than any other features of raising a disabled child per se (P.M. Ferguson, A. Gartner & D.K. Lipsky. 2000. The Experience of Disability in Families: A Synthesis of Research and Parent Narratives. In *Prenatal Testing and Disability Rights*. E. Parens & A. Asch, eds. Washington, DC: Georgetown University Press: 72-94).

90 Parens & Asch, op. cit. note 8.

91 V. Seavilleklein. 2007. The Values and Practice of Prenatal Screening in Canada. Doctoral Dissertation. Dalhousie University, Halifax, Nova Scotia.

33

MORAL OBLIGATIONS TO THE NOT-YET BORN:
THE FETUS AS PATIENT

Thomas H. Murray

SOURCE: *The Worth of a Child* (Berkeley: University of California Press, 1996), 96-114.

The health of the not-yet-born child—the fetus intended to be brought to live birth—periodically emerges as a subject of concern. From dramatic interventions such as fetal surgery through drugs and special diets on to efforts to get pregnant women to abstain from alcohol and tobacco or to bar them from workplaces possibly toxic to developing fetuses, there has been a recent surge of ideas on how to prevent, ameliorate, or remedy damage to the not-yet-born.

Many things might be done *with*, *by* or *to* a pregnant woman to benefit her not-yet-born child. They range from the most physically intrusive to the least, from the most technologically sophisticated to mundane efforts at education and persuasion, from those with clearly established benefit to the fetus to those of highly uncertain benefit. The ethical issues raised by interventions of all kinds designed to aid a fetus share essential features. Once some form of fetal surgery becomes established, the case of a woman who refuses it will raise many of the same moral questions as that of a woman whose alcoholism threatens her fetus's health to a point where incarceration or institutionalization are being considered. Although different in several respects, both of the cases require asking how far the state—and physicians as agents of the state—ought to go in coercively intervening in the life of a woman in order to benefit her fetus. And both presume at least a tentative answer to a difficult ethical question: What is the moral status of a fetus?

To answer such a question sensibly and with a modicum of wisdom is our ultimate goal. A burgeoning literature on fetal therapies, fetal surgery, fetal rights, and maternal-fetal conflicts has en-livened the argument. While technologically sophisticated interventions like fetal surgery are receiving the most attention, they will probably be relevant to only a minute proportion of all pregnancies. Yet most of the ethical questions raised by fetal surgery are equally pertinent to a host of other, less glamorous means to the same end. Some sample questions include the following:

- How far should we go in getting diabetic women to manage their disease during pregnancy? Should we inform them of the consequences to their fetus? Should we try to persuade them gently? Browbeat them? If they refuse to cooperate should we initiate civil or criminal proceedings to try and coerce them? Should we try to institutionalize them as has been done in some cases of drug addicted mothers, and then perhaps strip them of their children once they are born?
- What about a mother suspected of using drugs—legal or illegal—that might deleteriously affect the fetus? What of the mother who smokes or drinks? How hard do we try to discourage her smoking or drinking during pregnancy? If she continues to do either or both heavily, at what point if any do we move beyond persuasion to coercion?
- If we think that low levels of a potentially embryotoxic or fetotoxic substance are present in a workplace, should all pregnant women be kept out? What about "potentially pregnant," that is, nonsterile women? Many United States companies have "Fetal Protection Policies" that do just that.[1]

Key Issues

Given the present, chaotic state of the debate over fundamental issues of ethics, law, and public policy regarding the fetus, offering simple answers to questions such as the ones just asked would require ignoring even more important questions. It is more valuable in the long run to clarify some of the fundamental issues now. Five are discussed in this article.

1. Whether there are any moral duties to a fetus.
2. Whether viability affects those duties.
3. How the concept of duties to a fetus is frequently misused.
4. What pitfalls must be avoided in moving from moral judgments to public policy.
5. The importance of the social and historical context of the current debate.

Do We Have Moral Duties to a Fetus?

The moral status of those fetuses who will never be born alive is problematic. Right-to-life advocates claim that even the fertilized ovum is a person, entitled to all the protections and respect due every person. Many other people, including many of those with qualms about abortion, believe that the fetus, especially in its early stages of development, has a lesser moral stature than adults, infants, or even late-term fetuses. No consensus exists on such fetuses. Fortunately, we can discuss the fetus as patient without becoming bogged down in the mire of the abortion debate. All we need is a simple distinction between those fetuses destined to be brought to live birth, and those who will not know extrauterine life.

The Not-Yet-Born Child

The situation is quite different for fetuses who will be born alive. A few theorists argue that the fetus, or even the infant and young child, has no moral status, or else an inferior one.[2] Some writers, while not directly addressing the question, argue that whatever moral claims the fetus might have are always secondary to those of the woman in whose body the fetus lies.[3] Nonetheless, there is good reason to believe that we have moral obligations to the fetus destined to be born, who we will call the not-yet-born child to distinguish it from both the already-born child and from the fetus who will not be born alive. Further, this view has considerable popular support, as evidenced by the efforts aimed at preserving fetal health through antenatal medical care, public health education of pregnant women, and the like.

The Timing of a Harm Is Irrelevant

Imagine two different cases. In the first, a man assaults a woman with the intention of inflicting grave harm on her fetus. He succeeds, causing permanent, irreparable—but not fatal—damage to the fetus's spinal cord, resulting in paralysis. In the second case, all the circumstances are identical, except that the man attacks an infant rather than a fetus, with the same result—permanent, irreparable paralysis. Was the first act any less wrong than the second? In both cases, lifelong harm was done to humans who, whatever your beliefs about when personhood begins, would eventually cross that line and attain full moral status.

My thesis, in short, is that the timing of a harm, in itself, is not morally relevant. An act resulting in harm to a not-yet-born person (who will eventually be a full-fledged person according to everyone's moral theory) is as great a harm as if it were done later. The morally relevant factors are the usual ones: the actor's intentions; excuses; mitigating circumstances, and so on. In practice, a fetus is rarely harmed intentionally; typically, harm to a fetus occurs as a result of intentional or unintentional harm to its mother. The lack of intention to harm then is what affects our judgment about the wrongness of the act, and not the fact that it was a not-yet-born person who was harmed. We would judge unintended harm to a child or adult in a similar manner. The debate over the ethics of abortion aside, then, we can talk sensibly and without inherent contradiction about moral duties to the fetus destined to become a person—to the not-yet-born person. There will be duties to avoid harm, and there may be duties to render aid.

We can discuss moral duties to not-yet-born persons without becoming hopelessly trapped in the abortion debate. Before moving on to discuss the scope of our duties to the fetus, we need to consider whether viability affects these duties.

The Moral Relevance of Viability

Viability is, at best, a slippery concept. For one thing it is a moving front. As our ability to save younger and smaller newborns improves, the so-called age of viability is reached earlier. Physicians frequently use viability as a statistical concept: the age at which some unspecified percentage of newborns will survive. Sometimes the concept is used with reference to specific infants. We could describe survival possibilities as a probabilistic function of weight or gestational age. For example, the BW or GA 10 would be the birthweight or gestational age at which 10 per cent of infants survive. The GA 50 would be the level at which 50 per cent live, and so on. These numbers would change as our ability to save these infants change.

Viability and Abortion

The central question is whether our moral obligations to the fetus change as a function of viability. Viability as a determinant of our duties to a fetus was given great importance by its inclusion in the well-known Supreme Court abortion decision, *Roe v. Wade*.[4] The complex ruling says in its summary: "For the stage subsequent to viability, the State in promoting its interest in the potentiality of human life may, if it chooses, regulate, and even proscribe, abortion except where it is necessary, in appropriate medical judgment, for the preservation of the life or health of the mother."[5]

Viability serves as a threshold in *Roe v. Wade*. Even though the Court uses the ambiguous phrase "potentiality of human life," behind their decision must lie some notion of the fetus growing in legal and presumably moral stature as it approaches term. Otherwise, there would be no justification for linking the State's interest in protecting that potential life with viability which, at the time of that decision (1973), roughly coincided with the end of the second trimester for most fetuses.

Attempting to uncover the moral reasoning underlying a legal decision can be perilous because one may simply be wrong and because it may encourage the unfortunate tendency to see moral disapproval as a sufficient reason for taking legal action, something we will take up later. Bearing that caution in mind, we nonetheless must try to determine what moral ideas underlie the legal reasoning in *Roe v. Wade*. The court appears to believe that, prior to viability, whatever claim the fetus may have not to be killed is outweighed by a woman's right to choose whether or not to bear and give birth to a child, with all that those activities bring in their wake. After viability, the fetus's increasing nearness to actual rather than merely potential life strengthens its moral claim against being killed to the point where it overrides the mother's right to choose not to bear a child, though not so far as to force her to risk her own life in doing so.

Viability Is Irrelevant for Nonfatal Harms

In other words, for the problem of deciding whether a woman can abort her fetus, it may be important to know what the fetus's moral status is *at that particular moment*: whether or not it is a person or how close it is to becoming a full-fledged person may be important in this context. In stark contrast, the fetus's moral standing at that moment in its development is not relevant to judging our duties to avoid or avert nonfatal harms, since, as far as we know, the fetus will some day be a full person, and the timing of such nonlethal harms is not pertinent to determining their wrongfulness. Interestingly, the law itself seems to agree.

Until 1946, a child injured prenatally then born alive but impaired rarely found a court willing to sustain a suit for damages. But in that year began what Prosser, who wrote the standard reference work on tort law, called "the most spectacular abrupt reversal of a well settled rule in the whole history of the law of torts. The child, provided that he is born alive, is permitted to maintain an action for the consequences of prenatal injuries, and if he dies of such injuries after birth an action will lie for his wrongful death."[6] Prosser believed that the earlier denials of claims on behalf of children injured while they were still fetuses were based on invalid reasoning, and he approved of the reversal.

With the concept of prenatal injuries established as a valid one, does it matter whether the fetus was viable at the time of injury? Some courts have required that the fetus have been viable, or at least "quickened" at the time of injury.[7] But many courts have rejected viability as a relevant factor in determining whether the born child may recover from prenatal injury.[8] One critic of the concept of fetal rights says pointedly: "[V]iability is a meaningless distinction in the fetal rights context because the state's interest in the health of its future citizens is equally strong throughout pregnancy."[9] Prosser himself says, "[c]ertainly the [previable] infant may be no less injured; and all logic is in favor of ignoring the stage at which it occurs." Acknowledging that proving injury early in pregnancy might be difficult, he concludes, "[t]his, however, goes to proof rather than principle; and if, as is undoubtedly the case there are injuries as to which reliable medical proof is possible, it makes no sense to deny recovery on any such arbitrary basis."[10] The moral principle, that is, does not depend on the arbitrary criterion of viability.

While most cases have focused on recovering damages for harms already done, a number of recent cases attempt to prevent harm by affecting the pregnant woman's behavior, even to the point of outright coercion. The forced caesarean cases discussed elsewhere in this volume [*The Worth of a Child*] are one sort of example.[11] In another case (reported by a newspaper) a physician accused a woman, seven months pregnant, of endangering her fetus's development by abusing drugs. The woman was ordered to enter a drug rehabilitation program and undergo regular urinalyses until the child was born.[12] Whether this is a reasonable response to the problem is the subject of the next section.

Misusing the Idea of Duties to a Fetus

A recurrent theme in this essay is the danger of making moral judgments or public policy without sufficient regard for context. Just this sort of misuse of the concept of duties to a fetus occurs with unsettling frequency.

The Dangers of Oversimplifying Moral Decisions

The moral world we inhabit is one marked by a multiplicity of interests and duties. We are certainly entitled to give good moral weight to our own interests. Then there are duties to those with whom we have special relationships, relationships that prescribe even strenuous moral duties in certain domains. Finally, we have duties to "strangers"—those with whom no special moral relationship exists. Most significant moral decisions have implications for many of these interests and relationships simultaneously. For example, a woman who must decide whether to place her fetus at risk of harm by working in a factory with low levels of a suspected fetotoxin must weigh her own interests in having a job with the psychological and material benefits that it may bring against the risks imposed on herself as well as her fetus. She must also consider possible benefits to her fetus that the job makes possible, such as improved nutrition for herself and prenatal care facilitated by health insurance. Then there may be others dependent on her working: a spouse, other children, perhaps elderly parents. When we portray the ethical dimensions of her decision as beginning and ending with the question of whether or not she has duties to avoid exposing her fetus to risks, we rip such a complex decision out of its moral, as well as its social and political, context. Yet, this is commonly done. Or, not much better, the woman's "right" to do whatever she desires is counterposed to the fetus's right to protection from harm. Once the problem is framed this way, giving a nuanced answer becomes impossible. A more complex view of the moral life, one that encompasses a multiplicity of legitimate moral concerns, of interests and duties, of roles and relationships, allows us to frame the question in a way that can be answered, if not more easily, at least more satisfactorily.

Warning of Fearful Consequences

In a clash of rights, complex issues can become stripped of their nuances and turned into simplistic all-or-none contests. On either extreme, we can imagine bleak consequences. If, on the one hand, we give pre-eminence to the fetus's right to avoid being harmed, then must pregnant women structure every detail of their lives in order to avoid all suspected risks to their not-yet-born child? Such an attitude appears to have influenced some companies to adopt so-called "Fetal Protection Policies," or FPPs, that deny employment opportunities to women.[13] Fears of what would happen should fetal rights gain the upper hand generate a litany of nightmarish possibilities:

> A woman could be held civilly or criminally liable for fetal injuries caused by accidents resulting from maternal negligence, such as automobile or household accidents. She could also be held liable for any behavior during her pregnancy having potentially adverse effects on her fetus, including failure to eat properly, using prescription, non-prescription and illegal drugs, smoking, drinking alcohol, exposing herself to infectious disease or to any workplace hazards, engaging in immoderate exercise or sexual intercourse, residing at high altitudes for prolonged periods, or using a general anesthetic or drugs to induce rapid labor during delivery. If the current trend in fetal rights continues, pregnant women would live in constant fear that any accident or "error" in judgment could be deemed "unacceptable" and become the basis for a criminal prosecution by the state or a civil suit....[14]

On the other hand, if we give full sway to the woman's right to control her body, can we even level moral criticism against a case such as the one of a woman who at 40 weeks gestation, in labor with abruptio placenta with fetal distress, refused a caesarean section? After the infant was delivered stillborn, she explained to a nurse that "the death of the fetus solved complicated personal problems."[15] The language of rights in conflict may not permit us to give full and weighty consideration to a host of factors that we believe are important in making moral judgments. Examining relationships, legitimate interests, and duties may give us a more adequate picture of the moral choices people face.

Obligations to the Not-Yet-Born Are Not All or None

Take, for example, the case of the woman who must decide whether to accept a job that might pose some risk to her fetus. Let us suppose that she intends to bring the child to birth, so we do not have to worry about the ethics of abortion. As far as we know, this is a not-yet-born child; therefore the woman has some obligation to avoid harming it while it is still a fetus. What is the scope and intensity of this obligation? Must she refuse the job?

Because of the link between most discussions of the fetus's moral status and abortion, there is an unfortunate tendency to think of our obligations to the fetus as all-or-none. But there are other creatures dependent on us, to whom we have obligations, but where those duties do not unequivocally overwhelm all other considerations—our children for example. We certainly have a duty to do what is reasonable to protect our young children from harm. That requires keeping them from known and probable dangers. But we are not required to sacrifice everything else to this task. We should teach them not to play in busy streets, and offer them a protected play-area. But must we build crash-proof barriers around their playground, strong enough to stop a cement truck run wild? Obviously not. That would be beyond "reasonable" responsibility. Anytime we take them in a car, there is a risk of injury or death. Responsible parents should provide a secure carseat for their infant or toddler. But we are not forbidden from going for a drive, even though no matter how carefully we drive there is always the distinct possibility of an accident.

What is it that makes certain risks reasonable, and others the kind that responsible parents would not take? The probability of harm and its severity should it occur are certainly relevant. Also significant is the importance of the purpose for which the risk is run and the avoidability of the risk. If we want the children to see their grandparents, a long car ride may be unavoidable. And exposing our child to the considerable risks of cytotoxic drugs is clearly justifiable if and only if our purpose is to treat them for cancer.

My purpose here is to put us on more familiar ground than the exotic situations in which questions of fetal status typically arise. Two points come out of the discussion. First, whatever moral duties we might have to a fetus—a not-yet-born child—they may equal but not exceed our duties to already-born children. The circumstances of a fetus's physical enclosure within and link to its mother's body confuses many discussions. This linkage may mean that a broader range of actions might affect the fetus, and the facts of the case will be accordingly affected. But the same moral considerations apply equally to both the not-yet-born and the already-born—considerations such as intentions, probability and severity of risk, and duties to others. Second, duties to the not-yet-born, like duties to the already-born, are usually just one of many factors to be considered in judging the moral acceptability of an act.

Another advantage of discussing our obligations to the not-yet-born and already-born together is that it enables us to talk about fathers and not just mothers. To the extent that cultural blinders distort our view of a mother's responsibility to her fetus, then looking at a case with comparable morally relevant features, but one that asks about a father's responsibility to his child, may restore some moral clarity.

A Father-Child Analogy

Take the plausible case of a man who lost his job in the oil fields of west Texas. He has two children counting on him for support; his wife is also out of work. An offer comes of a job in a petrochemical plant near Houston. Taking that job will mean moving his family to a part of Texas crawling with petrochemical complexes where toxic releases into the air, ground, and water are not unknown, and where the risk of cancer is somewhat, though not drastically, higher than in their current community. There are a number of good reasons to take the job. He will be able to afford better food, clothing, and housing for his family and himself. Being unemployed threatens his sense of self-worth, which depresses him and incidentally also makes him a less thoughtful parent and spouse. Like most unemployed Americans, when he lost his job he also lost his health insurance; the new job will assure better access to health care for himself and his family. Perhaps the schools are better in the new community. Suppose he accepts the job even though he knows and regrets the increased risk that will mean for his children. Decisions such as this are all-things-considered choices: by their nature they involve weighing and balancing many things. Would we say that this man's choice was immoral? That he should not have exposed his children to the slightly increased risk of cancer whatever else was involved? It would make better sense to say that he made a responsible, morally defensible decision, even if we share his regret about the increased risk to which his children as well as his wife and himself will be exposed.

How was this man's decision any different from that of a woman who chooses to accept a job, knowing that her fetus will be exposed to some low but nonetheless increased risk of harm because of exposures there? Perhaps she too is without health insurance. Perhaps having a job is important to her sense of self-worth. Perhaps there are other children and a spouse at home who are dependent on her. The fact that she carries a fetus within her, a not-yet-born child, that she has moral duties to protect that fetus from harm, and that the workplace increases slightly the probability of harm does not make her decision immoral. Exactly the same considerations were relevant to the man's decision. To the extent that the morally relevant factors are comparable—and in this case they might well be identical—the decisions are equally justified. And if the circumstances vary, at least we know the kinds of morally significant considerations that will influence our judgments.[16] Whether it is a man or a woman is not relevant. Nor, I have argued, does it matter whether it is a not-yet-born or already-born child.

From Ethical Judgments to Public Policy

We do not ban all conduct we regard as morally suspect, nor do we compel people to carry out every moral duty. Many things are left to personal conscience, to moral suasion, or to social pressure. For good reasons, including moral ones, we are reluctant to allow the state to force its view of correct conduct on individuals unless the harm to be avoided is grave, especially when doing so requires coercion, bodily invasion, or incarceration. These means are among the most repugnant and are reserved for extreme circumstances. If we conclude then that a woman morally ought to quit smoking during pregnancy, moderate or eliminate her consumption of alcohol, and do likewise with caffeine, this does not automatically justify heavy-handed state intervention to assure that she does these things. Some wrongs are minimally so. The state should not exercise its often great power on such things. Sometimes the effort to correct a wrong itself creates new moral problems. The moral and other costs of enforcement may outweigh the good that might be done.

The fetus becomes a "patient" when its welfare becomes the physician's concern. The obstetrician caring for a mother and not-yet-born child has two patients. In much the way that a pediatrician advises parents about their newborn's diet, monitors the infant's health, and prescribes needed medication or other therapeutic interventions, an obstetrician routinely does the same for the mother and the fetus-patient. How extensive is the obstetrician's duty to assure that the fetus-patient's welfare is being protected?

The "Child-as-Maximum" Principle

One useful guideline might be called the "child-as-maximum" principle. The principle says that our obligations to ensure the fetus's welfare can equal but not exceed our obligations to a born child. If a pediatrician would not be obliged to do more than try to persuade parents to do a certain thing—say observe a special diet—then under conditions of comparable burdens and benefits, obstetricians cannot be obliged to do more to protect a fetus, although they may be required to do less.

One inescapable difference between the obstetrician's and the pediatrician's case is of course that the former's second patient, the fetus, is encased in the body of the first patient, the mother. All interventions directed at the fetus literally must go through its mother. The burdens created, therefore, generally will be much greater, as will be the potential for morally wronging one person in the effort to aid another. This is why the child-as-maximum principle emphasizes that our duties to a born child constitute an upper-bound for our duties to a not-yet-born child rather than a strict equivalence. A drug that might benefit a fetus but that will be harmful to the mother can be refused. That same drug for that same being, now born, should probably be administered. The pediatrician in the latter instance is justified in pushing harder for consent from the parents than was the obstetrician.

A Variety of Needs, a Range of Interventions

One study shows that women who smoke a pack of cigarettes or more a day have babies on average about 180 gm smaller at birth than women who do not smoke. The same study found that women who drank twenty or more beers per month sacrificed roughly 100 gm of birthweight, while those who consumed 300 or more grams of caffeine daily (three or four cups of coffee or seven cola beverages) had babies 40 to 50 gm smaller on average.[17] What should physicians do? When the risks are small, we usually employ education and persuasion. That is the typical and appropriate response to maternal smoking, diet, nutritional supplements, and the like. These anchor one end of a continuum of possible "interventions." We can move to stronger measures, such as New York City has done, by requiring that signs be posted in public places serving alcohol warning pregnant women that alcohol may endanger their fetus's health. This is a public policy that relies as much on shame as on the educative effect of the signs.

Beyond this is a broad range of more traditionally "medical" interventions: managing maternal diabetes in pregnancy;[18] placing women with PKU on low-phenylalanine diets when they wish to become pregnant;[19] treating fetal methylmelonic acidemia by giving vitamin B-12 to the mother;[20] treating congenital hypothyroidism by injections into the amniotic fluid;[21] drug therapy for fetal ventricular tachycardia,[22] and other possibilities.

There are surgical routes as well. In addition to the familiar exchange transfusions for erythroblastosis fetalis, a variety of still-experimental fetal surgeries are under triculomegaly,[23] diaphragmatic hernia,[24] and hematopoietic stem cell transplantation for severe immunologic deficiencies.[25] (The law and ethics of fetal surgery have been amply discussed elsewhere.)[26]

Our ethical analysis of any proposed interventions to benefit a fetus intended to be brought to birth should include at least the following considerations:

1. How certain is the benefit to the fetus? (Is the intervention experimental? Is it well-established? Does it carry substantial risks to the fetus?)

2. How great are the benefits? (Will a successful intervention make a large or small difference in the fetus's prognosis?)

3. How intrusive, coercive, or harmful will it be to the mother?

4. Will anything be lost or gained by waiting until after the child is born?

Even if we are convinced that the mother has a moral responsibility to agree to the intervention, the question of how far we should go in attempting to persuade or coerce her raises an entirely new set of issues at the intersection of ethics and public policy. Once we move to the level of policy, political and historical considerations become very important. At this point, a brief look at another era's concern for the health of the not-yet-born is appropriate.

Alcohol and "Race-Decay" in Edwardian England

This is not the first time that parental behavior has been held responsible for harm to the not-yet-born or the already-born. The oldest prenatal health advice of which I am aware is in the Old Testament. In Judges 13:7 the mother of Samson is told "Behold, thou shalt conceive and bear a son: and drink no wine or strong drink."

Many women today are fearful and suspicious of the movement towards ascribing moral status to the fetus. For women who aspire to compete in the economic marketplace on an equal footing with men, those fears and suspicions have substantial historical validity. Past social movements to protect helpless infants and not-yet-born children have had something less than pure and altruistic motives. One illuminating example comes from England at the turn of the century—the Edwardian era.

In the first decade of this century, England found itself losing its empire abroad and awash with immigrants at home: immigrants, moreover, whose children were more likely to survive infancy than their British neighbors. A number of laypeople and physicians believed they understood the problem—alcohol. A campaign to arouse public ire against parents who drank flourished in the first decade of the 1900s. While it was directed largely against women

who drank, men came in for their share of the blame as well. Indeed, one highly influential Swiss study reported that 78 per cent of women unable to breast-feed had fathers who drank, heavily. But for the most part women were faulted.

In 1906, a British physician wrote:

Undoubtedly much of the high infant mortality is due to alcoholism, and conditions directly ... or indirectly arising from this morbid condition. The widespread prevalence of alcoholism among women, especially during the reproductive period of life, is one of the most important factors making for racial-decay.[27]

"Race-decay" is but one of many dubious reasons given for worrying about women and drink. George Sims, a prominent journalist of the time, had a related concern: "What can be the future of our Empire, if on a falling birth rate 120,000 infants continue to die annually in the first year of their lives ...!"[28] And he knew the cause: "Bad motherhood is the first great cause of our appalling infant morality."[29] No less an exemplar of success than Andrew Carnegie, the American industrialist, pointed to the drunken worker as a central threat to British productivity.[30]

For the most part, this was a campaign waged by the upper classes, including a number of male physicians, against working class women. They were not doing their national duty by outreproducing the immigrants—Jews, Italians, Scots, and Irish. Theophilus Hyslop, a physician active in the anti-drink movement, referred to immigrants derogatorily and declared that if the British worker would give up alcohol, he could "drive the foreigner from our midst."[31]

Perhaps Dr. Robert Jones best expressed the sentiment feared by contemporary women: "Women are now the companions of men in ... industrial pursuits, and the freedom to work on equal terms with men has caused ... the same depressing physical and mental influences ..., for which stimulants offer a temporary relief."[32] Women, that is, as vessels of reproduction, as the assurers of racial integrity, as the saviors of the empire, as the protectors of the innocent must be made to look after their offspring, and not be contaminated in the labor marketplace.

Many women understand any contemporary movement emphasizing their biologic role as bearers of children to be a threat to their economic liberty and equality—"fetal rights" being no exception. The need to control reproduction so that they could compete in the job market emerged as a major theme among pro-choice activists in Kristin Luker's study of anti- and pro-abortion activists. Conversely, having and raising children were crucial sources of self-value for many who worked against abortion.[33] Because it focuses attention on women's reproductive capacities, it is not surprising that the trend toward regarding the fetus as a patient has evoked concern and controversy. And with the long history of efforts to keep women in roles defined by and in the interests of men, it is no less surprising that women regard the current trend with suspicion. Legitimate concerns for fetal rights can also be carried along by other, questionable, motives and may carry with them other destructive social consequences.

Conclusions

Five points emerge from this analysis. First, we can discuss moral duties to the fetus destined to be born—to the not-yet-born child—without logical contradiction and without becoming hopelessly mired in debate over abortion.

Second, whether the fetus is viable may be regarded as morally significant in the context of abortion decisions, but it is not directly relevant to our duties to not-yet-born children. This is so because of the irrelevance of the timing of a harm.

Third, that we do have moral duties to fetuses, viable and previable alike, may not have the horrendous consequences for women that is typically thought. Our common error has been to focus exclusively on a pregnant woman's duty to avoid harming her fetus, without regard for the multitude of other moral considerations she ought to include in her decision. A more complex and adequate view of the moral life understands that in such decisions a host of factors may be relevant such as promises made, the woman's own interests, her obligations to other family members, and the welfare of her not-yet-born child. Seeing the mother's moral relationship to the fetus as morally analo-

gous to a father's relationship to his child will help avoid oversimplification.

Fourth, establishing that women have moral duties to their not-yet-born children does not justify automatically coercive public policies to force them to fulfill those obligations. Again, the analogy to fathers and children may be helpful. The state must be very cautious in using its power to enforce particular notions of maternal duties. Effective enforcement might necessitate forcible invasion of a woman's body or prolonged incarceration. These are usually "last resorts" used only under very restricted circumstances. We must be careful to assure that they are not used more casually against pregnant women.

Fifth, women have ample reason to be suspicious of the growing tendency to focus on the welfare of the fetus-as-patient and, by implication, on the woman's role as bearer of children. Historically, movements allegedly directed toward aiding fetuses and children have often been motivated as much by other, less praiseworthy concerns, including racism, and especially by men's fear of women's political, social, and economic equality.

Rather than arguing for "fetal rights," let us use the less heated language of moral obligations to not-yet-born children. We must not oversimplify complex moral decisions, especially our tendency to focus on a pregnant woman's obligations to her not-yet-born child as the only morally important factor in her decisions. We would not tolerate such oversimplification when discussing parents' duties toward their children, and we must not tolerate it in the difficult decisions we now face regarding the welfare of the not-yet-born. History provides forceful reminders of the dangers of thinking of women as mere "vessels of reproduction." Finally, we must continue the work of clarifying our obligations toward both the fetus destined to be born and the mother who retains her full moral individuality and interests, and in whose body that developing person exists for a time.

Notes

1   US Congress, Office of Technology Assessment: Reproductive Health Hazards in the Workplace. US Government Printing Office: Washington, DC, 1985.

2 Tooley M.: *Abortion and Infanticide*. New York, Oxford University Press, 1983.

3 Engelhardt H.T.: *The Foundation of Bioethics*. New York, Oxford, 1986.

4 Roe v Wade, 410 U.S. 113, 1973.

5 Ibid.

6 Prosser W.L.: *Handbook of the Law of Torts*. Edition 3. St Paul, MN, West Publishing Co, 1964.

7 Ibid.

8 Keeton W.P., Dobbs D., Keeton R., et al: *Prosser and Keeton on the Law of Torts*. Edition 5. Mineola, NY, West Publishing Co, 1984.

9 Johnsen D.E.: The creation of fetal rights: Conflicts with women's constitutional rights to liberty, privacy, and equal protection. *Yale Law J* 95:599-625, 1986.

10 See note 6.

11 Trong C.: Ethical conflicts between mother and fetus in obstetrics. *Clin Perinatol* 14(2).

12 Shaw M.W.: Conditional prospective rights of the fetus. *J Leg Med* 5:63-116, 1984.

13 US Congress, Office of Technology Assessment: Reproductive Health Hazards in the Workplace. US Government Printing Office: Washington, DC, 1985.

14 Johnsen D.E.: The creation of fetal right: Conflicts with women's constitutional rights to liberty, privacy, and equal protection. *Yale Law J* 95:599-625, 1986.

15 Leiberman J.R., Mazor M., Chaim W., et al: The fetal right to live. *Obstet Gynecol* 53:515-517, 1979.

16 Murray T.H.: Who do fetal protection policies really protect? *Tech Rev* 88(7):12-13, 20, 1985.

17 Kuzma J.W., Sokol R.J.: Maternal drinking behavior and decreased intrauterine growth. *Alcohol Clin Exp Res* 6:396-402, 1982.

18 Gabbe S.G.: Management of diabetes mellitus in pregnancy. *AM J Obstet Gynecol* 153:824-827, 1985.

19 Robertson J.A., Schulman J.D.: PKU women and pregnancy: The limits of reproductive autonomy. Unpublished manuscript.

20 Schulman J.D.: Prenatal treatment of biochemical disorders. *Sem Perinatol* 9:75-78, 1985.

21 Weiner S., Scharf J.F., Bolognese P.J., et al: Antenatal diagnosis and treatment of fetal goiter. *J Reprod Med* 24:39-42, 1980.

22 Kleinman C.S., Copel J.A., Weinstein E.M., et al: In utero diagnosis and treatment of fetal supraventricular tachycardia. *Sem Perinatol* 9:113-129, 1985.

23 Clewell W.H., Meier P.R., Manchester D.K., et al: Ventriculomegaly: Evaluation and management. *Sem Perinatol* 9:98-102, 1985.

24 Harrison M.R., Adzick N.S., Nakayama D.K., et al: Fetal diaphragmatic hernia: Fatal but fixable. *Sem Parinatol* 9:103-112, 1985.

25 Simpson T.J., Golbus M.S.: In utero fetal hematopoietic stem cell transplantation. *Sem Perinatol* 9:68-74, 1985.

26 Fletcher, J.C.: Ethical considerations in and beyond experimental fetal therapy. *Sem Perinatol* 9:130-135, 1985; Murray T.H.: Ethical issues in fetal surgery. *Bull Am Col Surg* 70(6):6-10, 1985; Robertson J.A.: Legal issues in fetal therapy. *Sem Perinatol* 9:136-142, 1985.

27 Gutzke D.W.: "The cry of the children": The Edwardian medical campaign against maternal drinking. *Br J Addiction* 79:71-84, 1984.

28 Ibid.

29 Ibid.

30 Ibid.

31 Ibid.

32 Ibid.

33 Luker K.: *Abortion and the Politics of Motherhood*. University of California, Berkeley, 1984.

34.
DECISIONS REGARDING DISABLED NEWBORNS

Mary B. Mahowald

SOURCE: *Women and Children in Health Care: An Unequal Majority* (Oxford: Oxford University Press, 1996).

During the 1980s, both the media and the federal government focused their consideration of infants on a few controversial cases, possibly to the neglect of ethical issues involving other children, and larger social and ethical problems affecting all of us.[1] In this chapter, I broaden the perspective on neonatal dilemmas by providing a brief account of the historical, cultural, and medical contexts in which they arise, and a description of alternative approaches to their resolution. I also discuss cases in which nontreatment of extremely ill, impaired, and low birth weight infants may be morally justified. Although these conditions are often addressed separately, in practice they often occur in the same patient. From an egalitarian perspective, each infant should be treated as an individual, just as older patients are to be treated as individuals. In both situations, the patient represents a unique embodiment of limitations, abilities, possibilities, and relationships.[2]

Historical and Current Context

Facilities and technologies for neonatal intensive care are a relatively recent phenomenon, still comparatively unavailable or inaccessible to the populations of less developed nations. The first treatment center for newborn care in the United States was established early in this century, when infant deaths were primarily associated with infection or malnutrition.[3] At that time, rudimentary incubators provided necessary warmth for preterm infants, and oxygen supplementation was introduced to combat respiratory difficulties due to immature lung development. Progress in survival rates was not devoid of setbacks. For example, by 1954 it was recognized that the high oxygen concentrations that had saved some preterm newborns had also caused blindness. Subsequent curtailment of this treatment was accompanied by a corresponding rise in the rate of infant mortality.[4] Similarly, diethylstilbestrol (DES) was initially thought by some to be effective in bringing problematic pregnancies to term, but the drug was later implicated in carcinogenic and reproductive problems of the offspring.[5]

Further advances produced sophisticated techniques for prenatal diagnosis and treatment, monitoring neonatal heart rate, blood gases, and chemistries, and microsurgical procedures for newborn anomalies. Neonatology became a major pediatric specialty, spawning a huge and ongoing research effort with impressive clinical results.[6] Techniques introduced during the 1960s facilitated successful treatment of infants weighing less than 1,500 grams. These methods included constant positive airway pressure monitoring, by which oxygen requirements are constantly measured without interruption, and hyperalimentation, a means of providing nutrition to those who cannot tolerate other types of feeding. By 1970, the mortality rate from hyaline membrane disease, a common problem of preterm newborns, had dropped from 60 percent to 20 percent of those affected. By 1978, the survival rate for very early and very small babies had improved to the point where those weighing less than 1,000 grams warranted treatment.[7] Since then, fetal viability has advanced earlier into pregnancy, resulting in smaller and younger survivors of preterm birth and even late abortions. Two new techniques, extracorporeal membrane oxygenation (ECMO) and surfactant therapy have decreased the mortality rates of newborns even further. ECMO has improved the outcome for newborns suffering from four common or highly lethal conditions: meconium aspiration, persistent pulmonary hypertension, beta streptococcal sepsis, and congenital diaphragmatic hernia.[8] Surfactant therapy has been remarkably successful in treatment of lung immaturity in preterm infants.[9]

The majority of very low birth weight babies (less than 1.5 kilograms) who survive sustain no serious permanent compromise to their motor or mental functions. For example, 65 percent of the 781 infants weighing less than 1,500 grams who were admitted to the Neonatal Intensive Care Unit at Rainbow Babies and Children's Hospital in Cleveland between 1975 and 1978 survived; 80 percent of these had normal neurodevelopmental outcomes.[10] As might be suspected, morbidity increases with decreasing birth weight. From 1982 to 1988 a study at the same institution showed an 18 to 20 percent survival rate for newborns weighing less than 750 grams. Among the survivors, 22 to 50 percent had moderate to severe neurodevelopmental impairment.[11] A multicenter study published in 1991 showed a 34 percent survival for infants weighing 750 grams or less and 66 percent for those from 751 through 1,000 grams.[12] Morbidity factors for survivors in this study include chronic lung disease, severe bowel infection, and brain hemorrhage, all of which may lead to long-term severe impairment. Despite the impressive technological developments, not everyone agrees that all critically ill newborns should be provided with lifesaving or life-prolonging treatment. Infanticide is a long-standing practice with which nontreatment decisions may be compared.

Anthropologists tell us that infanticide has been practiced throughout history in many cultures, including those of the western world.[13] At times, the practice was deemed acceptable because it was undertaken indirectly rather than directly. In other words, infants were not killed outright, but were left to die—often because they were defective, sometimes because they were twins or female or illegitimate. Since abandonment of an infant inevitably leads to death, there is little practical distinction between killing and letting a newborn die. Just as euthanasia is morally problematic, regardless of whether it is characterized as active or passive, so is infanticide, whether characterized as direct or indirect.[14] Refusing to institute respiratory support in a newborn whose lungs are not yet mature may be construed as indirect infanticide. The refusal to pro-vide intravenous nutrition to an infant who is incapable of normal digestion may be construed similarly.[15] The difficulty of maintaining a sharp distinction between direct and indirect termination of lifesaving treatment has led Robert Weir to argue that it is sometimes morally justified to terminate an infant's life directly and actively.[16]

Several factors in contemporary American society conspire to exacerbate moral problems regarding infants. One is the emphasis on patient autonomy, which is generally assumed to be captured in the concept of "informed consent." While this concept is obviously inapplicable to newborns, it is sometimes applied to parents who make decisions on behalf of their children. In fact, the distinction between informed consent and proxy or substitute consent is often overlooked, and parents are falsely assumed to provide the former rather than the latter.[17] Legal and moral grounds for requiring informed consent of competent patients are stronger than those for substitute consent. Nonetheless, parental rights regarding their children have generally been perceived as primary, requiring practitioners to respect their decisions even when these involve the refusal of life-prolonging treatment.[18] Since the Baby Doe controversies of the 1980s, this emphasis has shifted to a situation where some physicians see themselves as advocates for infants even if this pits them against parents.[19]

In the past, a variety of treatment options were unavailable for many infants, regardless of whether they were disabled. Reversible life-threatening medical problems, which occur more frequently in permanently impaired newborns than in other infants, are now routinely repaired through surgery. The development of antibiotic therapy, feeding techniques, and fluid exchange procedures has greatly increased the actual number of disabled children who survive to adulthood. Moreover, while greater numbers of preterm infants now survive to live normal lives, some pay for their survival with iatrogenically induced permanent disabilities. There is thus an inevitable connection between very low birth weight babies and disabled infants.[20]

Two conflicting social phenomena make neonatal ethical dilemmas even more prevalent and complicated. One is the "premium baby" mentality that has resulted from the trend toward reduced family size, as well as the availability of contraceptive measures and abortion, discussed in earlier chapters. Allowing severely compromised infants to die is consistent with this mentality. In contrast, the "right to life" ideology and movement affirm the primacy of fetal interests over those of other individuals. Not surprisingly, "right to life" activists have joined the government and organizations representing the disabled in arguing that infants should not be denied treatment on the basis of their disabilities.[21] Either of these positions is supportable by an egalitarian perspective. Which position weighs more than the other depends on whether survival of a severely disabled newborn is of greater value than parental autonomy, or whether the obligation to respect parental autonomy overrides that of beneficence toward their infant. The cases considered next are well-known illustrations of this dilemma.

The Doe Babies

In the spring of 1982, an infant afflicted with Down syndrome and esophageal atresia was born at Bloomington Hospital in Indiana. Surgical repair is usually undertaken to correct the latter problem, but the former condition, with its concomitant mental retardation, is not correctable. For individuals with Down syndrome, the degree of mental retardation is not predictable at birth. The obstetrician informed the mother that she might choose between two "medical options" regarding her newborn: (1) consent to the surgery necessary for survival, or (2) decline that consent and request that the baby not be fed so as not to prolong his dying. The parents chose the latter course. Hospital personnel respected their choice, and local and state courts reviewed and approved their decision. Local attorneys attempted to reverse the decision through appeal to the U.S. Supreme Court. When the child died while the attorneys were en route to Washington for a special hearing of the court, the case became moot.[22]

Although his parents had him baptized, presumably giving him a name, the public came to know this infant as "Baby Doe." During his six days of life, he became uniquely but anonymously famous because of media coverage and public reaction to it.

As a resident of Bloomington at the time, I knew several of the principals associated with the case (the obstetrician, the pediatrician, the lawyer for the parents, the priest who baptized the baby, and the pathologist who performed the autopsy), but never learned the identity of the infant or his parents. To their credit, the press respected the family's privacy.

Following the infant's death, the government notified all federally supported institutions caring for infants that funding would be denied if they discriminated against the disabled, as had allegedly occurred with Baby Doe. In March of 1983, the Department of Health and Human Services issued a ruling that required all such institutions to post signs citing both the government statute prohibiting discrimination against the disabled and a phone number to use in reporting suspected violations of the statute.[23] This ruling was overturned one month later by U.S. District Judge Gerhard A. Gesell, who described it as conceived in "haste and inexperience," and "based on inadequate consideration of the regulation's consequences."[24]

The second Baby Doe was born in Port Jefferson, New York, in fall of 1983, this one distinguished from the other by being called "Jane Doe." Like her predecessor, she too became a subject of public controversy within her first days of life. Unlike him, her name (Keri-Lynn) was eventually revealed by the media, and the child survived despite her parents' initial refusal of treatment.

Baby Jane Doe was born with spina bifida (an open spine), hydrocephalus (excess fluid on the brain), and microcephaly (reduced brain size), conditions predictive of paralysis in her lower extremities, incontinence, and retardation. According to reports published during her first weeks of life, surgical intervention might allow the child to survive for approximately twenty years; without the surgery she was likely to die within two years. A physician who counseled the father told him that his daughter was so neurologically compromised that she "would never experience joy, never experience sorrow."[25] When both parents declined consent for the surgery, their decision was reviewed and approved at local and state levels, and supported by their priest counselor. Lawrence Washburn, an attorney from New Jersey, brought the case to the attention of federal authorities, who attempted unsuccessfully to obtain the medical records. As with the Bloomington case, the government considered nontreatment of Baby Jane Doe to be a violation of the 1973 statute prohibiting discrimination against the handicapped.[26]

Litigation relevant to the second Baby Doe case led to a denial of the government's right to require the surrender of medical records in order to investigate treatment decisions regarding disabled infants. During the summer of 1984, the government's Baby Doe regulations were permanently enjoined by the U.S. District Court in New York. However, in fall of the same year Congress passed legislation requiring state child protection agencies to intervene in cases where severely disabled infants are refused "medically indicated treatment." Exceptions to this requirement are situations where "the infant is irreversibly comatose or the treatment would be futile and inhumane or would only prolong dying."[27] According to Betty W. Levin, pediatric professionals tend to overestimate the degree of interventions required by this legislation.[28]

Conflicting positions regarding the role of government in "Baby Doe" cases reflect different constituencies: medical organizations, associations for the disabled, the Department of Health and Human Services, and the President's Commission for the Study of Ethical Problems in Medicine and Biomedical and Behavioral Research (hereafter, President's Commission). However, the documents in which these positions are articulated all invoke the same criterion, namely, the best interests of infants.[29] While disagreement continues about interpretation of, and procedures for implementing, the "best interest" criterion,[30] broader agreement may be reached through an examination of its meaning. Before addressing this, however, I wish to deal with an equally controversial question relevant to guideline 4: who should decide the fate of severely disabled newborns?

Who Should Decide?

"Informed consent" is often seen as a sine qua non of justification for medical interventions.[31] Competent adults may legally decline even lifesaving therapy by removing themselves from hospital treatment programs against medical advice. Exceptions have been based on the patient's responsibilities to others, or the claim that hospital personnel are not obliged to violate their own professional standards or commitments.[32] Since newborns are incapable of providing informed consent, their parents usually act as proxy or surrogate decision makers in their behalf. The right of parents to act as proxies may be overruled, however, if their decision opposes their child's best interest. For example, if a Jehovah's Witness parent declines a blood transfusion essential to the life of his child, hospital authorities will obtain a court order allowing hospital personnel to intervene in the child's behalf. Thus, the parents' right to decide about their infant's treatment is legally less binding than their right to decide about their own treatments.

The distinction between informed and proxy consent is also significant from a moral point of view. It suggests that a priority of decision makers be observed, based on the degree to which each decision maker is related to the infant. Typically, the child's parents hold first place. However, the child's caretakers are also related to the child through their professional commitment, as well as the personal and contractual relationships they maintain with the infant and family.

Despite the legal and moral requirement of informed or proxy consent, long standing practice assigns the role of principal decision maker of medical dilemmas to the physician.[33] The justification for this priority is sometimes comparable to the argument presented by the cardinal in Dostoyevsky's story of "The Grand Inquisitor."[34] By assuming control of people's lives, the cardinal claimed that his church had gradually removed the burden of freedom that Christ brought to the world. Similarly, the physician or the health care team may accept sole responsibility for difficult decisions in order to spare families the anguish and unnecessary guilt that often occurs in such situations. Despite its plausibility and appeal, this paternalistic reasoning has several crucial flaws. One is the failure to acknowledge that a sense of guilt may be experienced regardless of how a decision is made. If this is true, it is more helpful to focus on the moral justification for a decision to prolong or discontinue treatment—that is, the intent to do what is best for the patient. Both families and practitioners may need explicit reassurance that relinquishing the hold on another's life is sometimes the most loving and caring alternative available.

Another flaw in arguments favoring decisions made solely by physicians (or parents) is the fact that responsibility for decision making is inevitably shared by all of the autonomous participants in a dilemma. Even if an attending physician writes an order or parents indicate their wishes, others choose to implement, ignore, or challenge those decisions. At times, a practitioner does not consider her actions to be a matter of choice; rather, she may simply be following the order of the attending physician or supervisor. At other times, a practitioner may subtly, perhaps even inadvertently, interpret an "order" in a manner that compromises its intent. For example, in a situation where a physician has instructed staff to resuscitate a critically ill patient if necessary, a nurse or resident who disagrees with that decision may respond with deliberate slowness to a signal that the patient has suffered cardiac arrest.

In many cases regarding neonates, there is neither ambiguity nor controversy about what constitutes morally appropriate behavior. For example, the vast majority of pediatricians and pediatric surgeons agree that an anencephalic newborn who is afflicted with intestinal atresia should not have corrective surgery for the latter condition.[35] The invasiveness of surgery cannot be justified on the basis of benefit to the patient because the infant is already dying. In cases where agreement has been reached about moral aspects of treatment or nontreatment, it is probably neither necessary nor helpful to extend the decision base beyond the delivery room or nursery. In fact, involving others in the decision process increases the possibility of violating confidentiality for family privacy.

Moreover, treatment deferral sometimes involves a real risk of harming the patient. Possibly the most common example of such a situation involves intubation of very small (e.g., less than 650 grams) or very early (e.g., less than 24 weeks gestation) preterm newborns. Without intubation, the infant cannot survive. At such times, whoever is competent to provide the treatment is justified in making the decision on the patient's behalf. Subsequently, how-

ever, and in most chronic cases, there is time for discussion and broader input, which ought to be obtained in cases where ambiguity or disagreement continues. Since most decisions to terminate lifesaving treatment are irrevocable, treatment should continue until the conflict is resolved.

Why should there be broader input? Mainly because neither health care practitioners nor parents have any special moral expertise, and the possibility of arriving at well-reasoned moral decisions is increased by the collaborative efforts of reasonable people. Those who maintain a distance from the situation can sometimes provide a more objective perspective, which may complement and supplement the view of those whose involvement in the situation may preclude a totally rational analysis. Extending the decision base in unclear or controversial cases may also be reassuring to those closest to the patient because it represents one more attempt at responsible resolution of a difficult dilemma.

A decision base may be extended beyond the physician or parents through consultation with other clinicians, the entire health care team, a hospital-based review committee, or recourse to the courts. In the interests of maintaining confidentiality and family privacy, it is preferable to use the least public forum in which ambiguity or disagreement may be resolved. The widespread endorsement of the health care team's effectiveness in providing basic health care suggests that it might also be effective in dealing with medically related moral problems.[36] Hospital-based review committees are a newer phenomenon whose efficacy deserves to be tested.[37] Recourse to the courts is a particularly troublesome means of extending the decision base for ethical dilemmas. The legal system introduces an adversarial dimension into a set of relationships that should ideally be based on trust, openness, and consensus. Litigation threatens, and sometimes severs, those relationships, thwarting the therapeutic purpose of the practitioner-patient alliance. There are times when legal recourse may be the only way of resolving ambiguity and disagreement—for example, in cases involving blood transfusions for children of Jehovah's Witnesses. But court decisions are not necessarily morally correct. In the case of Bloomington's Baby Doe, for example, there is widespread agreement that the court's concurrence with the parents' decision to decline treatment was morally unjustified.[38]

Recent government attempts to impose investigative procedures on federally funded facilities that care for newborns seem to be intrusions on the right of privacy and the confidentiality of the physician-patient relationship, and may even be harmful to the patients affected. After investigating many anonymous reports of suspected neglect of impaired newborns, the Department of Health and Human Services concluded that appropriate medical, legal, and moral decisions had already been made in the vast majority of cases. In cases at Vanderbilt University in Nashville, Tennessee, and Strong Memorial Hospital in Rochester, New York, however, it was reported that the government investigation obstructed care of the infants who had allegedly been neglected as well as other patients. The time required for personnel to respond to the queries of investigators could only be purchased at the price of time spent in caring for patients.[39]

In January, 1984, the Department of Health and Human Services strongly encouraged the formation of hospital ethics review committees to consider cases of suspected neglect of disabled infants through denial of treatment.[40] In addition to health care professionals from various disciplines, it was recommended that representatives of the disabled also serve on these committees. In general, the government's encouragement of the committee review mechanism supported the recommendation of the President's Commission.[41] The American Academy of Pediatrics also recommended the formation of local review committees and suggested appropriate procedures and principles.[42] However, the Commission had proposed the local review mechanism as an alternative to federal investigative procedures, arguing that the latter was unlikely to promote the best interests of infants and might actually impede the achievement of that purpose.

The continuing legal controversy surrounding "Baby Doe" cases evoked fairly widespread interest in the use of hospital review committees to address difficult cases. The extent of this interest and the influence of committees on practice remain to be seen.[43] Regardless of how decisions are made, however, we must also deal with the substantive issue of criteria for ethical decisions regarding disabled neonates. These reflect egalitarian considerations and traditional principles of biomedical ethics. An emphasis on the best interests of others also reflects an ethic of care for them.

Prolonging Life in Others' Interests

Since life is commonly perceived as a great gift, it may credibly be maintained that loss of life is always negative for the patient, and therefore the loss can only (possibly) be justified on the basis of others' interests. Indeed, in certain cases, the interests of others may be primarily served through the prolongation of an infant's life. Consider, for example, the fact that fees paid to neonatologists, hospitals, and hospital personnel are partly dependent on the patient population, which is incremented through preservation of lives, no matter what their quality. So long as infants survive, the possibility of obtaining new knowledge through experimental therapies and further clinical data also continues. Beyond these results, there are more subtle rewards that accrue to clinicians who succeed in prolonging infants' lives. First is the feeling of accomplishment borne of the experience of doing rather than just letting go. Most doctors, after all, are activists, more inclined to cure than sustained caring. As one neonatologist put it, "It is easier for me to live with the consequences of something I've done than it is to worry about something I have not done which might have given better results."[44] Second is a perceived consistency between the end of health care and the prolongation of life. Conversely, for some clinicians the death of any patient evokes a sense of professional failure.[45] And third, effective ties build up between clinicians and child (as well as between parents and child, and clinicians and parents), sometimes reaching a point where the emotional needs of the concerned adults obfuscate their recognition of the infant's interests. A nurse thus made a pertinent and poignant comment concerning an infant whose life had been prolonged for two years, despite a preponderance of anguish to him with no expectation of ultimate relief or survival: "We have been doing this for ourselves rather than for him."[46]

Legally it may well be in the interests of clinicians and parents to prolong the life of an infant. Although malpractice suits may be pressed for prolonging life, suits are more likely when treatment has been withdrawn.[47] Even in that case, however, the probability of a successful suit is very slim so long as "letting die" (passive euthanasia) is distinguished from active euthanasia. It is also possible that efforts to prolong the lives of severely disabled infants serve the interests of politicians or political parties. Support for the Reagan administration was surely enhanced in some quarters by the steps it took to prevent a "Baby Doe" situation from recurring.

While motives for prolonging life are sometimes mixed, it may still be maintained that the prolongation is always in the infant's interests. This position is justified if life is assumed to be an absolute value, separable from any quality of life consideration. The assumption has often been associated with an essentially religious perspective, such as that of the Roman Catholic Church in its teaching regarding abortion. Yet religious reasons may also be given, from that tradition as well as from others, for the contrary view, namely, that life is an important but relative value.[48] Christian Science argues against any kind of medical intervention as impeding the natural course of God's plan among human beings.[49] Jehovah's Witnesses argue more selectively against blood transfusions, allowing that deaths which occur through loss of blood fulfill God's will.[50] If faith in divine omniscience and omnipotence is assumed, it may in fact be blasphemous to maintain that human beings can either prolong or shorten life. If faith in an afterlife is affirmed, death may sometimes be construed as preferable to life on earth.

Several nonreligious factors also support an assertion of the absolute value of an infant's life. One may be described as "the uncertainty principle," which applies to infancy more than to other periods of (extrauterine) human existence. While neonatology has achieved wondrous things in recent years, and programs for facilitating maximum development of disabled children have yielded impressive results, it remains impossible to predict with certainty what the subjective or objective future experience of a particular newborn will be.[51] Most clinicians have in their reservoir of experience recollections of minor and

major "miracles," that is, cases whose happy outcome was totally unexpected in light of the facts known at the time and the technology available. I think, for example, of an infant born with heart defects so grave that none similarly afflicted had ever been known to survive, whose recovery after surgery changed the mortality rate applicable to others. However, in this particular case, the issue was mainly a choice between probable death and an extremely slim chance of survival with neurological normalcy (or relative normalcy), rather than a choice between death and survival at a level of extreme neurological compromise.

Another relevant feature of newborn status or the status of children in general is the obvious contrast between them and adults with regard to the span of life already lived and that anticipated. The "right to life" is sometimes more compelling when asserted on behalf of those who have scarcely lived, which partly explains why children's deaths seem more tragic than those of the elderly. In some respects, new life signifies the fullness of hope, which may be dashed through death. On the other hand, in the case of a neonate, there has been little time and opportunity to build the affective ties that make death so painful for a loved one's survivors.

If the interests of the infant are primary, I do not believe that features peculiar to infants provide adequate justification for the preservation of any and every newborn's life. Nonetheless, these features do argue persuasively for a conservative approach to the irreversible decision to terminate or not initiate life-prolonging treatment. By "conservative" approach I mean one that seeks to prolong life if there is some real, although small, chance that the continuation is in the infant's own interests. Where there is high probability that this will not be the case, then the same criterion argues against prolonging life. To the extent that prolongation is likely to increase suffering for the child, a decision not to prolong life through technological support may be morally mandatory. It reflects our realization that those that can suffer should not be caused to suffer (guideline 3), and that individuals should not be treated as other than who or what they are (guideline 5). Just as the right to die may be construed as part of an adult's right to life, the same claim may be made with regard to infants. To deny this right to children is to practice what Richard McCormick has called a "racism of the adult world."[52]

An Infant's Right to Die

While the priority of the infant's interests suggests that decisions to prolong life will be made much more frequently than decisions to the contrary, that priority also suggests the relevance of "quality of life" considerations. Three types of cases are relevant in this regard. The first and simplest type is where therapy is futile because the underlying condition is irremediably fatal, and therapy would in no way reduce pain to the infant. In other words, survival beyond a few hours or days or weeks is not expected, no matter what is done or not done. Anencephaly, a condition where the infant's brain has failed to develop, is a commonly accepted example of this situation. Even those who claim "quality of life" factors are irrelevant agree that the life of an anencephalic infant need not be prolonged.

The second type of case is less simple: one where repeated, intrusive, painful interventions would prolong the infant's life, possibly for years, but continued life is of dubious benefit to the child. In such a situation, efforts to preserve life are likely to result in a preponderance of negative experiences for the infant without realistic expectation of improvement. The prolongation itself can only occur through multiple medical and surgical intrusions that are sometimes iatrogenic, and generally interfere with the natural course of the body's function. Not infrequently, despite use of analgesics and anesthesia, the interventions are also painful.

Consider, for example, an infant with the chromosomal abnormality Trisomy 13, which involves profound mental retardation and frequent seizures for the 18 percent who survive beyond the first year of life.[53] Often, these infants face immediate life-threatening problems such as severe heart defects. Correction of these and concomitant problems requires multiple surgeries, medical and orthopedic interventions, and permanent hospitalization. To prolong life through invasive procedures might serve the interests of parents and clinicians, but can scarcely be judged to serve those of the infants themselves. The decision to let such an infant die is usually based on the fallible judgment that prolonging life will cause the child a preponderance of suffering.

The third type of case is more problematic than the preceding: one where the required therapy is not itself a source of pain, but neither is it curative, and the life thus prolonged is probably devoid of any qualitative satisfaction for the infant. Consider, for instance, a newborn who has had a Grade IV cranial hemorrhage (bleeding into the cerebral tissues) with uncontrollable seizures, whose intestines have necrotized. The child can only be fed through parenteral hyperalimentation, a process by which predigested food is infused into the body. The combination of the hemorrhage and seizures indicates high probability that the child might survive but only at a vegetative level of existence, that is, without any cognitive function or capacity for social interchange. Although such a child might survive for years, it is doubtful that his survival is in anyone's interest, including his own. Unless life is an end in itself, rather than a necessary condition for the actualization of human values and potential, maintaining life in these circumstances may be exploiting the child, that is, using him as a means of furthering others' ends.

A claim that infants' interests include the right to die may be based on a conception of life that is not merely quantitative.[54] Life is then perceived as a crucial but relative value, extremely significant as the basis of all other human values, but not absolute. This view necessarily involves the notion that quality of life factors are essential to any full affirmation of the value of human life. However, which factors are relevant, and how they are relevant, remains problematic.

Decisions made in behalf of incompetent or unconscious adults may enlighten us with regard to infants. Either of two approaches is generally followed with adults: (1) the decision is based on the patient's history, that is, an understanding of the patient's desires or values as applicable to such a situation (as expressed, for example, in a living will or other form of advance directive), or (2) utilization of the "reasonable person" standard, that is, determination of treatment and nontreatment on the basis of what any competent, conscious person would reasonably choose in similar circumstances. Obviously the first approach is inapplicable to newborns, but the second seems appropriate even though infants may not be described as "reasonable persons."[55] If, for example, a reasonable person would decline surgery that could in no way benefit her, and might in fact prolong a predominantly painful existence, why might we not invoke this criterion to justify a similar decision for an infant? In all three types of cases, that criterion would apply. Thus, in situations where (1) therapy is futile, (2) where it would prolong a life of predominant anguish, or (3) where the patient has suffered irreparable neurological devastation, the decision not to prolong life beyond its natural limits is reasonable, and should be respected as such. To reject the applicability of this standard to infants or children suggests complicity in what we have already described as adult racism. It thus stands opposed to an egalitarian perspective.

Giving Priority to Infants' Interests

Where individuals attempt to observe the priority of infants' interests, the nuances of particular cases may be interpreted in light of certain distinctions. For example, natural law theology has long invoked the distinction between "ordinary" and "extraordinary" treatment, claiming that the former is obligatory while the latter is not. Ordinary and extraordinary treatment is explained as relative to the unique circumstances of the case, including the accessibility of necessary technology and therapy.[56] Thus, what might count as extraordinary treatment of a cancer-ridden elderly patient who has indicated a desire to die may be ordinary in dealing with a newborn, whether seriously ill or not. Similarly, a distinction between optimal and maximal care is pertinent: maximal care means prolonging life no matter what the cost to the patient; optimal care means prolonging life only to the extent that the prolongation is in the patient's interests.[57] Maximal care may (inadvertently) serve the interests of others—for example, students who can gain more clinical experience by continuing care for the dying; it may simultaneously impede optimal care for the patient. An obligation to provide optimal care implies that others' interests do not constitute a sufficient criterion for refusal of treatment, while those interests may be relevant in applying the ordinary versus extraordinary distinction.

Clinical interpretations that have served as guides for individuals addressing problematic cases include a distinction between "coercing" and "helping" someone to live, and between "doing to" and "doing for" a patient.[58] Roughly, "coercing" and "doing to" constitute unjustifiable intrusions, while "helping" and "doing for" are justifiable because they are oriented toward the patient's own interests. Determination of where the distinctions apply remains difficult, and may never be made with absolute certainty, but some cases involve a very high expectation that survival will mean prolonged and unmitigated misery for a particular patient, child or adult. An example of coercing someone to live might be a situation where a patient experiencing the terminal stage of an incurable cancer has suffered kidney failure that is treatable by dialysis. Performing corrective cardiac surgery on an infant with an incurable and fatal genetic abnormality may be another. In such cases, the right to die, as part of the right to life, seems an undeniable component of patient rights.

Another relevant distinction is between "defensive" and patient-centered medicine. Increasingly and unfortunately, "defensive medicine" (that is, medicine practiced to avoid legal entanglements) has motivated clinicians to prolong lives in cases where there is persuasive evidence that this is not in the best interests of the patient. In 1983, James Strain, as president of the American Academy of Pediatrics, wrote that today's pediatricians have a different view from those interviewed for a 1977 national survey that disclosed that the majority would acquiesce to parental refusal of lifesaving surgery for seriously disabled infants.[59] At this point in time, he alleged, physicians would not accede to the refusal. A 1988 survey of pediatricians in Massachusetts by I. David Todres confirmed Strain's thesis.[60] Todres found that physicians were less inclined to give priority to parents' wishes and more inclined to treat disabled infants than they were ten years earlier. Unfortunately, some erroneously believe they are legally obliged to treat disabled infants more aggressively than others. In the interest of "defensive medicine," disabled newborns are then subjected to the discrimination of overtreatment.

Medical as well as moral decisions continually need to be reassessed in light of the changing condition of the patient. Thus a decision to prolong life may be reversed because a patient's condition has so gravely deteriorated that the prognosis is one of overwhelming misery for him. For example, extremely premature or very low birth weight babies who have been kept alive through intubation immediately after birth may fail to develop independent respiratory function, and suffer further internal malfunction such as renal failure and cerebral hemorrhage. As already suggested, such instances, which are increasing in our neonatal intensive care units, argue that a distinction between a very ill and impaired infant is not a clear one; in fact, illnesses that can be cured may induce permanent and profound disabilities through the very process by which the infant's life is prolonged.[61]

Similarly, decisions not to prolong life need to be continually reassessed in light of the infant's progress. Because clinical judgments are fallible, certain patients may outlive (both qualitatively and quantitatively) a decision not to provide lifesaving treatment in their behalf. Where that occurs, a decision to terminate or not to initiate treatment needs to be reviewed, and aggressive treatment instituted, continuing so long as there is reasonable expectation that the infant's interests will thus be served. The fact that mistakes in judgment occur in ethical as well as clinical dilemmas in no way argues that the judgments themselves are wrong or right in the context of what was known at the time. Only in the long run do such results justifiably exert an influence on subsequent decisions. They do so then because of the knowledge built up over time, providing the rational basis for a general way of acting.

Baby Doe Revisited

The decision to allow Bloomington's Baby Doe to die could not be justified on the basis of the priority criterion discussed here. In light of what we know about children with Down syndrome, it is more likely that this infant's interests would be best served by overriding the parents' refusal of lifesaving treatment for him. The therapy was not futile, the prognosis was not one of neurological devastation, and

the predominant future experiences of the child might well have been positive for him. Moreover, while the parents preferred not to raise the child, adoption was a viable option. In fact, a number of couples, two of whom already had children with Down syndrome, offered to adopt Baby Doe before he died. This is a significant factor because actual promotion of infants' interests depends on the attitudes and resources of those who might (or might not) care for them, including government agencies. If a challenge to parental preference for withholding treatment does not address ways by which ongoing care will be provided, the challenge itself may pose a threat to the child's best interests.

In contrast to the Bloomington situation, the case of Baby Jane Doe was one where the priority of the infant's interests may have justified refusal of treatment. *If* the reported facts were correct (e.g., the prognosis that the child "would never experience joy, never experience sorrow"),[62] the option here was between intervention that would allow an extended period of life in a neurologically devastated state; and nonintervention that would permit gradual deterioration, with death occurring sometime during infancy. Obviously, the degree of uncertainty regarding these possibilities was a critical factor. Whether the child's medical problems and condition predicted a predominantly negative experience for her was crucial in determining the applicability of the criterion. However, if there were a high probability that this was so, the priority of the child's interests would be observed by foregoing medical interventions. In other words, the infant's right to life in such circumstances might best be respected by supporting her right to die. The parents' decision to respect that right was apparently motivated by a desire to place the interests of their child before their own: their ethic of care reasoned that love (especially parental love) occasionally means letting go of the one loved.

If the facts reported are correct, then the main difference between these cases is the probability that the future experience of one child would be predominantly positive for him, and the other child's future experience would probably be predominantly negative for her. Because of their differing prognoses, one infant's right to life had priority, and the other's right to die had priority. From an egalitarian perspective that respects differences among individual infants, each deserves to be treated differently.

Notes

1   "Nondiscrimination on the Basis of Handicaps; Procedures and Guidelines Relating to Health Care for Handicapped Infants," *Federal Register* (Jan. 12, 1984) 49: 1622-54; "Big Brother Doe," *Wall Street Journal* (Oct. 31, 1983), 20; "Baby Jane's Big Brothers," *New York Times* (Nov. 4, 1983), 28; and Mary B. Mahowald and Jerome Paulson, "The Baby Does: Two Different Situations," *The Cleveland Plain Dealer* (Dec. 31, 1983), 9-A.

2   Much of the material in this chapter is adapted from two of my earlier articles: "Ethical Decisions in Neonatal Intensive Care," in *Human Values in Critical Care Medicine*, ed. Stuart Youngner (Philadelphia: Praeger Publishers, 1986), and "In the Interest of Infants," *Philosophy in Context* 14, no. 9 (1984): 9-18.

3   William H. Tooley and Roderick H. Phibbs, "Neonatal Intensive Care: The State of the Art," in *Ethics of Newborn Intensive Care*, ed. Albert R. Jonsen and Michael J. Garland (San Francisco: Health Policy Program, University of California, 1976), 11-15.

4   Tooley and Phibbs, 11-15.

5   Barbara C. Tilley, "Assessment of Risks from DES," in *The Custom-Made Child?* ed. Helen B. Holmes, Betty B. Hoskins, and Michael Gross (Clifton, New Jersey: Humana Press, 1981), 29-39. Concerning ineffectiveness of the therapy, see W.J. Dieckmann, M.D. Davis, L.M. Rynkiewiez, et al., "Does Administration of Diethylstilbestrol During Pregnancy Have Therapeutic Value?" *American Journal of Obstetrics and Gynecology* 66, no. 5 (Nov. 1953): 1062-81. Concerning cancer and reproductive complications in offspring, see Arthur L. Herbst and Diane Anderson, "Clear Cell Adenocarcinoma of the Vagina and Cervix Secondary to Intrauterine Exposure to Diethylstilbestrol," *Seminars in Surgical Oncology* 6 (1990): 343-46; and Raymond H. Kaufman, Kenneth Noller, Ervin Adam, et al., "Upper Genital Tract Abnormalities and Pregnancy Outcome in Diethylstilbestrol-Exposed Progeny," *American Journal of Obstetrics and Gynecology*, 148, no. 7 (April 1, 1984): 973-82.

6   Marshall H. Klaus and Avroy Fanaroff, *Care of the High-Risk Neonate* (Philadelphia: W.B. Saunders, 1973), xi.

7   Mildred T. Stahlman, "Neonatal Intensive Care: Success or Failure," *Journal of Pediatrics* 105 (1984): 162-67.

8   Jay Goldsmith and Robert Arensman, "Predicting the Failure of Mechanical Ventilation: New Therapeutic Options," *Neonatal Intensive Care* 3 (1990): 40-47. Data supporting success rates in treatment of all four conditions are available through the Extracorporeal Life Support Registry, University of Michigan, 1991.

9   Richard Martin, "Neonatal Surfactant Therapy—Where Do We Go from Here?" *Journal of Pediatrics* 118, no. 4 (April 1991): 555-56; and T. Allen Merritt, Mikko Hallman, Charles Berry, et al., "Randomized, Placebo-Controlled Trial of Human Surfactant Given at Birth Versus Rescue Administration in Very Low Birth Weight Infants with Lung Immaturity," *Journal of Pediatrics* 118, no. 4 (April 1991): 581-94.

10 Maureen Hack, B. Caron, Ann Rivers, and Avroy Fanaroff, "The Very Low Birth Weight Infant: The Broader Spectrum of Morbidity during Infancy and Early Childhood," *Journal of Developmental and Behavioral Pediatrics* 4, no. 4 (Dec. 1983): 243-49.

11 Maureen Hack, Ann Rivers, and Avroy Fanaroff, "Outcomes of Extremely Low Birth Weight Infants between 1982 and 1988," *New England Journal of Medicine* 321, no 24 (Dec. 14, 1989): 1642-47.

12 See Maureen Hack, Jeffery D. Horbar, Michael H. Malloy, et al., "Very Low Birth Weight Outcomes of the National Institute of Child Health and Human Development Neonatal Network," *Pediatrics*, 87, no. 5 (May 1991): 587-97.

13 Laila Williamson, "Infanticide: An Anthropological Analysis," in *Infanticide and the Value of Life*, ed. Marvin Kohl (Buffalo, New York: Prometheus Books, 1978), 61-75.

14 James Rachels, "Active and Passive Euthanasia," *New England Journal of Medicine* 292, no. 2 (Jan. 9, 1975): 78-80.

15 John J. Paris and Anne B. Fletcher, "Infant Doe Regulations and the Absolute Requirement to Use Nourishment and Fluids for the Dying Infant," *Law, Medicine and Health Care* 11 (1983): 210-13.

16 Robert Weir, *Selective Nontreatment of Handicapped*

Infants: Moral Dilemmas in Neonatal Medicine (New York: Oxford University Press, 1984), 215-21.

17 Anthony Shaw, "Dilemmas of 'Informed Consent' in Children," *New England Journal of Medicine* 289, no 17 (Oct. 25, 1973): 885-90.

18 President's Commission for the Study of Ethical Problems in Medicine and Biomedical and Behavioral Research, *Making Health Care Decisions*, vol. 3, Appendices: Studies on the Foundations of Informed Consent (Washington DC: U.S. Government Printing Office, 1982), 175-245.

19 Gina Kolata, "Parents of Tiny Infants Find Care Choices Are Not Theirs," *New York Times* (Sept. 30, 1991), 1 and A11.

20 Hack, Rivers, and Fanaroff, 243-49.

21 H.E. Ehrhardt, "Abortion and Euthanasia: Common Problems—The Termination of Developing and Expiring Life," *Human Life Review* 1 (1975): 12-31.

22 See articles in *The Herald-Telephone*, Bloomington, Indiana, April 23 and May 1-3, 1982, and *The Criterion*, Indianapolis, Indiana, April 23, 1982. Also see Weir, 128-29.

23 U.S. Department of Health and Human Services, "Interim Final Rule 45 CFR Part 84, Nondiscrimination on the Basis of a Handicap," *Federal Register* 48 (March 7, 1983), 9630-32.

24 Barbara J. Culliton, "Baby Doe Regs Thrown Out by Court," *Science* 220 (April 29, 1983): 479-80.

25 It should be noted that the reported facts and media coverage of this case have been disputed, and the infant fared better than had been anticipated. In time, the parents consented to surgery for treatment of the hydrocephalus, her spinal lesion closed naturally, and her parents took her home from the hospital the following spring. See Steven Baer, "The Half-told Story of Baby Jane Doe," *Columbia Journalism Review* (Nov./Dec., 1984), 35-38; and "Baby Doe at Age 1: A Joy and Burden," *New York Times* (Oct. 14, 1984), Sect. 1, 56.

26 See note 1.

27 U.S. Department of Health and Human Services, "Child Abuse and Neglect Prevention and Treatment Program; Final Rule," *Federal Register* 50 (Jan. 11, 1985), 1487-92.

28 Betty W. Levin, "Consensus and Controversy in the Treatment of Catastrophically Ill Newborns," in *Which Babies Shall Live?* (Clifton, NJ: Humana Press, 1985), 169-205.

29 See President's Commission for the Study of Ethical Problems in Medicine and Biomedical and Behavioral Research, *Deciding to Forego Life-Sustaining Treatment, A Report of the Ethical, Medical, and Legal Issues in Treatment Decisions* (Washington, DC: Government Printing Office, March 1983), 214-22; James Strain, "The American Academy of Pediatrics' Comments on the 'Baby Doe II' Regulations," *New England Journal of Medicine* 309, no. 7 (Aug. 18, 1983): 443-44; and *Handicapped Americans Report* (July 14, 1983), 6.

30 That neonatologists' interpretations of the best interest standard are widely divergent is evident in statements attributed to them by Elisabeth Rosenthal in "As More Tiny Infants Live, Choices and Burden Grow," *New York Times* (Sept. 29, 1991), 1. John Arras has addressed the limitations of this standard in his "Toward an Ethic of Ambiguity," *Hastings Center Report* 14, no. 2 (April 1984): 30-31.

31 See, for example, Paul Ramsey, *The Patient as Person* (New Haven, CT: Yale University Press, 1970), 1-11; see also note 18.

32 Bernard M. Dickens, "Legally Informed Consent," in *Contemporary Issues in Biomedical Ethics*, ed. John W. Davis, Barry Hoffmaster, and Sarah Shorten (Clifton, NJ: Humana Press, 1978), 199-204.

33 David Thomasma, "Beyond Medical Paternalism and Patient Autonomy: A Model of Physician-Patient Relationship," *Annals of Internal Medicine* 98 (Feb. 1983): 243-48; and Thomas S. Szasz and Marc H. Hollender, "The Basic Models of the Doctor-Patient Relationship," *Archives of Internal Medicine* 97 (1956): 585-92.

34 Fyodor Dostoyevsky, "The Grand Inquisitor," in *The Brothers Karamazov* (New York: Modern Library, 1950), 255-74.

35 Anthony Shaw, Judson G. Randolph, and Barbara B. Manard, "Ethical Issues in Pediatric Surgery: A National Survey of Pediatricians and Pediatric Surgeons," *Pediatrics* 60 (1977): 590

36 Lawrence A. Rosini, Mary C. Howell, David Todres and John J. Dorman, "Group Meetings in a Pediatric Intensive Care Unit," *Pediatrics* 53 (1974): 371-74.

37 Richard A. McCormick, "Ethics Committees: Promise or Peril?" *Law, Medicine and Health Care* 12 (1984): 150-55; and Mary B. Mahowald, "Hospital Ethics Committees: Diverse and Problematic,"

Newsletter on Philosophy and Medicine (American Philosophical Association) 88, no. 2 (March 1989): 88-94, reprinted in HEC *Forum* 1 (1989): 237-46 and in *Bioethics News* 2 (1990): 4-13.

38   Alan R. Fleischman and Thomas Murray, "Ethics Committees for Infants Doe?" *Hastings Center Report* 13, no. 6 (Dec. 1983): 5-9.

39   James Strain, "The American Academy of Pediatrics' Comments on the 'Baby Doe II' Regulations," *New England Journal of Medicine* 309, no. 7 (Aug. 18, 1983): 443-44.

40   U.S. Department of Health and Human Services, "Nondiscrimination on the Basis of Handicap: Procedures and Guidelines Relating to Health Care for Handicapped Infants," *Federal Register* 49 (Jan. 12, 1984), 1651.

41   President's Commission for the Study of Ethical Problems in Medicine and Biomedical and Behavioral Research, 227.

42   American Academy of Pediatrics, *Guidelines for Infant Bioethics Committees* (Evanston, IL: American Academy of Pediatrics, 1984).

43   See Mary B. Mahowald, "Hospital Ethics Committees: Diverse and Problematic," 88-94. I have attempted to evaluate infant ethics committees in "Baby Doe Committees: A Critical Evaluation," *Current Controversies in Perinatal Care* 15, no. 4 (Dec. 1988), 789-800.

44   Joan E. Hoggman, "Withholding Treatment from Seriously Ill Newborns: A Neonatologist's View," in *Legal and Ethical Aspects of Treating Critically and Terminally Ill Patients*, ed. A. Edward Doudera, J.D., and J. Douglas Peters, J.D. (Ann Arbor, MI: AUPHA Press, 1982), 243. Note, however, that living more *easily* with the consequences of something one has done is not equivalent to moral justification for doing it.

45   See August Kasper, "The Doctor and Death," in *Moral Problems in Medicine*, ed. Samuel Gorowitz, Andrew L. Jameton, Ruth Macklin, John M. O'Connor, Eugene V. Perrin, Beverly Page St. Clair, and Susan Sherwin (Englewood Cliffs, NJ: Prentice Hall, Inc., 1976), 69-72.

46   Brenda Miller, at a health care team meeting, Pediatric Intensive Care Unit, Rainbow Babies and Children's Hospital, Cleveland, Ohio, September 27, 1983.

47   See Susan Schmidt, "Wrongful Life," *Journal of the American Medical Association* 250, no. 16 (Oct. 28, 1983): 2209-10: "Of all the birth-related legal theories, wrongful life, and action filed on behalf of the infant born with a genetic or other congenital birth defect, has met with the most disapproval."

48   For example, Richard McCormick, "To Save or Let Die," *Journal of the American Medical Association* 229, no. 2 (July 8, 1974): 172-76.

49   *Academic American Encyclopedia*, vol. 4 (Danbury, CT: Grolier Press, 1983), 412.

50   *Academic American Encyclopedia* vol. 11, 394.

51   See Carson Strong, "The Tiniest Newborns," *Hastings Center Report* 13, no. 1 (Feb. 1983): 14-19.

52   Richard McCormick, "Experimental Subjects—Who Should They Be?" *Journal of the American Medical Association* 235, no. 20 (May 17, 1976): 2197.

53   Kenneth Lyons Jones, *Smith's Recognizable Patterns of Human Malformation,* 4th ed. (Philadelphia: W.B. Saunders, 1988), 20-21.

54   See Hans Jonas, "The Right to Die," *Hastings Center Report* 8, no. 4 (Aug. 1978): 36: "Fully understood, it [i.e., the right to life] also includes the right to death."

55   Norman Fost applies this standard to infants under the aegis of "ideal observer theory" in "Ethical Issues in the Treatment of Critically Ill Newborns," *Pediatric Annals* 10, no.10 (Oct. 1981): 21. Jonathan Glover has a similar suggestion for dealing with infants. He claims that the best substitute for asking whether they wish to go on living (since they cannot register their own preferences) is "to ask whether we ourselves would find such a life preferable to death." See Jonathan Glover, *Causing Death and Saving Lives* (New York: Penguin, 1977), 161.

56   See Gerald Kelly, *Medico-Moral Problems* (St. Louis, MO: The Catholic Hospital Association, 1958), 129. For an excellent critique of this distinction, see James Rachels, *The End of Life* (New York: Oxford University Press, 1986), 96-100.

57   My formulation here is different from that of David Smith, who identifies "maximal" with "extraordinary," and "optimal" with "ordinary." See David H. Smith, "On Letting Some Babies Die," *Hastings Center Studies* 2, no. 2 (May 1974): 44. I return to the concept of "optimal care" in Chapter 15 [*Women and Children in Health Care*].

58   These are distinctions employed by pediatricians with whom I have worked: the first by Donald Schussler,

M.D., the second by Jeffery Blumer, M.D., Ph.D., both working in the Division of Critical Care, Rainbow Babies and Children's Hospital, Cleveland, Ohio, during the 1980s.

59 James Strain, "The Decision to Forego Life-Sustaining Treatment for Seriously Ill Newborns," *Pediatrics* 72, no. 4 (Oct. 1983): 572. Strain was comparing the pediatricians of 1983 with those interviewed for studies published in 1977 based on data obtained several years earlier. See, for example, Shaw, Randolph, and Manard, 588; and I. David Todres, Diane Krane, Mary C. Howell, et al., "Pediatricians' Attitudes Affecting Decision-Making in Defective Newborns," *Pediatrics* 6, no. 2 (Aug. 1977), 197-201.

60 Kolata, 1, A11; and I. David Todres, Jeanne Guillemin, Michael A. Grodin, and Dick Batten, "Life-Saving Therapy for Newborn: A Questionnaire Survey in the State of Massachusetts," *Pediatrics* 81, no. 5 (May 1988): 643.

61 See Note 7.

62 My analysis here is crucially dependent on the accuracy of the reported facts and of the prognosis associated with them. As indicated in note 25, both were disputed in subsequent accounts of the case.

CHAPTER SIX

DEATH, DYING, AND EUTHANASIA

35.
EUTHANASIA: THE FUNDAMENTAL ISSUES

Margaret P. Battin

SOURCE: Donald VanDeVeer and Tom Regan (eds.), *Health Care Ethics: An Introduction*
(Philadelphia: Temple University Press, 1987).

[handwritten marginalia: 1987 + passive = "allowing to die" ± active = voluntary — involuntary euthanasia = rejected]

Author's Note: When this article was first published in 1987, the meaning of the term 'euthanasia' as used in the United States had both positive and negative connotations. 'Passive euthanasia,' understood as 'allowing to die,' was generally accepted; 'active (voluntary) euthanasia' was controversial; involuntary euthanasia was rejected. 'Euthanasia' was sometimes understood in the original Greek sense of 'good death,' as it is in the Netherlands, sometimes in the post-Nazi sense of killing on ulterior grounds having nothing to do with the interests of the patient. However, as this article is republished in 2012, a quarter-century after its first appearance, the term 'euthanasia' as it is used in the U.S. has come to have almost exclusively negative connotations. The reader of this article is asked to keep this linguistic change in mind. —MPB

Because it arouses questions about the morality of killing, the effectiveness of consent, the duties of physicians, and equity in the distribution of resources, euthanasia is one of the most acute and uncomfortable contemporary problems in medical ethics. It is not a new problem; euthanasia has been discussed—and practiced—in both Eastern and Western cultures from the earliest historical times to the present. But because of medicine's new technological capacities to extend life, the problem is much more pressing than it has been in the past, and both the discussion and practice of euthanasia are more widespread. Despite this, much of contemporary Western culture remains strongly opposed to euthanasia: doctors ought not kill people, its public voices maintain, and ought not let them die if it is possible to save life.

I believe that this opposition to euthanasia is in serious moral error—on grounds of mercy, autonomy, and justice. I shall argue for the rightness of granting a person a humane, merciful death, if he or she wants it, even when this can be achieved only by a direct and deliberate killing. But I think there are dangers here. Consequently, I shall also suggest that there is a safer way to discharge our moral duties than relying on physician-initiated euthanasia, one

that nevertheless will satisfy those moral demands upon which the case for euthanasia rests.

The Case for Euthanasia, Part I: Mercy

The case for euthanasia rests on three fundamental moral principles: mercy, autonomy, and justice.

The principle of mercy asserts that *where possible, one ought to relieve the pain or suffering of another person, when it does not contravene that person's wishes, where one can do so without undue costs to oneself, where one will not violate other moral obligations, where the pain or suffering itself is not necessary for the sufferer's attainment of some overriding good, and where the pain or suffering can be relieved without precluding the sufferer's attainment of some overriding good.*[1] (This principle might best be called the principle of medical mercy, to distinguish it from principles concerning mercy in judicial contexts.)[2] Stated in this relatively weak form, and limited by these provisos, the principle of (medical) mercy is not controversial, though the point I wish to argue here certainly is: contexts that require mercy sometimes require euthanasia as a way of granting mercy—both by direct killing and by letting die.

321

Although philosophers do not agree on whether moral agents have positive duties of beneficence, including duties to those in pain, members of the medical world are not reticent about asserting them. "Relief of pain is the least disputed and most universal of the moral obligations of the physician," writes one doctor. "Few things a doctor does are more important than relieving pain," says another.[3] These are not simply assertions that the physician ought "do no harm," as the Hippocratic Oath is traditionally interpreted, but assertions of positive obligation. It might be argued that the physician's duty of mercy derives from a special contractual or fiduciary relationship with the patient, but I think that this is in error: rather, the duty of (medical) mercy is generally binding on all moral agents,[4] and it is only by virtue of their more frequent exposure to pain and their specialized training in its treatment that this duty falls more heavily on physicians and nurses than on others. Hence, though we may call it the principle of *medical* mercy, it asserts an obligation that we all have.

This principle of mercy establishes two component duties:

1. the duty not to cause further pain or suffering; and
2. the duty to act to end pain or suffering already occurring.

Under the first of these, for a physician or other caregiver to extend mercy to a suffering patient may mean to refrain from procedures that cause further suffering—provided, of course, that the treatment offers the patient no overriding benefits. So, for instance, the physician must refrain from ordering painful tests, therapies, or surgical procedures when they cannot alleviate suffering or contribute to a patient's improvement or cure. Perhaps the most familiar contemporary medical example is the treatment of burn victims when survival is unprecedented;[5] if with the treatments or without them the patient's chance of survival is nil, mercy requires the physician not to impose the debridement treatments, which are excruciatingly painful, when they can provide the patient no benefit at all.

Although it is increasingly difficult to determine when survival is unprecedented in burn victims,

other practices that the principles of mercy would rule out remain common. For instance, repeated cardiac resuscitation is sometimes performed even though a patient's survival is highly unlikely; although patients in arrest are unconscious at the time of resuscitation, it can be a brutal procedure, and if the patient regains consciousness, its aftermath can involve considerable pain. (On the contrary, of course, attempts at resuscitation would indeed be permitted under the principle of mercy if there were some chance of survival with good recovery, as in hypothermia or electrocution.) Patients are sometimes subjected to continued unproductive, painful treatment to complete a research protocol, to train student physicians, to protect the physician or hospital from legal action, or to appease the emotional needs of family members; although in some specific cases such practices may be justified on other grounds, in general they are prohibited by the principle of mercy. Of course, whether a painful test or therapy will actually contribute to some overriding good for the patient is not always clear. Nevertheless, the principle of mercy directs that where such procedures can reasonably be expected to impose suffering on the patient without overriding benefits for him or her, they ought not be done.

In many such cases, the patient will die whether or not the treatments are performed. In some cases, however, the principle of mercy may also demand withholding treatment that could extend the patient's life if the treatment is itself painful or discomforting and there is very little or no possibility that it will provide life that is pain-free or offers the possibility of other important goods. For instance, to provide respiratory support for a patient in the final, irreversible stages of a deteriorative disease may extend his or her life but will mean permanent dependence and incapacitation; though some patients may take continuing existence to make possible other important goods, for some patients continued treatment means the pointless imposition of continuing pain. "Death," whispered Abe Perlmutter, the Florida patient with amyotrophic lateral sclerosis—"Lou Gehrig's Disease"—who pursued through the courts his wish to have the tracheotomy tube connecting him to a respirator removed, "can't be any worse than what I'm going through now."[6] In such cases, the principle of mercy demands that the "treatments" no longer be imposed, and that the patient be allowed to die.

But the principle of mercy may also demand "letting die" in a still stronger sense. Under its second component, the principle asserts a duty to act to end suffering that is already occurring. Medicine already honors this duty through its various techniques of pain management, including physiological means such as narcotics, nerve blocks, acupuncture, and neurosurgery, and psychotherapeutic means such as self-hypnosis, conditioning, and good old-fashioned comforting care. But there are some difficult cases in which pain or suffering is severe but cannot be effectively controlled, at least as long as the patient remains sentient at all. Classical examples include tumors of the throat (where agonizing discomfort is not just a matter of pain but of inability to swallow); "air hunger," or acute shortness of breath; tumors of the brain or bone; and so on. Severe nausea, vomiting, and exhaustion may increase the patient's misery. In these cases, continuing life—or, at least, continuing consciousness—may mean continuing pain. Consequently, mercy's demand for euthanasia takes hold here: mercy demands that the pain, even if with it the life, be brought to an end.

Ending the pain, though with it the life, may be accomplished through what is usually called "passive euthanasia": withholding or withdrawing treatment that could prolong life. In the most indirect of these cases, the patient is simply not given treatment that might extend his or her life—say, radiation therapy in advanced cancer. In the more direct cases, lifesaving treatment is deliberately withheld in the face of an immediate, lethal threat—for instance, antibiotics are withheld from a cancer patient when an overwhelming infection develops; either the cancer or the infection will kill the patient, but the infection does so sooner and in a much gentler way. In all of the passive euthanasia cases, properly so called, the patient's life could be extended; it is mercy that demands that he or she be "allowed to die."

But the second component of the principle of mercy may also demand the easing of pain by means more direct than mere allowing to die; it may require *killing*. This is usually called "active euthanasia," and despite borderline cases (for instance, removing a respirator or a lifesaving IV), it can in general be conceptually distinguished from passive euthanasia. In passive euthanasia, treatment is withheld that could support failing bodily functions, either in warding off external threats or in performing its own processes; active euthanasia, in contrast, involves the direct interruption of ongoing bodily processes that otherwise would have been adequate to sustain life. However, although it may be possible to draw a conceptual distinction between passive and active euthanasia, this provides no warrant for the ubiquitous view that killing is morally worse than letting die.[7] Nor does it support the view that withdrawing treatment is worse than withholding it. If the patient's condition is so tragic that continuing life brings only pain, and there is no other way to relieve the pain than by death, then the more merciful act is not one that merely removes support for bodily processes and waits for eventual death to ensue; rather, it is one that brings the pain—and the patient's life—to an end *now*. If there are grounds on which it is merciful not to prolong life, then there are also grounds on which it is merciful to terminate it at once. The easy overdose, the lethal injection (successors to the hemlock used for this purpose by non-Hippocratic physicians in ancient Greece[8]), are what mercy demands when no other means will bring relief.

But, it may be objected, the cases I have mentioned to illustrate intolerable pain are classical ones; such cases are controllable now. Pain is a thing of the medical past, and euthanasia is no longer necessary, though it once may have been, to relieve pain. Given modern medical technology and recent remarkable advances in pain management, the sufferings of the mortally wounded and dying can be relieved by less dramatic means. For instance, many once-feared or painful diseases—tetanus, rabies, leprosy, tuberculosis—are now preventable or treatable. Improvements in battlefield first aid and transport of the wounded have been so great that the military coup de grace is now officially obsolete. We no longer speak of "mortal agony" and "death throes" as the probable last scenes of life. Particularly impressive are the huge advances under the hospice program in the amelioration of both the physical and emotional pain of terminal illness,[9] and our culture-wide fears of pain in terminal cancer are no longer justified: cancer pain, when it occurs, can now be controlled in virtually all cases. We can now end the pain without also ending the life.

This is a powerful objection, and one very frequently heard in medical circles. Nevertheless, it does not succeed. It is flatly incorrect to say that all pain, including pain in terminal illness, is or can be controlled. Some people still die in unspeakable agony. With superlative care, many kinds of pain can indeed be reduced in many patients, and adequate control of pain in terminal illness is often quite easy to achieve. Nevertheless, complete, universal, fully reliable pain control is a myth. Pain is not yet a "thing of the past," nor are many associated kinds of physical distress. Some kinds of conditions, such as difficulty in swallowing, are still difficult to relieve without introducing other discomforting limitations. Some kinds of pain are resistant to medication, as in elevated intracranial pressure or bone metastases and fractures. For some patients, narcotic drugs are dysphoric. Pain and distress may be increased by nausea, vomiting, itching, constipation, dry mouth, abscesses and decubitus ulcers that do not heal, weakness, breathing difficulties, and offensive smells. Severe respiratory insufficiency may mean—as Joanne Lynn describes it—"a singularly terrifying and agonizing final few hours."[10] Even a patient receiving the most advanced and sympathetic medical attention may still experience episodes of pain, perhaps alternating with unconsciousness, as his or her condition deteriorates and the physician attempts to adjust schedules and dosages of pain medication. Many dying patients, including half of all terminal cancer patients, have little or no pain,[11] but there are still cases in which pain management is difficult and erratic. Finally, there are cases in which pain control is theoretically possible but for various extraneous reasons does not occur. Some deaths take place in remote locations where there are no pain-relieving resources. Some patients are unable to communicate the nature or extent of their pain. And some institutions and institutional personnel who have the capacity to control pain do not do so, whether from inattention, malevolence, fears of addiction, or divergent priorities in resources.

In all these cases, of course, the patient can be sedated into unconsciousness; this does indeed end the pain. But in respect of the patient's experience, this is tantamount to causing death: the patient has no further conscious experience and thus can achieve no goods, experience no significant communication, satisfy no goals. Furthermore, adequate sedation, by depressing respiratory function, may hasten death. Thus, although it is always technically possible to achieve relief from pain, at least when the appropriate resources are available, the price may be functionally and practically equivalent, at least from the patient's point of view, to death. And this, of course, is just what the issue of euthanasia is about.

Of course, to see what the issue is about is not yet to reach its resolution, or to explain why attitudes about this issue are so starkly divergent. Rather, we must examine the logic of the argument for euthanasia and observe in particular how the principle of mercy functions in the overall case. The canon "One ought to act to end suffering," the second of the abstract duties generated by the principle of mercy, can be traced to the more general principle of beneficence. But its application in a given case also involves a minor premise that is ostensive in character: it points to an alleged case of suffering. This person is suffering, the applied argument from mercy holds, in a way that lays claim on us for help in relieving that pain.

It may be difficult to appreciate the force of this argument if its character is not adequately recognized. By asserting the abstract duty of mercy and pointing to specific occasions of pain, the argument generates the conclusion that we ought not let these cases of pain occur: not only ought we to prevent them from occurring if we can, but also we ought to bring them to an end if they do. In practice, most arguments for euthanasia on grounds of mercy are pursued by the graphic evocation of cases: the tortures suffered by victims of awful diseases.

But this argument strategy is problematic. The evocation of cases may be very powerful, but it is also subject to a certain unreliability. After all, pain is, in general, not well remembered by those not currently suffering it, and though bystanders may be capable of very great sympathy, no person can actually feel another's pain. Suffering that does not involve pain may be even harder for the bystander to assess. Conversely, however, bystanders sometimes seem to suffer more than the patient: pain, particularly in those for whom one has strong emotional attachments, is notoriously difficult to watch. Furthermore, sensitivity on the part of others to pain and suffering is very much subject to individual differences in experience with pain, beliefs concerning the purpose of suffering and pain, fears about pain, and physical sensitivity to painful stimuli. Yet there is no objective way to establish how seriously the ostensive premise of the argument from mercy should be taken in any specific case, or how one should respond. Clearly, such a premise can be taken too seriously—so that concern for another's pain or suffering outweighs all other considerations—or one can be far too cavalier about the facts. To break a promise to a patient—say, not to intubate him—because you perceive that he is in pain may be to overreact to his suffering. However, it is morally repugnant to stand by and watch another person suffer when one could prevent it; it is a moral failing, too, to be insensitive, when there is no overriding reason for doing so, to the fact that another person is in pain.

The principle of mercy holds that suffering ought to be relieved—unless, among other provisos, the suffering itself will give rise to some overriding benefit or unless the attainment of some benefit would be precluded by relieving the pain. But it might be argued that life itself is a benefit, always an overriding one. Certainly life is usually a benefit, one that we prize. But unless we accept certain metaphysical assumptions, such as "life is a gift from God," we must recognize that life is a benefit because of the experiences and interests associated with it. For the most part, we prize these, but when they are unrelievedly negative, life is not a benefit after all. Philippa Foot treats this as a conceptual point: "Ordinary human lives, even very hard lives, contain a minimum of basic goods, but when these are absent the idea of life is no longer linked to that of good."[12] Such basic goods, she explains, include not being forced to work far beyond one's capacity; having the support of a family or community, being able to more or less satisfy one's hunger, having hopes for the future; and being able to lie down to rest at night. When these goods are missing, she asserts, the connection between *life* and *good* is broken, and we cannot count it as a benefit to the person whose life it is that his or her life is preserved.

These basic goods may all be severely compromised or entirely absent in the severely ill or dying patient. He or she may be isolated from family or community, perhaps by virtue of institutionalization or for various other reasons; he or she may be unable to eat, to have hopes for the future, or even to sleep undisturbed at night. Yet even for someone lacking all of what Foot considers to be basic goods, the experiences associated with life may not be unrelievedly negative. We must be very cautious in asserting of someone, even someone in the most abysmal-seeming conditions of the severely ill or dying, that life is no longer a benefit, since the way in which particular experiences, interests, and "basic goods" are valued may vary widely from one person to the next. Whether a given set of experiences constitutes a life that is a benefit to the person whose life it is, is not a matter for *objective* determination, though there may be very good external clues to the way in which that person is in fact valuing them; it is, in the end, very much a function of subjective preference and choice. For some persons, life may be of value even in the grimmest conditions, for others, not. The crucial point is this: when a suffering person is conscious enough to have any experience at all, whether that experience counts as a benefit overriding the suffering or not is relative to that person and can be decided ultimately only by him or her.[13]

If this is so, then we can no longer assume that the cases in which euthanasia is indicated on grounds of mercy are infrequent or rare. It is true that contemporary pain-management techniques do make possible the control of pain to a considerable degree. But unless pain and discomforting symptoms are eliminated altogether without loss of function, the underlying problem for the principle of mercy remains: how does *this* patient value life, how does he or she weigh death against pain? We are accustomed to assume that only patients suffering extreme, irremediable pain could be candidates for euthanasia at all and do not consider whether some patients might choose death in preference to comparatively moderate chronic pain, even when the condition is not a terminal one. Of course, a patient's perceptions of pain are extremely subject to stress, anxiety, fear, exhaustion, and other factors, but even though these perceptions may vary, the underlying weighing still demands respect. This is not just a matter of differing sensitivities to pain, but of differing values as well: for some patients, severe pain may be accepted with resignation or even pious joy, whereas for others mild or moderate discomfort is simply not worth enduring. Yet, without appeal to religious beliefs about the spiritual value of suffering, we have no objective way to determine how much pain a person *ought* to stand. Consequently, we cannot assume that euthanasia is justified, if at all, in only the most severe cases. Thus, the issue of euthanasia looms larger, rather than smaller, in the contemporary medical world.

That we cannot objectively determine whether life is a benefit to a person or whether pain outweighs its value might seem to undermine all possibility of appeal to the principle of mercy. But I think it does not. Rather, it shows simply that the issue is more complex, and that we must recognize that the principle of mercy itself demands recognition of a second fundamental principle relevant in euthanasia cases: the principle of autonomy. If the sufferer is the best judge of the relative values of that suffering and other benefits to him- or herself, then his or her own choices in the matter of mercy ought to be respected. To impose "mercy" on someone who insists that despite his or her suffering life is still valuable to him or her would hardly be mercy; to withhold mercy from someone who pleads for it, on the basis that his or her life could still be worthwhile for him or her, is insensitive and cruel. Thus, the principle of mercy is conceptually tied to that of autonomy, at least insofar as what guarantees the best application of the principle—and hence, what guarantees the proper response to the ostensive premise in the argument from mercy—is respect for the patient's own wishes concerning the relief of his or her suffering or pain.

To this issue we now turn.

The Case for Euthanasia, Part II: Autonomy

The second principle supporting euthanasia is that of (patient) autonomy: one ought to respect a competent person's choices, where one can do so without undue costs to oneself, where doing so will not violate other moral obligations, and where these choices do not threaten harm to other persons or parties. This principle of autonomy, though limited by these provisos, grounds a person's right to have his or her own choices respected in determining the course of medical treatment, including those relevant to euthanasia: whether the patient wishes treatment that will extend life, though perhaps also suffering, or whether he or she wants the suffering relieved, either by being killed or by being allowed to die. It would of course also require respect for the choices of the person whose condition is chronic but not terminal, the person who is disabled though not dying, and the person not yet suffering at all, but facing senility or old age. Indeed, the principle of autonomy would require respect for self-determination in the matter of life and death in any condition at all, provided that the choice is freely and rationally made and does not harm others or violate other moral rules. Thus, the principle of autonomy would protect a much wider range of life-and-death acts than those we call euthanasia, as well as those performed for reasons of mercy.

Support for patient autonomy in matters of life and death is partially reflected in U.S. law, in which a patient's right to passive voluntary euthanasia (though it is not called by this name) is established in a long series of cases. In 1914, in the case of *Schloendorff v. New York Hospital*,[14] Justice Cardozo asserted that "every human being of adult years and sound mind has a right to determine what shall be done with his own body" and held that the plaintiff, who had been treated against his will, had the right to refuse treatment; more recent cases, including *Yetter*,[15] *Perlmutter*,[16] and *Bartling*,[17] establish that the competent adult has the right to refuse medical treatment, on religious or personal grounds, even if it means he or she will die. (Exceptions include some persons with dependents and persons who suffer from communicable diseases that pose a risk to the public at large.) Furthermore, the patient has the right to refuse a component of a course of treatment, even though he or she consents to others; this is established in the Jehovah's Witnesses cases in which patients refused blood transfusions but accepted surgery and other care. In many states, the law also recognizes passive voluntary euthanasia of the no longer competent adult who has signed a refusal-of-treatment document while still competent; such documents, called "natural death directives" or living wills, protect the physician from legal action for failure to treat if he or she follows the patient's antecedent request to be allowed to die. Additionally, the durable power of attorney permits a person to designate a relative, friend, or other person to make treatment decisions on his or her behalf after he or she is no longer competent; these may include decisions to refuse life-sustaining treatment. Many hospitals have adopted policies permitting the writing of orders not to resuscitate, or "no-code" orders, which stipulate that no attempt is to be made to revive a patient following a cardiorespiratory arrest. These policies typically are stated to require that such orders be issued only with the concurrence of the patient, if competent, or the patient's family or legal guardian. In theory, at least, living wills, no-code orders, durable powers of attorney, and similar devices are designed to protect the patient's voluntary choice to refuse life-prolonging treatment.

These legal mechanisms for refusal of treatment all protect individual autonomy in matters of euthanasia: the right to choose to live or to die. But it is crucial to see that they all protect only passive euthanasia, not any more active form. The Natural Death Act of California, like similar legislation in other states, expressly states that "nothing in this [Act] shall be construed to condone, authorize, or approve mercy killing."[18] Likewise, the living will directs only the withholding or cessation of treatment, in the absence of which the patient will die.[19] A durable power of attorney permits the same choices on behalf of the patient by a designated second party. These legal mechanisms are sometimes said to protect the "right to die," but it is important to see that this is only the right to be *allowed* to die, not to be helped to die or to have death actively brought about. However, we have already seen that allowing to die is sometimes less merciful than direct, humane killing: the principle of mercy demands the right to be killed, as well as to be allowed to die. Thus, the protections offered by the legal mechanisms now available may be seen as truncated conclusions from the principle of patient autonomy that supports them;

this principle should protect not only the patient's choice of refusal of treatment but also a choice of a more active means of death.

It is often objected that autonomy in euthanasia choices should not be recognized in practice, whether or not it is accepted in principle, because such choices are often erroneously made. One version of this argument points to physician error. Physicians make mistakes, it holds, and since medicine in any case is not a rigorous science, predictions of oncoming, painful death with no possibility of cure are never wholly reliable. People diagnosed as dying rapidly of inexorable cancers have survived, cancer-free, for dozens of years; people in cardiac failure or long-term irreversible coma have revived and regained full health. Although some of this can be attributed simply to physician error, we must also guard against the more pernicious phenomenon of the "hanging of crepe," in which the physician (usually not intentionally) delivers a prognosis dimmer than is actually warranted by the facts. If the patient succumbs, the physician cannot be blamed, since that is what was predicted; but if the patient survives, the physician is credited with the cure.[20] Other factors interfering with the accuracy of a diagnosis or prognosis include impatience on the part of a physician with a patient who is not doing well, difficulties in accurately estimating future complications, ignorance of a treatment or cure that is about to be discovered or is on the way, and a host of additional factors arising when the physician is emotionally involved, inexperienced, uninformed, or incompetent.[21]

A second argument pointing to the possibility of erroneous choice on the part of the patient asserts the very great likelihood of impairment of the patient's mental processes when seriously ill. Impairing factors include depression, anxiety, pain, fear, intimidation by authoritarian physicians or institutions, and drugs used in medical treatment that affect mental status. Perhaps a person in good health would be capable of calm, objective judgments even in such serious matters as euthanasia, so this view holds, but the person as patient is not. Depression, extremely common in terminal illness, is a particular culprit: it tends to narrow one's view of the possibilities still open; it may make recovery look impossible, it may screen off the possibilities, even without recovery, of significant human relationships and important human experience in the time that is left.[22] A choice of euthanasia in terminal illness, this view holds, probably reflects largely the gloominess of the depression, not the gravity of the underlying disease or any genuine intention to die.

If this is so, ought not the euthanasia request of a patient be ignored for his or her own sake? According to a limited paternalist view (sometimes called "soft" or "weak" paternalism), intervention in a person's choices for his or her own sake is justified if the person's thinking is impaired. Under this principle, not every euthanasia request should be honored; such requests should be construed, rather, as pleas for more sensitive physical and emotional care.

It is no doubt true that many requests to die are pleas for better care or improved conditions of life. But this still does not establish that all euthanasia requests should be ignored, because the principle of paternalism licenses intervention in a person's choices just *for his or her own good*. Sometimes the choice of euthanasia, though made in an impaired, irrational way, may seem to serve the person's own good better than remaining alive. Thus, since the paternalist, in intervening, must act for the sake of the person in whose liberty he or she interferes, the paternalist must take into account not only the costs for the person of failing to interfere with a euthanasia decision when euthanasia was not warranted (the cost is death, when death was not in this person's interests) but also the costs for that person of interfering in a decision that was warranted (the cost is continuing life—and continuing suffering—when death would have been the better choice).[23] The likelihood of these two undesirable outcomes must then be weighed. To claim that "there's always hope" or to insist that "the diagnosis could be wrong" in a morally responsible way, one must weigh not only the cost of unnecessary death to the patient but also the costs to the patient of dying in agony if the diagnosis is right and the cure does not materialize. But cases in which the diagnosis is right and the cure does not materialize are, unfortunately, much more frequent than cases in which the cure arrives or the diagnosis is wrong. The "there's always hope" argument, used to dissuade a person from choosing euthanasia, is morally irresponsible unless there is some quite good reason to

think there actually *is* hope. Of course, the "diagnosis could be wrong" argument against euthanasia is a good one in areas or specialities in which diagnoses are frequently inaccurate (the chief of one neurology service admitted that on initial diagnoses "we get it right about 50 percent of the time"), or where there is a systematic bias in favor of unduly grim prognoses—but it is not a good argument against euthanasia in general. Similarly, "a miracle cure may be developed tomorrow" is also almost always irresponsible. The paternalist who attempts to interfere with a patient's choice of euthanasia must weigh the enormous suffering of those to whom unrealistic hopes are held out against the benefits to those very few whose lives are saved in this way.

As with limited paternalism, extended "strong" or "hard" paternalism—permitting intervention not merely to counteract impairment but also to avoid great harm—provides a special case when applied to euthanasia situations. The hard paternalist may be tempted to argue that because death is the greatest of harms, euthanasia choices must always be thwarted. But the initial premise of this argument is precisely what is at issue in the euthanasia dispute itself, as we've seen: is death the worst of harms that can befall a person, or is unrelieved, hopeless suffering a still worse harm? The principle of mercy obliges us to relive suffering when it does not serve some overriding good; but the principle itself cannot tell us whether sheer existence—life—is an overriding good. In the absence of an objectively valid answer, we must appeal to the individual's own preferences and values. Which is the greater evil—death or pain? Some persons may adopt religious answers to this question, others may devise their own; but the answer always is tied to the person whose life it is, and cannot be supplied in any objective way. Hence, unless he or she can discover what the suffering person's preferences and values are, the hard paternalist cannot determine whether intervening to prolong life or to terminate it will count as acting for that person's sake.

Of course, there are limits to such a claim. When there is no evidence of suffering or pain, mental or physical, and no evidence of factors like depression, psychoactive drugs, or affect-altering disease that might impair cognitive functioning, an external observer usually can accurately determine whether life is a benefit: unless the person has an overriding commitment to a principle or cause that requires sacrifice of that life, life *is* a benefit to him or her. (But such a person, of course, is probably not a patient.) Conversely, when there is every evidence of pain and little or no evidence of factors that might outweigh the pain, such as cognitive capacities that might give rise to other valuable experience, then an external observer generally can also accurately determine the value of this person's life: it is a disbenefit, a burden, to him or her. (Given pain and complete cognitive incapacity, such a person is almost always a patient.) It is when both pain and cognitive capacities are found that the person-relative character of the value of life becomes most apparent, and most demanding of respect.

Thus, if we view the spectrum of persons from fully healthy through severely ill to decerebrate or brain dead, we may assert that the principle of autonomy operates most strongly at the middle of this range. The more severe a person's pain and suffering, when his or her condition is not so diminished as to preclude cognitive capacities altogether, the stronger the respect we must accord his or her own view of whether life is a benefit or not. At both ends of the scale, however, paternalistic considerations come into play: if the person is healthy and without pain, we will interfere to keep him or her alive (preventing, for instance, suicide attempts); if his or her life means *only* pain, we act for the person's sake by causing him or her to die (as we should for certain severely defective neonates who cannot survive, but are in continuous pain). But when the patient retains cognitive capacities, the greater is his or her suffering, and the more his or her choices concerning it deserve our respect. When the choice that is faced is death or pain, it is the patient who must choose which is worse.

We saw earlier that in euthanasia issues the principle of mercy is conceptually tied to the principle of autonomy, at least for its exercise; we now see that the principle of autonomy is dependent on the principle of mercy in certain sorts of cases. It is *not* dependent in this way, however, in those cases most likely to generate euthanasia requests. That someone voluntarily and knowingly requests release from

what he or she experiences as misery is sufficient, other things being equal, for the request to be honored; although this request is rooted in the patient's desire for mercy, we cannot insist on independent, objective evidence that mercy would in fact be served, or that death is better than pain. We can demand such evidence to protect a perfectly healthy person, and we can summon it to end the sufferings of someone who can no longer choose; but we cannot demand it or use it for the seriously ill person in pain. To claim that an incessantly pain-racked but conscious person cannot make a rational choice in matters of life and death is to misconstrue the point: he or she, better than anyone else, can make such a choice, based on intimate acquaintance with pain and his or her own beliefs and fears about death. If the patient wishes to live, despite such suffering, he or she must be allowed to do so; or the patient must be granted help if he or she wishes to die.

But this introduces a further problem. The principle of autonomy, when there are no countervailing considerations on paternalistic grounds or on grounds of harm to others, supports the practice of voluntary euthanasia and, in fact, any form of rational, voluntary suicide. We already recognize a patient's right to refuse any or all medical treatment and hence correlative duties of noninterference on the part of the physician to refrain from treating the patient against his or her will. But does the patient's right of self-determination also give rise to any positive obligation on the part of the physician or other bystander to actively produce death? Pope John Paul II asserts that "no one may ask to be killed";[24] Peter Williams argues that a person does not have a right to be killed even though to kill him might be humane.[25] But I think that both the Pope and Williams are wrong. Although we usually recognize only that the principle of autonomy generates rights to noninterference, in some circumstances a right of self-determination does generate claims to assistance or to the provision of goods.

We typically acknowledge this in cases of handicap or disability. For instance, the right of a person to seek an education ordinarily generates on the part of others only an obligation not to interfere with his or her attendance at the university, provided the person meets its standards; but the same right on the part of a person with a severe physical handicap may generate an obligation on the part of others to provide transportation, assist in acquiring textbooks, or provide interpretive services. The infant, incapable of earning or acquiring its own nourishment, has a right to be fed. There is a good deal of philosophic dispute about such claims, and public policies vary from one administration and court to the next. But if, in a situation of handicap or disability, a right to self-determination can generate claim rights (rights to be aided) as well as noninterference rights, the consequences for euthanasia practices are far-reaching indeed. Some singularly sympathetic cases—like that of Elizabeth Bouvier, who is almost completely paralyzed by cerebral palsy—have brought this issue to public attention. But notice that in euthanasia situations, *most* persons are handicapped with respect to producing for themselves an easy, "good," merciful death. The handicaps are occasionally physical, but most often involve lack of knowledge of how to bring this about and lack of access to means for so doing. If a patient chooses to refuse treatment and so die, he or she still may not know what components of the treatment to refuse in order to produce an easy rather than painful death; if the person chooses death by active means, he or she may not know what drugs or other methods would be appropriate, in what dosages, and in any case he or she may be unable to obtain them. Yet full autonomy is not achieved until one can both choose and act upon one's choices. It is here, in these cases of "handicap" that afflict many or most patients, that rights to self-determination may generate obligations on the part of physicians (provided, perhaps, that they do not have principled objections to participation in such activities themselves[26]). The physician's obligation is not only to respect the patient's choices but also to make it possible for the patient to act upon those choices. This means supplying the knowledge and equipment to enable the person to stay alive, if he or she so chooses; this is an obligation physicians now recognize. But it may also mean providing the knowledge, equipment, and help to enable the patient to die, if that is his or her choice; this is the other part of the physician's obligation, not yet recognized by the medical profession or the law in the United States.[27]

This is not to say that any doctor should be forced to kill any person who asks that: other contravening considerations—particularly that of ascertaining that the request is autonomous and not the product of coerced or irrational choice, and that of controlling abuses by unscrupulous physicians, relatives, or patients—would quickly override. Nor would the physician have an obligation to assist in "euthanasia" for someone not severely ill. But when the physician is sufficiently familiar with the patient to know the seriousness of the condition and the earnestness of the patient's request, when the patient is sufficiently helpless, and when there are no adequate objections on grounds of personal scruples or social welfare, then the principle of autonomy—like the principle of mercy—imposes on the physician the obligation to help the patient in achieving an easy, painless death.

The Case for Euthanasia, Part III: Justice

Although the term euthanasia originates from Greek roots meaning "good death," especially the avoidance of suffering, in recent years use of the term has been extended to cover cases in which the patient is neither suffering nor capable of choosing to die. Ruth Russell, for instance, includes among cases of euthanasia the ending of "a meaningless existence."[28] For Tom Beauchamp and Arnold Davidson, euthanasia can be the termination of an irreversibly comatose state.[29] Termination of the lives of the brain dead, the permanently comatose, and those who are, as Paul Ramsey puts it, "irretrievably inaccessible to human care"[30] is justified, it is argued, under the principle of justice: euthanasia permits fairer distribution of medical resources in a society that lacks sufficient resources to provide maximum care for all. Once this principle is invoked, however, it may seem that it also applies in cases in which the patient is still competent: to permit earlier, easier dying will be favored not only on grounds of mercy and autonomy but on grounds of justice as well.

Drawing on the principle of mercy advanced earlier, we may assert that each person, by virtue of his or her medical illness, injury, disability, or other medical abnormality that causes pain or suffering, has a claim on whatever medical resources might be effective in the full treatment of his or her condition:

because we have an obligation (subject to the provisos mentioned previously) to relieve the person's suffering, he or she has a correlative claim (subject to corresponding provisos) to whatever medical treatment can be used. But since there are not enough resources to supply full treatment for every condition for every person, and since the resources typically cannot be subdivided in a way that makes equal apportionment of them possible (half an operation will do you no good), full treatment can be devoted only to some conditions, or only to some persons. In a scarcity situation, not all competing claims can be satisfied, and a principle of distributive justice must be invoked to adjudicate among them.

Various principles can be proposed for allocating medical resources: to those in greatest medical need, to those for whom restoration of function would be most complete; to those who can pay; to those whose societal contributions are or have been greatest; to those who have been most deprived of medical care in the past; to those whose conditions are not self-induced (this might rule out people suffering from smokers' diseases, conditions exacerbated by obesity, suicide attempts, and perhaps venereal diseases and high-risk sports injuries); or to those who are the winners in a coin toss, lottery, or other system of random selection. Alternatively, treatment could be allocated on the basis of the medical condition involved; to end-stage kidney patients, for instance, but not to those with deteriorative heart disease. But, unless we expand the size of the resources pool, treatment will still be denied to some, *whatever* distributive principle is adopted. Hence, whatever the principle (except perhaps one that allocates all available resources simply to staving off death for the last few minutes in every medical condition), some of those denied treatment will die sooner than otherwise would be the case. But this, it can be argued, would be unjust, since it would impose earlier death on some persons on the basis of characteristics that are not legitimate grounds for death—ability to pay, and so on. Rather, it is often argued, if treatment is to be denied to some people with the result that they will die, it is better to deny it just to those people who are (loosely speaking) medically unsalvageable and will die soon anyway: the terminally ill, the extremely aged, and the seriously defective neonate. The practices of

euthanasia in accord with this principle—which can be called the salvageability principle—are justified, this argument then concludes, by the demands of justice in a scarcity situation.

Of course, to deny treatment to a dying patient on grounds of justice cannot properly be called euthanasia in the traditional sense, since it is not done for the sake of the patient or to provide a "good death." A congressional decision not to fund artificial heart research or not to provide Medicaid/Medicare payments for heart transplants can hardly be called euthanasia for those heart patients who will die. However, as we saw at the outset of this section, policies involving withholding treatment are frequently called euthanasia when practiced on the permanently comatose, the brain dead, the profoundly retarded, or others in nonsapient states. Despite the abuse of the term under the Nazi regime, our linguistic usage is again undergoing rapid change, and it is apparent that we are coming to use the term euthanasia not just for pain-sparing deaths but for resource-conserving deaths as well. It is in this newer sense that we can consider whether justice requires the practice of euthanasia in certain kinds of scarcity situations.

The argument from justice, though not always put forward in a coherent, comprehensive way, is often initiated with a recitation of facts. The hospital bill [in 1985] for a 500 gram newborn with serious deficits, it is said, may run somewhere between $60,000 and $80,000, or even more than $100,000; this does not by any means guarantee that the infant will survive or live a normal life. The cost of a coronary bypass, a procedure frequently employed even when it does not extend life expectancy (though it greatly increases the quality of life) is somewhere around $30,000. The bill for a series of bone marrow transplants may run to $80,000, even though the transplants may not succeed in staving off death. According to a study published late in 1981, the average intensive care unit bill (total hospital charges, plus ancillary charges) was $7,112—for patients who survived.[31] But for patients who died, the bill was more than double, a staggering $15,874. A vast proportion of medical costs are incurred during the final year of life (this includes unsalvageable neonates as well as adults), most of it in the last few weeks or days. Justice, under the distributive principle articulated previously, demands that the dying be allowed to die, and these resources be given instead to other, salvageable competitors for full health care.

This is not to suggest that the dying should be denied palliative and comfort care: indeed, if their claims to therapeutic treatment diminish, the principle of mercy demands that their claims to palliative care increase. Nor is it to suggest that the dying "do not deserve" medical care that could prolong their lives. *All* parties in the distribution have prima facie claims to care, under the principle of justice, but the claims of the dying are weakest.

This argument from justice is usually employed only to justify the denial of treatment, that is, to justify passive euthanasia, but similar considerations also favor active euthanasia. Passive euthanasia is often practiced upon unsalvageable patients by withholding treatment if a medical crisis occurs: for instance, no-code orders are issued, or pneumonias are not treated, or electrolyte imbalances not corrected if they occur. If justice demands that, despite the prima facie claims of these patients, the resources allocated to their care are better assigned somewhere else, then we must notice that *passive* euthanasia does not provide the most just redistribution of these resources. To "allow" the patient to die may still involve enormous expenditures of money, scarce supplies, or caregiver time. This is most evident in cases of "irretrievably inaccessible" patients, for whom no considerations of mercy or autonomy override the demands of justice in weighing claims. The cost [in 1985] of maintaining a coma patient in a nursing home without heroic treatment is somewhere around $15,000 a year; the cost for a profoundly retarded resident of a state institution is more than $20,000. Whole-brain dead patients may survive on life supports in hospital settings from several hours to a few days or more; upper-brain dead patients may live for years. The total cost of maintaining a permanently comatose woman, who was injured in a riding accident in 1956 at age twenty-seven and died eighteen years later, has been estimated at just over $6,000,000; this care provided her with not a single moment of conscious life.[32] The record survival for a coma patient is 37 years and 111 days.[33] The argument from justice demands that

these patients, since their claims for care are so weak as to have virtually no force at all, be killed, not simply allowed to die.

Objection to the Argument from Justice: The Slippery Slope

But if justice, under the salvageability principle considered here, licenses the killing of permanently comatose patients, will it not also license the killing of still-conscious, still-competent dying patients, perhaps still salvageable, close or not so close to death? What extensions of the scope of this principle might be made, should resources become still more scarce? These concerns introduce the "wedge" or "slippery slope" argument, which holds that although some acts of euthanasia may be morally permissible (say, on grounds of mercy or autonomy), to allow them to occur will set a logical precedent for, or will causally result in, consequences that are morally repugnant.[34] Just as Hitler's 1938 "euthanasia" program for mentally defective, senile, and terminally ill Aryans paved the way for the establishment of the extermination camps several years later, it is argued, so permissive euthanasia policies invite irreversible descent down that slippery slope that leads to mass murder. Indeed, to permit even the most humane euthanasia may do more than set a precedent: by accustoming doctors to ending life, by supplying death technology, by changing the expectations of family members or other guardians of those who become candidates for death, and by changing the expectations of patients themselves, the practice of euthanasia even in humane cases may lead to moral holocaust.

As it is usually posed, the form of the argument that points to the Nazi experience does not succeed: the forces that brought the mass extermination camps into being were not *caused* by the earlier euthanasia program, and, other things being equal, the extermination camps for Jews would no doubt have been established had there been no euthanasia program at all. To argue that permitting euthanasia now will lead to death camps like Hitler's is to overlook the many other political, social, and psychological factors of the Nazi period. Yet the wedge argument cannot be simply discarded; the factors operating to favor the slide from morally warranted euthanasia to murder are probably much stronger than we realize. They are best seen, I think, as misunderstandings or corruptions of the very principles that favor euthanasia: mercy, autonomy, and perhaps most prominently, justice.

A contemporary version of the wedge argument holds that to permit euthanasia at all—including cases justified on grounds of mercy, autonomy, or justice—will in the presence of strong financial incentives lead to circumstances in which people are killed who are not suffering or who do not wish to die. Furthermore, to permit some doctors to allow their patients to die or to kill them would invite cavalier attitudes concerning the lives of the patients and, in addition to financial incentives, ordinary greed, insensitivity, hastiness, and self-interest, would cause some doctors to let their patients die—or kill them—when there was no moral warrant for doing so.[35] Doctors treating difficult or unresponding patients would find an easy way out. Medical blunders could be more easily covered up, and doctors might use euthanasia as a way of avoiding criticism in cases that were medically difficult to treat. Particularly important, perhaps, are societal and political pressures, most evident in cost-containment policies, to which doctors might respond. After all, to permit earlier, less expensive death would ease the enormous pressure on third-party insurers, hospitals, and the Medicaid/Medicare system: euthanasia is less expensive than continuing medical care. The diagnosis-related group reimbursement system would particularly favor this since a hospital profits most from the patient who remains hospitalized for the shortest amount of time, but loses money on the one who remains longer than what is average for the DRG. Although passive euthanasia is cheaper than continuing life-prolonging treatment, active euthanasia is cheaper still: killing is the least expensive, most resource-conserving treatment of intractable disease.

Is there any reason to think such practices would actually occur? The reasons are closer to hand than one might imagine. Rather than predicting the future, we need simply look to our present practices for evidence that violations of the moral limits to euthanasia can occur. It is tempting to reply to a wedge argument against any social practice that we will always be able to draw a moral line when the time comes, but the clear evidence in the case of euthanasia is that we are not managing to do so now.

First, contemporary euthanasia practices sometimes involve violations of the principle of mercy. These violations are of two forms, neither conspicuous because neither involves evident physical cruelty. Nevertheless, both are cases of euthanasia that the principle of mercy does not endorse. First, there are cases in which the rhetoric of euthanasia, with its concept of painless, easy death, is used though considerations of mercy cannot possibly apply: these are the cases of the permanently comatose or brain dead. Since these persons do not suffer, euthanasia as the granting of mercy cannot be practiced upon them, and we mislead ourselves if we claim that they are "better off" dead. Second, there are cases in which the principle of mercy is violated when more than enough relief is given to those who do suffer. The principle of mercy demands euthanasia *only* when no other means of relieving pain will suffice. Yet we fail to acknowledge that the continuous, very heavy use of narcotizing drugs can be functionally equivalent to mercy killing itself: when used in a sustained way, without drug-free, conscious intervals or careful titration against alertness, such therapy effectively ends the patient's sentient life: his or her existence as a person ends when the drugging begins.[36] Of course, it may sometimes be difficult to obtain adequate and effective narcotics; nevertheless, because we do not recognize such drugging as equivalent in some respects to *active* euthanasia, we may be incautious and hasty in its use.

Contemporary euthanasia practices sometimes also involve violations of the principle of autonomy. It is true that much euthanasia, both passive and active, occurs at the request or with the consent of the individual who dies; passive euthanasia practices are provided for in natural death legislation and the use of durable powers of attorney and living wills. But we are also beginning to see the widespread development of hospital policies concerning nonresuscitation, and more frequent, routine physician exercise of this practice. It may even be fair to speak of a widespread consensus that in certain cases, nonresuscitation is the appropriate response. Official policies require that the patient—if competent—or his or her legal guardian be consulted before nonre-suscitation orders are written. But such directives are by no means always followed. In Salt Lake City recently (though the story is universal), a physician reminded the granddaughter of an alert, competent eighty-nine-year-old nursing home patient, "You can always have 'do not resuscitate' orders written into her record." ("Why don't you ask her if that's what she wants?" was the granddaughter's reply.) A cardi-ologist at a major university says, in contrast, that he would not make such a suggestion to the family—because he "wouldn't want to put them through that"; this physician writes no-code orders on his own, without consulting either patient or family. In some places, no-code orders are written in pencil, so that they can be erased from records if desired; or circumlocutions not intelligible to laypersons ("con-sult primary physician before initiating treatment") are used.

Most significant among our current euthanasia practices may be the violations of justice. The argu-ment from justice, as discussed so far, favors permit-ting euthanasia on the grounds that denial of treat-ment is morally permissible in certain specific cases: those in which the claims of a dying individual to medical resources are overridden by the claims of others in medical need. However, we often see the use of distributive policies that deny treatment to some but do not involve either the weighing of claims between the dying and others or the assurance that resources conserved would in fact be redistrib-uted in accord with justice. The congressional deci-sions concerning artificial and transplant heart care may be one kind of example; arbitrary age mini-mums and ceilings for transplants, pacemakers, and dialysis, when they are not medically appropriate, may be another. Yet distributive justice concerns the point at which a dying person's right to medical treatment is outweighed by the claims of others; and the salvageability principle considered here does not hold that dying deprives one altogether of rights to medical care. In a situation of dire scarcity, such as urgent organ transplants, denying a transplant to one person usually means granting a transplant to some-one else; if without it each person would die, the dis-tributive principle of salvageability considered here

holds that the person more likely to survive and ben-efit from the procedure has the stronger claim. But many distributive policies do not involve this kind of direct weighing of claims or assurances of realloca-tion, and much denial of treatment is done simply for thrift. *Thrift*, however, is not the same as *justice in distribution*. To deny treatment to the dying to "con-serve resources" to "save money" is not to show that the claims of the dying are overridden by stronger claims on the part of someone else, or a group of per-sons, to whom such resources would in fact be redis-tributed; yet it is this point that is essential in pre-serving the principle of justice as applied to euthanasia.

In all these areas, then, there is evidence of "euthanasia" practices not justified by moral princi-ple. Given these facts, the wedge argument and its objection to permitting euthanasia may loom larger. The wedge argument forecasts a slide down the slip-pery slope from morally permissible practices to impermissible ones; but even if we accept its model, there is no reason to assume that we are still at the top of this slope. Indeed, the evidence available sug-gests that we are already slipping. We already engage in "euthanasia" practices not justified on grounds of mercy, autonomy, or justice, and there is no reason to think that such abuses will not become still more widespread.

Nevertheless, I do not agree with the conclusion of the slippery slope argument: that because permis-sible euthanasia practices would lead (or are leading) to impermissible ones, we ought not allow them at all. We should not cease no-coding; mercy demands it. We should not restrict refusal of treatment or insist that all who can conceivably benefit be given as much treatment as possible; respect for autonomy requires that the patient be permitted to determine what is done to him or her. We should not resist leg-islative protections for passive euthanasia, like living wills and natural death laws, or oppose legislation permitting voluntary active euthanasia: justice, mercy, and autonomy all demand that euthanasia—both passive and active—be legally protected. Although the wedge argument is a serious one, pro-hibiting euthanasia is not the appropriate conclusion.

Most advocates of the wedge argument overlook a crucial feature of the structure of the argument itself.

The wedge argument is teleological in character: it points to the bad consequence of permitting a morally acceptable type of action (call it A), namely, that morally unacceptable type (B) occurs. But users of the wedge argument err in failing to recognize that B's occurrence is not the sole outcome of A; A and B are *distinct* actions, each with its own set of consequences. Thus, in deciding whether to permit A, one must reckon in the bad consequences of the occurrence of B, but must also reckon in the other, possibly good consequences of A. Or, if one is deciding to prohibit A, the reckoning will include the (good) effects of avoiding B, but must also include the other (bad) effects of not having A occur. The wedge argument against euthanasia usually takes the form of an appeal to the welfare or rights of those who would become victims of later, unjustified practices. Usually, however, when the conclusion is offered that euthanasia therefore ought not be permitted, no account is taken of the welfare or rights of those who are to be denied the benefits of this practice. Hence, even if the causal claims advanced in the wedge argument are true and we are not able to hold the line or avoid the slide, they still do not establish the conclusion. Rather, the argument sets up a conflict. Either we ignore the welfare and abridge the rights of persons for whom euthanasia would clearly be morally permissible in order to protect those who would be the victims of corrupt euthanasia practices, or we ignore the potential victims in order to extend mercy and respect for autonomy to those who are the current victims of euthanasia prohibitions.

Thus, this conflict itself reveals an issue of justice still more fundamental than the distributive problems with which I began. The wedge argument assumes, without adequate justification, that the rights of those who may become the victims of abuses of a practice outweigh the rights of those who become victims if a practice is prohibited to whose benefits they are morally entitled and urgently needed.

To protect those who might wrongly be killed or allowed to die might seem a stronger obligation than to satisfy the wishes of those who desire release from pain, analogous perhaps to the principle in law that "better ten guilty men go free than one be unjustly convicted."[37] However, the situation is not in fact analogous and does not favor protecting those who might wrongly be killed. To let ten guilty men go free in the interests of protecting one innocent man is not to impose harm on the ten guilty men. But to require the person who chooses to die to stay alive in order to protect those who might unwillingly be killed sometime in the future is to impose an extreme harm—intolerable suffering—on that person, which he or she must bear for the sake of others. Furthermore, since, as I have argued, the question of which is worse, suffering or death, is person-relative, we have no independent, objective basis for protecting the class of persons who might be killed at the expense of those who would suffer intolerable pain; perhaps our protecting ought to be done the other way around. Thus, I return to the recurrent problem throughout this discussion: which is the worse of two evils, death or pain? Since there are no prior agreements or claims that are relevant here, justice requires that rights to avoid the worse of the two evils be honored first, before others come into play. This, however, may be an obligation that, because it is person-relative and hence resistant to policy construction, we do not know how to meet.

Justice and Realistic Desire

Is there a workable solution to the problem that euthanasia poses? Certainly we can make some progress by attending to the violations of principle we have discovered. First, we must improve the conditions of dying; mercy will not demand euthanasia, nor will the autonomous person choose it, when the conditions of dying are humane. Cicely Saunders, the founder of St. Christopher's Hospice in England and an ardent opponent of euthanasia, is perfectly right when she says of euthanasia, "one should be working to see that it is not needed."[38] Second, we need to improve the quality of the mercy we extend by attending to the element of autonomy in it: we must learn to respond to suffering in a way that takes account of the patient's own wishes and tolerances for pain, so that we give neither too little relief nor too much. Third, we must broaden our respect of autonomy in matters of dying by recognizing that the patient may choose active as well as passive means of coming to die—or none at all. It is crucial that the dying person receive full information about the consequences of accepting treatment or refusing it, so that he or she can rationally choose the way of dying—or staying alive—most in accord with his or her own values.[39] After all, a "good death" must always be a death that counts as good *for the patient*. For some it is the least painful, for others it is the quickest, for others one that permits final communication with family, and for still others the one that can be delayed the longest possible time. In this most personal of matters, a person's choice deserves the greatest respect.

But attention to mercy and autonomy does not yet seem to solve the problem of justice: the problems of whose rights are to be honored, and who is to be denied care. I mentioned earlier that all the workable distributive principles we might adopt would have the effect of forcing death on some persons who do not want it—those who cannot pay, those who have made no societal contributions, etc. Even the most plausible of these principles—the salvageability principle—would force earlier death upon the already dying, some of whom may wish to die but some of whom, under their own conception of the relative disvalue of suffering and death, want to continue as long as they possibly can. Thus, I think that the salvageability principle too is in error. Rather, we should favor a distributive principle that would allocate medical resources to those who *want* treatment, where "wanting" is interpreted as "realistic desire." This is to say, realistic desire ought to be considered both a necessary and a sufficient condition for providing treatment for those who are seriously ill.

To desire medical treatment in a realistic, reasonable, or rational way, the patient must not only actually have or be about to contract the condition for which treatment is proposed but also must understand the treatment's intended purposes, its possible side effects, the probability of success or failure, and the possible end condition to which the treatment would lead. For, say, an appendectomy, the patient must not only have appendicitis but also must understand at least roughly the nature of the procedure, what could go wrong, the approximate likelihood of success, and the end condition: relief of the acute pain in the abdomen, avoidance of death, and a small scar on the side. In most cases of acute appendicitis, an appendectomy will be the object of realistic

desire. In a few cases, however, it is not, such as when the patient believes on religious grounds that the end condition of accepting medical treatment or a blood transfusion includes eventual damnation. Although religious cases are comparatively rare, there are many cases in which the principle of realistic desire would require substantial changes in our current distribution of medical care. Life-prolonging care given to the permanently comatose, decerebrate, profoundly brain damaged, and others who lack cognitive function is not, even in the case of antecedently executed directives, realistically desired, since such patients cannot want it, they are not entitled to life-prolonging care. Not even supportive care—such as feeding or routine hygiene—should be supplied, since this too cannot be realistically desired, patients in these extreme conditions should be allowed—or perhaps caused—to die.

Withholding care from permanently comatose patients may not seem morally problematic. But in a serious illness in which a cure cannot be guaranteed yet the patient remains competent, the problem becomes much more complex. Do patients with cancer of the larynx, for instance, *want* surgical treatment that, while providing a better-than-half chance of survival three years later, entails the permanent destruction of the normal voice? Most do, but, according to one study, at least 20 percent do not.[40] In such situations, the new distributive principle articulated here apportions treatment solely on the basis of a patient's desires, not on characteristics such as age or social worth. Most patients will receive appendectomies; four-fifths will have surgery on the larynx; permanently comatose patients will receive no care at all.

Would a distributive principle of realistic desire be effective in a scarcity situation? Although one's initial impression may be to the contrary, I believe that it would. It is crucial to remember that medical treatment is not like any ordinary consumer good; getting more of it does not entail that your advantages are increased. (Indeed, in an ideal lifetime, the amount of therapeutic medical treatment a person realistically wants is zero; this is the mark of the perfectly healthy life.) The treatments that are less likely to be realistically desired are, generally speaking, precisely those likely to occur at the end of life—the heroic, last-ditch, odds-against measures, undertaken because nothing else has worked. The chances are that the procedures will be painful, that they will introduce new limitations, and that they will not succeed. And the chance is also that these treatments will be extremely expensive. It is not possible to tell whether the savings in treatment costs under such a distributive policy would make it possible to provide full treatment for all who do want it, but there is no reason to *assume* that such savings would not: we need only recall the huge financial costs for nonsurvivors in an intensive care unit, for severely defective, unsalvageable neonates, or for permanently comatose patients in a nursing home or institution. A vast proportion of medical costs, as stated before, occurs in the last year of life. Most of this can be described as "needed" treatment. No doubt much of this is also "wanted" treatment, but much of it is not.

If use of the distributive principle of realistic desire should prove inadequate to solve the scarcity problem, then an additional distributive principle would need to be adopted to resolve conflicting claims among competitors who all realistically desire treatment: the salvageability principle, denying treatment to those who will die soon anyway, might then be brought into play. But those who will die soon may nevertheless want every moment of life they can possibly get, and it is unacceptable to adopt a distributive principle that has the effect of depriving some persons of wanted life before there is clear need to do so.

Of course, a distributive principle of realistic desire must have built into it paternalistic proxy procedures for providing medical care for incompetents of a variety of sorts, including infants and children, unconscious accident victims, the mentally ill, and the retarded. But I believe that these procedures should *not* include persons who are capable of realistic desire in the matter of terminal care but who have failed to consider and articulate their desires. Rather, it is becoming apparent that the individual has an obligation, increasingly evident as advances in medical technology both exacerbate the scarcity situation and offer heroic life-prolonging treatment that may not be desired, to stipulate in advance which modes of treatment he or she will accept and which he or she will decline, insofar as the patient's

probable future can be foreseen. Only about one death in ten is wholly unexpected, and most result from prolonged, chronic illnesses.[41] Thus, most deaths can be predicted, within a fairly limited range of possibilities, before the event, and the course of the dying in certain general ways anticipated. What, most basically, the patient is obliged to do is indicate, as fully as possible, which he or she takes to be worse in situations that can be foreseen: pain or death. From this basic choice the treatment alternatives appropriate to the patient's condition can be deduced. By failing to exercise this obligation, the individual may force others—his or her physician, family members, or the courts—to make what are often morally precarious euthanasia decisions for him or her, perhaps on the basis of self-interest, societal pressure, or distributive principles for which there is no moral warrant. Because the patient has rights to medical treatment that he or she realistically desires and because it is the corresponding obligation of others to distribute treatment in accord with these desires, it is in turn the obligation of the patient to make his or her desires known whenever it is possible to do so.

However, it is particularly important to notice that continuous sedation is *not* an option the patient may choose, nor is it a defensible general solution to the problem of euthanasia. The patient's autonomous requests must still conform to the demands of justice, particularly as specified for medical situations by the principle of realistic desire. It is true that continuous sedation may satisfy both the principles of mercy and autonomy, but because there is no ongoing experience or sentient end state to which the treatment leads, the patient cannot realistically desire the treatment that would maintain him or her. Of course, there may be many cases in which the patient's condition is potentially reversible or the sedation can be interrupted to permit further personal experience, and in these circumstances sedation may indeed be realistically preferred to either pain or death (given the difficulty of accurately predicting circumstances in which continuous sedation will be permanently required without any hope of intervening lucidity, such cases may be the rule rather than the exception); in these cases the patient retains his or her claim to care. There may also be certain special situations in which the needs of, say, family members or transplant recipients outweigh the claims of other patients competing for resources, so that justice will permit maintaining a patient in continuous sedation on the same basis as it might in rare cases permit maintaining a patient who is permanently comatose. But when such conditions do not obtain, even the patient who articulates his or her choices in advance is not entitled to request *permanent* sedation, since the principle of realistic desire prohibits him or her, like the proverbial dog in the manger, from laying claim to resources he or she cannot possibly enjoy. Nor may physicians turn to continuous sedation as a way of avoiding difficult moral dilemmas in terminal care (except, of course, in the frequent situations in which they think that their predictions may be wrong); they are bound to honor the choices of a patient made in accord with the principle of realistic desire, but this principle does not permit such a choice. At least in any scarcity situation, the patient must choose either death or periodically sentient life, though this may involve pain; he or she cannot morally choose to be maintained in a permanently sedated or unconscious state when that means depriving someone else of care.

Conclusion: Euthanasia and Suicide

It may be objected that requiring the patient to choose between death and life, insofar as the patient must antecedently consider treatment decisions that affect the circumstances and timing of his or her own demise, is equivalent to requiring the patient's consideration of suicide. In a sense, it is; but this is also the more general solution to the euthanasia problem. Although euthanasia is indeed warranted on grounds of mercy, autonomy, and justice, these principles can be more effectively and safely honored by permitting suicide, perhaps assisted by the physician who has care of the patient or a family member under the advice of the physicians,[42] and supplemented by nonvoluntary euthanasia *only* when the patient is permanently comatose or otherwise irretrievably inaccessible. Not only do practical reasons like avoiding greed and manipulation on the part of physicians or the institutions controlling them speak for preferring physician-assisted suicide

to physician-initiated euthanasia, but there are conceptual reasons as well. The conditions that distinguish morally permissible euthanasia from impermissible murder all involve matters that the patient, not the physician, is in a privileged position to know. To extend mercy, the physician must know how the patient weighs suffering against death, and at what point *for the patient* death becomes the lesser of two evils. To respect the patient's autonomy, the physician must know what his or her preferences are, given the alternatives available, in the matter of dying. And to exercise justice, the physician must know what treatment the patient realistically desires. Perhaps the physician who is painstakingly careful in listening to an articulate and self-aware patient may discover these things, but he or she cannot have the patient's knowledge. Consequently, since the risk of misinterpretation is great and the possibility of manipulation or coercion high, the physician should not be the one to *initiate* the choice. Rather, he or she must be prepared to assist the patient who chooses death, just as he or she is prepared to assist the patient who chooses continuing life. In physician-assisted suicide, it is the person whose death is in question who is responsible for the death; he or she originates and chooses this course of action, rather than having death chosen for him or her. Of course, to permit suicide in these situations may seem to increase the risk of encouraging ill-considered suicide among emotionally disturbed or mentally ill persons, but here the physician serves as a check: in the role of assistant to the suicide, the physician will refuse to assist whenever in his or her professional perception the circumstances clearly do not warrant such an act (such as in cases in which there is neither pain nor approaching death, but not in those exhibiting one or both). This is by no means a foolproof policy; the physician will no doubt often influence the patient. But this intrusion is still a far cry from having the physician decide when or why euthanasia is appropriate and initiate the act.

Furthermore, physician-assisted suicide is less subject to the erection of policy requirements than are euthanasia practices. The choices of patients about whether and how to die will vary widely; but then, there is no reason why they should not. These choices are influenced by an enormous range of individual values, past experiences, and moral and religious beliefs. Euthanasia policies developed by physicians or medical institutions may overlook individual differences in patients' wishes by establishing routine, common procedures for dealing with terminal illness, and in this way invite the continuing slide down the slippery slope. We must be prepared to permit and perform mercy killing when the patient desires it and when there is no other way to avoid the sufferings of death. But we do not want doctors to assume the responsibility for such killings, or to appeal to standardized, court-approved procedures, made under economic constraints, for determining when such killings are appropriate. Rather, mercy killing must ideally always be mercy killing of the patient by him- or herself, in which the patient is entitled to the assistance of the physician he or she has chosen. When proxy procedures are required, we must be sure that they approximate as nearly as possible what the person's own decision would have been. It is crucial to exercise mercy; it is essential to respect autonomy, and though we must submit to the demands of justice, we can hope to do so at no one's expense. It is extremely important to avoid any further slide down the involuntary thrift-euthanasia slope. Recognition of physician-aided suicide, as distinguished from physician-directed euthanasia, comes closest to satisfying all of these moral demands.

After all, we must not forget that we already practice euthanasia on quite a wide scale, but we do not always practice it in a morally defensible way. We practice passive euthanasia by withholding and withdrawing treatment, and we practice active quasi-euthanasia by using sedation sufficient to terminate the personal existence of a human being. Some of this is in accord with the principles of mercy, autonomy, and justice, but much of it is not. What grows dimmer in contemporary practice is the sense that euthanasia, as "good death," must be good *for the person whose death it is*; we are losing any sense that mercy must play a major role or that the patient's choice is crucial in determining whether that death counts as good. Already we are beginning to count resource-conserving deaths under this term. Paul Ramsey remarks that "it is better if you do not know

the Greek language or the root meaning of the word";[43]—but, of course, knowing these things permits us to see the shifts in our use of the term, shifts that are perhaps symptomatic of the slide already under way down the slippery slope. Our very language invites us to overlook distinctions that we ought to make. The concept of euthanasia has come to include letting patients die and killings that are not required by mercy, autonomy, or justice, but are simply the product of thrift in medical affairs. Yet at the same time our discomfort with this fact leads us to claim, at least officially, that we reject any practice of euthanasia at all, though of course this is not true. In this way, the increasing distortion of the term itself leads us to overlook a double moral fault: often, we practice "euthanasia" when we should not, and very often, we fail to practice euthanasia when we should.

Author's Note

I'd like to thank Arthur G. Lipmand, Pharm.D., and Howard Wilcox, M.D., as well as my colleagues in philosophy, Bruce Landesman and Leslie Francis, for comments on earlier drafts of this chapter.

Notes

1 Perhaps the principle of (medical) mercy is stronger than this and asserts a duty to relieve the suffering of others even at some substantial cost to oneself, or in violation of others of these provisos. The quite weak form of the principle, as I have stated it here, requires, for instance, that one ought not stand idly by (all other things being equal) when one could easily help an injured person but does not require feats of physical or financial heroism or self-sacrifice. This is not to say that I think a stronger version of the duty to relieve suffering (as defended, for instance, by Susan James, "The Duty to Relieve Suffering," *Ethics* [October 1982] 93:4-21), could not be supported, but that the stronger version is not necessary for the case I am making here: a prima facie duty to participate in both passive and active euthanasia, at least in a more permissive legal climate, is entailed even by the very weak form of the principle of mercy.

Incidentally, although much of the medical literature distinguishes between pain and suffering, I have not chosen to do so here: it would raise difficult mind/body problems, and in any case the two are clearly intertwined. I grant, however, that the principle of (medical) mercy would meet still broader assent if phrased to require the relieving of physical pain alone.

2   It is important not to confuse the principle of (medical) mercy with a principle permitting or requiring judicial mercy. In judicial and political contexts, such as pardons or amnesties, the individual on whom penalties have been or are about to be imposed may have no claim to benevolent treatment, and the issue concerns whether mercy may or should be granted. Many authors treat judicial mercy as a work of individual supererogation, not a requirement or duty, and some suggest that it is morally forbidden: one ought not excuse a person guilty of a crime. However, we are concerned here not with judicial mercy, but rather with mercy as it arises primarily in medical contexts: injuries, illnesses, disabilities, degenerative processes, and genetic defect or disease. Unlike pain or suffering inflicted in judicial contexts, in the medical context these are not warranted by the past actions of the suffering individual, but are usually of natural or accidental origin and in most cases are beyond the individual's control: pain and suffering are something that happen to him or her, not something the patient has earned. The principle of medical mercy is usually taken to apply even in cases in which a medical condition is caused or exacerbated by the individual's voluntary behavior, as in smokers' diseases or injuries from attempted suicide. It is consistent to hold that mercy is supererogatory (or perhaps morally forbidden) in judicial or political contexts, but also that it is required in medical ones.

3   Edmund D. Pellegrino, M.D., "The Clinical Ethics of Pain Management in the Terminally Ill," *Hospital Formulary* 17 (November 1982): 1495-96; and Marcia Angell, "The Quality of Mercy," *New England Journal of Medicine* 306 (January 1982): 98-99.

4   For instance, I take it to be a moral duty, and not merely a nice thing to do, to help a child remove a painful splinter from a finger when the child cannot do so alone and when this can be done without undue costs to oneself. (I assume that the splinter case satisfies the other provisos of the principle of medical

mercy.) Similarly, I take it to be a moral duty to stop the bleeding of a person who has been wounded or to pull someone from a fire, though in very many of the cases in which such circumstances arise (wars, accidents) this duty is abrogated because we cannot do so without risks to ourselves. The duty of medical mercy is not simply equivalent to either nonmaleficence or beneficence, though perhaps derived from them, since the former is understood as a duty to refrain from causing harm and the latter to do good in a positive sense; the duty of medical mercy requires one to counteract harms one did not cause, though it may not require conferring additional positive benefits.

5   See Sharon H. Imbus and Bruce E. Zawacki, "Autonomy for Burned Patients When Survival Is Unprecedented," *New England Journal of Medicine* 297 (August 11, 1977): 309-311.

6   See Mary Voboril, *Miami Herald*, Saturday, July 1, 1978, see also note 17.

7   An extensive discussion of the conceptual and moral distinctions between killing and letting die begins with Jonathan Bennett, "Whatever the Consequences," *Analysis* 26 (1966): 83-97, and, after the American Medical Association's stand prohibiting mercy killing but permitting cessation of treatment, continues in James Rachels's "Active and Passive Euthanasia," *New England Journal of Medicine* 292 (January 9, 1975): 78-80, and many subsequent papers.

8   See Ludwig Edelstein, "The Hippocratic Oath," in *Ancient Medicine: Selected Papers of Ludwig Edelstein*, ed. Owsei Temkin and C. Lilian Temkin (Baltimore: The Johns Hopkins University Press, 1967), esp. 9-15, on the Greek physician's role in euthanasia.

9   Hospice, founded and directed by Cicely Saunders, is a movement devoted to the development of institutions for providing palliative but medically nonaggressive care for terminal patients. In addition to its extraordinary contribution in developing methods of prophylactic pain control, according to which analgesics are administered on a scheduled basis in advance of experienced pain, Hospice has also emphasized attention to the emotional needs of the patient's family. An account of the theory and methodology of Hospice can be found in various publications by Saunders, including "Terminal Care in Medical Oncology," in *Medical Oncology*, ed. K.D. Bagshawe (Oxford: Blackwell, 1975), 563-576.

10 Joanne Lynn, M.D., "Supportive Care for Dying Patients: An Introduction for Health Care Professionals," Appendix B of the President's Commission for the Study of Ethical Problems in Medicine and Biomedical and Behavioral Research, *Deciding to Forego Life-Sustaining Treatment* (Washington, DC: Government Printing Office, 1983), 295.

11 . Robert G. Twycross, "Voluntary Euthanasia," in *Suicide and Euthanasia: The Rights of Personhood*, ed. Samuel E. Wallace and Albin Eser (Knoxville: The University of Tennessee Press, 1981), 89.

12 Phillippa Foot, "Euthanasia," *Philosophy & Public Affairs* 6 (Winter 1977): 95.

13 To discover what one's own views are, try the following thought experiment. Imagine that you have been captured by a gang of ruthless and superlatively clever criminals, whom you know with certainty will never be caught or change their minds. They plan either to execute you now, or to torture you unremittingly for the next twenty years and then put you to death. Which would be worse? Does your view change if the length of the torture period is reduced to twenty days or twenty minutes, and if so, why? How severe does the torture need to be?

14 211 N.Y. 127, 129; 105 N.E. 92, 93 (1914).

15 *In re Yetter*, 62 Pa. D. & C. 2d 619 (1973).

16 *Satz v. Perlmutter*, 362 S. 2d 160 (Fla. App. 1978), affirmed by Florida Supreme Court 379 So. 2d 359 (1980).

17 *Bartling v. Superior Court,* 2 Civ. No. B007907 (Calif. App. 1984).

18 California Health & Safety Code, Sections 7195-7196.

19 The living will and durable power of attorney forms valid in different states are distributed by Choice in Dying, 200 Varig Street, New York, NY 10014. Copies are also available from hospitals and attorneys.

20 M. Siegler, "Pascal's Wager and the Hanging of Crepe," *The New England Journal of Medicine* 293 (1975): 853-857.

21 See also a study of other factors associated with differences in prognosis and treatment decisions: R. Pearlman, T. Inui, and W. Carter, "Variability in Physician Bioethical Decision-Making," *Annals of Internal Medicine* 97 (September 1982): 420-425.

22 The effects of depression on the choice concerning whether to live or die are described by Richard B. Brandt, "The Morality and Rationality of Suicide," in *A Handbook for the Study of Suicide*, ed. Seymour Perlin (New York: Oxford University Press, 1975), 61-76, and reprinted in part in M. Pabst Battin and David J. Mayo, eds., *Suicide: The Philosophical Issues* (New York: St. Martin's Press, 1980), 117-132.

23 I've considered elsewhere the symmetrical argument that if death is in some circumstances actually better than life, the paternalist should be prepared to override a patient's choice of life. See M. Pabst Battin, *Ethical Issues in Suicide* (Englewood Cliffs, NJ: Prentice-Hall, 1982), 160-175.

24 Vatican Congregation for the Doctrine of the Faith, "Declaration on Euthanasia," June 26, 1980; see Section II, "Euthanasia."

25 Peter C. Williams, "Rights and the Alleged Right of Innocents to Be Killed," *Ethics* 87 (1976-77): 383-394.

26 This proviso may appear to resemble similar provisos exempting physicians, nurses, and other caregivers who have principled objections to participating in abortions. But I am much less certain that weight should be given to the scruples of physicians in euthanasia cases, at least at the time of need. As I will suggest in the final section of this chapter, the patient has an obligation to make his or her wishes concerning euthanasia known in advance in a foreseeable decline; if the physician objects, it is his or her duty to excuse himself or herself from the case and from the care of the patient altogether *before* the patient's deteriorating condition prevents or makes it difficult to transfer to another physician; the doctor cannot simply voice his or her objections when the patient finally reaches the point of requesting help in dying. The physician should of course object if, for instance, he or she believes that the patient is acting on faulty information; but the physician ought not introduce a principled objection to participation in euthanasia in general at this late date.

27 To this end, the British and Scottish voluntary euthanasia societies have published booklets of explicit information concerning methods of suicide for distribution to their members; the Dutch voluntary euthanasia society has published a handbook intended specifically for physicians, and voluntary physician-assisted euthanasia is legally tolerated in Holland. In the United States, Hemlock, a society

advocating legalization of voluntary euthanasia and assisted suicide, also makes available similar information.

28 O. Ruth Russell, *Freedom to Die: Moral and Legal Aspects of Euthanasia*, rev. ed. (New York: Human Sciences Press, 1977), 19.

29 Tom L. Beauchamp and Arnold I. Davidson, "The Definition of Euthanasia," *The Journal of Medicine and Philosophy* 4 (September 1979): 301.

30 Paul Ramsey, *The Patient as Person* (New Haven: Yale University Press, 1970), 161.

31 Allan S. Detsky et al., "Prognosis, Survival, and the Expenditure of Hospital Resources for Patients in an Intensive-Care Unit," *The New England Journal of Medicine* 305 (September 17, 1981): 667-672; figures from Table 1.

32 This case, originally presented in the *Illinois Medical Journal* and reprinted in *Connecticut Medicine* with commentary from medical, ethical, and legal experts, is summarized in *Concern for Dying* 8 (Summer 1982): 3. This patient did receive treatment for intervening infections, pneumonia, dermatitis, and convulsions, and for the ten days before her death was maintained on oxygen, respiratory therapy, and antibiotics.

33 President's Commission for the Study of Ethical Problems in Medicine and Biomedical and Behavioral Research, *Defining Death: Medical, Legal, and Ethical Issues in the Determination of Death* (Washington, DC: Government Printing Office, 1981), 18, citing the *Guinness Book of World Records* regarding the case of Elaine Esposito.

34 See the useful discussion of the form of the wedge argument in Tom L. Beauchamp and James F. Childress, *Principles of Biomedical Ethics* (New York: Oxford University Press, 1979), 109-117. I am concerned primarily with the second, empirical form of the argument here, but disagree with the conclusions Beauchamp and Childress reach.

35 As one physician has pointed out, objecting to the wedge argument's contention that greed would bring doctors to kill their patients, there is "not much financial incentive with a dead patient." In fact, greed may work the other way around: doctors strive to keep their patients alive, whatever the physical or financial costs to the patients, because their income is derived from services provided. As another physician has pointed out, however, not all patients are profitable, and the physician who has enough profitable ones will find that killing off the unprofitable ones further improves the bottom line. Needless to say, greed in any of these varieties will violate the principles of mercy, autonomy, and justice.

36 See the position of Pope Pius XII on the use of painkillers in "The Prolongation of Life," an address to an international congress of anesthesiologists, reprinted in Dennis J. Horan and David Mall, eds., *Death, Dying, and Euthanasia* (Frederick, MD: University Publications of America, 1980), 281-287. The view of Pius XII is reemphasized by Pope John Paul II (see note 24). Although both permit the use of painkillers that shorten life, provided they are intended to relieve pain, not intended to produce death, both also warn against the casual use of painkillers that cause unconsciousness, since, in the words of the latter, "a person not only has to be able to satisfy his or her moral duties and family obligations; he or she also has to prepare himself or herself with full consciousness for meeting Christ" (Section III). Advanced pain-management techniques may be able to reduce the problem, but in practice the excessive use of painkillers remains common.

37 See the discussion of this analogy in John D. Arras, "The Right to Die on the Slippery Slope," *Social Theory and Practice* 8 (Fall 1982): 301 ff.

38 Cicely Saunders, "The Moment of Truth: Care of the Dying Person," in *Confrontations of Death: A Book of Readings and a Suggested Method of Instruction*, ed. Francis G. Scott and Ruth M. Brewer (Corvalis, OR: A Continuing Education Book, 1971), 119, quoted in Paul Ramsey, *Ethics at the Edges of Life* (New Haven: Yale University Press, 1978), 152. Dame Saunders is the founder and medical director of St. Christopher's Hospice near London, which has provided the stimulus and model for the contemporary hospice movement.

39 See chapter 1 of this book [*Least Worth Death: Essays on the End of Life* (Philadelphia: Temple University Press, 1994)].

40 Barbara J. McNeil, Ralph Weichselbaum, and Stephen G. Pauker, "Speech and Survival: Tradeoffs between Quality and Quantity of Life in Laryngeal Cancer," *New England Journal of Medicine* 305 (October 22, 1981): 982-987. The study, how-

ever, was performed with healthy volunteers, not actual patients. See Correspondence, *New England Journal of Medicine* 306 (February 25, 1982): 482-483, for other criticisms of this study, including evidence that rehabilitation of speech may be quite satisfactory.

41 See Courtney S. Campbell, "'Aid-in-Dying' and the Taking of Human Life," *Journal of Medical Ethics* 18 (1992): 128-134, for an estimate that 76-84 percent of deaths are caused by chronic conditions.

42 It is sometimes argued that physician assistance in a patient's suicide would violate the Hippocratic Oath. It is true that the oath, in its original form, does contain an explicit injunction that the physician shall not give a lethal potion to a patient who requests it, nor make a suggestion to that effect (to do so was apparently common Greek medical practice at the time). But the oath in its original form also contains explicit prohibitions of the physician's accepting fees for teaching medicine, and of performing surgery—even on gallstones. These latter prohibitions are not retained in modern reformulations of the oath, and I see no reason why the provision against giving lethal potions to patients who request it should be. What is central to the oath and cannot be deleted without altering its essential character is the requirement that the physician shall come "for the benefit of the sick." Under the argument advanced here, physician assistance in patient suicide may in some cases indeed be for the benefit of the patient. What the oath would continue to prohibit is physician assistance in a suicide for the physician's own gain or to serve other institutional or societal ends.

43 Ramsey, *The Patient as Person*, 145.

36.
WHEN SELF-DETERMINATION RUNS AMOK

Daniel Callahan

SOURCE: *The Hastings Center Report* 22.2 (1992).

The euthanasia debate is not just another moral debate, one in a long list of arguments in our pluralistic society. It is profoundly emblematic of three important turning points in Western thought. The first is that of the legitimate conditions under which one person can kill another. The acceptance of voluntary active euthanasia would morally sanction what can only be called "consenting adult killing." By that term I mean the killing of one person by another in the name of their mutual right to be a killer and killed if they freely agree to play those roles. This turn flies in the face of a longstanding effort to limit the circumstances under which one person can take the life of another, from efforts to control the free flow of guns and arms, to abolish capital punishment, and to more tightly control warfare. Euthanasia would add a whole new category of killing to a society that already has too many excuses to indulge itself in that way.

The second turning point lies in the meaning and limits of self-determination. The acceptance of euthanasia would sanction a view of autonomy holding that individuals may, in the name of their own private, idiosyncratic view of the good life, call upon others, including such institutions as medicine, to help them pursue that life, even at the risk of harm to the common good. This works against the idea that the meaning and scope of our own right to lead our own lives must be conditioned by, and be compatible with, the good of the community, which is more than an aggregate of self-directing individuals.

The third turning point is to be found in the claim being made upon medicine: it should be prepared to make its skills available to individuals to help them achieve their private vision of the good life. This puts medicine in the business of promoting the individualistic pursuit of general human happiness and well-

being. It would overturn the traditional belief that medicine should limit its domain to promoting and preserving human health, redirecting it instead to the relief of that suffering which stems from life itself, not merely from a sick body.

I believe that, at each of these three turning points, proponents of euthanasia push us in the wrong direction. Arguments in favor of euthanasia fall into four general categories, which I will take up in turn: (1) the moral claim of individual self-determination and well-being; (2) the moral irrelevance of the difference between killing and allowing to die; (3) the supposed paucity of evidence to show likely harmful consequences of legalized euthanasia; and (4) the compatibility of euthanasia and medical practice.

Self-Determination

Central to most arguments for euthanasia is the principle of self-determination. People are presumed to have an interest in deciding for themselves, according to their own beliefs about what makes life good, how they will conduct their lives. That is an important value, but the question in the euthanasia context is, What does it mean and how far should it extend? If it were a question of suicide, where a person takes her own life without assistance from another, that principle might be pertinent, at least for debate. But euthanasia is not that limited a matter. The self-determination in that case can only be effected by the moral and physical assistance of another. Euthanasia is thus no longer a matter only of self-determination, but of a mutual, social decision between two people, the one to be killed and the other to do the killing.

How are we to make the moral move from my right of self-determination to some doctor's right to kill me—from *my* right to *his* right? Where does the doctor's moral warrant to kill come from? Ought doctors to be able to kill anyone they want as long as permission is given by competent persons? Is our right to life just like a piece of property, to be given away or alienated if the price (happiness, relief of suffering) is right? And then to be destroyed with our permission once alienated?

In answer to all those questions, I will say this: I have yet to hear a plausible argument why it should be permissible for us to put this kind of power in the hands of another, whether a doctor or anyone else. The idea that we can waive our right to life, and then give to another the power to take that life, requires a justification yet to be provided by anyone.

Slavery was long ago outlawed on the ground that one person should not have the right to own another, even with the other's permission. Why? Because it is a fundamental moral wrong for one person to give over his life and fate to another, whatever the good consequences, and no less a wrong for another person to have that kind of total, final power. Like slavery, dueling was long ago banned on similar grounds: even free, competent individuals should not have the power to kill each other, whatever their motives, whatever the circumstances. Consenting adult killing, like consenting adult slavery or degradation, is a strange route to human dignity.

There is another problem as well. If doctors, once sanctioned to carry out euthanasia, are to be themselves responsible moral agents—not simply hired hands with lethal injections at the ready—then they must have their own *independent* moral grounds to kill those who request such services. What do I mean? As those who favor euthanasia are quick to point out, some people want it because their life has become so burdensome it no longer seems worth living.

The doctor will have a difficulty at this point. The degree and intensity to which people suffer from their diseases and their dying, and whether they find life more of a burden than a benefit, has very little directly to do with the nature or extent of their actual physical nature or extent of their actual physical condition. Three people can have the same condition, but only one will find the suffering unbearable. People suffer, but suffering is as much a function of the values of individuals as it is of the physical caus-

es of that suffering. Inevitably in that circumstance, the doctor will in effect be treating the patient's values. To be responsible, the doctor would have to share those values. The doctor would have to decide, on her own, whether the patient's life was "no longer worth living."

But how could a doctor possibly know that or make such a judgment? Just because the patient said so? I raise this question because, while in Holland at [a] euthanasia conference ... the doctors present agreed that there is no objective way of measuring or judging the claims of patients that their suffering is unbearable. And if it is difficult to measure suffering, how much more difficult to determine the value of a patient's statement that her life is not worth living?

However one might want to answer such questions, the very need to ask them, to inquire into the physician's responsibility and grounds for medical and moral judgment, points out the social nature of the decision. Euthanasia is not a private matter of self-determination. It is an act that requires two people to make it possible, and a complicit society to make it acceptable.

Killing and Allowing to Die

Against common opinion, the argument is sometimes made that there is no moral difference between stopping life-sustaining treatment and more active forms of killing, such as lethal injection. Instead I would contend that the notion that there is no morally significant difference between omission and commission is just wrong. Consider in its broad implications what the eradication of the distinction implies: that death from disease has been banished, leaving only the actions of physicians in terminating treatment as the cause of death. Biology, which used to bring about death, has apparently been displaced by human agency. Doctors have finally, I suppose, thus genuinely become gods, now doing what nature and the deities once did.

What is the mistake here? It lies in confusing causality and culpability, and in failing to note the way in which human societies have overlaid natural causes with moral rules and interpretations. Causality (by which I mean the direct physical causes of death) and culpability (by which I mean our attribution of moral responsibility to human actions) are confused under three circumstances.

They are confused, first, when the action of a physician in stopping treatment of a patient with an underlying lethal disease is construed as *causing* death. On the contrary, the physician's omission can only bring about death on the condition that the patient's disease will kill him in the absence of treatment. We may hold the physician morally responsible for the death, if we have morally judged such actions wrongful omissions. But it confuses reality and moral judgment to see an omitted action as having the same causal status as one that directly kills. A lethal injection will kill both a healthy person and a sick person. A physician's omitted treatment will have no effect on a healthy person. Turn off the machine on me, a healthy person, and nothing will happen. It will only, in contrast, bring the life of a sick person to an end because of an underlying fatal disease.

Causality and culpability are confused, second, when we fail to note that judgments of moral responsibility and culpability are human constructs. By that I mean that we human beings, after moral reflection, have decided to call some actions right or wrong, and to devise moral rules to deal with them. When physicians could do nothing to stop death, they were not held responsible for it. When, with medical progress, they began to have some power over death—but only its timing and circumstances, not its ultimate inevitability—moral rules were devised to set forth their obligations. Natural causes of death were not thereby banished. They were, instead, overlaid with a medical ethics designed to determine moral culpability in deploying medical power.

To confuse the judgments of this ethics with the physical causes of death—which is the connotation of the word *kill*—is to confuse nature and human action. People will, one way or another, die of some disease; death will have dominion over all of us. To say that a doctor "kills" a patient by allowing this to happen should only be understood as a moral judgment about the licitness of his omission, nothing more. We can, as a fashion of speech only, talk about a doctor *killing* a patient by omitting treatment he should have provided. It is a fashion of speech precisely because it is the underlying disease that brings

death when treatment is omitted; that is its cause, not the physician's omission. It is a misuse of the word *killing* to use it when a doctor stops a treatment he believes will no longer benefit that patient—when, that is, he steps aside to allow an eventually inevitable death to occur now rather than later. The only deaths that human beings invented are those that come from direct killing—when, with a lethal injection, we both cause death and are morally responsible for it. In the case of omissions, we do not cause death even if we may be judged morally responsible for it.

This difference between causality and culpability also helps us see why a doctor who has omitted a treatment he should have provided has "killed" that patient while another doctor—performing precisely the same act of omission on another patient in different circumstances—does not kill her, but only allows her to die. The difference is that we have come, by moral convention and conviction, to classify unauthorized or illegitimate omissions as acts of "killing." We call them "killing" in the expanded sense of the term: a culpable action that permits the real cause of death, the underlying disease, to proceed to its lethal conclusion. By contrast, the doctor who, at the patient's request, omits or terminates unwanted treatment does not kill at all. Her underlying disease, not his action, is the physical cause of death; and we have agreed to consider actions of that kind to be morally licit. He thus can truly be said to have "allowed" her to die.

If we fail to maintain the distinction between killing and allowing to die, moreover, there are some disturbing possibilities. The first would be to confirm many physicians in their already too powerful belief that, when patients die, or when physicians stop treatment because of the futility of continuing it, they are somehow both morally and physically responsible for the deaths that follow. That notion needs to be abolished, not strengthened. It needlessly and wrongly burdens the physician, to whom should not be attributed the powers of the gods. The second possibility would be that, in every case where a doctor judges medical treatment no longer effective in prolonging life, a quick and direct killing of the patient would be seen as the next, most reasonable step, on grounds of both humaneness and economics. I do not see how that logic could easily be rejected.

Calculating the Consequences

When concerns about the adverse social consequences of permitting euthanasia are raised, its advocates tend to dismiss them as unfounded and overly speculative. On the contrary, recent data about the Dutch experience suggests that such concerns are right on target. From my own discussions in Holland, and from the articles on that subject in this issue and elsewhere, I believe we can now fully see most of the *likely* consequences of legal euthanasia.

Three consequences seem almost certain, in this or any other country: the inevitability of some abuse of the law; the difficulty of precisely writing, and then enforcing, the law; and the inherent slipperiness of the moral reasons for legalizing euthanasia in the first place.

Why is abuse inevitable? One reason is that almost all laws on delicate, controversial matters are to some extent abused. This happens because not everyone will agree with the law as written and will bend it, or ignore it, if they can get away with it. From explicit admissions to me by Dutch proponents of euthanasia, and from the corroborating information provided by the Remmelink Report and the outside studies of Carlos Gomez and John Keown, I am convinced that in the Netherlands there are a substantial number of cases of nonvoluntary euthanasia, that is, euthanasia undertaken without the explicit permission of the person being killed. The other reason abuse is inevitable is that the law is likely to have a low enforcement priority in the criminal justice system. Like other laws of similar status, unless there is an unrelenting and harsh willingness to pursue abuse, violations will ordinarily be tolerated. The worst thing to me about my experience in Holland was the casual, seemingly indifferent attitude toward abuse. I think that would happen everywhere.

Why would it be hard to precisely write, and then enforce, the law? The Dutch speak about the requirement of "unbearable" suffering, but admit that such a term is just about indefinable, a highly subjective matter admitting of no objective standards. A requirement for outside opinion is nice, but it is easy to find complaisant colleagues. A requirement that a medical condition be "terminal" will run aground on the notorious difficulties of knowing when an illness is actually terminal.

Apart from those technical problems there is a more profound worry. I see no way, even in principle, to write or enforce a meaningful law that can guarantee effective procedural safeguards. The reason is obvious yet almost always overlooked. The euthanasia transaction will ordinarily take place within the boundaries of the private and confidential doctor-patient relationship. No one can possibly know what takes place in that context unless the doctor chooses to reveal it. In Holland, less than 10 percent of the physicians report their acts of euthanasia and do so with almost complete legal impunity. There is no reason why the situation should be any better elsewhere. Doctors will have their own reasons for keeping euthanasia secret, and some patients will have no less a motive for wanting it concealed.

I would mention, finally, that the moral logic of the motives for euthanasia contain within them the ingredients of abuse. The two standard motives for euthanasia and assisted suicide are said to be our right of self-determination, and our claim upon the mercy of others, especially doctors, to relieve our suffering. These two motives are typically spliced together and presented as a single justification. Yet if they are considered independently—and there is no inherent reason why they must be linked—they reveal serious problems. It is said that a competent, adult person should have a right to euthanasia for the relief of suffering. But why must the person be suffering? Does not that stipulation already compromise the principle of self-determination? How can self-determination have any limits? Whatever the person's motives may be, why are they not sufficient?

Consider next the person who is suffering but not competent, who is perhaps demented or mentally retarded. The standard argument would deny euthanasia to that person. But why? If a person is suffering but not competent, then it would seem grossly unfair to deny relief solely on the grounds of incompetence. Are the incompetent less entitled to relief from suffering than the competent? Will it only be affluent, middle-class people, mentally fit and savvy about working the medical system, who can qualify? Do the incompetent suffer less because of their incompetence?

Considered from these angles, there are no good moral reasons to limit euthanasia once the principle of taking life for that purpose has been legitimated. If we really believe in self-determination, then any competent person should have a right to be killed by a doctor for any reason that suits him. If we believe in the relief of suffering, then it seems cruel and capricious to deny it to the incompetent. There is, in short, no reasonable or logical stopping point once the turn has been made down the road to euthanasia, which could soon turn into a convenient and commodious expressway.

Euthanasia and Medical Practice

A fourth kind of argument one often hears both in the Netherlands and in this country [the US] is that euthanasia and assisted suicide are perfectly compatible with the aims of medicine. I would note at the very outset that a physician who participates in another person's suicide already abuses medicine. Apart from depression (the main statistical cause of suicide), people commit suicide, because they find life empty, oppressive, or meaningless. Their judgment is a judgment about the value of continued life, not only about health (even if they are sick). Are doctors now to be given the right to make judgments about the kinds of life worth living and to give their blessing to suicide for those they judge wanting? What conceivable competence, technical or moral, could doctors claim to play such a role? Are we to medicalize suicide, turning judgments about its worth and value into one more clinical issue? Yes, those are rhetorical questions.

Yet they bring us to the core of the problem of euthanasia and medicine. The great temptation of modern medicine, not always resisted, is to move beyond the promotion and preservation of health into the boundless realm of general human happiness and wellbeing. The root problem of illness and mortality is both medical and philosophical or religious. "Why must I die?" can be asked as a technical, biological question or as a question about the meaning of life. When medicine tries to respond to the latter, which it is always under pressure to do, it moves beyond its proper role.

It is not medicine's place to lift from us the burden of that suffering which turns on the meaning we assign to the decay of the body and its eventual death. It is not medicine's place to determine when lives are not worth living or when the burden of life is too great to be borne. Doctors have no conceivable way of evaluating such claims on the part of patients, and they should have no right to act in response to them. Medicine should try to relive human suffering, but only that suffering which is brought on by illness and dying as biological phenomena, not that suffering which comes from anguish or despair at the human condition.

Doctors ought to relieve those forms of suffering that medically accompany serious illness and the threat of death. They should relive pain, do what they can to allay anxiety and uncertainty, and be a comforting presence. As sensitive human beings, doctors should be prepared to respond to patients who ask why they must die, or die in pain. But here the doctor and the patient are at the same level. The doctor may have no better an answer to those old questions than anyone else; and certainly no special insight from his training as a physician. It would be terrible for physicians to forget this, and to think that in a swift, lethal injection, medicine has found its own answer to the riddle of life. It would be a false answer, given by the wrong people. It would be no less a false answer for patients. They should neither ask medicine to put its own vocation at risk to serve their private interest, nor think that the answer to suffering is to be killed by another. The problem is precisely that, too often in human history, killing has seemed the quick, efficient way to put aside that which burdens us. It rarely helps, and too often simply adds to one evil still another. That is what I believe euthanasia would accomplish. It is self-determination run amok.

37.

RODRIGUEZ V. THE ATTORNEY GENERAL OF CANADA AND THE ATTORNEY GENERAL OF BRITISH COLUMBIA [1993] SUPREME COURT OF CANADA

Case Summary by C. Morano

SOURCE: http://scc.lexum.org/en/1993/1993scr3-519/1993scr3-519.html.

[Rodriguez v. The Attorney General of Canada and the Attorney General of British Columbia highlights the conflict between the state's interest in protecting the sanctity of life, and the individual who wishes for the assistance of a physician in committing suicide as her health deteriorates.]

Present: Lamer C.J. and La Forest, L'Heureux-Dubé, Sopinka, Gonthier, Cory, McLachlin, Iacobucci and Major JJ.

On appeal from the court of appeal for British Columbia.

Background

The appellant, a 42-year-old mother, is suffering from amyotrophic lateral sclerosis. Her condition is deteriorating and she will soon lose the ability to swallow, speak, walk and move her body without assistance. When she can no longer enjoy life, she wishes that a physician be able to assist her in ending her life. Section 241(b) of the *Criminal Code* prohibits giving assistance to commit suicide. The appellant applied to the Supreme Court of British Columbia for an order that Section 241(b) be declared invalid on the ground that it violates her Charter rights under ss. 7, 12 and 15(1). The trial judges dismissed the appellant's application and the Court of Appeal agreed with that decision.

The Supreme Court of Canada

A majority of the Supreme Court dismissed Sue Rodriguez's appeal and concluded that Section 241(b) of the Criminal Code is constitutional. Speaking on behalf of the majority, Sopinka J. stated that the prohibition does deprive Ms. Rodriguez of the security interest as well as her liberty interest, but the violation is in accordance with the principles of fundamental justice, because it relates to the state's interest in protecting the vulnerable and is reflective of fundamental values at play in our society: "Section 241(b) is grounded in the state interest in protecting life and reflects the policy of the state that human life should not be depreciated by allowing life to be taken. This state policy is part of our fundamental conception of the sanctity of life." Sopinka J. claimed that an infringement of Section 15 of the Charter can be saved under section 1 and, as a result, he immediately considered the application of Section 1 and assumed that there had been a violation of Ms. Rodriguez's right to equality. He concluded that "in order to effectively protect life and those who are vulnerable in society a prohibition without exception on the giving of assistance to commit suicide is the best approach. Attempts to fine tune this approach by creating exceptions have been unsatisfactory and have tended to support the theory of the 'slippery slope.'" Furthermore, Sopinka J. stated that "Parliament's repeal of the offence of attempted suicide from the *Criminal Code* was not recognition that suicide was to be accepted within Canadian society. Rather, this action merely reflected the recognition that the criminal law was an ineffectual and inappropriate tool for dealing with suicide attempts."

38.
GENDER, FEMINISM, AND DEATH:
PHYSICIAN-ASSISTED SUICIDE AND EUTHANASIA

Susan M. Wolf

SOURCE: Susan M. Wolf (ed.), *Feminism and Bioethics: Beyond Reproduction* (Oxford University Press, 1996).

The debate in the United States over whether to legitimate physician-assisted suicide and active euthanasia has reached new levels of intensity. Oregon has become the first state to legalize physician-assisted suicide, and there have been campaigns, ballot measures, bills, and litigation in other states in attempts to legalize one or both practices.[1] Scholars and others increasingly urge either outright legalization or some other form of legitimation, through recognition of an affirmative defense of "mercy killing" to a homicide prosecution or other means.[2]

Yet the debate over whether to legitimate physician-assisted suicide and euthanasia (by which I mean active euthanasia, as opposed to the termination of life-sustaining treatment)[3] is most often about a patient who does not exist—a patient with no gender, race, or insurance status. This is the same generic patient featured in most bioethics debates. Little discussion has focused on how differences between patients might alter the equation.

Even though the debate has largely ignored this question, there is ample reason to suspect that gender, among other factors, deserves analysis. The cases prominent in the American debate mostly feature women patients. This occurs against a backdrop of a long history of cultural images revering women's sacrifice and self-sacrifice. Moreover, dimensions of health status and health care that may affect a patient's vulnerability to considering physician-assisted suicide and euthanasia—including depression, poor pain relief, and difficulty obtaining good health care—differentially plague women. And suicide patterns themselves show a strong gender effect: women less often complete suicide, but more often attempt it.[4] These and other factors raise the question of whether the dynamics surrounding physician-assisted suicide and euthanasia may vary by gender.

Indeed, it would be surprising if gender had no influence. Women in America still live in a society marred by sexism, a society that particularly disvalues women with illness, disability, or merely advanced age. It would be hard to explain if health care, suicide, and fundamental dimensions of American society showed marked differences by gender, but gender suddenly dropped out of the equation when people became desperate enough to seek a physician's help in ending their lives.

What sort of gender effects might we expect? There are four different possibilities. First, we might anticipate a higher incidence of women than men dying by physician-assisted suicide and euthanasia in this country. This is an empirical claim that we cannot yet test; we currently lack good data in the face of the illegality of the practices in most states[5] and the condemnation of the organized medical profession.[6] The best data we do have are from the Netherlands and are inconclusive. As I discuss below, the Dutch data show that women predominate among patients dying through euthanasia or administration of drugs for pain relief, but not by much. In the smaller categories of physician-assisted suicide and "life-terminating events without request," however, men predominate. And men predominate too in making requests rejected by physicians. It is hard to say what this means for the United States. The Netherlands differs in a number of relevant respects, with universal health care and a more homogeneous society. But the Dutch data suggest that gender differences in the United States will not necessarily translate into higher numbers of women dying. At least one author speculates that there may in fact be

350

a sexist tendency to discount and refuse women's requests.[7]

There may, however, be a second gender effect. Gender differences may translate into women seeking physician-assisted suicide and euthanasia for somewhat different reasons than men. Problems we know to be correlated with gender—difficulty getting good medical care generally, poor pain relief, a higher incidence of depression, and a higher rate of poverty—may figure more prominently in women's motivation. Society's persisting sexism may figure as well. And the long history of valorizing women's self-sacrifice may be expressed in women's requesting assisted suicide or euthanasia.

The well-recognized gender differences in suicide statistics also suggest that women's requests for physician-assisted suicide and euthanasia may more often than men's requests be an effort to change an oppressive situation rather than a literal request for death. Thus some suicidologists interpret men's predominance among suicide "completers" and women's among suicide "attempters" to mean that women more often engage in suicidal behavior with a goal other than "completion."[8] The relationship between suicide and the practices of physician-assisted suicide and euthanasia itself deserves further study; not all suicides are even motivated by terminal disease or other factors relevant to the latter practices. But the marked gender differences in suicidal behavior are suggestive.

Third, gender differences may also come to the fore in physicians' decisions about whether to grant or refuse requests for assisted suicide or euthanasia. The same historical valorization of women's self-sacrifice and the same background sexism that may affect women's readiness to request may also affect physicians' responses. Physicians may be susceptible to affirming women's negative self-judgments. This might or might not result in physicians agreeing to assist; other gender-related judgments (such as that women are too emotionally labile, or that their choices should not be taken seriously) may intervene.[9] But the point is that gender may affect not just patient but physician.

Finally, gender may affect the broad public debate. The prominent U.S. cases so far and related historical imagery suggest that in debating physician-assisted suicide and euthanasia, many in our culture may envision a woman patient. Although the AIDS epidemic has called attention to physician-assisted suicide and euthanasia in men, the cases that have dominated the news accounts and scholarly journals in the recent renewal of debate have featured women patients. Thus we have reason to be concerned that at least some advocacy for these practices may build on the sense that these stories of women's deaths are somehow "right." If there is a felt correctness to these accounts, that may be playing a hidden and undesirable part in catalyzing support for the practices' legitimation.

Thus we have cause to worry whether the debate about and practice of physician-assisted suicide and euthanasia in this country are gendered in a number of respects. Serious attention to gender therefore seems essential. Before we license physicians to kill their patients or to assist patients in killing themselves, we had better understand the dynamic at work in that encounter, why the practice seems so alluring that we should court its dangers, and what dangers are likely to manifest. After all, the consequences of permitting killing or assistance in private encounters are serious, indeed fatal. We had better understand what distinguishes this from other forms of private violence, and other relationships of asymmetrical power that result in the deaths of women. And we had better determine whether tacit assumptions about gender are influencing the enthusiasm for legalization.

Yet even that is not enough. Beyond analysing the way gender figures in our cases, cultural imagery and practice, we must analyse the substantive arguments. For attention to gender, in the last two decades particularly, has yielded a wealth of feminist critiques and theoretical tools that can fruitfully be brought to bear. After all, the debate over physician-assisted suicide and euthanasia revolves around precisely the kind of issues on which feminist work has focused: what it means to talk about rights of self-determination and autonomy; the reconciliation of those rights with physicians' duties of beneficence and caring; and how to place all of this in a context including the strengths and failures of families, professionals, and communities, as well as real differentials of power and resources.

The debate over physician-assisted suicide and euthanasia so starkly raises questions of rights, caring, and context that at this point it would take determination *not* to bring to bear a literature that has been devoted to understanding those notions. Indeed, the work of Lawrence Kohlberg bears witness to what an obvious candidate this debate is for such analysis.[10] It was Kohlberg's work on moral development, of course, that provoked Carol Gilligan's *In a Different Voice*, criticizing Kohlberg's vision of progressive stages in moral maturation as one that was partial and gendered.[11] Gilligan proposed that there were really two different approaches to moral problems, one that emphasized generalized rights and universal principles, and the other that instead emphasized conceptualized caring and the maintenance of particular human relationships. She suggested that although women and men could use both approaches, women tended to use the latter and men the former. Both approaches, however, were important to moral maturity. Though Gilligan's and others' work on the ethics of care has been much debated and criticized, a number of bioethicists and health care professionals have found a particular pertinence to questions of physician caregiving.[12]

Embedded in Kohlberg's work, one finds proof that the euthanasia debate in particular calls for analysis in the very terms that he employs, and that Gilligan then critiques, enlarges, and reformulates. For one of the nine moral dilemmas Kohlberg used to gauge subjects' stage of moral development was a euthanasia problem. "Dilemma IV" features "a woman" with "very bad cancer" and "in terrible pain." Her physician, Dr. Jefferson, knows she has "only about six months to live." Between periods in which she is "delirious and almost crazy with pain," she asks the doctor to kill her with morphine. The question is what he should do.[13]

The euthanasia debate thus demands analysis along the care, rights, and context axes that the Kohlberg-Gilligan debate has identified.[14] Kohlberg himself used this problem to reveal how well respondents were doing in elevating general principles over the idiosyncrasies of relationship and context. It is no stretch, then, to apply the fruits of more than a decade of feminist critique. The problem has a genuine pedigree.

The purpose of this chapter thus is twofold. First, I explore gender's significance for analysing physician-assisted suicide and euthanasia. Thus I examine the prominent cases and cultural images, against the background of cautions recommended by what little data we have from the Netherlands. Finding indications that gender may well be significant, I investigate what that implies for the debate over physician-assisted suicide and euthanasia. Clearly more research is required. But in the meantime, patients' vulnerability to requesting these fatal interventions because of failures in health care and other background conditions, or because of a desire not to die but to alter circumstances, introduces reasons why we should be reluctant to endorse these practices. Indeed, we should be worried about the role of the physician in these cases, and consider the lessons we have learned from analysing other relationships that result in women's deaths. What we glean from looking at gender should lead us to look at other characteristics historically associated with disadvantage, and thus should prompt a general caution applicable to all patients.

My second purpose is to go beyond analysis of gender itself, to analysis of the arguments offered on whether to condone and legitimate these practices. Here is where I bring to bear the feminist literature on caring, rights, and context. I criticize the usual argument that patients' rights of self-determination dictate legitimation of physician-assisted suicide and euthanasia, on the grounds that this misconstrues the utility of rights talk for resolving this debate, and ignores essential features of the context. I then turn to arguments based on beneficence and caring. It is no accident that the word "mercy" has figured so large in our language about these problems; they do involve questions of compassion and caring. However, a shallow understanding of caring will lead us astray and I go on to elaborate what a deep and conceptualized understanding demands. I argue that physicians should be guided by a notion of "principled caring." Finally, I step back to suggest what a proper integration of rights and caring would look like in this context, how it can be coupled with attention to the fate of women and other historically disadvantaged groups, and what practical steps all of this counsels.

This chapter takes a position. As I have before, I oppose the legitimation of physician-assisted suicide and euthanasia.[15] Yet the most important part of what I do here is urge the necessity of feminist analysis of this issue. Physician-assisted suicide and euthanasia are difficult problems on which people may disagree. But I hope to persuade that attending to gender and feminist concerns in analysing these problems is no longer optional.

Gender in Cases, Images, and Practice

The tremendous upsurge in American debate over whether to legitimate physician-assisted suicide and euthanasia in recent years has been fueled by a series of cases featuring women. The case that seems to have begun this series is that of Debbie, published in 1988 by the *Journal of the American Medical Association (JAMA)*.[16] *JAMA* published this now infamous, first-person, and anonymous account by a resident in obstetrics and gynecology of performing euthanasia. Some subsequently queried whether the account was fiction. Yet it successfully catalyzed an enormous response.

The narrator of the piece tells us that Debbie is a young woman suffering from ovarian cancer. The resident has no prior relationship with her, but is called to her bedside late one night while on call and exhausted. Entering Debbie's room, the resident finds an older woman with her, but never pauses to find out who that second woman is and what relational context Debbie acts within. Instead, the resident responds to the patient's clear discomfort and to her words. Debbie says only one sentence, "Let's get this over with." It is unclear whether she thinks the resident is there to draw blood and wants that over with, or means something else. But on the strength of that one sentence, the resident retreats to the nursing station, prepares a lethal injection, returns to the room, and administers it. The story relates this as an act of mercy under the title "It's Over, Debbie," as if in caring response to the patient's words.

The lack of relationship to the patient; the failure to attend to her own history, relationships, and resources; the failure to explore beyond the patient's presented words and engage her in conversation; the sense that the cancer diagnosis plus the patient's

words demand death; and the construal of that response as an act of mercy are all themes that recur in the later cases. The equally infamous Dr. Jack Kevorkian has provided a slew of them.

They begin with Janet Adkins, a 54-year-old Oregon woman diagnosed with Alzheimer's disease.[17] Again, on the basis of almost no relationship with Ms. Adkins, on the basis of a diagnosis by exclusion that Kevorkian could not verify, prompted by a professed desire to die that is a predictable stage in response to a number of dire diagnoses, Kevorkian rigs her up to his "Mercitron" machine in a parking lot outside Detroit in what he presents as an act of mercy.

Then there is Marjorie Wantz, a 58-year-old woman without even a diagnosis.[18] Instead, she has pelvic pain whose source remains undetermined. By the time Kevorkian reaches Ms. Wantz, he is making little pretense of focusing on her needs in the context of a therapeutic relationship. Instead, he tells the press that he is determined to create a new medical specialty of "obitiatry." Ms. Wantz is among the first six potential patients with whom he is conferring. When Kevorkian presides over her death there is another woman who dies as well, Sherry Miller. Miller, 43, has multiple sclerosis. Thus neither woman is terminal.

The subsequent cases reiterate the basic themes.[19] And it is not until the ninth "patient" that Kevorkian finally presides over the death of a man.[20] By this time, published criticism of the predominance of women had begun to appear.[21]

Kevorkian's actions might be dismissed as the bizarre behavior of one man. But the public and press response has been enormous, attesting to the power of these accounts. Many people have treated these cases as important to the debate over physician-assisted suicide and euthanasia. Nor are Kevorkian's cases so aberrant—they pick up all the themes that emerge in "Debbie."

But we cannot proceed without analysis of Diane. This is the respectable version of what Kevorkian makes strange. I refer to the story published by Dr. Timothy Quill in the *New England Journal of Medicine*, recounting his assisting the suicide of his patient Diane.[22] She is a woman in her forties diagnosed with leukemia, who seeks and obtains from

Dr. Quill a prescription for drugs to take her life. Dr. Quill cures some of the problems with the prior cases. He does have a real relationship with her, he knows her history, and he obtains a psychiatric consult on her mental state. He is a caring, empathetic person. Yet once again we are left wondering about the broader context of Diane's life—why even the history of other problems that Quill describes has so drastically depleted her resources to deal with this one, and whether there were any alternatives. And we are once again left wondering about the physician's role—why he responded to her as he did, what self-scrutiny he brought to bear on his own urge to comply and how he reconciled this with the arguments that physicians who are moved to so respond should nonetheless resist.[23]

These cases will undoubtedly be joined by others, including cases featuring men, as the debate progresses. Indeed, they already have been. Yet the initial group of cases involving women has somehow played a pivotal role in catalyzing reexamination of two of the most fundamental and long-standing prohibitions in medicine. These are prohibitions that have been deemed by some constitutive of the physician's role: above all, do no harm; and give no deadly drug, even if asked. The power of this core of cases seems somehow evident.

This collection of early cases involving women cries out for analysis. It cannot be taken as significant evidence predicting that more women may die through physician-assisted suicide and euthanasia; these individual cases are no substitute for systematic data. But to understand what they suggest about the role of gender, we need to place them in context.

The images in these cases have a cultural lineage. We could trace a long history of portrayals of women as victims of sacrifice and self-sacrifice. In Greek tragedy, that ancient source of still reverberating images, "suicide ... [is] a woman's solution."[24] Almost no men die in this way. Specifically, suicide is a wife's solution; it is one of the few acts of autonomy open to her. Wives use suicide in these tragedies often to join their husbands in death. The other form of death specific to women is the sacrifice of young women who are virgins. The person putting such a woman to death must be male.[25] Thus "[i]t is by men that women meet their death, and it is for men, usu-

ally, that they kill themselves."[26] Men, in contrast, die by the sword or spear in battle.[27]

The connection between societal gender roles and modes of death persists through history. Howard Kushner writes that "Nineteenth-century European and American fiction is littered with the corpses of ... women.... [T]he cause was always ... rejection after an illicit love affair.... If women's death by suicide could not be attributed to dishonor, it was invariably tied to women's adopting roles ... assigned to men."[28] "By the mid-nineteenth century characterizations of women's suicides meshed with the ideology described by Barbara Welter as that of 'True Womanhood.... Adherence to the virtues of piety, purity, submissiveness and domesticity' translated into the belief that a 'fallen woman' was a 'fallen angel.'"[29] Even after statistics emerged showing that women completed suicide less often than men, the explanations offered centered on women's supposedly greater willingness to suffer misfortune, their lack of courage, and less arduous social role.[30]

Thus, prevailing values have imbued women's deaths with specific meaning. Indeed, Carol Gilligan builds on images of women's suicides and sacrifice in novels and drama, as well as on her own data, in finding a psychology and even an ethic of self-sacrifice among women. Gilligan finds one of the "conventions of femininity" to be "the moral equation of goodness with self-sacrifice."[31] "[V]irtue for women lies in self-sacrifice...."[32]

Given this history of images and the valorization of women's self-sacrifice, it should come as no surprise that the early cases dominating the debate about self-sacrifice through physician-assisted suicide and euthanasia have been cases of women. In Greek tragedy only women were candidates for sacrifice and self-sacrifice,[33] and to this day self-sacrifice is usually regarded as a feminine not masculine virtue.

This lineage has implications. It means that even while we debate physician-assisted suicide and euthanasia rationally, we may be animated by unacknowledged images that give the practices a certain gender logic and felt correctness. In some deep way it makes sense to us to see these women dying, it seems right. It fits an old piece into a familiar, ancient puzzle. Moreover, these acts seem good;

they are born of virtue. We may not recognize that the virtues in question—female sacrifice and self-sacrifice—are ones now widely questioned and deliberately rejected. Instead, our subconscious may harken back to older forms, reembracing those ancient virtues, and thus lauding these women's deaths.

Analysing the early cases against the background of this history also suggests hidden gender dynamics to be discovered by attending to the facts found in the accounts of these cases, or more properly the facts not found. What is most important in these accounts is what is left out, how truncated they are. We see a failure to attend to the patient's context, a readiness on the part of these physicians to facilitate death, a seeming lack of concern over why these women turn to these doctors for deliverance. A clue about why we should be concerned about each of these omissions is telegraphed by data from exit polls on the day Californians defeated a referendum measure to legalize active euthanasia. Those polls showed support for the measure lowest among women, older people, Asians, and African Americans, and highest among younger men with post-graduate education and incomes over $75,000 per year.[34] The *New York Times* analysis was that people from more vulnerable groups were more worried about allowing physicians actively to take life. This may suggest concern not only that physicians may be too ready to take their lives, but also that these patients may be markedly vulnerable to seeking such relief. Why would women, in particular, feel this?

Women are at greater risk for inadequate pain relief.[35] Indeed, fear of pain is one of the reasons most frequently cited by Americans for supporting legislation to legalize euthanasia.[36] Women are also at greater risk for depression.[37] And depression appears to underlie numerous requests for physician-assisted suicide and euthanasia.[38] These factors suggest that women may be differentially driven to consider requesting both practices.

That possibility is further supported by data showing systematic problems for women in relationship to physicians. As an American Medical Association report on gender disparities recounts, women receive more care even for the same illness, but the care is generally worse. Women are less likely to receive dialysis, kidney transplants, cardiac catheterization, and diagnostic testing for lung cancer. The report urges physicians to uproot "social or cultural biases that could affect medical care" and "presumptions about the relative worth of certain social roles."[39]

This all occurs against the background of a deeply flawed health care system that ties health insurance to employment. Men are differentially represented in the ranks of those with private health insurance, women in the ranks of the others—those either on government entitlement programs or uninsured.[40] In the U.S. two-tier health care system, men dominate in the higher-quality tier, women in the lower.

Moreover, women are differentially represented among the ranks of the poor. Many may feel they lack the resources to cope with disability and disease. To cope with Alzheimer's, breast cancer, multiple sclerosis, ALS, and a host of other diseases takes resources. It takes not only the financial resource of health insurance, but also access to stable working relationships with clinicians expert in these conditions, in the psychological issues involved, and in palliative care and pain relief. It may take access to home care, eventually residential care, and rehabilitation services. These are services often hard to get even for those with adequate resources, and almost impossible for those without. And who are those without in this country? Disproportionately they are women, people of color, the elderly, and children.[41]

Women may also be driven to consider physician-assisted suicide or euthanasia out of fear of otherwise burdening their families.[42] The dynamic at work in a family in which an ill member chooses suicide or active euthanasia is worrisome. This worry should increase when it is a woman who seeks to "avoid being a burden," or otherwise solve the problem she feels she poses, by opting for her own sacrifice. The history and persistence of family patterns in this country in which women are expected to adopt self-sacrificing behavior for the sake of the family may pave the way too for the patient's request for death. Women requesting death may also be sometimes seeking something other than death. The dominance of women among those attempting but not completing suicide in this country suggests that women may differentially engage in death-seeking behavior with a goal other than death. Instead, they may be seeking to change their relationships or circumstances.[43] A psychiatrist at Harvard has speculated about why those women among Kevorkian's "patients" who were still capable of killing themselves instead sought Kevorkian's help. After all, suicide has been decriminalized in this country and step-by-step instructions are readily available. The psychiatrist was apparently prompted to speculate by interviewing about twenty physicians who assisted patients' deaths and discovering that two-thirds to three-quarters of the patients had been women. The psychiatrist wondered whether turning to Kevorkian was a way to seek a relationship.[44] The women also found a supposed "expert" to rely upon, someone to whom they could yield control. But then we must wonder what circumstances, what relational context, led them to this point.

What I am suggesting is that there are issues relating to gender left out of the accounts of the early prominent cases of physician-assisted suicide and euthanasia or left unexplored that may well be driving or limiting the choices of these women. I am not suggesting that we should denigrate these choices or regard them as irrational. Rather, it is the opposite, that we should assume these decisions to be rational and grounded in a context. That forces us to attend to the background failures in that context.

Important analogies are offered by domestic violence. Such violence has been increasingly recognized as a widespread problem. It presents some structural similarities to physician-assisted suicide and especially active euthanasia. All three can be fatal. All three are typically acts performed behind closed doors. In the United States, all three are illegal in most jurisdictions, though the record of law enforcement on each is extremely inconsistent. Though men may be the victims and women the perpetrators of all three, in the case of domestic violence there are some conceptions of traditional values and virtues that endorse the notion that a husband may beat his wife. As I have suggested above, there are similarly traditional conceptions of feminine self-sacrifice that might bless a physician's assisting a woman's suicide or performing euthanasia.

Clearly there are limits to the analogy. But my point is that questions of choice and consent have been raised in the analysis of domestic violence against women, much as they have in the case of physician-assisted suicide and active euthanasia. If a woman chooses to remain in a battering relationship, do we regard that as a choice to be respected and reason not to intervene? While choosing to remain is not consent to battery, what if a woman says that she "deserves" to be beaten—do we take that as reason to condone the battering? The answers that have been developed to these questions are instructive, because they combine respect for the rationality of women's choices with a refusal to go the further step of excusing the batterer. We appreciate now that a woman hesitating to leave a battering relationship may have ample and rational reasons: well-grounded fear for her safety and that of her children, a justified expectation of economic distress, and warranted concern that the legal system will not effectively come to her aid. We further see mental health professionals now uncovering some of the deeper reasons why some women might say at some point they "deserve" violence. Taking all of these insights seriously has led to development of a host of new legal, psychotherapeutic, and other interventions meant to address the actual experiences and concerns that might lead women to "choose" to stay in a violent relationship or "choose" violence against them. Yet none of this condones the choice of the partner to batter or, worse yet, kill the woman. Indeed, the victim's consent, we should recall, is no legal defense to murder.

All of this should suggest that in analysing why women may request physician-assisted suicide and euthanasia, and why indeed the California polls indicate that women may feel more vulnerable to and wary of making that request, we have insights to bring to bear from other realms. Those insights render suspect an analysis that merely asserts women are choosing physician-assisted suicide and active euthanasia, without asking why they make that choice. The analogy to other forms of violence against women behind closed doors demands that we ask why the woman is there, what features of her context brought her there, and why she may feel there is no better place to be. Finally, the analogy counsels us that the patient's consent does not resolve the question of whether the physician acts properly in deliberately taking her life through physician-assisted suicide or active euthanasia. The two people are separate moral and legal agents.[45]

This leads us from consideration of why women patients may feel vulnerable to these practices, to the question of whether physicians may be vulnerable to regarding women's requests for physician-assisted suicide and euthanasia somewhat differently from men's. There may indeed be gender-linked reasons for physicians in this country to say "yes" to women seeking assistance in suicide or active euthanasia. In assessing whether the patient's life has become "meaningless," or a "burden," or otherwise what some might regard as suitable for extinguishing at her request, it would be remarkable if the physician's background views did not come into play on what makes a woman's life meaningful or how much of a burden on her family is too much.[46]

Second, there is a dynamic many have written about operating between the powerful expert physician and the woman surrendering to his care.[47] It is no accident that bioethics has focused on the problem of physician paternalism. Instead of an egalitarianism or what Susan Sherwin calls "amicalism,"[48] we see a vertically hierarchical arrangement built on domination and subordination. When the patient is female and the doctor male, as is true in most medical encounters, the problem is likely to be exacerbated by the background realities and history of male dominance and female subjugation in the broader society. Then a set of psychological dynamics are likely to make the male physician vulnerable to acceding to the woman patient's request for active assistance in dying. These may be a complex combination of rescue fantasies[49] and the desire to annihilate. Robert Burt talks about the pervasiveness of the ambivalence, quite apart from gender: "Rules governing doctor-patient relations must rest on the premise that anyone's wish to help a desperately pained, apparently helpless person is intertwined with a wish to hurt that person, to obliterate him from sight."[50] When the physician is from a dominant social group and the patient from a subordinate one, we should expect the ambivalence to be heightened. When the "help" requested *is* obliteration, the temptation to enact both parts of the ambivalence in a single act may be great.

This brief examination of the vulnerability of women patients and their physicians to collaboration on actively ending the women's life in a way reflecting gender roles suggests the need to examine the woman's context and where her request for death comes from, the physician's context and where his accession comes from, and the relationship between the two. We need to do that in a way that uses rather than ignores all we know about the issues plaguing the relations between women and men, especially suffering women and powerful expert men. The California exit polls may well signal both the attraction and the fear of enacting the familiar dynamics in a future in which it is legitimate to pursue that dynamic to the death. It would be implausible to maintain that medicine is somehow exempt from broader social dynamics. The question, then, is whether we want to bless deaths driven by those dynamics.

All of this suggests that physician-assisted suicide and euthanasia, as well as the debate about them, may be gendered. I have shown ways in which this may be true even if women do not die in greater numbers. But exploring gender would be incomplete without examining what data we have on its relationship to incidence. As noted above, those data, which are from the Netherlands, neither support the proposition that more women will die from these practices, nor provide good reason yet to dismiss the concern. We simply do not know how these practices may play out by gender in the United States. There are no good U.S. data, undoubtedly because these practices remain generally illegal.[51] And the Dutch data come from another culture, with a more homogeneous population, a different health care system providing universal coverage, and perhaps different gender dynamics.[52]

The status of physician-assisted suicide and euthanasia in the Netherlands is complex. Both practices remain criminal, but both are tolerated under a series of court decisions, guidelines from the Dutch medical association, and a more recent statute that carve out a domain in which the practices are accepted. If the patient is competent and contemporaneously requests assisted suicide or euthanasia, the patient's suffering cannot be relieved in any other way acceptable to the patient, a second physician concurs that acceding to the request is appropriate, and the physician performing the act reports it to permit monitoring and investigation, then the practices are allowed.

Dutch researchers have been reporting rigorous empirical research on the practices only in the past several years.[53] The team led by Dr. Paul van der Maas and working at governmental request published the first results of their nationwide study in 1991.[54] They found that "medical decisions concerning the end of life (MDEL)" were made in 38 percent of all deaths in the Netherlands, and thus were common. They differentiated five different types of MDELs: non-treatment decisions (which are neither physician-assisted suicide nor active euthanasia) caused 17.5 percent of deaths; administration of opioid drugs for pain and symptomatic relief (which would be considered active euthanasia in the United States if the physician's intent were to end life, rather than simply to relieve pain or symptoms with the foreseeable risk of hastening death) accounted for another 17.5 percent; active euthanasia at the patient's request (excluding the previous category) accounted for 1.8 percent; physician-assisted suicide (in which the patient, not physician, administers the drugs) covered 0.3 percent. Finally there was a category of "life-terminating events without explicit and persistent request" accounting for 0.8 percent. In more than half of these cases, the patient had expressed a desire for euthanasia previously, but was no longer able to communicate by the time a decision had to be made and effectuated.

Women predominated in all of these categories except for the two rarest, but not by a great deal.[55] Thus, the ratio of females to males is 52:48 for euthanasia,[56] the same for death from drugs for pain and symptomatic relief, and 55:45 for non-treatment decisions.[57] This is against a background ratio of 48:52 for all deaths in the Netherlands.[58] However, in the much smaller categories of physician-assisted suicide and "life-terminating events without explicit and persistent request," men predominated by 68:32 and 65:35 respectively.[59] Why would men predominate in these two categories? In the case of physician-assisted suicide, the researchers suggest that we are talking about younger, urbanized males who have adopted a more demanding style as patients[60] and may be seeking control.[61] Perhaps women, in contrast, are more often surrendering to their fate and relinquishing control to the physicians whom they ask to take their lives. Unfortunately, the researchers do not venture an explanation of why males predominate in the category of people who die from "life-terminating events without explicit and persistent request." This is numerically the smallest category and one that should not occur at all under the Dutch guidelines because these are not contemporaneously competent patients articulating a request. Thus the numbers may be particularly unreliable here, if there is reluctance to report this illicit activity. Finally, the researchers report that more males than females made requests for physician-assisted suicide and euthanasia that physicians refused (55:45).[62]

What can we learn from the Dutch data that is relevant to the United States? There are causes for caution in making the cross-cultural comparison. There may be fewer reasons to expect a gender difference in the Dutch practices of euthanasia and physician-assisted suicide (as we would define these terms, that is, including the administration of drugs for pain relief and palliation, when the physician's purpose is to end life). First, the Netherlands provides universal health care coverage, while the United States's failure to provide universal coverage and tolerance of a two-tier health care system differentially disadvantages women (and other historically oppressed groups), leaving them with fewer means to cope with serious illness and more reason to consider seeking death. Second, the Netherlands presents greater homogeneity in race and ethnicity.[63] Again, this means that the United States presents more opportunities for and history of oppression based on difference. Third, we have to wonder whether elderly women in the United States face more difficulties and thus more reason to consider physician-assisted suicide and euthanasia than those in the Netherlands. A significant number in the United States confront lack of financial resources and difficulties associated with the absence of universal health coverage. Older women in the United States may also find themselves disvalued. "[T]here is evidence that the decision to kill oneself is viewed as most 'understandable' when it is made by an older women."[64] Finally, it is worth speculating whether gender dynamics differ in the Netherlands.

Apart from that speculation, the differences in Dutch demographics and health care would be reasons to expect no gender differential in the Netherlands in the practices we are examining. The fact that we nonetheless see something of a gender difference in the case of most deaths intentionally caused by a physician at the patient's request should heighten our concern about gender differences in the United States. Given the general illegality of euthanasia and physician-assisted suicide currently in this country, decent data would be difficult to gather. Yet there seems to be reason to attend to gender in what studies we can do, and in our analysis of these problems. Studies planned for Oregon, the one American jurisdiction to legalize physician-assisted suicide so far, should surely investigate gender.

Attending to gender in the data available for the Netherlands, in the images animating the American debate, and in the cases yielding those images thus suggests that our customarily gender-neutral arguments about the merits of physician-assisted suicide and euthanasia miss much of the point. Though one can certainly conceive of a gender-neutral practice, that may be far from what we have, at least in the United States, with our history and inequalities.

Equally troubling, our failure thus far to attend to gender in debating these practices may represent more than mere oversight. It may be a product of the same deep-rooted sexism that makes the self-destruction of women in Greek tragedy seem somehow natural and right. Indeed, there is something systematic in our current submerging of gender. The details left out of the usual account of a case of assisted suicide or euthanasia—what failures of relationship, context, and resources have brought the woman to this point; precisely why death seems to her the best remaining option; what elements of self-sacrifice motivate her choice—are exactly the kind of details that might make the workings of gender visible.

They are also the kind of details that might make the workings of race, ethnicity, and insurance status visible as well. The sort of gender analysis that I have pursued here should also provoke us to other analyses of the role played by these other factors. To focus here on just the first of these, there is a long history of racism in medicine in this country as vividly demonstrated by the horrors of the Tuskegee Syphilis Study.[65] We now are seeing new studies showing a correlation between race and access to cardiac procedures, for instance.[66] Although analysis of the meaning of these correlations is in progress, we have ample reason to be concerned, to examine the dynamic at work between patients of color and their physicians, and to be wary of expanding the physician's arsenal so that he or she may directly take the patient's life.

This sort of analysis will have to be detailed and specific, whether exploring gender, race, or another historic basis for subordination. The cultural meaning, history, and medical profession's use of each of those categories is specific, even though we can expect commonalities. The analysis will also have to pay close attention to the intersection, when a patient presents multiple characteristics that have historically occasioned discrimination and disadvantage.[67] How all of these categories function in the context of physician-assisted suicide and euthanasia will bear careful examination.

Probably the category of gender is the one we actually know most about in that context. At least we have the most obvious clues about that category, thanks to the gendered nature of the imagery. We would be foolish not to pursue those clues. Indeed, given grounds for concern that physician-assisted suicide and euthanasia may work in different and troubling ways when the patient is a woman, we are compelled to investigate gender.

Feminism and the Arguments

Shifting from the images and stories that animate debate and the dynamics operating in practice to analysis of the arguments over physician-assisted suicide and euthanasia takes us further into the concerns of feminist theory. Arguments in favor of these practices have often depended on rights claims. More recently, some authors have grounded their arguments instead on ethical concepts of caring. Yet both argumentative strategies have been flawed in ways that feminist work can illuminate. What is missing is an analysis that integrates notions of physician caring with principled boundaries to physician action, while also attending to the patient's broader context and the community's wider concerns. Such an analysis would pay careful attention to the dangers posed by these practices to the historically most vulnerable populations, including women.

Advocacy of physician-assisted suicide and euthanasia has hinged to a great extent on rights claims. The argument is that the patient has a right of self-determination or autonomy that entitles her to assistance in suicide or euthanasia. The strategy is to extend the argument that self-determination entitles the patient to refuse unwanted life-sustaining treatment by maintaining that the same rationale supports patient entitlement to more active physician assistance in death. Indeed, it is sometimes argued that there is no principled difference between termination of life-sustaining treatment and the more active practices.

The narrowness and mechanical quality of this rights thinking, however, is shown by its application to the stories recounted above. That application suggests that the physicians in these stories are dealing with a simple equation: given an eligible rights bearer and her assertion of the right, the correct result is death. What makes a person an eligible rights bearer? Kevorkian seems to require neither a terminal disease nor thorough evaluation of whether the patient has non-fatal alternatives. Indeed, the Wantz case shows he does not even require a diagnosis. Nor does the Oregon physician-assisted suicide statute require evaluation or exhaustion of non-fatal alternatives; a patient could be driven by untreated pain, and still receive physician-assisted suicide. And what counts as an assertion of the right? For Debbie's doctor, merely "Let's get this over with." Disease plus demand requires death.

Such a rights approach raises a number of problems that feminist theory has illuminated. I should note that overlapping critiques of rights have been offered by Critical Legal Studies,[68] Critical Race Theory,[69] and some communitarian theory.[70] Thus some of these points would be echoed by those critiques.[71] Yet as will be seen, feminist theory offers ways to ground evaluation of rights and rights talk[72] in the experiences of women.

In particular, feminist critiques suggest three different sorts of problems with the rights equation

offered to justify physician-assisted suicide and euthanasia. First, it ignores context, both the patient's present context and her history. The prior and surrounding failures in her intimate relationships, in her resources to cope with illness and pain, and even in the adequacy of care being offered by the very same physician fade into invisibility next to the bright light of a rights bearer and her demand. In fact, her choices may be severely constrained. Some of those constraints may even be alterable or removable. Yet attention to those dimensions of decision is discouraged by the absolutism of the equation: either she is an eligible rights bearer or not; either she has asserted her right or not. There is no room for conceding her competence and request, yet querying whether under all the circumstances her choices are so constrained and alternatives so unexplored that acceding to the request may not be the proper course. Stark examples are provided by cases in which pain or symptomatic discomfort drives a person to request assisted suicide or euthanasia, yet the pain or discomfort is treatable. A number of Kevorkian's cases raise the problem as well: Did Janet Adkins ever receive psychological support for the predictable despair and desire to die that follow dire diagnoses such as Alzheimer's? Would the cause of Marjorie Wantz's undiagnosed pelvic pain have been ascertainable and even ameliorable at a better health center? In circumstances in which women and others who have traditionally lacked resources and experienced oppression are likely to have fewer options and a tougher time getting good care, mechanical application of the rights equation will authorize their deaths even when less drastic alternatives are or should be available. It will wrongly assume that all face serious illness and disability with the resources of the idealized rights bearer—a person of means untroubled by oppression. The realities of women and others whose circumstances are far from that abstraction's will be ignored.

Second, in ignoring context and relationship, the rights equation extols the vision of a rights bearer as an isolated monad and denigrates actual dependencies. Thus it may be seen as improper to ask what family, social, economic, and medical supports she is or is not getting; this insults her individual self-governance. Nor may it be seen as proper to investigate alternatives to acceding to her request for death; this too dilutes self-rule. Yet feminists have reminded us of the actual embeddedness of persons and the descriptive falseness of a vision of each as an isolated individual.[73] In addition, they have argued normatively that a society comprised of isolated individuals, without the pervasive connections and dependencies that we see, would be undesirable.[74] Indeed, the very meaning of the patient's request for death is socially constructed; that is the point of the prior section's review of the images animating the debate. If we construe the patient's request as a rights bearer's assertion of a right and deem that sufficient grounds on which the physician may proceed, it is because we choose to regard background failures as irrelevant even if they are differentially motivating the requests of the most vulnerable. We thereby avoid real scrutiny of the social arrangements, governmental failures, and health coverage exclusions that may underlie these requests. We also ignore the fact that these patients may be seeking improved circumstances more than death. We elect a myopia that makes the patient's request and death seem proper. We construct a story that clothes the patient's terrible despair in the glorious mantle of "rights."

Formulaic application of the rights equation in this realm thus exalts an Enlightenment vision of autonomy as self-governance and the exclusion of interfering others. Yet as feminists such as Jennifer Nedelsky have argued, this is not the only vision of autonomy available.[75] She argues that a superior vision of autonomy is to be found by rejecting "the pathological conception of autonomy as boundaries against others," a conception that takes the exclusion of others from one's property as its central symbol. Instead, "if we ask ourselves what actually enables people to be autonomous, the answer is not isolation but relationships ... that provide the support and guidance necessary for the development and experience of autonomy." Nedelsky thus proposes that the best "metaphor for autonomy is not property but childrearing. There we have encapsulated the emergence of autonomy through relationship with others."[76] Martha Minow, too, presents a vision of autonomy that resists the isolation of the self, and instead tries to support the relational context in which the rights bearer is embedded.[77] Neither author counsels abandonment of autonomy and rights. But they propose fundamental revisions that would rule out the mechanical application of a narrow rights equation that would regard disease or disability, coupled with demand, as adequate warrant for death.[78]

In fact, there are substantial problems with grounding advocacy for the specific practices of physician-assisted suicide and euthanasia in a rights analysis, even if one accepts the general importance of rights and self-determination. I have elsewhere argued repeatedly for an absolute or near-absolute moral and legal right to be free of unwanted life-sustaining treatment.[79] Yet the negative right to be free of unwanted bodily invasion does not imply an affirmative right to obtain bodily invasion (or assistance with bodily invasion) for the purpose of ending your own life.

Moreover, the former right is clearly grounded in fundamental entitlements to liberty, bodily privacy, and freedom from unconsented touching; in contrast there is no clear "right" to kill yourself or be killed. Suicide has been widely decriminalized, but decriminalizing an act does not mean that you have a positive right to do it and to command the help of others. Indeed, if a friend were to tell me that she wished to kill herself, I would not be lauded for giving her the tools. In fact, that act of assistance has *not* been decriminalized. That continued condemnation shows that whatever my friend's relation to the act of suicide (a "liberty," "right," or neither), it does not create a right in her sufficient to command or even permit my aid.

There are even less grounds for concluding that there is a right to be killed deliberately on request, that is, for euthanasia. There are reasons why a victim's consent has traditionally been no defense to an accusation of homicide. One reason is suggested by analogy to Mill's famous argument that one cannot consent to one's own enslavement: "The reason for not interfering ... with a person's voluntary acts, is consideration for his liberty.... But by selling himself for a slave, he abdicates his liberty; he foregoes any future use of it...."[80] Similarly, acceding to a patient's request to be killed wipes out the possibility of her future exercise of her liberty. The capacity to command or permit another to take your life deliberately, then, would seem beyond the bounds of those things to which you have a right grounded in notions of liberty. We lack the capacity to bless another's enslavement of us or direct killing of us. How is this compatible then with a right to refuse life-sustaining treatment? That right is not grounded in any so-called "right to die," however frequently the phrase appears in the general press.[81] Instead, it is grounded in rights to be free of unwanted bodily invasion, rights so fundamental that they prevail even when the foreseeable consequence is likely to be death.

Finally, the rights argument in favor of physician-assisted suicide and euthanasia confuses two separate questions: what the patient may do, and what the physician may do. After all, the real question in these debates is not what patients may request or even do. It is not at all infrequent for patients to talk about suicide and request assurance that the physician will help or actively bring on death when the patient wants;[82] that is an expected part of reaction to serious disease and discomfort. The real question is what the doctor may do in response to this predictable occurrence. That question is not answered by talk of what patients may ask; patients may and should be encouraged to reveal everything on their minds. Nor is it answered by the fact that decriminalization of suicide permits the patient to take her own life. The physician and patient are separate moral agents. Those who assert that what a patient may say or do determines the same for the physician, ignore the physician's separate moral and legal agency. They also ignore the fact that she is a professional, bound to act in keeping with a professional role and obligations. They thereby avoid a necessary argument over whether the historic obligations of the physician to "do no harm" and "give no deadly drug even if asked" should be abandoned.[83] Assertion of what the patient may do does not resolve that argument.

The inadequacy of rights arguments to legitimate physician-assisted suicide and euthanasia has led to a different approach, grounded on physicians' duties of beneficence. This might seem to be quite in keeping with feminists' development of an ethics of care.[84] Yet the beneficence argument in the euthana-

sia context is a strange one, because it asserts that the physician's obligation to relieve suffering permits or even commands her to annihilate the person who is experiencing the suffering. Indeed, at the end of this act of beneficence, no patient is left to experience its supposed benefits. Moreover, this argument ignores widespread agreement that fears of patient addiction in these cases should be discarded, physicians may sedate to unconsciousness, and the principle of double effect permits giving pain relief and palliative care in doses that risk inducing respiratory depression and thereby hastening death. Given all of that, it is far from clear what patients remain in the category of those whose pain or discomfort can only be relieved by killing them.

Thus this argument that a physician should provide so much "care" that she kills the patient is deeply flawed. A more sophisticated version, however, is offered by Howard Brody.[85] He acknowledges that both the usual rights arguments and traditional beneficence arguments have failed. Thus he claims to find a middle path. He advocates legitimation of physician-assisted suicide and euthanasia "as a compassionate response to one sort of medical failure," namely, medical failure to prolong life, restore function, or provide effective palliation. Even in such cases, he does not advocate the creation of a rule providing outright legalization. Instead, "compassionate and competent medical practice" should serve as a defense in a criminal proceeding.[86] Panels should review the practice case by case; a positive review should discourage prosecution.

There are elements of Brody's proposal that seem quite in keeping with much feminist work: his rejection of a binary either-or analysis, his skepticism that a broad rule will yield a proper resolution, his requirement instead of a case-by-case approach. Moreover, the centrality that he accords to "compassion" again echoes feminist work on an ethics of care. Yet ultimately he offers no real arguments for extending compassion to the point of killing a patient, for altering the traditional boundaries of medical practice, or for ignoring the fears that any legitimation of these practices will start us down a slippery slope leading to bad consequences. Brody's is more the proposal of a procedure—what he calls "not resolution but adjudication," following philosopher Hilary Putnam—than it is a true answer to the moral and legal quandaries.

What Brody's analysis does accomplish, however, is that it suggests that attention to method is a necessary, if not sufficient, part of solving the euthanasia problem. Thus we find that two of the most important current debates in bioethics are linked—the debate over euthanasia and the debate over the proper structure of bioethical analysis and method.[87] The inadequacies of rights arguments to establish patient entitlement to assisted suicide and euthanasia are linked to the inadequacies of a "top-down" or deductive bioethics driven by principles, abstract theories, or rules. They share certain flaws: both seem overly to ignore context and the nuances of cases; their simple abstractions overlook real power differentials in society and historic subordination; and they avoid the fact that these principles, rules, abstractions, and rights are themselves a product of historically oppressive social arrangements. Similarly, the inadequacies of beneficence and compassion arguments are linked to some of the problems with a "bottom-up" or inductive bioethics built on cases, ethnography and detailed description. In both instances it is difficult to see where the normative boundaries lie, and where to get a normative keel for the finely described ship.

What does feminism have to offer these debates? Feminists too have struggled extensively with the question of method, with how to integrate detailed attention to individual cases with rights, justice, and principles. Thus in criticizing Kohlberg and going beyond his vision of moral development, Carol Gilligan argued that human beings should be able to utilize both an ethics of justice and an ethics of care. "To understand how the tension between responsibilities and rights sustains the dialectic of human development is to see the integrity of two disparate modes of experience that are in the end connected.... In the representation of maturity both perspectives converge...."[88] What was less clear was precisely how the two should fit together. And unfortunately for our purposes, Gilligan never took up Kohlberg's mercy killing case to illuminate a care perspective or even more importantly how the two perspectives might properly be interwoven in that case.

That finally, I would suggest, is the question. Here we must look to those feminist scholars who have struggled directly with how the two perspectives might fit. Lawrence Blum has distinguished eight different positions that one might take, and that scholars have taken, on "the relation between impartial morality and morality of care":[89] (1) acting on care is just acting on complicated moral principles; (2) care is mot moral but personal; (3) care is moral but secondary to principle and generally adds mere refinements or supererogatory opportunities; (4) principle supplies a superior basis for moral action by ensuring consistency; (5) care morality concerns evaluation of persons while principles concern evaluation of acts; (6) principles set outer boundaries within which care can operate; (7) the preferability of a care perspective in some circumstances must be justified by reasoning from principles; and (8) care and justice must be integrated. Many others have struggled with the relationship between the two perspectives as well.

Despite this complexity, the core insight is forthrightly stated by Owen Flanagan and Kathryn Jackson: "[T]he most defensible specification of the moral domain will include issues of both right and good."[90] Martha Minow and Elizabeth Spelman go further. Exploring the axis of abstraction versus context, they argue against dichotomizing the two and in favor of recognizing their "constant interactions."[91] Indeed, they maintain that a dichotomy misdescribes the workings of context. "[C]ontextualists do not merely address each situation as a unique one with no relevance for the next one.... The basic norm of fairness—treat like cases alike—is fulfilled, not undermined, by attention to what particular traits make one case like, or unlike, another."[92] Similarly, "[w]hen a rule specifies a context, it does not undermine the commitment to universal application to the context specified; it merely identifies the situations to be covered by the rule."[93] If this kind of integration is available, then why do we hear such urgent pleas for attention to context? "[T]he call to context in the late twentieth century reflects a critical argument that prevailing legal and political norms have used the form of abstract, general, and universal prescriptions while neglecting the experiences and needs of women of all races and classes, people of color, and people without wealth."[94]

Here we find the beginning of an answer to our dilemma. It appears that we must attend to both context and abstraction, peering through the lenses of both care and justice. Yet our approach to each will be affected by its mate. Our apprehension and understanding of context or cases inevitably involves categories, while our categories and principles should be refined over time to apply to some contexts and not others.[95] Similarly, our understanding of what caring requires in a particular case will grow in part from our understanding of what sort of case this is and what limits principles set to our expressions of caring; while our principles should be scrutinized and amended according to their impact on real lives, especially the lives of those historically excluded from the process of generating principles.[96]

This last point is crucial and a distinctive feminist contribution to the debate over abstraction versus context, or in bioethics, principles versus cases. Various voices in the bioethics debate over method—be they advocating casuistry, specified principlism, principlism itself, or some other position—present various solutions to the question of how cases and principles or other higher-order abstractions should interconnect. Feminist writers too have substantive solutions to offer, as I have suggested. But feminists also urge something that the mainstream writers on bioethics method have overlooked altogether, namely the need to use cases and context to reveal the systematic biases such as sexism and racism built into the principles or other abstractions themselves. Those biases will rarely be explicit in a principle. Instead, we will frequently have to look at how the principle operates in actual cases, what it presupposes (such as wealth or life options), and what it ignores (such as preexisting sexism or racism among the very health care professionals meant to apply it).[97]

What, then, does all of this counsel in application to the debate over physician-assisted suicide and euthanasia? This debate cannot demand a choice between abstract rules or principles and physician caring. Although the debate has sometimes been framed that way, it is difficult to imagine a practice of medicine founded on one to the exclusion of the

other. Few would deny that physician beneficence and caring for the individual patient are essential. Indeed, they are constitutive parts of the practice of medicine as it has come to us through the centuries and aims to function today. Yet that caring cannot be unbounded. A physician cannot be free to do whatever caring for or empathy with the patient seems to urge in the moment. Physicians practice a profession with standards and limits, in the context of a democratic polity that itself imposes further limits.[98] These considerations have led the few who have begun to explore an ethics of care for physicians to argue that the notion of care in that context must be carefully delimited and distinct from the more general caring of a parent for a child (although there are limits, too, on what a caring parent may do).[99] Physicians must pursue what I will call "principled caring."

This notion of principled caring captures the need for limits and standards, whether technically stated as principles or some other form of generalization. Those principles or generalizations will articulate limits and obligations in a provisional way, subject to reconsideration and possible amendment in light of actual cases. Both individual cases and patterns of cases may specifically reveal that generalizations we have embraced are infected by sexism or other bias, either as those generalizations are formulated or as they function in the world. Indeed, given that both medicine and bioethics are cultural practices in a society riddled by such bias and that we have only begun to look carefully for such bias in our bioethical principles and practices, we should expect to find it.

Against this background, arguments for physician-assisted suicide and euthanasia—whether grounded on rights or beneficence—are automatically suspect when they fail to attend to the vulnerability of women and other groups. If our cases, cultural images, and perhaps practice differentially feature the deaths of women, we cannot ignore that. It is one thing to argue for these practices for the patient who is not so vulnerable, the wealthy white male living on Park Avenue in Manhattan who wants to add yet another means of control to his arsenal. It is quite another to suggest that the woman of color with no health care coverage or continuous physician relationship, who is given a dire diagnosis in the city hospital's emergency room, needs then to be offered direct killing.

To institute physician-assisted suicide and euthanasia at this point in this country—in which many millions are denied the resources to cope with serious illness, in which pain relief and palliative care are by all accounts woefully mishandled, and in which we have a long way to go to make proclaimed rights to refuse life-sustaining treatment and to make advance directives working realities in clinical settings—seems, at the very least, to be premature. Were we actually to fix those other problems, we have no idea what demand would remain for these more drastic practices and in what category of patients. We know for example, that the remaining category is likely to include very few, if any, patients in pain, once inappropriate fears of addiction, reluctance to sedate to unconsciousness, and confusion over the principle of double effect are overcome.

Yet against those background conditions, legitimating the practices is more than just premature. It is a danger to women. Those background conditions pose special problems for them. Women in this country are differentially poorer, more likely to be either uninsured or on government entitlement programs, more likely to be alone in their old age, and more susceptible to depression. Those facts alone would spell danger. But when you combine them with the long (indeed, ancient) history of legitimating the sacrifice and self-sacrifice of women, the danger intensifies. That history suggests that a woman requesting assisted suicide or euthanasia is likely to be seen as doing the "right" thing. She will fit into unspoken cultural stereotypes.[100] She may even be valorized for appropriate feminine self-sacrificing behavior, such as sparing her family further burden or the sight of an unaesthetic deterioration. Thus she may be subtly encouraged to seek death. At the least, her physician may have a difficult time seeing past the legitimating stereotypes and valorization to explore what is really going on with this particular patient, why she is so desperate, and what can be done about it. If many more patients in the Netherlands ask about assisted suicide and euthanasia than go through with it,[101] and if such inquiry is a routine part of any patient's responding to a dire diagnosis or improperly managed symptoms and pain, then were

the practices to be legitimated in the United States, we would expect to see a large group of patients inquiring. Yet given the differential impact of background conditions in the United States by gender and the legitimating stereotypes of women's deaths, we should also expect to see what has been urged as a neutral practice show marked gender effects.

Is it possible to erect a practice that avoids this? No one has yet explained how. A recent article advocating the legitimation of physician-assisted suicide, for example, acknowledges the need to protect the vulnerable (though it never lists women among them).[102] But none of the seven criteria it proposes to guide the practice involves deeply inquiring into the patient's life circumstances, whether she is alone, or whether she has health care coverage. Nor do the criteria require the physician to examine whether gender or other stereotypes are figuring in the physician's response to the patient's request. And the article fails to acknowledge the vast inequities and pervasive bias in social institutions that are the background for the whole problem. There is nothing in the piece that requires we remedy or even lessen those problems before these fatal practices begin.

The required interweaving of principles and caring, combined with attention to the heightened vulnerability of women and others, suggests that the right answer to the debate over legitimating these practices is at least "not yet" in this grossly imperfect society and perhaps a flat "no." Beneficence and caring indeed impose positive duties upon physicians, especially with patients who are suffering, despairing, or in pain. Physicians must work with these patients intensively; provide first-rate pain relief, palliative care, and symptomatic relief; and honor patients' exercise of their rights to refuse life-sustaining treatment and use advance directives. Never should the patient's illness, deterioration, or despair occasion physician abandonment. Whatever concerns the patient has should be heard and explored, including thoughts of suicide, or requests for aid or euthanasia.

Such requests should redouble the physician's efforts, prompt consultation with those more expert in pain relief or supportive care, suggest exploration of the details of the patient's circumstance, and a host of other efforts. What such requests should not do is prompt our collective legitimation of the physician's saying "yes" and actively taking the patient's life. The mandates of caring fail to bless killing the person for whom one cares. Any such practice in the United States will inevitably reflect enormous background inequities and persisting societal biases. And there are special reasons to expect gender bias to play a role.

The principles bounding medical practice are not written in stone. They are subject to reconsideration and societal renegotiation over time. Thus the ancient prohibitions against physicians assisting suicide and performing euthanasia do not magically defeat proposals for change. (Nor do mere assertions that "patients want it" mandate change, as I have argued above.)[103] But we ought to have compelling reasons for changing something as serious as the limits on physician killing, and to be rather confident that change will not mire physicians in a practice that is finally untenable.

By situating assisted suicide and euthanasia in a history of women's deaths, by suggesting the social meanings that over time have attached to and justified women's deaths, by revealing the background conditions that may motivate women's requests, and by stating the obvious—that medicine does not somehow sit outside society, exempt from all of this—I have argued that we cannot have that confidence. Moreover, in the real society in which we live, with its actual and for some groups fearful history, there are compelling reasons not to allow doctors to kill. We cannot ignore that such practice would allow what for now remains an elite and predominantly male profession to take the lives of the "other." We cannot explain how we will train the young physician both to care for the patient through difficult straits and to kill. We cannot protect the most vulnerable.

Conclusion

Some will find it puzzling that elsewhere we seek to have women's voices heard and moral agency respected, yet here I am urging that physicians not accede to the request for assisted suicide and euthanasia. Indeed, as noted above, I have elsewhere maintained that physicians must honor patients' requests to be free of unwanted life-sustaining treatment. In fact, attention to gender and feminist argument would urge some caution in both realms. As Jay Katz has suggested, any patient request or decision of consequence merits conversation and exploration.[104] And analysis by Steven Miles and Alison August suggests that gender bias may be operating in the realm of the termination of life-sustaining treatment too.[105] Yet finally there is a difference between the two domains. As I have argued above, there is a strong right to be free of unwanted bodily invasion. Indeed, for women, a long history of being harmed specifically through unwanted bodily invasion such as rape presents particularly compelling reasons for honoring a woman's refusal of invasion and effort to maintain bodily intactness. When it comes to the question of whether women's suicides should be aided, however, or whether women should be actively killed, there is no right to command physician assistance, the dangers of permitting assistance are immense, and the history of women's subordination cuts the other way. Women have historically been seen as fit objects for bodily invasion, self-sacrifice, and death at the hands of others. The task before us is to challenge all three.[106]

Certainly some women, including some feminists, will see this problem differently. That may be especially true of women who feel in control of their lives, are less subject to subordination by age or race or wealth, and seek yet another option to add to their many. I am not arguing that women should lose control of their lives and selves. Instead, I am arguing that when women request to be put to death or ask help in taking their own lives, they become part of a broader social dynamic of which we have properly learned to be extremely wary. These are fatal practices. We can no longer ignore questions of gender or the insights of feminist argument.

Author's Notes

My thanks to Arthur Applbaum, Larry Blum, Alta Charo, Norman Daniels, Johannes J.M. van Delden, Rebecca Dresser, Jorge Garcia, Henk ten Have, Warren Kearney, Elizabeth Kiss, Steven Miles, Christine Mitchell, Remco Oostendorp, Lynn Peterson, Dennis Thompson, and Alan Wertheimer for help at various stages, to the *Texas Journal on Women and the Law* at the University of Texas Law School for the opportunity to elicit comments on an earlier version, and to participants in the University of Minnesota Law School Faculty Workshop for valuable suggestions. Kent Spies and Terrence Dwyer of the University of Minnesota Law School provided important research assistance. Work on this chapter was supported in part by a Fellowship in the Program in Ethics and the Professions at Harvard University.

Notes

1   See, for example, Pamela Carroll, "Proponents of Physician-Assisted Suicide Continuing Efforts," *ACP Observer*, February 1992, p. 29 (describing state initiatives in Washington, California, Michigan, New Hampshire, and Oregon). Subsequently, Oregon voters made that state the first to legalize physician-assisted suicide. See 1995 Oregon Laws, Ch. 3, I. M. No. 16. But see also Lee V. Oregon, 869 F. Suppl. 1491. (DOOR. 1994), entering an injunction preventing the statute from going into effect. Further legal proceedings will decide the statute's fate. For attempts to legalize physician-assisted suicide through litigation, see Compassion in Dying v. Washington, 850 F. Supp. 1454 (W.D. Wash. 1994), *rev'd*, 49 F. 3d 586 (9th Cir. 1995); Quill v. Koppel, 870 F. Supp. 78 (S. D.N.Y., 1994). See also Hobbins v. Attorney General, 527 N. W. 2d 714 (Mich. 1994).

2   See, for example, Howard Brody, "Assisted Death—A Compassionate Response to a Medical Failure," *New England Journal of Medicine* 327 (1992): 1384-88; Timothy E. Quill, Christine K. Cassel, and Diane E. Meier, "Care of the Hopelessly Ill: Proposed Clinical Criteria for Physician-Assisted Suicide," *New England Journal of Medicine* 327 (1992): 1380-84; Guy I. Benrubi, "Euthanasia—The Need for Procedural Safeguards," *New England Journal of Medicine* 326 (1992): 197-99; Christine K. Cassel and Diane E. Meier, "Morals and Moralism in the Debate Over Euthanasia and Assisted Suicide," *New England Journal of Medicine* 323 (1990): 750-52; James Rachels, *The End of Life* (Oxford, England: Oxford University Press, 1986).

3   I restrict the term "euthanasia" to active euthanasia, excluding the termination of life-sustaining treatment, which has sometimes been called "passive euthanasia." Both law and ethics now treat the termination of treatment quite differently from the way they treat active euthanasia, so to use "euthanasia" to refer to both invites confusion. See generally "Report of the Council on Ethical and Judicial Affairs of the American Medical Association," *Issues in Law & Medicine* 10 (1994): 91-97, 92.

4   See Howard I. Kushner, "Women and Suicide in Historical Perspective," in Joyce McCarl Nielsen, ed., *Feminist Research Methods: Exemplary Readings in the Social Sciences* (Boulder, CO: Westview Press, 1990), 193-206, 198-200.

5   See Alan Meisel, *The Right to Die* (New York, NY: John Wiley & Sons, 1989), 62, & *1993 Cumulative Supplement* No. 2, 50-54.

6   See Council on Ethical and Judicial Affairs, Code of Medical Ethics: Current Opinions with Annotations (Chicago, IL: American Medical Association, 1994): 50-51; "Report of the Board of Trustees of the American Medical Association," *Issues in Law & Medicine* 10 (1994): 81-90; "Report of the Council on Ethical and Judicial Affairs," Report of the Council on Ethical and Judicial Affairs of the American Medical Association: Euthanasia (Chicago, IL: American Medical Association, 1989). There are U.S. data on public opinion and physicians' self-reported practices. See, for example, "Report of the Board of Trustees." But the legal and ethical condemnation of physician-assisted suicide and euthanasia in the United States undoubtedly affect the self-reporting and render this a poor indicator of actual practices.

7   See Nancy S. Jecker, "Physician-Assisted Death in the Netherlands and the United States: Ethical and Cultural Aspects of Health Policy Development," *Journal of the American Geriatrics Society* 42 (1994): 672-78, 676.

8   See generally Howard I. Kushner, "Women and Suicidal Behavior: Epidemiology, Gender, and Lethality in Historical Perspective," in Silvia Sara Canetto and David Lester, eds., *Women and Suicidal Behavior* (New York, NY: Springer, 1995).

9   Compare Jecker, "Physician-Assisted Death," 676, on reasons physicians might differentially refuse women's requests.

10 See Lawrence Kohlberg, *The Philosophy of Moral Development: Moral Stages and the Idea of Justice*, vol. I (San Francisco, CA: Harper & Row, 1981);

Lawrence Kohlberg, *The Psychology of Moral Development: The Nature and Validity of Moral Stages*, vol. II (San Francisco, CA: Harper & Row 1984).

11   See Carol Gilligan, *In a Different Voice: Psychological Theory and Women's Development* (Cambridge, MA: Harvard University Press, 1982).

12   Gilligan's work has prompted a large literature, building upon as well as criticizing her insights and methodology. See, for example, the essays collected in Larrabee, ed., *An Ethic of Care*. On attention to the ethics of care in bioethics and on feminist criticism of the ethics of care, see my Introduction to this volume [*Feminism and Bioethics*].

13   See Kohlberg, *The Psychology of Moral Development*, 644-47.

14   On the Kohlberg-Gilligan debate, see generally Lawrence A. Blum, "Gilligan and Kohlberg: Implications for Moral Theory" in Larrabee, ed., *An Ethic of Care*, 49-68; Owen Flanagan and Kathryn Jackson, "Justice, Care, and Gender: The Kohlberg-Gilligan Debate Revisited," in Larrabee, ed., *An Ethic of Care*, 69-84; Seyla Benhabib, "The Generalized and the Concrete Other: The Kohlberg-Gilligan Controversy and Feminist Theory," in Seyla Benhabib and Drucilla Cornell, eds., *Feminism as Critique: On the Politics of Gender* (Minneapolis, MN: University of Minnesota Press, 1987), 77-95.

15   See, for example, Susan M. Wolf, "Holding the Line on Euthanasia," *Hastings Center Report* 19 (Jan./Feb. 1989): special supp. 13-15.

16   See "It's Over, Debbie," *Journal of the American Medical Association* 259 (1988): 272.

17   See Timothy Egan, "As Memory and Music Faded, Oregon Woman Chose Death," *New York Times*, June 7, 1990, p. A1; Lisa Belkin, "Doctor Tells of First Death Using His Suicide Device," *New York Times*, June 6, 1990, p. A1.

18   See "Doctor Assists in Two More Suicides in Michigan," *New York Times*, October 24, 1991, p. A1 (Wantz and Miller).

19   See "Death at Kevorkian's Side Is Ruled Homicide," *New York Times*, June 6, 1992, p. 10; "Doctor Assists in Another Suicide," *New York Times*, September 27, 1992, p. 32; "Doctor in Michigan Helps a 6th Person to Commit Suicide," *New York Times*, November 24, 1992, p. A10; "2 Commit Suicide, Aided by Michigan Doctor," *New York Times*, December 16, 1992, p. A21.

20   See "Why Dr. Kevorkian Was Called In," *New York Times*, January 25, 1993, p. A16.

21   See B.D. Colen, "Gender Question in Assisted Suicides," *Newsday*, November 25, 1992, p. 17; Ellen Goodman, "Act Now to Stop Dr. Death," *Atlanta Journal and Constitution*, May 27, 1992, p. A11.

22   See Timothy E. Quill, "Death and Dignity—A Case of Individualized Decision Making," *New England Journal of Medicine* 324 (1991): 691-94.

23   On Quill's motivations, see Timothy E. Quill, "The Ambiguity of Clinical Intentions," *New England Journal of Medicine* 329 (1993): 1039-40.

24   Nicole Loraux, *Tragic Ways of Killing a Woman*, Anthony Forster, trans. (Cambridge, MA: Harvard University Press, 1987), 8.

25   *Ibid.*, 12.

26   *Ibid.*, 23.

27   *Ibid.*, 11.

28   Kushner, "Women and Suicidal Behavior," 16-17 (citations omitted).

29   Kushner, "Women and Suicide in Historical Perspective," 195, citing Barbara Welter, "The Cult of True Womanhood: 1820-1860," *American Quarterly* 18 (1966): 151-55.

30   *Ibid.*, 13-19.

31   Gilligan, *In a Different Voice*, 70.

32   *Ibid.*, 132.

33   Loraux in *Tragic Ways of Killing a Woman* notes the single exception of Ajax.

34   See Peter Steinfels, "Help for the Helping Hands in Death," *New York Times*, February 14, 1993, sec. 4, pp. 1, 6.

35   See Charles S. Cleeland et al., "Pain and Its Treatment in Outpatients with Metastatic Cancer," *New England Journal of Medicine* 330 (1994): 592-96.

36   See Robert J. Blendon, U.S. Szalay, and R.A. Knox, "Should Physicians Aid Their Patients in Dying?" *Journal of the American Medical Association* 267 (1992): 2658-62.

37   See William Coryell, Jean Endicott, and Martin B. Keller, "Major Depression in a Non-Clinical Sample: Demographic and Clinical Risk Factors for First Onset," *Archives of General Psychiatry* 49 (1992): 117-25.

38   See Susan D. Block and J. Andrew Billings, "Patient Requests to Hasten Death: Evaluation and Manage-

ment in Terminal Care," *Archives of Internal Medicine* 154 (1994): 2039-47.

39 Council on Ethical and Judicial Affairs, American Medical Association, "Gender Disparities in Clinical Decision Making," *Journal of the American Medical Association* 266 (1991): 559-62, 561-62.

40 See Nancy S. Jecker, "Can an Employer-Based Health Insurance System Be Just?" *Journal of Health Politics, Policy & Law* 18 (1993): 657-73; Employee Benefit Research Institute (EBRI), *Sources of Health Insurance and Characteristics of the Uninsured: Analysis of the March 1992 Current Population Survey*, EBRI Issue Brief No. 133 (Jan. 1993).

41 The patterns of uninsurance and underinsurance are complex. See, for example, Employee Benefit Resources Institute, *Sources of Health Insurance*. Recall that the poorest and the elderly are covered by Medicaid and Medicare, though they are subject to the gaps and deficiencies in quality of care that plague those programs.

42 Lawrence Schneiderman et al. purport to show that patients already consider burdens to others in making termination of treatment decisions, and—more importantly for this chapter—that men do so more than women. See Lawrence J. Schneiderman et al., "Attitudes of Seriously Ill Patients toward Treatment that Involves High Cost and Burdens on Others," *Journal of Clinical Ethics* 5 (1994): 109-12. But Peter A. Ubel and Robert M. Arnold criticize the methodology and dispute both conclusions in "The Euthanasia Debate and Empirical Evidence: Separating Burdens to Others from One's Own Quality of Life," *Journal of Clinical Ethics* 5 (1994): 155-58.

43 See, for example, Kushner, "Women and Suicidal Behavior."

44 See Colen, "Gender Question in Assisted Suicides."

45 Another area in which we do not allow apparent patient consent or request to authorize physician acquiescence is sex between doctor and patient. Even if the patient requests sex, the physician is morally and legally bound to refuse. The considerable consensus that now exists on this, however, has been the result of a difficult uphill battle. See generally Howard Brody, *The Healer's Power* (New Haven, CT: Yale University Press, 1992), 26-27; Nanette Gartrell et al., "Psychiatrist-Patient Sexual Contact: Results of a National Survey, Part 1. Preva-

lence," *American Journal of Psychiatry* 143 (1986): 1126-31.

46 As noted above, though, Nancy Jecker speculates that a physician's tendency to discount women's choices may also come into play. See Jecker, "Physician-Assisted Death," 676. Compare Silvia Sara Canetto, "Elderly Women and Suicidal Behavior," in Canetto and Lester, eds., *Women and Suicidal Behavior* 215-33, 228, asking whether physicians are more willing to accept women's suicides.

47 See, for example, Susan Sherwin, *No Longer Patient: Feminist Ethics and Health Care* (Philadelphia, PA: Temple University Press, 1992); Barbara Ehrenreich and Deirdre English, *For Her Own Good: 150 Years of the Experts' Advice to Women* (New York, NY: Doubleday, 1978).

48 Sherwin, *No Longer Patient*, 157.

49 Compare Brody "The Rescue Fantasy," in *The Healer's Art*, ch.9.

50 Robert A. Burt, *Taking Care of Strangers* (New York, NY: Free Press, 1979), vi. See also Steven H. Miles, "Physicians and Their Patients' Suicides," *Journal of the American Medical Association* 271 (1994): 1786-88. I discuss the significance of the ambivalence in the euthanasia context in Wolf, "Holding the Line on Euthanasia."

51 In an article advocating the legitimation of physician-assisted suicide, the authors nonetheless note the lack of good data on U.S. Practice: "From 3 to 37 percent of physicians responding to anonymous surveys reported secretly taking active steps to hasten a patient's death, but these survey data were flawed by low response rates and poor design." Quill, Cassel, and Meier, "Care of the Hopelessly Ill," 1381 (footnotes with citations omitted).

52 On relevant differences between the United States and the Netherlands, see Jecker, "Physician-Assisted Death: Report of the Board of Trustees"; Margaret Battin, "Voluntary Euthanasia and the Risks of Abuse: Can We Learn Anything from the Netherlands?" *Law, Medicine & Health Care* 20 (1992): 133-43.

53 There have been two major teams of researchers. The first, conducting research at governmental request, has produced publications including Loes Pijnenborg, Paul J. van der Maas, Johannes J.M. van Delden, and Caspar W.N. Looman, "Life-terminating

acts without explicit request of patient," *Lancet* 341 (1993): 1196-99. Paul J. van der Maas, Johannes J.M. van Delden, and Loes Pijnenborg, "Euthanasia and other medical decisions concerning the end of life: An investigation performed upon request of the Commission of Inquiry into the Medical Practice concerning Euthanasia," *Health Policy* 22 (1992): 1-262; and Paul J. van der Maas, Johannes J.M. van Delden, Loes Pijnenborg, and Caspar W.N. Looman, "Euthanasia and other medical decisions concerning the end of life," *Lancet* 338 (1991): 669-74. The second team's publications include G. van der Wal, J.T. van Eijk, H.J. Leenen, and C. Spreeuwenberg, "The use of drugs for euthanasia and assisted suicide in family practice" (Medline translation of Dutch title), *Nederlands Tijdschrift Voor Geneeskunde* 136 (1992): 1299-305; same authors, "Euthanasia and assisted suicide by physicians in the home situation. 2. Suffering of the patients" (Medline translation of Dutch title), same journal 135 (1991): 1599-603; and same authors, "Euthanasia and assisted suicide by physicians in the home situation. I. Diagnoses, age and sex of patients," same journal 135 (1991): 1593-98. More recently the latter group has published Gerrit van der Wal and Robert J.M. Dillmann, "Euthanasia in the Netherlands," *British Medical Journal* 308 (1994): 1346-49. M.T. Muller et al., "Voluntary Active Euthanasia and Physician-Assisted Suicide in Dutch Nursing Homes. Are the Requirements for Prudent Practice Properly Met?" *Journal of the American Geriatrics Society*, 42 (1994): 624-29. G. van der Wal et al., "Voluntary Active Euthanasia and Physician-Assisted Suicide in Dutch Nursing Homes: Requests and Administrations," *Journal of the American Geriatrics Society* 42 (1994): 620-23.

54　van der Maas et al., "Euthanasia," *Lancet*.

55　Henk ten Have has pointed out to me that women have also predominated in the court cases on physician-assisted suicide and euthanasia in the Netherlands. Personal communication, April 1993. Ideally those judicial opinions will be translated into English or be analyzed by someone bilingual, permitting comparison to the textual analysis of U.S. judicial opinions in Steven Miles and Alison August, "Courts, Gender, and 'the Right to Die,'" *Law, Medicine & Health Care* 18 (1990): 85-95.

56　van der Maas, van Delden, and Pijnenborg, "Euthanasia," *Health Policy*, 50.

57　van der Maas et al., "Euthanasia," *Lancet*, 671.

58　Johannes J.M. van Delden, personal communication, April 2, 1993.

59　Pijnenborg et al., "Life-terminating acts without explicit request of patient"; van der Maas, van Delden, and Pijnenborg, "Euthanasia," *Health Policy*, 50; Johannes J.M. van Delden, personal communication, April, 1993. Note that the 1991 *Lancet* article combines euthanasia, physician-assisted suicide, and "life-terminating events without explicit and persistent request," labeling the combination "euthanasia and related MDEL," and reporting a combined gender ratio of 61:39 with males predominating. See van der Maas et al., "Euthanasia," *Lancet*, 670-71. However, as I indicate in text, when you separate the three subcategories, women predominate for euthanasia.

60　Note that in *Lancet*, the researchers addressed both euthanasia and physician-assisted suicide in stating that, "Euthanasia and assisted suicide were more often found in deaths in relatively young men and in the urbanised western Netherlands, and this may be an indication of a shift towards a more demanding attitude of patients in matters concerning the end of life." van der Maas et al., "Euthanasia," *Lancet*, 673. See also Pijnenborg et al., "Life-terminating acts without explicit request of patient." However, in their subsequent *Health Policy* publication, they reported that euthanasia was *not* more often found in men, though physician-assisted suicide was. van der Maas, van Delden, and Pijnenborg, "Euthanasia," *Heathy Policy*, 50.

61　Johannes J.M. van Delden, personal communication, April 1993.

62　See van der Maas, van Delden, and Pijnenborg, "Euthanasia," *Health Policy*, 52.

63　Compare, for example, "Netherlands: Ethnic Minority Population to Reach One Million by 2000," *Financieele Dagblad*, March 3, 1994 (ethnic minority population will then be 6.6 percent), with U.S. Department of Commerce, Bureau of the Census, *Statistical Abstract of the United States* 1993, 113th ed., 18 (20 percent of the 1990 population was non-white).

64　Canetto, "Elderly Women and Suicidal Behavior," 225-26 (citation omitted). I am grateful to Alta Charo for suggesting I also consider the preponderance of women in American nursing homes. See *Census of the Population, 1990: General Population Characteristics of the United States* (Washington, DC: Government Printing Office, 1992), 48 (1,278,433 women in nursing homes versus 493,609 men). On suicidal behavior, both attempted and completed, in U.S. nursing homes see Nancy J. Osgood, Barbara A. Brant, and Aaron Lipman, *Suicide Among the Elderly in Long-Term Care Facilities* (New York, NY: Greenwood Press, 1991).

65 There is a substantial literature on the Tuskegee study. See, for example, Arthur L. Caplan, "When Evil Intrudes," Harold Edgar, "Outside the Community," Patricia King, "The Dangers of Difference," and James H. Jones, "The Tuskegee Legacy: AIDS and the Black Community," all in "Twenty Years After: The Legacy of the Tuskegee Syphilis Study," *Hastings Center Report* 22 (Nov.-Dec. 1992): 29-40; James H. Jones, *Bad Blood: The Tuskegee Syphilis Experiment* (New York, NY: Free Press, 1981); Allan M. Brandt, "Racism and Research: The Case of the Tuskegee Syphilis Study," *Hastings Center Report* 8 (Dec. 1978): 21-28.

66 See Mark B. Wenneker and Arnold M. Epstein, "Racial Inequalities in the Use of Procedures for Patients with Ischemic Heart Disease in Massachusetts," *Journal of the American Medical Association* 261 (1989): 233-57. See also Robert J. Blendon et al., "Access to Medical Care for Black and White Americans: A Matter of Continuing Concern," *Journal of the American Medical Association* 261 (1989): 278-81, Craig K. Svensson, "Representation of American Blacks in Clinical Trials of New Drugs," *Journal of the American Medical Association* 261 (1989): 263-65.

67 On the intersection of race and gender, for example, see Kimberle Crenshaw, "Demarginalizing the Intersection of Race and Sex: A Black Feminist Critique of Antidiscrimination Doctrine, Feminist Theory and Antiracist Politics," *Chicago Legal Forum* 1989: 139-67. See also Patricia Hill Collins, *Black Feminist Thought: Knowledge, Consciousness, and the Politics of Empowerment* (New York, NY: Routledge, 1991). On the intersection of race and gender in health, see Evelyn C. White, ed., *The Black Women's Health*

Book: Speaking for Ourselves (Seattle, WA: Seal Press, 1990).

68 See, for example, Morton J. Horowitz, "Rights," *Harvard Civil Rights-Civil Liberties Law Review* 23 (1988): 393-406; Mark Tushnet, "An Essay on Rights," *Texas Law Review* 62 (1984): 1363-403.

69 Though there is an overlap in the rights critiques of Critical Legal Studies (CLS) and Critical Race Theory, "[t]he CLS critique of rights and rules is the most problematic aspect of the CLS program, and provides few answers for minority scholars and lawyers." Richard Delgado, "The Ethereal Scholar: Does Critical Legal Studies Have What Minorities Want?" *Harvard Civil Rights-Civil Liberties Law Review* 22 (1987): 301-22, 304 (footnote omitted). Patricia Williams, indeed, has argued the necessity of rights discourse: "[S]tatements ... about the relative utility of needs over rights discourse overlook that blacks have been describing their needs for generations.... For blacks, describing needs has been a dismal failure...." Patricia J. Williams, *The Alchemy of Race and Rights* (Cambridge, MA: Harvard University Press, 1991), 151.

70 See, for example, Mary Ann Glendon, *Rights Talk: The Impoverishment of Political Discourse* (New York, NY: Free Press, 1991).

71 Margaret Farley has helpfully traced commonalities as well as distinctions between feminist theory and other traditions, noting that it is wrong to demand of any one critical stream that it bear no relation to the others. See Margaret A. Farley "Feminist Theology and Bioethics," in Earl E. Shelp, ed., *Theology and Bioethics: Exploring the Foundations and Frontiers* (Boston, MA: D. Reidel, 1985), 163-85.

72 I take the term "rights talk" from Glendon, *Rights Talk.*

73 See, for example, Jean Grimshaw, *Philosophy and Feminist Thinking* (Minneapolis, MN: University of Minnesota Press, 1986), 175.

74 See, for example, Naomi Scheman, "Individualism and the Objects of Psychology" in Sandra Harding and Merrill B. Hintikka, eds., *Discovering Reality: Feminist Perspectives on Epistemology, Metaphysics, Methodology, and the Philosophy of Science* (Boston, MA: D. Reidel, 1983), 225-44, 240.

75 See Jennifer Nedelsky "Reconceiving Autonomy:

Sources, Thoughts and Possibilities," *Yale Journal of Law and Feminism* 1 (1989): 7-36.

76   *Ibid.*, 12-13.

77   See Martha Minow, *Making All the Difference: Inclusion, Exclusion, and American Law* (Ithaca, NY: Cornell University Press, 1990).

78   Another author offering a feminist revision of autonomy and rights is Diana T. Meyers in "The Socialized Individual and Individual Autonomy: An Intersection between Philosophy and Psychology," in Eva Feder Kittay and Diana T. Meyers, eds., *Women and Moral Theory* (Savage, MD: Rowman & Littlefield, 1987), 139-53. See also Elizabeth M. Schneider, "The Dialectic of Rights and Politics: Perspectives from the Women's Movement," *New York University Law Review* 61 (1986): 589-652. There is a large feminist literature presenting a critique of rights, some of it rejecting the utility of such language. See, for example, Catharine MacKinnon, "Feminism, Marxism, Method and the State: Toward Feminist Jurisprudence," *Signs* 8 (1983): 635-58,658 ("Abstract rights will authorize the male experience of the world").

79   See, for example, Susan M. Wolf, "Nancy Beth Cruzan: In No Voice at All," *Hastings Center Report* 20 (Jan.-Feb. 1990): 38-41, *Guidelines on the Termination of Life-Sustaining Treatment and the Care of the Dying* (Bloomington, IN: Indiana University Press & The Hastings Center, 1987).

80   John Stuart Mill, "On Liberty," in Marshall Cohen, ed., *The Philosophy of John Stuart Mill: Ethical, Political and Religious* (New York, NY: Random House, 1961), 185-319, 304.

81   Leon R. Kass also argues against the existence of a "right to die" in "Is There a Right to Die?" *Hastings Center Report* 23 (Jan.-Feb. 1993): 34-43.

82   The Dutch studies show that even when patients know they can get assisted suicide and euthanasia, three times more patients ask for such assurance from their physicians than actually die that way. See van der Maas et al., "Euthanasia," *Lancet*, 673.

83   On these obligations and their derivation, see Leon R. Kass, "Neither for Love nor Money: Why Doctors Must Not Kill," *The Public Interest* 94 (Winter 1989): 25-46; Tom L. Beauchamp and James F. Childress, *Principles of Biomedical Ethics*, 4th ed. (New York, NY: Oxford University Press, 1994), 189, 226-27.

84   See Leslie Bender, "A Feminist Analysis of Physician-Assisted Dying and Voluntary Active Euthanasia," *Tennessee Law Review* 59 (1992): 519-46, making a "caring" argument in favor of "physician-assisted death."

85   Brody, "Assisted Death."

86   James Rachels offers a like proposal. See Rachels, *The End of Life*.

87   For a summary of the debate over the proper structure of bioethics, see David DeGrazia, "Moving Forward in Bioethical Theory: Theories, Cases, and Specified Principlism," *Journal of Medicine and Philosophy* 17 (1992): 511-40. There have been several different attacks on a bioethics driven by principles, which is usually taken to be exemplified by Beauchamp and Childress, *Principles of Biomedical Ethics*. Clouser and Gert argue for a bioethics that would be even more "top-down" or deductive, proceeding from theory instead of principles. See K. Danner Clouser and Bernard Gert, "A Critique of Principlism," *Journal of Medicine and Philosophy* 15 (1990): 219-36. A different attack is presented by Ronald M. Green, "Method in Bioethics: A Troubled Assessment," *Journal of Medicine and Philosophy* 15 (1990): 179-97. Hoffmaster argues for an ethnography driven, "bottom-up" or inductive bioethics. Barry Hoffmaster, "The Theory and Practice of Applied Ethics," *Dialogue* XXX (1991): 213-34. Jonsen and Toulmin have urged a revival of casuistry built on case-by-case analysis. Albert R. Jonsen and Stephen Toulmin, *The Abuse of Casuistry: A History of Moral Reasoning*, (Berkeley, CA: University of California Press, 1988). Beauchamp and Childress discuss these challenges at length in the 4th edition of *Principles of Biomedical Ethics*.

88   See Gilligan, *In a Different Voice*, 174. Lawrence Blum points out that Kohlberg himself stated that "the final, most mature stage of moral reasoning involves an 'integration of justice and care that forms a single moral principle,'" but that Kohlberg, too, never spelled out what that integration would be. See Lawrence A. Blum, "Gilligan and Kohlberg: Implications for Moral Theory," *Ethics* 98 (1988): 472-91, 482-83 (footnote with citation omitted).

89   See Blum, "Gilligan and Kohlberg," 477.

90   Owen Flanagan and Kathryn Jackson, "Justice, Care, and Gender: The Kohlberg-Gilligan Debate Revisited," in Larrabee, ed., *An Ethic of Care*, 69-84, 71.

91 Martha Minow and Elizabeth V. Spelman, "In Context," *Southern California Law Review* 63 (1990): 1597-652, 1625.

92 *Ibid.*, 1629.

93 *Ibid.*, 1630-31.

94 *Ibid.*, 1632-33.

95 There are significant similarities here to Henry Richardson's proposal of "specified principlism." See DeGrazia, "Moving Forward in Bioethical Theory."

96 On the importance of paying attention to who is doing the theorizing and to what end, including in feminist theorizing, see Maria C. Lugones and Elizabeth V. Spelman, "Have We Got a Theory for You! Feminist Theory, Cultural Imperialism and the Demand for 'The Woman's Voice,'" *Women's Studies International Forum* 6 (1983): 573-81.

97 I have elsewhere argued that health care institutions should create processes to uncover and combat sexism and racism, among other problems. See Susan M. Wolf, "Toward a Theory of Process," *Law, Medicine & Health Care* 20 (1992): 278-90.

98 On the importance of viewing the medical profession in the context of the democratic polity, see Troyen Brennan, *Just Doctoring: Medical Ethics in the Liberal State* (Berkeley, CA: University of California Press, 1991).

99 See, for example, Howard J. Curzer, "Is Care a Virtue for Health Care Professionals?" *Journal of Medicine and Philosophy* 18 (1993): 51-69. Nancy S. Jecker and Donnie J. Self, "Separating Care and Cure: An Analysis of Historical and Contemporary Images of Nursing and Medicine," *Journal of Medicine and Philosophy* 16 (1991): 285-306.

100 Compare Canetto, "Elderly Women and Suicidal Behavior," finding evidence of this with respect to elderly women electing suicide.

101 See van der Maas, van Delden, and Pijnenborg, "Euthanasia," *Health Policy*, 51-55, 145-46; van der Wal et al., "Voluntary Active Euthanasia and Physician-Assisted Suicide in Dutch Nursing Homes."

102 See Quill, Cassel, and Meier, "Care of the Hopelessly Ill."

103 In these two sentences, I disagree both with Kass's suggestion that the core commitments of medicine are set for all time by the ancient formulation of the doctor's role and with Brock's assertion that the core commitment of medicine is to do whatever the patient wants. See Kass, "Neither for Love Nor Money." Dan Brock, "Voluntary Active Euthanasia," *Hastings Center Report* 22 (Mar.-Apr. 1992): 10-22.

104 See Jay Katz, *The Silent World of Doctor and Patient* (New York, NY: Free Press, 1984), 121-22.

105 See Miles and August, "Gender, Courts, and the 'Right to die.'"

106 While a large literature analyzes the relationship between terminating life-sustaining treatment and the practices of physician-assisted suicide and euthanasia, more recently attention has turned to the relationship between those latter practices and abortion. On the question of whether respect for women's choice of abortion requires legitimation of those practices, see, for example, Seth F. Kreimer, "Does Pro-choice Mean Pro-Kevorkian? An Essay on *Roe, Casey,* and the Right to Die," *American University Law Review* 44 (1995): 803-54. Full analysis of why respect for the choice of abortion does not require legitimation of physician-assisted suicide and euthanasia is beyond the scope of this chapter. However, the courts themselves are beginning to argue the distinction. See Compassion in Dying v. Washington, 49 F. 3d 586 (9th Cir. 1995). On gender specifically, there are strong arguments that gender equity and concern for the fate of women demand respect for the abortion choice, whereas I am arguing that gender concerns cut the other way when it comes to physician-assisted suicide and euthanasia.

39.
WHY GENDER MATTERS TO THE EUTHANASIA DEBATE: ON DECISIONAL CAPACITY AND THE REJECTION OF WOMEN'S DEATH REQUESTS

Jennifer A. Parks

SOURCE: *Hastings Center Report* 30.1 (2000): 30-36.

Are women's requests for aid in dying honored more often than men's, or less? Feminist arguments can support conclusions either that gendered perceptions of women as self-sacrificing predispose physicians to accede to women's requests to die—or that cultural understandings of women as not fully rational agents lead physicians to reject their requests as irrational.

The euthanasia debate has typically addressed the tension between patient autonomy and physician obligations. Where physician-assisted suicide and active euthanasia are concerned, ethicists balance a patient's request to die against both the physician's role as healer and her duty of nonmaleficence. The physician is seen to be in a moral dilemma in which her commitments to healing and saving lives conflict with her commitment to serving her patients' needs, respecting their autonomy, and maintaining their trust. The focal question for ethical debate has thus been: how much should patient autonomy govern the practices of physician-assisted suicide and active euthanasia?

Such questions are too narrowly formulated because they fail to address the background conditions that may affect a patient's death request. Besides individual agency, we must take into account the ways gender roles and social circumstances affect patients' requests to die, and the way those requests are received by our culture. Feminist approaches raise such contextual and cultural questions, yet there is little available feminist literature on physician-assisted suicide and euthanasia. Although feminists are concerned about the cultural context within which women make medical decisions, they have primarily focused on women's reproductive decisions; only recently have feminist bioethicists turned to issues beyond reproduction.

Susan Wolf offers one of the few feminist treatments to date of euthanasia. She argues that women are more likely to request euthanasia and physician-assisted suicide in an attempt to avoid burdening their families—a perversion of the feminine ethic of care that takes women's caring for and about others to the extreme—and that physicians are simultaneously more likely to fulfill women's death requests, based on "the same historical valorization of women's self-sacrifice and the same background sexism."[1] In a culture that valorizes their altruism and caring for others, women who suffer from severe pain or terminal illness may perceive themselves as failing in their appointed duties; unable to care for others, they may see themselves as actually burdening them. For Wolf, the authenticity and rationality of a woman's request to die seems suspect at the very least, given the extent to which cultural expectations about not burdening others have likely affected her. Indeed, Wolf chastens physicians "not to accede to the request for assisted suicide and euthanasia" for this very reason (p. 308).

Wolf also discusses the unequal social conditions that may encourage women to seek death, such as poverty, higher incidences of depression, poor pain relief, lack of good medical care, and poor social support networks—essential topics in any ethical analysis of physician-assisted suicide and active euthanasia. While other feminists have shared these concerns for women's social conditions, Wolf is the first to relate them to the issue of euthanasia. Her analysis thus ushers in important theoretical and practical concerns regarding women's death requests and their implementation.

I have isolated Wolf as an influential feminist voice because she brings depth to a debate that has, until recently, focused almost exclusively on the issue of patient autonomy. I suggest, however, that Wolf's reasoning may actually lead to very different conclusions. While some women in particular can exhibit a preoccupation with and overemphasis on relationships, terminally ill women's death requests can also, like men's, stem from basic personal concerns for pain, psychic suffering, and the determination that their lives have become meaningless or burdensome to them. In taking Wolf's feminist account seriously, I suggest that women's requests to die may be discounted, trivialized, and ignored for the same reasons that Wolf claims they are too likely to be heeded. By virtue of the expectation that women will be altruistic, self-abnegating caregivers, women's own voices, and their claims to autonomy in requesting death, are easily dismissed. I conclude that women's choices, their capacity to reason, and their ability to accurately represent their own interests are undermined in our culture and as a consequence that women's claims to pain and suffering are often disregarded. Yet in cases of intolerable pain and suffering, a woman's request to die should not be questioned on the grounds that she is incapable of determining her own good; women, like men, should be extended the right to decide when their life is burdensome, meaningless, and no longer worth living.

Some Background

Both in Canada and the United States there has been growing support for social policies that would legalize active euthanasia and physician-assisted suicide. This increasing support is not surprising given North Americans' commitment to an individualistic ethic: the primary focus, socially, politically, and medically, is on the individual, and the protection of his or her autonomy. Ethicists are also primarily concerned with the individual and his rights: their debates largely concern the conflict between patient and physician and how to navigate the tensions between these two parties and their conflicting goals. For example, Dan Brock argues that the patient has a right to choose active euthanasia or physician-assisted suicide because, "If self-determination is a funda-

mental value, then the great variability among people on this question makes it especially important that individuals control the manner, circumstances, and timing of their dying and death."[2]

Conversely, arguments against euthanasia have also taken the individual's self-governance to be the main issue. Gay-Williams argues against euthanasia on the ground that, "Because death is final and irreversible, euthanasia contains within it the possibility that we will work against our own interest if we practice it or allow it to be practiced on us."[3] Plainly, traditional liberal concerns for protecting individual autonomy remain the primary focus of debates over euthanasia.

Autonomy is valued in a liberal society because it secures the interest that each citizen has in directing her life; it dominates liberal theories because self-government is an essential feature of a nonoppressive society. Autonomy is a cornerstone of the euthanasia debate because our interest in directing our own lives has special force when it comes to determining our mode and time of death. The choice of how and when to die is indeed a deeply personal decision. As Wolf critically states,

> Advocacy of physician-assisted suicide and euthanasia has hinged to a great extent on rights claims. The argument is that the patient has a right of self-determination or autonomy that entitles her to assistance in suicide or euthanasia. The strategy is to extend the argument that self-determination entitles the patient to refuse unwanted life-sustaining treatment by maintaining that the same rationale supports patient entitlement to more active physician assistance in death. Indeed, it is sometimes argued that there is no principled difference between termination of life-sustaining treatment and more active practices.[4]

On the autonomy model, if the rights-bearer asserts her right to die, then the appropriate response is to secure her death. And while this model intends the positive goal of individuals pursuing their own good as they see fit, the liberal conception of the individual as a rational, independent, rights-bearing agent choosing her own time and mode of death is impoverished. By contrast, a feminist approach to the euthanasia debate regards women's experiences in a gendered culture as relevant to determinations regarding the legitimacy of their death requests.

The Importance of Context

The demand for euthanasia, and the interaction between the patient requesting death and the physician considering the request, is largely understood as a private matter. Timothy Quill, for example, relates a case involving Diane, a patient who is dying of cancer and who is requesting his assistance in securing a painless death. He entitles this case "Death and Dignity: A Case of Individualized Decision-Making."[5] But feminist ethicists argue that practices like active euthanasia and physician-assisted suicide are not merely cases of individualized decision-making: such individual decisions are made within a social context that informs and affects individuals' choices. Thus unlike liberal accounts of the self, feminist approaches view the individual as a socially embedded, interdependent, relational subject whose choices are made within a complex web of social relationships. Where the euthanasia debate is concerned, the situated subject is not an isolatable, independent, atomistic subject: her choice to die has implications for both self and society, and her choices can be either upheld or undermined by the prevailing social ethos.[6]

That gender matters where physician-assisted suicide and active euthanasia are concerned is contentious. The individual expression of autonomy is held to be a right in which we all share an objective, equal interest. Thus the particular features of a patient's life are considered irrelevant once we have determined that her choices are unconstrained by coercion, irrationality, ignorance, or the limited options available to her. But here a feminist account of euthanasia departs from traditional liberal accounts; feminists assert that deep social inequalities affect individual agents in ways not recognized on traditional liberal approaches to autonomy. For example, liberal accounts of euthanasia fail to address the widespread sexism that serves to undermine respect for women's choices.

It is imperative that a feminist account of euthanasia consider the feminine ethic of care to which

women have been held, an ethic that requires women's unselfish commitment to the nurturance and care of others, especially their husbands, children, and elderly parents. The imperative to care for others—to the point of giving up their sense of self completely—encourages people to dismiss women's self-concerns, and it makes society less willing to consider euthanasia for women. A liberal, rights-based account of euthanasia fails to account for such difficulties because it does not countenance contextual features of this sort. A feminist account, however, can show how sexism may lead to the medical and social rejection of a woman's request for death.

As Wolf indicates, the valorization of women's self-sacrifice and self-abnegation has been criticized by feminist ethicists. Bonnelle Lewis Strickling, for example, argues that women's self-abnegation is such that there is often no "self" beyond their identification with others. Strickling recognizes two forms of self-abnegation: in its virtuous form, it accomplishes a "sympathetic understanding between and among persons" in which both parties' interests and feelings are taken into consideration.[7] In its negative form, the self-abnegator abandons any sense of being a particular self outside of her relationships with others. Self-abnegation in this form demands no less than that women renounce, discount, and deny the self: only if one has no self (or no conception of self) can one commit entirely to the service of others. And service to others is exactly what is expected of women in our culture. As Strickling claims,

> traditionally women have been asked to be helpful, loving without expectation of return, emotionally dependable, supportive, and generally nurturing to both children and husband both physically and in the sense of nurturing their respective senses of self, all without complaining ... taken together, these expectations comprise the expectation of self-renunciation on an extremely large scale. (p. 197)

Furthermore, women have been held to a feminine ethic of care, a conception of "womanly" virtues according to which it is part of women's moral obligation to care for and nurture others. This feminine ethic is rooted in women's traditional roles of homemaking, child-bearing and rearing, and the care and nurturing activities that accompany these roles.

That "womanly" virtues require caring for and nurturing others to the detriment of women's self-concern relates to my worries about gender and euthanasia. For if women are expected to be deferential to others, self-effacing, and caring to the point of sacrificing their own happiness, then any self-interested and self-directed claims they make (in this case, the request to die) may be more easily discounted or dismissed as irrational. A woman's capacity for reason and self-determination is not validated in our culture (since women have been historically viewed as emotional, not rational, beings); the presence of severe pain or terminal illness may be used as further support for the view that women are particularly incompetent when it comes to making even deeply personal life and death decisions.

For Daniel Callahan, the acceptance of voluntary active euthanasia and physician-assisted suicide minimally requires that the physician fulfilling or denying the patient's request have her own moral grounds for helping (or refusing to help) a patient to die. As Callahan states,

> If doctors, once sanctioned to carry out euthanasia, are to be themselves responsible moral agents—not simply hired hands with lethal injections at the ready—then they must have their own independent moral grounds to kill those who request such services.... The doctor would have to decide, on her own, whether the patient's life was "no longer worth living."[8]

If doctors have their own independent moral grounds for implementing euthanasia then we must question what those moral grounds are and whence they stem. On a feminist account, physicians' values are informed by a social context within which the undermining of women's self-regarding choices has a long history. One might expect physicians' judgments about patient competence to be more objective because of their medical training, but this is not so. Valerie Hartouni has recently offered an account of the subtle ways in which our vision is "trained," "impaired," and "partial." What we see, and the way we see it, is not merely a physiological event or a mechanical process, but is learned. As she claims, "Seeing is an act of immense construction.... Seeing is a set of learned practices and processes that allow us to organize the visual field and that engage us in producing the world we seem to greet and take in only passively."[9] On this account, our view of euthanasia, and those who have a legitimate claim to it, is not objectively determined, but is strongly influenced by the preorganized world through which our social and ethical vision is trained. The apparent illegitimacy of a woman's claim to euthanasia is effected by a social world in which her voice is silenced and her capacity for self- or other-regarding choices is questioned.

So a physician's moral grounds for rejecting euthanasia or physician-assisted suicide will—at least partially—reflect a social refusal to acknowledge the legitimacy of such feelings of burdensomeness and meaninglessness in a culture that denies women's competency. Not only does our culture view women as self-abnegating caregivers who lack reason and autonomy: physicians discount or dismiss women's reasoning capacity and ability to govern themselves, making it easier for them to reject women's death requests. For determining that a patient's life has become "meaningless" or "burdensome" involves making a value judgment that, like most value judgments, reflects dominant cultural prejudices, among them (in our society) the assumption that women are primarily nurturers and caregivers who lack the competency to self-govern. That a man may experience his life as "meaningless" or "burdensome" is considered a rational self-evaluation so long as his life is marked by intolerable pain, personal suffering, or terminal illness. But women's similar experiences are much more likely to be rejected, discounted, or unheeded because their capacity for such determinations of personal suffering are questioned. Perhaps, as Kathryn Morgan claims, the denial of women's full moral agency stems from the view that, "simply by virtue of their embodiment as women, women just are closer to nature and, hence, not capable of the kind of thought that is necessary for human moral life."[10]

Further Considerations

I have offered some theoretical worries about the background inequalities that lead doctors to discount or dismiss women's death requests. These worries lead in the opposite direction of Wolf's concerns that women are more likely to be euthanized in our gendered society.

Wolf's feminist account is also not supported by strong empirical evidence, although, as she points out, research on gender and euthanasia remains in its infancy.[11] Until we have strong empirical data relating to gender and euthanasia, and given that the theory alone can lead in different directions, we have equally good reason to suppose that women's legitimate death requests (that is, requests stemming from experiences of intolerable pain, human suffering, and negative experiences of terminal illness) are likely to go unheeded.

In support of her women-at-risk thesis Wolf cites the case of Dr. Jack Kevorkian, an American pathologist who has helped a preponderance of women to die, and the recent data from the Netherlands that has been collected from the Dutch experience with euthanasia. Kevorkian helped eight women to die before fulfilling a man's death request. That a large number of Kevorkian's "patients" have been women is telling on Wolf's account: Kevorkian may be acting out a cultural stereotype that demands women's commitment to caregiving and that rejects women's claims to be cared for in times of sickness or terminal illness. Kevorkian's actions are particularly heinous, then, when placed in the context of women's traditional role expectations as caregivers, nurturers, and self-abnegators.

Like Wolf, I have concerns about Kevorkian's actions and the context within which he is helping people to die. The demand for Kevorkian arises because individuals are not receiving help from a trusted physician in securing their deaths. Kevorkian-esque deaths do not derive from a long-standing relationship with one's physician. On the contrary, what the Kevorkian deaths indicate is not that women in particular are at a high risk of being put to death, but that social conditions for a socially accepted, dignified death through physician-assisted suicide or active euthanasia do not obtain, either at home or in care facilities. Kevorkian's practice does not provide evidence of a widespread social bias in favor of killing women; rather, his actions are witness to the sad position into which both women and men who are seeking death are placed.

Furthermore, the Dutch data that support her women-at-risk thesis are problematic; Wolf indicates that available data from the Netherlands are not decisive and may not be generalizable to the United States. Nevertheless, Wolf argues that the Dutch data indicate a slightly greater percentage of women than men being euthanized, and that we ought to be concerned about the difference since "the differences in Dutch demographics and health care would be reasons to expect no gender differential in the Netherlands in the practices we are examining" (p. 296). Given the differences in health care systems and demographics between the two counties, however, we can draw no conclusions from the Dutch data that would be relevant to the context of the United States. Furthermore, the Dutch data in fact neither support nor undermine Wolf's claim.

Wolf is justified in her concern that gender role socialization and ubiquitous cultural stereotypes may lead women to define themselves—and be defined by others—according to their caregiving role. Yet she errs in concluding that women are therefore more likely than men to have their death requests fulfilled when they are terminally ill or suffering and no longer capable of fulfilling their caregiving duties. On the contrary, a woman's death request—based as it is on her own knowledge claims and experiences of her own pain and suffering—is more easily dismissed. Evidence both inside and outside the medical arena indicates that women's knowledge claims and their claims to self-concern tend to be denied, not (as Wolf argues) too easily upheld. This evidence stems from a variety of sources; and while the data is not entirely conclusive, it suggests that for social reasons, physicians are less likely to heed women's death requests than those made by men.

Our social rejection of women's knowledge has a long history, a history too long to account for in this paper. But consider an early indicator that a female's attempts at independence and independent thinking is socially rejected: the American classroom. A report by Myra and David Sadker indicates that as early as preschool, sexism prevails in the classroom. As they note in their survey of studies done on classroom dynamics,

> teachers gave boys more attention, praised them more often and were at least twice as likely to have extended conversations with them.... [T]eachers were twice as likely to give male students detailed instructions on how to do things for themselves. With female students, teachers were more likely to do it for them instead. The result was that boys learned to become independent, girls learned to become dependent.[12]

The import of such a study is difficult to overestimate. It addresses a concern that feminists have been voicing for a very long time: that women's knowledge, independence, and self-promotion are systemically undermined in our culture. From an early age females are denied the opportunity to think and act independently. It would be unsurprising, then, if later in their lives women's death requests, which would be based on their own perspectives and experiences, were rejected because they were denied the capacity to make such determinations.

Consider also the case of abortion, where women's decisional capacity, their right to self-regarding choices, and their personal experiences have been questioned. Arguments against a woman's right to abortion turn on her alleged moral responsibility for others and her incapacity for rational decision-making at a time of great distress. Both non-feminists and pro-life feminists alike have argued that pregnant women are not entitled to consider only themselves as the subjects of concern: they are chided to place their families, their communities, and in particular their fetuses at the center of their moral deliberations. In the case of abortion, we again see a cultural predilection for imposing an other-oriented ethic on women that is not extended to men: a woman's right to make a self-regarding decision based on her own experiences (for example, her claim that she cannot financially or emotionally support a child at this particular time) comes under heavy attack. As Sidney Callahan claims, "A woman, involuntarily pregnant, has a moral obligation to the now-existing fetus whether she explicitly consented to its existence or not."[13]

In addition, critics of abortion argue that a pregnant woman has questionable decision-making capacities and should not be the final arbiter of her own good. Again, to quote Callahan, "It also seems a travesty of just procedures that a pregnant woman now, in effect, acts as the sole judge of her own case under the most stressful conditions" (p. 13).

Commentators on the abortion debate have perverted the ethic of care in order to deny women the right to place their interests ahead of others and to have their decisions respected. A woman's knowledge about her body, her financial situation, her social context, and her own emotional state—knowledge claims that find counterparts in the claims made by terminally ill women requesting death—are dismissed or discounted.

Even women's reports of coronary pain have, until fairly recently, been dismissed as being "all in their heads," resulting in many unnecessary deaths because of late detection of heart disease. Indeed, coronary research (like most other medical research) has targeted white men to the serious detriment of women. Heart disease has historically been understood as a man's affliction, and with physicians guiding their thinking on the subject, women have misunderstood their own symptoms. Since there has been little study of women's own particular experiences with heart disease, their reported symptoms have gone largely unrecognized. Instead, women's knowledge about their condition, their experiences of symptoms, and their request for medical attention tend to be rejected, and their complaints set aside as hyperbole or attributed to emotional causes.[14] If this conception of women is operating in the area of heart disease, one can only imagine how it affects consideration of women's requests to die.

That women have been treated differently from men is borne out by some directly relevant statistics. In a review of "right to die" cases, researchers found that courts honored the death requests of men in 75 percent of reported cases but respected similar requests by women in only 14 percent of reported cases.[15] More recently, the *New England Journal of Medicine* cites a national study of physician-assisted suicide and euthanasia in the United States, according to which men largely outnumber women in receiving undercover prescriptions for lethal doses of medication.[16] The survey reveals that 97 percent of those receiving undercover prescriptions were men, while of those who received an undercover lethal injection—active euthanasia—57 percent were men and 43 percent women. Significantly, in 95 percent of cases in which patients received the means for physician-assisted suicide it was the patient himself who made the request for the prescription (in the remaining 5 percent the request came from a family member or partner); by contrast 54 percent of all active euthanasia requests were made by family members. Such data suggest that in cases of physician-assisted suicide, where the patient characteristically makes the request and terminates his life at a time and place he deems appropriate, men are deemed capable of making such significant choices while women are not. Conversely, in cases of active euthanasia, which usually take place within institutions and are requested by family members, women are far more likely to have death requests fulfilled.[17]

Interestingly, the national survey supports both the thesis that women's death requests are less likely to be heeded than those of men and Wolf's claim that women are typically viewed as "expendable." It is largely when the death request is made *for* women by their family members that the request is fulfilled by physicians. Arguably, when family members request active euthanasia for a kinswoman, the broader society might understand that she is no longer capable of providing the care, nurturing, and self-sacrifice that is expected of women.

Dismissing Suffering

While Wolf's feminist account provides a foundation for a rich ethical analysis of euthanasia, it is not clear that women are more likely than men to be euthanized or extended the means for physician-assisted suicide. Indeed, there is reason to think, and statistical evidence to support the thought, that women are far less likely to be taken seriously, listened to, and supported in their end of life choices than are their male counterparts. While I share

Wolf's concern for the way in which the debate over euthanasia and physician-assisted suicide has been decontextualized and governed by an individualistic model, I believe that contextual considerations should lead us to question why women's death requests are taken less seriously and acted on less often than those of men.

Wolf acknowledges that some feminists "will see this problem differently. That may be especially true of women who feel in control of their lives, are less subject to subordination by age or race or wealth, and seek yet another option to add to their many."[18] She makes an important point: contingencies such as poverty, poor education, age, and race are important to a feminist account of euthanasia. But rather than making a woman's death request more likely to be respected, these contingencies make it less so: the less social weight a woman carries, the less likely she is to have her death requests taken seriously. A woman who is white, well educated, articulate, wealthy, or politically powerful is far less likely to be denied decisionmaking capacity than is her uneducated, poor, powerless counterpart. The more a woman is like the autonomous, rational, independent agent that is the traditional focus of the euthanasia debate, the more likely her death request will be taken seriously.

A person's access to euthanasia and physician-assisted suicide should not be affected by conditions over which she has no control: it is alarming to think that in a sexist society, only some members' claims to pain and psychic suffering will be taken seriously.

Notes

1   S. Wolf, "Gender, Feminism, and Death: Physician-Assisted Suicide and Euthanasia," in *Feminism & Bioethics: Beyond Reproduction*, ed. S. Wolf (New York: Oxford University Press, 1996), pp. 282-317, at 284.

2   D. Brock, "Voluntary Active Euthanasia," *Hastings Center Report* 22, no. 2 (1992): 11-21, at 11.

3   J. Gay-Williams, "The Wrongfulness of Euthanasia," reprinted in *Intervention and Reflection: Basic Issues in Medical Ethics*, ed. Ronald Munson, 5th ed. (Belmont, CA: Wadsworth Publishing Co., 1996), pp. 168-71, at 170.

4 See ref. 2, Wolf, "Gender, Feminism, and Death," p. 298.

5 T. Quill, "Death and Dignity: A Case of Individualized Decision-Making," reprinted in *Ethical Issues in Modern Medicine*, ed. J.D. Arras and B. Steinbock, (London: Mayfield Publishing Co., 1991), pp. 292-95.

6 Note, however, that feminists are concerned with both under-contextualizing and over-contextualizing women's lives. While ethicists should not ignore the situational aspects of women's lives, they also should not subordinate women's self-regarding choices to the requirements of maintaining social relationships.

7 B.L. Strickling, "Self-Abnegation," in *Feminist Perspectives: Philosophical Essays on Method and Morals*, ed. C. Overall, L. Code, and S. Mullet (Toronto: University of Toronto Press, 1988), pp. 190-201, at 194.

8 D. Callahan, "When Self-Determination Runs Amok," in *Ethical Issues in Modern Medicine*, ed. J. Arras and B. Steinbock, 4th ed. (London: Mayfield Publishing Co, 1996): 295-309, at 301.

9 V. Hartouni, *Cultural Conceptions: On Reproductive Technologies and the Remaking of Life* (Minneapolis: University of Minnesota Press, 1997), pp. 12-13.

10 K. Morgan, "Women and Moral Madness," in *Feminist Perspectives: Philosophical Essays on Method and Morals*, ed. C. Overall, L. Code, and S. Mullet (Toronto: University of Toronto Press, 1988), pp. 146-67, at 150.

11 See ref. 2, Wolf, "Gender, Feminism, and Death," p. 294.

12 M. Sadker and D. Sadker, "Sexism in the Schoolroom of the '80s," *Psychology Today* 19, no. 3 (1985): 54-57, at 55.

13 S. Callahan, "Abortion and the Sexual Agenda: A Case for Prolife Feminism," *Commonweal*, 25 April 1986: 9-17, at 15.

14 E. Nechas and D. Foley, *Unequal Treatment: What You Don't Know About How Women Are Mistreated by the Medical Community* (New York: Simon & Schuster, 1994), p. 66.

15 S.H. Miles and A. August, "Courts, Gender and the 'Right to Die,'" *Journal of Law, Medicine and Health Care* 18 (1990): 85-95.

16 D.E. Meier et al., "A National Survey of Physician-Assisted Suicide and Euthanasia in the United States," *NEJM* 338 (1998): 1193-200.

17 This study also indicates that when patients received a prescription for a lethal dose of medication (that is, the means to implement physician-assisted suicide), 90 percent of lethal prescriptions were given to patients who were at home, and only 5 percent were given to patients in nursing homes. However, in cases of active euthanasia, 99 percent of patients were hospitalized at the time of lethal injection (p. 1197).

18 See ref. 2. Wolf, "Gender, Feminism, and Death," p. 308.

40.
IS IT TIME TO ABANDON BRAIN DEATH?

Robert D. Truog

SOURCE: *Hastings Center Report* 27.1 (1997).

Over the past several decades, the concept of brain death has become well entrenched within the practice of medicine. At a practical level, this concept has been successful in delineating widely accepted ethical and legal boundaries for the procurement of vital organs for transplantation. Despite this success, however, there have been persistent concerns over whether the concept is theoretically coherent and internally consistent.[1] Indeed, some have concluded that the concept is fundamentally flawed, and that it represents only a "superficial and fragile consensus."[2] In this analysis I will identify the sources of these inconsistencies, and suggest that the best resolution to these issues may be to abandon the concept of brain death altogether.

Definitions, Concepts, and Tests

In its seminal work "Defining Death," the President's Commission for the Study of Ethical Problems in Medicine and Biomedical and Behavioral Research articulated a formulation of brain death that has come to be known as the "whole-brain standard."[3] In the Uniform Determination of Death Act, the President's Commission specified two criteria for determining death: (1) irreversible cessation of circulatory and respiratory functions, or (2) irreversible cessation of all functions of the entire brain, including the brainstem.

Neurologist James Bernat has been influential in defending and refining this standard. Along with others, he has recognized that analysis of the concept of brain death must begin by differentiating between three distinct levels. At the most general level, the concept must involve a *definition*. Next, *criteria* must be specified to determine when the definition has been fulfilled. Finally, *tests* must be available for

evaluating whether the criteria have been satisfied.[4] As clarified by Bernat and colleagues, therefore, the concept of death under the whole-brain formulation can be outlined as follows:[5]

> *Definition of Death:* The "permanent cessation of functioning of the organism as a whole."
> *Criterion for Death:* The "permanent cessation of functioning of the entire brain."
> *Tests for Death:* Two distinct sets of tests are available and acceptable for determining that the criterion is fulfilled:

(1) The cardiorespiratory standard is the traditional approach for determining death and relies upon documenting the prolonged absence of circulation or respiration. These tests fulfill the criterion, according to Bernat, since the prolonged absence of these vital signs is diagnostic for the permanent loss of all brain function.

(2) The neurological standard consists of a battery of tests and procedures, including establishment of an etiology sufficient to account for the loss of all brain functions, diagnosing the presence of coma, documenting apnea and the absence of brainstem reflexes, excluding reversible conditions, and showing the persistence of these findings over a sufficient period of time.[6]

Critique of the Current Formulation of Brain Death

Is this a coherent account of the concept of brain death? To answer this question, one must determine whether each level of analysis is consistent with the others. In other words, individuals who fulfill the tests must also fulfill the criterion, and those who satisfy the criterion must also satisfy the definition.[7]

First, regarding the tests-criterion relationship, there is evidence that many individuals who fulfill all of the tests for brain death do not have the "permanent cessation of functioning of the entire brain." In particular, many of these individuals retain clear evidence of integrated brain function at the level of the brainstem and midbrain, and may have evidence of cortical function.

For example, many patients who fulfill the tests for the diagnosis of brain death continue to exhibit intact neurohumoral function. Between 22 percent and 100 percent of brain-dead patients in different series have been found to retain free-water homeostasis through the neurologically mediated secretion of arginine vasopressin, as evidenced by serum hormonal levels and the absence of diabetes insipidus.[8] Since the brain is the only source of the regulated secretion of arginine vasopressin, patients without diabetes insipidus do not have the loss of all brain function. Neurologically regulated secretion of other hormones is also quite common.[9]

In addition, the tests for the diagnosis of brain death requires the patient not to be hypothermic.[10] This caveat is a particularly confusing Catch 22, since the absence of hypothermia generally indicates the continuation of neurologically mediated temperature homeostasis. The circularity of this reasoning can be clinically problematic, since hypothermic patients cannot be diagnosed as brain-dead but the absence of hypothermia is itself evidence of brain function.

Furthermore, studies have shown that many patients (20 percent in one series) who fulfill the tests for brain death continue to show electrical activity on their electroencephalograms.[11] While there is no way to determine how often this electrical activity represents true "function" (which would be incompatible with the criterion for brain death), in at least some cases the activity observed seems fully compatible with function.[12]

Finally, clinicians have observed that patients who fulfill the tests for brain death frequently respond to surgical incision at the time of organ procurement with a significant rise in both heart rate and blood pressure. This suggests that integrated neurological function at a supraspinal level may be present in at least some patients diagnosed as brain-dead.[13] This evidence points to the conclusion that there is a significant disparity between the standard tests used to make the diagnosis of brain death and the criterion these tests are purported to fulfill. Faced with these facts, even supporters of the current statutes acknowledge that the criterion of "whole-brain" death is only an approximation."[14]

If the tests for determining brain death are incompatible with the current criterion, then one way of solving the problem would be to require tests that always correlate with the "permanent cessation of functioning of the entire brain." Two options have been considered in this regard. The first would require tests that correlate with the actual destruction of the brain, since complete destruction would, of course, be incompatible with any degree of brain function. Only by satisfying these tests, some have argued, could we be assured that all functions of the entire brain have totally and permanently ceased.[15] But is there a constellation of clinical and laboratory tests that correlate with this degree of destruction? Unfortunately, a study of over 500 patients with both coma and apnea (including 146 autopsies for neuropathologic correlation) showed that "it was not possible to verify that a diagnosis made prior to cardiac arrest by any set or subset of criteria would invariably correlate with a diffusely destroyed brain."[16] On the basis of these data, a definition that required total brain destruction could only be confirmed at autopsy. Clearly, a condition that could only be determined after death could never be a requirement for declaring death.

Another way of modifying the tests to conform with the criterion would be to rely solely upon the cardiorespiratory standard for determining death. This standard would certainly identify the permanent cessation of all brain function (thereby fulfilling the criterion), since it is well established by common knowledge that prolonged absence of circulation and respiration results in the death of the entire brain (and every other organ). In addition, fulfillment of these tests would also convincingly demonstrate the cessation of function of the organism as a whole (thereby fulfilling the definition). Unfortunately, this approach for resolving the problem would also make it virtually impossible to obtain vital organs in a viable condition for transplantation, since under current laws it is generally necessary for these organs to be removed from a heart-beating donor.

These inconsistencies between the tests and the criterion are therefore not easily resolvable. In addition to these problems, there are also inconsistencies between the criterion and the definition. As outlined above, the whole-brain concept assumes that the "permanent cessation of functioning of the entire brain" (the criterion) necessarily implies the "permanent cessation of functioning of the organism as a whole" (the definition). Conceptually, this relationship assumes the principle that the brain is responsible for maintaining the body's homeostasis, and that without brain function the organism rapidly disintegrates. In the past, this relationship was demonstrated by showing that individuals who fulfilled the tests for the diagnosis of brain death inevitably had a cardiac arrest within a short period of time, even if they were provided with mechanical ventilation and intensive care.[17] Indeed, this assumption had been considered one of the linchpins in the ethical justification for the concept of brain death.[18] For example, in the largest empirical study of brain death ever performed, a collaborative group working under the auspices of the National Institutes of Health sought to specify the necessary tests for diagnosing brain death by attempting to identify a constellation of neurological findings that would inevitably predict the development of a cardiac arrest within three months, regardless of the level or intensity of support provided.[19]

This approach to defining brain death in terms of neurological findings that predict the development of cardiac arrest is plagued by both logical and scientific problems, however. First, it confuses a prognosis with a diagnosis. Demonstrating that a certain class of patients will suffer a cardiac arrest within a defined period of time certainly proves that they are *dying*, but it says nothing about whether they are *dead*.[20] This conceptual mistake can be clearly appreciated if one considers individuals who are dying of conditions not associated with severe neurological impairment. If a constellation of tests could identify a subgroup of patients with metastatic cancer who invariably suffered a cardiac arrest within a

short period of time, for example, we would certainly be comfortable in concluding that they were dying, but we clearly could not claim that they were already dead.

Second, this view relies upon the intuitive notion that the brain is the principal organ of the body, the "integrating" organ whose functions cannot be replaced by any other organ or by artificial means. Up through the early 1980s, this view was supported by numerous studies showing that almost all patients who fulfilled the usual battery of tests for brain death suffered a cardiac arrest within several weeks.[21]

The loss of homeostatic equilibrium that is empirically observed in brain-dead patients is almost certainly the result of their progressive loss of integrated neurohumoral and autonomic function. Over the past several decades, however, intensive care units (ICUs) have become increasingly sophisticated "surrogate brainstems," replacing both the respiratory functions as well as the hormonal and other regulatory activities of the damaged neuraxis.[22] This technology is presently utilized in those tragic cases in which a pregnant woman is diagnosed as brain-dead and an attempt is made to maintain her somatic existence until the fetus reaches a viable gestation, as well as for prolonging the organ viability of brain-dead patients awaiting organ procurement.[23] Although the functions of the brainstem are considerably more complex than those of the heart or the lungs, in theory (and increasingly in practice) they are entirely replaceable by modern technology. In terms of maintaining homeostatic functions, therefore, the brain is no more irreplaceable than any of the other vital organs. A definition of death predicated upon the "inevitable" development of a cardiac arrest within a short period of time is therefore inadequate, since this empirical "fact" is no longer true. In other words, cardiac arrest is inevitable only if it is allowed to occur, just as respiratory arrest in brain-dead patients is inevitable only if they are not provided with mechanical ventilation. This gradual development in technical expertise has unwittingly undermined one of the central ethical justifications for the whole-brain criterion of death.

In summary, then, the whole brain concept is plagued by internal inconsistencies in both the test-criterion and the criterion-definition relationships, and these problems cannot be easily solved. In addition, there is evidence that this lack of conceptual clarity has contributed to misunderstandings about the concept among both clinicians and laypersons. For example, Stuart Youngner and colleagues found that only 35 percent of physicians and nurses who were likely to be involved in organ procurement for transplantation correctly identified the legal and medical criteria for determining death.[24] Indeed, most of the respondents used inconsistent concepts of death, and a substantial minority misunderstood the criterion to be the permanent loss of consciousness, which the President's Commission had specifically rejected, in part because it would have classified anencephalic newborns and patients in a vegetative state as dead. In other words, medical professionals who were otherwise knowledgeable and sophisticated were generally confused about the concept of brain death. In an editorial accompanying this study, Dan Wikler and Alan Weisbard claimed that this confusion was "appropriate," given the lack of philosophical coherence in the concept itself.[25] In another study, a survey of Swedes found that laypersons were more willing to consent to autopsies than to organ donation for themselves or a close relative. In seeking an explanation for these findings, the authors reported that "the fear of not being dead during the removal of organs, reported by 22 percent of those undecided toward organ donation, was related to the uncertainty surrounding brain death."[26]

On one hand, these difficulties with the concept might be deemed to be so esoteric and theoretical that they should play no role in driving the policy debate about how to define death and procure organs for transplantation. This has certainly been the predominant view up to now. In many other circumstances, theoretical issues have taken a back seat to practical matters when it comes to determining public policy. For example, the question of whether tomatoes should be considered a vegetable or a fruit for purposes of taxation was said to hinge little upon the biological facts of the matter, but to turn primarily upon the political and economic issues at stake.[27] If this view is applied to the concept of brain death, then the best public policy would be that which best served the public's interest, regardless of theoretical concerns.

On the other hand, medicine has a long and respected history of continually seeking to refine the theoretical and conceptual underpinnings of its practice. While the impact of scientific and philosophical views upon social policy and public perception must be taken seriously, they cannot be the sole forces driving the debate. Given the evidence demonstrating a lack of coherence in the whole-brain death formulation and the confusion that is apparent among medical professionals, there is ample reason to prompt a look at alternatives to our current approach.

Alternative Approaches to the Whole-Brain Formulation

Alternatives to the whole-brain death formulation fall into two general categories. One approach is to emphasize the overriding importance of those functions of the brain that support the phenomenon of consciousness and to claim that individuals who have permanently suffered the loss of all consciousness are dead. This is known as the "higher-brain" criterion. The other approach is to return to the traditional tests for determining death, that is, the permanent loss of circulation and respiration. As noted above, this latter strategy could fit well with Bernat's formulation of the definition of death, since adoption of the cardiorespiratory standard as the test for determining death is consistent with both the criterion and the definition. The problem with this potential solution is that it would virtually eliminate the possibility of procuring vital organs from heart-beating donors under our present system of law and ethics, since current requirements insist that organs be removed only from individuals who have been declared dead (the "dead-donor rule").[28] Consideration of this later view would therefore be feasible only if it could be linked to fundamental changes in the permissible limits of organ procurement.

The Higher-Brain Formulation

The higher-brain criterion for death holds that maintaining the potential for consciousness is the critical function of the brain relevant to questions of life and death. Under this definition, all individuals who are permanently unconscious would be considered to be dead. Included in this category would be (1) patients who fulfill the cardiorespiratory standard, (2) those who fulfill the current tests for whole-brain death, (3) those diagnosed as being in a permanent vegetative state, and (4) newborns with anencephaly. Various versions of this view have been defended by many philosophers, and arguments have been advanced from moral as well as ontological perspectives.[29] In addition, this view correlates very well with many commonsense opinions about personal identity. To take a stock philosophical illustration, for example, consider the typical reaction of a person who has undergone a hypothetical "brain switch" procedure, when one's brain is transplanted into another's body, and vice versa. Virtually anyone presented with this scenario will say that "what matters" for their existence now resides in the new body, even though an outside observer would insist that it is the person's old body that "appears" to be the original person. Thought experiments like this one illustrate that we typically identify ourselves with our experience of consciousness, and this observation forms the basis of the claim that the permanent absence of consciousness should be seen as representing the death of the person.

Implementation of this standard would present certain problems, however. First, is it possible to diagnose the state of permanent unconsciousness with the high level of certainty required for the determination of death? More specifically, is it currently possible to definitively diagnose the permanent vegetative state and anencephaly? A Multi-Society Task Force recently outlined guidelines for diagnosis of permanent vegetative state and claimed that sufficient data are now available to make the diagnosis of permanent vegetative state in appropriate patients with a high degree of certainty.[30] On the other hand, case reports of patients who met these criteria but who later recovered a higher degree of neurological functioning suggest that use of the term "permanent" may be overstating the degree of diagnostic certainty that is currently possible. This would be an especially important issue in the context of diagnosing death, where false positive diagnoses would be particularly problematic.[31] Similarly, while the Medical Task Force on Anencephaly has concluded that most cases of anencephaly can be diagnosed by a compe-

tent clinician without significant uncertainly, others have emphasized the ambiguities inherent in evaluating this condition.[32]

Another line of criticism is that the higher-brain approach assumes the definition of death should reflect the death of the *person* rather than the death of the *organism*.[33] By focusing on the person, this theory does not account for what is common to the death of all organisms, such as humans, frogs, or trees. Since we do not know what it would mean to talk about the permanent loss of consciousness of frogs or trees, then this approach to death may appear to be idiosyncratic. In response, higher-brain theorists believe that it is critical to define death within the context of the specific subject under consideration. For example, we may speak of the death of an ancient civilization, the death of a species, or the death of a particular system of belief. In each case, the definition of death will be different, and must be appropriate to the subject in order for the concept to make any sense. Following this line of reasoning, the higher-brain approach is correct precisely because it seeks to identify what is uniquely relevant to the death of a person.

Aside from these diagnostic and philosophical concerns, however, perhaps the greatest objections to the higher brain formulation emerge from the implications of treating breathing patients as if they are dead. For example, if patients in a permanent vegetative state were considered to be dead, then they should logically be considered suitable for burial. Yet all of these patients breathe, and some of them "live" for many years.[34] The thought of burying or cremating a breathing individual, even if unconscious, would be unthinkable for many people, creating a significant barrier to acceptance of this view into public policy.[35]

One way of avoiding this implication would be to utilize a "lethal injection" before cremation or burial to terminate cardiac and respiratory function. This would not be euthanasia, since the individual would be declared dead before the injection. The purpose of the injection would be purely "aesthetic." This practice could even be viewed as simply an extension of our current protocols, where the vital functions of patients diagnosed as brain-dead are terminated prior to burial, either by discontinuing mechanical ventilation or by removing their heart and/or lungs during the process of organ procurement. While this line of argumentation has a certain logical persuasiveness, it nevertheless fails to address the central fact that most people find it counterintuitive to perceive a breathing patient as "dead." Wikler has suggested that this attitude is likely to change over time, and that eventually society will come to accept that the body of a patient in a permanent vegetative state is simply that person's "living remains."[36] This optimism about higher-brain death is reminiscent of the comments by the President's Commission regarding whole-brain death: "Although undeniably disconcerting for many people, the confusion created in personal perception by a determination of 'brain-death' does not ... provide a basis for and ethical objection to discontinuing medical measures on these dead bodies any more than on other dead bodies."[37] Nevertheless, at the present time any inclination toward a higher brain death standard remains primarily in the realm of philosophers and not policymakers.

Return to the Traditional Cardiorespiratory Standard

In contrast to the higher-brain concept of death, the other main alternative to our current approach would involve moving in the opposite direction and abandoning the diagnosis of brain death altogether. This would involve returning to the traditional approach to determining death, that is, the cardiorespiratory standard. In evaluating the wisdom of "turning back the clock," it is helpful to retrace the development of the concept of brain death back to 1968 and the conclusions of the Ad Hoc Committee that developed the Harvard Criteria for the diagnosis of brain death. They began by claiming:

There are two reasons why there is need for a definition [of brain death]: (1) Improvements in resuscitative and supportive measures have led to increased efforts to save those who are desperately injured. Sometimes these efforts have only partial success so that the result is an individual whose heart continues to beat but whose brain is irreversibly damaged. The burden is great on patients who suffer permanent loss of intellect, on

their families, and on those in need of hospital beds already occupied by these comatose patients. (2) Obsolete criteria for the definition of death can lead to controversy in obtaining organs for transplantation.[38]

These two issues can be subdivided into at least four distinct questions:

1. When is it permissible to withdraw life support from patients with irreversible neurological damage for the benefit of the patient?
2. When is it permissible to withdraw life support from patients with irreversible neurological damage for the benefit of society, where the benefit is either in the form of economic savings or to make an ICU bed available for someone with a better prognosis?
3. When is it permissible to remove organs from a patient for transplantation?
4. When is a patient ready to be cremated or buried?

The Harvard Committee chose to address all of those questions with a single answer, that is, the determination of brain death. Each of these questions involves unique theoretical issues, however, and each raises a different set of concerns. By analyzing the concept of brain death in terms of the separate questions that led to its development, alternatives to brain death may be considered.

Withdrawal of Life Support

The Harvard Committee clearly viewed the diagnosis of brain death as a necessary condition for the withdrawal of life support: "It should be emphasized that we recommend the patient be declared dead before any effort is made to take him off a respirator ... [since] otherwise, the physicians would be turning off the respirator on a person who is, in the present strict, technical application of law, still alive" (p. 339).

The ethical and legal mandates that surround the withdrawal of life support have changed dramatically since the recommendations of the Harvard committee. Numerous court decisions and consensus statements have emphasized the rights of patients or their surrogates to demand the withdrawal of life-sustaining treatments, including mechanical ventilation. In the practice of critical care medicine today, patients are rarely diagnosed as brain-dead solely for the purpose of discontinuing mechanical ventilation. When patients are not candidates for organ transplantation, either because of medical contraindications or lack of consent, families are informed of the dismal prognosis, and artificial ventilation is withdrawn. While the diagnosis of brain death was once critical in allowing physicians to discontinue life-sustaining treatments, decision making about these important questions is now appropriately centered around the patient's previously stated wishes and judgements about the patient's best interest. Questions about the definition of death have become virtually irrelevant to these deliberations.

Allocation of Scarce Resources

The Harvard Committee alluded to its concerns about having patients with a hopeless prognosis occupying ICU beds. In the years since that report this issue has become even more pressing. The diagnosis of brain death, however, is of little significance in helping to resolve these issues. Even considering the unusual cases where families refuse to have the ventilator removed from a brain-dead patient, the overall impact of the diagnosis of brain death upon scarce ICU resources is minimal. Much more important to the current debate over the just allocation of ICU resources are patients with less severe degrees of neurological dysfunction, such as patients in a permanent vegetative state or individuals with advanced dementia. Again, the diagnosis of brain death is of little relevance to this central concern of the Harvard Committee.

Organ Transplantation

Without question, the most important reason for the continued use of brain death criteria is the need for transplantable organs. Yet even here, the requirement for brain death may be doing more harm than good. The need for organs is expanding at an ever-increasing rate, while the number of available organs has essentially plateaued. In an effort to expand the limited pool of organs, several attempts have been made to circumvent the usual restrictions of brain death on organ procurement.

At the University of Pittsburgh, for example, a new protocol allows critically ill patients or their surrogates to offer their organs for donation after the withdrawal of life-support, even though the patients never meet brain death criteria.[39] Suitable patients are taken to the operating room, where intravascular monitors are placed and the patient is "prepped and draped" for surgical incision. Life-support is then withdrawn, and the patient is monitored for the development of cardiac arrest. Assuming this occurs within a short period of time, the attending physician waits until there has been two minutes of pulselessness, and then pronounces the patient dead. The transplant team then enters the operating room and immediately removes the organs for transplantation.

This novel approach has a number of problems when viewed from within the traditional framework. For example, after the patient is pronounced dead, why should the team rush to remove the organs? If the Pittsburgh team truly believes that the patient is dead, why not begin chest compressions and mechanical ventilation, insert cannulae to place the patient on full cardiopulmonary bypass, and remove the organs in a more controlled fashion? Presumably, this is not done because two minutes of pulselessness is almost certainly not long enough to ensure the development of brain death.[40] It is even conceivable that patients managed in this way could regain consciousness during the process of organ procurement while supported with cardiopulmonary bypass, despite having already been diagnosed as "dead." In other words, the reluctance of the Pittsburgh team to extend their protocol in ways that would be acceptable for dead patients could be an indication that the patients may really not be dead after all.

A similar attempt to circumvent the usual restrictions on organ procurement was recently attempted with anencephalic newborns at Loma Linda University. Again, the protocol involved manipulation of the dying process, with mechanical ventilation being instituted and maintained solely for the purpose of preserving the organs until criteria for brain death could be documented. The results were disappointing, and the investigators concluded that "it is usually not feasible, with the restrictions of current law, to procure solid organs for transplantation from anencephalic infants."[41]

Why do these protocols strike many commentators as contrived and even somewhat bizarre? The motives of the individuals involved are certainly commendable: they want to offer the benefits of transplantable organs to individuals who desperately need them. In addition, they are seeking to obtain organs only from individuals who cannot be harmed by the procurement and only in those situations where the patient or a surrogate requests the donation. The problem with these protocols lies not with the motive, but with the method and justification. By manipulating both the process and the definition of death, these protocols give the appearance that the physicians involved are only too willing to draw the boundary between life and death wherever it happens to maximize the chances for organ procurement.

How can the legitimate desire to increase the supply of transplantable organs be reconciled with the need to maintain a clear and simple distinction between the living and the dead? One way would be to abandon the requirement for the death of the donor prior to organ procurement and, instead, focus upon alternative and perhaps more fundamental ethical criteria to constrain the procurement of organs, such as the principles of consent and nonmaleficence.[42]

For example, policies could be changed such that organ procurement would be permitted only with the consent of the donor or appropriate surrogate and only when doing so would not harm the donor. Individuals who could not be harmed by the procedure would include those who are permanently and irreversibly unconscious (patients in a persistent vegetative state or newborns with anencephaly) and those who are imminently and irreversibly dying.

The American Medical Association's Council on Ethical and Judicial Affairs recently proposed (but has subsequently retracted) a position consistent with this approach.[43] The council stated that, "It is ethically permissible to consider the anencephalic as a potential organ donor, although still alive under the current definition of death," if, among other requirements, the diagnosis is certain and the parents give their permission. The council concluded, "It is normally required that the donor be legally dead before removal of their life-necessary organs.... The use of the anencephalic neonate as a live donor is a limited exception to the general standard because of the fact that the infant has never experienced, and will never experience, consciousness" (pp. 1617-18).

This alternative approach to organ procurement would require substantial changes in the law. The process of organ procurement would have to be legitimated as a form of justified killing, rather than just as the dissecting of a corpse. There is certainly precedent in the law for recognizing instances of justified killing. The concept is also not an anathema to the public, as evidenced by the growing support for euthanasia, another practice that would have to be legally construed as a form of justified killing. Even now, surveys show that one-third of physicians and nurses do not believe brain-dead patients are actually dead, but feel comfortable with the process of organ procurement because the patients are permanently unconscious and/or imminently dying.[44] In other words, many clinicians already seem to justify their actions on the basis of nonmaleficence and consent, rather than with the belief that the patients are actually dead.

This alternative approach would also eliminate the need for protocols like the one being used at the University of Pittsburgh, with its contrived and perhaps questionable approach to declaring death prior to organ procurement. Under the proposed system, qualified individuals who had given their consent could simply have their organs removed under general anesthesia, without first undergoing an orchestrated withdrawal of life support. Anencephalic newborns whose parents requested organ donation could likewise have the organs removed under general anesthesia, without the need to wait for the diagnosis of brain death.

The Diagnosis of Death

Seen in this light, the concept of brain death may have become obsolete. Certainly the diagnosis of brain death has been extremely useful during the last several decades, as society has struggled with a myriad of issues that were never encountered before the era of mechanical ventilation and organ transplantation. As society emerges from this transitional period, and as many of these issues are more clearly understood as questions that are inherently unrelated to the distinction between life and death, then the concept of brain death may no longer be useful or relevant. If this is the case, then it may be preferable to return to the traditional standard and limit tests for the determination of death to those based solely upon the permanent cessation of respiration and circulation. Even today we uniformly regard the cessation of respiration and circulation as the standard for determining when patients are ready to be cremated or buried.

Another advantage of a return to the traditional approach is that it would represent a "common denominator" in the definition of death that virtually all cultural groups and religious traditions would find acceptable.[45] Recently both New Jersey and New York have enacted statutes that recognize the objections of particular religious views to the concept of brain death. In New Jersey, physicians are prohibited from declaring brain death in persons who come from religious traditions that do not accept the concept.[46] Return to a cardiorespiratory standard would eliminate problems with these objections.

Linda Emanuel recently proposed a "bounded zone" definition of death that shares some features with the approach outlined here.[47] Her proposal would adopt the cardiorespiratory standard as a "lower bound" for determining death that would apply to all cases, but would allow individuals to choose a definition of death that encompassed neurologic dysfunction up to the level of the permanent vegetative state (the "higher bound"). The practical implications of such a policy would be similar to some of those discussed here, in that it would (1) allow patients and surrogates to request organ donation when and if the patients were diagnosed with whole-brain death, permanent vegetative state, or anencephaly, and (2) it would permit rejection of the diagnosis of brain death by patients and surrogates opposed to the concept. Emanuel's proposal would not permit organ donation from terminal and imminently dying patients, however, prior to the diagnosis of death.

Despite these similarities, these two proposals differ markedly in the justifications used to support their conclusions. Emanuel follows the President's Commission in seeking to address several separate questions by reference to the diagnosis of death, whereas the approach suggested here would adopt a single and uniform definition of death, and then seek to resolve questions around organ donation on a different ethical and legal foundation.

Emanuel's proposal also provides another illustration of the problems encountered when a variety of diverse issues all hinge upon the definition of death. Under her scheme, some individuals would undoubtedly opt for a definition of death based on the "higher bound" of the permanent vegetative state in order to permit the donation of their vital organs if they should develop this condition. However, few of these individuals would probably agree to being cremated while still breathing, even if they were vegetative. Most likely, they would not want to be cremated until after they had sustained a cardiorespiratory arrest. Once again, this creates the awkward and confusing necessity of diagnosing death for one purpose (organ donation) but not for another (cremation). Only by abandoning the concept of brain death is it possible to adopt a definition of death that is valid for all purposes, while separating questions of organ donation from dependence upon the life/death dichotomy.

Turning Back

The tension between the need to maintain workable and practical standards for the procurement of transplantable organs and our desire to have a conceptually coherent account of death is an issue that must be given serious attention. Resolving these inconsistencies by moving toward a higher-brain definition of death would most likely create additional practical problems regarding accurate diagnosis as well as introduce concepts that are highly counterintuitive to the general public. Uncoupling the link between organ transplantation and brain death, on the other hand, offers a number of advantages. By shifting the ethical foundations for organ donation to the principles of nonmaleficence and consent, the pool of potential donors may be substantially increased. In addition, by reverting to a simpler and more traditional definition of death, the long-standing debate over fundamental inconsistencies in the concept of brain death may finally be resolved.

The most difficult challenge for this proposal would be to gain acceptance of the view that killing may sometimes be a justifiable necessity for procuring transplantable organs. Careful attention to the principles of consent and nonmaleficence should provide an adequate bulwark against slippery slope concerns that this practice would be extended in unforeseen and unacceptable ways. Just as the euthanasia debate often seems to turn less upon abstract theoretical concerns and more upon the empirical question of whether guidelines for assisted dying would be abused, so the success of this proposal could also rest upon factual questions of societal acceptance and whether this approach would erode respect for human life and the integrity of clinicians. While the answers to these questions are not known, the potential benefits of this proposal make it worthy of continued discussion and debate.

Acknowledgments

The author thanks numerous friends and colleagues for critical readings of the manuscript, with special acknowledgments to Dan Wikler and Linda Emanuel.

Notes

1 Some of the more notable critiques include Robert M. Veatch, "The Whole-Brain-Oriented Concept of Death. An Outmoded Philosophical Formulation," *Journal of Thanatology* 3 (1975): 13-30; Michael B. Green and Daniel Wikler, "Brain Death and Personal Identity," *Philosophy and Public Affairs* 9 (1980): 105-33; Stuart J. Youngner and Edward T. Bartlett, "Human Death and High Technology: The Failure of the Whole-Brain Formulations," *Annals of Internal Medicine* 99 (1983): 252-58; Amir Halevy and Baruch Brody, "Brain Death: Reconciling Definitions, Criteria, and Tests," *Annals of Internal Medicine* 119 (1993): 519-25.

2 Stuart J. Youngner, "Defining Death: A Superficial and Fragile Consensus," *Archives of Neurology* 49 (1992): 570-72.

3 Presidents's Commission for the Study of Ethical Problems in Medicine and Biomedical and Behavioral Research, *Defining Death* (Washington, DC: Government Printing Office, 1981).

4 Karen Gervais has been especially articulate in defining these levels. See Karen G. Gervais, *Redefining Death* (New Haven: Yale University Press, 1986); "Advancing the Definition of Death: A Philosophical Essay," *Medical Humanities Review* 3, no. 2 (1989): 7-19.

5 James L. Bernat, Charles M. Culver, and Bernard Gert, "On the Definition and Criterion of Death," *Annals of Internal Medicine* 94 (1981): 389-94; James L. Bernat, "How Much of the Brain Must Die in Brain Death?" *Journal of Clinical Ethics* 3 (1992): 21-26.

6 Report of the Medical Consultants on the Diagnosis of Death, "Guidelines for the Determination of Death," *JAMA* 246 (1981): 2184-86.

7 Aspects of this analysis have been explored previously in, Robert D. Truog and James C. Fackler, "Rethinking Brain Death," *Critical Care Medicine* 20 (1992); 1705-13: Halevy and Brody, "Brain Death."

8 H. Schrader et al., "Changes of Pituitary Hormones in Brain Death," *Acta Neurochirurgica* 52 (1980): 239-48; Kristen M. Outwater and Mark A. Rockoff, "Diabetes Insipidus Accompanying Brain Death in Children," *Neurology* 34 (1984): 1243-46; James C. Fackler, Juan C. Troncoso, and Frank R. Gioia, "Age-Specific Characteristics of Brain Death in Children," *American Journal of Diseases of Childhood* 142 (1988): 999-1003.

9 Schrader et al., "Changes of Pituitary Hormones in Brain Death"; H.J. Gramm et al., "Acute Endocrine Failure after Brain Death," *Transplantation* 54 (1992): 851-57.

10 Report of Medical Consultants on the Diagnosis of Death, "Guidelines for the Determination of Death," p. 339.

11 Madeleine M. Grigg et al., "Electroencephalographic Activity after Brain Death," *Archives of Neurology* 44 (1987): 948-54; A. Earl Walker, *Cerebral Death*, 2nd ed. (Baltimore: Urban & Schwarzenberg, 1981), pp. 89-90; and Christopher Pallis, "ABC of Brain Stem Death. The Arguments about the EEG," *British Medical Journal [Clinical Research]* 286 (1983): 284-87.

12   Ernst Rodin et al., "Brainstem Death," *Clinical Elec-troencephalography* 16 (1985): 63-71.

13   Randall C. Wetzel et al., "Hemodynamic Responses in Brain Dead Organ Donor Patients," *Anesthesia and Analgesia* 64 (1985): 125-28; S.H. Pennefather, J.H. Dark, and R.E. Bullock, "Haemodynamic Responses to Surgery in Brain-Dead Organ Donors," *Anaesthesia* 48 (1993): 1034-38; and D.J. Hill, R. Munglani, and D. Sapsford, "Haemodynamic Responses to Surgery in Brain-Dead Organ Donors," *Anaesthesia* 49 (1994): 835-36.

14   Bernat, "How Much of the Brain Must Die in Brain Death?"

15   Paul A. Byrne, Sean O'Reilly, and Paul M. Quay, "Brain Death—An Opposing Viewpoint," *JAMA* 242 (1979): 1985-90.

16   Gaetano F. Molinari, "The NINCDS Collaborative Study of Brain Death: A Historical Perspective," in U.S. Department of Health and Human Services, *NINCDS monograph No. 24 NIH publication NO. 81-2286* (1980): 1-32.

17   Pallis, "ABC of Brain Stem Death," pp. 123-24; Bryan Jennett and Catherine Hessett, "Brain Death in Britain as Reflected in Renal Donors," *British Medical Journal* 283 (1981): 359-62; Peter M. Black, "Brain Death (first of two parts)," *NEJM* 299 (1978): 338-44.

18   President's Commission, *Defining Death*.

19   "An Appraisal of the Criteria of Cerebral Death, A Summary Statement: A Collaborative Study," *JAMA* 237 (1977): 982-86.

20   Green and Wikler, "Brain Death and Personal Identity."

21   President's Commission, *Defining Death*.

22   Green and Wikler, "Brain Death and Personal Identity"; Daniel Wikler, "Brain Death: A Durable Consensus?," *Bioethics* 7 (1993): 239-46.

23   David R. Field et al., "Maternal Brain Death During Pregnancy: Medical and Ethical Issues," *JAMA* 260 (1988): 816-22; Masanobu Washida et al., "Beneficial Effect of Combined 3, 5, 3'—Triiodothyronine and Vasopressin Administration on Hepatic Energy Status and Systemic Hemodynamics after Brain Death," *Transplantation* 54 (1992): 44-49.

24   Stuart J. Youngner et al., "'Brain Death' and Organ Retrieval: A Cross-Sectional Survey of Knowledge and Concepts among Health Professionals," *JAMA* 261 (1989): 2205-10.

25   Daniel Wikler and Alan J. Weisbard "Appropriate Confusion over 'Brain Death,'" *JAMA* 261 (1989): 2246.

26   Margareta Sanner, "A Comparison of Public Attitudes toward Autopsy, Organ Donation, and Anatomic Dissection: A Swedish Survey," *JAMA* 271 (1994): 284-88, at 287.

27   Green and Wikler, "Brain Death and Personal Identity."

28   Robert M. Arnold and Stuart J. Youngner, "The Dead Donor Rule: Should We Stretch It, Bend It, or Abandon It?" *Kennedy Institute of Ethics Journal* 3 (1993): 263-78.

29   Some of the many works defending this view include: Green and Wikler, "Brain Death and Personal Identity"; Gervais, *Redefining Death*; Truog and Fackler, "Rethinking Brain Death," and Robert M. Veatch, *Death, Dying, and the Biological Revolution* (New Haven: Yale University Press, 1989).

30   The Multi-Society Task Force on PVS, "Medical Aspects of the Persistent Vegetative State," *NEJM* 330 (1994): 1499-1508 and 1572-79; D. Alan Shewmon, "Anencephaly: Selected Medical Aspects," *Hastings Center Report* 18, no. 5 (1988):11-19.

31   Nancy L. Childs and Walt N. Mercer, "Brief Report: Late Improvement in Consciousness after Post-Traumatic Vegetative State," *NEJM* 334 (1996): 24-25; James L. Bernat, "The Boundaries of the Persistent Vegetative State," *Journal of Clinical Ethics* 3 (1992): 176-80.

32   Medical Task Force on Anencephaly, "The Infant with Anencephaly," *NEJM* 322 (1990): 669-74; Shewmon, "Anencephaly: Selected Medical Aspects."

33   Jeffery R. Botkin and Stephen G. Post, "Confusion in the Determination of Death: Distinguishing Philosophy from Physiology," *Perspectives in Biology and Medicine* 36 (1993): 129-38.

34   The Multi-Society Task Force on PVS. "Medical Aspects of the Persistent Vegetative State."

35   Marcia Angell, "After Quinlan: The Dilemma of the Persistent Vegetative State," *NEJM* 330 (1994): 1524-25.

36   Wikler, "Brain Death: A Durable Consensus."

37   President's Commission, *Defining Death*, p. 84.

38   Report of the Ad Hoc Committee of the Harvard Medical School to Examine the Definition of Brain

Death, "A Definition of Irreversible Coma," *JAMA* 205 (1968): 337-40.

39   "University of Pittsburgh Medical Center Policy and Procedure Manual: Management of Terminally Ill Patients Who May Become Organ Donors after Death," *Kennedy Institute of Ethics Journal* 3 (1993): A1-A15; Stuart Youngner and Robert Arnold, "Ethical, Psychosocial, and Public Policy Implications of Procuring Organs from Non-Heart-Beating Cadaver Donors," *JAMA* 269 (1993): 2769-74. Of note, the June 1993 issue of the *Kennedy Institute of Ethics Journal* is devoted to this topic in its entirety.

40   Joanne Lynn, "Are the Patients Who Become Organ Donors Under the Pittsburgh Protocol for 'Non-Heart-Beating Donors' Really Dead?" *Kennedy Institute of Ethics Journal* 3 (1993): 167-78.

41   Joyce L. Peabody, Janet R. Emery, and Stephen Ashwal, "Experience with Anencephalic Infants as Prospective Organ Donors," *NEJM* 321 (1989): 344-50.

42   See for example, Norman Fost, "The New Body Snatchers: On Scott's 'The Body as Property,'" *American Bar Foundation Research Journal* 3 (1983): 718-32; John A. Robertson, "Relaxing the Death Standard for Organ Donation in Pediatric Situations," in *Organ Substitution Technology: Ethical, Legal, and Public Policy Issues*, ed. D. Mathieu (Boulder, CO: Westview Press, 1988), pp. 69-76; Arnold and Youngner, "The Dead Donor Rule."

43   AMA Council on Ethical and Judicial Affairs, "The Use of Anencephalic Neonates as Organ Donors," *JAMA* 273 (1995): 1614-18. After extensive debate among AMA members, the Council retracted this position statement. See Charles W. Plows, "Reconsideration of AMA Opinion on Anencephalic Neonates as Organ Donors," *JAMA* 275 (1996): 443-44.

44   Youngner et al., "'Brain Death' and Organ Retrieval."

45   Jiro Nudeshima, "Obstacles to Brain Death and Organ Transplantation in Japan," *Lancet* 338 (1991): 1063-64.

46   Robert S. Olick, "Brain Death, Religious Freedom, and Public Policy: New Jersey's Landmark Legislative Initiative," *Kennedy Institute of Ethics Journal* 1 (1991): 275-88.

47   Linda L. Emanuel, "Reexamining Death: The Asymptotic Model and a Bounded Zone Definition," *Hastings Center Report* 25, no. 4 (1995): 27-35.

41.
DEATH AND ORGAN DONATION: BACK TO THE FUTURE

F.G. Miller

SOURCE: *Journal of Medical Ethics* 35:10 (2009): 616-20.

The practice of transplantation of vital organs from "brain-dead" donors is in a state of theoretical disarray. Although the law and prevailing medical ethics treat patients diagnosed as having irreversible total brain failure as dead, scholars have increasingly challenged the established rationale for regarding these patients as dead. To understand the ethical situation that we now face, it is helpful to revisit the writings of the philosopher Hans Jonas, who forcefully challenged the emerging effort to redefine death in the late 1960s.

The President's Council on Bioethics recently issued a report entitled, "Controversies in the determination of death."[1] The title signifies the unsettled state of current thinking regarding the determination of death, with fundamental implications for the ethics of vital organ transplantation. A 1981 publication by a predecessor public bioethics body—The President's Commission for the Study of Ethical Problems in Medicine and Biomedical and Behavioral Research—consolidated a consensus regarding the determination of death on neurological criteria and articulated what was then seen as a persuasive rationale for regarding patients diagnosed as having "brain death" as biologically dead.[2] The acceptance of brain death as death of the human being legitimated the practice of procuring viable vital organs from patients with devastating neurological injury who were still breathing (and perfusing their organs) with the aid of mechanical ventilators. By the late 1990s, however, the equation of brain death with death of the human being was increasingly challenged by scholars, based on evidence regarding the array of biological functioning displayed by patients correctly diagnosed as having this condition who were maintained on mechanical ventilation for substantial periods of time.[3-5] These patients maintained the ability to sustain circulation and respiration, control temperature, excrete wastes, heal wounds, fight infections and, most dramatically, to gestate fetuses (in the case of pregnant "brain-dead" women).[6,7]

The thesis propounded by the President's Commission that the "death" of the brain constituted death of the human being, because the integrated functioning of the organism as a whole had ceased, no longer seemed credible to critics of the "whole brain" standard of death. This scholarly criticism was instrumental in prompting the President's Council on Bioethics to re-examine the determination of death, to reject the rationale of the President's Commission for neurological criteria defining death, and to attempt a new (but unpersuasive) account of why patients with "total brain failure" are biologically dead.

Nevertheless, the practice of transplantation with vital organs procured from brain-dead donors has proceeded on the basis of "business as usual," with death declared before extracting organs, consistent with the "dead donor rule." Moreover, the scholarly controversy over determining death has yet to disturb the prevailing understanding within the medical establishment of vital organ donation as based solidly on the thesis that brain death equals death. A recent commentary in the *JAMA* Classics series, reviewing the landmark 1968 article promulgating the criteria for defining brain death, declared that "The criteria for brain death enumerated in this article have surely held up during the past 40 years."[8] The author goes on to observe that "identification of an irreversible state of coma has made possible the ethical and practical donation of living organs from patients with brain death." Remarkably, there is no mention of any controversy over whether the clinical state denominated as "brain death" constitutes death of the human being.

In this article I endeavour to illuminate the ethical situation that we now face with respect to the determination of death and vital organ donation by revisiting the perspective of the philosopher Hans Jonas—a pioneer in bioethics. In two papers written between 1968 and 1970, Jonas rejected the emerging concept of brain death and the prospect of procuring vital organs for transplantation from those designated as brain dead. By going back to the thinking of Jonas, during an era when neurological criteria for determining death had yet to be established and organ transplantation was a novel procedure, we can obtain fresh insight into where we are and where we might be going in understanding the connection between death and vital organ donation.

Setting the Stage

Before examining the details of the position staked out by Jonas, it helps to set the stage. In the 1960s intensive care units had been established and organ transplantation was under development. Medicine faced a problem and an opportunity in the intersection between these two areas of clinical practice.[9] The problem was how to respond appropriately to the situation of patients with devastating and permanent neurological injury who were hooked up to mechanical ventilators in intensive care units. The opportunity was to take advantage of the fact that these patients, who had no prospect of return to a meaningful human life, were ideal sources of organs for transplantation. In 1968, an Ad Hoc Committee of the Harvard Medical School, headed by the distinguished anaesthesiologist Henry Beecher, produced an article, published in *JAMA*, defining brain death.[10] This article noted two purposes for establishing "a new criterion for death": "(1) improvements in resuscitative and supportive measures have led to increased efforts to save those who are desperately injured. Sometimes these efforts have led to partial success so that the result is an individual whose heart continues to beat but whose brain is irreversibly damaged. The burden is great on patients who suffer permanent loss of intellect, on their families, on the hospitals, and on those in need of hospital beds already occupied by these comatose patients. (2) Obsolete criteria for

definition of death can lead to controversy in obtaining organs for transplantation."

Historical commentators have diverged in evaluating the real motivations of Beecher and the Harvard committee. Some have argued, following the committee's stated position, that organ transplantation was only a secondary concern. The primary motivation was to overcome reluctance on the part of physicians to stop intensive care treatment for brain-dead patients, as continued treatment was of no value for them, a needless burden on their families and a waste of scarce resources.[11] Others have contended that the first-mentioned and emphasised concern about life-sustaining treatment was a smokescreen masking the primary motivation to legitimate and facilitate organ transplantation—a smokescreen because physicians were already comfortable with stopping treatment for brain-dead patients.[12]

From the dual perspective of examining the views of Jonas and illuminating our current situation, there is no need to take sides on this dispute about the true motivation of the Harvard committee. Jonas was especially concerned with the prospect of using brain-injured patients as a source of organs for transplantation. However matters stood in 1968, by the early 1980s the legality and ethics of withdrawing life-sustaining treatment was not in question. Based on the evolution of law and medical ethics, clinicians became comfortable with withdrawing life-sustaining treatment in a wide range of circumstances that were not predicated on determining that the patient is already dead.[13] (Ethicists, however, continue to disagree about how to characterise the act of treatment withdrawal—is it merely allowing to die or does it cause death?—and, accordingly, how it differs from or resembles active euthanasia.) Instead, we currently face the challenge of providing a coherent and cogent justification of vital organ transplantation in view of the controversy over the status of donors diagnosed as being brain dead.

Jonas on Death and Organ Donation

Jonas was one of the first philosophers to engage with the issue of the ethics of human experimentation. In a now classic article on this topic, published in 1969, he devoted the penultimate section to "On the redefinition of death."[14] He seized the opportunity to express his strong opposition to the implications for organ donation of the position of the Harvard Ad Hoc Committee. Looking back from the present—from a time when transplantation of vital organs procured from brain-dead patients has become routinised as a standard life-saving procedure—this section looks tacked on and out of place. Indeed, in a later essay elaborating his views on the definition of death and organ transplantation, Jonas[15] noted that his discussion of this topic in the previous essay was "marginal to the discussion of 'experimentation on human subjects.'" Yet in 1968, organ transplantation was essentially experimental and unsuccessful as a longer-term treatment, as a result of an inability to solve the problem of organ rejection by the recipient. Moreover, the famous conclusion of Jonas's essay on human experimentation[14] was apparently also meant to apply to the effort to redefine death in order to facilitate organ transplantation: "Let us not forget that progress is an optional goal, not an unconditional commitment ... Let us also remember that a slower progress in the conquest of disease would not threaten society, grievous as it is to those who have to deplore that their particular disease be not yet conquered, but that society would indeed be threatened by the erosion of those moral values whose loss, possibly caused by too ruthless a pursuit of scientific progress, would make its dazzling triumphs not worth having."

In a nutshell, Jonas argued that "brain-dead" patients remained alive, and that using them as a source of vital organs for transplantation was just the sort of erosion of moral values that would threaten the normative foundations of social life.

Jonas contended that there were no grounds for regarding the patient diagnosed as being "brain dead" as a dead human being. We need absolute certainty of death to treat the human body as a corpse or cadaver, from which it may be appropriate to extract organs with the aim of saving the life of another. This, however, is not afforded by the condition of "irreversible coma" that the Harvard committee described as satisfying a new criterion for death. In addition, the nascent rationale that the organism as a whole failed to function in these patients did not hold water according to Jonas. He correctly saw res-

piration and circulation as central organismic functions, albeit driven by artificial means. Indeed, he opined that the brain-dead organism was capable of "pretty much everything not involving neural control," a thesis that has been borne out by more recent evidence.[15] In this vein, Shewmon[16] has demonstrated that, setting aside the capacity for consciousness, the brain-dead patient essentially displays the same pattern of biological functioning and dysfunction as ventilator-dependent quadriplegic patients with high level cervical damage, who unquestionably are alive.

Jonas took pains to emphasise that he had no objection to stopping life-sustaining treatment in these patients—"to cease the artificial prolongation of certain functions (like heartbeat) traditionally regarded as signs of life," and thus to allow them to die.[14] Allowing to die by stopping treatment is one thing and the lethal act of extracting vital organs in still-living patients is another. Thinking "against the stream"—the title of his follow-up essay explaining his position on the new definition of death—Jonas got it right concerning the living status of "brain-dead" patients. They neither appear to be, nor are, corpses or cadavers—a conclusion that has become all the more apparent with greater knowledge about the biological functioning that they maintain with the aid of mechanical ventilation and other measures of routine support. Does it follow that it is wrong to extract vital organs from these patients, as Jonas eloquently contended?

Jonas adduced three arguments against procuring organs from patients in the irreversible coma described as "brain death." First, we cannot be confident that these still heart-beating and breathing human beings are immune from suffering. Indeed, he notes that the prospect of organ extraction from these patients would amount to what would have previously been called "vivisection" and "would be torture and death to any living body."[14] He acknowledges, however, that this point "is merely a subsidiary and not the real point of my argument."[14] Second, it is wrongful exploitation to extract vital organs from living patients, no matter how neurologically compromised they may be. Jonas states, "When only permanent coma can be gained with the artificial sustaining of functions, by all means turn off the respirator ... and let the patient die; but let him die all the way. Do not, instead, arrest the process and start *using him as a mine*" (italics added).[14] Extracting organs before death treats the living being as a thing. In his later essay, Jonas invokes the Kantian injunction against using people merely as a means. The patient in an irreversible coma retains the "sacrosanctity" of a living human being: "That sacrosanctity decrees that it must not be used as a mere means."[15] Third, for physicians to engage in a practice of lethal organ donation is contrary to the moral vocation of medicine. Consistent with his penchant for strong rhetoric, exhibited in the quotes above, Jonas remarks, "The patient must be absolutely sure that his doctor does not become his executioner, and that no definition authorises him ever to become one."[14]

Critique

What are the merits of these arguments? I set aside the first relating to suffering. The neurological condition of patients satisfying the clinical criteria for brain death makes it highly doubtful that they retain the capacity for feeling pain; moreover, any doubts on that score could be addressed by using anaesthesia during the process of organ extraction. With respect to exploitation, Jonas presumably would have had no objection to procuring organs from individuals who were genuinely dead, provided that proper consent to do so was obtained. As Paul Ramsey observed, "Let it be said at once that after it has been determined that a patient has died and doctors and the family are in the presence of an unburied corpse, the corpse itself can certainly be used as a 'vital organ bank.'"[17] However, if "brain-dead" patients remain alive, as Jonas contended, are they necessarily being exploited when their organs are procured for transplantation to save the lives of others? In a non-moral sense of the word, they certainly are being exploited, as their vital organs are being used for the purpose of transplantation. The key issue is whether they are merely being used—whether the use is wrongful. In many areas of interpersonal conduct, consent marks the difference between wrongfully using a person merely as a means and morally permissible interaction, as in the differences between slavery and employment, theft

and borrowing, rape and permissible sexual intercourse, and treating patients as human guinea pigs and ethical clinical research.

Consider the situation of healthy individuals who donate blood, bone marrow, or a kidney. When they validly consent for such donation, we do not regard them as being wrongfully exploited. They are being used, with their consent, to help save the lives of others; but they are not being treated as a "mine," from which precious resources can be extracted for profit. Why, then, should vital organ procurement from still-living but brain-dead patients be understood as wrongful exploitation? Although individuals who have the irreversible coma known as brain death are not able to give contemporaneous informed consent, many may have expressed previously their preferences for organ donation. When no previous preferences have been registered or expressed, family members are entitled to consent for organ donation on behalf of the brain-dead individual. To be sure, currently the choice of becoming a "cadaveric" organ donor in the event of brain death is predicated on the premise that to be diagnosed as having this condition is to be dead. The issue here is exploitation, not the justification of causing death in the act of procuring vital organs. Setting aside concerns about whether consent to be killed, in some circumstances, should be regarded as validly authorising a lethal process of organ procurement, with respect to the charge of wrongful exploitation it is difficult to see why it matters whether the donating individual is alive or dead, provided there is genuine consent.

The crux of the matter ethically centres on the possible legitimacy of lethal organ donation, in which vital organs are extracted from irreversibly comatose but still-living individuals before a planned withdrawal of life-sustaining treatment. Describing the transplant surgeon as an "executioner" does not serve moral clarity in approaching this issue. Jonas apparently saw a moral bright line between stopping life-sustaining treatment, thus (merely) allowing the patient to die and causing death by extracting vital organs. In this respect his position reflects prevailing medical ethics. Some ethicists, however, regard stopping life support for those who require it to continue living as patently a matter of causing death.[18] According to this perspective, insisting that withdrawing life-sustaining treatment is a passive omission of treatment that merely allows the patient to die amounts to a "moral fiction"—a morally motivated false belief—endorsed in order to preserve the absolute validity of the traditional norm that doctors must not kill patients. Given the ethical legitimacy of stopping life-sustaining treatment (despite causing death) on the grounds of self-determination and nonmaleficence, it is far from obvious that any harm or wrong is done to patients diagnosed as having irreversible apnoeic coma (brain death) if their vital organs are donated, with proper consent, before stopping life-sustaining treatment.[19] As the imminent and legitimate outcome from withdrawing life support is the patient's death, whether caused or allowed to occur, should we not be concerned about wasting the precious life-saving resource of vital organs? This concern about the consequences of failing to use an available resource might be considered the obverse of the charge of exploitation.

Is the life-saving medical progress represented by vital organ transplantation an optional goal? Jonas undoubtedly is right that progress is not morally imperative if it comes at the expense of violating human rights. Scientific and technological interventions aimed at promoting human well-being must be subject to deontological constraints. However, it is important not to beg the question concerning the wrongfulness of vital organ procurement from braindead but still-living patients—whether it is the sort of grave moral wrong that would make the "dazzling triumphs" of scientific progress "not worth having." In 1968 the progress from organ transplantation was anticipated but not achieved. However, if Jonas's position had prevailed, substantial medical progress in saving lives would have been deterred. This progress was ostensibly justified by means of invoking the moral fiction that brain death equals death of the human being—a fiction that Jonas presciently exposed. Whether we are prepared to persist in the practice of vital organ donation without the support of this fiction is the ethical situation that we now face.

Where We Stand Today

Revisiting the still-provocative essays of Jonas on brain death and organ donation helps in mapping present and future ethical and policy options. Four options seem most salient. First, we can follow the lead of Jonas by adopting a stance of deontological rectitude that abandons vital organ procurement from brain-dead, but still-living patients. This position is logically tidy and unassailable if its major premise is endorsed: (1) doctors must not kill patients; (2) brain-dead patients are alive; (3) procuring vital organs from brain-dead patients would cause their death; therefore, (4) this practice is wrong and must cease. However, the validity of the first premise is debatable; and if applied consistently, it would have drastic consequences. For not only would it put a stop to the life-saving practice of vital organ transplantation using the organs of brain-dead individuals; it also arguably would rule out the routine practice of deliberately stopping life-sustaining treatment, assuming the reasonable, but unorthodox, view that this practice involves causing death. (A partial way out of this latter impasse might be afforded by putting timers on life-support technology, such as ventilators, as is practised in Israel, thus permitting a genuine omission of treatment that does not cause death by virtue of deciding not to restart life support.)[20] In any case, the deleterious consequences of this position limited to vital organ donation from brain-dead patients are sufficient to give pause to anyone seriously considering its adoption. Beyond foregoing life-saving transplantations, these consequences include thwarting the preferences of people interested in organ donation in the event of catastrophic neurological injury such as brain death and of family members interested in making some good come out of an unexpected tragedy.

A second position attempts to justify vital organ donation while maintaining (at least nominally) the dead donor rule by appealing to a distinction between the death of the human being and the death of the biological organism. According to this position, Jonas is right that the brain-dead patient is biologically alive; however, what matters ethically with respect to vital organ procurement is whether the human being has ceased to exist. In this "higher brain" position, the permanent loss of consciousness is regarded as the death of the human being.[21-23] Once human life has ceased, stopping life-sustaining treatment is appropriate (or imperative), and there can be no ethical objection to extracting vital organs beforehand.

Although attractive to some philosophers, this position is unlikely to garner a wide consensus. It was rejected by both the President's Commission in 1981 and the President's Council on Bioethics in 2008. Advocates of the mainstream whole brain standard of death have insisted that there is only one (essentially biological) concept of death, which encompasses both neurological and cardiopulmonary criteria. They have claimed, although unpersuasively, that the brain-dead body is really a breathing corpse or cadaver because it is truly a dead organism. The purpose of a standard for the determination of death has been to indicate decisively when a human body is a corpse, making it suitable for burial or cremation as well as a source of organs to benefit others. The higher brain position, by contrast, entirely severs the concept of death of the human being from the status of being a corpse, making it decidedly counterintuitive. Moreover, it faces diagnostic problems. When can we be certain that biologically alive human beings are dead because they have irreversibly lost the capacity for consciousness? Any move beyond the diagnostic criteria for brain death is fraught with peril, in view of emerging data on the neural functioning of patients in a persistent vegetative state.[8] Nor is this position free of philosophical difficulties. It at least appears to conflate loss of personhood, or the loss of all value in existence, with death. Advocates of this position may respond that there is no conflation because death is not a univocal concept: the death of the human being does not equate to the death of the organism.[23] However, apart from the strategic effort to uphold the dead donor rule while permitting vital organ donation from permanently unconscious patients, it is not clear why it is necessary or desirable to invoke two kinds of death on the human level, as distinct from the unitary concept of death that applies to the rest of the biological world. The concept of the death of the human being based on permanent loss of consciousness is not needed to justify stopping life-sustaining treatment, as this can be appropriate for mentally intact patients who view continued living in their condition as intolerable.[24,25]

A third position justifies vital organ donation while retaining the traditional cardiopulmonary criteria for determining death by biting the bullet of abandoning the dead donor rule.[19] As suggested above, this position sees vital organ procurement from "brain-dead" but still-living patients as exposing them neither to harm nor violating their rights as long as it is connected with a previous plan to stop life-sustaining treatment and proper consent, both for stopping treatment and organ donation. Stopping life-sustaining treatment when justified is a legitimate act of causing the patient's death; procuring vital organs before treatment withdrawal is justified on essentially the same ethical grounds of self-determination and nonmaleficence.[19]

Regardless of its theoretical and practical merits, this position will be staunchly resisted by all those who endorse the "sanctity" of human life and the related traditional norm of medical ethics that doctors must never kill (cause the death of) patients. Whether openly procuring vital organs from living patients would be accepted by the public is also in question. However, if press reports indicate how lay persons think about this issue, there is reason to think that many members of the public do not believe that brain death constitutes death, despite support for organ donation. For example, a recent news report of policemen killed in the line of duty, stated that "A police officer shot during a traffic stop was pronounced brain-dead but remained on life support. Oakland police spokesman Jeff Thomason ... said that [officer] Hege was being kept alive while a final decision was made about donating his organs."[26] The public by and large may consider brain-dead patients alive but "as good as dead," making it legitimate to procure their organs, with proper consent.[27]

It is important to acknowledge that informed consent for lethal organ donation under this third position differs from the current practice of informed consent for organ donation that is predicated on the assumption that the "brain-dead" patient is dead. Prospective consent of donors or contemporaneous consent of surrogates would need to be based on recognition that the donor diagnosed as "brain dead" remains alive and will die as the result of the process of organ procurement and/or stopping life-sustaining treatment. Would it be harder to obtain consent for vital organ donation from such patients who are recognised as still living? It is not clear that facing the truth about the status of "brain-dead" individuals would affect the willingness to provide consent, in view of the evidence suggesting that many people currently do not regard them as genuinely dead.

Finally, a fourth position upholds the status quo by insisting that brain death constitutes biological death of the human organism, despite powerful evidence to the contrary. No plausible and coherent account has been advanced to explain why brain-dead patients are dead, making this position the least intellectually satisfactory of the various options; however, it is likely to be the one that will prevail in the near future. This position can take the form of articulating some rationale that gives the appearance of making sense of dual neurological and cardiopulmonary criteria for death, as in the case of the novel account presented in the President's Council recent report, or simply insisting on the fact that brain death constitutes death has been established, as in the recent *JAMA* commentary on the 1968 report of the Harvard committee.[8] The other positions, although superior in internal coherence, are apt to seem unpalatable. On the one hand, for most people it would be morally intolerable to put a stop to, or drastically curtail, vital organ donation. On the other hand, neither the higher brain standard nor openly abandoning the dead donor rule are likely to be acceptable to most ethicists and to professionals involved in critical care and transplantation.

Nevertheless, any semblance of a consensus over death and vital organ donation will be fragile and theoretically weak. Brain dead patients do not appear to be dead, and arguments that they really are dead do not inspire conviction. Hans Jonas got it right in 1968 regarding the living status of these patients; and he correctly discerned that efforts to explain their being dead on the grounds that the organism as a whole ceased to exist were dubious. Where do we go from here? We face an unsettled and unsettling situation characterised by the moral imperative to continue vital organ transplantation, the entrenched norm that doctors must not kill, and the increasingly transparent fiction that the brain dead are really dead. In at least the near future it is probable that we will continue to muddle through. In the longer run, the medical profession and society may, and should, be prepared to accept the reality and justifiability of life-terminating acts in medicine in the context of stopping life-sustaining treatment and performing vital organ transplantation.

The opinions expressed are the views of the author and do not necessarily reflect the policy of the National Institutes of Health, the Public Health Service, or the US Department of Health and Human Services.

References

1   President's Council on Bioethics. 2008. *Controversies in the determination of death*. Washington, DC. www.bioethics.gov (accessed July 2009).

2   President's Commission for the Study of Ethical Problems in Medicine and Biomedical and Behavioral Research. *Defining death: medical, legal and ethical issues in the determination of death*. Washington, DC: Government Printing Office, 1981.

3   Veatch RM. The impending collapse of the whole-brain definition of death. *Hastings Center Report* 1993;23:18-24.

4   Truog RD. Is it time to abandon brain death? *Hastings Center Report* 1997;27:29-37.

5   Shewmon DA. Chronic 'brain death': meta-analysis and conceptual consequences. *Neurology* 1998;51:1538-45.

6   Souza JP, Oliveria-Neto A, Surita FG, et al. The prolongation of somatic support in a pregnant woman with brain-death: a case report. *Reproductive Health* 2006;3:3 doi:10.1186/1742-4755-3-3.

7   Yeung P, McManus C, Tchabo J-G. Extended somatic support for a pregnant woman with brain death from metastatic malignant melanoma: a case report. *J Maternal-Fetal Neonatal Med* 2008;21:509-11.

8   Rosenberg RN. Consciousness, coma and brain death—2009. *JAMA* 2009;301:1172-74.

9   Youngner SJ. The definition of death. In: Steinbock B, ed. *The Oxford handbook of bioethics*. Oxford: Oxford University Press, 2007:285-303.

10 Ad Hoc Committee of the Harvard Medical School to Examine the Definition of Brain Death. A definition of irreversible coma. *JAMA* 1968;205:337-40.

11 Belkin GS. Brain death and the historical understanding of bioethics. *J Hist Med Allied Sci* 2003;58:325-61.

12 Stevens MLT. *Bioethics in America*. Baltimore: Johns Hopkins University Press, 2000:75-108.

13 President's Commission for the Study of Ethical Problems in Medicine and Biomedical and Behavioral Research. *Deciding to forego life-sustaining treatment*. Washington, DC: Government Printing Office, 1983.

14 Jonas H. Philosophical reflections on experimenting with human subjects. In: Freund PA, ed. *Experimentation with human subjects*. New York: George Braziller, 1970:1-31.

15 Jonas H. Against the stream: comments on the definition and redefinition of death. In: Jonas H, ed. *Philosophical essays*. Chicago: University of Chicago Press, 1974:132-40.

16 Shewmon DA. Spinal shock and 'brain death': Somatic pathophysiological equivalence and implications for the integrative-unity rationale. *Spinal Cord* 1999;37:313-24.

17 Ramsey P. On updating procedures for stating that a man has died. In: Ramsey P, ed. *The patient as person*, 2nd ed. New Haven: Yale University Press, 2002:69.

18 Miller FG, Truog RD, Brock DW. Moral fictions and medical ethics. *Bioethics* 2009; in press.

19 Miller FG, Truog RD. Rethinking the ethics of vital organ donation. *Hastings Center Report* 2008;38:38-46.

20 Ravitsky V. Timers on ventilators. *BMJ* 2005; 330:415-17.

21 Green MB, Wikler D. Brain death and personal identity. *Philos Public Affairs* 1980;9:105-33.

22 Gervais KG. *Redefining death*. New Haven: Yale University Press, 1986.

23 McMahan J. An alternative to brain death. *J Law, Med Ethics* 2006;34:44-48.

24 Powell T, Lowenstein B. Refusing life-sustaining treatment after catastrophic injury: ethical implications. *J Law, Med Ethics* 1996;24:54-61.

25 Miller FG. A planned death in the family. *Hastings Center Report* 2009;39:28-30.

26 Collins T, Leff L. Wounded Oakland officer brain-dead. *The Washington Post*, 23 March 2009, A4.

27 Siminoff LA, Burant C, Youngner SJ. Death and organ procurement: public beliefs and attitudes. *Soc Sci Med* 2004;59:2325-34.

CHAPTER SEVEN

RESEARCH INVOLVING
HUMAN PARTICIPANTS

Web Links

(1) Link to Declaration of Helsinki.

   http://www.wma.net/en/30publications/10policies/b3/17c.pdf

The Declaration of Helsinki was developed by the World Medical Association in 1964. It is a statement of ethical norms for conducting clinical research and experimentation involving human beings. These standards have been of particular importance since the Second World War, when a series of Nazi experiments were conducted on prisoners and resulted in death, disfigurement, and disability. The Helsinki Declaration modified the earlier Nuremberg Code and has undergone a series of revisions. It has informed the development of documents such as Canada's Tri-Council Policy Statement.

(2) Link to Tri-Council Policy Statement.

   http://www.pre.ethics.gc.ca/pdf/eng/tcps2/TCPS_2_FINAL_Web.pdf

The Tri-Council includes the Canadian Institutes of Health Research (CIHR), the Natural Sciences and Engineering Research Council (NSERC), and the Social Sciences and Humanities Research Council (SSHRC). The statement sets out the principles and standards for maintaining ethical behaviour in research with humans.

* For an up-to-date list of the web links in this book, please visit:
http://sites.broadviewpress.com/healthcare.

42.

MISUNDERSTANDING IN CLINICAL RESEARCH: DISTINGUISHING THERAPEUTIC MISCONCEPTION, THERAPEUTIC MISESTIMATION, AND THERAPEUTIC OPTIMISM

Sam Horng and Christine Grady

SOURCE: *IRB: Ethics and Human Research* 25.1 (2003): 11-16.

Understanding is a requirement of informed consent,[1] which is itself fundamental to ethical clinical research.[2] Data show that many research subjects misunderstand various aspects of the research in which they participate, and investigators, study coordinators, and IRBs are also suspected to share these misunderstandings. Interview studies with subjects in phase I cancer trials, for example, reveal that many of them confuse the aims of research with the aims of clinical care,[3,4,5,6] and both subjects and investigators overestimate the expected benefit of phase I trial participation.[7,8,9,10] Ethicists have pointed to these misunderstandings as cause for alarm by invoking the therapeutic misconception.[11] Unfortunately, therapeutic misconception has been used loosely to refer to any number of misunderstandings that subjects may have in the research context. This imprecise use of the term can itself cloud our assessment of when informed consent is compromised. Different types of misunderstanding are possible, and in this paper, we distinguish and discuss two of them in order to demonstrate how misunderstandings of different components of research carry distinct ethical implications for informed consent. We further distinguish the concepts of misunderstanding and optimism.

Illustrative Cases

Mark is a 63-year-old retired engineer with advanced colon cancer. He wishes to participate in a phase I clinical trial that is testing the safety of a new chemotherapeutic agent. Before enrollment, as the primary investigator interviews Mark in order to assess his understanding of the research, Mark reports that the purpose of the trial is to find out how well the chemotherapy will shrink his tumor. Even though the actual purpose of the trial is to discover the maximum tolerated dose of the agent in humans, he claims that the trial "is designed to help people who have no other options," and that the research doctors "have [his] best interests in mind." While the risks of the untested agent exceed those of standard chemotherapy, he feels that the possible risks are "no worse than the treatment [he has] already tried." He estimates the probability of benefit to be at least 30%. The investigator's estimate of potential benefit is 5%, based on previous meta-analyses of similar phase I cancer trials.

Susan is a 45-year-old journalist who also suffers from advanced colon cancer. She volunteers for the same phase I cancer trial as Mark. In the pre-enrollment interview, Susan states correctly that the purpose of the trial is "to find the highest dose of the drug that is safe in humans." Moreover, she mentions that she has considered the possibility of being assigned either to a dose that is too low to have a therapeutic effect on her cancer or to a dose that is high enough to cause severe side effects. Nevertheless, she states that this is a "low risk research trial," and estimates the probability of benefit to be around 30%.

Thomas, a 57-year-old painter with advanced colon cancer, wishes to enroll in the phase I trial as well. He recognizes that safety testing is the purpose of the trial and estimates harm and benefit with probabilities similar to those of the investigator. However, he hopes that he is "one of the 5%" to receive benefit from the tested agent.

Which, if any these cases, is ethically problematic? Mark, Susan, and Thomas demonstrate differ-

Figure 1.

Concept	Definition	Ethical Significance	Example
Therapeutic Misconception	The research subject conflates research with clinical care.	*Rarely* tolerable because understanding the nature of research is necessary for an autonomous decision to participate in research.	Mark believes that the purpose of the phase I cancer trial is to help him personally.
Therapeutic Misestimation	The research subject under-estimates risk, overestimates benefit, or both.	*Sometimes* tolerable because under-standing the exact probability of harm and benefit may not be necessary for an autonomous decision to participate in research.	Susan estimates that she has a 30% chance of benefit in the phase I cancer trial. A meta-analysis of similar studies shows that benefit accrues to 5% of subjects.
Therapeutic Optimism	The research subject hopes for the best personal outcome.	*Always* tolerable because hope does not compromise the autonomy of a decision to participate in research.	Thomas hopes that he will be one of the 5% who benefit from the phase I cancer trial.

ent degrees of understanding. Both Susan and Thomas have a better understanding of the research and its differences from clinical care than Mark does. Mark and Susan seem to be overestimating the probability of benefit and underestimating the probability of harm in the trial. Thomas appears to have an accurate understanding of the probabilities, but is optimistic that he will beat the odds. What approach should IRBs or investigators take in addressing these misunderstandings?

Understanding in Informed Consent

To approach these questions, we must recognize why informed consent is important as well as how under-standing contributes to it. Informed consent is important because of the value we place on respect-ing individuals' autonomous decision-making.[12] This respect involves making sure that an individ-ual's decision to volunteer for research includes four elements: 1) competence, 2) provision of informa-tion, 3) understanding, and 4) voluntariness.[13]

For the sake of conceptual analysis, let us assume that Mark, Susan, and Thomas were competent enough to make decisions, their decisions to partici-pate were voluntary, and the research team provided accurate information on the purpose of the phase I trial, its high risk, and its low probability of benefit. Under these hypothetical conditions, understanding is

the critical concern. What kind or degree of under-standing must Mark, Susan, or Thomas have to autonomously decide to participate in the trial? Under-standing in the context of informed consent includes having an accurate grasp of the available options and the consequences of choosing one option over any oth-ers. To deliberate meaningfully over options, research subjects should understand what those options entail. If they misunderstand aspects of the research and its consequences, these misunderstandings are ethically salient insofar as they compromise an autonomous decision to participate in research.

Therapeutic Misconception: A Warning Flag

In clinical research, patient-subjects often confuse research with clinical care. Appelbaum and col-leagues have termed this misunderstanding "the therapeutic misconception."[14] The therapeutic mis-conception operates when a subject believes that "every aspect of the research project ... [is] designed to benefit him [or her] directly." Although a subject may benefit directly from research participation, the primary purpose of clinical research is always the production of generalizable knowledge.[15] Failure to understand this fact is ethically troubling, especially when the design of a trial is inconsistent with the research subject's expectation that personal care will be maximized and individualized.

In their original characterization of the therapeutic misconception, Appelbaum and colleagues invoke experience from a randomized, placebo-controlled trial for schizophrenia.[16] In this trial, some subjects understood the abstract concept of randomization to a placebo, but did not apply this concept to their *own* group assignment within the trial. Because they believed that the investigator would provide them with the best possible care, they could not conceive of being personally assigned to the placebo group. The subjects' expectation for personalized care conflicted with the actual design of the trial.[17]

In a similar way, Mark has a therapeutic misconception that conflicts with the design of the phase I cancer trial. He states that the purpose of the trial is to test whether the chemotherapeutic agent will shrink his tumor, when in fact the purpose is to test for safety. While a doctor in the clinical setting might adjust the dose of Mark's medication in order to increase efficacy or minimize side effects, the research investigator is restricted from doing so by the trial's dose escalation design. There is incongruence between Mark's beliefs that decisions about his medications and care will be made according to his personal best interests and the reality of research procedures that are required to answer a scientific question.

A decision to participate in research when the nature of the research has been misunderstood raises concerns about the autonomy of that decision. If a person does not understand the nature of research and how it differs from clinical care, then that person has a distorted representation of the research project and is making a decision about something that is different from the actual project at hand. Thus in most cases we want subjects to understand the nature of research and its distinction from clinical care for their enrollment to be ethically acceptable.

A solid understanding of a study's purpose and design can reinforce an understanding of the difference between research and clinical care. While subjects often need not understand the scientific or procedural details, the more features of the trial diverge significantly from what one would expect in clinical care, the more fully subjects should understand the purpose and procedures of the trial. For example, the use of procedures such as randomization to a place-bo or dose-escalation might conflict with what the subject would expect in the clinical care context. The same holds for such research aims as determining toxicity or provoking psychiatric symptoms.

Conversely, as features of a research trial more closely resemble those of clinical care, the less important it may be that a subject understand the specific research purpose and procedures. There may even be circumstances in which the therapeutic misconception, that is, a genuine conflation of research with clinical care, may be tolerated. For instance, in a phase III trial testing the comparative efficacy of a new agent against standard treatment, procedures and care may be close to or no different from those provided in the clinical care context. Thus even if the subject does not fully understand the research nature of the trial, the differences between what the subject experiences in the trial and in the clinical care setting are small. Although a genuine effort should still be made to redress this therapeutic misconception, if unsuccessful, it may be acceptable in some cases to tolerate the misunderstanding.[18] Additionally, a high prospect of personal benefit from the trial may support tolerating a subject's therapeutic misconception, since significant health benefits are most likely to be consistent with the subject's overarching goals.

Although a therapeutic misconception compromises the autonomy of a subject's decision to participate in research, because, by definition, it represents inaccurately the object of that decision, may not always be unacceptable. When efforts to correct a therapeutic misconception have failed, the compromised decisional autonomy of the subject may in some cases be compensated for by other factors, such as a high prospect of benefit and/or a lack of substantial conflict between the subject's expectations and the various features of research participation.

Therapeutic Misestimation: Another Form of Misunderstanding

The therapeutic misconception is not the only type of misunderstanding that subjects may have in research, however. In the case above, Susan did not misunderstand the research purpose or difference between research and clinical care, but rather overestimated the probability that she would receive benefit in the trial and downplayed the risks of the experimental agent.

Studies demonstrating that subjects in phase I cancer trials are motivated by expectations of benefit suggest that participants may overestimate the probability of benefit and underestimate risk in a similar way.[19] This form of misunderstanding is descriptively and ethically distinct from the therapeutic misconception. We call it the "therapeutic misestimation." While the therapeutic misconception involves misunderstanding the *nature* or *intent* of clinical research, the therapeutic misestimation involves misunderstanding the *probability* of direct benefit or harms that may result from participating in research.[20] We suspect that the therapeutic misestimation may manifest itself as an overestimation of benefit, an underestimation of risk, or both together.[21]

The therapeutic misestimation is frequently combined or confused with the therapeutic misconception. Macklin characterizes the therapeutic misconception as "the belief that ... research is a promising treatment intended to benefit subjects,"[22] while King claims that the therapeutic misconception results from the assumption that "clinical research offers a reasonable potential for direct benefit to subjects."[23] Distinguishing the two concepts is useful when considering instances in which one exists without the other, as in Susan's case.

A therapeutic misestimation can exist along with a reasonably accurate representation of the nature and purpose of a research project. Conversely, a therapeutic misconception might exist despite a realistic expectation of risks and benefits. Although the therapeutic misconception and misestimation can coexist in the minds of subjects, recognizing two separate elements of misunderstanding allows one to identify the different ways in which those elements can compromise the autonomous decisionmaking of patient-subjects.

How Do Research Subjects Understand Probability?

Is the "therapeutic misestimation" a misunderstanding per se or merely an optimistic interpretation of probability data? To answer this question, it is help-ful to consider the possible ways in which research subjects understand and interpret concepts of probability. Currently, little is understood about how research subjects understand probability and the role it plays in their decision to participate in clinical research.[24] However, the existing literature on presentation of risk in *clinical* settings suggests that both patients and clinicians commonly misunderstand statistical data expressed in the form of percentages.[25] Certain modes of presentation increase understanding, but patient preferences do not always include these modes.[26]

Given the complexity of understanding probability and the dearth of empirical data in the research setting, we suspect that investigators and research participants may interpret probability data differently and that participants may be predisposed to interpret probability data in their own favor.

First, subjects may question whether a probability estimate applies to themselves as individuals.[27] When using group data to predict the chances of an event happening to an individual, the assumption is that the individual and all members of the group are similar. However, there is always the possibility either that an individual has certain qualities that members of the group lacked, or that the group was heterogeneous for important, as yet undiscovered traits that affect the outcome. In clinical research, the usual outcome measures are physical responses, and subjects' intuitive awareness of factors that separate them from other people may make them reluctant to accept the probabilities that investigators provide. Whether or not they have actual reason to disregard a probability estimate, subjects may be inclined to interpret those estimates to reflect a more optimistic outlook.

Second, it is also possible that subjects interpret a probability estimate in terms of odds, whereas researchers interpret it in terms of frequency.[28] While both interpretations are statistically "correct," it seems as if the odds interpretation might lead subjects either to "spin" a probability estimate in their favor or simply to be more willing to accept risk. For example, for a 50% chance of liver damage, from an odds perspective a subject may believe rightly that there is no greater confidence in an outcome of liver damage than there is in an outcome of no liver damage, and thus may be more willing to accept the risk. In contrast, an investigator may view the data as the expected frequency of liver damage in her subject pool, expecting approximately half of her subjects to experience this side effect. From this perspective, she may feel that subjects should be less willing to accept the risk. We speculate that an odds interpretation leaves more room for individual subjects to "hedge their bets."

Of course, the intuition that patient-subjects tend to disregard or misestimate probabilities is empirically unproven and we should be careful not to support any ethical conclusions with nonexistent data. In any case, even if subjects *do* tend to misunderstand probability data, this tendency is a weak justification for tolerating it. A better understanding of how subjects (and investigators) understand probability should serve to make IRBs and investigators more attuned to misestimation and more informed about possible strategies to correct it.

Therapeutic Misestimation: A Threat to Informed Consent?

The ethical importance of a therapeutic misestimation should be assessed in regard to two important elements: the magnitude of misestimation and the personal relevance of a misestimated risk or benefit to the subject. There are cases when a therapeutic misestimation is indeed problematic. For example, in a chemotherapy protocol that presents a 90% chance of hearing loss, a cellist should demonstrate a reasonable expectation that his participation will most likely result in deafness. If he expects a 10% chance of hearing loss, this estimate may be so unrealistic as to compromise the choice that he has made.

We suspect that the larger the misestimation, the more likely it is to misinform the subject's decision to participate. In addition, the relevance of a particular harm (or benefit) to an individual's life, such as hearing loss to a musician, augments the importance of that risk in the decision-making process. When the likelihood of an outcome is grossly misestimated and/or that outcome holds special significance for the individual, the subject most likely chooses among misrepresented options and the validity of his or her consent may be compromised. A large or personally meaningful misconstrual of risk/benefit probabilities can be an ethically significant concern, and should be met by further efforts to ensure that the patient-subject comprehends the actual risks and benefits of participating. One might plausibly argue that Susan's expectation of harms and benefit from the phase I cancer trial was not so large or personally meaningful as to compromise her decision.

The therapeutic misestimation may be especially problematic in trials in which the risk is high or severe and the probability of benefit is low. Because it is possible that individuals may interpret probability estimates in problematic ways, the onus of risk-benefit calculation is more appropriately placed on the research team and the IRB. Ethically and by regulation, research should be designed in a way that minimizes risk and enhances the possibility of benefit. The need to carry out high-risk, low-benefit studies, especially when they involve subjects who might understandably have therapeutic expectations, as in phase I cancer research, requires that researchers recognize and address the possibility that subjects— and investigators themselves—may engage in therapeutic misestimation.

Optimism versus Misunderstanding

Misunderstanding, especially in the form of misestimation, can be confused with personal optimism. In both clinical care and research settings, patients and subjects naturally hope for the best outcome. In practice, it may be difficult to separate this sense of hope from a therapeutic misconception or misestimation. Yet it is possible, and may be therapeutically important, for patient-subjects to maintain optimism, while demonstrating an understanding of both the nature of research and the probability of important risks and benefits. In the third case above, Thomas appears to have neither therapeutic misconception nor a therapeutic misestimation, but maintains a personally optimistic outlook.

Optimism alone should never be ethically problematic. An optimistic outlook likely makes a positive contribution to the healing process.[29] A patient-subject is still a patient, even in the context of research,[30] and if participating willingly and with understanding, she or he can hope for the best

Figure 2.
Critical questions and strategies for IRBs and Investigators

Type of Misunderstanding	Factors that increase the possibility of misunderstanding	Strategies for minimizing the possibility of misunderstanding	When persistent misunderstanding might be tolerated after efforts have been made to correct it
Therapeutic Misconception	• Studies in which the research design approximates clinical care • Subjects who have limited options for treatment • Subjects who are invited to participate in research by regular medical physician or team	• Explicit and clear descriptions of research purpose, procedures, and features and their difference from clinical care, e.g., placebo-controls, randomization, dose-escalation, extra bloods or scans • Careful and comprehensive discussion of alternatives and voluntary nature of participation • An explicit plan for assessing subject understanding of research purpose and procedures • In some cases, recommendation for consent to be obtained from a researcher uninvolved in patients' care or for consent monitoring	• High similarity to clinical care in research design or procedures, e.g., Phase III trials • High or exclusive chance for personal benefit, especially when there is low risk
Therapeutic Misestimation	• Studies in which the prospect of benefit is low or unlikely • Subjects who are hoping for treatment	• Specific information about the probability and magnitude of possible risk and benefit, when data are available • A clear distinction between uncertainty due to lack of data and uncertainty associated with evidence-based probabilities • Comparison with risks and benefits of other options • Presentation of probability data in a variety of forms • A clear plan for assessing subject understanding of various risks and the prospect of benefit and distinguishing misestimation from optimism	• When the misestimation of benefit or risk is not too large and not the primary factor in the subject's decision to participate

medical outcome without compromising the research partnership. In this way, personal optimism should be supported and encouraged in the research setting.

Nevertheless, optimism can contribute to misunderstanding, just as misunderstanding can sustain optimism. In reality, it may be extremely difficult to ascertain whether a research subject misunderstands the prospect of benefit or has simply adopted an optimistic outlook along with an awareness of the facts. An awareness of these concepts and careful discussion with subjects can help a research team identify and preserve hope in the process of improving patient-subjects' understanding of research.

A Three-Way Ethical Distinction

We have distinguished three separate but related concepts: therapeutic misconception, that is, conflating research with clinical care; therapeutic misestimation, misunderstanding the probability of benefits and/or harms in research; and therapeutic optimism which refers to hope for the best outcome. (See Figure 1.) We offer some critical questions for IRBs to consider in reviewing protocols, as well as strategies to prevent and minimize a therapeutic misconception or misestimation (Figure 2).

Both the nature of research and the probability of harms/benefits are important to a person in deciding to participate in research. But misunderstanding these elements can compromise the individual's decision to participate in research in different ways or to different degrees. Whereas understanding the nature of research is integral to understanding research as an option, the probability of harms/benefits is merely one aspect of that option, and misunderstandings here may be less problematic. A therapeutic misconception fundamentally misrepresents the choice of research participation, whereas a therapeutic misestimation affects the subject's decision to participate only insofar as it shapes significantly his or her expectations about personal health outcome.

Therapeutic misconception undermines the autonomy of subject decisionmaking and thus is ethically problematic. Therapeutic misestimation compromises a subject's decisionmaking when it involves a large alteration of probability or when it concerns a personally significant outcome of the research. Therapeutic misconception should be tolerated only when factors counterbalance the compromised autonomy of the decision, as when there is significant prospect of individual benefit and/or the study is procedurally similar to clinical care. Therapeutic misestimation should be tolerated in situations when modest misestimates do not compromise a reasonable awareness of possible outcomes. Therapeutic optimism should be tolerated in most cases, and even actively preserved.

Despite our willingness to tolerate therapeutic misconception or therapeutic misestimation in some cases, it is always preferable that participants not misunderstand at all what they are getting into. Efforts should always be made to minimize misunderstanding. And even when therapeutic misconception or therapeutic misestimation might be ethically tolerable, neither should be encouraged. To actively contribute to misunderstanding on the grounds of its presumed therapeutic effect or administrative convenience violates our commitment to partnership with subjects in research.

Encouraging Meaningful Consent

Researchers should encourage patient-subjects to make a meaningful choice when deciding to participate in research. Attaining this goal requires that investigators promote clear understanding of the nature of research as well as realistic estimates of risk and benefit. Current empirical data on research subjects' understanding of research participation does not sufficiently distinguish between therapeutic misconception and therapeutic misestimation, which may confuse efforts to correct these different forms of misunderstanding. Studies to date also obscure the difference between misunderstanding and optimism. By utilizing more precisely the concepts of therapeutic misconception, therapeutic misestimation, and therapeutic optimism, we can begin to differentiate more precisely when misunderstanding is ethically problematic and how to tailor our efforts to correct it.

Acknowledgment

We thank Dan Brock, Ezekiel Emanuel, and Frank Miller for their helpful comments. The opinions expressed in this article are those of the authors and do not represent the view or policies of the Department of Health and Human Services or the National Institutes of Health.

Notes

1 Faden RR and Beauchamp TL. *A History and Theory of Informed Consent*. New York: Oxford University Press, 1986: 235-73.

2 Emanuel EJ, Wendler D, and Grady C. What makes clinical research ethical? *JAMA* 2000; 283: 2701-11.

3 Daugherty C, Ratain MJ, Grochowski E, et al. Perceptions of cancer patients and their physicians involved in phase I trials. *Journal of Clinical Oncology* 1995; 13(5): 1062-72.

4 Joffe S, Cook EF, Cleary PD, et al. Quality of informed consent in cancer clinical trials: A cross-sectional survey. *Lancet* 2001; 358: 1772-77.

5 Daugherty CK, Danik DM, Janish L, et al. Quantitative analysis of ethical issues in phase I trials: A survey interview study of 144 advanced cancer patients. *IRB* 2000; 22(3): 6-13.

6 Yoder LH, O'Rourke TJ, Etnyre A, et al. Expectations and experiences of patients with cancer participating in phase I clinical trials. *Onc Nurse Forum* 1997; 24(5): 891-96.

7   Itoh K, Sasaki Y, Miyata Y, et al. Therapeutic response in phase I clinical trials of anticancer agents conducted in Japan. *Cancer Chemotherapy & Pharmacology* 1994; 34: 451-44.

8   Von Hoff D, Turner J. Response rates, duration of response, and dose response effects in phase I studies of antineoplastics. *Investigational New Drugs* 1991; 9: 115-22.

9   Miller M. Phase I cancer trials: A collusion of misunderstanding. *Hastings Center Report* 2000; 30(4): 34-42.

10 Kodish E, Stocking C, Ratain MJ, Kohrman A, Siegler M. Ethical issues in phase I oncology research: A comparison of investigators and institutional review board chairpersons. *Journal of Clinical Oncology* 1992; 10(11): 1810-16.

11 Appelbaum PS, Roth LH, Lidz CW, Benson P, Winslade W. False hopes and best data: Consent to research and the therapeutic misconception. *Hastings Center Report* 1987; 12(2): 20-24.

12 Beauchamp TL, Childress JF. *Principles of Biomedical Ethics*, 4th ed. New York: Oxford University Press, 1994.

13 See ref. 1, Faden & Beauchamp 1986.

14 See ref. 11, Appelbaum et al. 1987.

15 The National Commission for the Protection of Human Subjects of Biomedical and Behavioral Research. *The Belmont Report*. Washington, DC: U.S. Government Printing Office, 1979.

16 See ref. 11, Appelbaum et al. 1987.

17 Berg and colleagues have distinguished between concepts of understanding, the "ability to acquire information," and appreciation, the "ability to evaluate information," or apply it to oneself. We are incorporating this notion of appreciation into our account of understanding. Berg J, Appelbaum PS, Lidz CW, Parker LS. *Informed Consent: Legal Theory and Clinical Practice*, 2nd ed. New York: Oxford University Press, 2001: 102.

18 Freedman argues that a subject's 'ignorant consent' because of a refusal to receive information may be similarly tolerated in cases when that information is not "serious" to the decision to participate in research. Freedman B. The validity of ignorant consent to medical research. *IRB* 1982. 4(2): 1-5.

19 See: ref. 3, Daugherty et al. 1995; ref. 4, Joffe et al. 2001; ref. 5, Daugherty et al. 2000; ref. 6, Yoder et al. 1997; ref. 7, Itoh et al. 1994; ref. 8, Von Hoff & Turner 1991.

20 A therapeutic misestimation could conceivably exist in the clinical care setting as well, although we focus here on the therapeutic misestimation in research.

21 It is also possible for potential subjects to underestimate the chance of benefit or overestimate risk. In these cases, 'misestimation' may contribute to a decision not to participate in research. This situation may occur in individuals or populations that are suspicious of research. In this paper, we only discuss the decision of subjects to participate in research.

22 Macklin R. Understanding informed consent. *Acta Oncologica* 1999; 38: 83-87.

23 King NMP. Defining and describing benefit appropriately in clinical trials. *Journal of Law Medicine & Ethics* 2000; 28: 332-43.

24 Redeimeier DA, Rozin P, Kahneman D. Understanding patients' decisions: Cognitive and emotional perspectives. *JAMA* 1993; 270: 72-76.

25 Hoffrage U, Lindsey S, Hertwig R, Gigerenzer G. Communicating statistical information. *Science* 2000; 290: 2261-62.

26 Edwards A, Elwyn G, and Mulley A. Explaining risks: Turning numerical data into meaningful pictures. *British Medical Journal* 2002; 324: 827-30.

27 Walker, VR. Direct inference, probability, and a conceptual gulf in risk communication. *Risk Analysis* 1995; 15: 603-09.

28 See ref. 27, Walker 1995.

29 Hickey SS. Enabling hope. *Cancer Nursing* 1986; 9: 133-37.

30 Miller FG, Rosenstein DL, DeRenzo EG. Professional integrity in clinical research. *JAMA* 1998; 280: 1449-54.

43.
A CRITIQUE OF CLINICAL EQUIPOISE: THERAPEUTIC MISCONCEPTION IN THE ETHICS OF CLINICAL TRIALS

Franklin G. Miller and Howard Brody

SOURCE: *Hastings Center Report* 33.3 (2003): 19-31.

The Hypericum Depression Trial Study Group published in 2002 the results of a randomized trial comparing hypericum (St. John's Wort), sertraline (Zoloft), and placebo in the treatment of major depression.[1] In the study, funded by the National Institutes of Health, 340 subjects from twelve participating centers were randomized to three trial arms for an eight-week period, with careful monitoring to assure that patients who worsened significantly or who became suicidal were removed from the study and received adequate treatment. Neither hypericum nor sertraline was found to be superior to placebo on the primary outcome measures. The authors noted, "From a methodological point of view, this study can be considered an example of the importance of including inactive and active comparators in trials testing the possible antidepressant effects of medications. In fact, without a placebo, hypericum could easily have been considered as effective as sertraline."[2]

What can we conclude about the ethics of this trial? One dominant viewpoint in research ethics would have prohibited the study. On this viewpoint, a randomized trial is ethical only in circumstances of "clinical equipoise"—a genuine uncertainty within the medical community as to whether (in this case) any of the three treatment arms are superior to the other two. No such uncertainty exists. Approximately twenty-five clinically available antidepressants, including sertraline, have been shown to be superior to placebo.[3] Moreover, the majority opinion within psychiatry probably holds that sertraline is definitely superior to hypericum for major depression, even if hypericum has potential for the treatment of mild to moderate depression. But another widespread

viewpoint would hold that the trial was ethically sound. Depressed individuals widely use hypericum, a "natural" agent, despite the lack of proven efficacy. Accordingly, a rigorous evaluation offered scientific, clinical, and social value. According to the report of trial results, the study was approved by institutional review boards (IRBs) at twelve sites and subjects provided written informed consent.

But if clinical equipoise is a basic requirement for ethical research, how could all these review boards be blind to the unethical nature of this trial? And how could two such radically divergent viewpoints exist, without research ethics being widely regarded as in a state of crisis?

Therapeutic Misconceptions

The prevailing ethical perspective on clinical trials holds that physician-investigators can discharge their "therapeutic obligation" to patients in the context of randomized clinical trials (RCTs) as long as treatments being tested scientifically satisfy clinical equipoise. We contend that this ethical perspective is fundamentally flawed. An ethical framework that provides normative guidance about a practice should accurately characterize the practice. The prevailing ethical perspective fails this test: All sound ethical thinking about clinical research, and the regulatory framework for review of protocols for clinical investigation, depends on a basic distinction between research and therapy. But the claims in the prevailing ethical perspective on clinical trials conflate research and therapy. These claims are that the ethics of the physician-patient relationship must govern RCTs, that physicians who conduct these trials have a "therapeutic obligation" to patients enrolled in them, and that RCTs must be compatible with some form of equipoise.

Certainly, investigators and ethicists recognize that clinical trials are scientific experiments, which differ from standard medical care. They also recognize that they are subject to regulatory requirements which do not apply to routine medical practice. However, the prevailing ethical framework views clinical trials through a therapeutic lens. The mainstream ethical approach to clinical trials attempts to have it both ways: to view the clinical trial as a scientific experiment, aimed at producing knowledge that can help improve the care of future patients, and as treatment conducted by physicians who retain fidelity to the principles of therapeutic beneficence and therapeutic nonmaleficence that govern the ethics of clinical medicine. The doctrine of clinical equipoise has emerged as the bridge between medical care and scientific experimentation, allegedly making it possible to conduct RCTs without sacrificing the therapeutic obligation of physicians to provide treatment according to a scientifically validated standard of care. This constitutes a "therapeutic misconception" concerning the ethics of clinical trials, analogous to the tendency of patient volunteers to confuse treatment in the context of RCTs with routine medical care.[4] As Paul Appelbaum has recently observed, "In fact, this confusion between the ethics of research and of ordinary clinical care appears rampant in the world of clinical trials."[5]

The therapeutic misconception in the ethics of clinical trials is reflected in the language commonly used within the clinical research enterprise. Clinical trials are often described as "therapeutic research," and investigators are regarded as having a "therapeutic intent." Research participants who are being studied because they have a medical condition under investigation are referred to as "patients," and investigators as "physicians" or "doctors," without qualification.

To demonstrate our contention about the mainstream approach to the ethics of clinical trials, we will offer an intellectual reconstruction of some of the history of research ethics since the 1970s. This history is characterized by incoherence resulting from commitment to two incompatible positions, each approaching research ethics in a fundamentally different way. The therapeutic misconception about the ethics of clinical trials has emerged from the "similarity position," which argues that ultimately, the ethics of clinical trials rest on the same moral considerations that underlie the ethics of therapeutic medicine. The "difference position" argues that the ethics of clinical trials must start with the realization that medical research and medical treatment are two distinct forms of activity, governed by different ethical principles.

The reigning ethical paradigm for clinical trials has coexisted with clinical trials practice that departs from its guidance. Clinical equipoise, the cornerstone of the similarity position, rules out placebo-controlled trials whenever there is a proven effective treatment for the disorder under investigation.[6] However, IRBs have routinely approved such placebo-controlled trials. These two anomalies—unappreciated theoretical incoherence and conflict between the theoretical paradigm and the practice of ethical review of clinical trials—call for critical examination of the similarity position and the doctrine of clinical equipoise.

The Distinction between Research and Therapy

In 1979, Robert Levine summarized "the most important achievements of the National Commission" for the Protection of Human Subjects of Biomedical and Behavioral Research in "correcting the conceptual and semantic errors that had undermined virtually all previous attempts to develop rational public policy on research involving human subjects."[7] Two portions of Levine's summary capture the essential ingredients of the difference position: recognizing the distinction between research and therapy and, accordingly, abandoning the distinction between therapeutic and nontherapeutic research.

Clinical research shares with medical care the fact that both are performed by physicians in clinical settings, and both often use similar diagnostic and treatment interventions. When the commission began its work, physicians commonly regarded clinical research and medical therapy as inextricably connected. One authority quoted by Levine claimed that "Every time a physician administers a drug to a patient, he is in a sense performing an experiment." But the commission recognized the importance of determining the boundaries between routine medical practice and research. For Levine, the commission's conceptual breakthrough came with the realization that the physicians of the day were thinking about clinical research in the wrong way, and that the boundary between research and therapy was clear rather than fuzzy. The commission came to hold that clinical research is fundamentally different from medical practice.[8] Clinical medicine aims at providing optimal medical care for individual patients. Ethically, it is governed by the principles of therapeutic beneficence and therapeutic nonmaleficence.

Therapeutic beneficence directs physicians to practice medicine with primary fidelity to promoting the health of particular patients. According to therapeutic nonmaleficence, the risks of medical care to which a patient is exposed are to be justified by the prospect of compensating medical benefits for that patient. The physician uses scientific knowledge to care for the patient and engages in therapeutic experimentation with the aim only of finding optimal treatment. It is not part of the role of the physician in providing medical care to develop scientific knowledge that can help future patients.

Clinical research, in contrast, is not a therapeutic activity devoted to the personal care of patients. It is designed for answering a scientific question, with the aim of producing "generalizable knowledge." The investigator seeks to learn about disease and its treatment in groups of patients, with the ultimate aim of improving medical care. Scientific interest in any particular patient concerns what can be learned that is applicable to other patients. In view of the nature and purpose of clinical research, the principles of beneficence and nonmaleficence applicable to clinical research lack the therapeutic meaning that guides their application to medical care. Clinical research is dedicated primarily to promoting the medical good of future patients by means of scientific knowledge derived from experimentation with current research participants—a frankly utilitarian purpose.

A major reason for distinguishing research from therapy is to underscore that clinical research has an inherent potential for exploiting research participants.[9] Exploitation also may occur in clinical med-

icine—venal physicians sometimes perform medically unnecessary procedures for the sake of profit, for example. Yet when physicians of integrity practice medicine, physicians' and patients' interests converge. The patient desires to regain or maintain health or to relieve suffering; the physician is dedicated to providing the medical help that the patient needs.

In clinical research, by contrast, the interests of investigators and patient volunteers are likely to diverge, even when the investigator acts with complete integrity. Patient volunteers, especially in clinical trials, typically seek therapeutic benefit, though they also may be motivated by altruism.[10] Investigators are interested primarily in developing scientific knowledge about groups of patients. Regardless of investigators' motivations, patient volunteers are at risk of having their well-being compromised in the course of scientific investigation. Clinical research involves an inherent tension between pursuing rigorous science and protecting research participants from harm.[11]

Historically, the ethical distinction between research and therapy emerged out of concern about exploitive abuses of patients in clinical research. Reflection on this dark history gave rise to a major development in the ethics of clinical research: the requirement for independent, prospective review and approval of research protocols.[12] Prior independent review was considered necessary for clinical research because of the divergence between the interests of the investigator and the research participant. Self-regulation by physician-investigators could not be trusted in the research context to the same extent that self-regulation by physicians was appropriate in the therapeutic context. The basic rationale for prospective, independent research review depends on the distinction between research and therapy.

The point of distinguishing research and therapy is not to make an invidious comparison, implying that clinical trials are more risky or ethically problematic than routine clinical practice. Indeed, there is some evidence that patients receive more favorable medical outcomes in many clinical trials,[13] and clinical medicine is certainly rife with ethical problems. Further, since research is more carefully regulated than medical practice, it is quite likely that fewer ethical violations occur in research. To say that two activities are ethically different is not to say that either is inherently better than the other.

Abandoning the Distinction

The distinction between research and therapy is most likely to be obfuscated in the context of clinical trials, which test the safety or efficacy of investigational and standard treatments. Since patients may derive medical benefit from trial participation, especially in phase III RCTs (the final stage of testing, which many investigational drugs never even reach), clinical trials are often characterized as "therapeutic research."

Nonetheless, the process of treatment in RCTs differs radically from routine clinical practice.[14] Consider the contrast between the hypericumsertraline trial and routine medical care for depression. If a physician treated 340 patients for major depression, she would not decide which drug to administer by flipping a coin. If the physician elected to use sertraline, she would judge each case individually to determine dose, when to change the dose, and whether to prescribe a second antidepressant or recommend other treatment. We would expect to find considerable variation in the treatment administered to those 340 patients after eight weeks or so. From the vantage point of therapy, this is what it means to provide care to patients.

From the vantage point of research, such variation would wreak havoc on experimental design and the validity and generalizability of findings. So when patients are randomized to one or another experimental drug, and are treated according to relatively inflexible protocols, the activity is very different from therapeutic medicine.

In many other ways, too, routine aspects of research deviate from what would be required by the duties of therapeutic beneficence and nonmaleficence. Volunteer patients and physician investigators are often ignorant of assignment to the experimental or control treatment, which may be a placebo. Trials often include interventions such as blood draws, lumbar punctures, radiation imaging, or biopsies that measure trial outcomes but in no way benefit participants. RCTs often contain a drug "washout" phase

before randomization to avoid confounding the evaluation of the investigational treatment with the effects of medication that patients were receiving prior to the trial. These various features of research design promote scientific validity; they carry risks to participants without the prospect of compensating therapeutic benefit.

For these reasons, Levine argued that the second major contribution of the commission was to abandon the "illogical" distinction between therapeutic and nontherapeutic research, which previous policymakers thought was essential to the proper regulation of research and the protection of human subjects.[15] Because research and therapy are distinct activities, and the ethics of therapeutic medicine therefore cannot be automatically extended to guide research, it is mistaken to label research as "therapeutic" or "nontherapeutic," as if that made any fundamental ethical difference. Many research trials consist of a complex mix of therapeutic and nontherapeutic elements—the placebo-controlled trial being only one obvious example—such that labeling the trial as a whole as "therapeutic" or "nontherapeutic" is misleading. In addition, the therapeutic-nontherapeutic distinction diverts attention from key ethical issues. Consider a nontherapeutic trial in which one interviews subjects and takes saliva samples, and a therapeutic trial in which one is testing a new cancer drug that has some promise for creating remission, but also has potentially life-threatening toxicity. Is the latter trial less in need of stringent regulatory oversight because it is "therapeutic"? Or does the therapeutic-nontherapeutic distinction distract the observer from those aspects of the trials that assume far greater moral weight, such as the level of risks and the potential vulnerability of subjects?

Once one understands the distinction between research and therapy, one realizes that "therapeutic" research is still research, and that the ethical rules appropriate to it are those appropriate for clinical research generally. Even though the patient may derive benefit from treatment being evaluated, the basic goal of the activity is not personal therapy, but rather the acquisition of generally applicable scientific knowledge. The basic goal and nature of the activity determines the ethical standards that ought to apply.

Writing in 1993, Jay Katz affirmed the vital importance of the distinction between research and therapy and deplored its blurring in practice: "The astronomical increase in clinical research has, in practice, not led to a clear demarcation between therapy and research, bioethical theories notwithstanding. This vital distinction remains blurred when physician investigators view subjects as patients, and then believe that patients' interests and not science's are being served by participation in randomized clinical trials that are so commonly conducted in today's world."[16] One of the reasons investigators (and bioethicists) have failed to appreciate the distinction between research and therapy is that the similarity position has conceived the ethics of clinical trials within the context of the physician patient relationship.

Charles Fried and the Similarity Position

In 1974, Fried published "Medical Experimentation: Personal Integrity and Social Policy," which launched the similarity position within bioethics.[17] Fried assumed that answers to ethical dilemmas in research would have to be found within the ethics of therapeutic medicine. He defended fidelity to the interests of the individual patient against a model in which "medicine is to be viewed as caring for populations."[18] What made the RCT ethically suspect was that it seemed to him a prime example of population focused—rather than individualized—and utilitarian medicine.

Fried devoted most of his book to defending patients' "rights in personal care."[19] Returning to medical research, he took issue with trials in which patients were randomized to receive either the experimental intervention or standard care. Fried coined the term "equipoise" to describe the ethically necessary condition for conducting an RCT: physician-investigators must be indifferent to the therapeutic value of the experimental and control treatments evaluated in the trial. The basic idea of equipoise had previously been articulated by Bradford Hill, a pioneer in the development of RCTs.[20] But what Fried objected to primarily in RCTs was not randomization per se, but the fact that no informed consent had been obtained. Fried saw the threat of "care for groups" (instead of "care for individuals") as residing primarily in the idea that it was legitimate to enroll subjects in an RCT without explicit, informed consent because the results of the trial would provide new medical knowledge that would improve the lot of future patients.[21] Because Fried was concerned chiefly about informed consent, an essential ingredient of both medical research and therapeutic medicine, he saw no problem in applying the ethics of medical therapy to medical research.

In the 1970s, the "respect for patient autonomy" movement was gaining steam as a replacement for the old Hippocratic ethic of paternalistic beneficence. Since both Fried and the National Commission seemed on the surface to be championing patient autonomy, it was easy to miss the point that they were proposing two fundamentally different strategies for approaching the ethics of clinical trials. Put another way, so long as the bioethics debate of the moment has to do with whether research ethics requires all competent subjects to give fully informed consent, any fundamental divergence between the similarity and the difference positions is likely to be obscured.

The Emergence of Clinical Equipoise

During the 1980s, philosophers interested in research ethics recognized a tension between the obligation of physicians to offer optimal care to their patients ("the therapeutic obligation") and the provision of medical treatment in the context of clinical trials. Don Marquis addressed this problem in a 1983 essay, "Leaving Therapy to Chance."[22] The title is significant, suggesting that the RCT is a form of therapy rather than an ethically distinct activity. Marquis began his essay, "Consider this dilemma: according to an argument that is hard to refute, the procedure for conducting randomized clinical trials of anticancer drugs is incompatible with the ethics of the physician-patient relationship. If this problem is to be resolved, then either a key procedure for achieving scientific knowledge in medicine must be given up or unethical behavior by physicians must be tolerated."[23] In framing this "RCT dilemma," Marquis assumed that the appropriate ethic for clinical trials was that of the (therapeutic) physician-patient relationship.

Fred Gifford, following the lead of Marquis, examined the RCT dilemma in greater depth: "The central dilemma concerning randomized clinical trials (RCTs) arises out of some simple facts about causal methodology (RCTs are the best way to generate the reliable causal knowledge necessary for optimally-informed action) and a prima facie plausible principle concerning how physicians should treat their patients (always do what it is most reasonable to believe will be best for the patient)."[24] Neither Marquis nor Gifford found what they regarded as a satisfactory solution, and neither considered the possibility that the difference position could dismiss the "RCT dilemma" as misguided to begin with.

In a landmark 1987 article, Benjamin Freedman offered a solution to the RCT dilemma that gained widespread acceptance within bioethics. He argued that the tension between ethically legitimate scientific experimentation and the therapeutic obligation of physicians could be overcome by the principle of "clinical equipoise."[25] Freedman agreed with Fried and Marquis that ethical clinical trials had to be compatible with therapeutic beneficence and nonmaleficence. But he argued that Fried's formulation of equipoise was too constraining. Freedman called Fried's original concept "theoretical equipoise" (sometimes called "individual equipoise") and contrasted it with his favored concept of "clinical equipoise" (sometimes called "collective equipoise"). In the latter sense of equipoise, any individual investigator or physician might have reasons to believe that one arm of the RCT offers a therapeutic benefit over the other arm, but the medical profession as a whole remains divided. According to Freedman, an RCT is ethical so long as the professional community has not yet reached a consensus, which recognizes that "medicine is social rather than individual in nature."[26] When, and only when, clinical equipoise is satisfied will patients enrolled in a clinical trial be assured that they will not be randomized to treatment known to be inferior. Freedman thus asserted in a later article that clinical equipoise is "grounded in the normative nature of clinical practice, the view that a patient is ethically entitled to expect treatment from his or her physician—an entitlement that cannot be sacrificed to scientific curiosity."[27]

The bioethics community perceived Freedman's concept of clinical equipoise as both a theoretical and a practical advance. Theoretically, it appeared to offer a more intellectually compelling argument than Fried's initial formulation. Practically, it would permit useful RCTs that would otherwise be ethically proscribed to go forward. Since it appeared to solve the RCT dilemma by accommodating the conduct of clinical trials with the therapeutic obligation of physicians to offer optimal medical care, clinical equipoise gained wide currency as a fundamental concept of the ethics of clinical trials.[28] The persuasive way in which Freedman fortified the similarity position diverted attention from the fact that clinical equipoise collapsed the distinction between research and therapy.

The similarity position and clinical equipoise have been popular not only among bioethicists, but also among investigators. We speculate that this ethical perspective helps to address investigators' psychological needs. Physician-investigators, after all, went to medical school, not investigator school. To think of research with patients outside the ethical framework of the physician-patient relationship, as the difference position requires, may be difficult and threatening to them. Clinical equipoise offers a formula that seems to allow them to mix both physician and investigator roles—even if the psychological comfort is purchased at the price of ethical obfuscation.

The anomaly therefore exists that much of today's bioethical thinking accepts clinical equipoise as an outgrowth of the similarity position, while the Federal regulations grew out of the work of the National Commission, which largely endorsed the difference position. One would imagine that sooner or later proponents of clinical equipoise would realize the need to defend this doctrine from the charge that it conflates the ethics of clinical trials with the ethics of medical care. But this is precisely what has not yet happened.

The Case of Placebo-Controlled Trials

Although the similarity position, bolstered by clinical equipoise, became the reigning paradigm in the ethics of clinical trials, its dominion over practice was limited. This divorce between theory and practice has been particularly pronounced in the case of placebo-controlled trials. Freedman and his colleagues argued that the use of placebo controls is unethical whenever proven effective treatment exists for the medical condition under investigation in a clinical trial because those randomized to placebo would receive treatment known to be inferior.[29]

Despite the clear implications of clinical equipoise for the ethics of placebo-controlled trials, numerous trials, such as the hypericum-sertraline trial, continued to use placebo controls despite proven effective treatment. Placebo controls have typically been used in trials of new treatments for a wide range of chronic conditions—including mood and anxiety disorders, asthma, stable angina, hypertension, and migraine headaches—all of which can be treated with medication of proven efficacy.

There are two explanations for this incoherence between theory and practice. First, the FDA has encouraged the use of placebo controls in trials concerning these and other chronic conditions.[30] Active-controlled trials designed to test the equivalence of the experimental treatment with a standard treatment suffer from serious methodological limitations. Whenever active-controlled trials show no statistically significant difference between the investigational treatment and an active comparator, two conclusions are possible. Either both were effective in the trial sample of patients, or neither was effective. Without the use of a placebo control, such trials lack internal validity. Accordingly, the FDA has insisted that pharmaceutical companies use placebo controls in trials of new treatments for conditions characterized by fluctuating symptoms and high rates of placebo response.[31] Second, the U.S. federal regulations governing human subjects research do not provide any explicit guidance on the use of placebo controls.[32] IRBs have been free to approve such placebo-controlled trials, provided that they meet regulatory requirements for a favorable risk-benefit ratio, including the potential value of knowledge to be gained and informed consent.

For the most part, this lack of fit between theory and practice received little critical attention until the publication in 1994 of an article in the *New England Journal of Medicine* entitled "The Continuing Unethical Use of Placebo Controls."[33] Kenneth Rothman and Karin Michels castigated the practice of placebo-controlled trials in the face of proven effective treatment and the role of the FDA in encouraging these trials. They cited the Declaration of Helsinki, which relies heavily on the similarity position, as prohibiting this widespread "unethical" practice.

Their article stimulated a lively debate over the ethics of placebo-controlled trials. Freedman and his colleagues attacked "the placebo orthodoxy" in a two-part article that challenged the scientific value of placebo-controlled trials and reiterated that they are unethical when proven effective treatments exist because they contravene clinical equipoise.[34] Other commentators, writing in leading medical journals, defended more or less extensive use of placebo-controlled trials on methodological and ethical grounds.[35] Without directly challenging the doctrine of clinical equipoise, they implied that clinical equipoise provides erroneous ethical guidance for placebo-controlled trials. Accordingly, the debate over placebo-controlled trials jeopardizes the reigning ethical paradigm of the similarity position and clinical equipoise.

Critique of the Similarity Position and Clinical Equipoise

Our reconstruction of the recent history of the ethics of clinical trials has traced the emergence and dominance of the similarity position. This history also reveals cracks in the foundation of this ethical paradigm. Simultaneous endorsement of the difference position, reflected in the federal regulatory system and the Belmont Report, and the similarity position, which invokes the doctrine of clinical equipoise, has left the ethics of clinical trials in a state of incoherence. Although this incoherence has not received critical attention, it becomes apparent once the assumptions underlying the similarity position and clinical equipoise are challenged. In addition, the divorce between research ethics theory and clinical trials practice in the case of placebo-controlled trials suggests that a critique of the similarity position and clinical equipoise is overdue.

We contend that clinical equipoise is fundamentally mistaken because "the RCT dilemma," for which it was proposed as a solution, is false. Clinical equipoise and all other forms of equipoise make sense as a normative requirement for clinical trials only on the assumption that investigators have a therapeutic obligation to the research participants. The "therapeutic obligation" of investigators, forming one horn of the RCT dilemma, constitutes a therapeutic misconception about the ethics of clinical trials. The presumption that RCTs must be compatible with the ethics of the physician-patient relationship assumes erroneously that the RCT is a form of therapy, thus inappropriately applying the principles of therapeutic beneficence and nonmaleficence that govern clinical medicine to the fundamentally different practice of clinical research. It is impossible to maintain fidelity to doing what is best medically for patients in the context of RCTs because these are not designed for, and may conflict with, personalized care. Although ethically appealing, the project of bridging the gap between therapy and research via the doctrine of clinical equipoise is doomed to fail.

The insight that the RCT contravenes the ethics of the physician-patient relationship led Samuel Hellman and Debra Hellman to argue that the RCT is unethical and that other methods of evaluating treatments should be employed.[36] This stance, however, would deprive patients and society of the benefits that flow from rigorous scientific evaluation of experimental and standard treatments. The more reasonable conclusion is that RCTs should be governed by ethical norms appropriate to clinical research, which are distinct from therapeutic beneficence and therapeutic nonmaleficence.

Clinical equipoise is neither necessary nor sufficient for ethically justifiable RCTs. The use of placebo controls when proven effective treatment exists violates clinical equipoise; however, when methodologically indicated, their use is no different in principle from any research intervention that poses risks to subjects without the prospect of benefiting them.[37] In many cases, the risks of withholding effective treatment are excessive, and the use of placebo controls would thus be unethical. Nevertheless, it is the unacceptable level of risk, not the violation of investigators' alleged "therapeutic obligation," that makes these trials unethical. In other cases, including the hypericum-sertraline trial, use of placebo controls when proven effective treatment exists is ethically justifiable.

By conflating the ethics of clinical trials with the ethics of therapeutic medicine, proponents of the similarity position may also contribute to the lack of adequate informed consent. If investigators view the ethics of clinical trials through a therapeutic lens, they may explicitly or implicitly foster the therapeutic misconception among research participants—that is, the tendency of participants in trials to confuse clinical trials with medical care. Research participants need to know that the overall activity is aimed not at their own ultimate benefit, but at discovering new knowledge to help future patients. If they think that clinical trial participation is a form of therapy, then they cannot give informed consent. Moreover, unlike the therapeutic context, the patient-subject cannot delegate the decision to the physician-researcher. In the therapeutic setting, a patient can decide to trust the physician to choose the best treatment because the physician has the patient's best interests at heart. The investigator has the interests of future patients at heart, and so cannot decide for the subject whether or not to participate in the research. To be trustworthy, investigators must themselves understand clearly the ways in which clinical research differs from clinical practice and convey this forthrightly to potential research subjects.

It is worth pondering, however, the practical consequences that might ensue if physicians, investigators, patients, and ethicists understood clinical trials without distortion by therapeutic misconceptions. Would recruitment of participants for valuable clinical trials become substantially more difficult, slowing progress in medical care? The fact that clinical trials are no longer seen as a mode of therapy leaves unchanged the real prospect of therapeutic benefits offered to patients from trial participation, including the opportunity to receive promising investigational agents, ancillary medical care, expert diagnostic evaluations, and education about their disorder. Nonetheless, some patients might be less inclined to participate in clinical trials when they appreciate the differences between these scientific experiments and medical care.

To attract enough subjects, researchers might have to pay people for their participation, as researchers in industry-sponsored clinical trials already do with increasing frequency. Payments would add to the cost of conducting clinical trials, but it might help prevent the therapeutic misconception among trial participants.[38] To be paid signifies that the trial participant is not merely a patient seeking therapy. If additional expenditure is necessary to motivate clinical trial participation, then this is a price worth paying for enhanced professional integrity and informed consent.

An Alternative Ethical Framework

In view of the theoretical and practical problems associated with the similarity position and its logical offspring, clinical equipoise, an alternative framework for the ethics of clinical trials is needed. The most promising recent treatment of research ethics has been developed by Ezekiel Emanuel, David Wendler, and Christine Grady.[39] They propose seven ethical requirements for all clinical research: (1) scientific or social value; (2) scientific validity; (3) fair subject selection; (4) favorable risk-benefit ratio; (5) independent review; (6) informed consent; and (7) respect for enrolled research participants. This framework is built on the difference between research and therapy and on the core value of protecting research participants from exploitation.

Yet even this formulation of an ethical framework appropriate to clinical research testifies to the hold of the similarity position. The authors endorse clinical equipoise, claiming it is implied by the requirements of value, validity, and risk-benefit ratio. We contend, by contrast, that the endorsement of clinical equipoise renders incoherent any account that arises from the difference position. The most important next step for research ethics is to develop this "non-exploitation" framework systematically in a way that avoids any conflation of clinical research with medical care.

Those who agree that physician investigators who conduct clinical trials are not governed by therapeutic beneficence still might argue that clinical equipoise provides important methodological guidance for justifying clinical trials. Freedman and his colleagues have argued that clinical equipoise is both an ethical and a scientific principle: "That principle can be put into normative or scientific language. As a normative matter, it defines ethical trial design as prohibiting any compromise of a patient's right to medical treatment by enrolling in a study. The same concern is often stated scientifically when we assert that a study must start with an honest null hypothesis, genuine medical uncertainty concerning the relative merits of the various treatment arms included in the trial's design."[40] Nevertheless, whatever is valid methodologically in clinical equipoise—the honest null hypothesis—can be stated more clearly and without confusion with the therapeutic obligation, by appeal to the requirement of scientific value: no research participants should be exposed to the risks of valueless research. Clinical trials must be designed to answer valuable scientific questions. If the answer is already known or the question is trivial, then there is no honest null hypothesis, and a clinical trial should not be conducted. But this is logically independent of whether all the patients enrolled in the trial would receive medical treatment that is believed by the expert medical community to be at least as good as the standard of care.

This alternative framework provides accurate ethical guidance concerning clinical research without presuming that the ethics of therapeutic medicine should govern clinical trials. We illustrate this by applying the seven ethical requirements to the example of the hypericum-sertraline trial.

Scientific or social value and scientific validity. The study has social value owing to the widespread use of herbal remedies. Since the efficacy of hypericum in treating depression (especially major depression) was uncertain, there was an honest null hypothesis that hypericum would be no better than placebo. It would have been unreasonable to design the trial as an active-controlled superiority trial, since it is highly unlikely that hypericum could be shown to be more effective than sertraline. An active-controlled equivalence trial would lack "assay sensitivity" because the finding that the reduction in symptoms of depression experienced by those trial participants receiving hypericum was not significantly different for those receiving sertaline would not validly support the inference that hypericum was effective.[41] It would remain possible that neither treatment was effective in the study sample—as was in fact shown. The study, therefore, was properly designed as a three-arm placebo-controlled trial.

Fair subject selection. There is no evidence to suggest that particularly vulnerable patients were recruited inappropriately for this study, which included a sample representative of depressed patients.

Favorable risk-benefit ratio. Risk-benefit assessment of research protocols ultimately comes down to a matter of judgment. With respect to the use of the placebo control—the aspect of the trial that violated clinical equipoise—the risks to participants from an eight-week trial, with careful exclusionary criteria and monitoring, were not excessive and were justifiable by the anticipated value of the knowledge to be gained from the research. Hence, the placebo component of the study had a favorable risk-benefit ratio. Eliminating the placebo would have made the risk-benefit ratio unfavorable by virtue of undermining the scientific validity of the research.

Independent review, informed consent, and respect for enrolled research participants. The report of the study asserted that IRB approval was obtained at all sites and that all subjects gave informed consent. In addition, the described procedures for monitoring subjects for possible risk of harm indicated an acceptable level of respect.

In sum, this study was ethically justifiable despite violating clinical equipoise; moreover, had it been designed in accordance with clinical equipoise, it would have been methodologically deficient and therefore ethically questionable.

Charles Weijer, a leading advocate of clinical equipoise and the similarity position, has recently claimed that "Placebo-controlled trials in the context of serious illnesses such as depression or schizophrenia are ethically egregious precisely because no competent physician would fail to offer therapy to a patient with the condition."[42] Although we agree that

depression is a serious illness, the hypericum-sertaline trial demonstrates that there is nothing "ethically egregious" about the use of placebo controls in trials of treatment for depression, as long as the ethical requirements for clinical research are satisfied. Whether or not one agrees that, all things considered, the placebo control was ethical in this trial, the ethical justification of placebo controls has nothing to do with the therapeutic practice of competent physicians. In any case, the alternative ethical framework with its seven requirements provides adequate guidance for clinical trials without appeal to the incoherent doctrine of clinical equipoise and without conflating the ethics of research with the ethics of therapy.

Notes

1   Hypericum Depression Trial Study Group, "Effect of Hypericum Perforatum (St John's Wort) in Major Depressive Disorder: A Randomized Controlled Trial," *JAMA* 287 (2002):1807-14.

2   Ibid., 1813.

3   S.M. Stahl, *Essential Psychopharmacology of Depression and Bipolar Disorder* (New York: Cambridge University Press, 2000).

4   P.S. Appelbaum, L.H. Roth, C.W. Lidz, P. Benson, and W. Winslade, "False Hopes and Best Data: Consent to Research and the Therapeutic Misconception," *Hastings Center Report* 17, no. 2 (1987):20-24.

5   P.S. Appelbaum, "Clarifying the Ethics of Clinical Research: A Path Toward Avoiding the Therapeutic Misconception," *American Journal of Bioethics* 2, no. 2 (2002):22.

6   B. Freedman, "Placebo-Controlled Trials and the Logic of Clinical Purpose," *IRB* 12, no. 6 (1990):1-6.

7   R.J. Levine, "Clarifying the Concepts of Research Ethics," *Hastings Center Report* 9, no. 3 (1979):21-26.

8   National Commission for the Protection of Human Subjects of Biomedical and Behavioral Research, *The Belmont Report* (Washington, DC: U.S. Government Printing Office, 1979) p. 3.

9   E.J. Emanuel, D. Wendler, and C. Grady, "What Makes Clinical Research Ethical?" *JAMA* 283 (2000):2701-11.

10 J. Sugarman, N.E. Kass, S.N. Goodman, P. Perentesis, P. Fernandes, and R.R. Faden, "What Patients Say About Medical Research," *IRB* 20, no. 4 (1998): 17.

11 E.G. Miller, D.L. Rosenstein, and E.G. DeRenzo, "Professional Integrity in Clinical Research," *JAMA* 280 (1998):1449-54.

12 R.R. Faden and T.L. Beauchamp, *A History and Theory of Informed Consent* (New York: Oxford University Press, 1986):200-32.

13 D.A. Braunholtz, S.J.L. Edwards, and R.J. Lilford, "Are Randomized Clinical Trials Good for Us (in the Short term)? Evidence for a Trial Effect," *Journal of Clinical Epidemiology* 54 (2001):217-24.

14 J.W. Berg, P.S. Appelbaum, C.W. Lidz, and L.S. Parker, *Informed Consent: Legal Theory and Clinical Practice*, 2nd edition (New York: Oxford University Press, 2001):280-83.

15 R. Levine, *Ethics and Regulation of Clinical Research*, 2nd ed. (New Haven: Yale University Press, 1986):8-10.

16 J. Katz, "Ethics and Clinical Research Revisited: A tribute to Henry K. Beecher," *Hastings Center Report* 23, no. 5 (1993):36.

17 C. Fried, *Medical Experimentation: Personal Integrity and Social Policy* (New York: American Elsevier, 1974).

18 Ibid., 5.

19 Ibid., 94.

20 A.B. Hill, "Medical Ethics and Controlled Trials," *British Medical Journal* 1 (1963):1043-49.

21 C. Fried, *Medical Experimentation: Personal Integrity and Social Policy* (New York: American Elsevier, 1974):8.

22 D. Marquis, "Leaving Therapy to Chance," *Hastings Center Report* 13, no. 4 (1983):40-47.

23 Ibid., 40.

24 F. Gifford, "The Conflict Between Randomized Clinical Trials and the Therapeutic Obligation," *Journal of Medicine and Philosophy* 11 (1986):347-66.

25 B. Freedman, "Equipoise and the Ethics of Clinical Research," *NEJM* 3,17 (1987):141-45.

26 Ibid., 144.

27 B. Freedman, "Placebo-Controlled Trials and the Logic of Scientific Purpose," *IRB* 12, no. 6 (1990):5.

28 T.L. Beauchamp, and J.E Childress, *Principles of Biomedical Ethics*, 5th edition (New York: Oxford University Press, 2001):323-27.

29 B. Freedman, K.C. Glass, and C. Weijer, "Placebo Orthodoxy in Clinical Research. II: Ethical, Legal and Regulatory Myths," *Journal of Law, Medicine & Ethics* 6, 24 (1996):252-59.

30 R. Temple and S.E. Ellenberg, "Placebo-Controlled Trials and Active-Control Trials in the Evaluation of New Treatments: Part 1: Ethical and Scientific Issues," *Annals of Internal Medicine* 1, 33 (2000):455-63.

31 T.P. Laughren, "The Scientific and Ethical Basis for Placebo-Controlled Trials in Depression and Schizophrenia: An FDA Perspective," *European Psychiatry* 16 (2001):418-23.

32 Department of Health and Human Services. Protection of Human Subjects. Code of Federal Regulations. 45CFR46, 1991.

33 K.J. Rothman and K.B. Michels, "The Continuing Unethical Use of Placebo Controls," *NEJM* 331 (1994):394-98.

34 See B. Freedman, K.C. Glass, and C. Weijer, "Placebo Orthodoxy in Clinical Research. I: Empirical and Methodological Myths," *Journal of Law, Medicine & Ethics* 24 (1996):243-51; and B. Freedman, K.C. Glass, and C. Weijer, "Placebo Orthodoxy in Clinical Research. II: Ethical, Legal and Regulatory Myths," *Journal of Law, Medicine & Ethics* 24 (1996):252-59.

35 R. Temple and S.E. Ellenberg, "Placebo-Controlled Trials and Active-Control Trials in the Evaluation of New Treatments: Part 1: Ethical and Scientific Issues," *Annals of Internal Medicine* 133 (2000):455-63; E.J. Emanuel and E.G. Miller, "The Ethics of Placebo-Controlled Trials—A Middle Ground," *NEJM* 345 (2001):915-19.

36 S. Hellman and D.S. Hellman, "Of Mice But Not Men: Problems of the Randomized Controlled Trial," *NEJM* 324 (1991):1585-89.

37 E.G. Miller and H. Brody, "What Makes Placebo-Controlled Trials Unethical?" *American Journal of Bioethics* 2, no. 2 (2002):3-9.

38 N. Dickert and C. Grady, "What's the Price of a Research Subject? Approaches to Payment for Research Participation," *New England Journal of Medicine* 341 (1999):198-203.

39 See E.J. Emanuel, D. Wendler, and C. Grady, "What Makes Clinical Research Ethical?" *JAMA* 283 (2000):2701-11.

40 B. Freedman, K.C. Glass, and C. Weijer, "Placebo Orthodoxy in Clinical Research. II: Ethical, Legal and Regulatory Myths," *Journal of Law, Medicine & Ethics* 24 (1996):253.

41 R. Temple and S.E. Ellenberg, "Placebo-Controlled Trials and Active-Control trials in the Evaluation of New Treatments: Part 1: Ethical and Scientific Issues," *Annals of Internal Medicine* 133 (2000):455-63.

42 C. Weijer, "When Argument Fails," *American Journal of Bioethics* 2, no. 2 (2002):10-11.

44.
PLACEBO CONTROLLED TRIALS: RESTRICTIONS, NOT PROHIBITIONS

Ana Smith Iltis

SOURCE: *Cambridge Quarterly of Health Care Ethics* 13:4 (2004): 380-93.

Introduction

The last two decades have witnessed intense debate over the ethical legitimacy of placebo controlled trials (PCTs).[1] Most of the arguments for and against the use of PCTs turn on one of the following issues: (1) the compatibility of the obligations of clinicians and researchers with PCTs, (2) the scientific merit of PCTs, and (3) the influence of patients' and subjects' perceptions, ability to consent, expectations, and rights on the permissibility of PCTs. I introduce each of these categories and assess the principal arguments in each group. I argue that, although some of the arguments against PCTs have limitations, they do inform the debate in significant ways by pointing to important constraints on PCTs. Those concerning patients' and subjects' perceptions, capacity to consent, expectations, and rights are particularly instructive. They do not, for the most part, sustain an absolute prohibition of PCTs, but they do suggest types of PCTs that are inappropriate and they indicate issues that must be addressed when PCTs are conducted. I argue that we should look to the reasonableness and permissibility of informed refusals of care (1) to evaluate the extent to which a trial is a legitimate PCT (e.g., cases in which clinicians would be highly suspect of accepting informed refusals may be more problematic than PCTs in situations in which clinicians would be comfortable accepting informed refusals); (2) to determine which potential subjects should be considered eligible to enroll in a PCT (e.g., those who would not be permitted to refuse treatment generally might not be eligible to enroll in a PCT); and (3) to inform the language that should be used in describing the study as part of the informed consent process (e.g., prospective subjects should be asked if they are willing to forgo treatment and not enroll in the trial).

There are numerous scenarios under which PCTs can be conducted. The different types of PCTs include some that do not seem morally problematic, others that seem highly problematic, and some that are difficult to assess. Perhaps the least morally problematic type of PCT is one that tests a new treatment for a condition for which no treatment is currently available. In this case, those who are receiving the placebo are in effect receiving the standard of care, and those receiving the new treatment may or may not benefit. These are the least problematic cases because even those who hold that researchers have a therapeutic obligation toward subjects recognize that, if no known treatment exists, the subjects receiving placebo are not receiving any less than they otherwise would. A second case is that in which the only known treatment is highly burdensome and the new one would be less burdensome. Third are those cases in which there is an established treatment, but it has never been subjected to rigorous scientific study. Fourth are PCTs for treatments for conditions for which there are proven, established treatments, but a company wants to test its own treatment against placebo. The last two categories, and especially the latter of the two, are the most controversial types of PCTs. The focus of this paper is on PCTs where established (both proven and unproven) treatments already exist, because this is the focus of much of the recent debate. In particular, this was the focus of Benjamin Freedman and his colleagues,[2] whose work is paradigmatic in the anti-PCT literature.

Assessing Arguments against PCTs

Arguments that PCTs are always or often unethical where an established therapy exists can be grouped into three areas of concern: physician obligations, scientific merit, and patient/subject expectations and capacity to consent.

Physician Obligations

Some of the most often discussed arguments against PCTs are those that suggest that to enroll individuals in PCTs when an established therapy exists violates a fundamental ethical obligation of physicians, especially the therapeutic obligation or the obligation of beneficence.

Therapeutic Obligation
to Provide Standard of Care

Perhaps the most well known argument against PCTs from therapeutic obligation is that of Benjamin Freedman and his colleagues.[3] Freedman et al. argue that only when clinical equipoise exists concerning a treatment is it appropriate to enroll patients in PCTs. That is, only when the medical community truly does not know if a proposed treatment is actually better or more effective than placebo is it ethical to enroll patients in a PCT. It is impermissible to use "placebos in the face of established treatment, because enrolling in a trial would imply that a proportion of enrollees will receive medical attention currently considered inferior by the expert community."[4] The use of the word "established" rather than "proven" or "well-tested" is interesting. There are numerous examples in which established treatments that were the standard of care later proved to be ineffective at best, and dangerous at worst. These cases include older examples, such as the practice of exposing premature infants to high concentrations of oxygen, which resulted in blindness, as well as more recent examples, such as rest and dietary restrictions to treat ulcers that were actually caused by bacteria and required antibiotic therapy, hormone replacement therapy for women in menopause, and arthroscopic knee surgery for osteoarthritis.[5] I will discuss this further later with regard to the scientific merit of PCTs.

Glass and Waring make similar claims regarding the obligations of researchers to provide subjects with at least the established treatment. They hold that, in physicians' codes of ethics, no exceptions are made to the obligation of physicians to consider their patients' well-being when the patients are research subjects: "Conducting a trial is not an invitation to practice sub-standard medicine."[6] Moreover, "physician researchers who fail to provide available effective treatment ... can be held to the same, or higher standards than the practitioner who is not involved in research."[7] The presumption underlying the claims of Freedman et al. is that physicians, including researchers, have the obligation to provide at least the standard of care to their patients and that research subjects are patients even in the research setting.

A number of authors have identified difficulties with this claim. Frank Miller and Howard Brody argue that Freedman et al. ignore the fact that sometimes research subjects are not patients at all and that clinical medical standards are not the only standards that exist in medicine.[8] The standards and goals that frame clinical research medicine differ in important ways and for important reasons. To suggest that all clinical standards hold in the research setting is to fail to see research medicine as a legitimate and worthy aspect of medicine. Miller and Brody concede to Freedman et al. that physicians should not enroll their own patients into PCTs they are conducting when proven, established therapies exist, because in such cases the ethics of clinical medicine, where the obligation to meet the standard of care, does hold. Even then, I argue, there could be exceptions, including cases in which patients refuse treatment. I will discuss this further later. Responses like that of Miller and Brody will not persuade those who share Freedman's view. The parties disagree precisely on the issue of what obligations researchers share with clinicians. Thus to stipulate that research and clinical ethics are not equivalent and discuss the implications of the difference will not advance the debate. An analysis of the concept of therapeutic obligation itself is necessary. In particular, we must examine first what precisely the therapeutic obligation requires; second, when a physician has fulfilled the obligation; and third, what a physician may do once the obligation has been fulfilled.

Even though those who offer therapeutic obligation as an argument against PCTs present the obligation as the obligation to actually provide patients with at least the standard of care, it should not be understood in this way. It is, instead, the obligation to offer standard treatments to patients, recommend a course of treatment, and then respect patients' choices. To treat therapeutic obligation as the obligation to actually provide treatment stands in opposition to the obligation to respect patients' autonomy, including their right to refuse care. Once a patient has refused treatment, provided that the refusal was an informed, competent, and voluntary refusal, the physician has fulfilled the therapeutic obligation even though the physician does not actually provide treatment. In fact, the physician is prohibited from forcibly providing the standard of care to such a patient. When a physician has fulfilled the therapeutic obligation as described by Freedman et al., it may be justifiable for the physician to conduct a PCT, though other restrictions may apply. This means that there may be cases in which it is permissible for physicians to enroll their own patients as subjects in PCTs. Those cases might be limited to those in which a patient has refused the standard treatment. Once the patient has refused the available treatment, the physician may offer the possibility of enrolling in a PCT. It seems likely that a patient who has refused the standard of care will not be interested in enrolling in such a trial, but that does not make it impermissible for the patient to be offered the opportunity to enroll, as long as the invitation is extended in a noncoercive manner. This situation points to Robert Veatch's argument that it is ethically legitimate for patients to enroll in a PCT if they are "approximately indifferent" between the available treatment and no treatment.[9] If a patient is approximately indifferent between treatment options, then the interest in making "a modest contribution to science" may lead him to decide to enroll in a PCT rather than merely refuse treatment.[10] His argument is that patients who are in a position to refuse treatment and do not feel strongly enough about either pursuing or refusing treatment may choose to enroll in a PCT out of an interest in contributing to science. This is a legitimate choice that should be recognized and respect-

ed. Thus even where there is a proven, established treatment, if a patient is approximately indifferent with regard to accepting or refusing treatment, it may be permissible for his clinician to invite him to participate in a PCT. This implies that, if the clinician is convinced that the standard treatment is superior to placebo and the patient does not show indifference toward receiving treatment or indicate a desire to refuse care, then the physician should not offer the PCT option to the patient. However, there may be situations in which it is permissible to do so.

As already noted, to understand therapeutic obligation as an obligation to actually provide treatment conflicts with the obligation to respect patient autonomy, including informed refusals of care. There is a further reason proponents of arguments against PCTs grounded in the therapeutic obligation should not refer to the therapeutic obligation as a requirement to treat. As Freedman et al. present therapeutic obligation, it might make not only PCTs but active-controlled trials (ACTs) impermissible, something they do not seem to intend. We can only measure the extent to which a researcher fulfills the obligation to provide "at least the established treatment" after the trial has been completed in the case of ACTs. If a researcher is testing an established treatment against a new one and, as Freedman et al. claim, the researcher must provide at least the established treatment to the subject, there is no way to know antecedently that the new agent is at least as effective as the established one. If it turns out that the new treatment is at least as good as the established one, then the researcher has satisfied this obligation. However, if it turns out that the new treatment is not as effective as the established one, then the researcher has failed to provide at least the standard of care to his subjects. The argument Freedman et al. offer is not that the researcher should try to provide at least the established treatment. Therapeutic obligation is the obligation to actually provide at least the standard of care. Thus Freedman et al. argue for attributing an obligation to physicians that can only be met some of the time even in ACTs. That hardly seems a plausible standard for research ethics, and it is one that imposes on researchers the burdens associated with moral luck.

The Obligation of Beneficence

Others have argued against PCTs with a focus on the obligations of physicians beyond therapeutic obligation. They, too, hold that researchers have obligations typically attributed to clinicians, but they focus on the obligation of beneficence. According to Trudo Lemmens and Paul Miller,[11] for example, the distinctions between research and clinical care as well as between research and clinical ethics are not morally relevant; researchers have the same obligation of beneficence clinicians have. In making their claim, Lemmens and Miller rely on the understanding of beneficence found in the Belmont Report[12] and argue that beneficence involves (1) not harming and (2) maximizing benefits while minimizing harms.

To understand the force of the argument for the absolute prohibition of PCTs where established therapies exist grounded in the obligation of beneficence, it is necessary to clarify the meaning of this obligation. Taken literally, the obligation of beneficence is outcomes based; it would require physicians to actually maximize benefits and minimize harms. If in fact physicians have the obligation to actually maximize benefits and minimize harms, they may be required to forcibly provide treatment to benefit persons who refuse care. Physicians can offer the best possible treatment to their patients, but they cannot always provide it. When patients refuse treatment or choose a therapy that is less than the best one available, physicians will be unable to maximize benefits and minimize harms if they respect patients' rights to refuse treatment. Moreover, physicians cannot guarantee outcomes even when patients pursue established treatments. This is not generally what is meant by beneficence. Instead, what is generally meant by beneficence is best described as the obligation of benevolence, which requires that physicians try or intend to benefit their patients and to not harm them. To what extent do physicians in general, and researchers in particular, have the obligation of beneficence understood as benevolence? What are the implications of this obligation for the permissibility of PCTs? There are forms of research generally held to be permissible that involve burdening a patient/subject without the intention of benefiting

the patient/subject. Consider research that involves drawing blood from participants to measure the percentage of people in a population that have high cholesterol. The results will not directly benefit subjects in the immediate future because they will not be linked to individuals and thus cannot be used for clinical care. If such studies are considered ethically permissible, it is not plausible to claim that physician-researchers always have an overriding obligation of beneficence. But to note that there are some exceptions to the obligation of beneficence does not tell us whether the exception ever applies to PCTs when established therapies exist and, if so, under what circumstances.

If the obligation of beneficence is understood as benevolence and if clinicians and researchers do in fact have this obligation, is it ever permissible to conduct a PCT when an established treatment is available? I argue that the answer is "yes," though the cases would be limited to those in which patients had refused the standard treatment and cases in which established treatments had not been proven. I will discuss the latter case more later. To enroll a patient who has refused the standard treatment in a PCT offers (1) the possibility of being treated and (2) an increased likelihood that the patient's condition will be monitored, both of which may be the best a physician can do for a patient who has already decided to forgo standard treatment. Thus if the obligation of beneficence applies to both clinicians and researchers, PCTs when established therapies exist may be permissible only when patients have refused treatment or, as I will argue, the standard treatment is not a proven treatment. This restriction does not prohibit PCTs altogether. Thus, even those who hold that clinicians and researchers have the same obligation of beneficence—as benevolence cannot claim an absolute prohibition of PCTs even when established therapies exist.

Scientific Merit

A second category of arguments against the ethics of PCTs concerns the lack of scientific merit of PCTs. It is a widely accepted standard in research ethics that studies that are lacking scientific merit should not be conducted, in part because it is wrong to expose subjects to any degree of risk, discomfort, or burden if the study is not expected to yield useful data. Some have claimed that PCTs where there is already an established treatment are not scientifically necessary and thus should not be conducted.[13] One major difficulty with this claim is that sometimes established treatments have not been thoroughly tested. The medical community acts as if they have been tested and uses them widely enough that they become the standard of care without rigorous analysis. To do this is to practice substandard medicine. To fail to conduct trials to test such established treatments when it is possible to do so without significant risk to subjects is wrong, rather than vice versa. Consider the debates during the past decade regarding the use of rest and dietary restrictions to treat peptic ulcers, hormone replacement therapy for women in menopause, and arthroscopic knee surgery to treat osteoarthritis in the knee. These were established treatments routinely applied, yet they turned out to be either harmful or ineffective.[14] Freedman's reliance on the notion that established treatments must always be provided is inappropriate when the established treatments have not been thoroughly tested. Those are cases in which clinicians should subscribe to the null hypothesis, yet often they do not. Their reliance on the established treatment is lacking in scientific merit.

A more difficult question is the case of proven, established treatments. Is it permissible to conduct a PCT when a proven, established therapy exists, or is it impossible in such cases to begin with the null hypothesis such that those trials would lack scientific merit because one can expect that the agent will be better than the placebo? Freedman, Glass, and Weijer, and Rothman and Michels have argued that, when proven, established treatments exist, PCTs lack scientific merit because the relevant question is whether the new treatment works better than the existing one.[15] A PCT cannot resolve this issue. There has been significant debate on this issue, and it is at least an open question. Temple and Ellenberg[16] have contrasted PCTs with ACTs and argue that there are methodological difficulties associated with ACTs that suggest that, when possible, PCTs should be pursued. PCTs are more rigorous, they argue, and thus generally have greater scientific

merit. Moreover, ACTs in which the goal is to show equivalence between the new and old treatment are more prone to show positive results that suggest equivalence where there is none, as a result of poor methodology or other research errors.[17] This is not to say that we have proof that PCTs are far superior scientifically, but the analysis of PCTs versus ACTs suggests that PCTs may be better, at least in some cases, such that they should not be categorically dismissed as lacking scientific merit in the face of proven treatments.

Second, some disorders seem to have high rates of placebo response, such as back pain and rheumatoid arthritis.[18] In those cases, it seems important to test against a placebo and not against another therapy.[19] This might not seem plausible initially. If an established treatment was shown in a PCT to be better than placebo and an ACT shows that the new treatment is equivalent to the established treatment, the new treatment should also be better than placebo such that a PCT is not necessary. This, however, is true only when the ACT is sufficiently powered. If the ACT is insufficiently powered, it may fail to detect a difference between the established and new treatments, so the new treatment appears to be as effective as the established one but may in fact not be more effective than placebo. This is not in itself an argument for PCTs. Instead, it suggests that, when ACTs are conducted, they must be sufficiently powered. If they cannot be sufficiently powered, then a PCT may be more appropriate. Or, if running an ACT that is sufficiently powered would be more risky and burdensome than a PCT, then a PCT may be more appropriate. The relevant ethical issue is determining when a high-powered ACT should be conducted rather than a PCT. The answer, I argue, is not always, as some might wish to claim, in favor of ACTs. To conduct a high-powered ACT may require many more subjects than a PCT, which can sometimes generate more data with fewer subjects.[20] This is ethically relevant. If one can generate information that is at least as good and burden fewer people, there is good reason to at least consider that approach. The burdens imposed on individual subjects and the number of subjects burdened overall are both relevant. There may be situations in which a high-powered ACT is appropriate and a PCT is not, such as situations in which forgoing treatment is highly risky. But this is not always the case.

If in fact it is shown that PCTs have no scientific merit when proven, established therapies already exist, then they should not be conducted, just as any trial lacking scientific merit, such as an underpowered one, should not be conducted. However, there is sufficient disagreement on this point to suggest that at least in some cases PCTs are scientifically merited. The history of medicine suggests that PCTs on established therapies that have not been thoroughly tested have scientific merit; this is not an open question. There need not always be a new treatment available for it to be appropriate to conduct a trial. If an established treatment has not been thoroughly tested and its efficacy can be tested without serious risk, it may be important to do so. To ask whether an established treatment is effective and is, all things considered, better than "doing nothing" is an important scientific question.

Patient Expectations and Consent

The third category of arguments against PCTs, and perhaps the one from which we can learn the most, are those that involve issues of patients' and subjects' ability to consent, their perspectives on healthcare and medical research, and their expectations. The possibility of therapeutic misconception, discussed by Appelbaum et al.,[21] whereby patients involved as subjects in biomedical research mistakenly think that in research the physician will act only with the intention of benefiting them, is often used to suggest that PCTs are inappropriate because subjects may erroneously think that they are receiving treatment even when they are not.[22] Even when told they are participating in research, that they may not be receiving any treatment at all, and that there are risks associated with being a research subject, they continue to see physicians as caregivers who will act only in their interests as patients. Therefore, the argument continues, PCTs are not permissible because subjects may enroll thinking that they are receiving treatment or that the researcher would not put them at more risk than they would encounter in the clinical setting. This is part of the argument offered by Lemmens and Miller against PCTs:

When meeting physicians in a medical context, patients expect that their best medical interests will be protected and promoted. They do not expect that physician-researchers will hold their therapeutic obligations in suspense at their discretion, whenever they believe they are involved in "research activities."[23]

The circumstance that patient expectations may not cohere with the reality of research medicine points to a serious issue in biomedical research, but it does not imply that PCTs are always inappropriate, even when established treatments exist. What an understanding of patient expectations and therapeutic misconception tells us is that the process of informed consent may need to be more rigorous and that perhaps stronger language must be used to reveal to potential subjects the reality of biomedical research. A more rigorous informed consent process would not only reduce the number of potential subjects who suffered from therapeutic misconception but it would also help distinguish between true therapeutic misconception and what Sam Horng and Christine Grady have called "therapeutic misestimation" and "therapeutic optimism."[24] These terms refer to situations in which subjects either underestimate risk or overestimate benefit (therapeutic misestimation) or hope for the best (therapeutic optimism). Unlike true therapeutic misconception where subjects do not realize that research is not equivalent to clinical care, therapeutic misestimation and therapeutic optimism are not always ethically problematic, according to Horng and Grady's analysis.

One problem with the argument against PCTs that relies on therapeutic misconception is that it does not prohibit PCTs as its proponents claim. The possibility of therapeutic misconception does require that recruitment and informed consent processes attend to the possibility of confusion among potential subjects and that subjects who suffer from therapeutic misconception not be enrolled.

Patient expectations inform the debate over PCTs to the extent that they increase our understanding of the requirements of informed consent and clarify some of the issues researchers must make sure that potential subjects understand. However, the argument from therapeutic misconception is not sufficiently robust to prohibit PCTs altogether.

A second set of arguments against PCTs that fall into this category are those that suggest that informed consent is not enough and that there are some actions or situations to which individuals should not be able to consent.[25] Prima facie, this seems to be a violation of patient autonomy and patient rights. It is true, I would argue, that physicians acting as clinicians or as researchers should not intentionally cause harm to persons for the purpose of causing harm. It is in many cases permissible to cause harm for the sake of the person's good with the person's permission; that is, after all, what surgeons routinely do. It is also recognized that, in the research context, subjects may be burdened even when they themselves are not benefited from the research, provided that the knowledge to be gained is sufficiently important, they freely consent to participate, and they understand the risks and burdens involved in research. To say that patients are never permitted to consent to harms or burdens, even when they are not going to benefit directly, is to go against one of the very basic tenets of clinical and research medicine. Moreover, generally patients must be permitted to refuse treatment as long as they are competent; to do otherwise is to grossly violate their rights as free persons. Certainly physicians, whether acting as clinicians or as researchers, have a role in ensuring that the quality of consent individuals offer is good and there are side constraints on what they may ask individuals to consent to—for example, it is not permissible for a sadistic physician to ask patients for permission to harm them for the sake of harming them. However, that is different, both morally and legally, from recognizing the right of patients to refuse care and recognizing the right of patients to endure risks or burdens for the greater good. In their capacity as physicians, clinicians and researchers have the obligation to ask persons to consent only to those things that are part of the legitimate ends of medicine.

The argument against PCTs from the insufficiency of consent is characterized by Glass and Waring:

Consent alone is an insufficient defense when a physician fails to act according to the established

standard. Prospective research subjects should not be invited to consent to what by law would constitute negligence in the practice of medicine. Physician researchers who fail to provide available effective treatment, or what has been judged to be the equivalent by pretrial clinical evidence, can be held to the same, or higher standards than the practitioner who is not involved in research.[26]

This has far-reaching implications. It is one thing to claim that physicians are obligated to explain to patients their options and recommend a treatment and to hold that researchers must tell potential subjects what alternatives exist to participating in a trial. To add to this the obligation to provide available, effective treatment is different, yet the statement above implies that even when patients refuse treatment or give their informed consent for treatment to be stopped, physicians must continue to provide whatever care they judge to be clinically best or risk the charge of negligence. Whereas this type of argument may be plausible in a very different cultural and legal milieu, it is foreign to Western medicine, where patient autonomy is considered highly important. Second, I maintain that physicians should always make it clear to patients who have the capacity to consent and refuse care, as part of the informed consent process, that they have the right to refuse treatment. To do otherwise is to give patients the sense that their only choice is to agree to what the physician recommends. This generally is not the case.

A fourth difficulty is that what Glass and Waring are willing to accept as "established treatment" includes not only proven therapies but those which "pretrial clinical evidence" suggests are effective. This is problematic scientifically. First, there are disorders that have high rates of response to placebos. In those cases, treatments may seem effective. However, for many of those patients, the placebo might have been just as effective but might have cost less or been less risky. Second, pretrial clinical evidence amounts to anecdotal evidence, which is not considered to be the most scientifically reliable. There are numerous examples of treatments that were widely used yet it was later discovered that they were either ineffective or dangerous. A third issue here is the claim that researchers have the same obligation, if not a greater obligation, than nonresearcher physicians to ensure that patients receive available effective treatment. Glass and Waring provide no support for the highly implausible claim that researchers have more of an obligation to provide standard treatment than do clinicians. Glass and Waring's claim is grossly paternalistic and would be subject to great criticism by those who have worked on the importance of respecting patient autonomy or patients' decisions, including advance directives. Physicians must accept that there are times when patients choose to pursue actions that they as physicians do not think are best for the patient. Physicians may not simply override patients' choices; consent limits what physicians may and may not do. In most cases, the competent refusal of patients is sufficient to prevent a physician from providing standard treatment or doing whatever else she deems necessary to benefit the patient. To suggest otherwise is to uphold a doctrine that supports significant violations of patients' rights.

Among this final set of arguments concerning PCTs are those that involve the capacity of potential subjects to consent to participate in a PCT. There may be types of patients who, because of their medical condition (e.g., the mentally ill), age (e.g., children), or social status (e.g., prisoners and sometimes pregnant women), are categorized as "vulnerable," are considered ineligible for PCTs, and routinely are denied the right to refuse treatment or to consent to participate in a PCT. The issues that arise because of patient vulnerability are interesting and rich. To attend to them in detail here would take our discussion in a different direction. I will say that there are types of patients who are not candidates for giving informed consent in the clinical setting, and those same individuals are not candidates for giving informed consent in the research setting. The threshold for consent may be even higher in the research setting, however, especially for PCTs where established treatments are available. It may be the case that there are persons whose consent to treatment we accept in the clinical setting but whom we would not permit to consent to participate in research because of their inability to weigh risks, for example. We can imagine that someone who is depressed and was offered drug therapy in the clinical setting could say

yes and we would support the physician in pursuing the treatment. That same person, however, if severely depressed, might not be in a position to weigh the additional issues associated with being involved in a PCT for antidepressants. There is extensive literature on PCTs for drugs for mental illness, particularly depression and schizophrenia.[27]

One way to evaluate the extent to which we think any one of these "vulnerable subjects" is eligible to enroll in a PCT is to ask whether we would accept his informed refusal in the clinical setting. If we would accept an informed refusal from the patient, then prima facie it seems that the patient would also be eligible to consent to participate in a PCT. If we hold that someone can choose between receiving treatment and not receiving treatment, and we are willing to accept the patient's refusal, then, as long as consent is informed and free and voluntary, we should generally be able to accept the patient's consent to participate in a PCT. If there are other risks involved, such as the risk to a fetus, this may not be a sufficient condition. If we think a person is capable of making the choice to refuse treatment and that we should respect it, then that person most likely is capable of understanding the implications of being in a PCT, presuming that the informed consent process for the PCT is rigorous. A further possibility to consider here is that persons on the placebo may be better off in the trial than if they had refused treatment altogether, because in the trial some of them will end up receiving treatment, all will be monitored, and there will be a rescue plan available to them if their condition worsens. The capacity to refuse treatment may be a minimum threshold for patients whom physicians wish to enroll in PCTs.

The concerns raised regarding patient expectations, their capacity to consent, and so on not only suggest that there are limits to the classes of patients who are candidates for PCTs but also teach us something about what the advertising and informed consent processes for PCTs must include. This is the focus of the next section.

Recommendations

This analysis of arguments for and against PCTs raises numerous issues that must be addressed for PCTs to be permissible when an established treatment is already available. First, the analysis demonstrates that there are cases when PCTs are in principle permissible despite the availability of an established treatment. At a minimum, the trials must have scientific merit and pose a prospect of benefit as governed by the Code of Federal Regulations. The benefits associated with research sometimes are not experienced until later by either the subjects in the future or by other persons or both. The benefits that PCTs generate can take many forms, including more conclusive data with fewer subjects. This is to say that we must take seriously the advantages PCTs sometimes have over ACTs. This is not to say that PCTs are always superior to ACTs or that PCTs are never inappropriate. For example, when patients have a condition that is life threatening without treatment, PCTs are generally inappropriate if there is an established treatment. However, there may be cases in which the only available treatment is highly burdensome and patients routinely refuse treatment. It might be possible to argue that, in such cases, when patients have already refused care, they can be invited to participate in a PCT even if the risks of not receiving treatment are higher. I will not argue this point here.

In addition to clarifying the types of cases in which PCTs may be scientifically beneficial, this analysis demonstrates that there may be limits on the types of patients whom it is ethical to invite to enroll in PCTs. The right to refuse treatment in particular informs the minimum conditions patients must meet to be eligible for PCTs. Patients whose right to refuse treatment is limited or nonexistent, perhaps because of the disorder from which they suffer, their age, or their status, generally are not good candidates to participate as subjects in PCTs when an effective treatment is already available. For example, if a patient suffers from a condition that makes it impossible to recognize as legitimate a refusal of treatment in the clinical setting, it may be inappropriate to accept his consent to participate in a PCT. There is the possibility that a proxy could consent for research, but the case is more difficult to make. There may be exceptions to this rule, but in general, we can use the right to refuse treatment as a minimum threshold patients must meet to be eligible to enroll in a PCT.

A third recommendation this study suggests is that researchers must clearly understand their roles. Physicians inviting potential subjects to enroll must not be confused about their roles as clinicians and researchers. Confusion on the part of the physician is likely to lead to confusion in the form of therapeutic misconception among potential subjects.[28] There is evidence that researchers do not always have an appropriate sense of the risks and benefits at stake in a trial.[29] Thus, part of what is necessary to provide sufficient information to allow for informed consent among subjects is that researchers understand their roles and the distinction between their clinical and research goals. Otherwise, they may make a PCT sound therapeutic to potential subjects.

Fourth, this analysis of PCTs points to certain kinds of information potential subjects must be offered. It also suggests ways in which the information can be delivered to improve their understanding of PCTs. The information physicians must provide to patients if they initially refuse care also should be provided to those who are considering enrollment in a PCT. To explain a PCT well, the language of "refusal of care" should be used in the informed consent process. Prospective subjects should be told that they may be refusing treatment. They can even be asked directly if they are willing to refuse treatment and not be in the trial. If the answer is "no," then the physician should continue to talk with the person to determine why the potential subject is willing to enroll in a PCT but is not willing simply to refuse care. The potential subject may in fact think that she is contributing something to science and may not care that much about the treatment such that she is willing to possibly forgo treatment if there is some benefit to science. She is not willing to forgo treatment if there is nothing to be gained by anyone. Or, it may turn out that the patient does suffer from therapeutic misconception, in which case the patient is not sufficiently informed to consent to participate in the PCT.

A fifth consideration involves subject recruitment. It may generally not be appropriate for physicians to enroll their own patients in PCTs they are conducting when established therapies are available because patients are more likely to suffer from therapeutic misconception. This may be the result of the fact that they see their physicians as clinicians and thus appropriately think of them as caregivers. They may also see enrollment in a PCT as one among other treatment options if the invitation comes from their own physicians. This can be prevented by permitting physicians to invite their own patients to participate in a PCT where established therapies exist only after they have refused care or have indicated in some way that they are what Veatch calls "approximately indifferent" about accepting care. A further consideration here, one that attenuates the strict prohibition of physicians enrolling their own patients in their own PCTs, is the radical shift in recent years among patients' attitudes toward biomedical research. This change, which Rebecca Dresser documents in *When Science Offers Salvation: Patient Advocacy and Research Ethics*,[30] has changed the relationship between physician-researchers and patients. Today, many patients see research trials as advantageous because they offer the opportunity to be on the cutting edge of medicine and to potentially receive the newest treatments. Even though in PCTs a significant number would receive placebo, on Dresser's account, many would fight for the right to be included. Among many patients, the fact that an established treatment exists for their disorder is not enough. If something new might be available, they want access to it. As Dresser notes, there are people who now advocate not for the protection of research subjects' rights to informed consent and refusal but for the right of patients to be research subjects. This is just to say that many patients today, especially among those suffering from certain disorders, hold that they have a right to participate in research. They would consider it a violation of this right for their physician to not tell them about a PCT she was conducting, even if there were already an established treatment.

Sixth, PCTs must have appropriate mechanisms for monitoring subjects and "rescuing" them. Patients who consent to enroll as subjects in PCTs when an established therapy exists essentially turn down the opportunity to definitely receive care. Should they suffer a setback that makes them desire treatment, or for any other reason wish to reclaim their right to consent to treatment, this option must be available to them.

Finally, much of what concerns those who argue against PCTs involves the expectations of patients. In addition to limiting the circumstances under which physicians may recruit their own patients into PCTs and using the language of treatment refusal in describing a trial and obtaining consent, advertisements for PCTs must be carefully worded to prevent confusion. Institutional review boards generally review advertisements for all trials, and they should review any PCT advertisements with special attention to the possibility that they may be misleading.

The debate over the permissibility of PCTs is instructive. Even where arguments against PCTs fail, they often provide insight into the difficulties associated with medical research in general and PCTs in particular. These insights should be used to strengthen our understanding of the conditions under which PCTs are permissible, who may recruit subjects, the conditions for recruitment, which types of patients are candidates for PCTs, and the information that must be provided to potential subjects.

Notes

1　See: Freedman B. Equipoise and the ethics of clinical research. *New England Journal of Medicine* 1987;317:141-45; Miller FD, Rosenstein DL, DeRenzo EG. Professional integrity in clinical research. *JAMA* 1998;280:1449-54; Rothman K, Michels K. The continuing unethical use of placebo controls. *New England Journal of Medicine* 1994;331:394-98; Freedman B, Glass K, Weijer C. Placebo orthodoxy in clinical research: part 1. empirical and methodological myths. *Journal of Law, Medicine, and Ethics* 1996a;24:243-51; Freedman B, Glass K, Weijer C. Placebo orthodoxy in clinical research: part 2. ethical, legal, and regulatory myths. *Journal of Law, Medicine, and Ethics* 1996b;24:252-59; Rothman K. Declaration of Helsinki should be strengthened. *BMJ* 2000;321:442-45; Emanuel E, Miller F. The ethics of placebo-controlled trials: a middle ground. *New England Journal of Medicine* 2001;345:915-19; Miller F, Brody H. What makes placebo-controlled trials unethical? *American Journal of Bioethics* 2002;2(2):3-9.

2　See note 1, Freedman 1987; Freedman, Glass, Weijer 1996a, 1996b.

3 See note 1, Freedman 1987; Freedman, Glass, Weijer 1996a, 1996b.

4 See note 1, Freedman, Glass, Weijer 1996b:253.

5 Cohen P. The placebo is not dead: three historical vignettes. *IRB: A Review of Human Subjects Research* 1998;20(2-3):6-8. For further discussion of this issue, see: Cohen P. Failure to conduct a placebo-controlled trial may be unethical. *American Journal of Bioethics* 2002;2(2):24; Helicobacter pylori in peptic ulcer disease. *NIH Consensus Statement* 1994;12(1):1-23; Writing Group for the Women's Health Initiative Investigators. Risks and benefits of estrogen plus progestin in healthy postmenopausal women: principal results from the Women's Health Initiative randomized controlled trial. *JAMA* 2002;288(3):321-33; Moseley JB, O'Malley K, Petersen NJ, Menke TJ, Brody BA, Kuykendall DH, et al. A controlled trial of arthroscopic surgery for osteoarthritis of the knee. *New England Journal of Medicine* 2002;247(2):81-88.

6 Glass KC, Waring D. Effective trial design need not conflict with good patient care. *American Journal of Bioethics* 2002;2(2):25-26.

7 See note 6, Glass, Waring 2002:26.

8 See note 1, Miller, Brody 2002.

9 See: Veatch R. Indifference of subjects: an alternative to equipoise in randomized clinical trials. *Social Philosophy and Policy* 2002;19(2):295-323.

10 See: Veatch R. Subject indifference and the justification of placebo-controlled trials. *American Journal of Bioethics* 2002;2(2):12-13.

11 Lemmens T, Miller P. Avoiding a Jekyll-Hyde approach to the ethics of clinical research and practice. *American Journal of Bioethics* 2002;2(2):14-17.

12 National Commission for the Protection of Human Subjects of Biomedical and Behavioral Research. The Belmont Report: Ethical Principles and Guidelines for the Protection of Human Subjects of Biomedical and Behavior Research. Washington, DC: National Commission for the Protection of Human Subjects of Biomedical and Behavior Research; 1979.

13 See note 1, Freedman, Glass, Weijer 1996b:253.

14 An interesting difficulty here is assigning blame. It is not clear we can say precisely who acts wrongly or who is blameworthy for the failure to study such treatments. However, we can say it is poor medical practice never to study them yet continue to use them.

15 See note 1, Freedman, Glass, Weijer 1996a; Rothman, Michels 1994.

16 Temple R, Ellenberg SE. Placebo-controlled trials and active-controlled trials in the evaluation of new treatments: part 1. ethical and scientific issues. *Annals of Internal Medicine* 2000a;133:455-63; Temple R, Ellenberg SE. Placebo-controlled trials and active-controlled trials in the evaluation of new treatments: part 2. practical issues and specific cases. *Annals of Internal Medicine* 2000b;133:464-70.

17 Hart C. The mysterious placebo effect. Modern Drug Discovery 1999;2(4):30-40.

18 Price DD, Fields HL. The contribution of desire and expectation to placebo analgesia: implications for new research strategies. In: Harrington A, ed. *The Placebo Effect: An Interdisciplinary Exploration.* Cambridge, MA: Harvard University Press; 1997:117-37; Kirsch I. Specifying nonspecifics: psychological mechanisms of placebo effects. In: Harrington A, ed. *The Placebo Effect: An Interdisciplinary Exploration.* Cambridge, MA: Harvard University Press; 1997:166-86.

19 See note 1, Emanuel, Miller 2001.

20 Leon A. Can placebo controls reduce the number of nonresponders in clinical trials? a power-analytic perspective. *Clinical Therapeutics* 2001;23:596-603; See note 1, Miller, Brody 2002:7.

21 Appelbaum P, Roth L, Lidz C. The therapeutic misconception: informed consent in psychiatric research. *International Journal of Law and Psychiatry* 1982;5:319-29; Appelbaum P, Roth L, Lidz C. False hopes and best data: consent to research and the therapeutic misconception. *Hastings Center Report* 1987;17(2):20-24.

22 Appelbaum recently has supported PCTs with some qualification, so discussion of the therapeutic misconception on his part should not be taken as an absolute criticism of PCTs. It should be understood as a warning and an indication of the need to be careful in informing potential subjects about a trial and the circumstances of medical research. See: Appelbaum P. Clarifying the ethics of clinical research: a path toward avoiding the therapeutic misconception. *American Journal of Bioethics* 2002;2(2):22-23.

23 See note 11, Lemmens, Miller 2002:15.

24 Horng S, Grady C. Misunderstanding in clinical

research: distinguishing therapeutic misconception, therapeutic misestimation, and therapeutic optimism. *IRB Ethics and Human Research* 2003;25(1):11-16.

25 See note 1, Freedman 1987; see note 11, Lemmens, Miller 2002:15.

26 See note 6, Glass, Waring 2002:25.

27 See: Elliot C. Caring about risks: are severely depressed patients competent to consent to research? *Archives of General Psychiatry* 1997;54:113-16; Weijer C. The ethical analysis of risk. *Journal of Law, Medicine, and Ethics* 2000;28:344-61; Healy D. Are concerns about the ethics of placebos a stalking horse for other issues? *American Journal of Bioethics* 2002;2(2):17-19.

28 See note 22, Appelbaum 2002.

29 Itoh K, Sasaki Y, Miyata Y, Fujii H, Ohtsu T, Wakita H et al. Therapeutic response in phase I clinical trials of anticancer agents conducted in Japan. *Cancer Chemotherapy and Pharmacology* 1994;34:451-54.

30 Dresser R. *When Science Offers Salvation: Patient Advocacy and Research Ethics.* London/New York: Oxford University Press; 2001.

45.
REFRAMING RESEARCH INVOLVING HUMANS

Françoise Baylis, Jocelyn Downie, and Susan Sherwin

SOURCE: The Feminist Health Care Research Network, *The Politics of Women's Health: Exploring Agency and Autonomy* (Philadelphia: Temple University Press, 1998).

In the Spring of 1994, in the wake of a number of research related controversies,[1] a Tri-council working group involving Canada's three major national funding agencies—the Medical Research Council (MRC), the Natural Sciences and Engineering Research Council (NSERC), and the Social Sciences and Humanities Research Council (SSHRC)—was convened at the initiative of the Ministry of Health and the Ministry of Industry and Commerce. The goal was to develop a common set of ethics guidelines (not legislation) that would govern research involving humans in Canada.[2] The task initially set by the Chair, however, was "more circumscribed, namely, to revise the '87 [MRC] guidelines where necessary." (Working Group on Ethics Guidelines for Research with Human Subjects 1994, 7). In the Fall of 1994, the Tri-council Working Group [hereafter, the Working Group] issued a call for input on its task.

Now, whereas many academics believe that they should try to remove themselves from the influence of any special interests in the pursuit of some abstract ideal of "truth," feminists believe that interestedness is more effective in inquiry than disinterestedness, and that knowledge is not incompatible with political and emotional interests. In our view, doing ethics well requires express moral commitments that are clearly visible when addressing ethical issues. Ethics is far more than an intellectual exercise or an application of certain philosophical skills; it is an effort to determine what sorts of behaviours are to be encouraged and what sorts condemned. For us, it also includes a commitment to promoting what is morally right and correcting what is morally wrong. Further, in our view, it is only when ethicists engage in public debate and attend to

the implications of their positions in actual policy that they are likely to develop sufficient understanding of the issues in question to decide on morally appropriate practices.[3] Thus, members of the Network on Feminist Health Care Ethics [hereafter, the Network], rejecting the view that ethical theory and political activism are and must remain distinct activities, chose to respond to the call for input and thereby to engage in the political process initiated by the Working Group (Baylis 1996). While our Network was organized around research activities, we determined that our research agenda required us to take the opportunity offered by the Working Group and to try to influence the guidelines for research involving humans, from a feminist perspective.

In this chapter we document the work of the Network as we participated in the public consultation process in an effort to ensure that the concerns of women and others who are systematically oppressed in society were not overlooked. First, we provide an overview of the theoretical views that informed the Network's participation. Second, we outline a number of specific feminist concerns regarding research involving humans. Third, we summarize and review the Network's various attempts to have an impact on the policy-making process. In conclusion, we focus explicitly on the themes of the book, namely autonomy, agency and politics, and reflect on the substance and process discussed previously.

Theoretical Framework

Our conception of a feminist approach to the ethical questions associated with research involving humans is rooted in both feminist ethics and feminist epistemology. Feminist ethics informs the view that in addition to the traditional questions about informed consent and respect for persons that bioethicists typically raise, questions of power—i.e., those involving patterns of oppression and of privilege—must also be raised. Feminist ethics begins with at least one clearly defined moral value, namely, a recognition that oppression is morally wrong. Feminist epistemology informs the view that research is a social activity that is conducted within a community of differently situated individuals that is best accomplished when all participants (including subject-participants and researcher-participants)[4] are clear about their own interests and engaged in forthright negotiations with others to ensure that no one's interests are subordinated to those of more powerful participants.

More specifically, our account is grounded in our understanding that feminist ethics explores questions about political relations as well as interpersonal ones. Unlike traditional (non-feminist) ethics which tends to focus on interactions among individuals (such as between physician and patient or researcher and subject) in isolation from the context in which they are situated, feminist ethics promotes an awareness of the various ways in which people's interpersonal relationships are also structured by larger social patterns; power attaches to people as members of social groups and not merely as a consequence of their own efforts in the world. Feminist ethics is especially concerned with systematic patterns of oppression in a society. This perspective encourages us to consider how expectations are derived from deeply entrenched social patterns that structure social institutions and practices. It also helps us to appreciate how these institutions and practices help to maintain oppressive patterns, for example, by serving some groups' interests at the expense of others. Finally, because it is ultimately committed to challenging and eliminating oppression, feminist ethics asks us to consider how these institutions and practices can be modified to reduce their oppressive impact and increase their liberatory potential.[5]

As such, feminist ethics provides us with a framework for reviewing the norms that govern research involving and affecting women and members of other oppressed groups in a way that invites us to consider how research practices have harmed women and oth-

ers (individually and collectively). By raising the familiar feminist questions of "whose interests are served?" and "whose interests are harmed?" the ways in which research has historically tended to serve the interests of privileged social groups and to subordinate those of oppressed groups is made visible. Further, feminist ethics' commitment to social change encourages us to consider how current research practices might be reformed to better serve the interests of those who have been disadvantaged, so as to improve their health status. Appealing to a concept of social justice that involves not only fair distribution of identifiable and quantifiable benefits and burdens in society, but also fair relations among social groups (see Young 1990), feminists ethics allows us to see the sorts of institutional changes necessary if the conduct of research in our society is to meet the standards of justice that it should.

Feminist epistemology provides us with an analysis that encourages us to challenge the traditional distinction between active researcher-participant and passive object of study. The traditional view is rooted in the belief that accurate scientific observation must be conducted by disinterested parties who study "pure" data that is "free" from the influence of personal interests. Particular interests and desires on the part of either the researcher-participant or the subject-participant are commonly thought to pose a risk of distortion since either or both parties might consciously or unconsciously manipulate the process and thereby skew the research results. Such interest-based distortion is considered to be especially risky in the case of subject-participants because they are typically assumed to be unknowledgeable about the technicalities and requirements of the research process. Hence, if subject-participants have reason to prefer one outcome to another, it is feared that they will modify their behaviour or reports to represent that outcome. It is also thought that even highly trained researcher-participants—who are well schooled in the importance of maintaining neutral, dispassionate postures, who appreciate the need to remain open to whatever results appear, and who are thoroughly committed to the necessity of minimizing the effect of their own personal preferences on their observations by erasing the details of their own status in the process of data collection—run the risk of unconsciously contaminating data whenever they have a personal stake in detecting one outcome over others. Hence, for generations scientists have been trained in the ideology of "the scientific method" which requires them to approach their work under norms of objectivity understood to mean that they conduct their research with no preferences as to the outcome(s) that results. This approach encourages them to discount the specificity of their own locations and concerns and it obscures rather than addresses the particular nature of each scientist's distinct agency in the research process.

Feminist epistemologists have been critical of such interpretations of objectivity (Harding 1991). They have argued that researcher-participants are seldom truly indifferent to the outcomes of their studies and that the inevitable personal interests involved are most dangerous when denied rather than made explicit. Science is not a value neutral activity in practice, nor should it aspire to be. The demands of disinterestedness do not promote better science, but rather science that preferentially serves some interests and neglects others while blocking efforts to expose that fact by denying and thereby hiding the interests that are operative. When the determinate interests are those of the dominant group(s) in society; they seem to be both natural and general since they blend seamlessly with the cultural dominance of those groups in all spheres of activity. It is only the particular interests of marginalized groups (i.e., those who are subject to oppression) that appear to be "special interests" which threaten to complicate or contaminate otherwise "pure" scientific methods. Feminist epistemology helps us to understand the importance of challenging the underlying assumptions about the conduct of research in order to ensure that research programs not perpetuate patterns of privilege and oppression, but rather serve to break down such forms of injustice. In such ways, scientific research can help to promote the well-being and autonomy of members of oppressed groups.

Some Feminist Concerns
Regarding Research Involving Humans

In this section, we apply the theoretical underpinnings of feminist ethics and epistemology more directly to concrete problems with research involving members of oppressed groups, and in particular women. These issues are discussed with particular (but not exclusive) attention to biomedical and pharmacological research, under the following headings: exclusion and under representation; exploitation; and research priorities.

Exclusion and Under Representation

The exclusion and under representation of women subject-participants is, at this time, the most visible and widely debated issue concerning women in the research process. As Rebecca Dresser notes, women's exclusion is "ubiquitous." For example, using age-standardized morality rates, coronary heart disease is the leading cause of death among North American women (Wilkins and Mark 1992) and yet,

> an NIH-sponsored study showing that heart attacks were reduced when subjects took one aspirin every other day was conducted on men, and the relationship between low cholesterol diets and cardiovascular disease has been almost exclusively studied in men.... (Dresser 1992, 24)

Two thirds of the elderly population are women (as on average women live eight years longer than men); and yet, "the first twenty years of a major federal study on health and aging included only men." In fact, until quite recently, issues pertinent to women and aging have been seriously understudied. Women suffer from migraines up to three times as often as men and yet, "the announcement that aspirin can help prevent migraine headaches is based on data from males only." Women are the fastest growing AIDS population and yet, "studies on AIDS treatment frequently omit women." Women, not men, get uterine cancer and yet, "a pilot project on the impact of obesity on breast and uterine cancer [was] conducted ... solely on men."[6] A direct consequence of this sort of exclusion is that the data necessary for making choices regarding prevention and treatment for women are unavailable and must be inferred from data collected about men, even though there are important physiological and psychosocial differences between men and women that make such inferences problematic.

In addition to the problem of complete exclusion, there are the related problems of significant under-representation and the failure to undertake appropriate gender-based analyses of the research data. Many of those who contest the claim that women have been excluded from research fail to appreciate that the issue is not just the inclusion of some women, but the inclusion of women in numbers proportionate to the population expected to benefit from the research results. Of equal concern is the way in which the data are collected and analyzed. In many instances in which women are included in research, the research is not designed to look for anything that is specific to women, or to specific groups of women (e.g., those who are elderly, pregnant, or poor).

In recent years the principle of inclusion and representation has been accepted by North American policy makers. In the United States, the National Institute of Health (NIH) and the Federal Drug Agency (FDA) recently passed guidelines concerning the inclusion and representation of women and minorities in most clinical research studies.[7] And, on September 25, 1996, a policy statement regarding the inclusion and representation of women in clinical trials during drug development was issued by the Drugs Directorate of Health Canada. The policy explicitly requires "the enrollment of a representative number of women into clinical trials for those drugs that are intended to be used specifically by women or in populations that are expected to include women" (Drugs Directorate, Health Canada 1996, 2pp.). Not surprisingly, however, political change has brought political resistance. This resistance is manifested in at least three ways. Some deny the claim that women have been excluded from and underrepresented in research; others deny that the exclusion and underrepresentation of women has harmed women; and others attempt to justify the exclusion and underrepresentation.[8]

The first form of resistance to the principle of required inclusion and representation is evident in the widespread movement among researcher-participants and others to deny that women have ever been (improperly) excluded from or underrepresented in research. This claim is difficult to rebut because data

regarding study composition typically are not reported in a manner that would facilitate the requisite analysis.[9] In the United States, at least, this was the finding of the Institute of Medicine Committee on Ethical and Legal Issues Relating to the Inclusion of Women in Clinical Studies (Mastroianni, Faden, and Federman 1994), which had considerable resources at its disposal to address this very issue. The Committee concluded that the full data were unavailable. It did find, however, examples of federal policies and particular protocols that had the effect of treating female subject-participants differently from male subject-participants. It also found evidence of gender inequity in at least two significant areas of research, namely coronary heart disease and AIDS (Mastroianni, Faden, and Federman 1994). In these areas of study, the exclusion and under representation of women were deemed to be significant because of known important differences between men and women in the disease presentation, progression and response to trial interventions. Whereas in some areas of research it is possible (and appropriate) to extrapolate data from one gender to another (e.g., studies on antibiotics), with cardiovascular and AIDS research the gender-based disparities are such that data from male-only studies cannot be appropriately generalized to females.

The second form of resistance to the principle of required inclusion and representation is the denial of the harm resulting from exclusion and underrepresentation. However, consider, for example, the exclusion of women from many of the studies on cardiovascular disease that have significantly influenced both prevention and treatment—MRFIT, Coronary Drug Project (CPD), Lipid Research Clinic, and the Physician's Health Study (Healy 1991). This exclusion has been harmful to women in at least two ways. First, it has resulted in "insufficient information about preventive strategies, diagnostic testing, responses to medical and surgical therapies, and other aspects of cardiovascular illness in women" (Wenger, Speroff, and Packard 1993). Second, as a result, women have been offered less effective or ineffective interventions. For example, the Physicians's Health Study (a male-only study) found that an aspirin every other day reduced heart attacks. Subsequent data has shown, however, that while aspirin is an effective primary preventative for men, it is not so for women (McAnally, Corn, and Hamilton 1992). Consider also, the exclusion of women from AIDS research. As late as 1991, there were "virtually no published, prospective data on the natural history of HIV infection in women or IVDUs (intravenous drug users)" (Modlin and Saah 1991, 39). Furthermore, "as with the natural history, the literature to date on the clinical management of HIV infection [was] necessarily based almost exclusively on reports involving male patients" (Modlin and Saah, 39). As the disease may manifest itself differently in women than men (Modlin and Saah 1991), there is no doubt that as a result of the male bias in the research, women's health care has been seriously compromised. Clearly, resulting knowledge gaps have limited women's ability to make informed choices about their health care and thus unjustly limited their ability to exercise full autonomy in the affected areas.

A similar male-bias prevails in occupational health research. A recent example is a study by Jack Siemiatycki and colleagues on cancer risks associated with certain occupational exposures (Siemiatycki et al. 1989). When challenged to defend the decision to exclude women from the research, Siemiatycki simply stated "It's a cost-benefit analysis; women don't get many occupational cancers" (Cited in Messing 1995, 231). However, arguably, Siemiatycki's analysis is invalid. Because of the exclusion of women from occupational health research, we simply don't know the incidence of occupational cancers among women. The absence of knowledge that he and others perpetuate through exclusionary studies is harmful to women as it is confused with absence of occupational cancers and then used to justify continued exclusion of women from relevant research. And, lest one think this is an isolated incident in the realm of occupational research, it is worth noting, that 73 percent of all research funded by the Quebec Institute for Research in Occupational Health and Safety during its first six years of operation involved absolutely no women workers (Tremblay 1990).

Further, in the realm of psychological research, we find the now infamous Kohlberg studies on moral development (Kohlberg 1984). As Carol Gilligan

demonstrated (to name his most influential critic), Kohlberg's work left invisible an entire supplementary, if not alternative, approach to moral decision-making. As with the other examples discussed above, the harms of the exclusion went beyond invisibility. In this case, they extended to what Kathryn Morgan has characterized as "moral madness" (Morgan 1987).

It is telling that many of the researcher-participants who deny the exclusion and underrepresentation of women from research are among those who object to the provisions aimed at ensuring adequate inclusion and representation. Arguably, this undercuts their denial of such exclusion and underrepresentation. If indeed women have not been excluded or underrepresented from research, and thus special provisions to ensure their appropriate inclusion and representation are unnecessary, then why the vigorous objections to initiatives that presumably would only codify existing practice? If, on the other hand, these initiatives do demand changes in current practice, the objections of researcher-participants would seem to suggest that they do indeed prefer to conduct their studies without the complications that may be created by including women in the subject-participant population. These complications may include dealing with the hormonal changes of the menstrual cycle (and the possible use of exogenous hormones), the need for a larger subject-participant population in order to ensure statistical significance, as well as the tracking of data along more variables.

The final form of resistance to the required inclusion and representation of women involves attempts to justify this exclusion and underrepresentation. For example, it is argued that women can be appropriately excluded from research that examines male-specific conditions. While there is no disagreement with this claim, disagreement arises when the justification for excluding women extends to research on conditions that occur disproportionately in males (e.g., spinal cord injuries), or research using a male population simply for reasons of convenience. Also suspect are claims based on the importance of a homogeneous research population, the need to protect women and fetuses from research harms, and the increased costs associated with the participation of women (see, for example, Baylis 1996).

Consider first the claim that "good science" requires the use of a homogeneous research population. In the realm of the biomedical sciences it is argued, from the perspective of researcher-participants, that "the more alike the [subject-participants], the more any variation can be attributed to the experimental intervention" (Dresser 1992, 25). On this basis it is argued that including women in specific research protocols unnecessarily "complicates" the research. Such "complications" are deemed unnecessary because women and men "have more biological similarities than differences" (Piantadosi and Wittes 1993, 565). Now, most often when women are excluded from research it is on the basis of stipulated inclusion/exclusion criteria. At times, however, they are included in the original subject-participant population and their data is later removed (i.e., not included in the final analysis). One striking example (amongst many) of the scientific elimination of women from a study is the research by Gladys Block and colleagues on cancer among phosphate-exposed workers in a fertilizer plant. One-hundred-and-seventy-three women were included among the 3,400 subject-participants. Their data was eliminated from the research results with the sole comment that "Females accounted for only about 5% of the study population, and were not included in these analyses" (Block et al. 1988, 7298).

There are a number of possible responses to the argument that researchers must keep the sample uniform. First, even if there are legitimate scientific reasons for studying populations that are as "uniform" as possible, it doesn't follow that the homogenous group to be studied should be white males. If women and men "have more biological similarities than differences" such that it is sufficient to study one gender, why assume that "the white male is the normal representative human being?" (Dresser 1992, 28). Second, it is well-documented that, in at least some areas of health care, drug trials for instance, there is good reason to believe that women and men will respond differently to the study intervention. Factors such as body weight, body surface, ratio of lean to adipose tissue can affect optimal doses as can the greater concentration of steroids in men's bodies, the differences in hormones, the use of artificial hormones by women (for birth control, control of

menopausal symptoms, fertility treatments), etc. Vanessa Merton writes: "Without good science that included the full range of human subjects, patients who depart from the white male norm will not have the advantage of good clinical medicine—medicine that addresses their problems and works safely and effectively for them" (Merton 1994, 276). Focusing on one type of human physiology reduces the generalizability of the experimental data and thus reduces the scientific utility of the research. The "best" approach should surely be linked to the promise of benefit to society (broadly construed).

Consider now the spectre of miscarriages and birth defects. Reference is frequently made to concerns about women who are or who could become pregnant while enrolled in clinical trials. This view is problematic in that it is both over-inclusive and under-inclusive. It is over-inclusive because, in the name of potential protection for potentially pregnant women and their fetuses, all women lose opportunities to improve their health and possibly extend their lives. Complete exclusion of women subject-participants is an unnecessarily blunt instrument to accomplish the goal of fetal protection. This approach is also under-inclusive because it ignores the fact that research participation can carry reproductive risks for men as well as women. For example, it is possible that the research intervention will genetically damage the sperm or, in the alternative, that a new substance will bind to the sperm without affecting motility. If the sperm is able to effectively fertilize an ovum, this could result in birth defects in the offspring. And yet, the spectre of birth defects is not used to justify a blanket exclusion of men. It should also be noted here that only a very small class of clinical studies are relevant to fetal well-being.

Finally consider the claim of the prohibitive cost of inclusion. One of the main reasons for the powerful resistance to the principle of inclusion is the fear that inclusion requirements will increase the costs of particular studies and hence make them more difficult to conduct. Unless there are known important gender differences, it is argued that there is no need to assume the additional costs of including women subject-participants. The short response to this is that when there is no anticipated statistical difference between men and women, it is appropriate to include both and inappropriate to exclude either. Such inclusion allows for the possibility of recognizing unanticipated differences provided that gender is coded for. More importantly, one must recognize that a potential increase in the financial cost of conducting a particular trial is not the only cost associated with the equal participation of men and women in research. As Merton notes, the question that must be asked is "cost to whom?" (Merton 1994, 273). Typically the costs considered are those borne by the researcher-participant (e.g., costs associated with recruiting and retaining a larger subject-participant population and costs associated with tracking and analysing data along more variables), not those borne by the persons whose health may be negatively affected by the absence of relevant health data. While it is likely that a principle of inclusion will involve some additional costs to the researcher-participants, these are legitimate costs to be incurred for the benefit of the subject-participants.

The Risk of Exploitation

It is important not to translate the call for greater research attention towards women and other oppressed groups into a wholesale endorsement of the use of members of oppressed groups as subject-participants in all studies. Clinal trials often expose subject-participants to significant risk, discomfort, or inconvenience without offering any special benefits to either the subject-participants or the groups from which they are recruited. Many shameful events in the history of clinical research testify to the ease with which researcher-participants have exploited the vulnerability of oppressed or devalued members of society for the ultimate benefit of others. The Nazi studies on concentration camp residents and the Tuskegee syphilis study are two of the most notorious examples in this category (Grodin 1992; Hones 1981). A more contemporary example of exploitation, one involving the exploitation of women, is the contraceptive research in the US on minority populations (e.g., Enovid studies on Puerto Rican and Mexican American women) (Hamilton 1996), and in the Third World (e.g., Norplant studies in Bangladesh, Sri Lanka, the Phillipines, the Dominican Republic, Chile and Nigeria) (Hamilton

1996). There is also the suggestion that experimental AIDS vaccines be tested in high risk populations in the Third World such as prostitutes in Thailand (Hamilton 1996).

While most ethics guidelines recognize the need to take special precautions with certain groups, such as children, prisoners, and very ill patients, none seem to have appreciated that members of oppressed groups also face unacceptable risks of exploitation in a society that values them less highly than members of other groups and so is more inclined to expose them to risk. To guard against such exploitation, clinical studies which propose to recruit women or members of other oppressed groups should be required to demonstrate that the results produced will be of specific benefit to the individuals or to the group in question (see Sherwin 1992, 159-65).

We recognize that some feminists are wary of this principle as it seems to invite paternalistic approaches to women's participation in research. Their argument against it might run as follows: it allows others to decide whether women should be invited to participate in certain studies; it implies that women are not capable of making such decisions for themselves; there is no reason to assume that women are any less qualified than other competent potential subject-participants to make these decisions independently and no need for special protections to be built in for them as they are for members of groups thought incompetent to make such decisions; moreover, given the historical tendency to exclude women from studies that promise benefits to the participants and to women generally (as discussed above), it is a mistake to build in a principle that serves as a license to disregard our first principle (of inclusion) and allows perpetuation of the historical pattern of exclusion of women from research.

We are sympathetic to this concern but ultimately are not convinced by the argument. We believe it rests on an individualistic view of autonomy that we reject in favour of a more nuanced relational approach (see Sherwin 1998). Specifically, we believe that it is important to keep in mind the role that oppression plays in the choices made by members of oppressed groups as potential subject-participants. Members of oppressed groups experience a far greater risk of exploitation than members of more privileged groups. In our view, the oppression of women is so deeply entrenched in our culture that it often goes unnoticed and women's training in self-sacrifice could mean that many women would be overly compliant with researcher-participants' efforts at recruitment and retention of women subject-participants. Hence, we believe it remains necessary to take steps to ensure that the exploitation of women is not operating in research context.

Two additional but closely related issues must be considered in the context of exploitation: first, the lack of clear distinctions between therapy and innovative practice on the one hand, and research and innovative practice on the other; and second, the resultant lack of norms for innovative practice.[10] Research, unlike innovative practice is governed by regulations and/or guidelines that require peer review (before the initiation of the study or the publication of its results), detailed disclosure of information to prospective subject-participants regarding potential harms and benefits, as well as careful monitoring and the implementation of other precautionary measures to reduce the risk of harm. In contrast, less rigorous controls exist for conventional therapies, and still less for innovative practices.

Historically, many interventions have been developed and offered to women as innovative practices without adequate prior research to establish their safety and efficacy. Consider, for example, contraceptives (Dalkon Shield, early doses of birth control pills), drugs prescribed in pregnancy (DES, thalidomide), and the ever-expanding practices in the area of new reproductive technologies. As a result of the failure to adequately research these "innovations" many women have been seriously harmed. Therapy, research, and innovative practice must be carefully distinguished and innovative practices must be subject to careful scrutiny. Moreover, when dealing with practices offered solely to members of an oppressed group it is especially important to rigorously scrutinize the proposed practices.

*Research Priorities: What They Are
and Who Sets Them*

The research agenda regarding the health needs of women and members of other oppressed groups has historically neglected many important questions. For example, even though the links between poverty and illness are well known, health research often focuses on ways of responding to illness rather than avoiding it in the first place. Also, it is noteworthy that many clinical studies explore expensive, highly technological innovations, even though such treatments will be economically inaccessible to most people in the world. In sharp contrast to the neglect of many of the health needs of women, there has been a substantial body of research directed at gaining control over women's reproduction. In this area, women have received a disproportionately large share of research attention, and, as a result, women must now assume an unfair share of the burden, risks, expenses, and responsibility for managing fertility, because that is where the knowledge base is. The concentration of medical attention on women's reproductive roles not only assumes but also reinforces the conventional view that women are, by nature, to be responsible and available for reproductive activities; it also legitimizes, reinforces, and further entrenches such views and the oppressive attitudes that accompany them.

This unacceptably narrow research focus underscores the importance of moving the control of the research agenda from the hands of an elite group of knowledgeable scientists to a more democratically representative group. In our view, the prevailing norms, according to which research subject-participants are reduced to passive objects of study, is unacceptable. Along with Sandra Harding, and other feminist scholars, we propose that research be pursued as a collegial activity; under this model, subject-participants and researcher-participants collectively negotiate the terms of participation and the goals of the activity (see, for example, Harding 1991). We believe that it is both possible and desirable to conduct scientifically valid research that involves subject-participants in the initial formulation of the research questions to pursue and the method of study, as well as the decision about whether to participate once all the terms of participation have been set. Provided that an effort is made to involve subject-participants with diverse perspectives and experiences, such engagement need not undermine the research endeavour or the validity of the research results. Relational autonomy demands that members of oppressed groups, in particular, be made active participants in the process of determining research priorities and approaches. Restricting a group's involvement to the opportunity to consent to or refuse subject status on a pre-determined project retains the focus on agency alone, and not the more encompassing notion of relational autonomy.

We recognize the moral and epistemological value of efforts aimed at reversing the traditional research pattern in which researcher-participants and those who support their work (funding agencies, publishers, colleagues), who are predominantly drawn from the most privileged sectors of society (white, male, middle class), decide what research projects to pursue and who to recruit to participate in them and on what terms. In place of the traditional pattern we envision a research program that is designed to ensure that the least powerful and most vulnerable participants—those who are, at best, typically afforded only the opportunity to agree or refuse to participate in a set protocol—gain an opportunity to ensure that the research to be pursued is responsible to their interests and needs.

[...]

Notes

1 See, for example: Division of Research Investigations, St. Luc Hospital 1993; Angell and Kassiner 1994; Cowan 1994.

2 Prior to this initiative, NSERC, which has the largest research budget of the three agencies, had not developed its own ethical guidelines for the research that it funded. The other two Councils had had such guidelines since the late 1970s. MRC developed its original guidelines in 1978 (*Medical Research Council of Canada, "MRC Report No. 6, Ethics in Human Experimentation," Ottawa, 1978*) and these were subsequently revised in 1987 (*Medical Research Council of Canada, Guidelines on Research Involving Human Subjects, 1987. Minister of Supply and Services Canada, Ottawa, 1987*). SSHRC adopted its first ethics guidelines in 1979 when it became independent of the Canada Council, at which time the Report of the Consultative Group of Ethics (*Report of the Consultative Group on Ethics, the Canada Council,*

Ethics, Canada Council, Ottawa, 1977) was officially endorsed. In 1980, an Ad Hoc Committee on Ethics was established and revised guidelines were published in booklet form in 1981 (*Social Sciences and Humanities Research Council of Canada, "Ethics: Guidelines for research with Human Subjects," Ottawa, 1981*). The content of these ethics guidelines has since been reordered and reformatted and minor changes have been introduced for clarification. The substance, however, has remained unchanged. The guidelines are reprinted annually in the annexes of the SSHRC applicant guides.

3 In Susan Sherwin, "Theory versus Practice in Ethics: Feminist Perspective on Justice in Health Care," (1996), the argument is developed as to why efforts to identify concepts and choose morally adequate policies cannot be complete if ethicists confine themselves to purely philosophical exercises.

4 Where appropriate, we use the expressions "subject-participant" and "researcher-participant" instead of the traditional terms "subject" and "researcher." We do this, despite the somewhat unwieldy nature of these expressions, because of negative connotations associated with the recognition that *both* researchers and subjects are participants in the research endeavour.

5 See Sherwin (1992) for an elaboration of these claims.

6 All examples are taken from Dresser.

7 The new NIH Guidelines ("*NIH Guidelines on the Inclusion of Women & Minorities as Subjects in Clinical Research*" 59 Fed. Reg. 14508 [28 March 1994]) require the inclusion of women and minorities in all NIH-funded research in numbers that would permit a valid analysis.

8 For a discussion of the recent U.S. backlash against feminist critiques of health research, see Baylis 1996, 235-39.

9 This being said, it is interesting to note that in 1995 an assistant to the MRC Advisory Council on Women and Clinical Trials searched the MRC archives in an effort to address this issue. He was able to retrieve 37 of the 129 MRC-funded clinical trials since 1985. He found that 15 of these proposals made no reference to gender. One specified all male subject-participants (this was a study on knee surgery funded in 1991). Fourteen proposals specified all female subject-participants (all of these studies were about reproduc-

tion and breast cancer). Five excluded women of child-bearing potential. Only two required proportional gender representation.

10   For a discussion of the differences between research, therapy, and innovative practice, see Baylis 1993, 52-53.

References

Angell, Marcia, and Jerome P. Kassirer. 1994. "Setting the Record Straight in the Breast Cancer Trials," *New England Journal of Medicine* 330(20): 1448-49.

Baylis, Francoise. 1993. "Assisted Reproductive Technologies: Informed Choice." In *New Reproductive Technologies*, Royal Commission on New Reproductive Technologies. Ottawa, Ministry of Supplies and Services.

——. 1996. "Women and Health Research: Working for Change." *Journal of Clinical Ethics* 7(3): 229-42.

Block, G., G. Matanowski, R. Seltser, and T. Mitchell. 1988. "Cancer Morbidity and Mortality in Phosphate Workers." *Cancer Research* 48: 7298-303.

Cowan, John Scott. 1994. "Lessons from the Fabrikant File: A Report to the Board of Governors of Concordia University." Paper prepared at Concordia University.

Division of Research Investigations. 1993. "Investigation Report: St. Luc Hospital." Office of Research Integrity, Report No. 91-08, Rockville, MD.

Dresser, Rebecca. 1992. "Wanted: Single, White Male for Medical Research." *Hastings Center Report* 22: 24-29.

Drugs Directorate, Health Canada. 1996. "Inclusion of Women in Clinical Trials during Pregnancy." Ottawa, September 25.

DuBose, E.R., R. Hamel, and L.J. O'Connell. 1994. *A Matter of Principles? Ferment in U.S. Bioethics*. Valley Forge, PA: Trinity Press International.

Engelhardt, T.H. 1996. *The Foundations of Bioethics*, 2nd ed. Oxford: Oxford University Press.

Grodin, M. 1992. *The Nazi Doctors and the Nuremberg Code: Human Rights in Human Experimentation*. New York: Oxford University Press.

Hamilton, J.A. 1996. "Women and Health Policy: On the Inclusion of Females in Clinical Trials." In *Gender and Health: An International Perspective*, ed. Carolyn Sargent and Caroline Bretall. Upper Saddle River, NJ: Prentice-Hall.

Harding, Sandra. 1991. *Whose Science? Whose Knowl-edge? Thinking from Women's Lives*. Ithaca, NY: Cornell University Press.

Healey, B. 1991. "The Yentl Syndrome." *New England Journal of Medicine* 325(4): 274-76.

Lohlberg, L. 1984. *Essays on Moral Development. Vol. 2: The Psychology of Moral Development: The Nature and Validity of Moral Stages*. San Francisco: Harper and Row.

Jonsen, A.R., and S. Toulmin. 1988. *The Abuse of Casuistry: A History of Reasoning*. Berkeley and Los Angeles: University of California Press.

Mastoianni, Anna C., Ruth Faden, and Daniel Federman, eds. 1994. *Women and Health Research: Ethical and Legal Issues of Including Women in Clinical Studies*. 2 vols. Washington, DC: National Academy Press.

McAnally, L.E., C.R. Corn, and S.F. Hamilton. 1992. "Aspirin for the Prevention of Vascular Death in Women." *Annals of Pharmacology* 26: 1530-34.

Merton, Vanessa. 1994. "Review Essay: Women and Health Research." *Journal of Law, Medicine and Ethics* 22(3): 272-79.

Messing, K. 1995. "Don't Use a Wrench to Peel Potatoes: Biological Science Constructed on Male Model Systems Is a Risk to Women Workers' Health." In *Changing Methods: Women Transforming Practice*, ed. S. Burt and L. Code. Peterborough, ON: Broadview Press.

Modlin, John, and Alfred Saah. 1991. "Public Health and Clinical Aspects of HIV Infestion and Disease in Women and Children in the United States." In *AIDS, Women and the Next Generation: Towards a Morally Acceptable Public Policy for HIV Testing of Pregnant Women and Newborns*, ed. Ruth Faden, Gail Geller, and Madison Powers. New York: Oxford University Press.

Morgan, C. 1987. "Women and Moral Madness." In Science, Morality and Feminist Theory, ed. Marsha Hanen and Kai Nielsen. *Canadian Journal of Philosophy* 13 (supplementary volume): 201-26.

Pellegrino, E., and D.C. Thomasma. 1988. *For the Patient's Good: The Restoration of Beneficence in Health Care*. New York: Oxford University Press.

Piantodosi, P., and J. Wittles. 1993. "Politically Correct Clinical Trials" (letter to the editor). *Controlled Clinical Trials* 14: 562-67.

Sherwin, Susan. 1992. *No Longer Patient: Feminist Ethics and Health Care*. Philadelphia: Temple University Press.

——. 1996. "Theory versus Practice in Ethics: A Feminist

Perspective on Justice in Health Care." In *Philosophical Perspectives on Bioethics*, ed. L.W. Sumner and Joseph Boyle. Toronto: University of Toronto Press.

Siemiatycki, J., R. Dewar, R. Lakhani, L. Nadon, L. Richardson, and M. Ferin. 1989. "Cancer risks Associated with Ten Organic Dusts: Results from a Case-Controlled Study in Montreal." *American Journal of Industrial Medicine* 16: 547-67.

Singer, P. 1993. *Practical Ethics*, 2nd ed. Cambridge: Cambridge University Press.

Tremblay, Celine. 1990. "Les particularitiés et les difficultés de l'intervention preventive dans le domaine de la santé et de la sécurité des femmes en lieu de travail." Paper presented at the 58th Annual Meeting of the Association canadienne-francaise pour l'avancement des sciences. Université Laval, Quebec City, May 14. Cited in Messing 1995.

Wenger, M.K., L. Speroff, and B. Packard. 1993. "Cardiovascular Health and Disease in Women." *New England Journal of Medicine* 329(4): 247.

Wilkins, K., and E. Mark. 1992. "Potential Years of Life Lost, Canada, 1990." *Chronic Disease in Canada* 13(6): 11-13.

Working Group on Ethics Guidelines for research with Human Subjects. 1994. Minutes of meeting, Toronto, June 30.

Young, Iris Marion. 1990. *Justice and the Politics of Difference*. Princeton, NJ: Princeton University Press.

46.
EVIDENCE-BASED MEDICINE AND WOMEN: DO THE PRINCIPLES AND PRACTICE OF EBM FURTHER WOMEN'S HEALTH?

Wendy Rogers

SOURCE: *Bioethics* 18.1 (2004): 50-71.

Clinicians and policy makers the world over are embracing evidence-based medicine (EBM). The promise of EBM is to use summaries of research evidence to determine which healthcare interventions are effective and which are not, so that patients may benefit from effective interventions and be protected from useless or harmful ones. EBM provides an ostensibly rational and objective means of deciding whether or not an intervention should be provided on the basis of its effectiveness, in theory leading to fair and effective healthcare for all.

In this paper I closely examine these claims from the perspective of healthcare for women, using relevant examples. I argue that the current processes of evidence-based medicine contain a number of biases against women. These biases occur in the production of the research that informs evidence-based medicine, in the methods used to analyse and synthesise the evidence, and in the application of EBM through the use of guidelines. Finally, the biomedical model of health that underpins most of the medical research used by EBM ignores the social and political context which contributes so much to the ill-health of women.

Introduction

Thirty years ago, a British epidemiologist called Archie Cochrane argued that medical care could be improved by greater use of research evidence. He drew attention to our collective ignorance about the effects of healthcare, saying that: 'It is surely a great criticism of our profession that we have not organised a critical summary, by specialty or subspecialty, adapted periodically, of all relevant randomized controlled trials.'[1]

Cochrane was concerned that without some kind of critical summary, important effects of healthcare (good and bad) will not be identified promptly, with the result that patients may receive useless or even harmful treatments whilst not receiving treatments which work. In addition, without systematic, up-to-date reviews of previous research, plans for new research will be ill informed, so that promising leads are missed or existing research duplicated.

Today, Cochrane's beliefs have become enshrined in an international phenomenon known as evidence-based medicine or EBM. EBM is the term coined to represent both a critical summary of relevant research and the use of that evidence to make decisions about medical care. EBM has become widely adopted around the world, with evidence playing a critical role in informing health policy, commissioning resources and directing clinical practice through mechanisms such as evidence-based clinical guidelines.[2] Governments in Europe, America and Australasia have created and funded institutions based upon the principles of EBM to synthesise evidence and produce evidence-based guidelines which may be used by policy makers and clinicians alike.

EBM promises an objective and rational basis for healthcare, a promise that has proved irresistible. And yet there are concerns. In this paper I briefly describe the nature and methods of EBM, and then explore the relationship between EBM and women's health.[3] Does EBM point the way to better healthcare for women, or are there significant flaws in its methods and application? I argue that despite the potential benefits of EBM, there are several reasons why EBM may not deliver better healthcare for women.

Evidence-Based Medicine

What is evidence-based medicine? EBM has been defined as 'the conscientious, explicit, and judicious use of current best evidence in making decisions about the care of individual patients.'[4] This involves tracking down the best available evidence from research in order to answer questions about healthcare. The research may be about diagnostic tests or prognosis, but to date the main focus of EBM has been on answering questions about the efficacy of therapeutic interventions.

Searching for evidence is time consuming and requires expertise. There are well-defined techniques, known as systematic reviews, which aim to collect all of the research evidence (published and unpublished) about specific interventions.[5] The results from randomised controlled trials (RCTs) can be pooled using meta-analyses so as to provide more conclusive evidence about the benefits and harms of interventions. Once results from multiple trials have been reviewed and combined, the final result is considered to be the best available evidence we have on the topic. This evidence can then be used to inform decisions about healthcare, either directly, as the basis for guideline recommendations, or at a policy level.

The process of searching the evidence can be done by individual practitioners, but a thorough systematic review may take several months and be costly. To make the process easier dedicated organisations, such as the Cochrane Collaboration,[6] perform systematic reviews and publish summaries of evidence, appraised according to 'uniform scientific principles.'[7]

A further synthesis of evidence occurs in the production of evidence-based clinical guidelines.[8] Guidelines are summaries of evidence on specific topics, produced with the aim of making the evidence accessible to busy practitioners. During the production of guidelines, decisions are made about what counts as effective treatment, and when the use of such treatment is appropriate, resulting in an often didactic list of instructions for the practitioner. Guidelines are the familiar face of EBM for many clinicians, as they provide a convenient way to access the products of systematic reviews.

Why do we need EBM? Many doctors do not use up to date research results to inform their clinical practice. Doctors use information that they learned at medical school, which may be twenty or thirty years out of date, or rely upon educated guesswork, tradition, or information from pharmaceutical representatives.[9] When new effective medical technology is developed or its efficacy recognised in research, it can take many years to be used in practice.[10] The use of antenatal steroids to prevent lung disease in premature babies and the use of thrombolytics after acute heart attacks are two examples of therapies that took many years to be adopted into practice after there was research evidence about their efficacy. Sometimes doctors use treatments that have never been proven to work, or which may actually be harmful. Also, there are wide variations in practice, for example in the rate of caesarean sections.[11] This means that some people are getting unnecessary surgery, or that others are not getting enough.

The rhetoric of EBM promises that doctors will use the best available evidence to provide medical care of proven effectiveness. People will receive treatments that benefit their problems, and will not receive futile or harmful treatments, thus meeting the ethical requirements of both beneficence and non-maleficence.[12] Explicit use of evidence can bring greater openness into clinical decision-making. EBM has the potential to enhance patient autonomy by providing evidence about the benefits and harms of different treatments to inform patients' choices.[13]

EBM has proved very attractive to policy makers.[14] The idea of using only proven, effective medical interventions is intrinsically appealing. EBM is also appealing as a basis for allocating health-care goods. Policy decisions based upon EBM encourage expenditure on effective treatments, with the understanding that money will not be wasted on treatments which have been shown not to work.[15] EBM provides an apparently clear and objective basis for decision making, based on evidence that may be less open to criticism than overtly political policies.[16]

In an ideal world, EBM would further the health of all people, including women. Effective treatments would be rapidly introduced into practice, whilst use of treatments with unknown or harmful effects would cease. Women would have better choices as there would be more high quality information about the efficacy of different treatments, and would not be subject to interventions with no benefits. There are some examples of this occurring. A Cochrane review shows that policies that advocate routine use of episiotomies are more harmful than policies that restrict the use of episiotomies.[17] This information allows women to challenge birthing units with routine episiotomy policies. Similarly, another Cochrane review shows that there are almost no benefits from continuous electronic heart rate monitoring for foetal assessment in labour.[18] Citing the evidence can be a powerful way for women to resist practices entrenched through tradition or physician preferences.

Despite these positive examples, EBM and its uses raise a number of issues for women's health. EBM is superimposed upon current medical practice, repeating and reinforcing existing biases against women, both in research and in treatment. The methods of EBM potentially disenfranchise women, both in defining 'the best evidence' and in developing guidelines. The model of health underpinning EBM neglects gendered differences in the causes of ill health. Despite these problems, EBM has become enormously influential in health policy, research and clinical practice. The effect of embracing EBM may be to further strengthen an already highly interventionist and reductionist healthcare system, at the risk of ignoring many aspects of women's ill health. I discuss each of these areas in turn.

Developing and Performing Research: Inherited Discrimination

Evidence-based medicine is reliant upon existing research, which is the raw material for its processes of summarising and synthesising evidence. This means that EBM reflects any gaps or bias in existing research. Current medical research programmes discriminate against women in two ways: the first is in developing research agendas and the second is in performing research.

Developing Research Agendas

Current research agendas reflect an uneasy combination of too much attention to gender in some areas, and too little in other areas; that is, there is both biological essentialism and gender blindness.

Biological essentialism refers to a focus on women as reproducers, so that research into women's health is primarily conceived in terms of reproductive capacity and function.[19] If we consider research into women's health, we can identify large numbers of studies into, for example, pharmaceutical treatments for the menopause and to control fertility, or interventions in pregnancy and childbirth. Breast cancer, gynaecological cancer and menstrual disorders all figure as major topics in 'women's health.' Undoubtedly, fertility related issues are a major cause of mortality and morbidity for women, with approximately 500,000 maternal deaths occurring each year world-wide.[20] However, defining women's health as a single risk category associated with reproductive biology ignores the ways in which the social, rather than the biological, effects of gender impact upon women's health.[21]

Biological essentialism marginalises women's health issues that are not related to biological aspects of reproduction. The focus on women as reproducers seems to exhaust interest in women's health, leading to gender blindness with regard to other health problems which have important gender dimensions, such as HIV/AIDS, coronary heart disease, depression, tropical infectious diseases and tuberculosis. There are recognised sex differences in the causes, incidence, response to treatment and prognosis of all these diseases, due to a combination of biological factors, social conditions or social processes, all of which may have important gender dimensions.[22] Research questions tend to be blind to the potential for gender related differences in aetiology, treatment, responses and experiences of any conditions not directly related to biological sex, with the result that the research base for EBM does not address many questions which are directly relevant to the health of women.

The burden of disease with HIV/AIDS is increasingly falling upon women, who now have a greater mortality from HIV/AIDS than men. There are also gender differences in the morbidity and mortality associated with cardiovascular disease (heart disease plus stroke), with nearly one million more women than men dying of cardiovascular diseases in 1999 (see Table 1).

Table 1
Death Rates by Cause and Gender, Estimates for 1999 (% of all causes of death)[23]

Disease	Males	Females
HIV/AIDS	1 302 000 (4.5%)	1 371 000 (5.1%)
Cardiovascular disease	8 059 000 (27.6%)	8 911 000 (33.2%)

These sex differences relate to complex differences in both biological and social risk factors and susceptibility. However, the research base in these two fields related specifically to gender differences remains small.[24] A further problem occurs when the results from various research projects are combined using the techniques of EBM. For example, of three recent reviews on heart disease in adults listed in the Cochrane library,[25] only one provides information about the gender of participants in the trials. Even where information about gender is provided, none of the reviews analyse by gender.[26] This means that we do not know how much being female matters with regard to aetiology, treatment, or response. The evidence as synthesised in these reviews is gender blind. A similar situation occurs in Cochrane reviews on depressive disorders, which omit mention of gender, with the exception of reviews of post-partum depression or use of anti-depressants in breast-feeding women.

The evidence currently produced by research about diseases that are major causes of morbidity and mortality in women may not be relevant to women. Instead, we have an over-abundance of evidence related to fertility and a lack of evidence about health problems in which gender plays an important role.

Obviously EBM cannot be held responsible for the contents of research agendas reaching back one or two decades. However, there is a responsibility for the authors and publishers of EBM reviews to highlight any deficiencies in the research base, and this is not apparent with regard to the lack of research into gender differences in diseases which are of major significance to women.

Gender Bias in Performing Research

Once a research agenda has been set, the specific details have to be sorted out, as to the nature of the interventions, the outcomes to be measured as proof of effectiveness, and the participants in the trials. How do women fare in these areas?

Many factors influence which interventions are investigated by research, with the source of funding being of prime importance. Pharmaceutical companies are major funders of medical research; unsurprisingly there is much research into drug treatments.[27] However, non-pharmaceutical interventions may be more useful than drugs for many women as they are more likely to be safer for pregnant or breast feeding women. In addition, women have good historical reasons to be suspicious of pharmaceutical solutions to their perceived health problems.[28] Interventions that cannot be patented, such as exercise programmes, are less attractive to commercial research funders.

Research to establish the efficacy of new interventions compares new treatments with existing treatments. Therefore research tends to cluster around a narrow range of interventions, reinforcing current patterns. It is much easier to run a double blind randomised controlled trial (RCT) comparing a new drug with an existing one, than it is to test the efficacy of two different interventions, such as acupuncture versus an established drug. Publicly funded research may be directed towards national health priority areas, set by government and responsive to what may be short-term political agendas.

Traditionally and practically, women have little control over the choice of interventions that are researched.[29] Women are poorly represented in positions of authority and power, both at the policy level and as leaders of research projects.[30] The research questions that interest women may not be considered relevant or interesting by research teams or may not be financially attractive to funders.

Bastian notes, of the research reviewed by the Cochrane Pregnancy and Childbirth group, that 'issues of obvious significance to women are often conspicuous by their absence.'[31] Many obstetrical interventions cause pain and discomfort for women, yet the research focuses upon neonatal well-being and tells us nothing of the comfort or otherwise of the women involved. Bastian cites the example of pain relief after caesarean section as an area with very little research despite the frequency of the operation and the complexities of pain relief for women who are breast-feeding.

The choice of outcomes also depends upon a number of factors. Hard outcomes, which are easy to measure, figure more prominently than less 'objective' measures such as patient wellbeing or pain, even though at times the latter may be more appropriate. For example, a Cochrane review of the effectiveness of enemas in childbirth used outcomes relating to foetal and maternal morbidity and mortality.[32] The aim of the review was to discover whether enemas actually decrease maternal and neonatal infection due to decreased contamination with faecal matter during delivery, which was the original rationale for enema use. The reviewers recognised that enemas are costly and uncomfortable, but looked only at outcomes related to maternal and neonatal morbidity and mortality, and did not include outcomes relating to maternal satisfaction (which may not have been available in the original research). The review found that there was insufficient evidence to recommend the routine use of enemas during labour. However, rather than comment upon the lack of relevant outcome measures, the reviewers ended with the recommendation that: 'Better quality and ideally blind, randomized clinical trials are needed to provide data to this review in order to give an evidence-based recommendation.'[33] This would require an RCT of many thousands of women in order to show either the presence or absence of significant effects of enemas on morbidity and mortality. In contrast, research using maternal satisfaction as a major outcome might provide a conclusive answer very swift-

ly. The quest for evidence appears to have blinded the reviewers about the relevance of their chosen outcomes to the women subjected to the enemas.

A similar problem occurred with research into heavy menstrual bleeding, a condition which can lead to hysterectomy. The main outcomes that have been used in research trials are change in measured blood loss and haemoglobin.[34] These outcomes ignore the fact that women with heavy periods have a constellation of symptoms, including the pattern of loss, flooding, and pain and discomfort, as well as total blood loss. The review concluded that a drug called norethisterone, which is very commonly prescribed, is not effective for reducing measured total blood loss. However, clinical experience indicates that many women find norethisterone to be helpful for the problem of heavy periods. The evidence seems to have targeted the wrong outcomes whilst ignoring outcomes of importance to women.

Choices about interventions and outcomes may relate as much to the relative power of consumers and researchers as to gender per se. However, given the way that divisions of power tend to mirror those of gender in our society, women are overrepresented amongst those who have little power to influence research. Whilst men as consumers may be underrepresented in positions of power, men in general undoubtedly benefit from the influence of the men who have commissioned and performed so much research into their own health needs, creating a solid evidence base about relevant interventions for coronary heart disease, lung cancer and peptic ulcer in men.[35]

The gender bias amongst participants in clinical trials is well known.[36] Women have been excluded from research for many years, for a variety of reasons including the alleged need for homogenous populations, the fear of harms to pregnant women, the cost of including women, and the purported difficulty of recruiting women.[37] Despite robust criticisms, the bias towards male participants in research trials remains. In the US, 85% of research participants are male; this rises to 95% in Canada.[38]

Reviews of gender bias in, for example, cardiovascular research consistently find under-representation of women.[39] The very large studies from the 1980s used exclusively men. Later trials have includ-

Box 1: Hierarchy of Evidence

Ia	Evidence obtained from meta-analysis of randomised controlled trials.
Ib	Evidence obtained from at least one randomised controlled trial.
IIa	Evidence obtained from at least one well designed controlled study without randomisation.
IIb	Evidence obtained from at least one other type of well-designed quasi-experimental study.
III	Evidence obtained from well-designed non-experimental descriptive studies, such as comparative studies, correlation studies and case studies.
IV	Evidence obtained from expert committee reports or opinions and/or clinical experiences of respected authorities.

ed women, in some trials up to 48% of the total, but the mean is only 24%.[40] Even when women are included, there is little or no analysis by gender. These imbalances remain despite the adoption of gender-related policies requiring equal numbers of male and female participants in research funded by government agencies.[41] There are no large-scale trials that are for women only. Reviews published in 2001 continue to identify the lack of data on cardiovascular interventions in women.[42]

Research into HIV/AIDS shows a similar pattern. Women were 5.4% of participants in relevant HIV trials between 1995-1998.[43] The situation is slowly changing with the initiation of research into HIV in women, however much of this focuses exclusively on maternal-foetal transmission.[44]

The potential for women to 'catch up' in terms of research data is low. Research that repeats previous investigations, albeit with different participants, is of lower status than new research. This makes it less attractive to investigators and funders, and less likely to be published.

A further gender bias occurs with the exclusion of elderly people from many clinical trials. Elderly people are excluded from trials for a variety of reasons, such as co-morbidity, leading to a lack of evidence about the efficacy of recognised interventions in this group.[45] Women form a greater proportion of the elderly population due to their relative longevity, with the result that a lack of evidence about effective interventions in the elderly has a greater impact upon the health of women.

So far, these sources of bias are pre-existing in medical research, rather than due to any flaws in the processes of EBM. Indeed, the identification of these gaps is facilitated by the existence of systematic reviews that collect information about research. If EBM is a tool to facilitate access to research, it may hardly be fair to blame EBM for what we find when we use that tool. However, if one of the roles of EBM is to identify gaps in the research base to inform new research, this must surely create a responsibility for those reviewing the evidence to be attentive to all omissions, including those related to gender. When evidence is presented as convincing, objective and authoritative, and yet pertains only to men, reviewers miss an opportunity to speak out about gender inequalities. In much of its reporting, the reviews of EBM continue the tradition that male bodies are the norm in our society, and that women only count in relation to their reproductive differences.

Bias in the Methods of EBM

The methods of EBM include collecting and reviewing evidence, and then the further synthesis of this evidence into guidelines suitable for use by practitioners. Both of these processes have gender implications.

What Kind of Evidence?

EBM draws much of its authority from its methods, which follow strict protocols for finding research results and combining them in specified ways to ensure that the end results are valid.[46] Part of the process, especially in the production of evidence-based guidelines, uses an internationally accepted hierarchy of evidence that has evidence from RCTs at the top.[47] (See Box 1.)

The use of this hierarchy privileges the results of RCTs over results from other research methods, implying that RCT results are more reliable or valid than other results. Of course, for some research questions RCTs do give the most reliable results, but this hierarchy does not acknowledge that research methods must be tailored to the question at hand, and that for some questions, the best evidence comes from other research designs. This ranking of research methods is significant, as there is considerable debate about the connections between gender and methods in research.[48] In the so-called paradigm wars, quantitative methods such as RCTs have been characterised as masculine, objective, experimental and controlling, in contrast with qualitative methods which are seen to be feminine, subjective, observational, and context-dependant. Qualitative methods are favoured by some feminist researchers for allowing the voices of women to be heard, in describing problems and in finding solutions.[49] For example, a qualitative research project is ideally suited to yield useful information about domestic violence against women, or the use of condoms to prevent transmission of HIV.[50]

Oakley argues that maintaining strict distinctions between masculine/quantitative and feminine/qualitative research can be difficult, as both kinds of research often contain elements of the other.[51] More importantly, both provide valuable and complementary sources of information. Yet the current evidence hierarchy makes it impossible for evidence from qualitative research to reach anything above level III, effectively making qualitative research a less powerful source of evidence than quantitative evidence. Given the current culture of research in which there are these gendered divisions along methodological lines, widespread use of an evidence hierarchy which discounts evidence from qualitative research has implications for women's health, both in terms of women as researchers influencing research agendas and women as participants in research.

Making Guidelines

As mentioned previously, an important part of EBM is the use of evidence to generate guidelines for clinical and policy use. These guidelines are the end products and visible face of EBM, developed by groups of dedicated individuals. The group defines the scope of the guidelines, the interventions to be assessed and the outcomes of interest. Guideline development groups combine the evidence-finding techniques of EBM with the group's considered judgement to develop recommendations. The final recommendations are influenced by the composition of the group, reflecting the interests of those involved.[52] However, despite a commitment to multi-disciplinary membership, women are under-represented in guideline development groups. Chart 1 shows the composition of seventeen recent guideline development groups working in the Scottish national guideline programme.

Men form the majority in fourteen out of these seventeen groups; there are only three female chairs. Given the importance of group composition upon guideline recommendations, this lack of women in the groups suggests that women's interests may be under-represented in guideline recommendations, unless the group pays particular attention to gender issues. In addition, guideline groups advise on areas requiring further research, indicating another way in which women's interests may be disenfranchised.

These biases in the methods of EBM are not insurmountable. There is a growing awareness of the need to fit the research method to the type of problem, and a recognition that RCTs cannot provide all of the answers. The Cochrane Collaboration has a 'Possible Cochrane Qualitative Research Methods Group.' The composition and functioning of guideline development groups are coming under increasing scrutiny.[53] Yet it is disappointing that a new and idealistic technique such as EBM has so faithfully repeated well-recognised patterns of discrimination against women.

Gender Bias in Using the Evidence

Once the research has been performed, reviewed into evidence and packaged into guidelines, it can be used for clinical practice and for policy. The lack of evidence about the effectiveness of interventions in women has two major implications: withholding treatment and inappropriate treatment.

A relative lack of evidence which is applicable to women may lead to the withholding of treatment

Percentage of women on SIGN guideline development groups 1999-2001

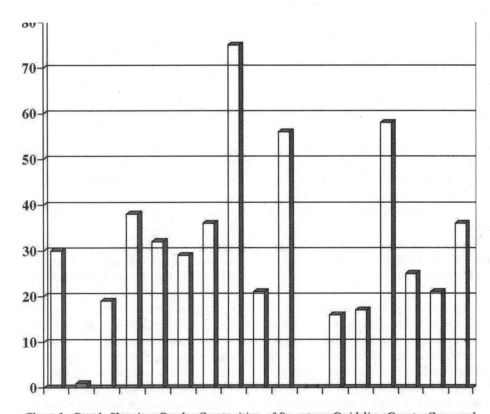

Chart 1: Graph Showing Gender Composition of Seventeen Guideline Groups Convened by the Scottish Intercollegiate Guidelines Network (SIGN)

because there is no proof that it will work in women.[54] Gender differences in the treatment of cardiovascular diseases are well recognised.[55] The reasons for the under treatment of women are not clear, but a belief that the evidence does not apply to women has been proposed as a possible reason for this.[56]

Sometimes lack of evidence may serve as an excuse not to introduce an intervention, diverting attention away from the underlying reason. Low dose oral contraceptives were not available to Japanese women for many years. One of the reasons cited for this was lack of evidence that these drugs were safe in Japanese women, despite the established safety record in women of other nationalities. This reasoning invoked an overtly objective basis to deci-

sion-making (i.e., lack of evidence), coupled with an apparent reluctance to expose Japanese women to possible harms from an 'untested' drug. However, it seems that other interests were at stake, as the pill was not approved for several years after the completion of Japanese trials.[57] This suspicion seems to be confirmed by the observation that when Viagra came on to the market, it was introduced immediately into Japan despite the lack of trials on Japanese men.

Lack of applicable evidence may lead to inappropriate treatment for women if they are given interventions that have been shown to be effective only in men. Despite the enormous amount of research into cardiovascular disease, we still have very little information about which interventions are effective in

Table 2
Risk of Dying in Poor Households Compared to Non-Poor Households[63]

Age group	Females in poverty	Males in poverty
Children aged under 15	4.8	4.3
Adults aged 15-59	4.3	2.2

modifying risk factors for cardiovascular disease in women.[58] The latest as yet unpublished research claims to provide the first clear evidence of the benefits of lowering cholesterol in women through the use of statins, but we are no further forward with non-pharmaceutical interventions.[59]

Bias in the Nature of EBM: Models of Health and Disease

There is a large body of research demonstrating the intimate connection between gender inequalities and health.[60] Gender inequality and discrimination harm girls' and women's health directly and indirectly, throughout the life cycle.[61] Female infanticide, inadequate food and medical care, physical abuse, genital mutilation, forced sex and early childbirth are directly responsible for the deaths of many women.[62] These factors are also implicated in the genesis of specific diseases such as heart disease, mental illness and infectious diseases. (See Box 2.)

Box 2: Health Effects of Being Female

Primary effects
Selective abortion, infanticide, genital mutilation, social neglect, medical neglect, sexual abuse, poverty, discrimination.

Secondary effects
Physical injury, malnutrition, sexually transmitted disease, forced pregnancy.

Tertiary effects
Early death, disability, acute infections, chronic infections, anaemia, heart disease, mental illness.

Poverty is also a major risk factor for ill health. Whilst poverty affects both men and women, pover-

ty itself and the effects of poverty are gendered.[64] Women are more likely than men to be poor, and thus to suffer the ill health consequences of poverty. In addition, within poor households, limited access to healthcare has a greater relative impact on women than men.

The health gap between poor and non-poor exists for both males and females, but the risks are greater for women. Poverty quadruples the risk of dying for women in poor households compared to women in non-poor households; for poor men the risk is doubled compared with non-poor men (see Table 2).

The adverse health effects of both female gender and poverty are mediated through society rather than biology, so that we must seek social rather than biological solutions. However, the efforts of EBM are by and large located within a biomedical model in which identifiable causes lead to disease outcomes, such as raised cholesterol increasing the risk of heart disease, or inoculation with the tuberculosis bacterium leading to TB. This way of defining problems lends itself to a research agenda in which the immediate and identifiable causes are investigated and treated. The focus is upon physical interventions acting on the diseased person, such as taking medicines to kill infectious agents or surgery to removed diseased parts. The problem with this model of disease is that it ignores the wider determinants of health such as poverty, discrimination and oppression, which are major causes of ill health in women.[65]

Measuring oppression and discrimination poses considerable methodological challenges. There are no scales or biological markers to indicate degree of oppression or level of discrimination. This does not mean that we cannot or should not investigate these topics, but points to the difficulty of devising interventions which can be investigated by research methods meeting the methodological requirements of EBM.[66] Evidence of efficacy is best proved by changes in well defined outcomes such as weight of babies, number of deaths or level of blood pressure; where it is not possible to define these kind of outcomes, it is more difficult for research to demonstrate effectiveness. A narrowly biomedical research programme receiving much of its funding from the pharmaceutical industry is unlikely to embrace research into effective social interventions, such as income support, or programmes to decrease violence against women.

A further problem with biomedical research is the focus on the individual. This allows researchers to ignore the social and political context leading to increased risks of ill health. If the aim is to provide interventions at the individual level, the wider context conveniently drops out of the picture.[67] Thus a campaign aiming to curb the transmission of HIV/AIDS may ignore the social and cultural situation of women in order to concentrate on the perceived risky behaviour of individual women, such as unprotected intercourse. This might lead to an intervention aimed at increasing condom use, ignoring sexual power relations that leave women little control over condom use or the promiscuity of their partners.[68]

EBM cannot be considered responsible for the biomedical model, which has long been criticised. Perhaps it is unreasonable to expect biomedical researchers to repudiate their traditional ways. However, EBM is a powerful influence upon the way we think about health and illness. Framing health problems in terms of the search for evidence of effective interventions tends to maintain discussions of health within the narrow biomedical model, diverting attention and resources away from alternative views.

The overall effect of EBM occurring within a biomedical framework is to provide evidence about the effectiveness of medical interventions for a narrowly defined range of disease states. This narrow focus is especially worrying when governments adopt policies based upon evidence.[69] A commitment to funding only health interventions which are supported by evidence legitimises governments' continued reluctance to tackle the wider causes of ill health. Treating the effects of poverty and discrimination rather than the causes allows perpetuation of the social structures that cause ill health.

Conclusion

Before the introduction of EBM, healthcare practices were often biased and unreliable. Prima facie, basing health interventions on evidence rather than limited experiences, hope or advice from an equally out of date colleague will benefit those receiving health-care. Research evidence can be a powerful tool for challenging and changing practice, for women as patients as well as amongst professionals. On balance, finding and using relevant evidence is surely better than not doing so. However, for EBM to make its full contribution towards improving the health of women, some changes are needed.

Attention to gender across all the processes of EBM is a necessary step. Ways to redress the gender imbalance in research might include withholding funding and ethical approval and refusal to publish the results for trials that do not include equal numbers of men and women. The evidence hierarchy should be revised to remove the implicit assumption that RCT evidence is always better than evidence from other research methods. Improving career structures for research staff is crucial, to avoid the pressure and insecurity of short-term contracts which are the fate of many women in research. Better employment conditions will facilitate the participation of women in all aspects of research. Encouraging, supporting and funding women (professional and lay) to participate in guideline development groups may overcome some of the barriers imposed by the largely voluntary nature of many of these groups.

All of these measures may lead to the production of evidence that is more relevant to women's health, which is to be welcomed. The larger question remains about the place of biomedical research within our healthcare systems. The quest for better evidence may blind both healthcare providers and policy makers as to the overall desirability and potential contribution to the health of women of narrowly biomedical interventions. No matter how good the evidence for specific interventions, if they are used in a world in which gender is a risk factor for women's health, their impact will remain limited.

Acknowledgement

Earlier versions of this paper were presented at the Beijing Symposium on Feminist Approaches to Bioethics, November 2001, and in the Department of Primary Care and General Practice at the University of Birmingham, February 2002. I would like to thank participants at those meetings for helpful comments. I would also like to thank colleagues working in EBM who offered constructive criticisms. During the preparation of this paper, I received financial support from the National Health and Medical Research Council of Australia in the form of a fellowship (ID 007129).

Notes

1   Cited on the Cochrane Collaboration website www.cochrane.org (accessed October, 2001).

2   S. Woolf, R. Grol, A. Hutchinson, M. Eccles & J. Grimshaw. Potential Benefits, Limitations, and Harms of Clinical Guidelines. *BMJ* 1999; 318: 527-530.

3   I use the term 'EBM' in its widest sense, including both methodological issues and practical applications such as evidence-based guidelines and evidence-based health policy.

4   D. Sackett. Evidence Based Medicine: What It Is and What It Isn't. *BMJ* 1996; 312: 71-72.

5   D. Sackett, W. Richardson, W. Rosenberg & R. Haynes. 1997. *Evidence-Based Medicine: How to Practice and Teach EBM*. New York. Churchill Livingstone; I. Chalmers & D. Altmann. 1995. *Systematic Reviews*. London. BMJ Publishing Group.

6   The Cochrane Collaboration is an international organisation with centres in 14 countries (Australia, Brazil, Canada, China, France, Germany, Iberoamerica, Italy, the Netherlands, New England, Scandinavia, San Francisco, South Africa, and the UK). Cochrane reviews are produced by a network of international review groups.

7   Sackett et al., op. cit. note 5, p. 15.

8   In the UK, the National Institute for Clinical Excellence (NICE) and the Scottish Intercollegiate Guidelines Network (SIGN) produce and disseminate evidence-based guidelines on a variety of topics.

9   A. Oakley. 2000. *Experiments in Knowing: Gender and Method in the Social Sciences*. Oxford. Polity Press.

10 Sackett et al., op. cit. note 5.

11 A. Coulter. Theory into Practice: Applying the Evidence across the Health Service. *Bailliere's Clinical Obstetrics and Gynaecology* 1996; 10: 715-729.

12 W.A. Rogers. Are Guidelines Ethical? Some Considerations for General Practice. *British Journal of General Practice* 2002; 52: 663-669.

13 W.A. Rogers. Evidence-Based Medicine in Practice: Limiting or Facilitating Patient Choice? *Health Expectations* 2002; 5: 95-103.

14 S. Macintyre, I. Chalmers, R. Horton & R. Smith. Using Evidence to Inform Health Policy: Case Study. *BMJ* 2001; 322: 222-225; L.W. Niessen, E. Grijseels & F. Rutten. The Evidence-Based Approach in Health Policy and Health Care Delivery. *Social Science and Medicine* 2000; 51: 859-869.

15 It is important to distinguish between evidence of lack of efficacy (i.e., demonstrated not to work) and lack of evidence of efficacy (i.e., unknown whether or not the intervention works) as a basis for decision-making. Only the first of these should count as EBM, however, it may be easy to gloss over the distinction when citing 'lack of evidence' as the reason for withholding an intervention or service. T. Hope. Evidence-Based Medicine and Ethics. *Journal of Medical Ethics* 1995; 21: 259-260.

16 S. Harrison. The Politics of Evidence-Based Medicine in the United Kingdom. *Policy and Politics* 1998; 26: 15-31.

17 Routine use of episiotomies compared to restricted use leads to more posterior perineal trauma, more suturing, and more complications. There are no benefits with regard to pain and severe vaginal or perineal trauma. G. Carroli & J. Belizan. Episiotomy for Vaginal Birth (Cochrane Review). *The Cochrane Library* 2001; 4. Oxford. Update Software.

18 S. Thacker, D. Stroup & M. Chang. Continuous Electronic Heart Rate Monitoring for Fetal Assessment during Labour (Cochrane Review). *The Cochrane Library* 2001; 4. Oxford. Update Software.

19 M. Inhorn & K. Whittle. Feminism Meets the 'new' Epidemiologies: Towards an Appraisal of Antifeminist Biases in Epidemiological Research on Women's Health. *Social Science and Medicine* 2001; 53: 553-567.

20 L. Doyal. Gender Equity in Health: Debates and Dilemmas. *Social Science and Medicine* 2000; 51: 931-939.

21 Inhorn & Whittle, op. cit. note 19.

22 Doyal, op. cit. note 20; Inhorn & Whittle, op. cit. note 19; S. Kjeldsen, R. Kolloch, G. Leonetti, J. Mallion, A. Zanchetti, D. Elmfeldt, I. Warnold & L. Hansson. Influence of Gender and Age on Preventing Cardiovascular Disease by Antihypertensive Treatment and Acetylsalicylic Acid. The HOT study. Hypertension Optimal Treatment. *Journal of Hypertension* 2000; 18: 629-642; D. Lawlor, S. Ebrahim & G. Davey Smith. Sex Matters: Secular and Geographical Trends in Sex Differences in Coronary Heart Disease Mortality. *BMJ* 2001; 323: 541-545; L. Mosca, C. McGillen & M. Rubenfire. Gender Differences in Barriers to Lifestyle Change for Cardiovascular Disease Prevention. *Journal of Women's Health* 1998; 7: 711-715; J. Ussher. 2000. Women and Mental Illness. In *Women, Health and the Mind*. L. Sherr & J. St Lawrence, eds. Chichester. John Wiley and Sons Ltd: 77-90.

23 WHO. 2000. *Statistics World Health Report 2000: Deaths by Cause, Sex and Mortality Stratum in WHO Regions, Estimates for 1999* (Annex Table 3).

24 Inhorn & Whittle, op. cit. note 19.

25 A search of the Cochrane library using the MeSH term HEART-DISEASESME, exploded term (accessed 6-9-01) gave 11 hits under Cochrane database of systematic reviews, three of which were about heart disease in adults: B. Mayosi, J. Volmink & P. Commerford. Interventions for Treating Tuberculous Pericarditis (Cochrane Review). The Cochrane Library 2001; 3. Oxford. Update Software; S. Ebrahim & G. Davey Smith. Multiple Risk Factor Interventions for Primary Prevention of Coronary Heart Disease (Cochrane Review). The Cochrane Library 2001; 3. Oxford. Update Software; M. Cucherat, E. Bonnefoy & G. Tremeau. Primary Angioplasty versus Intravenous Thrombolysis for Acute Myocardial Infarction (Cochrane Review). The Cochrane Library 2001; 3. Oxford. Update Software.

26 In the review by Mayosi et al., 3 trials were reviewed with a total of 411 participants. There was no analysis by gender and no reporting of gender in tables of study characteristics. Ebrahim and Davey Smith reviewed 18 trials, with a total of 141477 participants.

7 trials were men only, with 109 740 participants; 2 trials were women only, with 3428 participants, and for the remainder (28309 participants) the gender was not stated. There was no analysis by gender. Cucherat et al. reviewed 10 trials with a total of 2573 participants. There was no reporting of gender in the table of study characteristics, and no analysis by gender. Subgroup analysis by gender may not always be methodologically possible, and may increase the risk of errors, but if there is a reasonable belief that gender is significant, trials should be designed to allow for this.

27 T. Bodenheimer. Uneasy Alliance: Clinical Investigators and the Pharmaceutical Industry. *NEJM* 2000; 342: 1539-1540.

28 For example, many women suffered from the widespread prescription of the benzodiazopene anxiolytics.

29 S. Sherwin. 1992. *No Longer Patient: Feminist Ethics and Health Care*. Philadelphia. Temple University Press.

30 L. Sherr. 2000. Women and Clinical Trials. In *Women, Health and the Mind*, op. cit. note 22, pp. 47-58.

31 H. Bastian. 1994. The Power of Sharing Knowledge: Consumer Participation in the Cochrane Collaboration. Cochrane Consumer Network website: http://www.cochraneconsumer.com/index.asp?SHOW=HotTopics (accessed October, 2001).

32 L. Cuervo, M. Rodriguez & M. Delgado. Enemas During Labor (Cochrane Review). The Cochrane Library 2001; 3. Oxford. Update Software.

33 Ibid.

34 The Management of Menorrhagia. 1995. *Effective Health Care Bulletin*. York. NHS Centre for Reviews and Dissemination, University of York.

35 Inhorn & Whittle, op. cit. note 19.

36 R. Dresser. Wanted: Single, White Male for Medical Research. *Hastings Center Report* 1992; 22: 24-29; Sherr, op. cit. note 30.

37 Ibid.

38 Sherr, op. cit. note 30.

39 S. Ebrahim & G. Davey Smith. Systematic Review of Randomised Controlled Trials of Multiple Risk Factor Interventions for Preventing Coronary Heart Disease. *BMJ* 1997; 314: 1666-1674; R. Raine, T. Crayford, K. Chan & J. Chambers. Gender Differences in

the Treatment of Patients with Acute Myocardial Ischemia and Infarction in England. *International Journal of Technology Assessment in Health Care* 1999; 15: 136-146; P. Rochon, J. Clark, M. Binns, V. Patel & J. Gurwitz. Reporting of Gender-Related Information in Clinical Trials of Drug Therapy for Myocardial Infarction. Canadian *Medical Association Journal* 1998; 159: 321-327.

40 Rochon et al., ibid.

41 Ibid.

42 L. Hooper, C. Summerbell, J. Higgins, R. Thompson, N. Capps, G. Davey Smith & S. Ebrahim. Dietary Fat Intake and Prevention of Cardiovascular Disease: A Systematic Review. *BMJ* 2001; 322: 757-763; D. Krummel, D. Koffman, Y. Bronner, J. Davis, K. Greenlund, I. Tessaro, D. Upson & J. Wilbur. Cardiovascular Health Interventions in Women: What Works? *Journal of Women's Health & Gender-Based Medicine* 2001; 10: 117-136.

43 Sherr, op. cit. note 30.

44 Most of the women with HIV/AIDS live in developing countries, and thus are doubly disadvantaged both by their gender and by the lack of research in these countries.

45 K. Hall & R. Luepker. Is Hypercholesterolemia a Risk Factor and Should It Be Treated in the Elderly? *American Journal of Health Promotion* 2000; 14: 347-356.

46 Chalmers & Altmann, op. cit. note 5; Sackett et al., op. cit. note 5.

47 P.G. Shekelle, S.H. Woolf, M. Eccles & J. Grimshaw. Developing Guidelines. *BMJ* 1999; 318: 593-596. Note that the original descriptions of EBM (by, for example Sackett et al, op. cit. note 5) do not include a hierarchy of evidence, but this has now become widely incorporated into much of the literature and is linked to the strength of recommendations in many evidence-based guidelines.

48 See Oakley, op. cit. note 9, for a full review of these debates.

49 E. Annandale & K. Hunt. 2000 Gender Inequalities in Health: Research at the Crossroads. In *Gender Inequalities in Health*. E. Annandale & K. Hunt, eds. Buckingham. Open University Press: 1-35; Inhorn & Whittle, op. cit. note 19.

50 S. Craddock. 2001. Scales of Justice: Women, Equity and HIV in East Africa. In *Geographies of Women's Health*. I. Dyck, N.D. Lewis & S. McLafferty, eds. London. Routledge: 41-60; S. Ruangjiratain & J. Kendall. Understanding Women's Risk of HIV Infection in Thailand through Critical Hermeneutics. *Advances in Nursing Science* 1998; 21: 42-51.

51 Oakley, op. cit. note 9.

52 Woolf et al., op. cit. note 2.

53 C. Pagliari, J. Grimshaw & M. Eccles. The Potential Influence of Small Group Processes on Guideline Development. Journal of Evaluation in Clinical Practice 2001; 7: 191-199.

54 See also [note] 15 on blurring the distinction between lack of evidence of efficacy and evidence of lack of efficacy.

55 J. Brophy, J. Diodati, P. Bogaty & P. Theroux. The Delay to Thrombolysis: An Analysis of Hospital and Patient Characteristics. Quebec Acute Coronary Care Working Group. *Canadian Medical Association Journal* 1998; 158: 475-480; L. Davis, J. Evans, J. Strickland, L. Shaw & G. Wagner. Delays in Thrombolytic Therapy for Acute Myocardial Infarction: Association with Mode of Transportation to the Hospital, Age, Sex, and Race. *American Journal of Critical Care* 2001; 10: 35-42; R. Raine, T. Crayford, K. Chan & J. Chambers. Gender Differences in the Treatment of Patients with Acute Myocardial Ischemia and Infarction in England. *International Journal of Technology Assessment in Health Care* 1999; 15: 136-146.

56 Rochon et al., op. cit. note 39; I. Sharp. 1998. Gender Issues in the Prevention and Treatment of Coronary Heart Disease. In *Women and Health Services*. L. Doyal, ed. Buckingham. Open University Press: 100-112.

57 A. Goto, M. Reich & I. Aitken. Oral Contraceptives and Women's Health in Japan. *JAMA* 1999; 282: 2173-2177.

58 Hooper et al., op. cit. note 42; Kjeldsen et al., op. cit. note 22; Krummel et al., op. cit. note 42.

59 I am referring to the Heart Protection Study (lead investigator R. Collins, reported in the News section of the *BMJ* 2001: 323; 1145).

60 Reviewed by Doyal, op. cit. note 20.

61 L. Doyal. 1995. *What Makes Women Sick: Gender and the Political Economy of Health*. Basingstoke, Hampshire. Macmillan Press Ltd.

62 United Nations Population Fund. 2001. The State of

World Population 2000. Chapter 2 (accessed electronically: http://www.unfpa.org/swp/2000/english /index.html).

63   United Nations Population Fund op. cit. note 62, chapter 5.

64   M. Bartley, A. Sacker, D. Firth & R. Fitzpatrick. 2000. Dimensions of Inequality and the Health of Women. In *Understanding Health Inequalities*. H. Graham, ed. Buckingham. Open University Press: 58-78; Doyal, op. cit. note 20; Inhorn & Whittle, op. cit. note 19.

65   D. Acheson. 1998. Independent Inquiry into Inequalities in Health. London. Stationery Office.

66   M. Whitehead, F. Diderichsen & B. Burstrom. 2000. Researching the Impact of Public Policy on Inequalities in Health. In *Understanding Health Inequalities*. H. Graham, ed. Buckingham. Open University Press: 203-218.

67   Inhorn & Whittle, op. cit. note 19.

68   Ruangjiratain & Kendall, op. cit. note 50.

69   G. Davey Smith, S. Ebrahim & S. Frankel. How Policy Informs the Evidence. *BMJ* 2001; 322: 184-185.

47.
THE ETHICS OF GENETIC RESEARCH ON SEXUAL ORIENTATION

Udo Schüklenk, Edward Stein, Jacinta Kerin, and William Byne

SOURCE: *Hastings Center Report* 27.4 (1997).

Research on the origins of sexual orientation has received much public attention in recent years, especially findings consistent with the notion of relatively simple links between genes and sexual orientation. Investigation into the causes of same-sex attraction has, however, been ongoing for more than one hundred years.[1] Claims that such inquiry is dangerous, especially in certain social and political climates, are as old as the research itself. In this paper, we show that such genetic research in particular gives rise to serious ethical issues.

Genetic Research

Scientific research on sexual orientation has taken many forms. One early idea was to find evidence of a person's sexual orientation in such bodily features as amount of facial hair, size of external genitalia, and the ratio of shoulder width to hip width. Today's seemingly more sophisticated morphological research looks instead at neuroanatomical structures. Such inquiry usually assumes sexual orientation is a trait with two forms, one typically associated with males and the other typically associated with females. Researchers who accept this assumption expect particular aspects of an individual's brain or physiology to conform to either a male type that causes sexual attraction to women (shared by heterosexual men and lesbians) or a female type that causes sexual attraction to men (shared by heterosexual women and gay men). This assumption is scientifically unsupported and there are alternatives to it.

Another early approach was to find evidence of a person's sexual orientation in his or her endocrine system. The idea was that gay men would have less androgenic hormones (the so-called male-typical hormones) or more estrogenic hormones (the so-called female-typical sex hormones) than straight men and that lesbians would have more androgenic and less estrogenic sex hormones than straight women. However, an overwhelming majority of studies failed to demonstrate any correlation between sexual orientation and adult hormonal constitution.[2] According to current hormonal theories of sexual orientation, lesbians and gay men were exposed to atypical hormone levels early in their development. Such theories draw heavily on the observation that, in rodents, hormonal exposure in early development exerts organizational influences on the brain that determine the balance between male and female patterns of mating behaviors in adulthood. Extrapolating from behaviors in rodents to psychological phenomena in humans is, however, quite problematic. In rodents, a male who allows himself to be mounted by another male is counted as homosexual, while a male that mounts another male is considered heterosexual. This model defines sexual orientation in terms of specific postures and behaviors. In contrast, in the human case, sexual orientation is defined not by what "position" one takes in sexual intercourse but by one's pattern of erotic responsiveness and the sex of one's preferred sex partner.

Although early sex researchers reported that homosexuality runs in families, careful studies of this hypothesis are only beginning to be done. Several studies suggest that male homosexuality runs in families,[3] but they are not helpful in distinguishing between genetic and environmental influences because most related individuals share both genes and environmental variables. Further disentanglement of genetic and environmental influences requires adoption studies.

The only heritability study of male homosexuality that includes an adoption component is the highly publicized study of Bailey and Pillard.[4] The study suggests a significant environmental contribution to the development of sexual orientation in men in addition to a moderate generic influence. This study assessed sexual orientation not only in the identical and fraternal twins, but also in the nontwin biological brothers and the unrelated adopted brothers of the gay men who volunteered for the study. The concordance rate for identical twins (52 percent) was much higher than the concordance rate for the fraternal twins (22 percent). These concordance rates show that the environment must play a significant role in sex orientation because approximately half of the monozygotic twin pairs were discordant for sexual orientation despite sharing both their genes and familial environments. The higher concordance rate in the identical twins is *consistent* with a genetic effect because identical twins share all of their genes while fraternal twins, on average, share only half. Genes cannot, however, explain the remaining results of this study. In the absence of a significant environmental influence, the incidence of homosexuality among the adopted brothers of gay men should be equal to the rate of homosexuality in the general population, which recent studies place at somewhere between 2 and 5 percent. The observed concordance rate was 11 percent (two and five times higher than expected given the estimates); this suggests a major environmental contribution. Further, no genetic explanation can account for the fact that the concordance rate for homosexuality among nontwin brothers was about the same whether or not they were genetically related (the rate for homosexuality among nontwin biological brothers was 9 percent; among adopted brothers it was 11 percent).

When all the data from the twin study are considered, it appears that sexual orientation is the result of a combination of both genetic and environmental influences. Further, the combined effect of genetic and environmental influences might not simply be their sum; these factors could interact in a nonadditive or synergistic manner. In fact, recent heritability studies consistently find that almost half of the identical twin pairs are discordant for sexual orientations even though they share the same genes and similar familial environments. This finding underscores how little we know about the origins of sexual orientation.

Of all the recent biological studies, the genetic linkage study by Dean Hamer's group is the most conceptually complex. This study presents statistical evidence that genes influencing sexual orientation may reside in the q28 region of the X chromosome.[5] Females have two X chromosomes, but they pass a copy of only one to a son. The theoretical probability of two sons receiving a copy of the same Xq28 from their mother is thus 50 percent. Hamer found that of forty pairs of gay siblings, thirty-three instead of the expected twenty had received the same Xq28 region from their mother. Hamer's finding is often misinterpreted as showing that all sixty-six men from these thirty-three pairs shared the same Xq28 sequence. In fact, all he showed was that each member of the thirty-three concordant pairs shared his Xq28 region with his brother but not with any of the other sixty-four men. No single specific Xq28 sequence was common to all sixty-six men.

There are several problems with Hamer's study. First, a Canadian research team has been unable to duplicate the finding using a comparable experimental design.[6] Second, Hamer confined his search to the X-chromosome on the basis of family interviews, which seems to reveal a disproportionately high number of male homosexuals on the mothers' side of the family. Women might, however, be more likely to know details of family medical history, rendering these interviews less than objective in terms of directing experimental design.[7] Third, one of Hamer's coauthors has expressed serious concerns about the methodology of the study.[8] Fourth, there is some question about whether Hamer's results, correctly interpreted, are statistically significant. His conclusions rest on the assumption that the rate of homosexuality in the population at large (the base rate of homosexuality) is 2 percent. If the base rate is actually 4 percent or higher, then Hamer's results are not statistically significant. A leading geneticist argues that Hamer's own data support the four percent estimate.[9]

To understand what is at issue here, it is useful to contrast three models of the role genes might play in sexual orientation.[10] According to the "permissive effect model," genes or other biological factors influence the neural substrate on which sexual orientation is inscribed by formative experience. On this view, genetic factors might also delimit the period during which experience can affect a person's sexual orientation. According to the "indirect effect model," genes code for (or other biological factors influence) temperamental or personality factors that influence how one interacts with and shapes one's environment and formative experiences. On this view, the same gene (or set of genes) might predispose to homosexuality in some environments, to heterosexuality in others, and have no effect on sexual orientation in others. Finally, according to the "direct effect model," genes (or other biological factors) influence the brain structures that mediate sexual orientation. Hamer, LeVay, and most other researchers seem to favor the direct model.

One version of the direct model involves talk of "gay genes." It is important to remember that genes in themselves cannot directly specify any behaviors or psychological phenomena; rather, a gene directs a particular pattern of RNA synthesis that in turn specifies the amino acid sequence of a particular protein that may influence behavior. There are necessarily many intervening pathways between a gene and a behavior and even more between a gene and a pattern that involves both thinking and behaving. For the term "gay gene" to have a clear meaning, one needs to propose that a particular gene, perhaps through a hormonal mechanism, organizes the brain specifically to support the desire to have sex with people of the same sex. No one has, however, presented evidence in support of such a simple and direct link between genes and sexual orientation.

Importantly, "gay genes" are not required for homosexuality to be heritable. This is because heritability has a precise technical meaning; it refers to the ratio of genetic variation to total (phenotypic) variation. As such, heritability merely reflects the degree to which a given outcome is linked to genetic factors; it says nothing about the nature of those factors nor about their mechanism of action. Homosexuality would be heritable if genes worked through a very indirect mechanism. For example, if the indirect model is right and genes act on temperamental variables that influence how we perceive and interact

with our environment, then temperament could play an important role from the moment of birth in shaping the relationships and experience that influence how sexual orientation develops. The moral is that any genetic influence on sexual orientation might prove to be very indirect. In general, there is no convincing evidence to support the direct model; current biological evidence is equally compatible with both the direct and the indirect model.

Ethical Concerns

We have several ethical concerns about genetic research on sexual orientation. Underlying these concerns is the fact that even in our contemporary societies, lesbians, gay men, and bisexuals are subject to widespread discrimination and social disapprobation. Against this background, we are concerned about the particularly gruesome history of the use of such research. Many homosexual people have been forced to undergo "treatments" to change their sexual orientation, while others have "chosen" to undergo them in order to escape societal homophobia. All too often, scientifically questionable "therapeutic" approaches destroyed the lives of perfectly healthy people. "Conversion therapies" have included electroshock treatment, hormonal therapies, genital mutilation, and brain surgery.[11] We are concerned about the negative ramifications of biological research on sexual orientation, especially in homophobic societies. In Germany, some scholars have warned of the potential for abuse of such genetic research, while others have called for a moratorium on such research to prevent the possible abuse of its results in homophobic societies. These warnings should be taken seriously.

We are concerned that people conducting research on sexual orientation work within homophobic frameworks, despite their occasional claims to the contrary. A prime example is the German obstetrician Günter Dörner, whose descriptions of homosexuality ill-conceal his heterosexism. Dörner writes about homosexuality as a "dysfunction" or "disease" based on "abnormal brain development." He postulates that it can be prevented by "*optimizing*" natural conditions or by "*correcting* abnormal hormonal concentrations prenatally" (emphasis added).[12]

Another example is provided by psychoanalyst Richard Friedman, who engages in speculation about nongay outcome given proper therapeutic intervention.[13] Research influenced by homophobia is likely to result in significantly biased accounts of human sexuality; further, such work is more likely to strengthen and perpetuate the homophobic attitudes on which it is based.

Sexual Orientation Research Is Not Value Neutral

Furthermore, we question whether those who research sexual orientation can ever conduct their work in a value-neutral manner. One might think that the majority of American sex researchers treat homosexuality not as a disease, but rather as a variation analogous to a neutral polymorphism. To consider whether or not this is the case, one must look at the context in which interest in sexual orientation arises. Homophobia still exists to some degree in all societies within which sexual orientation research is conducted. The cultures in which scientists live and work influence both the questions they ask and the hypotheses they imagine and explore. Given this, we believe it is unlikely that the sexual orientation research of any scientist (even one who is homosexual) will escape some taint of homophobia. This argument is importantly different from one which claims that objective research can be used unethically in discriminatory societies. The latter logic implies that what should be questioned is the regulation of the application of technology, not the development of the technology in the first place. While we do provide arguments for questioning the efficacy of such regulations should they be developed, our deeper concerns are directed toward the institutional and social structures that constrain sex research. Attention to these contextual details shows that research into sexual orientation is different from research into most other physical/behavioral variations. Since sexual orientation is the focus of intense private and public interest, relevant inquiry cannot be studied independently of societal investment. It is naive to suggest that individual researchers might suddenly find themselves in the position of neutral inquirers. Social mores both con-

strain and enable the ways in which an individual's research is focused.

We are not claiming that all researchers are homophobic to some degree whether or not they are aware of it. Nor are we talking about the implicit or explicit intentions of individual sexual orientation researchers. Rather we are seeking to highlight that the very motivation for seeking the "origin" of homosexuality has its source within social frameworks that are pervasively homophobic. Recognition that scientific projects are constituted by, and to some degree complicit in, social structures does not necessarily entail that all such science should cease. At the very least, however, it follows that sexual orientation research and its use should be subject to critique. Such a critique will call into question the claim that, by treating homosexuality as a mere variation of human behavior, researchers are conducting neutral investigations into sexual orientation.

Predicting Sexual Orientation in Utero

We are also worried that an amniocentesis-like test will be developed that claims to detect genes or hormonal levels that might predispose for homosexuality. This concern may seem paradoxical, since the development of such a test seems to rely on the truth of the direct model of sexual orientation, which we describe as scientifically unsupported. Yet the development of such a test is, in principle, compatible with either the direct or indirect genetic model of sexual orientation. While current scientific results favor neither model, it is conceivable that future studies might clarify this impasse. Even evidence for the indirect model might inform the creation of a genetic screening technique that purports to influence sexual orientation in a given environment. Thus we are concerned that tests which do no more than suggest a predisposition for homosexuality would be favorably received in homophobic societies. If prospective parents believe they are able to predict the sexual orientation of a fetus by using a prenatal screening technique, it is possible that they would choose to abort a fetus that seemed to be "homosexually predisposed." In many countries, the preference for male versus female offspring leads to the abortion of female fetuses. This preference is clearly connected to sexism operating at a societal level. In such instances, science is subverted to serve the interests of discriminatory societies. Thus, discrimination can be institutionalized through genetic screening techniques.

Moreover, tests can be both developed and well received even if they are based on bad science. People might make use of genetic screening procedures that are supposed to select for heterosexual children even if such procedures did not work. This is partly for the general reason that the public can, in various ways, be lead to accept unsound scientific procedures. More specifically, potential users of sexual-orientation-selection procedures will have a difficult time assessing the efficacy of such procedures for at least three reasons. First, since some children turn out to be heterosexual even without the use of such a procedure, many parents who make use of it will believe that the procedure has worked, even though the procedure has done nothing. Second, many people take a long time to come to grips with their sexual orientation. Parents who made use of such a procedure might think that it had been successful, but only because their child had not yet figured out her or his sexual orientation. Third, because some lesbians, gay men, and bisexuals hide their sexual orientation, many parents will think that their attempt at selecting their child's sexual orientation has worked when in fact it has not. Further, if a lesbian, gay man, or bisexual knows that his or her parents used such a procedure, this would increase the likelihood that the person would hide his or her sexual orientation from them. For these reasons, such a procedure is likely to appear to work even if it does not. Given the appearance that such procedures work, as well as the widespread prejudice and discrimination against lesbians, gay men, and bisexuals, some people will attempt to select the sexual orientation of their children. This would likely engender and perpetuate attitudes that lesbians and gay men are undesirable and not valuable, policies that discriminate against lesbians and gay men, and the very conditions that give rise to such attitudes and policies.[14]

Replies to These Concerns

Given the wide-ranging abuse of the results of biological research on sexual orientation in the past, it is not surprising that people realize that ethical justifications for this work are needed. Some researchers say their work can provide answers to centuries-old questions surrounding religious propositions that homosexuality is abnormal or unnatural.[15] However, biological research on the causes of sexual orientation cannot possibly provide answers to questions concerning the nature and normality of homosexuality. As we will go on to illustrate, the only senses in which homosexuality can be said to be, or fail to be, natural or normal are of no ethical relevance. Given that some scientists claim their *empirical* research can provide answers to *normative* questions, the danger of committing a naturalistic fallacy in this context is very real.

Normativity of Naturalness and Normality

Why is there a dispute as to whether homosexuality is natural or normal? We suggest it is because many people seem to think that nature has a prescriptive normative force such that what is deemed natural or normal is necessarily good and therefore *ought* to be. Everything that falls outside these terms is constructed as unnatural and abnormal, and it has been argued that this constitutes sufficient reason to consider homosexuality worth avoiding.[16] Arguments that appeal to "normality" to provide us with moral guidelines also risk committing the naturalistic fallacy. The naturalistic fallacy is committed when one mistakenly deduces from the way things are to the way they ought to be. For instance, Dean Hamer and colleagues commit this error in their *Science* article when they state that "it would be fundamentally unethical to use such information to try to assess or alter a person's current or future sexual orientation, either heterosexual or homosexual, or other normal attributes of human behavior."[17] Hamer and colleagues believe that there is a major genetic factor contributing to sexual orientation. From this they think it follows that homosexuality is normal, and thus worthy of preservation. Thus they believe that genetics can tell us what is normal, and that the content of what is normal tells us what ought to be. This is a typical example of a naturalistic fallacy.

Normality can be defined in a number of ways, but none of them direct us in the making of moral judgments. First, normality can be reasonably defined in a *descriptive* sense as a statistical average. Appeals to what is usual, regular, and/or conforming to existing standards ultimately collapse into statistical statements. For an ethical evaluation of homosexuality, it is irrelevant whether homosexuality is normal or abnormal in this sense. All sorts of human traits and behaviors are abnormal in a statistical sense, but this is not a sufficient justification for a negative ethical judgment about them. Second, "normality" might be defined in a functional sense, where what is normal is something that has served an adaptive function from an evolutionary perspective. This definition of normality can be found in sociobiology, which seeks biological explanations for social behavior. There are a number of serious problems with the sociobiological project.[18] For the purposes of this argument, however, suffice it to say that even if sociobiology could establish that certain behavioral traits were the direct result of biological evolution, no moral assessment of these traits would follow. To illustrate our point, suppose any trait that can be reasonably believed to have served an adaptive function at some evolutionary stage is normal. Some questions arise that exemplify the problems with deriving normative conclusions from descriptive science. Are traits that are perpetuated simply through linkage to selectively advantageous loci less "normal" than those for which selection was direct? Given that social contexts now exert "selective pressure" in a way that nature once did, how are we to decide which traits are to be intentionally fostered?

Positions holding the view that homosexuality is unnatural, and therefore wrong, also inevitably develop incoherencies. They often fail to explicate the basis upon which the line between natural and unnatural is drawn. More importantly, they fail to explain why we should consider all human-made or artificial things as immoral or wrong. These views are usually firmly based in a nonempirical, *prescriptive* interpretation of nature rather than a scientific *descriptive* approach. They define arbitrarily what is natural and have to import other normative assumptions and premises to build a basis for their conclusions. For instance, they often claim that an entity called "God" has declared homosexuality to be unnatural and sinful.[19] Unfortunately, these analyses

have real-world consequences. In Singapore, "unnatural acts" are considered a criminal offence, and "natural intercourse" is arbitrarily defined as "the coitus of the male and female organs." A recent High Court decision there declared oral sex "unnatural," and therefore a criminal offence, unless it leads to subsequent reproductive intercourse.

Historical Evidence

In response to some of the ethical concerns about biological research on sexual orientation, some people have appealed to previous research on homosexuality that has *not* been used to the detriment of homosexuals. For example, Timothy Murphy invokes the work of Evelyn Hooker, which arguably provided evidence for the "normality" of homosexuals.[20] However, historical examples are often disanalogous to present-day biological research. Hooker's small-scale study, in fact, had nothing to do with the origins of sexual orientation. Rather, she sought to discover whether or not homosexual people were "well-adapted" (by assessing the degree to which their daily practices conformed with that of "normal" Americans). Showing that nonbiological research has not been used unethically does not show that biological research will be used ethically. It is important to discern which *sorts* of historical events can be considered relevant to the debate concerning the implications and applications of research on sexual orientation.

Another defense of genetic research on sexual orientation, offered by Simon LeVay, suggests that psychological and sociological research is even more dangerous. LeVay bases his argument on the assertion that, for ideological reasons, the Nazis did not generally consider homosexuality to be innate or a sign of degeneracy, but rather that they thought homosexuality was spread by seduction.[21] This is historically not true. The Nazis were as supportive of genetic research as they were of any other type of research designed to support the elimination of homosexuality.[22] Even if LeVay's assertions were historically correct, however, they would not provide any support (ethical or otherwise) for genetic research. Arguing that one type of research is ethically problematic does not legitimize the other;

indeed, it only provides further reason to question the whole enterprise.

U.S.-Specific Arguments

In the United States, several scholars and lesbian and gay activists have argued that establishing a genetic basis for sexual orientation will help make the case for lesbian and gay rights. The idea is that scientific research will show that people do not choose their sexual orientations and therefore they should not be punished or discriminated against in virtue of them. This general argument is flawed in several ways.[23] First, we do not need to show that a trait is genetically determined to argue that it is not amenable to change at will. This is clearly shown by the failure rates of conversion "therapies."[24] These failures establish that sexual orientation is resistant to change, but they do not say anything about its ontogeny or etiology. Sexual orientation can be unchangeable without being genetically determined. There is strong observational evidence to support the claim that sexual orientation is difficult to change, but this evidence is perfectly compatible with non-genetic accounts of the origins of sexual orientations. More importantly, we should not embrace arguments that seek to legitimate homosexuality by denying that there is any choice in sexual preference because the implicit premise of such arguments is that if there *was* a choice, then homosexuals would be blameworthy.

Relatedly, arguments for lesbian and gay rights based on scientific evidence run the risk of leading to impoverished forms of lesbian and gay rights. Regardless of what causes homosexuality, a person has to decide to publicly identify as a lesbian, to engage in sexual acts with another woman, to raise children with her same-sex lover, or to be active in the lesbian and gay community. It is when people make such decisions that they are likely to face discrimination, arrest, or physical violence. It is decisions like these that need legal protection. An argument for lesbian and gay rights based on genetic evidence is impotent with respect to protecting such decisions because it focuses exclusively on the very aspects of sexuality that might not involve choices.

Another version of this argument focuses on the specifics of U.S. law. According to this version, scientific evidence will establish the immutability of sexual orientation, which, according to one current interpretation of the Equal Protection Clause of the Fourteenth Amendment of the U.S. Constitution, is one of three criteria required of a classification if it is to evoke heightened judicial scrutiny. While this line of argument has serious internal problems,[25] such an argument, like a good deal of American bioethical reasoning, has limited or no relevance to the global context. Since the results of the scientific research are not confined within American borders, justifications that go beyond U.S. legislation are required.

The same sort of problem occurs in other defenses of sexual orientation research that discuss possible ramifications in U.S.-specific legislative terms. For instance, Timothy Murphy claims that, even if a genetic probe predictive of sexual orientation were available, mandatory testing would be unlikely.[26] He bases this claim on the fact that in some states employment and housing discrimination against homosexual people is illegal. In many countries, however, the political climate is vastly different, and legal anti-gay discrimination is widespread. And there is evidence that scientific research would be used in a manner that discriminates against homosexuals.[27] As already mentioned, in Singapore, homosexual sex acts are a criminal offense. The Singapore Penal Code sections 377 and 377A threaten sentences ranging from two years to life imprisonment for homosexual people engaging in same-sex acts. Not coincidentally, in light of our concerns, a National University of Singapore psychiatrist recently implied that "pre-symptomatic testing for homosexuality should be offered in the absence of treatment,"[28] thereby accepting the idea that homosexuality is something in need of a cure.

Genetic Screening

Several attempts to defend sexual orientation research against ethical concerns related to the selective abortion of "pre-homosexual" fetuses have been made. It has been claimed that this sort of genetic screening will not become commonplace because "diagnostic genetic testing is at present the exception rather than the rule."[29] While this may indeed be true in the U.S., it has far more to do with the types of tests currently offered than with a reluctance on the part of either the medical profession or the reproducing public to partake of such technology. For example, the types of tests available are diagnostic for diseases and are offered on the basis of family history or specific risk factors. The possibility of tests that are supposed to be (however vaguely) predictive of behavioral traits opens genetic technology to a far greater population, especially when the traits in question are undesired by a largely prejudiced society.

Furthermore, it has been claimed that the medical profession would not advocate such a test that does not serve "important state interests" (p. 341). This argument not only ignores the existence of homophobia among individuals within medicine,[30] it assumes also that public demand for genetic testing varies predominantly according to medical advice. However, should such a test become available, the media hype surrounding its market arrival would render its existence common knowledge, which, coupled with homophobic bias, would create a demand for the test irrespective of its accuracy and of any kind of state interest. Furthermore, this argument ignores the fact that genetic screening for a socially undesirable characteristic has already been greeted with great public demand in countries such as India, where abortion on the basis of female sex is commonplace, irrespective of its legality.[31] Techniques to select the sexual orientation of children, if made available, might well be widely utilized.[32]

Some have argued that orientation-selection techniques involving genetic screening will not succeed because environmental factors influencing sexual orientation would elude genetic screening.[33] While there are such environmental factors, we are still concerned about the potential effects of the availability of orientation-selection techniques, even if they fail to work. Further, if environmental factors are identified, their modification could be defended on the same grounds as the elimination of "gay genes." In fact, behavior modification techniques have been, and continue to be, used to prevent homosexuality in children with "gender identity disorder" (that is, "sissies" and "tom boys").[34]

It has also been claimed that if homosexual people themselves made use of orientation-selection techniques (whether to ensure homosexual or heterosexual offspring), the charge that such testing is inherently homophobic becomes "paradoxical."[35] However, just as the fact that homosexual people conduct scientific research on sexual orientation does not show that such research is ethically justifiable, the fact that some homosexuals might use such techniques would not prove that the technology does not serve to discriminate. To illustrate this point, consider that in a society like India in which widespread discrimination against women exists, there are many pragmatic reasons why one might prefer a male child. We would not argue, however, that prenatal sex selection is no longer discriminatory against females because women sometimes seek abortions for the purpose of having male offspring. Similarly, in societies with entrenched homophobia, a heterosexual child might be preferable for reasons that might appear most salient to homosexuals themselves in lieu of the discrimination they have encountered. The use of a technology by people against whom it may discriminate (even if they attempt to use it to their benefit) does not establish its neutrality. It does, however, highlight the pervasive biases within a given society that should be addressed directly rather than be fostered with enabling technology. Discriminated-against users of discriminatory technology might have a variety of motives, none of which necessarily diffuse the charge of bias.

The Value of Knowing the Truth

Finally, various scholars appeal to the value of the truth to defend research on sexual orientation in the face of ethical concerns. Scientific research does, however, have its costs and not every research program is of equal importance. Even granting that, in general, knowledge is better than ignorance, not all risks for the sake of knowledge are worth taking. With respect to sexual orientation, historically, almost every hypothesis about the causes of homosexuality led to attempts to "cure" healthy people. History indicates that current genetic research is likely to have negative effects on lesbians and gay men, particularly those living in homophobic societies.[36]

A Global Perspective

Homosexual people have in the past suffered greatly from societal discrimination. Historically, the results of biological research on sexual orientation have been used against them. We have analyzed the arguments offered by well-intentioned defenders of such work and concluded that none survive philosophical scrutiny. It is true that in some countries in Scandinavia, North America, and most parts of Western Europe the legal situation of homosexual people has improved, but an adequate ethical analysis of the implications of genetic inquiry into the causes of sexual orientation must operate from a global perspective. Sexual orientation researchers should be aware that their work may harm homosexuals in countries other than their own. It is difficult to imagine any good that could come of genetic research on sexual orientation in homophobic societies. Such work faces serious ethical concerns so long as homophobic societies continue to exist. Insofar as a socially responsible genetic research on sexual orientation is possible, it must begin with the awareness that it will not be a cure for homophobia and that the ethical status of lesbians and gay men does not in any way hinge on its results.

Notes

1   Rüdiger Lautmann, ed., *Homosexualität: Handbuch der Theorie und Forschungsgeschichte* (Campus Verlag: Frankfurt am Main, 1993); Vern Bullough, *Science in the Bedroom: The History of Sex Research* (Basic Books: New York, 1994).

2   Heino Meyer-Bahlburg, "Psychoendocrine Research on Sexual Orientation: Current Status and Future Options," *Progress in Brain Research* 71 (1984): 375-97.

3   For example, Richard Pillard and James Weinrich, "Evidence for a Familial Nature of Male Homosexuality," *Archives of General Psychiatry* 43 (1986): 808-12

4   J. Michael Bailey and Richard Pillard, "A Genetic Study of Male Sexual Orientation," *Archives of General Psychiatry* 48 (1991): 1089-96.

5   Dean Hamer et al., "A Linkage Between DNA Markers on the X Chromosome and Male Sexual Orientation," *Science* 261 (1993): 321-27.

6   G. Rice, C. Anderson, N. Risch, and G. Ebers, "Male Homosexuality: Absence of Linkage to Microsatellite Markers on the X Chromosome in a Canadian Study," presented at the 21st Annual Meeting of the International Academy of Sex Research 1995, Provincetown, Mass. This presentation is discussed in E. Marshall, "NIH 'Gay Gene' Study Questioned," *Science* 268 (1995): 1841.

7   Evan Balaban, quoted in V. D'Alessio, "Born to Be Gay?" *New Scientist* (28 September 1996): 32-35.

8   Marshall, "NIH's 'Gay Gene' Study Questioned," p. 1841.

9   Neil Risch, Elizabeth Squires-Wheeler, and Bronya Keats, "Male Sexual Orientation and Genetic Evidence," *Science* 262 (1993): 2063-65.

10 William Byne, "Biology and Sexual Orientation: Implications of Endocronological and Neuroanatomical Research," in *Comprehensive Textbook of Homosexuality*, ed. R. Labaj and T. Stein (Washington, DC: American Psychiatric Press, 1996), pp. 129-46.

11 Jonathan Ned Katz, *Gay American History* (New York: Thomas Crowell, 1976), pp. 197-422.

12 Günter Dörner, "Hormone-dependent Brain Development and Neuroendocrine Prophylaxis," *Experimental and Clinical Endocrinology* 94 (1989): 4-22.

13 Richard C. Friedman, *Male Homosexuality: A Contemporary Psychoanalytic Perspective* (New Haven: Yale University Press, 1988), p. 20.

14 Edward Stein, "Choosing the Sexual Orientation of Children," *Bioethics* (1998), forthcoming.

15 Udo Schüklenk and Michael Ristow, "The Ethics of Research into the Causes of Homosexuality," *Journal of Homosexuality* 31, nos. 3, 4 (1996): 5-30.

16 Michael Levin, "Why Homosexuality is Abnormal," *Monist* 67 (1984): 251-83.

17 Hamer et al., "A Linkage Between DNA Markers on the X Chromosome and Male Sexual Orientation," p. 326.

18 Philip Kitcher, *Vaulting Ambition: Sociobiology and the Quest for Human Nature* (Cambridge, MA: MIT Press, 1985).

19 Udo Schüklenk and David Mertz, "Christliche Kirchen und AIDS," in *Die Lehre des Unheils*, ed.

Edgar Dahl. (Hamburg: Carlsen, 1993), pp. 263-79 and 309-12.

20   Timothy Murphy, "Abortion and the Ethics of Genetic Sexual Orientation Research," *Cambridge Quarterly of Healthcare Ethics* 4 (1995): 340-50, especially p. 347.

21   Simon LeVay, *Queer Science: The Use and Abuse of Research on Homosexuality* (Cambridge, MA: MIT Press, 1996), pp. 38 and 113.

22   See, for example, Julius Deussen, "Sexualpathologie," in *Fortschritte der Erbpathologie, Rassenhygiene und ihrer Grenzgebiete* 2 (1939): 67-102. Interestingly, the British Eugenics Society showed a keen interest in the outcome of this research. Matthias Weber, Ernst Rüdin, *Eine kritische Biographie* (Berlin: Springer, 1993). See also Pauline M.H. Mazumdar, *Eugenics, Human Genetics and Human Failings: The Eugenics Society, Its Sources and Its Critics in Britain* (London: Routledge 1992). We thank Professor Hans-Peter Kröner, Institute for Theory and History of Medicine Westfälische Wilhelms-Universität Münster, for bringing this information to our attention.

23   Edward Stein, "The Relevance of Scientific Research Concerning Sexual Orientation to Lesbian and Gay Rights," *Journal of Homosexuality* 27 (1994): 269-308.

24   Charles Silverstein, "Psychological and Medical Treatments of Homosexuality," in *Homosexuality: Research Implications for Public Policy*, ed. J.C. Gonsiorek and J.D. Weinrich (Newbury Park, CA: Sage, 1991), pp. 101-14.

25   Janet Halley, "Sexual Orientation and the Politics of Biology: A Critique of the New Argument from Immutability," *Stanford Law Review* 46 (1994): 503-68.

26   Murphy, "Abortion and the Ethics of Genetic Sexual Orientation Research," p. 341.

27   Paul Billings, "Genetic Discrimination and Behavioural Genetics: The Analysis of Sexual Orientation," in *Intractable Neurological Disorders, Human Genome, Research and Society*, ed. Norio Fujiki and Darryl Macer (Christchurch and Tsukuba: Eubios Ethics Institute, 1993), p. 37; Paul Billings, "International Aspects of Genetic Discrimination," in *Human Genome Research and Society*, ed. Norio Fujiki and Darryl Macer (Christchurch and Tsukuba: Eubios Ethics Institute, 1992), pp. 114-17.

28   L.C.C. Lim, "Present Controversies in the Genetics of Male Homosexuality," *Annals of the Academy of Medicine Singapore* 24 (1995): 759-62.

29   Murphy, "Abortion and the Ethics of Genetic Sexual Orientation Research," p. 341.

30   Kevin Speight, "Homophobia Is a Health Issue," *Health Care Analysis* 3 (1995): 143-48.

31   Kusum, "The Use of Prenatal Diagnostic Techniques for Sex Selection: The Indian Scene," *Bioethics* 7 (1993): 149-65.

32   Richard Posner, *Sex and Reason* (Cambridge, MA: Harvard University Press, 1992), p. 308

33   Murphy, "Abortion and the Ethics of Genetic Sexual Orientation Research," p. 346. Indeed, the recently announced Environmental Genome Project launched by the NIH has begun with research on the interaction of genes and the environment.

34   See Richard Green, *The "Sissy Boy" Syndrome and the Development of Homosexuality* (New Haven: Yale University Press, 1987); Phyllis Burke, *Gender Shock: Exploding the Myths of Male and Female* (New York: Anchor Books, 1996).

35   Murphy, "Abortion and the Ethics of Genetic Sexual Orientation Research," p. 343.

36   For further elaborations on this argument see Edward Stein, Udo Schüklenk, and Jacinta Kerin, "Scientific Research on Sexual Orientation," in *Encyclopedia of Applied Ethics*, ed. Ruth Chadwick (San Diego: Academic Press, 1997).

48.
MOVING THE WOMB

Arthur L. Caplan, Constance Perry, Lauren A. Plante, Joseph Saloma, and Frances R. Batzer

SOURCE: *Hastings Center Report* 37.3 (2007): 18-20.

Recently, a team of physicians at the New York Downtown Hospital announced they had received approval from their institutional review board to attempt the first uterus transplant in the world from a cadaver donor.[1] Teams in the United Kingdom and Sweden have also publicly stated their interest in trying uterus transplantation in women.

Transplantation always involves serious risks for recipients, stemming both from the solid organ transplant surgery itself and from the immunosuppressive drugs that transplant recipients will have to take for the rest of their lives. These risks, however, have been generally viewed as acceptable by surgeons, third-party payers, government regulators, and patients because the success rate is high and the benefit of receiving a heart, kidney, lung, or liver—continued life—is self-evident.

The point of a uterus transplant would not be to save a life, however. Uterus transplants would be attempted only to improve the recipient's quality of life: they would allow her to give birth. This very different risk-benefit calculation raises many ethical questions that should be thoroughly aired and understood before the procedure is attempted.

The Need

Thousands of women in the United States cannot bear children. Disease, accidents, complications from earlier pregnancies, and congenital malformations can impair a woman's uterine function, and some women simply do not have a uterus at all. But not all women who cannot bear children are flatly barred from parenthood. In some states in the United States and in other nations, there has been for many years an active market in surrogate mothers—women who will "rent" their wombs for a fee to other women so they may bear children. Gestational surrogacy is not an option for all women who do not have a functioning uterus, however. It is illegal in some states and in some countries, and, even in states where it is legal, many ethical and legal uncertainties surround the practice. Some religions, including Islam, have specific prohibitions against surrogacy. It can also be very expensive, yet it may not even satisfy a woman's need to have her own baby. Many women wish to bear their children themselves as part of the parenting experience. Various cases of older women who have utilized donor embryos or donor sperm and egg to become pregnant, despite great risks to themselves and their potential children, show how strong this desire can be.[2]

Women who want to experience pregnancy and those for whom gestational surrogacy is out of reach (whether for religious or financial reasons) form a group who are willing, even eager, to subject themselves to experimental uterine surgery. Their eagerness puts these women—and those seeking to recruit them—at risk of the "therapeutic misconception": they need to be frequently and emphatically reminded that the women who first receive uterus transplants are subjects in a research study, not patients getting a new treatment. It is unlikely that they will benefit by delivering a baby. Their motivation for participating ought to be that they will shed light on the safety and practicality of uterus transplants.

The Experience So Far

Only one known uterus transplant using a living donor has been attempted in humans. Physicians at the King Fahd Hospital in Saudi Arabia performed the operation in 2002. The donor was a forty-six-year-old woman, and the recipient was a twenty-six-year-old who had undergone a hysterectomy. Doctors had to remove the transplanted uterus after three months due to circulatory problems.[3]

A number of attempts have also been made with different kinds of animals. The team of transplant researchers at New York Downtown Hospital has been experimenting with uterus transplants in pigs and rats for five years. The transplanted uteri reportedly survived and functioned for several months in the pigs, producing normal menstrual cycles.[4] However, none of the animals were able to become pregnant, and the researchers do not know why. A few attempts have been made to transplant uteri in sheep and monkeys, but no pregnancies have resulted. A Swedish team that has been working with mice for many years has achieved one pregnancy that produced a birth.[5]

This work is not enough. There are significant differences between the reproductive anatomy of humans and that of rodents, pigs, and sheep. The fact that so few experiments—much less successful ones—have been carried out in primates should generate considerable concern about the wisdom of moving to human trials any time soon.

Donor Issues

The New York team wants to obtain a uterus for transplant from a deceased donor, yet it makes more sense biologically to use a donor uterus from a tissue-matched sibling or relative. Such a donor would be able to consent to the donation knowing the risks and benefits. Living donation might also improve the quality of the organ to be transplanted, and close tissue matching might prolong its lifespan in the recipient, thereby decreasing the dose of immunosuppressive medications necessary to prevent rejection.

Obtaining the uterus from a deceased donor raises some unique ethical issues. The doctors in New York say they will use someone who has signed a donor card and whose family has no objection to uterus donation. But is this really enough? Few, if any, American women ever thought that the uterus might be one of the organs considered for donation when they signed a donor card. A woman might not prove as willing to donate her uterus as she would be to donate her heart or liver. The transplant team would

be on firmer moral ground if they used a donated uterus from a woman who had explicitly consented to donate that organ prior to her death, and who made it very clear that she and her family renounced any and all claims to a relationship with any child that might result.

However, while using a close relative or sibling may seem to be the better choice, it also increases the risk of coercion. There could also be potential problems if a family member initially consents to being a uterus donor and then changes her mind—a possibility that a transplant team considering living donors must be prepared to manage.

The desire to experience a pregnancy cannot be considered separately from the ultimate goal of pregnancy—a healthy child. The evidence on uterus transplant cannot yet assure that outcome.

Risks

Surgeons proposing uterus transplant have tended to dismiss concerns about risk to the prospective recipient by noting that, since the uterus is not a life-preserving organ, it can simply be removed if complications arise. But what if that uterus contains a fetus? What if the mother decides she is willing to die to try to give birth? What if the father or the mother decides they want the uterus removed even if it contains a fetus or an embryo? The surgical team has not said as much as they need to about their "exit" strategy if the experiment does not go as planned.

The New York surgical team says that risks to fetuses are not at issue because women who have had other types of transplants have given birth. This is not exactly true. Women have given birth following solid organ and bone marrow transplantation, which require the use of immunosuppressive agents during pregnancy. A national transplantation pregnancy registry provides some data as to the effects of immunosuppressive drugs on offspring.[6] The power of that data is limited, however, by the relatively small number of pregnancies tracked to date. There is no reliable data yet on the long-term health of children born post-transplant. When a woman has received a solid organ transplant, doctors usually recommend postponing pregnancy for two years to ensure that the graft survives. No one knows what guidelines to recommend concerning pregnancy after uterus transplantation.

A woman who has a transplanted liver and later undertakes a pregnancy presents a very different case from a woman who subjects both herself and her potential offspring to these drugs purely for the purpose of carrying a pregnancy. Also, the potential risk to a fetus or fetuses from the procedure is not solely that of exposure to immunosuppressive drugs. There is a risk of structural failure caused by clotting and thrombosis of major arteries supplying oxygen to the transplanted uterus. This could have a negative effect on fetal development, increasing the possibility not only of fetal death, but of preterm delivery and developmental problems associated with poor circulation, infection, and loss of fluid.

For uterus transplantation, the risks seem to be justifiable only if clinical equipoise exists—that is, if the risk-benefit ratio of the experimental procedure can reasonably be assumed to be equal to existing alternatives. Uterus transplants fail the clinical equipoise test. We lack solid animal data on the impact of uterus transplant on maternal health and fetal well-being, so we don't really know the risks. In addition, most women have the safe alternatives of gestational surrogacy, adoption, and foster care to allow them to experience parenthood. The desire to experience a pregnancy, while certainly legitimate, cannot be considered separately from the ultimate goal of pregnancy—namely, a healthy child. The available evidence cannot yet assure that outcome.

Finally, aside from the physical risks, a child born from a uterus transplant could also face some unique psychological issues. The child or adult might seek contact with the survivors of the woman who had donated the uterus. Children born after sperm donation, adoption, or surrogacy sometimes go to great lengths to find information about their conception; surely children gestated in a dead woman's uterus would wonder about their origins. Provisions must be made for handling these issues prior to undertaking the first cadaver uterus transplants.

Subject Selection

Many women who want a uterus transplant might not be candidates for one, but the selection process for identifying subjects has received very little discussion. Women born without a uterus or with certain congenital anomalies will not have the appropriate vascular connections for attachment. Women who had their uteri removed because of cancer—particularly cervical or childhood cancer—may not be candidates if the original cancer treatment involved radiation that led to scarring, which makes vascular reattachment difficult. And there are obvious questions that must be asked about the psychological stability and social support necessary to undergo an experimental transplant fraught with unknown risks.

The prospect of uterus transplant has also led to some discussion about the possibility of a male pregnancy.[7] While this idea may seem appealing to some, the physiological requirements for nourishing a uterus and maintaining a pregnancy make it exceedingly unlikely that a uterus transplant would work in a man. During a pregnancy, up to one-fifth of a woman's cardiac output goes to the pregnant uterus. Since the vascular connections for a uterus do not exist in males, they would have to be created. Hormonal supplementation would also be required, along with the immunosuppression. Obviously, the bodily incompatibilities are so daunting that to even try for a male pregnancy seems inappropriate. While it makes for some fascinating science fiction scenarios, the risks involved make the selection of a male subject for this experiment ethically dubious.

The Glory of Being First

There are transplant teams willing to undertake uterus transplants and women willing to undergo them. But this is an experiment that requires more than willingness. Multiple studies demonstrate the difficulty of achieving informed consent with desperate patients. The transplant team must manage conflicting roles and interests in order to ensure truly informed and voluntary consent from potential donors, donor families, and recipients. In the midst of all this, the prospect of being the first to successfully transplant a uterus—and win acclaim and publicity for the programs, doctors, and institutions involved in the effort—raises deep concerns about conflict of interest. The desire to be first could make it very difficult for the team to seriously consider whether sufficient evidence exists to support a favorable risk-benefit ratio for initiating a clinical trial. Society must be reassured that donation involving a cadaver donor will be done according to the highest standards of informed consent. The transplant team must be clear about how it will manage a pregnancy if the transplant goes wrong. And the risk to the fetus of being conceived and carried in a transplanted uterus must be carefully weighed against the woman's desire to have the experience of the gestational component of motherhood. Is that worth a lifetime of risk to a child? Until these questions are answered, it is not time to initiate experiments with uterus transplantation.

Notes

1 R. Stein, "First U.S. Uterus Transplant Planned," *Washington Post*, January 15, 2007.

2 A.L. Caplan, *Smart Mice, Not So Smart People* (Lanham, MD: Rowman & Littlefield, 2006).

3 W. Fageeh et al., "Transplantation of the Human Uterus," *International Journal of Gynecology & Obstetrics* 76 (2002): 245-51.

4 Stein, "First U.S. Uterus Transplant Planned."

5 D. Kingsley, "Swedes Achieve World's First Womb Transplant," ABC.net, July 2, 2003, http://www.abc.net.au/science/news/stories/s892281.htm.

6 http://www.temple.edu/NTPR/.

7 B. Radford, "Male Pregnancy," *Skeptical Inquirer* 31, no. 2 (2007): 22-23.

CHAPTER EIGHT

SCARCE MEDICAL RESOURCES
AND CATASTROPHIC CIRCUMSTANCES

Web Link

(1) Link to Trillium Gift of Life Network: Ontario's Organ and Tissue Donation Agency.

   http://www.giftoflife.on.ca/

Trillium manages the procurement, distribution, and delivery of organs and tissue in Ontario. The network also manages the wait lists for transplants, promotes awareness, and coordinates activities relating to organ and tissue donation.

* For an up-to-date list of the web links in this book, please visit:
http://sites.broadviewpress.com/healthcare.

49.
THE PROSTITUTE, THE PLAYBOY, AND THE POET: RATIONING SCHEMES FOR ORGAN TRANSPLANTATION

George J. Annas

SOURCE: *American Journal of Public Health* 75.2 (1985): 187-89.

In the public debate about the availability of heart and liver transplants, the issue of rationing on a massive scale has been credibly raised for the first time in United States medical care. In an era of scarce resources, the eventual arrival of such a discussion was, of course, inevitable.[1] Unless we decide to ban heart and liver transplantation, or make them available to everyone, some rationing scheme must be used to choose among potential transplant candidates. The debate has existed throughout the history of medical ethics. Traditionally it has been stated as a choice between saving one of two patients, both of whom require the immediate assistance of the only available physician to survive.

National attention was focused on decisions regarding the rationing of kidney dialysis machines when they were first used on a limited basis in the late 1960s. As one commentator described the debate within the medical profession:

Shall machines or organs go to the sickest, or to the ones with most promise of recovery; on a first-come, first-served basis; to the most "valuable" patient (based on wealth, education, position, what?); to the one with the most dependents; to women and children first; to those who can pay; to whom? Or should lots be cast, impersonally and uncritically?[2]

In Seattle, Washington, an anonymous screening committee was set up to pick who among competing candidates would receive the life-saving technology. One lay member of the screening committee is quoted as saying:

The choices were hard ... I remember voting against a young woman who was a known prostitute. I found I couldn't vote for her, rather than another candidate, a young wife and mother. I also voted against a young man who, until he learned he had renal failure, had been a ne'er do-well, a real playboy. He promised he would reform his character, go back to school and so on, if only he were selected for treatment. But I felt I'd lived long enough to know that a person like that won't do what he was promising at the time.[3]

When the biases and selection criteria of the committee were made public, there was a general negative reaction against this type of arbitrary device. Two experts reacted to the "numbing accounts of how close to the surface lie the prejudices and mindless clichés that pollute the committee's deliberations," by concluding that the committee was "measuring persons in accordance with its own middle-class values." The committee process, they noted, ruled out "creative nonconformists" and made the Pacific Northwest "no place for a Henry David Thoreau with bad kidneys."[4]

There are four major approaches to rationing scarce medical resources: the market approach; the selection committee approach; the lottery approach; and the "customary" approach.[5]

The Market Approach

The market approach would provide an organ to everyone who could pay for it with their own funds or private insurance. It puts a very high value on individual rights, and a very low value on equality and fairness. It has properly been criticized on a number of bases, including that the transplant tech-

479

nologies have been developed and are supported with public funds, that medical resources used for transplantation will not be available for higher priority care, and that financial success alone is an insufficient justification for demanding a medical procedure. Most telling is its complete lack of concern for fairness and equity.[6]

A "bake sale" or charity approach that requires the less financially fortunate to make public appeals for funding is demeaning to the individuals involved, and to society as a whole. Rationing by financial ability says we do not believe in equality, but believe that a price can and should be placed on human life and that it should be paid by the individual whose life is at stake. Neither belief is tolerable in a society in which income is inequitably distributed.

The Committee Selection Process

The Seattle Selection Committee is a model of the committee process. Ethic committees set up in some hospitals to decide whether or not certain handicapped newborn infants should be given medical care may represent another.[7] These committees have developed because it was seen as unworkable or unwise to explicitly set forth the criteria on which selection decisions would be made. But only two results are possible, as Professor Guido Calabrezi has pointed out: either a pattern of decision-making will develop or it will not. If a pattern does develop (e.g., in Seattle, the imposition of middle-class values), then it can be articulated and those decision "rules" codified and used directly, without resort to the committee. If a pattern does not develop, the committee is vulnerable to the charge that it is acting arbitrarily, or dishonestly, and therefore cannot be permitted to continue to make such important decision.[8]

In the end, public designation of a committee to make selection decisions on vague criteria will fail because it too closely involves the state and all members of society in explicitly preferring specific individuals over others, and in devaluing the interests those others have in living. It thus directly undermines, as surely as the market system does, society's view of equality and the value of human life.

The Lottery Approach

The lottery approach is the ultimate equalizer which puts equality ahead of every other value. This makes it extremely attractive, since all comers have an equal chance at selection regardless of race, color, creed, or financial status. On the other hand, it offends our notions of efficiency and fairness since it makes no distinctions among such things as the strength of the desires of the candidates, their potential survival, and their quality of life. In this sense it is a mindless method of trying to solve society's dilemma which is caused by its unwillingness or inability to spend enough resources to make a lottery unnecessary. By making this macro spending decision evident to all, it also undermines society's view of the pricelessness of human life. A first-come, first-served system is a type of natural lottery since referral to a transplant program is generally random in time. Nonetheless, higher income groups have quicker access to referral networks and thus have an inherent advantage over the poor in a strict first-come, first-served system.[9]

The Customary Approach

Society has traditionally attempted to avoid explicitly recognizing that we are making a choice not to save individual lives because it is too expensive to do so. As long as such decisions are not explicitly acknowledged, they can be tolerated by society. For example, until recently there was said to be a general understanding among general practitioners in Britain that individuals over age 55 suffering from end-stage kidney disease not be referred for dialysis or transplant. In 1984, however, this unwritten practice became highly publicized, with figures that showed a rate of new cases of end-stage kidney disease treated in Britain at 40 per million (versus the US figure of 80 per million) resulting in 1500-3000 "unnecessary deaths" annually.[10] This has, predictably, led to movements to enlarge the National Health Service budget to expand dialysis to meet this need, a more socially acceptable solution than permitting the now publicly recognized situation to continue.

In the US, the customary approach permits individual physicians to select their patients on the basis of medical criteria or clinical suitability. This, however, contains much hidden social worth criteria. For example, one criterion, common in the transplant literature, requires an individual to have sufficient family support for successful aftercare. This discriminates against individuals without families and those who have become alienated from their families. The criterion may be relevant, but it is hardly medical.

Similar observations can be made about medical criteria that include IQ, mental illness, criminal records, employment, indigency, alcoholism, drug addiction, or geographical location. Age is perhaps more difficult, since it may be impressionistically related to outcome. But it is not medically logical to assume that an individual who is 49 years old is necessarily a better medical candidate for a transplant than one who is 50 years old. Unless specific examination of the characteristics of older persons that make them less desirable candidates is undertaken, such a cut off is arbitrary, and thus devalues the lives of older citizens. The same can be said of blanket exclusions of alcoholics and drug addicts.

In short, the customary approach has one great advantage for society and one great disadvantage: it gives us the illusion that we do not have to make choices; but the cost is mass deception, and when this deception is uncovered, we must deal with it either by universal entitlement or by choosing another method of patient selection.

A Combination of Approaches

A socially acceptable approach must be fair, efficient, and reflective of important social values. The most important values at stake in organ transplantation are fairness itself, equity in the sense of equality, and the value of life. To promote efficiency, it is important that no one receive a transplant unless they want one and are likely to obtain significant benefit from it in the sense of years of life at a reasonable level of functioning.

Accordingly, it is appropriate for there to be an initial screening process that is based *exclusively* on medical criteria designed to measure the probability of a successful transplant, i.e., one in which the patient survives for at least a number of years and is rehabilitated. There is room in medical criteria for social worth judgments, but there is probably no way to avoid this completely. For example, it has been noted that "in many respects social and medical criteria are inextricably intertwined" and that therefore medical criteria might "exclude the poor and disadvantaged because health and socioeconomic status are highly interdependent."[11] Roger Evans gives an example. In the End Stage Renal Disease Program, "those of lower socioeconomic status are likely to have multiple comorbid health conditions such as diabetes, hepatitis, and hypertension" making them both less desirable candidates and more expensive to treat.[12]

To prevent the gulf between the haves and have nots from widening, we must make every reasonable attempt to develop medical criteria that are objective and independent of social worth categories. One minimal way to approach this is to require that medical screening be reviewed and approved by an ethics committee with significant public representation, filed with a public agency, and made readily available to the public for comment. In the event that more than one hospital in a state is offering a particular transplant service, it would be most fair and efficient for the individual hospitals to perform the initial medical screening themselves (based on the uniform, objective criteria), but to have all subsequent non-medical selection done by a method approved by a single selection committee composed of representatives of all hospitals engaged in the particular transplant procedure, as well as significant representation of the public at large.

As this implies, after the medical screening is performed, there may be more acceptable candidates in the "pool" than there are organs or surgical teams to go around. Selection among waiting candidates will then be necessary. This situation occurs now in kidney transplantation, but since the organ matching is much more sophisticated than in hearts and livers (permitting much more precise matching of organ and recipient), and since dialysis permits individuals to wait almost indefinitely for an organ without risking death, the situations are not close enough to permit use of the same matching criteria. On the other hand, to the extent that organs are specifically tissue- and size-matched and fairly distributed to the best matched candidate, the organ distribution system itself will resemble a natural lottery.

When a pool of acceptable candidates is developed, a decision about who gets the next available, suitable organ must be made. We must choose between using a conscious, value-laden, social worth selection criterion (including a committee to make the actual choice), or some type of random device. In view of the unacceptability and arbitrariness of social worth criteria being applied, implicitly or explicitly, by committee, this method is neither viable nor proper. On the other hand, strict adherence to a lottery might create a situation where an individual who has only a one-in-four chance of living five years with a transplant (but who could survive another six months without one) would get an organ before an individual who could survive as long or longer, but who will die within days or hours if he or she is not immediately transplanted. Accordingly, the most reasonable approach seems to be to allocate organs on a first-come, first-served basis to members of the pool but permit individuals to "jump" the queue if the second level selection committee believes they are in immediate danger of death (but still have a reasonable prospect for long-term survival with a transplant) and the person who would otherwise get the organ can survive long enough to be reasonably assured that he or she will be able to get another organ.

The first-come, first-served method of basic selection (after a medical screen) seems the preferred method because it most closely approximates the randomness of a straight lottery without the obviousness of making equity the only promoted value. Some unfairness is introduced by the fact that the more wealthy and medically astute will likely get into the pool first, and thus be ahead in line, but this advantage should decrease sharply as public awareness of the system grows. The possibility of unfairness is also inherent in permitting individuals to jump the queue, but some flexibility needs to be retained in the system to permit it to respond to reasonable contingencies.

We will have to face the fact that should the resources devoted to organ transplantation be limited (as they are now and are likely to be in the future), at some point it is likely that significant numbers of individuals will die in the pool waiting for a transplant. Three things can be done to avoid this: 1) medical criteria can be made stricter, perhaps by adding a more rigorous notion of "quality" of life to longevity and prospects for rehabilitation; 2) resources devoted to transplantation and organ procurement can be increased; or 3) individuals can be persuaded not to attempt to join the pool.

Of these three options, only the third has the promise of both conserving resources and promoting autonomy. While most persons medically eligible for a transplant would probably want one, some would not—at least if they understood all that was involved, including the need for a lifetime commitment to daily immunosuppression medications, and periodic medical monitoring for rejection symptoms. Accordingly, it makes public policy sense to publicize the risks and side effects of transplantation, and to require careful explanations of the procedure be given to prospective patients before they undergo medical screening. It is likely that by the time patients come to the transplant center they have made up their minds and would do almost anything to get the transplant. Nonetheless, if there are patients who, when confronted with all the facts, would voluntarily elect not to proceed, we enhance both their own freedom and the efficiency and cost-effectiveness of the transplantation system by screening them out as early as possible.

Conclusion

Choices among patients that seem to condemn some to death and give others an opportunity to survive will always be tragic. Society has developed a number of mechanisms to make such decisions more acceptable by camouflaging them. In an era of scarce resources and conscious cost containment, such mechanisms will become public, and they will be usable only if they are fair and efficient. If they are not so perceived, we will shift from one mechanism to another in an effort to continue the illusion that tragic choices really don't have to be made, and that we can simultaneously move toward equity of access, quality of services, and cost containment without any challenges to our values. Along with the prostitute, the playboy, and the poet, we all need to be involved in the development of an access model to extreme and expensive medical technologies with which we can live.

Notes

1   Calabresi G, Bobbit P: *Tragic Choices*. New York: Norton, 1978.

2   Fletcher J: Our shameful waste of human tissue. *In*: Cutler DR. (ed): *The Religious Situation*. Boston: Beacon Press, 1969; 223-252.

3   Quoted in Fox R, Swazey J: *The Courage to Fail. Chicago*: Univ of Chicago Press, 1974; 232.

4   Sanders and Dukeminier: Medical advance and legal lag: hemodialysis and kidney transplantation. *UCLA L Rev* 1968; 15: 357.

5   See note 1.

6   President's Commission for the Study of Ethical Problems in Medicine: *Securing Access to Health Care*. US Govt Printing Office, 1983; 25.

7   Annas GJ: Ethics committees on neonatal care: substantive protection or procedural diversion? *Am J Public Health* 1984; 74: 843-845.

8   See note 1.

9   Bayer R: Justice and health care in an era of cost containment: allocating scarce medical resources. *Soc Responsibility* 1984; 9:37-52; Annas GJ: Allocation of artificial hearts in the year 2002: Minerva v. National Health Agency. *Am J Law Med* 1977; 3: 59-76.

10 Commentary: UK's poor record in treatment of renal failure. *Lancet* July 7, 1984; 53.

11 Evans R: Health care technology and the inevitability of resource allocation and rationing decisions, Part II. *JAMA* 1983; 249: 2208, 2217.

12 See note 11.

50.
AS IF THERE WERE FETUSES WITHOUT WOMEN: A REMEDIAL ESSAY

Mary Mahowald

Source: Joan C. Callahan (ed.), *Reproduction, Ethics and the Law*
(Bloomington: Indiana University Press, 1995).

As with abortion, most of the moral controversy regarding fetal tissue transplantation focuses on fetuses rather than pregnant women. In both of these related issues, that focus needs to be corrected so as to avoid the fallacy of abstraction, that is, consideration of an object as if it exists without a context. For example, "pro-life" arguments are generally based on the claim that the fetus is a person, and "pro-choice" arguments are generally based on the claim that the fetus is not a person.[1] Assuming the validity of arguments on both sides, the truth status of their conclusions depends on whether the criteria for personhood have been met by the fetus. Despite the fact that fetuses do not exist apart from women, who are inevitably affected by decisions about fetuses, women are ignored by either side so long as fetuses are the pivotal focus of the argument.

With regard to fetal tissue transplantation, women are ignored to the extent that arguments supporting and opposing it are linked with abortion as the means through which the tissue is made available. Women are also ignored where the focus is solely on commercialization of fetal tissue, the experimental status of the technique, or the needs of possible recipients. Interestingly, the important parallel between this issue and others that principally and undeniably affect women (such as contract motherhood, egg provision, and prostitution) is that women have been neglected, and in some cases, flatly ignored.

In this chapter, I want to redress the omission that prevails by reviewing the issue of fetal tissue transplantation with a focus that explicitly includes women as necessary participants in the process. In doing so, I will compare and contrast this with other issues that particularly affect women, and examine different frameworks for ethical assessment of fetal tissue transplantation. First, however, I want to say why it is wrong to focus on fetuses apart from their relationship to women.

Fetuses as Such

The term "fetus" is defined as "the unborn young of an animal while still within the uterus."[2] Fortunately or unfortunately, medical technology has not yet produced an artificial uterus, and it may be biologically impossible to do so. To speak of the uterus without acknowledgment that it is within a woman is thus another example of prescinding from necessary context. According to *Stedman's Medical Dictionary*, the human fetus "represents the product of conception from the end of the eighth week to the moment of birth."[3] Human birth is understood to mean the emergence of a fetus from a woman's body. *Stedman's* defines the human embryo as "the developing organism from conception until approximately the end of the second month."[4] Since the advent of in vitro fertilization techniques, development of an embryo can be initiated and sustained for several days apart from a woman's body. By definition, nonviable fetuses cannot be so sustained. No matter how early the gestation, a viable fetus removed from a woman's body is no longer a fetus but a newborn. If a nonviable fetus is removed from a woman's body, it is an abortus. In other words, no fetus as such exists apart from a woman's body.

Two major (overlapping) feminist criticisms of traditional ethics are exemplified in our insistence that fetuses not be considered as if they were not present in women. First is the objection that traditional ethics calls for a deductive process through which universal principles are applied to cases.[5] Starting from different principles, whether these are a priori or a posteriori in their derivation, the process (if conducted correctly) leads inexorably to answers about what should be done in specific situations. Feminists argue that this type of deductive analysis cannot adequately attend to the complexity and uniqueness of real cases and issues. To rectify the inadequacy, attention to context is essential.[6]

Second is the objection that much of traditional ethics emphasizes the rights of individuals, neglecting the realm of relationships.[7] In fact, through its assumption that impartiality is a requirement of ethically justifiable judgments, traditional ethics eschews considerations based on particular relationships such as occur between pregnant women and their fetuses. Many of the arguments in which abortion is supported or opposed solely on grounds of the moral status of the fetus exemplify this. In contrast, feminists insist on the moral relevance of relationships, whether these are based on choice, chance, genetics, or affection.[8] The ethics of care elaborated by Carol Gilligan, Nel Noddings, and Sara Ruddick provide frameworks for understanding the essential role that relationships play in moral decision making.[9]

When it is consistently recognized that fetuses exist only in relationship to women who are inevitably affected by decisions regarding them, the above concerns are addressed. Inattention to this ongoing relationship is unscientific because it neglects an element of analysis that affects the validity of scientific interpretation. It is unethical because it ignores the interests and preferences of pregnant women, which may be at odds with the interests of the fetus.

Use of Fetal Tissue in Transplantation

An accurate understanding of reality can only be attained through analysis of the complexity of context. With regard to fetal tissue transplantation, the analysis involves at least the following variables: (1) the empirical status of fetuses or abortuses used for grafts, (2) different purposes and sites of tissue retrieval or implantation, (3) therapeutic potential for the recipient, (4) the means through which fetuses are made available for transplantation, and (5) possible motives, "donors," and recipients of fetal tissue.[10]

Regarding (1), human fetuses or abortuses used for tissue grafts may be living or dead. Living fetuses or abortuses may be viable, nonviable, or possibly viable, and they may be sentient, nonsentient, or possibly sentient, depending in part on the duration of gestation.[11] Viability is particularly relevant because it implies that others in addition to the pregnant woman can maintain the fetus ex utero if it is to be delivered or aborted. Sentience is relevant because the prima facie obligation to avoid inflicting pain on others applies to fetuses regardless of whether they are persons. While that obligation does not imply that killing is always wrong, it does imply that pain relief or prevention should be attempted for all sentient, or even possibly sentient, individuals.

Regarding (2), the procedure may be undertaken solely for research purposes, as experimental treatment, or (if and when the procedure becomes standard therapy) solely as therapy for recipients. Ordinarily, therapeutic reasons are more compelling than research reasons for medical procedures. Thus governmental and institutional regulations are more strict for research protocols than for therapeutic protocols.[12] Tissue may be retrieved from the brain or from other parts of a fetus, and implanted directly into a recipient's brain or into other regions of the recipient's body. Brain grafts are generally more problematic than nonbrain grafts because the brain is usually seen as, and may in fact be, the source of a person's identity as well as cognitive function. Nonetheless, the small amount and immaturity of tissue used in transplants serve to minimize this concern.

Regarding (3), non-neural fetal tissue has been transplanted for many years to treat diseases such as DeGeorge's syndrome and diabetes mellitus, without creating public controversy.[13] The prospects that have evoked public debate involve use of neural tissue for treatment of severe and previously incurable neurological disorders. Among the neurological conditions that are potentially treatable are Alzheimer's disease, Parkinson's disease, amyotrophic lateral sclerosis (Lou Gehrig's disease), Huntington's disease, multiple sclerosis, spinal-cord injury, epilepsy, and stroke.[14] The research is most advanced in treatment of Parkinson's disease, but this treatment is still experimental. Comparatively few Parkinson patients have thus far been treated.[15] One case of apparent success in treatment of Hurler's syndrome (through fetus-to-fetus transplant) has also been reported.[16] While preliminary results are promising, there are too little data as yet to generalize about the treatment's effectiveness.

Regarding (4), abortion is the means through which human fetal tissue becomes available for transplantation. Abortions may be spontaneous or induced, and induced abortions may be performed for medical or non-medical reasons. Medical reasons for induced abortion include those based on the pregnant women's health, those based on fetal anomaly, or both. While use of tissue obtained from spontaneous abortions may be less ethically controversial than use of tissue obtained from induced abortions, the tissue from spontaneously aborted fetuses is unlikely to be normal or suitable for transplantation.[17] Because of that likelihood, it may be argued that use of tissue from spontaneously aborted fetuses constitutes undue risk to the recipient. Nonetheless, the first reported human use of fetal neural tissue for treatment of Parkinson's patients involved tissue retrieved from a spontaneously aborted fetus. This work evoked criticism from researchers involved in neurografting.[18]

Regarding (5), fetal tissue may be "donated" for altruistic reasons, self-interested reasons, or both. Ordinarily, the recipient is unrelated and unknown to the pregnant woman. Anonymity has been proposed by at least two panels reviewing the issue as a requirement for donor status.[19] However, an ethic that emphasizes relationships supports a decision to donate the tissue on the part of someone such as a friend or spouse who is both known and related to the recipient. A care ethic may also support a decision to become pregnant in order to provide the tissue to someone with whom one has a special relationship.

Further, a pregnant woman might herself be the recipient, and could deliberately become pregnant in order to provide the fetal tissue that might lead to her own cure. There is one published report of a woman with severe aplastic anemia who was transplanted with the liver of her own fetus after an elective abortion.[20] Although the details of the case are sketchy, the pregnancy was probably not initiated with the intention of providing the fetal tissue for two reasons. First, pregnancy is a serious risk to women with this disease, and second, the fetus would not necessarily be an appropriate tissue match for the woman. Nonetheless, a woman's right to self-preservation supports such an attempt to provide the tissue for her own treatment.

From a feminist perspective, all of the above variables are morally relevant to determination of whether fetal tissue transplantation is justified in specific cases. Particularly important is the means through which fetal tissue is obtained, namely, abortion. In order to insure respect for women's autonomy, decisions to terminate pregnancies must be separable from decisions to provide fetal tissue for transplantation. (Note that I have used the word "separable" rather than "separate.") As we will see in the next section, however, the possibility of separating the two has been disputed.

Fetal Tissue Transplantation and Abortion

Although the connection between grafts of human fetal tissue and abortion might have triggered public controversy decades ago, this did not occur until reports circulated early in 1987 about the prospect of using the tissue for treatment of neurological disorders.[21] Apparent reasons for the shift include the fact that abortion was not the volatile issue that it is today when fetal tissue was first used for research or therapeutic purposes. Another reason is that the type of diseases that the tissue may potentially be used to treat afflict literally millions of people who are severely debilitated with otherwise incurable diseases. There seems to be little doubt that political interests were at work in establishing the moratorium on government funding in the United States for research projects involving use of fetal tissue obtained from abortions. Before the Clinton administration lifted the moratorium in 1993, researchers could only find support for use of electively aborted fetal tissue through private sources. Although the moratorium slowed progress in the United States, researchers in Colorado and Connecticut, states that permit research with electively aborted fetal tissue, pursued their projects through private funding.[22]

The problematic connection between fetal tissue transplantation and abortion was first noted by a group who met in Cleveland in 1986. In collaboration with neuroscientist Jerry Silver, I had organized the meeting to review the issue in order to facilitate informed public debate. In March 1987, a consensus statement of the group appeared in *Science*.[23] We maintained that the procedure held "the promise of great benefit to victims of serious neurological disorders." Despite the legality of abortion, fetal tissue transplantation "was acknowledged to be ethically controversial because of its association with abortion." In light of that controversy, we proposed "separation between decisions related to the acquisition of tissue and decisions regarding the transplantation of tissue into a recipient." Two years later, a panel of experts convened by the National Institutes of Health (NIH), several of whom had signed the earlier consensus statement, offered a similar recommendation.[24]

Feminist support for distinguishing between decisions about abortion and decisions about fetal tissue transplantation is mainly based on concerns about possibilities for exploiting women or pressuring them to undergo abortions, or to delay or modify abortion procedures in order to provide fetal tissue to prospective recipients. As yet, it has not been necessary to delay or modify abortion procedures in treatment by means of fetal tissue grafts. Preliminary data suggest that the gestational age optimal for successful transplants into Parkinson's patients is as early as seven weeks, using tissue obtained from abortions performed by standard clinical methods.[25]

While feminists generally support the right of women to terminate pregnancies, most see abortion as a "forced" and tragic option.[26] It is regrettable that a woman must choose between continuation and termination of her pregnancy because both alternatives involve burdens or harms. Accordingly, we would not like to see the option of providing fetal tissue for transplantation precipitate an increase in abortions. Ironically, this concern coincides with one of the concerns mentioned in minority reports of the NIH Human Fetal Tissue Transplantation Research panel

(hereafter, NIH panel). Several members of the NIH panel argued against government support for the procedure on grounds that it would constitute an inducement to abortion, at least for pregnant women who had not yet decided whether to terminate their pregnancies.[27] There are no data supporting this claim.

A further concern of a minority of the NIH panel was that participation in fetal tissue transplantation constitutes complicity in, and legitimation of, abortion. According to James Bopp and James Burtchaell,

> Whatever the researcher's intentions may be, by entering into an institutionalized partnership with the abortion industry as a supplier of preference, he or she becomes complicit, though after the fact, with the abortions that have expropriated the tissue for his or her purposes.[28]

They thus maintain that those who use fetal tissue from elective abortions ally themselves with the "evil" that abortion represents.

Bopp and Burtchaell further claim that legitimation occurs when pregnant women considering abortion construe the possibility of benefiting someone by donating fetal tissue as a positive endorsement of abortion. The abortion is then seen as a less tragic choice than it would otherwise be, and in some circumstances it might even be seen as virtuous. Legitimation would occur on a social level if the good of successful treatment through fetal tissue transplantation became so compelling that the means of achieving the success were never critically assessed. The end would then have justified the means, at least as perceived by those who pursue the end without scrutinizing the end in its own right.

The legitimation argument illustrates more general concerns about slippery slope reasoning. Questions such as the following are then raised: if we now approve use of fetal tissue for transplants under restrictive conditions, are we not likely in time to relax the conditions if the therapy proves highly successful or if the restrictive conditions limit its usefulness? Most people agree that some restrictions are necessary to avoid abuses that could accompany use of the technology; they disagree about where to place wedges along the slippery slope.[29]

Some have proposed less restrictive guidelines than those recommended by the NIH panel, particularly with regard to commercialization. For example, Lori Andrews argues that a woman should be allowed to sell the tissue of a fetus she has agreed to abort. Feminists, she maintains, are inconsistent with their commitment to promote women's right to control their own bodies if they oppose commercial surrogacy.[30] Most feminists, however, oppose both contract motherhood and commerce in fetal tissue because of the possibility they present for exploiting women. Unlike Andrews, we thus place greater emphasis on social equality than on individual liberty. Social equality is seen as a necessary condition for authentic choice. Until and unless general equality prevails, the liberty of individual women is inevitably curtailed.

Different views regarding abortion also give rise to different views regarding the consent necessary for fetal tissue transplantation. Those who are morally opposed to elective abortion generally deny that women who choose abortion have a right to donate fetal tissue.[31] Such women, they allege, have forfeited that right even as parents may forfeit their right to consent for their child if they abuse or abandon the child. On the other side of the issue are those who stress the importance of the pregnant woman's consent to use of fetal tissue because she has the right to abortion and because the tissue belongs to her.[32] Among those who consider abortion a separable issue from fetal tissue transplantation, some insist that the pregnant woman's consent is necessary because the timing and procedure for abortion may be altered in order to maximize the chance for a successful graft.[33] In other words, if the pregnant woman may herself be affected, her consent to use fetal tissue is morally indispensable.

On therapeutic grounds alone, a comparison of the potential advantages of using fetal tissue from electively aborted fetuses with the potential and actual disadvantages of treatment through other means provides a strong case for use of fetal tissue from elective abortions. Many of the diseases that are potentially curable with fetal tissue grafts are curable by no other known means. However, therapeutic efficacy alone doesn't constitute moral justification. This returns us, then, to the problem of whether the ques-

tion of induced abortion is morally separable from the question of fetal tissue transplantation. The issue calls for reexamination of the traditional moral dilemma involving the relationship between means and ends. Does the end justify the means in transplantation of fetal tissue for cure of otherwise incurable disorders?

A simplistic version of utilitarianism supports an affirmative answer to the question. In other words, the tremendous good that might be accomplished through the new technique outweighs the harm that might be done through elective abortion. However, if endorsement of the procedure led to widespread increase in elective abortions and to exploitation of women, such undesirable consequences might outweigh the potential benefit of the technique. So, even if ends can justify means, it is not clear that the end justifies the means in this case. Whether or not the overall consequences of treating debilitating disorders through fetal tissue transplantation will generally constitute a preponderance of harms over benefits is an empirical issue for which more data is needed to support a credible utilitarian position.

From a deontological point of view, the end does not justify means that are otherwise morally unacceptable, but this does not imply that fetal tissue transplantation is morally unjustified. The individual who knowingly and freely pursues a specific end, also knowingly and freely chooses the means to its fulfilment. Intention is thus crucial to the moral relevance of the relationship. If a woman were to deliberately become pregnant, choose abortion, or persuade another to become pregnant or choose abortion, solely for the sake of fetal tissue transplantation, she would then be responsible for both means and end because she would be intending both. As we already noted, the motive of the decision may be altruistic, self-interested, or both. Although worthy motives are morally relevant, they do not alter the fact that the intention in such cases applies to both ends and means.

In other situations involving fetal tissue transplantation, the individual who intends to use the tissue need not even be aware of the abortion through which the tissue becomes available. Presumably, she does intend the retrieval procedure. However, just as a transplant surgeon may retrieve essential organs

from the brain-dead victim of a drunk-driving accident, without any implication that she thus endorses
the behavior that led to the availability of the organs,
so may a neurosurgeon who is totally opposed to
abortion transplant neural tissue from an electively
aborted fetus into a severely impaired patient, without thereby compromising her moral convictions. In
fact, one may argue that a truly pro-life position
favors the saving or prolonging of life that the transplantation intends, while acknowledging the nega-
tion of life that abortion implies. When the abortion
decision has already been made by others, a decision
not to transplant seems less in keeping with a position that is genuinely pro-life than its opposite. One
opponent of abortion even found support for fetal tissue transplants in the biblical account of creation.
Barbara Culliton attributed the following statement
to the Baptist father whose infant had prenatally
been treated with cells obtained from an aborted
fetus: "God formed one human being from the tissue
of another. Not only does God approve of this [trans-
plantation], he himself performed the first one."[34]

Fetal Tissue Transplants and Use of Women's Bodies

If abortion and fetal tissue transplants are not separable issues, then the latter is parallel in important
respects to at least three other practices which can
only be undertaken through use of women's bodies.
Contract motherhood, egg provision, and prostitution are comparable practices because they all
involve both benefit to a third party and material
remuneration to the woman who provides the benefit through use of her body. The rationale by which
most feminists oppose these practices is also
applicable to the apparent tie between abortion and
fetal tissue grafts. However, this opposition does
not extend to fetal tissue grafts considered as an
issue distinct from abortion. From a feminist standpoint, it is possible to support a woman's right to
abortion while opposing the practice of fetal tissue
transplantation.

Contract motherhood necessarily involves the
commodification of a woman's body: she "rents" or
lends her womb, and may have contributed an egg to
the embryo that develops within her. In commercial

contracts, the woman accepts payment from an infertile couple for her "services." According to the final
ruling in the Mary Beth Whitehead case, payment
for such "services" is equivalent to baby selling.[35]
This is an interesting designation because it totally
ignores what pregnancy and birth meant to the
woman, focusing exclusively on the baby to whom
she gives birth. Adoption is the better analogue for
the act through which infertile women or couples
thus become parents. The woman has agreed to rent
her womb and donate or sell her egg, and a child has
been produced through the services rendered.
Whether or not she is genetically related to the fetus,
the surrogate is biologically related to it through
gestation.

If contract motherhood is equivalent to baby selling, payment to pregnant women for use of their
aborted fetuses may also be equivalent to baby selling.[36] In both cases, it is the use of the woman's body
before abortion or delivery that is remunerated by
someone to whom the fetus is valued. Neither case
necessarily involves financial remuneration because
both *may* be undertaken for altruistic reasons. Contract motherhood and use of fetal tissue may also be
undertaken by mutual agreement prior to the establishment of pregnancy. In neither case is there an
intent to keep the product of conception. In one case,
however, a living infant is provided for a third party;
in the other, the tissue of a dead fetus is obtained in
order to provide for the health of a third party. In
both situations, the intention of the pregnant women
may be both self-interested and altruistic, regardless
of whether payment is involved.

Egg donation may be compared with sperm
"donation" because both involve the provision of
gametes, usually for financial compensation. But
unlike the provision of sperm, providing eggs
involves considerable discomfort and risk. When the
procedure was first reported in Cleveland in 1987, it
required administration of superovulatory drugs and
laparoscopic retrieval of ova under general anaesthesia.[37] In most centers, retrieval is now undertaken
trough transvaginal aspiration with a local anaesthetic. As with sperm, the term "donation" is misleading
because individuals who agree to provide ova generally do so for the money. As a student who volunteered for the world's first egg donor program put it:

"I would never go through this if I were not a poor student."[38] The compensation provided to egg donors in the program in which she enrolled was $900-$1200. In 1992, compensation ranged from $1500 to $3000, depending on the clinic.[39]

The practice of egg donation is comparable to fetal tissue provision insofar as the woman in each case contributes genetic material and may receive compensation. Occasionally, the ova retrieved may simply be the product of a normal menstrual cycle, without requiring administration of superovulatory medication. When this occurs, the retrieval is comparable to retrieval of fetal tissue from women who undergo abortions to terminate unwanted pregnancies. Unlike fetuses, ova are regularly disposed of through menstruation. They may even be retrieved as a by-product of surgery undertaken for treatment purposes. In such circumstances, providing eggs for another is more like providing tissue from spontaneously aborted fetuses than providing tissue obtained from elective abortions.

As with contract motherhood and sperm donation, egg donation is oriented to the development of a new human life. Fetal tissue becomes available for transplantation only after the death of the embryo or fetus, which occurs in the context of either spontaneous or elective abortion. The tissue that thus becomes available constitutes the possibility of extending another human life. In all of these cases, therefore, another life is affirmed through birth or healing.

Prostitution is different from the other issues discussed because it does not involve a comparable goal. To some people, the very suggestion of a parallel between prostitution and egg provision or contract motherhood is offensive because the former practice is clearly illegal and immoral, while the latter two practices are not.[40] Another difference is that prostitution does not involve medical technology. Although contract motherhood through artificial insemination may be undertaken without the help of a medical expert, this is probably a rare event, and arrangements in which gestational and genetic roles are separate require in vitro fertilization.[41] Despite these differences, the parallel between prostitution and the other issues is valid insofar as all of them involve the use of women's bodies to satisfy the desires of another. So does fetal tissue transplantation.

By definition, prostitution is practiced for material remuneration, usually money, and not for altruistic reasons intended to benefit those who employ prostitutes.[42] In some cases, however, women sell the intimacy of their bodies in order to support their children; for many women, prostitution is a means of survival, and in some cases it is perceived as (and may in fact be) the only available means of survival.[43] From a moral point of view, prostitution to obtain funds necessary for one's own or others' survival is surely defensible. What is immoral in such a situation is the social situation that presents so tragic a limitation of alternatives to women.[44]

Because prostitution is always practiced for material gain for the prostitute, it is only comparable to fetal tissue transplantation when the latter procedure also procures material gain for the woman who provides the fetal tissue. As with prostitution, however, the material gain that is accessible through fetal tissue grafts may be sought indirectly, and the motive for providing the tissue may be altruistic rather than self-interested. It is possible, for example, for a woman to initiate and terminate a pregnancy to produce fetal tissue for someone from whom she hopes to inherit wealth because of that decision. It is also possible to sell fetal tissue that she develops through a pregnancy that is deliberately undertaken to obtain funds necessary for her own or others' sustenance. A woman could even sell a fetus conceived through intercourse as a prostitute. While there are long-standing social, moral, and religious objections to prostitution, the grounds for these objections are not substantively different from objections that may be raised to contract motherhood, at least when the woman who gives birth is not genetically related to the offspring. Both involve the use of a woman's intimate body parts for payment, and in both cases the woman is generally of considerably lower socioeconomic status than the payer.

If prostitution is practiced to promote one's own survival, it parallels the situation of a pregnant woman who wishes her fetal tissue to be used for treatment of her own devastating disease, that is, to insure her own survival. If a pregnant woman sells her fetus to obtain funds to support others, her act is comparable to that of the woman who prostitutes herself to support her children. Fetal tissue transplantation is more morally problematic than prostitution because it involves not only the use of women's bodies but also the use of human fetuses. The same argument can be made with regard to a comparison between prostitution and eggs provision or contract motherhood. The latter practices may be viewed as more problematic because they involve the use of gametes and fetuses or newborns as well as the use of women's bodies for remuneration.

Paradigms and Frameworks for Assessing Fetal Tissue Transplantation

Different paradigms and frameworks have been invoked to defend or oppose fetal tissue transplantation. The paradigms include transplantation from living donors, as in kidney transplants; transplantation from cadaver donors, as in heart transplants; and "surrogate motherhood."[45] The first two are familiar and generally accepted means of obtaining organs from tissue, so long as consent is obtained from the donor or proxy and the retrieval does not constitute a major threat to the donor's health. Use of tissue from living fetuses has generally been rejected, but it is sometimes difficult to determine whether a fetus is dead. Traditional means of assessing brain death are not applicable to early fetuses or abortuses. Although "surrogacy" is a more controversial paradigm for fetal tissue transplantation, it captures, as the other two paradigms do not, the unique possibilities for exploitation of women that fetal tissue transplantation represents. As I have already suggested, these possibilities are also present in egg provision and prostitution, which are also comparable to fetal tissue transplantation.

Dorothy Vawter and her colleagues at the University of Minnesota have proposed three "competing frameworks" that may be related to the above paradigms.[46] The first is based on the premise that the fetus from which tissue may be retrieved should be regarded as a human research subject. On this view, either of two rationales may prevail, depending on whether the aborted fetus is construed as living or dead. If the former, use of fetal tissue "should satisfy the federal regulations for research involving living fetuses, and be reviewed and approved by an institutional review board." If the aborted fetus is regarded as a cadaver, a proxy decision-maker should be required "to base a decision regarding participation either on the basis of what the dead fetus would have wanted or on some view of what is in the dead fetus' best interests." Not surprisingly, neither of these standards is explained, and the authors acknowledge that it is "extremely difficult to see how a proxy decision-maker could base a decision on [them]."[47]

The second ethical framework proposed by the Minnesota group is a view of the dead fetus as a cadaveric organ donor. This generally means following the standards of the Uniform Anatomical Gift Act, which is applicable in all 50 states in the United States. This Act allows either parent to provide the necessary consent for use of fetal tissue so long as the other parent does not object. Moreover, because the dead fetus can hardly be accredited with wishes or interests, parents may base their decision on their own needs, concerns, and interests. The consensus statement of the 1986 forum in Cleveland utilized this framework. According to the authors,

> retrieval of tissue from fetal remains is analogous to the transplantation of organs or tissue obtained from adult human cadavers. Similarities include the fact that the donor is dead, and the expectation that there will be significant benefits for the recipient. These similarities suggest the appropriateness of using the same ethical and legal criteria now followed for cadaver transplantation.[48]

The beginning point of the published reports from both the Cleveland group and the NIH panel is that fetal tissue should only be retrieved from *dead* fetuses. Only then does the analogy with retrieval of tissue from "adult human cadavers" work. Even so, the differences between transplantation from human fetal cadavers rather than mature human cadavers are to be addressed through added requirements, such as the exclusion of familial donors and the observance of anonymity between donors and recipients. Obviously, this excludes the possibility of a woman initiating or terminating pregnancy in order to provide tissue for herself or for another with whom she has a special relationship.

The third framework proposed by Vawter and her colleagues is one in which the dead fetus or abortus is equated with discarded tissue. In that context,

> fetal remains, whether the result of elective abortion, ectopic pregnancy, or spontaneous abortion, are treated as any other bodily tissue and fluid removed during a diagnostic or surgical procedure.[49]

Aborted tissue is thus construed as a tissue specimen of the woman from whose body it was removed. Permission from those whose discarded tissue may be examined for educative, research, or future treatment purposes is routinely obtained in the clinical setting. Typically, the consent forms include "boilerplate" language requesting blanket permission for use of any biological "waste materials" or "tissue specimens" removed during surgical procedures. Similar boilerplate language could be incorporated into the consent form for abortion procedures.

Whereas the first two frameworks proposed by the Minnesota Center focus on the fetus as a separate being from the pregnant woman, the third focuses on the fact that fetal tissue is in fact the woman's tissue, and ought to be treated as such even when aborted. It is appropriate, therefore, to ask the pregnant woman for consent to use of her fetal tissue prior to the abortion, and her consent alone is morally adequate. Some might argue that consent of the man who impregnated the woman should also be required for use of fetal tissue, but this suggests an unusual concept of "discarded tissue," and a departure from the usual manner of dealing with discarded tissue. Moreover, since abortion is a decision legally made by women and not by their male partners, men cannot effectively challenge pregnant women's decisions regarding disposition of their fetuses.

Like the "surrogacy" model, the discarded tissue framework emphasizes the essential tie between fetus and pregnant woman. The latter model is a means of avoiding the abuses that we have seen associated with contract motherhood. Because the discarded tissue model gives priority to the pregnant woman's autonomy, it serves as a check on the possibilities for exploitation of women that trans-

plantation of fetal tissue allows. Thus there are both conceptual and moral reasons for preferring this framework to the others: it takes account of the unique relationship between fetus and pregnant woman, and the practice it engenders is consistent with respect for patient autonomy in comparable situations.

Conclusion

Like abortion, and probably because of its association with abortion, the issue of fetal tissue transplantation is a volatile one. Ironically, both feminists and those opposed to elective abortion are concerned about its association with abortion because for the former it represents possible pressures on women to initiate or terminate pregnancies, and for the latter it expresses complicity in, and legitimation of, abortion. From a feminist standpoint, there is strong support for keeping the two issues separable, but not necessarily separate. "Separable" allows for the possibility that individual women may choose to connect their abortions with the provision of fetal tissue. If the issues are "separate," that connection is precluded.

Because fetuses do not exist apart from women, fetal tissue transplantation raises concerns that may be seen in other troublesome issues that centrally affect women: contract motherhood, egg provision, and prostitution. Examination of the similarities and dissimilarities among these issues facilitates a better grasp of problematic aspects of the involvement of women in fetal tissue transplantation. If abortion decisions are separable from decisions about use of fetal tissue, the problematic aspects are reduced.

Of the frameworks that have been proposed for moral assessment of fetal tissue transplantation, the use of fetal remains from abortions is more like use of discarded tissue than use of tissue from research subjects or from cadaver donors. Whether the abortion through which fetal tissue becomes available is spontaneous or induced, the tissue used for grafts is discarded from the body of the pregnant woman. However, even the analogy with use of discarded tissue misses the uniqueness and complexity of the relationship between pregnant women and fetuses.

The uniqueness and complexity of that relationship call for explicit attention to the fact that fetuses do not exist without women.

Notes

1 My use of the terms "pro-life" and "pro-choice" accords with popular usage. In another article I have noted that this usage is not fully affirmative of life and choice, respectively. See my "Abortion and Equality," in Sidney Callahan and Daniel Callahan, eds., *Abortion* (New York: Plenum Press 1984), 179-180. One notable exception to the tendency to base "pro-choice" arguments on the status of the fetus is Judith Jarvis Thomson's "A Defense of Abortion," in *Philosophy and Public Affairs* 1, 1 (1971), 47-66. Thomson defends a woman's right to abortion *even if* the fetus is a person.

2 E.g., see *Webster's New World Dictionary*, 2nd college ed. (New York: Simon and Schuster, 1982), 517; cf. *Churchill's Medical Dictionary* (New York: Churchill Livingston Inc., 1989), 693.

3 *Stedman's Medical Dictionary*, 25th ed. (Baltimore: Williams and Wilkins, 1990), 573. This calculation of the duration of gestation is based on the first day of the last menstrual period rather than fertilization. If duration of gestation is calculated from fertilization, the fetal stage of development commences at six weeks. See James Knight and Joan Callahan, *Preventing Birth* (Salt Lake City: University of Utah Press, 1989), 205.

4 *Stedman's*, 501. However, Knight and Callahan note that the term "embryo" refers to the developing human organism between weeks 2 and 6 of gestation (205). Implantation in the uterus occurs about two weeks after fertilization. Between fertilization and implantation, the conceptus may be referred to as "pre-implantation embryo." The term "pre-embryo" is sometimes used by in vitro fertilization specialists to refer to the conceptus before implantation. In popular usage, however, the term "embryo" is often used to characterize the conceptus from fertilization until fetal stage.

5 Susan Sherwin develops this criticism on the part of medical ethics as well as feminist ethics. See her "Feminist and Medical Ethics: Two different Approaches to Contextual Ethics," *Hypatia* 4, 2 (Summer 1989), 57-72.

6 Marilyn Friedman, "Care and Context in Moral Reasoning," *Women and Moral Theory*, ed. by Eva F. Kittay and Diana T. Meyers (Totowa, New Jersey: Rowman and Littlefield, 1987), 190-204.

7 See Friedman; see also Christina Sommers, "Filial Morality," in Kittay and Meyers, 69-84.

8 Some feminists argue that the genetic tie is hardly relevant in defining parental relationships. See, e.g., Barbara Katz Rothman, *Recreating Motherhood* (New York: W.W. Norton 1989), 37-40. In some cases, however, the law insists on the significance of the genetic tie. For example, known (genetic) fathers are legally responsible for support of their children. It is well known that statutes requiring such support are only occasionally enforced.

9 Carol Gilligan, *In a Different Voice* (Cambridge: Harvard University Press, 1982); Nel Noddings, *Caring* (Berkeley: University of California Press, 1984); Sara Ruddick, *Maternal Thinking* (New York: Ballantine Books 1989). While developing a model of maternal thinking that is applicable to men as well as women, Ruddick refers to the work of mothering as "caring labor" (46). See also Mary Jean Larrabee, ed., *An Ethic of Care* (New York: Routledge, 1993); Joan Tronto, *Moral Boundaries* (New York: Routledge, 1993); Rita C. Manning, *Speaking from the Heart* (Lanham, MD: Rowman and Littlefield, 1992).

10 I have discussed these variables at greater length in "Neural Fetal Tissue Transplantation—Should We Do What We Can Do?" *Neurologic Clinics* 7, 4 (November 1989), 745-753.

11 Technically, a viable or even a nonviable (living) "abortus" is a newborn. What is relevant here, however, is not that technical difference but the moral significance of viability and sentience for any developing organism.

12 Although research with human subjects, including fetuses, must be reviewed by an institutional review board, no such review is necessary for established therapies.

13 Dorothy E. Vawter, Warren Kearney, Karen G. Gervais et al., *The Use of Human Fetal Tissue: Scientific, Ethical and Policy Concerns* (Minneapolis: University of Minnesota Press, January 1990), 45-67, 2128-2129.

14 Cf. U.S. Congress, Office of Technology Assessment, *Neural Grafting: Repairing the Brain and Spinal*

Cord, OTA-BA-462 (Washington, DC: U.S. Government Printing Office, September 1990), 93-107.

15   Stanley Fahn, "Fetal-Tissue Transplants in Parkinson's Disease," *New England Journal of Medicine* 327, 22 (Nov. 26, 1992): 1550.

16   Barbara J. Culliton, "Needed: Fetal Tissue Research," *Nature* 355 (January 23, 1992), 295.

17   Vawter et al., 136-138.

18   Vawter et al., 109, 138.

19   These were the *Forum on Transplantation of Neural Tissue from Fetuses*, convened by the Case Western Reserve University School of Medicine, Cleveland, December 4-5, 1986, and the National Institutes of Health's *Human Fetal Tissue Transplantation Research Panel*, which met in Washington, DC late in 1988.

20   Cited in Vawter et al., 42, from E. Kelemen, "Recovery from Chronic Idiopathic Bone Marrow Aplasia of a Young Mother after Intravenous Injection of Unprocessed Cells from the Liver (and Yolk Sac) of Her 22 m CR-length Embryo. A Preliminary Report." *Scandinavian Journal of Haemotology* 10 (1973), 305-308.

21   The first of these was a letter in *Science* signed by Mary B. Mahowald, Judith Areen, Barry J. Hoffer, Albert R. Jonsen, Patricia King, Jerry Silver, John R. Sladek, Jr., and LeRoy Walters, "Transplantation of Neural Tissue from Fetuses," *Science* 235 (Mar. 13, 1987), 1307-1308.

22   Cf. Curt R. Freed, Robert E. Breeze, Neil L. Rosenberg et al., "Survival of Implanted Fetal Dopamine Cells and Neurologic Improvement 12 to 46 Months after Transplantation for Parkinson's Disease," *New England Journal of Medicine* 327, 22 (Nov. 26, 1992): 1549-1555; Dennis D. Spencer, Richard J. Robbins, Frederick Naftolin et al., "Unilateral Transplantation of Human Fetal Mesencephalic Tissue into the Caudate Nucleus of Patients with Parkinson's Disease," *New England Journal of Medicine* 327, 22 (Nov. 26, 1992), 1541-1548.

23   Mahowald et al., *Science*, 1308-1309.

24   Consultants to the Advisory Committee to the Director, National Institutes of Health, *Report of the Human Fetal Tissue Transplantation Research Panel* (hereafter NIH Report), vol. 2 (December 1988), A2.

25   Freed, Breeze, Rosenberg et al., 1550.

26   It is "forced" in the sense that William James delin-

eates one of the marks of a genuine option. In other words, choice is unavoidable. See "The Will to Believe," in William James, *Essays on Faith and Morals* (Cleveland: Meridian Books, 1962), 34.

27   In addition to its three chairs, the NIH panel consisted of 18 members, three of whom disagreed with the majority view.

28   *Report of the Human Fetal Tissue Transplantation Research Panel* (NIH Report), vol. 1 (December 1988), 70.

29   Cf. my "Placing Wedges along the Slippery Slope," *Clinical Research* 36, 3 (1988): 220-222.

30   Cf. NIH Report 1, 56 and Lori B. Andrews, "Feminism Revisited: Fallacies and Policies in the Surrogacy Debate," *Logos* 9 (1988), 81-96.

31   Cf. NIH Report 1, 47-50.

32   Cf. Lori Andrews, "My Body, My Property," *Hastings Center Report* 16, 5 (October 1986), 28-38, and John Robertson, "Rights, Symbolism, and Public Policy in Fetal Tissue Transplants," *Hastings Center Report* 18, 6 (December 1988), 9-10. A key point here is whether externalization of the fetus through birth or abortion terminates or reduces the woman's claims to ownership of the tissue. Mary Ann Warren distinguishes the rights of fetuses and infants, arguing that even late-term fetuses cannot have "the full and equal rights" to which newborns may be entitled. See her "The Moral Significance of Birth," *Hypatia* 4, 3 (Fall 1989), 63.

33   Cf. Mary B. Mahowald, Jerry Silver, and Robert A. Ratcheson, "The Ethical Options in Fetal Transplants," *Hastings Center Report* 17, 1 (February 1987), 13.

34   Culliton, 295. This statement was attributed to the Baptist father of a baby who had prenatally received grafted cells from an aborted fetus for treatment of Hurler's syndrome. Two older children had already died of the disease. Both parents were strongly opposed to abortion and remain so.

35   *In re Baby M.*, New Jersey Lexis 1, 79 (New Jersey Supreme Court No. A-39), Feb. 1988.

36   Admittedly, "baby selling" is different from sale of aborted fetuses insofar as "baby selling" involves living infants.

37   "Clinic in Ohio Starts Egg Donor Plan," *New York Times* (July 15, 1987), A16.

38   This was my student in a course on "Moral Problems

in Medicine" at Case Western Reserve University in 1987.

39 Paula Monarez, "Halfway There," *Chicago Tribune* (Feb. 2, 1992), sect. 6, 4.

40 Although commercial surrogacy is illegal in some states (e.g., New Jersey), most states have no legislation regarding the practice. The morality of contract motherhood remains a matter of public debate.

41 The practice of self-insemination is not new, but there is no reliable documentation of its incidence, in part because the insemination occurs in private, and through private arrangement with a semen provider. While the desire of some women to become parents without the involvement of men may increase the practice, concerns about the status of semen (especially its HIV status) now prompt women to seek technical assistance to test semen used for insemination. For a description of self-insemination, see Mary Barton, Kenneth Walker, and B. P. Wiesner, "Artificial Insemination," *British Medical Journal* 1 (1945), 40-43; Frederick E. Lane, "Artificial Insemination at Home," *Fertility and Sterility* 5 (1954), 372-373; and *Self Insemination* (London: The Feminist Self-Insemination Group, Sept. 1980). Infants born as a result of self-insemination without medical assistance have sometimes been referred to as "turkey baster babies." The technique allows lesbian couples to obtain sperm, and have one inseminate the other. Lori B. Andrews describes a case of surrogate gestation in which a friend of the infertile couple inseminated herself with the sperm of the husband. See her *New Conceptions* (New York: St. Martin's Press, 1984), 202.

42 E.g., Webster's New World Dictionary, 2nd college ed., thus defines "prostitute": "to sell the services of (oneself or another) for purposes of sexual intercourse" (New York: Simon and Schuster, 1982), 1140.

43 Marriage has been compared with prostitution because it similarly involves the use of women's bodies for material remuneration. According to Esther Vilar,

> By the age of twelve at the latest, most women have decided to become prostitutes. Or, to put it another way, they have planned a future for themselves which consists of choosing a man and letting him do all the work. In return for his support, they are prepared to let him make use of their vagina at certain given moments.

See Vilar, "What Is Woman?" in Mary Briody Mahowald, ed., *Philosophy of Woman: Classical to Current Concepts*, revised ed. (Indianapolis, IN: Hackett, 1983), 30.

44 Cf. Alison M. Jaggar, *Feminist Politics and Human Nature* (Totowa, NJ: Rowman and Allanheld, 1983), 263-264. Also, cf. Laurie Shrage, "Should Feminists Oppose Prostitution?" *Ethics* 99, 2 (January 1989), 347-361.

45 Mahowald et al., *Hastings Center Report*, 11-12. Although I here use the term "surrogate motherhood," I agree with Rosemarie Tong's criticism of the term because it implies that the woman who gives birth is not the child's mother. Tong initially preferred the term "contract motherhood," which more accurately reflects the arrangement through which a woman agrees to become a biological mother so that another person may become a social parent. See Tong, "The Overdue Death of a Feminist Chameleon: Taking a Stand on Surrogacy Arrangements," *Journal of Social Philosophy* XXI, 2 (Fall/Winter 1990), 40-56. [Tong now suggests the term "gestational motherhood," since it better captures non-commercial arrangements and it leaves OUT the notion of contract. See her paper....]

46 Vawter et al., 211-231.

47 Vawter et al., 212-213.

48 Mahowald et al., *Science*, 235, 1308.

49 Vawter et al., 211.

51.
CONSCRIPTION OF CADAVERIC ORGANS FOR TRANSPLANTATION: A STIMULATING IDEA WHOSE TIME HAS NOT YET COME

Aaron Spital

SOURCE: *Cambridge Quarterly of Healthcare Ethics* 14.1 (2005): 107-12.

Transplantation is now the best therapy for eligible patients with end-stage organ disease. For patients with failed kidneys, successful renal transplantation improves the quality and increases the quantity of their lives. For people with other types of organ failure, transplantation offers the only hope for long-term survival.

Unfortunately, the ability to deliver this medical miracle is limited by a severe worldwide shortage of organs that continues to worsen. Despite recent large increases in the number of organs transplanted from living donors, especially from genetically unrelated volunteers, supply continues to lag far behind demand. The result is a tragic situation in which some patients with end-stage organ disease die not because we don't know how to treat them, but rather because there are not enough organs for all who need them. Compounding this tragedy is the fact that many usable organs are being buried or burned instead of being transplanted. Clearly, something is wrong with our current procurement system for cadaveric organs. What can we do to improve it?

Part of the problem lies in overly conservative selection criteria, which now is being addressed through increasing acceptance of extended-criteria and nonheartbeating donors. But in the United States, the most common reason for lost cadaveric organs is family refusal to allow organ recovery from a recently deceased loved one; about 50% of families say no. Several plans designed to overcome this family consent barrier have been proposed. These include adopting a system of presumed consent or mandated choice, and offering financial incentives to families who agree to donate. Despite growing interest in these proposals, all remain highly controversial. Furthermore, it is extremely unlikely that any of them could come close to achieving 100% efficiency of cadaveric organ procurement that patients with end-stage organ disease desperately need. However, there is another alternative that could approach this lofty goal: conscription of all usable cadaveric organs.

What Does Conscription of Cadaveric Organs Mean?

Under this plan, usable organs would be removed from all cadavers soon after death and made available for transplantation. Consent would be neither required nor requested. With the possible exception of exemption on religious grounds, opting-out would not be possible. Like a draft of military recruits, this would be a draft of organs.

This proposal will be quickly rejected by those who believe that consent is an absolute requirement for cadaveric organ procurement. However, the ethical basis for this widely held view has not been well developed, perhaps because the need for consent has long been accepted as obvious and not in need of justification. But a careful look at the relevant issues will at the very least cast doubt on this seemingly immutable tenet of organ procurement and may even convince some that, given the severe organ shortage, conscription of cadaveric organs is ethically preferable to requiring consent.

Advantages of Conscription of Cadaveric Organs for Transplantation

The most important advantage of conscription is that under this plan, the efficiency of organ procurement should approach 100%, which would dramatically increase the number of organs available for transplantation. As previously noted, it is highly unlikely that any other approach could do nearly as well. As a result of the increased availability of organs that conscription would provide, the lives of many more patients with end-stage organ failure could be improved and extended.

Another advantage of conscription is that this system would be much simpler and less costly than other approaches to organ procurement. Under this plan there would be no need to search for the best approach for obtaining consent, no need for expensive, labor-intensive educational programs designed to encourage more people to say yes, no need to train requestors to obtain and document consent, no need to maintain donor registries, and no need for complex regulatory mechanisms to prevent abuse as would be required were financial incentives allowed.

A third advantage of conscription is that because permission from the family would no longer be sought, this plan would eliminate the added stress that devastated families now endure when asked to consider organ donation in the midst of the grief and shock that follow the sudden death of a loved one. Furthermore, delays in organ recovery that result from the current need to wait for family approval, and that jeopardize the quality of organs, would be eliminated.

A final advantage of conscription is that, in contrast to other approaches to organ procurement, it satisfies the principle of distributive justice, which refers to equitable sharing of burdens and benefits by members of the community. Under conscription, all people who die with usable organs would contribute to the cadaveric organ pool—there would be no more "free riders"[1]—and all people would stand to benefit should they ever need an organ transplant. This contrasts with our current system in which people can refuse to donate and yet compete equally for an organ with generous people who choose to give.

Concerns about Conscripting Cadaveric Organs for Transplantation

The major concern about conscription of cadaveric organs is that, because it eliminates the need for consent, it would be seen by some as usurping autonomy. But it does not make sense to talk about autonomy of dead people. As Jonsen points out: "consent is ethically important because it manifests and protects the moral autonomy of persons ... [and] it is a barrier to exploitation and harm. These purposes are no longer relevant to the cadaver which has no autonomy and cannot be harmed."[2]

Not everyone agrees with Jonsen. Those who disagree claim that people may have interests that survive their deaths. Glannon suggests that one example of a surviving interest is a desire for "bodily integrity after death."[3] He and others argue that thwarting this interest, by conscripting organs from the bodies of people who had, while alive, expressed opposition to posthumous organ donation, would harm these people after their deaths. To my mind the concepts of surviving interests and especially posthumous harm are difficult ones and I have yet to be convinced of their existence. But even if they are real, they cannot possibly be as important as the interests of the living. As Harris points out: "[T]here is almost universal agreement that death is usually the worst harm that can befall a human person who wants to live.... [R]ights or interests would have to be extremely powerful to warrant upholding such rights or interests at the cost of the lives of others.... [T]he interests involved after death are simply nowhere near strong enough [to justify doing this]."[4] Furthermore, it should be remembered, but often is not, that although some people wish to remain intact after death, this is impossible—the body always decays and returns to the "biomass."[5]

The possibility that surviving family members could be harmed is more tangible and concerning. But just as in the case of surviving interests, however much harm conscripting organs would impose on the family, the magnitude of such harm could never be large enough to justify allowing people with end-stage organ disease to die for lack of a transplant—a transplant that could have been performed had organs not been discarded in the name of respecting family wishes. In this regard, Harris argues: "If we can save or prolong the lives of living people and can only do so at the expense of the sensibilities of others, it seems clear to me that we should. For the alternative involves the equivalent of sacrificing people's lives so that others will simply feel better or not feel so bad, and this seems nothing short of outrageous."[6] Similarly, Emson claims that it is "morally unacceptable for the relatives of the deceased to deny utilisation of the cadaver as a source of transplantable organs. Their only claim upon it is as a temporary memorial of a loved one, inevitably destined to decay or be burned in a very short time. To me, any such claim cannot morally be sustained in the face of what I regard as the overwhelming and preemptive need of the potential recipient."[7] And note that society accepts that a military draft may sometimes be necessary even though the death of young soldiers would be much more traumatic to surviving family members than would be mandatory removal of organs for transplantation from relatives who are already dead.

Another concern is that allowing people to opt out on religious grounds could greatly reduce the efficacy of the program if many objectors would claim this exemption regardless of their religious beliefs. But this is unlikely if a strong burden of proof of religious objection is required of those who attempt to invoke this exclusion, as was true for conscientious objectors to military service. Furthermore, because conscription of cadaveric organs would cause little if any harm, it is likely that for many objectors the benefit of getting out of the program would not be worth the effort required to do so.

A final concern about conscription of cadaveric organs is that it would generate outrage among the public. Although there likely would be public resistance at the outset, people might become more accepting of the idea once they understood the very favorable risk/benefit ratio of the plan. Supporting this prediction is the observation that there already exist widely accepted coercive practices that are designed to benefit the public and that require participation of all citizens regardless of their wishes. Examples include mandatory autopsy when foul play or contagious disease may be the cause of death, a military draft during wartime, forced taxation, and the requirement to serve on juries. Just as is true of these examples, I suspect that had we been born into a society in which conscription of organs after death were an established practice, seen as serving the public interest at an acceptably low cost, very few of us would ever question it.

Further Justification for Conscription of Cadaveric Organs

There is a general consensus that there exists a moral obligation to rescue when there is little or no risk or cost for the rescuer—for example, throwing a life preserver to a person in danger of drowning. It has been argued cogently that posthumous organ donation is another example of an easy rescue of an endangered person because organ recovery and transplantation are often lifesaving for recipients and entail little if any risk for cadavers. Based on this reasoning, Peters claims that consenting to posthumous organ recovery "is not an act of charity. It is, rather, a moral duty of substantial stringency."[8] Unfortunately, under our current voluntary system, refusal rates for organ donation are high, which indicates that many people do not meet this obligation. Therefore, conscription of cadaveric organs can also be justified as necessary to ensure that people do what they should have done on their own but did not.

I recognize that there is a difference between a moral duty and a legal duty and that the law does not always require us to do the right thing. However, in the special case of easy rescue of an endangered person, where the potential benefit is enormous and the costs and risk of harm are negligible, I believe that our moral duty to help should be written into law. Good Samaritan laws that have been enacted in several states and many European countries provide precedent for this approach.

Synthesis

Careful consideration of the pros and cons of conscription of organs after death leads me to conclude that it is not only ethically acceptable but actually ethically preferable to our current voluntary approach to cadaveric organ procurement. In discussing this issue, Emson goes even further: "It is immoral to require consent for cadaver organ donation."[9] Of course, not everyone agrees, and this issue remains highly controversial. In general, controversies about policy proposals can only be resolved through actual experience. I believe that the arguments in favor of conscripting cadaveric organs for transplantation are strong enough to recommend a pilot study to see how well the system would work. At the same time, I recognize that any plan, no matter how seemingly sound in theory, is doomed to fail if it is widely opposed by the public. Furthermore, attempting to implement policies without public support risks damaging the system we have in place. Therefore, before undertaking a trial of conscription, it is essential to explore public attitudes.

Attitudes Toward Conscription of Cadaveric Organs for Transplantation among the U.S. Public

To investigate public attitudes toward conscription of cadaveric organs for transplantation, I contracted Harris Interactive, a national polling organization with many years of experience, to conduct a telephone survey about this issue. One thousand fourteen adults living in the continental United States, all at least 18 years of age, were interviewed in September 2003. The subjects were chosen by a random digit dialing technique that reaches people with listed and unlisted phone numbers. The responses were weighted to known proportions for age, geographic region, sex, and race among the U.S. adult population. This method is designed to produce a sample of respondents that is representative of the general public. The maximum margin of error for the response rates was plus or minus 3%. The introduction and questions were written by the author, reviewed by Harris to minimize the likelihood of bias, and pretested for understanding on ten members of the lay public. The relevant sections of the introduction and the question are reproduced below. (Another question that asked about the acceptability of a non-financial incentive to donate was included in the survey; because the arguments for and against that proposal differ so greatly from those of conscription, the results for that question will be reported in a separate publication.)

Introduction: "Transplantation is a highly successful life-saving treatment for people with failing organs. Most transplanted organs come from people who have just died. Unfortunately there are not enough of these organs for all who need them, in part because many families say no when asked for permission to take organs from a loved one who has just died. Several plans have been suggested in the hope of making more organs available. One of these ... is to allow hospitals to remove organs from people who have died without asking for permission. Like a military draft, this would be a draft of organs after death except for people who objected on religious grounds. What do you think about these ideas? As you answer, please keep in mind that the doctors who determine that someone has died are not the same doctors that remove organs for transplantation."

Question: "In view of the tremendous shortage of life-saving organs, would you be willing to accept a policy that allows trustworthy medical teams to remove organs from people who have died without asking for permission, unless they had objected on religious grounds?"

Participants could choose from the following possible responses: yes, probably yes, probably no, no, don't know, or refuse to answer.

Thirty-one percent of the respondents said they would likely accept a policy of cadaveric organ conscription; 19% definitely would and 12% probably would. Sixty-six percent said they would oppose conscription; 53% definitely would and 13% probably would. Three percent said they didn't know or refused to answer. Responses were similar among males and females and among blacks and whites, although the percentage of blacks that supported conscription was slightly higher than the percentage of supportive whites. College-educated participants were less supportive of conscription than were less educated groups, and younger respondents were more supportive of the plan than were older respondents. Among those aged 25-44, nearly 40% would likely accept conscription.

I recognize that surveys of the public may not always provide a valid representation of how the public would act when faced with a real situation. However, this is of greatest concern when one of the choices is more socially desirable than the others or when the issues are misunderstood. In the present study none of the choices was clearly socially desirable and the question was pretested for understanding. Furthermore, even if the results do not portray precisely how the public would respond if actually faced with the possibility of conscription of cadaveric organs, they probably represent the best estimate we can provide.

Conclusions

The results of this survey indicate that most of the U.S. public would oppose conscription of cadaveric organs for transplantation. This is not surprising given the individualistic nature of our society and the fact that so many families refuse to allow organ recovery when asked. Therefore, any attempt to implement a trial of conscription would probably not succeed at this time. On the other hand, the arguments in favor of conscription are compelling and a large minority of the public, especially young adults, would likely support it. Furthermore, only about half the respondents were definitely opposed. Therefore, I believe that it would be a mistake to conclude that conscription of cadaveric organs is not worth pursuing. On the contrary, it is possible that educational programs (aimed at professionals as well as the public) that outline the virtues of conscription, combined with attempts to understand and address concerns of the public, could increase levels of support to more than 50%, at which point a trial of conscription could perhaps be undertaken.

Notes

1   Jarvis R. Join the club: A modest proposal to increase availability of donor organs. *Journal of Medical Ethics* 1995; 21:199-204.

2   Jonsen AR. Transplantation of fetal tissue: An ethicist's viewpoint. *Clinical Research* 1988; 36:215-19, at 219.

3   Glannon W. Do the sick have a right to cadaveric organs? *Journal of Medical Ethics* 2003; 29:153-56.

4   Harris J. Organ procurement: Dead interests, living needs. *Journal of Medical Ethics* 2003; 29:130-34, at 132.

5   See note 4, Harris 2003. Also see Emson HE. It is immoral to require consent for cadaver organ donation. *Journal of Medical Ethics* 2003; 29:125-27.

6   Harris J. Wonderwoman and Superman. *The Ethics of Human Biotechnology*. Oxford: Oxford University Press; 1992:100-03, at 101.

7   See note 5, Emson 2003:126.

8   Peters DA. A unified approach to organ donor recruitment, organ procurement, and distribution. *Journal of Law and Health* 1989-90; 3:157-87, at 168.

9   See note 5, Emson 2003:125.

52.
THE ETHICS OF XENOTRANSPLANTATION

Michael J. Reiss

SOURCE: *Journal of Applied Philosophy* 17.3 (2000): 253-62.

Xenotransplantation entails moving (i.e., transplanting) one or more organs (e.g., a heart) or cells (such as pancreatic cells) from an individual of one species into an individual of another species. Since the 1980s a number of research groups have been attempting to genetically engineer domestic pigs so that their organs may be given to humans. From the perspective of applied philosophy, xenotransplantation is interesting in part because of the wide range of issues it raises. Is it necessary? Would it be safe? What are the animal welfare implications? Does it entail being disrespectful to non-human animals or involve violation of their telos or integrity? This paper cannot hope to provide definitive answers to all of these questions. However, it does aim to provide a map of the bioethical territory that needs to be traversed before such a set of answers can be arrived at.

I believe that such a map is now needed. There are several research groups which have actively been working in this field in a number of countries. Thousands of pigs genetically engineered with human genes have already been brought into existence and tens of millions of pounds have been spent in research. Since the research began, tens of thousands of people have died as a result of shortages of human organs for transplants. By the time this article appears, clinical trials of xenotransplants may have begun.[1] In any event, the first decade of the twenty-first century of the Common Era is likely to see whether this technology becomes a regular feature of Western medicine or not.

One way of trying to decide whether any practice (e.g., xenotransplantation, prostitution, insider dealing, capital punishment) is acceptable is to examine all possible arguments for and against the practice within a single ethical framework. An obvious difficulty, though, is to decide which framework to adopt. There is little to be gained in applied philosophy in plumping for one ethical framework—e.g., consequentialism—when there still exists no widespread agreement as to what such an ethical framework should be or even whether one overarching one exists. The approach that is therefore taken here is to put forward, and briefly examine, appropriate arguments within a variety of possible frameworks.[2] As will become apparent, there are a considerable number of frameworks within which xenotransplantation can be examined. But first, some relevant factual information is needed about the biology of xenotransplantation, about its safety and about whether there is a need for it.

The Biology of Xenotransplantation

Immunology is a complicated subject. The long and short of it, though, is that each of us as humans, in common with certain other animal species, has the physiological ability to recognise that our individual body and the organs therein are ours in a physical sense. The net result is that while our immune system (white blood cells, etc.) attacks foreign biological objects inside us, it does not normally attack ourselves. The advantage of this is obvious. Disease-causing organisms (e.g., viruses, harmful bacteria) can be attacked and destroyed without the body turning against itself.

The immune system can misfunction in various ways. For example, it may overreact to foreign bodies. This is what happens with allergies. In the worst case, such over-reaction can cause death (e.g., the fatal shock experienced by some people on eating nut products or being stung by a bee/wasp). The other main way the immune system can misfunction is by starting to attack parts of its own body. This seems to be what happens in a number of chronic diseases including rheumatoid arthritis.

It is because the immune system normally works so effectively that people receiving human-to-human transplants generally have to be given large doses of immunosuppressive drugs. As their name implies, these drugs suppress the immune system and so prevent it from rejecting the transplanted organ. Unfortunately, patients with suppressed immune systems are less able to fight off germs though with the latest generation of immunosuppressive drugs this is now less of a problem.

When it comes to transplanting non-human organs into humans, an extra difficulty arises. Within hours of the transplant, even if immunosuppressive drugs are used, so called hyperacute rejection sets in and the transplant fails. It is to try and overcome this problem that pigs are being genetically engineered to carry a single human gene. This gene results in the pigs producing a human protein on the surface of their internal organs. As a result, it is hoped that when these organs are used in transplants, hyperacute rejection will be avoided.

Would Xenotransplantation Be Safe?

A number of national and international ethical committees as well as individual scientists have looked at the question of xenotransplantation.[3] One of the particular foci of concern has been the issue of safety. We know that pigs carry what are called porcine endogenous retroviruses (engagingly abbreviated as 'PERVS'). In the light of BSE and AIDS it is unsurprising, and encouraging, that there is tremendous hesitancy in allowing any scientific/technological procedure to go ahead that might lead to new human infections.

The current (February 2000) position in the UK is that if (and it is a big 'if') xenotransplants are allowed, the safety requirements will be stringent. In particular, there is a great deal of work going on to reduce to near-zero levels the chance of any infectious agents, such as viruses, passing as a result of transplants from pigs to humans. The United Kingdom Xenotransplantation Interim Regulatory Authority is proposing that anyone receiving a xeno-

transplant must agree to provide lifelong post-operative compliance with a whole set of conditions including: (a) use of barrier contraception; (b) refraining from pregnancy/fathering a child; (c) allowing the relevant Health Authorities to be notified when moving abroad. In addition, all household members and sexual partners will need to be seen pre-xenotransplantation to ensure they are informed about possible risks, how to minimise them, and to have baseline blood samples taken for indefinite archiving.[4]

Some recent research suggests that the chances of porcine endogenous retroviruses passing from pigs to humans may be low. Perhaps surprisingly, worldwide there are several hundred people who have already been treated with various living pig tissues. Most commonly this has been done when a patient's blood is passed through a pig liver or spleen to 'clean' it—the pig organ remaining outside the patient's body. A careful study has shown that in none of the 160 patients who had been treated with a living pig tissue and from whom samples could be obtained was there any evidence of pig-to-human transmission of porcine endogenous retroviruses. This was the case despite the fact that 23 of the patients had living pig cells inside themselves, in some cases for over eight years.[5]

Of course, this study does not prove that pig viruses won't infect humans but it does suggest that the likelihood is lower than many experts had feared. What is still unclear is how serious the consequences would be if such infection(s) did occur.

Is There a Need for Xenotransplantation?

World-wide there are approximately 150,000 people waiting for an organ transplant.[6] Each year many thousands of people have their lives saved as a result of human-to-human transplants. However, each year many thousands of people die who would have lived had they received a transplant. Indeed, the majority of people waiting for a transplant never receive one. The purchase of human organs—a market-led 'solution' to the shortage—is, by-and-large, illegal. The qualification 'by-and-large' is necessary as some countries permit the sale of human eggs, sperm and blood. None, though, to my knowledge, allows the purchase of organs for transplants. Nevertheless, there are not infrequent reports in the media of organs being offered for sale and/or bought for transplants. In one case, US$5.7 million was apparently bid during an online auction of a human kidney before the auction was halted.[7] The original advertisement read:

> You can choose either kidney ... Buyer pays all transplant and medical costs. Of course only one for sale, as I need the other one to live. Serious bids only.

The reason that most people waiting for an organ transplant never receive one is simply that there aren't enough human organs to go around. There are three main reasons for this. First, the number of people who would benefit from a transplant continues to rise. In part this is because of advances in transplant surgery which mean that more organs (e.g., lungs) can now be transplanted than used to be the case. In part, too, this is because a greater range of medical conditions can now be treated by transplantation than used to be the case.

A second reason why there aren't enough human organs to go around is that only a very small proportion of deaths result in organs that are suitable for transplants. Deaths from motor vehicle accidents provide a high proportion of suitable organs, yet, thanks to improvements in road safety (seat belts, improved car design, better road layouts, greater use of motor cycle helmets), the number of people killed in such accidents is reducing in those countries—i.e., the West—where transplant surgery is numerically significant.

A final reason for the shortage of human organs is that many countries have some sort of 'opt in' rather than 'opt out' system for organ donation. This can mean that for a transplant organ to become available (a) the dead person needs previously to have expressed a wish for their organs to be used for transplantation; (b) a doctor must ask relatives to consent to this; (c) no close relative must object to the transplant.

Of course, the question 'Is there a need for X?' cannot be answered simply by demonstrating a use to which X could be put. The use must be deemed appropriate and many people (i.e., non-consequen-tialists) would also argue that the means required to effect X must also be acceptable in themselves. Most people are likely to accept that human-to-human transplants fulfil a need in that such transplants manifestly lead to many people each living for several to many more years of life, typically with a significantly enhanced quality of life too. It is difficult for anyone who has even watched a television programme about transplantation, let alone known someone who has benefited from one, to argue that human-to-human transplants aren't needed.

Nevertheless, it would, in principle, be possible for someone to argue that it would be a better world if (a) more people accepted that their lives should not be prolonged by human-to-human transplants; (b) the money spent on the procedures was put to better use elsewhere—whether within the medical services or, for instance, by employing more academics with a specialism in philosophy. However, even someone arguing thus would, I suspect, be hard pushed to maintain that human-to-human transplants should be forbidden by law. Even most vegetarians, in my experience, don't argue for all meat-eating to be outlawed. It should, though, be noted that there are some strong cultural differences between countries with regard to the acceptability of human-to-human transplants. In Japan, for example, heart transplants are virtually unheard of because death is only understood to have occurred once the heart stops beating. Such hearts cannot be used in transplants.

However, even if it is accepted that there is a need for human-to-human transplants, this is not to imply that there is necessarily a need for xenotransplantation. For one thing, it is very possible that, at least in the early stages of 'treatments' with xenotransplants, patient survival will be significantly lower when compared with human-to-human transplants. A cost-benefit analysis (for those who accept that cost-benefit analyses are the appropriate way to decide such ethical problems) might weigh against these xenotransplants. A separate point is that perhaps societies are wrong to ban the sale of human organs for transplants. Indeed, don't I have a duty to provide one of my two healthy kidneys for someone who has none?[8]

More prosaically, better health education might lead to less of a demand for hearts and other organs. Further, if only more of us carried donor cards and gave permission for our dead relatives' organs to be used in transplants the need for xenotransplants to meet the shortfall would be reduced. In addition, though it is still too early to be sure that they will ever have a widespread practical utility, significant advances are being made in artificial (metal and plastic) organs. Finally, advances in tissue culture, cloning and stem cell research hold out the hope that at least some human organs may be grown from a patient's own tissues. One advantage, should this ever become possible, is that there should be few or no rejection problems.

Welfare Considerations

Practically everyone agrees that welfare considerations need to be taken into account when deciding whether, and if so how, sentient animals such as pigs should be used for human ends. Suffering involves susceptibility to pain and an awareness of being, having been or being about to be in pain.[9] Pain here is used in its widest sense and includes stress, discomfort, distress, anxiety and fear. As every biologist knows, it is difficult to argue against the contention that vertebrates, and probably certain invertebrates such as octopuses, can experience pain.[10] The extent to which animals are aware of their pain is more open to question, but there is increasing acceptance that certain of our closest evolutionary relatives have the requisite degree of self-consciousness. A growing number of biologists and philosophers accept that, at the very least, most mammals can suffer.[11]

So would xenotransplantation lead to significant amounts of non-human animal suffering? Consider, first of all, the pigs that would be used. Companies involved in research on xenotransplantation maintain that their pigs are extremely well looked after. Indeed, in the UK, the pigs (both those which have been genetically engineered and those which have not) used in the research are, in my view, looked after better than are pigs on many pig farms. Imutran, for example, uses what is widely agreed to be a high quality animal welfare system (the Nurtinger system) to house its pigs.[12] This comprises a warm, insulated bed and a cooler area for loafing, feeding and drinking. It gives pigs a choice of environment and temperature and provides for social contact.

However, there is more to the welfare of the pigs than their housing.[13] For a start, the pigs are subjected to a number of surgical procedures. Laparatomies (to flush out eggs) are performed under general anaesthetic because of the convoluted nature of the uterine horns in the pig. In addition, if and when clinical trials begin, it seems likely that some so-called 'gnotobiotic' (germ-free) animals will be needed. Such animals would be obtained by what is sometimes euphemistically called 'surgical derivation.' This means that shortly before birth, the entire uterus with the piglets would be removed (surgical hysterectomy) from the mother. The piglets would then be raised in isolation and in sterile conditions. The current UK draft code of practice for the housing and care of pigs intended for use as xenotransplant source animals states:

> Due to the high welfare costs to the animals, in terms of being raised in a barren environment with little or no social contact, source animals must not be reared beyond four weeks of age in an isolator.[14]

Further, it is not only pig welfare that needs to be considered. Current research aimed at improving the success of xenotransplants has meant that many hundreds, possibly thousands, of primates (captive-bred cynomolgus monkeys and wild-caught baboons) have already been used in surgical operations. While many of these operations are deemed a research 'success,' this, of course, is to view the procedure from the perspective of the surgeons and scientists involved (and perhaps, ultimately, the patients and shareholders who may benefit). From the point of view of the non-human primates, every such operation leads to considerable pain and a dramatic shortening of lifespan.

It is difficult to be sure but, on balance, my prediction would be that while xenotransplantation raises significant animal welfare issues, these are unlikely to be perceived by regulators or, indeed, by most people, to be sufficient for xenotransplantation to be outlawed on these grounds. However, there are other issues to consider in addition to human safety and animal welfare.

Changing the Nature of Animals

Let us assume that xenotransplantation will require genetically engineering pigs through the insertion into pig DNA of one or more human genes. Manifestly this involves changing the 'nature' of the pigs in at least some sense. Is this acceptable? Imutran has argued that 'This involves changing only 0.001% of the genetic make-up of the pig.'[15] To some, though, the actual percentage of change is not of prime importance. If I am unfaithful to my spouse on only 0.5% of nights, is this ten times better than if I am unfaithful on 5% of nights? More mundanely, a change of x% at the genetic level may have a very different effect at the phenotypic level. A frequent cry against genetic engineering of any sort is that 'It's unnatural.' However, this objection is difficult to defend. After all, what is 'natural'? In everyday language smallpox, earthquakes and death are natural whereas vaccines, laptops and foreign holidays aren't. In other words, there doesn't seem to be much of a relationship between what is 'natural' and what is good.

Nevertheless, the 'It's unnatural' argument can be defended in a number of ways. For a start, a number of religions argue that, at least to some extent and in some sense, nature is good. In the Jewish and Christian traditions, the understanding is that on the sixth day 'God saw everything that he had made, and behold, it was very good.'[16] Death and decay entered the world through sin, but even after the Fall sufficiency of God's goodness is manifest in the creation for much that is natural to be good. Around this notion there has built up an entire theology of natural law.

Nor is it only within religions that nature has been seen as an indicator of goodness. Even Nietzsche at times suggested this while Heidegger criticised technology in that instead of allowing our purposes to find creative expression through the qualities of objects themselves we design things to suit our purposes.[17] To this day there is a considerable body of opinion holding that 'natural' practices are desirable in such separate activities as education (Rousseau onwards), child nutrition (e.g., 'breast is best'), agriculture (organic farming), food (non-artificial flavourings) and medicine (traditional medicines).

Aside from psychological reasons for the success of appeals to nature, one great advantage of nature is that it has been around for quite a while. Consciously or otherwise the thought may be 'Our ancestors successfully brought up their children, farmed and prepared their food in these ways so traditional approaches must be OK.' After all, and quite logically, one cannot be sure about the long-term consequences of any new technology (including genetic engineering), only of practices that have been around for a considerable time and so are now considered 'natural.'

However, to what extent does the genetic engineering in question in this particular technology really change the nature of pigs? From the pigs' point(s) of view, it can be argued 'not at all.' As considered above, the practicalities of genetic engineering have significant welfare implications but it seems difficult to argue from a pig's perspective that the genetic engineering itself has changed its nature. The pig's behaviour is no different; its mental capacities and experiences are unchanged. The only difference is that it produces an extra internal protein. Traditional breeding, on the other hand, has resulted in very significant changes to the natures of farm animals (increased tolerance of high stocking densities, increased tractability, massive changes in milk, wool and meat production, etc.).

Religious Considerations

Most religious writers are cautious about genetic engineering with some objecting to it outright on the grounds that it is tantamount to 'playing God.' Interestingly, though, some theologians have argued that part of what it is to be human is to accept our God-given creativity and use it wisely.[18] This would mean that genetic engineering, per se, is no more inadmissible than any other technology. Rather it should be judged by its fruits, by the way it is undertaken and by the intentions of those who undertake it.

At the same time, there have been significant movements within Judaism, Christianity and Islam in recent decades serving, as it were, to give greater voice to the perspectives of non-human animals.[19] After all, the Hebrew scriptures include a number of instructions relating to non-human animal welfare, with some of the Wisdom writings arguing that non-human animals have a purpose beyond that of human benefit.

Other religions have longer established or stronger teachings about the need for human duties towards non-human animals. In Buddhism, for example, there is a prohibition on the taking of animal life, while according to the Isa Upanishad, in the Hindu scriptures, the Earth does not belong to humanity. In Jainism, the concern for ahisma (non-injury) goes hand-in-hand with an insistence on a vegetarian diet. Lay members are encouraged to engage only in occupations that minimise the loss of life while it is the monastic practice to carry a small broom with which gently to remove any living creature before one sits or lies down.

Animal Rights, Respect, Telos, Genetic Integrity and Intrinsic Value

As has been very widely discussed, moral philosophers disagree as to whether even humans have rights.[20] Even if we do, it has been maintained, by many philosophers from Kant onwards, that non-humans have no rights. On the other hand, it has been argued, on grounds that derive from Rawls' veil of ignorance, that even contractarianism can allow non-rational, but sentient, agents to possess moral status and have rights.[21] Obviously those who believe that non-human animals have rights are likely to argue that xenotransplantation is ethically wrong.

A different approach is to ask whether xenotransplantation and the attendant research is disrespectful to pigs and the primates used in the research. It seems difficult to answer 'no.' After all, the pigs and primates are being used instrumentally as means to ends with many of their normal behaviours and 'intentions' thwarted. However, it could be argued that their lives are still worth living and that most of them would not even have lives were the research not being undertaken (the 'eating bacon is good for pigs' argument).

Other ethical frameworks put at centre stage the telos of animals (their ends in an Aristotelian sense), their genetic integrity or their intrinsic value (the worth organisms have in themselves, irrespective of their usefulness for humans).[22]

To consider each of these frameworks adequately would require a paper in itself. Suffice it to say that as yet no agreement exists as to the validity of any of them. To some extent, it may be that it is precisely because of the plethora of non-consequentialist frameworks which have been proposed that utilitarianism remains the dominant framework within which many of the regulations concerned with our use of animals are framed.

Changing the Nature of Humans

A further argument against xenotransplantation would be to maintain that in some way the practice changes human nature, that it breaks down the barrier(s) between ourselves and other species. From a purely ethical perspective this objection is difficult to substantiate. After all, our status as moral subjects is not dependent, surely, on the origin of our hearts or other internal organs. To suppose otherwise would be to commit the genetic fallacy in both its classical and current senses. Further, many evolutionary biologists and certain philosophers would welcome the breaching of what is often felt as too rigid a barrier between ourselves and other animals.[23] Nevertheless, the argument has psychological appeal and deserves serious consideration for this reason. To take an extreme instance, one could imagine—and the 1973 film *O Lucky Man!* did so imagine—a scenario in which a whole pig body (minus the head) is transplanted onto a human head.[24] Would we be in favour of such a practice? My supposition is that most people would find such a procedure abhorrent. Now such 'arguments from disgust,' as we might term them, cannot simply be accepted at face value; after all many people in previous generations found the notion of female doctors disgusting while many people today recoil from the idea of same-sex sexual relationships. Nevertheless, such arguments deserve serious consideration, if only because they are widely held. Indeed, I am surprised that, to my knowledge, no-one has yet cited the New Testament verse 'For not all flesh is alike, but there is one kind for men, another for animals, another for birds, and another for fish' in support of the notion that xenotransplantation—indeed, genetic engineering more generally—is wrong on the grounds that it blurs the distinction between humans and non-humans.[25]

Conclusion

Given this tremendous diversity of opinion, what are we to conclude? From the perspective of public policy and regulation—which cannot wait for agreement among moral philosophers—perhaps the only way forward is to try to reach decisions by consensus.[26] It is true that this does not solve everything. After all, what does one do when consensus cannot be arrived at? Nor can one be certain that consensus always arrives at the right answer—a consensus may once have existed that women should not have the vote. Nevertheless, there are highly desirable reasons both in principle and in practice in searching for consensus.

A consensus should be based on reason, take into account long established practices of ethical reasoning and be open to refutation and the possibility of change. Consensus should not be equated with majority voting. Special consideration needs to be given to minorities, particularly if they are especially affected by the outcomes, and to those—such as young children, the mentally infirm and non-humans—unable to participate in the decision-making process.

We cannot be certain that a consensus is absolutely valid. However, procedures can be put in place which increase the likelihood that a consensus is reliable and trustworthy. The issue is partly one of epistemology. For example, anyone arguing either for or against xenotransplantation from a utilitarian perspective would have their hand strengthened if they were able to produce rigorous conclusions based on the following three numbers:

- Some measure of the overall harm that would result from the research in terms of suffering to the animals used. (Strictly, this should include the upset caused to people who oppose the use of animals in this way.)
- Some measure of the overall benefit that is expected to result from the research if it succeeds. (Strictly, this should include the pleasure experienced by people as a result of the successful use of xenotransplants enabling their relatives and friends to live longer, more fulfilling lives.)
- An estimate of the chances of the research succeeding.

In the meantime, until widespread agreement as to the acceptability or otherwise of xenotransplantation is reached, a considerable amount of work remains to be done on its ethics.[27]

Notes

1   Unsurprisingly, companies, such as Imutran Ltd. (a Novartis Pharma Company) and Genzyme, involved in the production and breeding of pigs for xenotransplantation, are keen for clinical trials to be allowed without a delay of many years.

2   Most people who write on animal biotechnology, with the exception of certain philosophers, agree that the most fruitful way forward is to examine each issue within a variety of ethical frameworks. See, for example, Alan Hikkabd and Andrew Johnson (eds.) (1998) *Animal Biotechnology and Ethics* (London, Chapman & Hall); Peter Sandøe and Nils Holtung (1998) Ethical aspects of biotechnology in farm animal production, *Acta Agriculturae Scandinavica*, Section A, Animal Science, Supplementum, 29, 51; and Mike Appleby (1999) *What Should We Do about Animal Welfare?* (Oxford, Blackwell Science). See also Anne Maclean (1993) *The Elimination of Morality: Reflections on utilitarianism and bioethics* (London, Routledge).

3   See NUFFIELD COUNCIL ON BIOETHICS (1996) *Animal-to-Human Transplants: The ethics of xenotransplantation* (London, Nuffield Council on Bioethics); THE ADVISORY GROUP ON THE ETHICS OF XENOTRANSPLANTATION (1996) Animal Tissue into Humans (London, Department of Health); MAE-WAN HO (1998) *Genetic Engineering—Dream or Nightmare? The Brave New World of bad science and big business* (Bath, Gateway Books); Robert A. Weiss (1998) Transgenic pigs and virus adaptation, *Nature*, 391, 327; and Eve-Marie Engels (1999) Xenotransplantation: a doubtful prospect, *Biologist*, 46, 73. The World Health Organisation has an active electronic discussion group on xenotransplantation to which a number of philosophers, amongst others, contribute. To subscribe to it—there is no fee—send an e-mail with the subject line blank and with 'subscribe xenodiscussion' in the body of the message to <majordomo@who.int>. An archive website is supported by the OECD at

www.oecd.org./dsti /sti/s_t/biotech/xenosite/country .htm which also provides links to policy and consultation documents produced by individual countries. In 1999 the Council of Europe Parliamentary Assembly voted for an international moratorium on xenotransplantation but for further research to be undertaken.

4   UNITED KINGDOM XENOTRANSPLANTATION INTERIM REGULATORY AUTHORITY (1999) Draft Report of the Infection Surveillance Steering Group of the UKXIA (London, Department of Health). Similar stipulations are being proposed in some other countries.

5   Khazal Paradis, Gillian Langford, Zhifeng Long, Walid Heneine, Paul Sabd-Strom, William Switzer, Louisa E. Chapman, Chris Lockey, David Onions, The Xen 111 Study Group and Edward Otto (1999) Search for cross-species transmission of porcine endogenous retrovirus in patients treated with living pig tissue, *Science*, 285, 1236.

6   Novartis Imutran (1999) *Animal Welfare: Xenotransplantation—helping to solve the global organ shortage* (Cambridge, Imutran Ltd.).

7   Anon (1999) Online bidders' stake in kidney, *Monash Bioethics Review*, 18, 39.

8   For discussion of the ethical issues raised by the sale of human organs see Andrew Kimbrell (1993) *The Human Body Shop: The engineering and marketing of life* (London, HarperCollins Religious); and Nicole Gerrand (1999) The misuse of Kant in the debate about a market for human body parts, *Journal of Applied Philosophy*, 16, 59.

9   Michael J. Reiss and Roger Straughan (1996) *Improving Nature? The science and ethics of genetic engineering* (Cambridge, Cambridge University Press).

10   Jane A. Smith and Kenneth M. Boyd (eds.) (1991) *Lives in the Balance: The ethics of using animals in biomedical research—The Report of a Working Party of the Institute of Medical Ethics* (Oxford, Oxford University Press).

11   Marian Stamp Dawkins (1980) *Animal Suffering: The science of animal welfare* (London, Chapman and Hall); and Peter Singer (1993) *Practical Ethics*, 2nd edn (Cambridge, Cambridge University Press). For a review of attempts to determine the suffering of animals, including transgenic animals, used in experimental procedures see E.S. Jenkins and R.D. Combes (1999) The welfare problems associated with using transgenic mice to bioassay for bovine spongiform encephalopathy, *Animal Welfare*, 8, 421.

12   Novartis Imutran op. cit.

13   Gill Langley and Joyce D'silva (1998) *Animal Organs in Humans: Uncalculated risks & unanswered questions* (London, British Union for the Abolition of Vivisection & Petersfield, Compassion in World Farming); Tim O'biren (1998) *Farm Animal Genetic Engineering*, 2nd edn (Petersfield, Compassion in World Farming); and Home Office (1999) Draft Code of Practice for the Housing and Care of Pigs Intended for Use as Xenotransplant Source Animals (London, Home Office).

14   Home Office op. cit., p.18.

15   Novartis Imutran op. cit.

16   Genesis 1.31.

17   Martin Heidegger (1977) *The Question Concerning Technology and Other Essays*. Translated and with an Introduction by William Lovitt (New York, Harper Colophon).

18   Ted Peters (1997) *Playing God? Genetic determinism and human freedom* (New York, Routledge).

19   Reviewed by Reiss and Straughan op. cit. See also Andrew Linzey and Dorothy Yamamoto (eds.) (1998) *Animals on the Agenda: Questions about animals for theology and ethics* (London, SCM).

20   For a recent collection of essays on human rights situated within the field of genetics see Justine Burley (ed.) (1999) *The Genetic Revolution and Human Rights: The Oxford Amnesty Lectures 1998* (Oxford, Oxford University Press).

21   Mark Rowlands (1997) Contractarianism and animal rights, *Journal of Applied Philosophy*, 14, 235.

22   Henk Verhoog (1992), The concept of intrinsic value and transgenic animals, *Journal of Agricultural and Environmental Ethics*, 5, 147; Bernard E. Rollin (1995) *The Frankenstein Syndrome: Ethical and social issues in the genetic engineering of animals* (Cambridge, Cambridge University Press); and Holland and Johnson op. cit.

23   Peter Singer (1981) *The Expanding Circle: Ethics and sociobiology* (Oxford, Clarendon Press); and James Rachels (1991) *Created from Animals: The moral implications of Darwinism* (Oxford, Oxford University Press).

24 The script is available as Lindsay Anderson and David Sheerwin (1973) O Lucky Man! (Plexus, London). The original screenplay is © 1973 by SAM.

25 1 Corinthians 15.39.

26 Jonathan D. Moreno (1995) *Deciding Together: Bioethics and moral consensus* (Oxford, Oxford University Press); and Michael Reiss (1998) Building animals to order, *Biologist*, 45, 161.

27 This paper is based in part on talks given at the 3rd World Congress on Alternatives and Animal use in the Life Sciences (Bologna, 1999) and at the British Association Annual Festival of Science (Sheffield, 1999). I am very grateful to Roger Straughan who first instructed me in bioethics and who provided valuable comments on an earlier draft of this paper.

53.
PANDETHICS

M.J. Selgelid

SOURCE: *Public Health* 123.3 (2009): 255-59.

This paper explains the ethical importance of infectious diseases, and reviews four major ethical issues associated with pandemic influenza: the obligation of individuals to avoid infecting others, healthcare workers' 'duty to treat,' allocation of scarce resources, and coercive social distancing measures. In each case, ways in which the ethical issues turn on both philosophical and empirical questions are highlighted. The paper concludes that ethicists should play a greater role in identifying ethically important empirical questions, and that scientists should take the ethical as well as the scientific importance of such questions into consideration when choosing research projects.

Introduction

The ethical importance of infectious diseases is partly revealed by the fact that their consequences are almost unrivalled.[1] Historically, they have caused more morbidity and mortality than any other cause, including war.[2] The Black Death eliminated one-third of the European population over the course of a few years during the mid-fourteenth century;[3] tuberculosis killed 1 billion people from 1850 to 1950;[4] the 1918 flu killed between 20 and 100 million people;[5] and smallpox killed between 300 and 500 million people during the twentieth century alone, i.e., three times more than were killed by all the wars of that period.[6] Infectious diseases are currently the biggest killers of children and young adults, and the continuing threat of infectious diseases is revealed by the emergence of many new infectious diseases during recent decades [including human immunodeficiency virus/acquired immunodeficiency syndrome (HIV/AIDS), Ebola, severe acute respiratory syndrome (SARS) and avian influenza], the growing problem of drug resistance and the spectre of bioterrorism.

Second, infectious diseases raise difficult ethico-philosophical questions of their own. Although measures such as surveillance, mandatory treatment and vaccination, isolation and quarantine may sometimes be important to the protection of public health, they may each involve infringement of basic rights and liberties, i.e., the right to privacy, informed consent to medical intervention, and freedom of movement. Given that most deny that either the goal to promote public health or the goal to protect individual rights and liberties should always take absolute priority over the other, a difficult ethical question is how to strike a balance between these two types of goals in cases of conflict.

Third, the topic of infectious disease is closely connected to the topic of justice. Malnutrition, dirty water, overcrowded living and working conditions, lack of sanitation and hygiene, poor education, and lack of access to health care make poor people more likely to become infected and more likely to suffer poor outcomes when infection occurs. As bad health, in turn, exacerbates poverty, a vicious cycle promotes both poverty and disease.

Fourth, infectious diseases are prone to promote fear, panic, stigma, discrimination, and emotional and irrational decision and policy making.[7]

Fifth, and finally, infectious diseases pose threats to security. Security dangers are associated with fast-moving infectious disease outbreaks that overwhelm response capacity and cause chaos. In 2007, the World Health Organization described pandemic influenza as 'the most feared security threat,'[8] and former US President George W. Bush suggested that a military response may be necessary in the event of a flu pandemic. Security may also be jeopardized for economic reasons in the case of slower-moving epidemics. HIV/AIDS, for example, has brought numerous African societies to the verge of economic collapse. Historical studies reveal that factors such as high infant mortality, low life expectancy and decreasing life expectancy—especially salient in sub-Saharan Africa at present, largely as a result of HIV/AIDS—are among the most reliable indicators of societal upheaval.[9]

Given the ethical importance of infectious disease, it is encouraging that public health ethics has emerged as a rapidly growing subdiscipline of bioethics, and that an increasing body of literature is focusing on ethical issues associated with infectious disease in particular. A majority of the ethics and infectious disease literature has focused on HIV/AIDS, SARS, pandemic influenza and bioterrorism. This article will review four major ethical issues associated with pandemic influenza: the obligation of individuals to avoid infecting others, healthcare workers' 'duty to treat,' allocation of scarce resources, and the use of coercive social distancing measures. In each case, ways in which the ethical issues turn on both philosophical and empirical questions are highlighted.

Obligation to Avoid Infecting Others

While bioethics has traditionally focused on the dyadic relationship between healthcare workers and patients and/or health-care policy making, contagious infectious diseases raise issues of individual morality. In the event of a major flu pandemic, the failure of an individual to take precautionary infection control measures may endanger the lives of others. Such dangers are, of course, most obvious when an individual knows he/she is infected and contagious, but they also arise when an individual has reason to believe that he/she might be infected (and contagious) because he/she was or may have been exposed to someone else who was contagious. While the widely accepted 'duty to do no harm' would appear to require that infected or potentially infected individuals should take action to avoid (potentially lethally) endangering others, there surely must be limits to such a duty. We cannot, that is, expect everyone who is or just might be infected to do everything that they can to avoid the infection of others; that would unnecessarily bring too many lives to a standstill. What, then, are the limits to the duty in question? And to what extent should the duty be enforced by law? Although these questions are both interesting and difficult, they have received surprisingly little discussion to date. The author is only familiar with two papers on this particular topic.[10,11] No attempt will be made to answer such questions fully in this article, although a number of suggestions are offered. First, it is safe to say that the strength of an individual's duty to take precautionary infection control measures, e.g., submitting oneself to voluntary quarantine, limiting interaction with others, wearing a mask, etc., should be proportional to the risk that one is actually infected: the greater the probability that someone is infected, the more he/she should do to avoid exposing him-/herself to others. Second, more research should aim to establish evidence regarding the effectiveness of infection control measures. If evidence reveals that masks, for example, provide highly effective means of infection prevention, then the duty (of even those not especially likely to be infected) to wear masks would be higher than would otherwise be the case. Such research is scientifically important, but there is also an ethical imperative that more of this type of research take place. Third, there is a need to raise greater public awareness of both the ethical imperative to avoid infecting others and the available means of preventing infection. Fourth, when an individual fails to voluntarily take morally required precautions against the infection of others, legal sanctions and/or the use of force may be justified. This follows from Dworkin's suggestion that if actions are immoral, 'then the freedom to pursue them counts for less.'[12]

Duty to Treat

An issue which has received considerably more attention, especially in the context of HIV/AIDS, SARS and pandemic influenza, concerns a healthcare worker's 'duty to treat' contagious patients when this poses risks of infection, and perhaps death, to the healthcare worker him-/herself.[13] Many believe that facing such risks is part of a healthcare worker's job, just as it is a fire-fighter's job to face risks fighting fires, and that healthcare workers implicitly consent to such risk taking when they take up this type of employment. The duty in question is also often explicitly stated in health professions' codes of conduct. It is sometimes additionally argued that the duty is established via social contract. Healthcare workers receive special, often exclusive, education and training, and they are granted other privileges by society; the expectation is that they will provide health care, when needed, in return.[14] If trained health professionals refuse to provide care in times of emergency, there is no one else to turn to.

Although it is plausible that healthcare workers do, in fact, have such duties, they often have other, potentially conflicting, duties as well. If a healthcare worker becomes ill or dies as a result of treating this particular patient, for example, then he/she may not be able to treat other patients to whom he/she also has duties, and he/she may not be able to fulfil duties to family members or other loved ones. Healthcare workers also have duties to co-workers. Health-care provision involves teamwork, and if a worker refuses to work, someone else will be called in to do the job. If all workers refuse, the healthcare system will no longer function. Solidarity is, therefore, called for.[15] While duties to other patients and family members may conflict with the duty to treat a particular (contagious) patient, the duty to fellow co-workers may support it. How to resolve conflict between duties is a difficult philosophical question.

Another philosophical question concerns the limit to the duty to treat. Like the obligation to avoid infecting others, the duty to treat should not be considered absolute (even if there were, by hypothesis, no conflicting duties). Virtually everyone denies that a healthcare worker should be expected to treat if it is known that treating would (likely) be a death sentence for the healthcare worker. But what if the risk of death for the healthcare worker was 50%, 20%, 10% or 1%? For what X should a healthcare worker be expected to treat, so long as the risk of death for the healthcare worker is less than X%? The answer presumably depends on the expected effectiveness of treatment.[16] The more likely that treatment would save the patient's life, the greater the level of risk that healthcare workers should be

expected to face to provide treatment (which is not to say that healthcare workers should be expected to provide treatment even when the risks are especially high). However, they should not be expected to face as much risk when treatment would likely be futile or merely palliative.

Assessing the duty to treat in the event of a major flu pandemic would apparently require assessment of: (1) the risk to the healthcare worker in light of the particular strain of flu involved; and (2) the likely efficacy of treatment. In the context of HIV/AIDS, Daniels persuasively argued that refusal to treat AIDS patients involved invidious discrimination because the risks were less than those already routinely faced by healthcare workers.[17] In the event of a flu pandemic, it will be important to assess whether or not, or the extent to which, risks exceed those which are already tolerated. Given that the duty also depends on effectiveness of treatment, evidence regarding likely efficacy of treatment against the particular strain of flu will be wanted. Early in a pandemic involving a novel strain of pathogen, however, such evidence may be unavailable. Even if it was possible to specify the limits of the duty to treat, it is unclear what expectations should be in cases involving uncertainty, i.e., about whether or not the limits to the duty to treat have actually been exceeded.

Some of these quandaries could be avoided if working conditions were safer to begin with. Improving infection control in hospitals by increasing availability of respirators and isolation wards with negative pressure ventilation systems, for example, would make healthcare provision less dangerous. If society expects healthcare workers to provide care during times of emergency, it is reasonable for healthcare workers to expect health systems to minimize dangers. Healthcare workers willing to face dangers may also deserve higher pay and/or priority in the provision of drugs, vaccines and ventilators. Harmed healthcare workers—or their families, in the event of death—should likewise receive financial compensation. These are matters for reciprocity.[18]

Allocation of Scarce Medical Resources

In the event of a major flu pandemic, it is likely that there will be insufficient supplies of drugs, vaccines and ventilators for everyone who needs them. What principle(s) should determine allocation of resources under such circumstances, and who, if anyone, should receive priority? Resources might, for example, be allocated by lottery or on a first come, first served basis. Or allocation decisions might aim to save the most lives, to treat those who are 'worst-off,' to treat those who are most likely to recover, or to treat those who are most socially productive.[19]

The Australian Health Management Plan for Pandemic Influenza gives vaccine priority 'first to people at high risk of exposure to the virus and providing essential services, then to people most vulnerable to severe illness from infection.'[20] During the maintenance phase of a pandemic, healthcare workers at high risk of exposure would receive antivirals (for prophylactic purposes) continuously. It is estimated that this would consume 65% of (2006) stockpiles in just 12 weeks.[20]

There are numerous reasons for thinking that healthcare workers should be prioritized in the allocation of scarce medical resources in the event of a pandemic. As indicated above, this may compensate them for providing services under risky conditions and/or for harms suffered as a result. Prioritizing healthcare workers might also be justified on the grounds of social utility, i.e., because healthy healthcare workers will be needed in order to fight a pandemic. It is true that many others, including politicians and bus drivers, also play important social roles, but it would be impractical to prioritize each according to the importance of his/her social function.[21] However, if it is practical and appropriate to prioritize those who play special roles regarding the pandemic emergency under consideration, in addition to healthcare workers, we might aim to prioritize 'pandemic responders' more generally. Grave-diggers, for example, would play an especially important role, and those familiar with the history of the 1918 pandemic (when there was a serious shortage of such people) would recognize reasons for keeping them healthy too.

Supposing that healthcare workers and/or other pandemic responders should receive priority in the allocation of medicine, a further question is how much priority they should receive. If a major rationale behind the Australian plan is that healthcare workers should be prioritized because they are needed to fight the pandemic, then it may be counterproductive to have them consume such a large portion of the medicine supply. If the bulk of the medicine supply is used up by healthcare workers, they would not be able to fight the pandemic after all because there would be little or no medicines for them to provide treatment with!

Another popular idea is that the young should receive priority when allocation of resource decisions are made. Emanuel and Wertheimer, for example, argue for prioritization of the young on the grounds of a 'life-cycle allocation principle, based on the idea that each person should have an opportunity to live through all the stages of life.'[19] A similar idea underlies what is sometimes referred to as the 'fair innings' argument, which suggests that everyone is entitled to some 'normal' span of life years. According to this argument, younger people have stronger claims to life-saving interventions than older people because they have had fewer opportunities to experience life.[22] The idea that everyone should get the chance to enjoy a normal span of years, or to live through all the stages of life, appeals to considerations of fairness. The suggestion that one might be 'entitled' or have a right to such things, however, is controversial.

It is therefore important to recognize an additional, perhaps more powerful, reason for prioritizing the young when making allocation of resource decisions. As, other things being equal, saving a young person would generally lead to greater reduction in the burden of disease, there are straightforward utilitarian reasons for prioritizing the young. Burden of disease is usually measured in DALYs (disability adjusted life years).[23] The DALY is a 'health gap' measure of the number of years of healthy life lost to morbidity and mortality. The earlier in life a disease kills someone, the greater the number of life years that are lost (assuming that, as in the most recent Global Burden of Disease study, age weighting is not used in DALY calculations). Other things being equal, saving a younger person rather than an older person will avert a greater number of DALYs. If (as seems plausible) distribution of resource decisions should aim at maximal disease burden reduction, then fair innings considerations could play a role in age weighting, i.e., years of life lost in early life could be weighted more heavily than years of life lost later in life when DALY calculations are made. Without going into a technical discussion of DALYs, the point being made here is that there may be two distinct important reasons for prioritizing the young: (1) saving the young will save more years of healthy life; and (2) 'saving one year of life for a young person is valued more than saving one year of life for an older person'[22] (if the fair innings argument and/or the 'life-cycle allocation principle' is sound).

Coercive Social Distancing

Coercive social distancing measures such as isolation and quarantine raise some of the most controversial ethical issues associated with pandemic disease. As noted above, such measures are sometimes important to the protection of public health, but they conflict with basic rights/liberties. How should a balance be struck between the two?

Although rights to liberties such as freedom of movement are important, they must sometimes be over-ridden when the danger to society as a whole is sufficiently severe. How great, then, must the threat to public health be for confinement of an individual to be justified? For what disease burden X would confinement of an individual be justified (for a given period of time), so long as the free movement of the individual would (on average be expected to) lead to disease burden X?[24] This is the key philosophical question raised by coercive social distancing measures, but it is rarely identified in such terms. Although answering this question with precision would be difficult, for now it suffices to say that the stakes would need to be high for coercion to be justified. Contra utilitarianism, rights should not be violated whenever this would benefit society as a whole.

Second, for coercive social distancing measures to be justified, there would need to be good evidence that they are likely to be effective in the context under consideration. The effectiveness of such measures, however, is notoriously difficult to study, and effectiveness will vary from context to context. Gostin claims that isolation and quarantine would probably only have an early and limited role in the case of a major flu pandemic.[25] This might usually

be true on large continents, but islands (and other isolated environments) may be a different story. History suggests that long-term social distancing was highly effective in American Samoa during the 1918 flu pandemic.[26] As the ethical acceptability of coercive social distancing depends on evidence regarding efficacy, there is an ethical imperative to carry out more research that explores the empirical basis for these policies.

How much evidence would be needed to justify the use of coercive social distancing measures? Kass argues that '[a]s a rule of thumb, the greater the burdens posed by a [public health] programme for example in terms of cost [or] constraints on liberty, the stronger the evidence must be to demonstrate that the program will achieve its goals.'[27] The more basic the right or liberty at stake, therefore, the higher the level of evidence that should be needed before imposing intrusive public health measures. As freedom of movement is one of the most basic rights, one might conclude that isolation and quarantine require the highest level of evidentiary justification, i.e., systematic review/meta-analysis on the Cochrane scale of evidence-based medicine.[28] Although it is plausible that (other things being equal) higher levels of evidence should be attained before infringing upon the most basic rights, the magnitude of utility threatened is another relevant consideration. If anecdotal evidence strongly suggests that isolation and quarantine may be necessary to save thousands or millions of lives, and if this is all the evidence there is to go on, it may be imprudent to insist on the highest level of evidence (which would be especially difficult to come by during early stages of an epidemic involving a novel strain of disease). The greater the amount of utility that is threatened, therefore, the lower the level of evidence that should be demanded before imposing coercive social distancing measures.

Third, it is commonly argued that the 'least restrictive' means should be used to achieve healthcare goals. A related idea is that coercive isolation and quarantine should only be used as a 'last resort.' If the latter entails that all other (less restrictive) measures must be tried before resorting to isolation and quarantine, this may not be feasible, because in the event of a public health emergency, there might not be time to try everything else that just might have worked. It is plausible, however, that we should use the least restrictive means that there is good reason to believe will be effective in achieving the goal in question. If there is reason to believe that voluntary quarantine would be just as effective as coercive quarantine, then we should not resort to the latter. Again, more research is needed to establish evidence about what would be the least restrictive (effective) means in various circumstances. Fourth, if it is determined that their use is necessary, coercive social distancing measures must be used in an equitable manner. One idea is that they should not be used, as they have in the past, in a discriminatory fashion against the marginalized and dis-empowered. Another idea is that the grounds for their use must be strongest when those being considered for confinement are among the worst-off groups of society. Just as research ethics aims to provide special protection for vulnerable members of society, the ethics of isolation and quarantine should arguably do the same.

Fifth, confinement should be minimally burdensome. Those subjected to isolation and quarantine should be made as comfortable as possible, and they should be provided with basic necessities and health care insofar as possible. A related point is that those who are coerced should receive financial compensation for inconvenience, lost wages (if they are unable to work), and simply for having their liberty restricted. Coercive social distancing is only justified if it results in net benefits to society as a whole. Some of these benefits should be returned to the victims of coercive measures. In the absence of compensation, those coerced would suffer a disproportionate share of the burdens required to benefit society, and this would be unfair. Compensation is a matter of reciprocity.[28] In addition to promoting fairness, a system of compensation would likely promote trust in the public health system and cooperation with public health policy.[29] Given the importance of trust to the success of public health programmes, compensation may have substantial health benefits.

Conclusion

This review of ethical issues associated with pandemic disease highlights ways in which the issues turn on both empirical and philosophical questions in need of further research and analysis. Although those with an interest in health ethics have traditionally focused on philosophical and/or legal questions, the importance of the empirical questions that the ethical questions turn on should not be underestimated. This suggests that those concerned with health ethics should, in addition to engaging in philosophical analysis, play a greater role in identifying ethically important empirical questions and advocating that relevant research gets done. A message for scientists is that there are many empirical questions which are not only scientifically important but also crucial to the making of ethically sound policy. This should be taken into consideration when scientific/empirical research projects are chosen. Given the potential consequences of a major flu pandemic, for individuals and society as a whole, the need for sound policy is especially pressing.

Notes

1 Selgelid MJ. Ethics and infectious disease. *Bioethics* 2005;19:272-89.

2 Price-Smith AT. *The health of nations: infectious disease, environmental change, and their effects on national security and development*. Cambridge, MA: MIT Press; 2001.

3 Ziegler P. *The black death*. 2nd ed. London: Penguin; 1998.

4 Iseman MD. Evolution of multi-drug resistant tuberculosis: a tale of two species. *Proc Natl Acad USA* 1994;91:2428-29.

5 Kolata G. *Flu*. London: Pan Books; 2001.

6 Oldstone MBA. *Viruses, plagues, and history*. New York: Oxford University Press; 1998.

7 Smith CB, Battin MP, Jacobson JA, Francis LP, Botkin JR, Asplund EP, et al. Are there characteristics of infectious disease that raise special ethical issues? *Dev World Bioeth* 2004;4:1-16.

8 World Health Organization. A safer future: global public health security in the 21st century. *World Health Report* 2007. Geneva: World Health Organization; 2007. p. 5.

9 National Intelligence Council. The global infectious disease threat and its implications for the United States. National Intelligence Council. Available at:

http://www.cia.gov/cia/reports/nie/report/nie99-17d .html; 2000 [accessed 18.11.2003].

10 Harris J, Holm S. Is there a duty not to infect others? *BMJ* 1995;311:1215-17.

11 Verweij M. Obligatory precautions against infection. *Bioethics* 2005;19:323-35.

12 Dworkin R. *Taking rights seriously*. Cambridge, MA: Harvard University Press; 1977.

13 Malm H, May T, Francis LP, Omer SB, Salmon DA, Hood R. Ethics, pandemics, and the duty to treat. *Am J Bioeth* 2008;8:4-19.

14 Huber SJ, Wynia MK. When pestilence prevails: physician responsibilities in epidemics. *Am J Bioeth*:W5-11. Available at: http://www.bioethics .net/journal/ j_articles.php?aid¼463, 2004;4 [accessed 10.12.2007].

15 Reid L. Diminishing returns? Risk and the duty to care in the SARS epidemic. *Bioethics* 2005;19:348-61.

16 Selgelid MJ, Chen YC. Specifying the duty to treat. *Am J Bioeth* 2008;8:26-27.

17 Daniels N. Duty to treat or right to refuse. *Hastings Cent Rep* 1999;21:36-46.

18 University of Toronto Joint Centre for Bioethics. Stand on guard for thee: ethical considerations in preparedness planning for pandemic influenza. University of Toronto Joint Centre for Bioethics Pandemic Influenza Working Group. Available at: http://www .utoronto.ca/jcb/home/documents/pandemic .pdf;2005 [accessed 10.12.2007].

19 Emanuel EJ, Wertheimer A. Who should get influenza vaccine when not all can? *Science* 2006;312:854-55.

20 Australian health management plan for pandemic influenza. Commonwealth of Australia. p. 37. Available at: http://www.health.gov.au/internet/main/publishing.nsf/Content/851B7469ADF70118CA257202 001E8989/$File/ahmppiprint.pdf; 2006 [accessed 01.06.2008].

21 Verweij M. Equitable access to therapeutic and prophylactic measures. Draft paper for Working Group One (20 October 2006), WHO Project on Addressing Ethical Issues in Pandemic Influenza. Available at: http://www.who.int/eth/ethics/PIEthicsdraftpaper WG12oct06.pdf [accessed 26.12.2008].

22 World Health Organization. Ethical considerations in developing a public health response to pandemic influenza. Available at: http://www.who.int/csr/ resources/publications/WHO_CDS_EPR_GIP_2007 _2/en/index.html [accessed 01.06.2008].

23 Murray CJL. Rethinking DALYs. In: Murray CJL, Lopez AD, editors. *The global burden of disease: a comprehensive assessment of mortality and disability from diseases, injuries and risk factors in 1990 and projected to 2020*. Cambridge, MA: Harvard School of Public Health on Behalf of the World Health Organization and the World Bank; 1996. p. 1-98.

24 Selgelid MJ. Ethics, tuberculosis and globalization. *Public Health Ethics* 2008;1:10-20.

25 Gostin L. Public health strategies for pandemic influenza: ethics and the law. *J Am Med Assoc* 2006; 295:1700-04.

26 Crosby AW. *America's forgotten pandemic: the influenza of 1918*. 2nd ed. Cambridge: Cambridge University Press; 2003.

27 Kass NE. An ethics framework for public health. *Am J Public Health* 2001;91:1776-82.

28 Verma G, Upshur REG, Rea E, Benatar SR. Critical reflections on evidence, ethics and effectiveness in the management of tuberculosis: public health and global perspectives. *BMC Med Ethics*:2. Available at: http://www.biomedcentral.com/1472-6939/5/2, 2004; 5 [accessed 01.06.2008].

29 Ly T, Selgelid MJ, Kerridge I. Pandemic and public health controls: toward an equitable compensation system. *J Law Med* 2007;15:318-24.

54.
MEDICINE'S DUTY TO TREAT PANDEMIC ILLNESS: SOLIDARITY AND VULNERABILITY

Howard Brody and Eric N. Avery

SOURCE: *Hastings Center Report* 39.1 (2009): 40-48.

In the wake of SARS and with the possibility of bioterror, pandemic avian influenza, and other emerging infections looming, bioethicists are exploring the extent of a health professional's duty to treat the victims of such an infectious outbreak, even at some substantial risk to the caregiver's own health or life. The World Health Organization announced in August 2003 that 20 percent of all persons known to have been infected with SARS were health care workers. Three of the forty-one people who died of SARS in Canada were health professionals, as were six of the 180 who died in Taiwan.[1] Dr. Carlo Urbani of Médecins Sans Frontières, who with others initially identified SARS as a new infectious disease in Hanoi, voluntarily quarantined himself and eventually died of SARS, leaving a widow and three children.[2] Should we regard Dr. Urbani as a medical hero, or as a physician simply doing his duty?

Physicians' moral duties arise from at least two sources. As members of society, they owe the same general duties to others as any citizen. In addition— as one of us has previously argued—they assume a further set of moral duties connected with the nature of medicine as a practice. By announcing to the community that they are practitioners of medicine, physicians implicitly accept and undertake these duties.[3] Although the core features of the internal morality of medicine persist over time, the interpretations of these duties are not static and are implicitly renegotiated with society as the practice of medicine evolves.[4]

The internal morality of medicine consists of both goals and ethical side constraints. The goals of medicine, which physicians ought to promote, include healing and curing but also extend to prevention, rehabilitation, palliation, reassurance, and health education. The side constraints distinguish the appropriate from the inappropriate ways of pursuing those goals. Physicians should be technically competent and truthful about the nature of their craft, avoid causing harm that is disproportionate to anticipated benefits, and serve as loyal patient advocates.[5]

Our account of the internal morality of medicine provides a prima facie answer to whether physicians have a duty to treat pandemic illness. All members of society have an ethical duty to rescue others in dire need of help when they are in a position to do so. Physicians arguably have a role-specific duty of rescue by virtue of their medical competence to provide the help that victims of infectious outbreaks require. The goals of medicine include curing when possible and minimizing patients' suffering when curing is not possible. Physicians are duty-bound as fiduciaries to the interests of their patients. It therefore appears that physicians cannot, with integrity, refuse to serve the victims of an infectious outbreak out of fear of contracting the disease. This duty to treat is strengthened by organizational structures related to professional status that assign to physicians exclusive control over many resources and skills needed to assist patients, such as the right to prescribe medication. Having effectively denied non-physicians the means to assist victims of pandemics, physicians appear even more duty-bound to help. This prima facie account, however attractive initially, turns out on further exploration to be insufficient to sustain a robust duty to treat. Recent work that attempts to apply lessons from the SARS outbreak to a possible avian influenza pandemic provides some illumination. The discussion must be broadened from physicians to include not only all health professionals, but also the nonprofessional service workers without whom any hospital would soon cease to function.[6] The health care worker's other obligations, especially for the care of family members, must be considered alongside duties owed to patients. Finally, a deeper account of the professional's duty to treat will eventually have to address in detail important concerns of social solidarity. Three levels must be addressed: Solidarity among health workers within institutions, solidarity between health professionals and the community, and the commitment of the community as a whole to its most vulnerable members.

Justifying a Duty to Treat

Despite the strong prima facie case for a robust duty to treat, providing an ethical justification for this duty has proved more daunting than many anticipated. Laurence McCullough, for instance, offers one of the few systematic treatments of physicians' legitimate self-interests that counterbalance their professional responsibilities. He includes among these interests sufficient time to engage in hobbies and other leisure activities.[7] If hobbies constitute an ethically acceptable self-interest, preserving one's own life would seem to be a more compelling one. But recognizing that interest would pull the rug out from under any meaningful duty to treat in the face of substantial risks to life and health.

Many assume that the historical traditions of medicine provide at least a partial justification for a strong duty to treat. Careful analysis of the historical record, however, reveals a decidedly mixed picture.[8] Between the early nineteenth and the mid-twentieth centuries in the United States, a duty to treat even at considerable personal risk was widely accepted by physicians. Before that, from late medieval times into the eighteenth century, physicians commonly fled the city when an epidemic struck.

If the historical record is univocal on any point, it would seem to be that the duties that physicians accepted were contingent upon the physicians' place and role in society, and on a negotiation between the medical profession and the community at large. Usually this negotiation was implicit, but occasionally it was conducted explicitly. For example, when plagues afflicted Europe between the fourteenth and seventeenth centuries, the civic authorities often compensated for the flight of the town's regular physicians by paying enough to attract a cadre of "plague doctors" to replace them.[9]

The AIDS crisis of the 1980s surprised those who had assumed that the duty to treat still held. They did not anticipate the effect of the soothing myth, promulgated during the 1960s, that epidemics had been conquered and so risking death while treating patients was no longer a part of the physician's job description. Told that there was a small chance of contracting a disease thought then to be 100 percent fatal from treating an HIV-positive patient, at least some younger physicians said in effect, "Wait a minute—I never signed up for this." This disconnect between traditionally accepted ethical obligations and actual physician behavior led to a flurry of ethical analysis. Data showing that the risk of patient-to-physician transmission was very low quickly provided justification to those arguing for a strong duty to treat.[10] But because of this, when a disease like SARS struck, carrying a much higher risk of falling ill and dying from patient contact, the ethical dialogue around HIV/AIDS turned out largely to be beside the point. The advent of SARS revealed another serious limitation to the ethical tradition of a strong duty to treat. When American physicians endorsed this duty as it was expressed in early versions of the American Medical Association Code of Medical Ethics, they took a number of things for granted. For instance, they assumed physicians would be male. If they had families, then they also had wives, who were presumed to be primarily responsible for the care of hearth and home while the men attended to professional duties and business interests. If an epidemic struck the town, men could remain at their posts while their wives took the children to a place of safety.[11] Physicians who share equal duties for the care of dependents and possible travel restrictions that might keep an entire family at home or within the confines of the city were not contemplated as part of the ethical "contract" between physicians and society.

The SARS epidemic also highlights the ethical importance of the notion of emerging infectious diseases. In the case of a future pandemic, some health professionals (like Dr. Urbani in Hanoi) will become involved at the earliest stages simply because they are on duty; they will care for the first patients unaware that a pandemic has even begun. Others will be expected to commit themselves to serve at an early stage of the outbreak and to follow through on that commitment, especially if an entire hospital is quarantined and staff are prohibited from leaving. At the time a commitment to treat is made, either by circumstance or by choice, the data on the disease's actual rates of transmission and mortality will not yet be known.[12] These circumstances suggest how slippery it is to try to base a duty to treat on the precise extent of the risks, even if in principle the degree of risk seems highly relevant to the extent of the ethical duty.

Duty to Treat: Current Status

Neither our initial prima facie statement of physician obligation nor the account of the historical ethical tradition has proven sufficient to ground a robust duty to treat in the face of significant risks. In the face of this relative ethical disarray, a number of analyses have now appeared that examine the health professional's duty in the face of an infectious disease posing risks comparable to SARS or to the threatened pandemic of avian influenza.[13] To focus our discussion we will look particularly at two works derived from the SARS experience in Canada.[14]

The Pandemic Influenza Working Group of the Joint Centre for Bioethics at the University of Toronto addressed a health worker's duty to treat by appealing to substantive and procedural values. Of ten substantive values that generally should inform a community's response to the threat of pandemic influenza, it selected four as specifically informing the duty-to-treat issue. The four values it identified were the duty to provide care; reciprocity, or society's duty to support those who assume disproportionate burdens to protect the public good; trust, both between patients and providers and between the community and public health authorities; and solidarity among health professionals, within the community, and among nations when fighting a pandemic. It defined this last value specifically as "collaborative approaches that set aside traditional values of self-interest or territoriality among health care professionals, services, or institutions."[15]

The remaining six substantive values that the working group identified were individual liberty, protection of the public from harm, proportionality, privacy, equity, and stewardship. It stated that though these values may be very helpful when applied to other ethical issues such as quarantine and allocating scarce resources, they are not directly pertinent to a duty to treat. In contrast, the group found the procedural values it identified to be equally applicable to all ethical issues that arise in a pandemic, including the duty to treat. These values specify that a community's pandemic policy should reflect procedures that are reasonable, open and transparent, inclusive, responsible, and accountable. The group further recommended that professional organizations should instruct their members regarding their duty to treat in pandemic via codes of ethics. Government and the health sector, in turn, should guarantee that all means are used to protect health workers' safety, that risks are spread among workers equitably, and that provision is made for workers and their families, including disability and death benefits.

At first glance, the working group's approach appears consistent with the model of physicians' moral duties with which we began. Relying on codes of ethics promulgated by professional organizations suggests that discernment of duties is in some sense internal to the various health professions. The values of reciprocity, trust, and solidarity recognize that this internal discernment is nevertheless in tension with a process of negotiation between health professionals and the larger community. The list of procedural values suggests that, ideally, this negotiation would occur explicitly instead, assuring its openness, transparency, and accountability. The group argues that this, in turn, would engender enhanced trust, which it highlights as one of the substantive values directly informing a duty to treat.

Nevertheless, one might object to several features of the working group's account. Readers—especially those in the United States—will note that the group's overall list of substantive values includes "individual liberty" and "proportionality." Individual liberty is invoked to assure that in a public health emergency, coercive measures such as quarantine are used only when absolutely necessary.[16] Proportionality dictates that individual liberty is compromised only to the extent necessary to address the true threat. It would seem implicit in this analysis that when risk is high and public health measures cannot adequately protect the individual from it, the individual then has a right to remove herself from the risk situation, provided that she can do so without directly causing excess risks to others around her. If this reading is correct, then health providers might well wonder why the working group has seen individual liberty and proportionality as relevant only to members of the public, and not to health workers themselves. Why did it not include these two values on the list of values relevant to the duty to treat?

The working group similarly appears ambivalent in invoking solidarity and the procedural values. The existence of a duty to treat and whatever limits of qualifications might apply to it do not appear to be a matter for negotiation; professional societies will simply instruct practitioners that this duty exists and must be adhered to. While it might well be true that the general public expects health professionals to adhere to such a duty, is there nothing to be said about its expected limits? We assume, for instance, that in the case of firefighters, community representatives can agree on a level of immediate risk to life that would countermand the duty to reenter a burning building to try to rescue those trapped inside.[17] If the success of the rescue is highly unlikely, the risk cannot be justified—there is, after all, no advantage simply to having more dead firefighters. But the model presented by the working group envisions no such negotiation between health professionals and the public that they serve.

The suggested model, moreover, appears potentially destructive to one key level of solidarity—the solidarity that exists among health workers within a facility such as a hospital. If each separate professional group must individually instruct its members on the duty to treat, how can we assure that these duties are articulated in complementary ways for all the workers who must cooperate if care is to be effective? How can we assure that kitchen staff, housekeepers, and others who are unlikely to be members of a professional organization feel a similar duty to stay at their posts, since the work of the hospital would quickly grind to a halt without them? A professional balkanization of

an ethical duty to treat does not appear to be a promising start.

The Toronto working group's analysis takes us only part way toward an adequate defense of a duty to treat on the part of all essential health workers. The group has identified the key moral values at stake. Yet the application and implications of all the relevant values remain only partially developed.

Solidarity within Institutions

Lynette Reid proposes that Canadian health workers faced with the risk of SARS generally provided exemplary patient care, in many cases rising to a level we would term heroic. They did so not by carefully calculating that the risk of SARS fell within some prespecified boundary where the duty to treat took precedence over self-preservation. Instead, Reid attributes the workers' behavior primarily to a sense of solidarity within the institution—what one might paraphrase as "we are all in this together." Any worker who contemplated avoiding duty in the name of personal safety could look over and see the fellow professional whose workload would be doubled as a result. When one of these workers then fell sick, her fellows took pride in being the first to offer care to her.[18]

Despite the aptness of the term in this situation, Reid is concerned about the label "hero" because she thinks that it is bad policy to rely on heroism to get us through foreseeable crises. She writes:

> We must not expect individual moral heroism to do work that is best spread around: the obligation is on all of us to create and sustain a healthcare system that does not leave the provision of our care dependent upon extreme actions of self-sacrifice by a limited group. Epidemics do create occasions for moral heroism—but it is incumbent upon us as a society not to multiply unnecessarily the conflicts between self-interest and altruism or beneficence that our healthcare system presents individuals with, in order to enjoy the sight of a great deal of moral heroism.[19]

To this end, it is worth noting that organizations, as well as individuals, can be virtuous. A virtuous organization encourages and nurtures the virtuous behavior of the individuals within it. At the very least, the virtuous organization avoids creating unnecessary barriers to the virtuous behavior of individuals. Generally, an individual is morally accountable for her own level of virtue. If she is forced to work within a peculiarly vicious organization, however, we may withhold much of the blame that we would otherwise attach to her failure to act virtuously.

Reid argues that within optimally virtuous health care systems, we will see many more professionals and other staff freely assuming a duty to care, thus assuring that we do not exploit a small cadre of heroes.[20] The working group continues this line of thought, stating that both government and health systems have a role to play in promoting this level of virtue. When institutions and the surrounding community step forward to assure workers that their own needs and the needs of their families will be looked after, workers will presumably be much more likely to provide care.[21]

Consider the example of a nurse who is caring for an elderly parent in her home.[22] Told to come to work in the face of a pandemic that could result in her being quarantined within the hospital for an indefinite period of time, and where her life would be put at risk, is she a bad person if she weighs her professional obligations against her duties to care for those who depend upon her at home? According to McCullough's analysis, a health provider who could simply abandon her mother at home in the name of adhering to an abstract professional duty might not be the sort of human being we would wish to care for us, at least in normal times.[23] If, on the other hand, the hospital and the surrounding community had put a good deal of effort into organizing an assistance program that would provide care for the mother in such a situation, there is a much greater likelihood that the nurse would show up for work.[24] Within a virtuous institutional and community setting, she would not need to swim against a stiff current in order to act virtuously herself.

In one touching anecdote related by Dianne Godkin and Hazel Markwell in their 2003 report, *The Duty to Care of Healthcare Professionals*, a hospital staff member who faced the dual challenges of caring for SARS patients and being unable to leave the facility due to quarantine reported that the most meaningful event of her day was a phone call from a member of the Department of Family Medicine who simply asked how she was and if she needed anything.[25] This anecdote suggests how relatively simple the actions required to sow a sense of solidarity may be that can move people toward exemplary care of the sick in the face of personal risk and considerable inconvenience.

Solidarity between Profession and Community

Sociologists of the professions have long employed a conceptual model by which "society" and "the profession" enter into an implicit negotiation. Society grants the profession powers and privileges—notably monopoly control over its practice and considerable freedom from outside regulation. Laypeople look up to members of the profession. In exchange, the profession agrees to accept some degree of sacrifice—it places the interest of its patients and the general public above its own. A crude expression of this concept as pertains to physicians could be put this way: You run the risk of dying in the event of an infectious outbreak; we will admire you for it, and incidentally allow you to achieve an income level considerably above the average.

Samuel Huber and Matthew Wynia adopt this basic sociologic model and employ a value of reciprocity similar to the Toronto working group's when they suggest that "expectation of some reciprocal social obligations" are one factor that "should contour the duty to treat."[26] They hold that the reciprocal social obligations are: 1) provision of adequate protective precautions and equipment to prevent the disease from spreading to caregivers and their families; 2) guarantees of care for professionals who become ill; 3) reduced malpractice threats for physicians who accept the duty to treat; and 4) reliable compensation for the families of caregivers who die in the line of duty.[27]

The professional-society relationship may play a crucial role in determining the presence and scope of a duty to treat. It is especially distressing to read that in Taiwan—and to a lesser extent in Canada—health workers who rose to their professional responsibilities and cared for SARS patients later encountered social ostracism because others in the community feared that they and their families were potential sources of contagion.[28] It may seem quaint to us today to read the section of the American Medical Association 1847 code of ethics that lists ethical duties owed by the patient and the community to the physician. Yet these Taiwanese and Canadian communities failed in their ethical duties to their health workers in a significant way. A society or a community cannot make fearful people act sensibly. But it can express, in no uncertain terms, the appreciation felt toward the workers and the irrationality and indecency of community ostracism.

Reid, as we have seen, accepts the desirability of these reciprocal measures. But she also argues that at least two things are wrong with this standard sociologic model. The first is the dual problem of the threatened balkanization of the different professions and the exclusion of nonprofessional but essential health workers that would undermine the value of solidarity among workers within the health care institution. Second, she claims that the standard model of the "social contract" between society and profession is too constraining. She suggests that the core question is:

> Does any of us, knowing our own human vulnerability to disease and death, prefer to live in a society that provides healthcare to people with infectious disease, or in a society that leaves epidemics to run their course and devastate the population, or in a society that practices a form of quarantining of the ill without treatment, leaving them to die in isolation?[29]

This more basic question—What sort of a society do we want to live in?—cannot be negotiated between the society and a professional group. It is a question for the society to answer in some fashion as a whole, and professionals must participate in the decision as members of society first and foremost.

Social Solidarity and Care of the Vulnerable

The question of what sort of society we want to live in challenges all of us, including the health profes-

sionals, to decide whether we will pull together in the face of pandemic threats, or whether we will allow our communities to deteriorate into what Hobbes called "the war of all against all." In the United States, the answer so far is that we wish to promote community solidarity when such threats arise. But doubt still remains as to whether by this we mean the entire community, or only those segments of the community that are, under normal circumstances, already best served by both the health care sector and other governmental services. At a time when resources are scarce and the public is eager for scapegoats, vulnerable populations who have all along been least well served by the health care system are in danger of being even further neglected and victimized.[30]

The response to Hurricane Katrina in 2005 is not reassuring in this regard. It seems clear in hindsight that government planning focused on those who had the means to flee on their own. Planning was woefully deficient for those who lacked such means. Within the regional health system, it also seems clear in hindsight that disaster and evacuation planning took inadequate account of the needs and obstacles experienced by vulnerable and minority populations.[31] For these reasons, a critical test of true social solidarity and social justice is whether we are willing to put the needs of vulnerable, underserved populations first. Dr. Margaret Chan of Hong Kong, upon being confirmed as the new head of the World Health Organization in 2007, implicitly suggested such a commitment: "I want us to be judged by the impact we have on the health of the people of Africa and the health of women."[32]

Two ethical theories converge to require this primary attention to the needs of the most vulnerable. Rawls's difference principle, a critical component of his overall scheme of "justice as fairness," stipulates that social and economic inequalities can be justified only when they specifically work to improve the lot of the least-advantaged classes of citizens. To say that a rising tide lifts all boats is not enough. One is obligated to pay attention to the boats that carry the least advantaged to be sure that they indeed rise and are not swamped by the rising waters; otherwise the advantages enjoyed by the yachts of the better-off classes must be condemned as unjust.[33]

A similar view, justified on very different grounds, is conveyed by the teachings of liberation theology.[34] According to this version of Christian moral perspective, people will ultimately be judged primarily according to how well they treat the most vulnerable and neglected among society.

On either of these views, a just system of pandemic preparedness planning would begin by cataloguing all the ways in which vulnerable populations are likely to be neglected and stigmatized. It would then create provisions to prevent those outcomes even before it begins to plan to serve the larger number of more-advantaged people in need.[35] The health professional's duty to treat is enhanced and deepened when placed upon such a foundation of social solidarity. Health workers now can be confident that they are not tending to the needs of a privileged slice of the population while a much needier group of potential patients has been excluded from their care.

Concern for social solidarity, as evidenced by plans to care for the most vulnerable, returns us to both the procedural values argued for by the Toronto working group, and to one of its substantive values that we have not yet discussed—trust.[36] A common characteristic of populations neglected by the health care system in the past is their greater distrust of that system. This is a potentially dangerous situation in a pandemic. If the public health authorities announce ways to prevent the spread of the emerging infection, but members of the vulnerable community have no trust in these authorities, they are unlikely to act as directed. The lack of trust will lead both to excess death and morbidity in the vulnerable community, and to a reservoir of infection that can spread to other communities as well.[37]

By contrast, suppose that the public health officials are motivated by the model of social solidarity we have described. To assure that the actual needs of the vulnerable are addressed in the preparedness planning, they must engage the community in a process of open dialogue and inquiry. This process, adhering to the five procedural values recommended by the working group, will go a long way toward reestablishing trust between the authorities and the previously neglected communities. Moreover, this approach to preparedness planning will engender a greater level of trust across the entire society. Each

person will see that even if he loses his job or his money or whatever status now gives him assurance that he can get what he needs out of the health care system, he will not be neglected in a pandemic. Yet so far, the process of pandemic preparedness planning utilized in the United States and elsewhere fails to include the level of community involvement and dialogue that would lay the groundwork for optimal trust and solidarity in the face of an infectious outbreak.[38]

A Duty Shared

A solid ethical basis for the health professional's duty to treat the victims of emerging infectious diseases, even at some level of personal risk, has proven elusive. We began by arguing that some moral obligations of physicians could be discerned as part of an internal morality, rooted in medicine's nature and goals. We stipulated also that this internal morality was not eternal and static, but, rather, responsive to medicine's changing social environment.

A more careful analysis of the duty to treat has provided us with an illustration of what this "social responsiveness" might entail. A full account, we claim, will have to incorporate the various types or levels of social solidarity that are important in a duty to treat. This understanding, in turn, will create a central role for social justice and for the care of vulnerable populations. We also see the importance of social reciprocity in facilitating the virtuous behavior of individual health care workers and their institutions.

The analysis has also shown the limitations of addressing a duty to treat as if it were the exclusive province of any individual health profession. If an institution like a hospital is to respond satisfactorily to a pandemic, a duty to treat will have to be accepted by its physicians, by other health professionals, and by service and support personnel who are not usually viewed as professionals and who have no professional codes of ethics to refer to. We began this discussion with an account of medical morality that encouraged physicians to look inward at the fundamental goals and means that made them a unique profession. If each occupational group in health care looked only inward in this fashion, it is very unlikely that we would arrive at a satisfactory conclusion.

All health care providers need to look outward, both at themselves collectively and at society as a whole.

In sum, we have discovered no single ethical foundation for a duty to treat that would be commensurate with the needs posed by an emerging infectious disease pandemic. The model of the internal morality of a profession, the historical account of physicians' duties, and considerations of solidarity each provide a necessary element. We have focused on the importance of solidarity because it seems to have been neglected in the literature until quite recently.

The examples of community-wide pandemic preparedness planning with which we are familiar have not, for the most part, been conceived of as exercises in ethics and solidarity-building.[39] The materials we have reviewed on pandemic preparedness too often speak of the need to "instruct" or "educate" health workers or members of the community, rather than engaging them in dialogue in order to consider seriously their views and concerns. We argue that this dimension of preparedness should be emphasized in future efforts. If the more pessimistic predictions of when we may face an avian influenza or similar outbreak are correct, we do not have much time.

Notes

1   D.H. Hsin and D.R. Macer, "Heroes of SARS: Professional Roles and Ethics of Health Care Workers," *Journal of Infection* 49 (2004): 210-15.

2   B. Reilley, M. Van Herp, D. Sermand, and N. Dentico, "SARS and Carlo Urbani," *New England Journal of Medicine* 348 (2003): 1951-52.

3   E.D. Pellegrino, "Toward a Reconstruction of Medical Morality: The Primacy of the Act of Profession and the Fact of Illness," *Journal of Medicine and Philosophy* 4 (1979): 32-56; H. Brody and F.G. Miller, "The Internal Morality of Medicine: Explication and Application to Managed Care," *Journal of Medicine and Philosophy* 23 (1998): 384-410.

4   F.G. Miller and H. Brody, "The Internal Morality of Medicine: An Evolutionary Perspective," *Journal of Medicine and Philosophy* 26 (2001): 581-99.

5   Miller and Brody, "The Internal Morality of Medicine: An Evolutionary Perspective." The discussion in that article is restricted to therapeutic medicine and excludes medical research and public health. Our

main focus in this article is the duty to treat among physicians (and other health care practitioners) involved in the clinical care of individual patients. Naturally, in a pandemic situation, public health efforts will play a very important role, and cleanly distinguishing the therapeutic from the public-health roles of physicians and nurses will be difficult.

6   The wide range of workers involved is suggested in a recent report by the U.S. Occupational Safety and Health Administration (OSHA): "The delivery of healthcare services requires a broad range of employees, such as first responders, nurses, physicians, pharmacists, technicians and aides, building maintenance, security and administrative personnel, social workers, laboratory employees, food service, housekeeping, and mortuary personnel. Moreover, these employees can be found in a variety of workplace settings, including hospitals, chronic care facilities, outpatient clinics (e.g., medical and dental offices, schools, physical and rehabilitation therapy centers, health departments, occupational health clinics, and prisons), free-standing ambulatory care and surgical facilities, and emergency response settings." Occupational Safety and Health Administration, U.S. Department of Labor, Pandemic Influenza Preparedness and Response Guidance for Healthcare Workers and Healthcare Employees (OSHA 3328-05, 2007), 5, http://www.osha.gov/Publications/OSHA_pandemic _health.pdf.

7   L.B. McCullough, "The Physician's Virtues and Legitimate Self-Interest in the Patient-Physician Contract," *Mount Sinai Journal of Medicine* 60 (1993): 11-14.

8   A.R. Jonsen, *A Short History of Medical Ethics* (New York: Oxford University Press, 2000), esp. p. 46; A. Zuger and S.H. Miles, "Physicians, AIDS, and Occupational Risk. Historic Traditions and Ethical Obligations," *Journal of the American Medical Association* 258 (1987): 1924-28; D.M. Fox, "The Politics of Physicians' Responsibility in Epidemics: A Note on History," *Hastings Center Report Special Supplement* 18, no. 2 (1988): S5-S10.

9   Fox, "The Politics of Physicians' Responsibility."

10 J.H. Kim and J.R. Perfect, "To Help the Sick: An Historical and Ethical Essay Concerning the Refusal to Care for Patients with AIDS," *American Journal of Medicine* 84 (1988): 135-38. It seems evident today

that the unwillingness of many physicians to treat AIDS victims in the 1980s actually had little to do with the statistical risk of infection, and much more to do with the social stigma attached to the groups among which the victims were disproportionately found. We will not address this aspect of the historical record. The ways in which diseases like SARS and influenza spread tend to minimize the element of social stigma in the public response to an epidemic, but we should not underestimate the tendency of a society under threat to degenerate into stigmatization and ostracism, as evidenced by recent calls in the United States to exclude illegal immigrants as a potential source of infection.

11 We are grateful to Laurence McCullough for stressing this point in a personal communication.

12 L.O. Gostin, R. Bayer, and A.L. Fairchild, "Ethical and Legal Challenges Posed by Severe Acute Respiratory Syndrome: Implications for the Control of Severe Infectious Disease Threats," *Journal of the American Medical Association* 290 (2003): 3229-37.

13 C. Ruderman, C.S. Tracy, C.M. Bensimon, et al., "On Pandemics and the Duty to Care: Whose Duty? Who Cares?" *BMC Medical Ethics* 7, no. 1 (2006): E5; C.C. Clark, "In Harm's Way: AMA Physicians and the Duty to Treat," *Journal of Medicine and Philosophy* 30 (2005): 65-87; S.E. Straus, K. Wilson, G. Rambaldini, et al., "Severe Acute Respiratory Syndrome and Its Impact on Professionalism: Qualitative Study of Physicians' Behavior During an Emerging Healthcare Crisis," *BMJ* 329 (2004): 83; D. Godkin and H. Markwell, *The Duty to Care of Healthcare Professionals: Ethical Issues and Guidelines for Policy Development* (Toronto, Ontario, Canada: University of Toronto Joint Centre for Bioethics, December 2003); G.C. Alexander and M.K. Wynia, "Ready and Willing? Physicians' Sense of Preparedness for Bioterrorism," *Health Affairs* 22 (2003): 189-97; S. Huber and M.K. Wynia, "When Pestilence Prevails ... Physician Responsibilities in Epidemics," *American Journal of Bioethics* 4, no. 1 (2004): W5-W11; P.A. Singer, S.R. Benatar, M. Bernstein, et al., "Ethics and SARS: Lessons from Toronto," *BMJ* 327 (2003): 1342-44; R. Jones, "Declining Altruism in Medicine" (Editorial), *BMJ* 324 (2002): 624-25; M.W. Chaffee, "Making the Decision to Report to Work in a Disaster: Nurses May Have Conflicting Obligations,"

American Journal of Nursing 106, no. 9 (2006): 54-57; D.K. Sokol, "Virulent Epidemics and Scope of Healthcare Workers' Duty of Care," *Emerging Infectious Diseases* 12 (2006): 1238-41.

14 Pandemic Influenza Working Group, Stand on Guard for Thee: Ethical Considerations in Preparedness Planning for Pandemic Influenza (Toronto, Ontario, Canada: University of Toronto Joint Centre for Bioethics, November 2005), http://www.utoronto.ca/jcb/home/documents/pandemic.pdf; L. Reid, "Diminishing Returns? Risk and the Duty to Care in the SARS Epidemic," *Bioethics* 19 (2005): 348-61. See also University Health Network, University of Toronto, "SARS Key Learnings from the Perspective of the University Health Network: Notes for the Campbell Commission," http://www.uhn.ca/About_UHN/what_is_UHN/docs/campbell_presentation_100103.pdf (accessed June 2, 2007). The entire Campbell Commission report on the Canadian SARS experience can be found at http://www.sarscommission.ca/report/index.html.

15 Solidarity as a value might also be characterized as an alternative to an exclusive focus on individual rights and choices; see, for example, S.R. Benatar, A.S. Daar, and P.A. Singer, "Global Health Ethics: The Rationale for Mutual Caring," *International Affairs* 79 (2003): 107-138.

16 While quarantine may be the first disease containment strategy that comes to mind, experts on emerging infections such as avian influenza argue that generally more effective strategies might be decreased social mixing and increased social distancing, such as closing large public gathering places, schools, and so forth. Civil confinement, including quarantine, would be a more intrusive measure to be restricted to special needs. See, for example, L.O. Gostin, "Public Health Preparedness and Ethical Values in Pandemic Influenza," in *The Threat of Pandemic Influenza: Are We Ready?* Workshop Summary, ed. S.L. Knobler, A. Mack, A. Mahmoud, and S.M. Lemon (Washington, DC: National Academies Press, 2005), 357-71.

17 Singer et al., "Ethics and SARS"; Sokol, "Virulent Epidemics"; E.J. Emanuel, "Do Physicians Have an Obligation to Treat Patients with AIDS?" *New England Journal of Medicine* 318 (1988): 1686-90.

18 Reid, "Diminishing Returns?" Reid herself speaks less of "solidarity" and more of broad vs. narrow

social contracts, virtues, and just systems. Nevertheless, we believe that the term is apt.

19 Reid, "Diminishing Returns?" 359. The Canadian SARS Commission agreed: "The health system's capacity to protect its workers was in a state of neglect.... There was no system in place to prevent SARS or to stop it in its tracks. The only thing that saved us from a worse disaster was the courage and sacrifice and personal initiative of those who stepped up—the nurses, the doctors, the paramedics and all the others—sometimes at great personal risk, to get us through a crisis that never should have happened. Underlying all their work was the magnificent response of the public at large: patient, cooperative, supportive." SARS Commission Executive Summary: Spring of Fear, volume one, 2-3, http://www.sarscommission.ca/report/v1-pdf/Volume1.pdf (accessed June 2, 2007).

20 Reid, "Diminishing Returns?"

21 Pandemic Influenza Working Group, Stand on Guard for Thee.

22 Chaffee, "Making the Decision to Report"; B.P. Ehrenstein, F. Hanses, and B. Salzberger, "Influenza Pandemic and Professional Duty: Family or Patients First? A Survey of Hospital Employees," BMC Public Health 6 (2006): 311.

23 McCullough, "The Physician's Virtues."

24 The OSHA report notes that current assumptions used for a national pandemic influenza strategy include a 30 percent attack rate across the United States. Of those who are ill, half will seek medical attention, and they will have a work absentee rate of up to 40 percent. The report seems to view the 40 percent absentee figure as applying to health care workers along with the rest of the population. OSHA, Pandemic Influenza Preparedness, 37-38.

25 Godkin and Markwell, The Duty to Care.

26 Huber and Wynia, "When Pestilence Prevails," W9.

27 Ibid.

28 M.A. Rothstein, M.G. Alcalde, N.R. Elster, et al. Quarantine and Isolation: Lessons Learned from SARS. A Report to the Centers for Disease Control and Prevention (Louisville, KY: University of Louisville School of Medicine Institute for Bioethics, Health Policy and Law, November 2003), http://louisville.edu/bioethics/public-health/SARS.pdf; L.M. Hall, J. Angus, E. Peter, et al. "Media Portrayal of Nurses' Perspectives and Concerns in the SARS Crisis in Toronto," Journal of Nursing Scholarship 35 (2003): 211-16; D. H-C. Hsin, "SARS: An Asian Catastrophe Which Has Challenged the Relationships between People in Society—My Experience in Taiwan," Eubios Journal of Asian and International Bioethics 13 (2003):106-08.

29 Reid, "Diminishing Returns?" 354.

30 Bellagio Group, "The Bellagio Meeting on Social Justice and Influenza. Bellagio Statement," (Baltimore, MD: Johns Hopkins Berman Institute of Bioethics, July 2006), http://www.hopkinsmedicine.org/bioethics/bellagio/statement.html.

31 D.P. Eisenman, K.M. Cordasco, S. Asch, et al., "Disaster Planning and Risk Communication with Vulnerable Communities: Lessons from Hurricane Katrina," American Journal of Public Health 97, Suppl. 1 (2007): S109-S115.

32 M. Shuchman, "Improving Global Health—Margaret Chan at the WHO," New England Journal of Medicine 356 (2007): 653-56, at 655.

33 J. Rawls, A Theory of Justice (Cambridge, MA: Harvard University Press, 1971), 75-83.

34 P. Farmer, Pathologies of Power: Health, Human Rights, and the New War on the Poor (Berkeley, CA: University of California Press, 2003): 139-59.

35 Bellagio Group, "Bellagio Statement."

36 Pandemic Influenza Working Group, Stand on Guard for Thee.

37 American observers of the Canadian SARS experience have emphasized the importance of trust: "When containment measures such as quarantines must be put in place, establishing the trust of the public is crucial to their effectiveness. Social cohesion and compliance with the SARS quarantine in Toronto, for example, has been attributed in part to a combination of clear communication and practical guidance by public health authorities." Learning from SARS: Preparing for the Next Disease Outbreak. Workshop Summary, ed. S. Knobler, A. Mahmoud, S. Lemon, et al. (Washington, DC: National Academies Press, 2004), 207.

38 J. Kotalik, "Preparing for an Influenza Pandemic: Ethical Issues," Bioethics 19 (2005): 422-31.

39 Trust for America's Health, Ready or Not? Protecting the Public's Health from Diseases, Disasters, and Bioterrorism (Washington, DC: Trust for America's Health, December 2006), http://healthyamericans.org/reports/bioterror06/BioTerrorReport2006.pdf.

55.
DIMINISHING RETURNS?
RISK AND THE DUTY TO CARE IN THE SARS EPIDEMIC

Lynette Reid

SOURCE: *Bioethics* 19.4 (2005): 348-61.

SARS placed healthcare workers' lives and health at risk to a degree that has not been seen in generations. It tested public health systems[1] and it tested the courage of many individual medical professionals.[2] Such a crisis also tests the ethical self-understanding of healthcare professionals and the general public: are the stories we tell ourselves about the nature of our moral obligations and the frameworks we employ for moral reasoning consonant with the reality of situations where our obligations come into play and we make moral choices?

Bioethicists and healthcare professionals have debated the duty to care both in particular cases and in its general outlines. The emergence of HIV/AIDS in the late 1980s was the occasion of a vigorous debate that sought to define the framework for evaluating the existence of a particular duty to care.[3] More broadly, ethicists have reflected on the nature of the duty to care as related to professional virtues or principles, such as beneficence and altruism. Reflection on the experience of healthcare workers during the SARS epidemic offers valuable new lessons about the importance of context in our understanding of the relationship between risk and duty; attention to context is helpful as well in developing a measured understanding of the roles altruism and heroism might play in the social and medical response to an epidemic.

The Legacy of the HIV/AIDS Debate: Defining Acceptable Levels of Risk

Debates concerning risk and obligation usually revolve around a certain hypothetical moral agent: an autonomous individual who pursues immediate self-interest by natural inclination and enlightened self-interest by rational conviction. The questions that we might suppose such an autonomous individual would want answered to establish his or her duty to care for infectious patients would be, first, what is the degree of risk entailed by occupational exposure? And second, is that level of risk the same as or lower than the level implicitly accepted in the choice for employment as a healthcare professional?[4]

With such an agent presupposed in the debates around duty to care in the early days of HIV/AIDS, a consensus emerged that any risk comparable to the risk of an infectious disease to which healthcare professionals were already exposed would fall within their duty to care.[5] It was established that the risk was in fact equal to or well below the known risk of Hepatitis B infection (the risk of contraction being much lower but the risk of death if contracted being much higher); such a risk was sufficiently minimal to establish a duty of care for the American Nursing Association, but the American Medical Association still had to wrestle with the question of how that duty to accept a certain risk fit with the right they claim as autonomous professionals to accept or reject patients at will. The resolution of the dilemma came through the definition of HIV-infected persons as persons with disability: it would be invidious discrimination to refuse them medical care, according to the AMA's final stand on the issue in 1987.[6]

Huber points out that the duty to care articulated in the HIV/AIDS debate was a weak one, strong enough only to do the political job in the face of HIV/AIDS.[7] Such an appeal to minimal risk, as Freedman argues, leaves open the question of whether healthcare professionals are obligated to accept more than a minimal risk.[8]

According to the framework of the HIV/AIDS debate, obligation sinks with rising levels of risk and there is a level of risk at which the duty to care no longer holds. It is surprising then to read bioethicists presenting the unquestioning assumption of a duty to care on the part of healthcare workers during SARS as an affirmation of the outcome of the HIV/AIDS debate. Emanuel claims that healthcare workers rose to the occasion in SARS as the direct result of the HIV/AIDS debate:[9] as he tells the story, a generation of medical students was brought up under sway of the outcome of the HIV/AIDS debate, hence in full consciousness that adopting their chosen profession implies the willingness to take personal risks in the line of duty. Clark, writing in a similar vein, casually subsumes SARS under 'some degree of risk' that commitment to a medical profession implies.[10] However, if one understands the relationship between risk and obligation as inversely proportionate, as the HIV/AIDS debate claimed, the most striking feature of the SARS epidemic is that healthcare professionals did not abandon their posts en masse in the face of strong evidence that their service placed them at significant risk of illness and death.[11] While healthcare workers in the US actually report a lower level of HIV infection than the general population,[12] and 23% of American residents surveyed would nonetheless, if given the choice, avoid the very small risk of HIV infection,[13] in SARS, anywhere from 3% (in the United States) to 43% (in Canada) of those falling prey to the deadly infectious disease were healthcare workers—with a case fatality ratio of approximately 15%, but much higher for those over 65.[14]

The lesson of SARS is in fact contrary to the conclusion drawn from the HIV/AIDS debate: risk and obligation do not stand in an inverse relationship. The factors playing into ethical decision-making are not exhausted by an 'implicit contract' defined by past risk level accepted. A debate about duty to care in the context of an epidemic asks whether it is fair to expect of healthcare workers that they take on a risk of personal injury or death and the burden of psychological stress associated with that risk in order to provide care.[15] There are two constraining features given in the context of such a debate that were not evident during HIV/AIDS. One constraining feature is that the risk has its source in something that does not itself respond to claims of fairness: the biological reality of an epidemic. The individual and autonomous risk-calculator is also a biologically vulnerable human being, and as such encounters risk not only by choice but also by chance. The other constraining feature is the social context: to a significant extent, the risk refused by one individual is left to be absorbed by someone else, whether within the healthcare professions or in the society as a whole. In this sense, the individual and autonomous risk-calculator negotiating a fair distribution of risks does confront agents who do respond to claims of fairness, but these agents ipso facto assert their own claims of fairness in turn.[16]

Writers in the HIV/AIDS debate imagined that the limits of obligation would be reached when we reached a certain level of risk. SARS took us to vastly increased levels of risk, but at the same time showed that risk is both biologically given and socially distributed. The choice is not between past risk levels and current risk levels, but between accepting current risk levels and passing them on to someone else—and particularly because of the elevated risk for healthcare workers, that 'someone else' in SARS was not a hypothetical doctor, whom the HIV-positive patient was left to find on his own, but a known colleague in the hospital setting. SARS did raise the question of duty to care for each individual healthcare worker but ipso facto raised the question: if not me, then who?

Such a question points to the issue of distribution of risk within the healthcare community. It also points to the broader question of the social response to medical necessity: if physicians and nurses do not care for those who are critically ill, then who will? Is there supposed to be some other group in our society who are more appropriately trained and more deeply obligated to serve in case of a medical emergency? If the choice instead is for quarantine and abandonment to death, then on what basis are the military or police, who presumably would carry out such a policy, any more obligated to risk their lives in carrying it out than medical personnel are obligated to risk theirs in providing care?

Professionalism and Duty to Care: Broadening the Social Contract

It has been argued traditionally that the special commitment of doctors to a high standard of altruism and beneficence, and hence to a duty to care even at risk to themselves, is one side of the social contract between the profession and society at large. Contracts offer benefits in exchange for services rendered: the benefits doctors seek in exchange for recognizing a duty to care have been proposed to be self-regulation,[17] or the high status and generous remuneration of the profession, such as it is in wealthy societies. Clark, for instance, writing from (but not officially on behalf of) the ethics office of the AMA, praises the selfless service of doctors in the face of SARS,[18] but alerts us in the subsequent exchange of letters[19] that this service is perhaps not as selfless as it appears: he characterizes this 'selfless service' as something of a bargaining tool, and claims that the good that doctors bargain for with this service is their status as independent practitioners, self-regulating, and beholden to no outside social body. This issue of professional self-image played a role in the HIV/AIDS debate, as we saw, making it more difficult for the AMA than the ANA to arrive at a policy statement affirming duty to care. The determination of some physicians to preserve their independent status and avoid any arrangement that might turn them into 'employees' makes it difficult for them to accept politically an articulation of a duty to fulfil social needs at all. It is more agreeable, after all, to do good out of generosity than because one is expected or compelled to.[20]

While such arguments present self-regulation and status as the professional privileges offered in exchange for physicians' trust-inspiring recognition of the duty to care, surely the professional privilege most relevant to duty to care is exclusive scope of practice. Why would society grant exclusive scope of practice in relation to an essential human service to a professional group not prepared to guarantee provision of that service in an emergency? The social contract forming the professions leaves us no one but licensed healthcare professionals to turn to in an emergency.

While the existence of exclusive scope of practice speaks for a strong duty to care, it does not capture the whole basis of duty to care. An approach that focuses on the social contract defining the physicians' profession neglects the fact that doctors are not the only ones who are called upon to accept risk and psychological distress while serving in the face of an infectious epidemic like SARS. Nurses, paramedics, and hospital janitorial staff served and died alongside doctors in the SARS epidemic.[21] A basis for duty to care founded only on doctors' or other licensed health professionals' narrow professional self-interests would be inadequate to underwrite the provision of healthcare more broadly. It would also give doctors a motivation for purportedly moral actions that is in fact very thin. Is it plausible that a commitment to the one form of professional governance over another would be a stronger motivation for risk-taking than a commitment to patients or to a social vision about the value of caring for the ill?[22]

A more basic and universal social contract emerges from reflection on the following question: does any of us, knowing our own human vulnerability to disease and death, prefer to live in a society that provides healthcare to people with infectious disease, or in a society that leaves epidemics to run their course and devastate the population, or in a society that practises a form of quarantining of the ill without treatment, leaving them to die in isolation?[23]

The advantage of recognizing a broader social contract underlying the duty to care is that it brings all involved in supporting, maintaining, and running a healthcare facility under its umbrella, so that we can recognize that all healthcare workers—from medical to administrative to maintenance staff—face a common risk and burden of psychological distress, and face relevant moral dilemmas. Indeed, some of them face these dilemmas with less luxury of choice, less economic and social reward, less information and hence less safety derived from information, than the doctors whose special moral obligations bioethicists have traditionally sought to define.

In addition, such basic social reflection extends to the general public in our role of supporting the healthcare system both during an epidemic and in times where there is no crisis. The public supports a world where the ill are cared for when they pay taxes or vote for governments that support the healthcare system, or pay into an insurance fund. Similarly, we support the provision of care in an epidemic when we trust public health's risk assessment enough to greet and shake the hand of our neighbour who works in healthcare and is not in quarantine. Health-care workers felt it deeply when their neighbours avoided and isolated them and their families.[24] We expected them, at considerable personal risk, to trust public health and infection control measures in accepting their workplaces as 'safe enough' under the circumstances; when the general public infor-mally quarantined those who were not quarantined, we failed to extend such trust, at very slight risk to ourselves, to express our support of them in concrete and human ways. In doing so, we violated what ought to be a shared commitment to enacting a social value.

Virtues, Principles, and Duty to Care: Heroism and Altruism

It is undeniable that healthcare workers exhibited the virtues of heroism and altruism in the face of danger during the SARS epidemic. Nonetheless, a critical perspective is needed on the theoretical and practical work we expect personal commitment to high moral standards to do. Are altruism and heroism particular virtues of medical professionals? What role should we expect them to play in ensuring care during infec-tious epidemics?

In a paper that set the tone for decades of debate in ethics, J.O. Urmson argued that moral theory needs to be able to make the distinction between the good that we expect of one another (our duties) and the good that one may hope for or aspire to or admire in others but that is above and beyond the call of duty and outside the realm of ordinary socially-enforced obligations, i.e., the supererogatory.[25] Although Urmson intended the example of heroism to make a meta-ethical point by establishing the existence in ordinary moral thought of a category awkward for philosophy, philosophers responded by vigorously debating the existence, character, and implications of the supererogatory: the heroic or saintly as such came under critical scrutiny.

Some philosophers who might be counted as advocates of heroism have argued that Urmson was mistaken in claiming that the actions of saints ought not of necessity inspire us to emulate them, either to do acts that express the same virtues though perhaps more modestly than the extreme acts of heroes,[26] or to become heroes ourselves.[27] Others have argued for a more critical attitude towards the heroic, argu-ing that supererogatory acts are not always com-mendable,[28] that the heroes and saints who perform them are not necessarily exhibiting a superior variant of ethical agency,[29] and, following Kant, that an eth-ical theory that places an emphasis on heroic acts endorses a dubious form of ethics where one makes up for day to day neglect of duty with the occasion-al large magnanimous gesture.[30] Saints may be bent on developing their own moral perfection to the point where other important human qualities are lost. Acts that appear to be supererogatory may be fool-ish, self-destructive, or indicative of a lack of healthy self-esteem.

Urmson himself distinguished the doctor who works long hours and tends to her fiduciary obliga-tions in the ordinary course of her practice, i.e., the doctor acting out of duty where the duty of the pro-fession is (arguably) onerous in comparison with other professions, from the doctor acting above and beyond the call of duty in joining Doctors Without Borders. While philosophers are circumscribed and critical in their discussions of supererogation, and distinguish beneficence as a professional virtue of medicine from a heroic degree of beneficence, some bioethicists and healthcare professionals have taken up the notion of supererogation to argue that doctors should understand their adoption of the profession as the adoption of a supererogatory level of commit-ment to the altruistic ideals of medicine,[31] even to the point of arguing that accepting pay for one's work is dubious and taking holidays suspect.[32]

R.S. Downie, on the other hand, has long disputed the notion that doctors have a special moral calling, and that the practice of medicine is in any sense especially beneficent or altruistic. We expect our doctors to work to the best of their ability to benefit rather than harm us just as we expect this of our auto mechanics, and the fact that they are reasonably remunerated for their efforts means that it strains language to describe the practice of medicine in itself as 'altruistic.'[33] It is not uncommon to identify ethics entirely with one's obligations to others, in effect construing one form of moral failure (selfishness) as expressing the basic character of all moral failure. Judith Andre has argued, contrary to this assumption about the nature of morality, that one's obligations to oneself are no less moral in character than one's obligations to others.[34] Just as one can be unjust towards others, or dishonest with them, so one can be unjust towards oneself, or dishonest with oneself, and that would constitute moral failing. Carol Gilligan has argued that there are two directions of moral growth: for the person to whom self-regarding actions come more easily, to learn to take the needs of others into account; for the one to whom other-regarding actions come more easily, to learn to treat oneself as equally worthy of care and respect.[35]

The supererogation debate alerts us to the dangers of heroism; other developments in moral philosophy offer a tempered view of altruism. The fabled noble sacrifice of doctors in eras past may have come at too high a cost to family commitments and personal health.[36] Medicine is for the most part no longer practised by individual doctors in private settings; emergency care in a deadly epidemic in particular could never be handled on such a model. The provision of healthcare is the task of a complex sector involving many agents. Where the culture at large once expected the individual charity of individual doctors to meet the healthcare needs of those who might otherwise go without treatment for financial reasons, insurance systems, governments, and taxpayers have taken on the responsibility of enabling access to care by means that do not require healthcare professionals to face a stark conflict between the promptings of conscience and the necessities of earning a living. We also need systems-level responses to the needs of those who may go without treatment for reason of the danger of infection that they pose to others. To treat the duty to care as a matter of individual moral commitment to altruism, beneficence, or supererogatory action is to ignore the responsibility we all share to create and maintain structures that support people in fulfilling their duties as healthcare professionals and workers in the healthcare sector.

These considerations do not imply that healthcare workers ought to be selfish rather than altruistic, but that the simple opposition between altruism and selfishness impedes rather than aids our understanding of duty to care. Nor is it to deny that the challenge SARS posed for the healthcare system was in fact met by acts of heroism and altruism on the part of healthcare professionals and all workers involved in the operation of the healthcare system, or even to claim that such crises can be met without heroes. The point is rather to place these acts of heroism in a broader context where the strengths and limitations of heroism can be appreciated. Posing the issue of duty to care solely in terms of an obligation to others in conflict with self-interest[37] fails to capture the real moral dilemmas faced by healthcare workers in an infectious epidemic.

While accepting risk in the line of duty was not controversial among healthcare workers during SARS, moral dilemmas arose for those who felt their obligations as healthcare professionals conflicted with their obligations to others as family members and caregivers.[38] In addition, infection control measures were not only physically stressful,[39] but also gave staff the very difficult requirement, contrary for many of them to temperament and to their training in professional ethics, that they delay or deny treatment to patients in order to take the time to suit up and protect themselves.[40] Identification of duty to care with altruism makes invisible moral conflicts between the various parties to whom a person may owe care, and interferes with the need of healthcare professionals to understand and accept that they must take all possible measures consistent with the social need for a functioning healthcare system to protect themselves in an epidemic. The obligation to noble self-sacrifice seems incompatible with insisting on proper protective equipment and psychologically sustainable working arrangements.[41] Medical ethics should not make invisible that learning to care for oneself can for some people at some moments be an ethical task, in the way we more commonly assume that learning to care for others is, and that acting in concert with others to ensure that the group to which one belongs is not unfairly burdened can likewise be the expression of a social value that is to be lauded.

I have argued above that the duty to care arises from a broad rather than narrow social contract: the systems that care for the ill, both in the ordinary course of things and in epidemics, are the creation of a broad range of workers and stakeholders. If we as taxpayers vote consistently for governments that cut healthcare budgets, or as consumers in market systems make choices that drive healthcare professionals into unsustainable working situations—and then expect the individual, morally-mandated heroic effort of overworked healthcare workers in over-burdened systems to save us from the consequences of such policies and choices in the event of emergencies, then we are not fulfilling our duties as a society. We must not expect individual moral heroism to do work that is best spread around: the obligation is on all of us to create and sustain a healthcare system that does not leave the provision of our care dependent upon extreme actions of self-sacrifice by a limited group. Epidemics do create occasions for moral heroism—but it is incumbent upon us as a society not to multiply unnecessarily the conflicts between self-interest and altruism or beneficence that our healthcare system presents individuals with, in order to enjoy the sight of a great deal of moral heroism. The ordinary course of life and the contingencies of natural and biological disasters can generally be counted on to supply a sufficient number of opportunities for supererogatory deeds, however much support we offer health-care workers.

Just Systems

We need a range of ethical concepts that enable us to distinguish social and individual decisions, and to relate the social and the individual in a sophisticated and realistic manner. To consider the social question is to ask what range of options we have for response as a society to infectious epidemics. What is our ideal? In SARS we were able to approximate an ideal in which full medical care was provided for all those who fell ill. What would be the constraints that might, in more severe situations, prevent us from attaining that ideal? Those constraints include but are not limited to the degree of risk to which individual workers within the healthcare system are prepared to subject themselves. Crucially, they will include weighing the possibilities against alternative options and the costs of those alternatives, a theme remarkably absent from the HIV/AIDS debates.[42] What are the consequences of not providing medical care to the ill? Who would manage the spread of an epidemic if healthcare professionals could not do so, how would they manage it, and how would we understand their obligations to do so?

The question of how that risk is to be distributed is a complex mix of pragmatics and considerations of justice: Fox reminds us that traditionally epidemics have not been met with the expectation that all doctors serve equally, but with the financing of cadres of 'plague doctors,' or with the exploitation of existing pools of military medical personnel (in the flu epidemic after the First World War) who are habituated to following orders and accepting risk.[43] During SARS, the hospitals adopted a variety of voluntary and compulsory means of fulfilling their duty to care for SARS patients.[44]

Within a social response to infectious epidemic, decisions on the individual level and the ethics of these decisions remains a live topic: what levels of risk are we prepared to ask individuals to suffer, and what levels of risk are they or we prepared to accept? How much risk individuals are prepared to assume will depend less on the past level of risk assumed than the HIV/AIDS debate led us to believe. SARS taught us that elevated levels of risk strengthen rather than weaken duty to care—insofar as the question is one of a social distribution of a biologically-given risk within the workplace, and in society at large.

Notes

1   A. Campbell. 2004. The SARS commission interim report: SARS and public health in Ontario. Toronto. Commission to investigate the introduction and spread of SARS in Ontario; D. Walker. 2003. For the public's health: initial report of the Ontario expert panel on SARS and infectious disease control. Toronto. Ministry of Health; D. Naylor. 2003. Learning from SARS: renewal of public health in Canada: a report of the National Advisory Committee on SARS and Public Health. Ottawa. Health Canada.

2   D.H. Hsin et al. Heroes of SARS. *Journal of Infectious Diseases* 2004; 49: 210-215.

3 See for instance G.J. Annas. Legal risks and responsibilities of physicians in the AIDS epidemic. *Hastings Center Report* 1988; 18: S26-S32; J.D. Arras. The fragile web of responsibility. *Hastings Center Report* 1988; 18: S10-S20; D.M. Fox. The politics of physicians' responsibility in epidemics. *Hastings Center Report* 1988; 18: S5-S10; A. Zuger et al. Physicians, AIDS, and occupational risk. *JAMA* 1987; 258: 1924-1928.

4 See for instance N. Daniels. Duty to treat or right to refuse? *Hastings Center Report* 1991; 21: 36-46; E.J. Emanuel. Do physicians have an obligation to treat patients with AIDS? *NEJM* 1988; 318: 1686-1690. I leave aside the well-known philosophical difficulties of the notion of implicit consent.

5 This standard for acceptable levels of risk does not stand up to rigorous philosophical scrutiny: Why should someone's acceptance of a risk level x imply acceptance of a risk level 2x? The calculation did establish that the right to turn away an HIV/AIDS patient on the basis of risk was no greater than the right to turn away a Hepatitis B patient, hence giving credence to the charge that refusing care to an HIV/AIDS patient would be an act of discrimination.

6 B. Freedman. Health professions, codes, and the right to refuse to treat HIV-infectious patients. *Hastings Center Report* 1988; 18: S20-S25.

7 S.J. Huber et al. When pestilence prevails. *American Journal of Bioethics* 2004; 4: W5-W11.

8 Freedman, op. cit. note 6, p. 22.

9 E.J. Emanuel. The lessons of SARS. *Annals of Internal Medicine* 2003; 139: 589-591.

10 C.C. Clark. In harm's way. *Hastings Center Report* 2003; 33: inside back cover.

11 G. Farrow. SARS in health care workers. *CMAJ* 2003; 169: 1147; S.E. Straus et al. Severe acute respiratory syndrome and its impact on professionalism. *BMJ* 2004; 329: 83.

12 D.M. Bell. Occupational risk of human immunodeficiency virus infection in healthcare workers: an overview. *American Journal of Medicine* 1997; 102: 9-15.

13 M.F. Shapiro et al. Residents' experiences in, and attitudes toward, the care of persons with AIDS in Canada, France, and the United States. *JAMA* 1992; 268: 510-515; D. Smolkin. HIV infection, risk taking, and the duty to treat. *Journal of Medicine and Philosophy* 1997; 22: 55-74.

14 World Health Organization. 2003. Consensus document on the epidemiology of severe acute respiratory syndrome (SARS). Geneva. World Health Organization.

15 Literature on the psychosocial effects of SARS on healthcare workers includes S. Chan. Nurses fighting against severe acute respiratory syndrome (SARS) in Hong Kong. *Journal of Nursing Scholarship* 2003; 35: 209; R. Maunder et al. The immediate psychological and occupational impact of the 2003 SARS outbreak in a teaching hospital. *CMAJ* 2003; 168: 1245-1251; K. Sim et al. The psychological impact of SARS. *CMAJ* 2004; 170: 811-812.

16 While I present no gender analysis in this essay, this perspective is learned from feminist bioethics. See S. Sherwin. A relational approach to autonomy in health care in S. Sherwin and the Feminist Healthcare Ethics Network, eds. 1998. *The politics of women's health: exploring agency and autonomy*. Philadelphia. Temple University Press: 19-47.

17 C.C. Clark. Trust in Medicine. *Journal of Medicine and Philosophy* 2002; 27: 11-29.

18 Clark, op. cit. note 10.

19 C.C. Clark. Reply. *Hastings Center Report* 2004; 34: 4.

20 Some data on medical students' appreciation of this point: F.W. Hafferty. What medical students know about professionalism. *Mount Sinai Journal of Medicine* 2002; 69: 385-397.

21 D. Koh et al. SARS: health care work can be hazardous to health. *Occupational Medicine* (London) 2003; 53: 241-243.

22 Several physicians who commented on drafts of this paper found distressing the suggestion that duty to care was a professional trade-off rather than a response to human need.

23 The Kantian (universalizing) style of the reflection invited in this question is evident.

24 L.A. Nickell et al. Psychosocial effects of SARS on hospital staff. *CMAJ* 2004; 170: 793-798; D. Walker. op. cit. note 2, pp. 175-176.

25 J.O. Urmson. 1958. *Saints and heroes. In Essays in moral philosophy*. A.I. Melden, ed. Seattle. University of Washington Press: 198-216.

26 Pybus. 'Saints and Heroes.' *Philosophy* 1982; 57: 193-199.

27 D. Heyd. 1982. *Supererogation*. Cambridge. Cambridge University Press.

28 J. Hampton. Selflessness and the loss of self. *Social Philosophy and Policy* 1993; 10: 135-165.

29 S. Wolf. Moral saints. *Journal of Philosophy* 1982; 79: 419-439.

30 M. Baron. Kantian ethics and supererogation. *Journal of Philosophy* 1987; 84: 237-262.

31 A.C. McKay. Supererogation and the profession of medicine. *Journal of Medical Ethics* 2002; 28: 70-73; S.A. McLean. Commentary on Glannon and Ross, and McKay. *Journal of Medical Ethics* 2002; 28: 74.

32 D.C. Thomasma et al. A dialogue on compassion and supererogation in medicine. *Cambridge Quarterly for Healthcare Ethics* 1995; 4: 415-425.

33 See R.S. Downie. Supererogation and altruism: a comment. *Journal of Medical Ethics* 2002; 28: 75-76, and Downie and Gillon's lively 1986 exchange in the pages of the same journal: R.S. Downie. Professional ethics. *JME* 1986; 12: 64-66; *JME* 1986; 12: 195-196; R. Gillon. More on professional ethics. *JME* 1986; 12: 59-60; Do doctors owe a special duty of beneficence to their patients? *JME* 1986; 12: 171-173. W.C. McGaghie et al. Altruism and compassion in the health professions. *Medical Teacher* 2002; 24: 374-378.

34 J. Andre. The equal moral weight of self- and other-regarding acts. *Canadian Journal of Philosophy* 1987; 17: 155-166.

35 C. Gilligan. 1993. *In a different voice*. Cambridge, MA. Harvard University Press.

36 M. Winerip. Did you hear about Doc Ogden? *New York Times Magazine*. May 5, 2004; 42.

37 See, for instance, R. Jones. Declining altruism in medicine. *BMJ* 2002; 324: 624-625.

38 M. Bernstein et al. Challenging beliefs and ethical concepts. *Critical Care* 2003; 7: 269-271; Nickell et al., op. cit. note 24; P.A. Singer et al. Ethics and SARS. *BMJ* 2003; 327: 1342-1344.

39 Nickell et al., op. cit. note 24.

40 Straus et al., op. cit. note 11; Bernstein et al., op. cit. note 38.

41 B. Sibbald. Right to refuse work becomes another SARS issue. *CMAJ* 2003; 169: 141.

42 A substantive consequentialist argument around duty to care in HIV/AIDS did not emerge until 1997, in Smolkin, op. cit. note 13, p. 61.

43 Fox, op. cit. note 3, pp. S5-S10.

44 Sibbald, op. cit. note 41, p. 141.

56.
HIV/AIDS CLINICAL RESEARCH, AND THE CLAIMS OF BENEFICENCE, JUSTICE, AND INTEGRITY

Deborah Zion

SOURCE: *Cambridge Quarterly of Healthcare Ethics* 13.4 (2004): 404-13.

In a recent edition of the *Medical Journal of Australia*, Greg Dore and David Cooper called on persons in developed nations like Australia to bridge the divide between resource-rich countries to nations in the developing world, where therapies to ease or halt the ravages of the virus are nonexistent or in short supply.[1]

Indeed, Rob Moodie has suggested that HIV is an issue that pertains above all to development. He states:

> In sub-Saharan Africa, the single most important risk factor for women is simply being married. For young women in rural Thailand and Laos or Myanmar, the main risk factor is being poor. (p. 6)[2]

HIV is a disease that reveals much to us about both the best and worst of human behavior. About manly courage among gay men, many of whom were themselves unwell, but who cared compassionately for their friends, while establishing sophisticated mechanisms to supply treatment and halt the spread of the disease. But it also reveals the worst, as the virus spreads most rapidly among disempowered persons.

When we consider the world of HIV medical research, we also see the best of ethical practice and, conversely, studies that must be described as ethically questionable. The purpose of this paper is to ask two questions:

1. On what basis can we ground duties that some or all persons here might have toward persons who are participants in HIV clinical trials in the developing world?

2. If we can, how can we go about fulfilling our obligations toward them?

Before I attempt to answer these questions, I want to establish why I think that a great deal of the research in question is, at best, ethically questionable. To do so, I will briefly look at two recent trials that epitomize what is wrong with HIV clinical research in the developing world.

Rakai

The first of the trials in question took place in the Rakai district of Uganda. There were two objectives:

1. to see how other kinds of sexually transmitted diseases affected HIV transmission in heterosexual couples.
2. to see how HIV transmission was affected by viral load.[3]

To test these hypotheses, a cluster of ten villages in the Rakai district of Uganda were selected, and within them 415 couples, in which one partner was negative and the other positive. Investigators gave residents of five of the ten villages antibiotic treatment every ten months, whereas the persons in the control group were given an anthelmintic drug, an iron-folate tablet, and from the second survey round, a single low-dose vitamin pill.[4] At the same time, viral load was monitored and correlated with the rate of new infection. Participants in the trial were provided with condoms and safe sex counseling.

What Then Is Unethical about These Trials?

Subjects who were HIV positive were observed for up to 30 months but not treated. Seropositive partners were interviewed but not informed of their partners' serostatus. Finally, those in the control arm who had treatable sexually transmitted diseases were left to seek their own treatment.[5] But most importantly, the results of the second part of the trial—that the level of viral load has a direct bearing on the rate of new infections—is of absolutely no use to the subjects of the study or their communities, as they cannot afford treatments that will halt the virus or reduce its levels. This trial, on the other hand, is of great use to people in developed countries, where effective antiretroviral treatment is available.

A trial of this kind could not be carried out in a developed country, where a fatal but treatable illness—be it HIV or syphilis—would have had to be treated as part of the trial. But when investigators can rely on the best local standards of treatment, the way is left open for trials that exploit populations in developing countries for the good of the developed world.

The Mombassa Non-Oxynol 9
Phase 3 Preventative Trial

In early 1997, the World Health Organization began a phase 3 trial of vaginal gels to determine their effect in lowering the transmission of HIV among women in Kenya.[6] Consent was obtained from the largely illiterate population. The trial was a double-blind placebo controlled trial, and organizers relied on providing treatment to participants at the best local standard rather than the best international standard. One investigator wrote:

> Anti-retroviral therapy is not routinely available in Kenya. We provide a basic level of primary care to all women in the trial. As the women who acquire HIV-1 are recent seroconverters, they are not yet having HIV related illnesses.[7]

Given that a placebo was used, it is clear that, even if the gels had proved to be 100 percent efficacious, some people would have contracted HIV, for which no treatment was then offered to them. Clinical researchers, however, relied on the idea that the participants were personally responsible for their exposure to the virus, as they received counseling about the importance of condoms, and the condoms most liked by the women were provided free of charge. Women kept a coital log, on which the use of gel and condoms was recorded. Women who were inconsistent in gel and condom use were counseled to use gels and condoms at each sexual encounter.[8]

Despite these interventions, it is clear that cultural practices and economic desperation undermined the provision of condoms. In a recent study, Jackson et al. implied that African women do not receive much cooperation concerning the use of condoms.[9] Their study also points out that "seropositive male partners may be less likely to use condoms if they knew that the woman was participating in a vaccine trial."[10] This last point is particularly pertinent to the argument that being on a trial could actually increase the risk of infection. As well, recent research suggests that the product in question actually increased the women's chances of contracting the virus, as the gel seems to contribute to the development of lesions.[11]

Summary of Ethical Problems

- The trials exploited the desperation of subjects.
- The trials, although applying a formal definition of informed consent, did not take into account a different understanding of the fallibility of Western medicine.
- They did not take into account the power structures inherent within the communities in question, particularly as related to gender.
- The trials produced results that were more applicable for the Western world than the trial population (Rakai).
- The trials actually increased the risk of HIV transmission for some participants, without backup care being offered to them (non-oxynol 9).

The Duty of Beneficence

Let me return to my original questions. How can we establish that we owe anything to persons taking part in such trials? If we can establish such a claim, what is it that we should do? On whom should they fall? To answer these questions I will begin with a discussion of the duty of beneficence.

In his formulation of the duty of beneficence, Peter Singer suggests that:

> if it is in our power to prevent something bad from happening, without thereby sacrificing anything of comparable moral importance, we ought, morally, to do it. (p. 28)[12]

If, for example, we see a child drowning in a shallow pond and have only to sacrifice a few minutes and the slight inconvenience of wet clothes, then we have a duty to give assistance. Singer uses this example as a kind of paradigm, suggesting that in many other situations, such as helping the severely impoverished, rendering aid would cost as little effort, and do as much good, as rescuing the drowning child.

Singer is responding to the assertion that "charity begins at home"—that is, the argument that people close to us either physically or emotionally have some special claim. He argues, on the contrary, that particular attachments of this kind are irrelevant when considering our obligations to others. The only important issue, according to Singer, is that our rendering assistance does not exacerbate a bad situation or in itself bring about comparable harm. Singer's "obligation to assist"[13] has been criticized by many on the basis that it is unrealistically overdemanding.[14] John Arthur, for example, suggests that Singer's formulation produces a duty for healthy people to donate one eye or one kidney, on the grounds that the inconvenience caused to the donating agent is seriously outweighed by the good such organs might do to the blind or dying. What is problematic about this kind of argument is best summed up by Michael Slote, in his discussion of Singer's "duty to assist" when he suggests that persons should not have their major life plans disrupted by the duty to help others.[15] Slote's limitation of the duty makes more sense if we consider the lives of the moderately well off than if we apply it to exploitative millionaires. However, his point—that limits must be set to beneficence—is significant.

The Duty of Beneficence and Collectivity

How then do we set such limits when considering what we might owe others? The bioethicists Beauchamp and Childress respond to the excessive burden objection in their formulation of the duty of beneficence by discussing the way in which collectivity is an important factor in fulfilling the obligation to help others, pointing out that group action both lessens the burden on each individual and also increases the chance that the action undertaken will actually make some difference.

The importance of collective action is also central to Robert Goodin's work *Protecting the Vulnerable*, especially in his discussion of foreign aid and world hunger.[16] He suggests that personal donations to schemes that target individuals like "sponsor a child" do not take into account the massive restructuring that is needed in impoverished communities. Thus, Goodin contends that, when considering aid to the severely impoverished, giving money is not enough—individuals must also engage in political action to organize efficacious schemes.[17] The main advantages of collective action are, therefore, efficacy and an easing of the burden on individual donors, thus once again answering to some degree the "overdemandingness" objection.

The relationship between collectivity and the duty of beneficence is particularly significant because the problems raised by HIV/AIDS trials in developing countries are not limited to research alone and do indeed have the potential to impose a significant burden. I suggest that chronic poverty, and in many cases the lack of political freedoms, meant that a considerable number of subjects were deprived of basic rights and were thus easily exploitable. If we consider Singer's account, then it is easy to establish a duty to donate aid that is logically prior to any obligation that might be engendered by the trials themselves, in the same way that we might have a duty to help any chronically impoverished and deprived population. In the creation of a just world, where basic rights were intact, many of the problems that vex clinical trials would cease to exist. The question of the need to create a more equitable world, however, distracts us from specific problems that beset clinical trials and the important ways in which specific groups of people might respond to them.

Without such a focus, the ongoing issues of exploitation of research subjects might be lost among claims that relate to other kinds of deprivation.

Justice

Singer's work alerts us to the possibility of a different way of functioning in the world, whereas writers like Goodin show us that collective action might resolve some of the "overdemandingness" objection. However, if we focus on issues related to justice, we might see more clearly why some of us might have specific duties to those engaged in the trials in question and what they might look like.

The political philosopher Kok-Chor Tan suggests that "[t]he intricate economic, social, and political interdependencies of the global community draw virtually everyone, some more deeply than others, into social arrangements with each other" (p. 62).[18]

In the case of HIV/AIDS clinical trials, I have already argued that decisions made in the developed world have an important part to play in the ongoing development of unethical research, particularly patents and generic antiretroviral therapy. It follows, then, that those who have benefited from such research have a duty to redress the imbalance that such involvement has caused. Tan, for example, suggests that, if I witness a bank robbery and the thief hands me a wad of $100 bills, I have gained from an unjust act, even though I was neither involved in the robbery nor its intended beneficiary.

This argument is significant in the case of HIV/AIDS trials under discussion, not only because those using the results in question benefit but also because their use of the results—in some cases—is an incentive for such research to continue. Before we can draw such a conclusion, however, we must examine carefully the issue of justice as it is related to HIV/AIDS research and consider some competing formulations of justice that challenge the assumption that there are indeed grounds for the existence of such claims.

Justice: The Problem of Distribution

Many formulations of justice are pertinent to HIV/AIDS research. One of the most significant is that which Allen Buchanan refers to as "justice as fair reciprocity."[19] According to this version of justice, we are entitled to social resources only if we can contribute to the cooperative surplus.[20] Thus, by this account, severely disabled persons, for example, would not be entitled to be allocated resources, as they would never be in a position to enter into schemes that might generate goods.

Other formulations of justice pertinent to clinical trials in developing countries rely on the idea that justice can be equated with compensating people for ill fortune.[21] As Richard Arneson suggests:

> The concern of distributive justice is to compensate individuals for misfortune. Some people are blessed with good luck, some are cursed with bad luck, and it is the responsibility of society—all of us regarded collectively—to alter the distribution of goods and evils that arises from the jumble of lotteries that constitute human life as we know it.[22]

This view of justice as fair distribution is based on the work of John Rawls and has at its heart the idea that persons have intrinsic moral worth and entitlements, regardless of their actual or potential contributions. Central to Rawls's formulation of justice as fairness is the creation of a level playing field, on which equitable relationships can be built. He states:

> All social primary goods—liberty and opportunity, income and wealth, and the bases of self-respect—are to be distributed equally unless an unequal distribution of any or all of these goods is to the advantage of the least favoured.[23]

In many situations, justice as fair reciprocity and the allocation of goods based on a system of equitable distribution can coexist. Buchanan points out that the generation of special rights might come about "through voluntary participation in cooperative schemes."[24] That is, everyone would be entitled to basic rights simply by virtue of personhood, and reciprocal rights when they entered into certain schemes.

When we consider the guidelines that govern clinical trials, we see both of these versions of justice. For example, the Committee for International Organization of Medical Sciences (CIOMS) guideline 10 states that:

> Individuals or communities to be invited to be subjects of research will be selected in such a way that the burdens and benefits of the research will be equally distributed. Special justification is required for inviting vulnerable individuals, and if they are selected, the means of protecting their rights and welfare must be particularly strictly applied. (p. 600)[25]

This particular guideline sought to redress the exploitative practice of using vulnerable populations, such as prisoners, to test therapies that were to be used by others. It also states that, should such persons become research subjects, they must share in the goods created through their participation. However, what is not clearly explained in the CIOMS guidelines is that justice as fair reciprocity—a share in the profits of an enterprise—is not a substitute for the kinds of basic rights that help to ensure that such trials do not exploit the subjects taking part in them in the first place. Nor does it ensure that research is carried out so that clinical investigators know exactly which rights and goods participants consider to be important. Significantly, there are almost no follow-up studies that are routinely done after clinical trials.

If the claims of justice cannot be met by simply repaying subjects for their participation with drugs that have been developed by the trials in which they have been involved, then my original questions need further attention; that is, what obligations and duties might persons in a first world country like Australia have toward those involved in HIV/AIDS research in the developing world? To whom might these duties apply?

Negative and Positive Duties

In the first instance, those who have profited from unfair bargains in the production of HIV/AIDS drugs can be seen to have a particular duty. Kok-Chor Tan suggests that Kantian duties based on justice can be extended to "preventing pending violations."[26] He states:

> Because everyone is inadvertently a participant in an economic bargaining scheme and some of these participants are particularly vulnerable to coercion and deception, there is a duty of justice on the part of other participants to render them less vulnerable to coercion and deception.[27]

This view of justice is somewhat different from the idea of redressing past wrongs. Instead, it bears some resemblance to the idea of "subject centred justice,"[28] as expressed by writers like John Rawls. In particular, Tan seems to be suggesting that it is incumbent on everyone to create a just foundation on which other enterprises can be negotiated. The kinds of positive duties that we might have then would be to ensure that all enterprises in which we were involved began on a just basis.

In a similar vein, the political theorist Henry Shue describes the way in which collectivity might also give claims based on justice more force. Although negative duties—that is, duties not to harm others—are relatively easy to maintain, positive duties, according to Shue, require some "division of labour."[29] One reason for this is to do with the "overdemandingness" objection that I discussed in relation to the Utilitarian formulation of the duty of beneficence. Another is the degree of efficacy that institutions can achieve in fulfilling basic needs. However, Shue goes further. He also describes an important relationship between institutions and the fulfilment of positive duties through the story of two men, Benny and Al. Benny is relatively wealthy, whereas Al is deprived of the most basic of rights and goods. In his commentary on their situation, Shue asks the important question: why should Benny, who shares neither culture nor any institutions with Al, have a duty to protect and fulfill his rights?[30]

Shue's answer to this question is that these two men do indeed share crude and primitive institutions connected to the global economy. However, these institutions do not assign rights and duties. According to Shue, individuals therefore have duties "for the design and creation of positive-duty-performing institutions" in order for rights to be fulfilled.[31]

The idea that there might be some duty to create "mediating institutions" is an important one when we consider HIV/AIDS research.[32] It might create a duty for those involved in the research at every level and those who use the drugs created by it. In particular, those involved in conducting pretrial research into the communities from which subjects could be drawn, as well as the medical researchers, might be seen to have particular duties to create mechanisms through which some problems relating to vulnerability might be addressed. Moreover, the rights of subjects should be protected, and issues related to justice addressed before and after the commencement of clinical trials. Tessa Tan-Torres Edejer puts it as follows:

> Increasingly, there is an awareness that the success of North-South research collaboration should not be judged solely on the results of scientific research activities. This awareness must be coupled with a learning approach to create a sustainable, mutually beneficial working relationship, that aside from advancing science must address inequity and put local priorities first, develop capacity with a long term perspective and preserve the dignity of local people by ensuring that the benefits of research will truly uplift their status.[33]

A discussion of the kinds of claims justice might generate help us to not only define more specifically the nature of claims but go some way to fulfilling them. I want briefly to add a final argument and illustrate it with a case study. This argument relates to integrity and shows us why some persons might feel particular duties to the research subjects under discussion.

AFAO and Bangkok HIV Preventative Vaccine Preparation

In 2003 the Australian federation of AIDS organizations received a commission from NIH to run the social research arm of the HIV preventative phase 2 trial that will start shortly in Bangkok. It seems that this kind of organization has particularly strong duties to make sure that the trial in question is ethical—duties that are, in fact, reflected in the care that they are taking to involve genuine community representatives and ensure distribution of any drugs produced.

Why, then, is the issue of integrity particularly important in relation to AFAO? Those working for this organization are accountable to many activist groups who have been involved in negotiating new ways to conduct HIV/ AIDS clinical trials in which research subjects were able to enter into a just partnership with clinical investigators. Therefore, it would seem inconsistent for persons engaged in creating such a research tradition to fail to apply its principles elsewhere.[34] The kind of integrity I am talking about is reliant on the work of Cheshire Calhoun. Calhoun talks about integrity as both an interactive and a social virtue, rather than merely a personal one.

According to Calhoun, integrity is a social virtue because when a subject sticks by her best judgment about "what is worth doing" she stands for something. Thus, "[h]er standing for something is not just something she does for herself. She takes a stand for, and before, all deliberators who share her goal of determining what is worth doing" (p. 257).[35] Central to Calhoun's argument is also the idea that a person who acts with integrity must treat others' best judgments in the same way. She suggests that "[i]ntegrity calls us simultaneously to stand behind our convictions and to take seriously others' doubts about them."[36]

This view seems important because it is also directive about how to act. That is, to act with integrity on this definition and in this context is to enter into a true negotiation with research subjects, so that they can reveal exactly which rights and goods they consider to be important. In this way, we move toward a view of justice that is reliant not on goods but on empowering all persons engaged in the research process. As the philosopher Elizabeth Anderson puts it:

> The proper negative aim of equalitarian justice is not to eliminate the impact of brute bad luck from

human affairs, but to end oppression, which by definition is socially imposed. Its proper positive aim is not to ensure that everyone gets what they morally deserve, but to create a community in which people stand in relations of equality to others.[37]

Notes

1 Dore G, Cooper D. Bridging the divide: global inequalities in access to HIV/AIDS therapy. *Medical Journal of Australia* 2001;175:570-72.

2 Moodie R. Should HIV be on the development agenda? *Development Bulletin* 2000;52:6-8.

3 Quinn TC, Wawer MJ, Sewankambo N, Serwadda D, Li C, Wabwire-Mangen F et al. Viral load and heterosexual transmission of human immunodeficiency virus type 1. *New England Journal of Medicine* 2000;342:921-29. See also: Wawer MJ, Sewankambo NK, Serwadda D, Quinn TC, Paxton LA, Kiwanuka N et al. Control of sexually transmitted diseases for AIDS prevention in Uganda: a randomised community trial. *Lancet* 1999;353(9512):525-35. For commentaries on this trial, see: Angell M. Investigator's responsibilities for human subjects in developing countries. *New England Journal of Medicine* 2000;342(13)967-69; and Groopman J. In an AIDS study, the devil is in the details. *New York Times* 2 Apr 2000.

4 See note 3, Wawer, Sewankambo, Serwadda, Quinn, Paxton, Kiwanuka et al. 1999; see note 3, Quinn, Wawer, Sewankambo, Serwadda, Li, Wabwire-Mangen et al. 2000:921; see note 3, Angell 2000:967.

5 See note 3, Angell 2000:967.

6 See: Zion D. "Moral taint" or ethical responsibility? unethical information and the problem of HIV clinical trials in developing countries. *Journal of Applied Philosophy* 1998;15(3):231-41.

7 Personal correspondence from Hal Martin, clinical investigator, non-oxynol 9 trial, Kenya, University of Washington. 11 Feb 1997.

8 See note 7, Martin 1997.

9 Jackson DJ, Martin H Jr, Bwayo J, Nyange P, Rakwar J, Kashonga F et al. Acceptability of HIV vaccine trials in high-risk heterosexual cohorts in Mombassa, Kenya. *AIDS* 1995;9(11):1279-83, at 1282.

10 See note 9, Jackson, Martin, Bwayo, Nyange, Rakwar, Kashonga et al. 1995:1282.

11 Microbicide may increase risk of HIV. *Business Day* 13 Jul 2000.

12 Singer P. Famine, affluence, and morality. In: Aiken W, LaFollette H, eds. *World Hunger and Morality*, 2nd ed. Englewood Cliffs, NJ: Prentice Hall; 1996:26-38.

13 Singer P. *Practical Ethics*. New York: Cambridge University Press; 1979:128ff. See also: Beauchamp TL, Childress J. *Principles of Biomedical Ethics*, 3rd ed. New York: Oxford University Press, 1989.

14 Arthur J. Rights and the duty to bring aid. In: Aiken W, LaFollette H, eds. *World Hunger and Morality*, 2nd ed. Englewood Cliffs, NJ: Prentice Hall; 1996:39-50, at 43-44.

15 Slote M. The morality of wealth. In: Aiken W, LaFollette H, eds. *World Hunger and Moral Obligation*. Englewood Cliffs, NJ: Prentice Hall; 1977:124-47, at 125-27.

16 Goodin R. *Protecting the Vulnerable: A Reanalysis of Our Social Responsibilities*. Chicago: University of Chicago Press; 1985:163.

17 See note 16, Goodin 1985:164.

18 Tan KC. Kantian ethics and global justice. *Social Theory and Practice* 1997;23(1):53-73. See also: Shue H. Mediating duties. *Ethics* 1988;98:687-704, at 693.

19 Buchanan A. Justice as reciprocity versus subject centred justice. *Philosophy and Public Affairs* 1990;19(3):227-52, at 229-31.

20 See note 19, Buchanan 1990:230.

21 Buchanan refers to this as "subject centred justice." See note 19, Buchanan 1990:230.

22 Arneson R. Rawls, responsibility, and distributive justice. In: Salles M, Weymark JA, eds. *Justice, Political Liberalism, and Utilitarianism: Themes from Harsanyi and Rawls*. New York: Cambridge University Press; forthcoming. Quoted in: Anderson ES. What is the point of equality? *Ethics* 1999; 109(2):287-337. See also: Rawls J. *A Theory of Justice*. Cambridge, MA: Harvard University Press; 1971:100-04; see also: Anderson 1999.

23 See note 22, Rawls 1971:303.

24 See note 19, Buchanan 1990:231.

25 CIOMS, WHO. International ethical guidelines for biomedical research involving human subjects. In: Arras J, Steinbock B, eds. *Ethical Issues in Modern Medicine*, 5th ed. Mountain View, CA: Mayfield Publishing; 1999:597-601.

26 See note 18, Tan 1997:66.

27 See note 18, Tan 1997.

28 This term is Allen Buchanan's. See note 19, Buchanan 1990.

29 See note 18, Shue 1988:690.

30 See note 18, Shue 1988:700-04.

31 See note 18, Shue 1988:703.

32 In fact, I am suggesting that the trials themselves, if properly designed, become mediating institutions. For an example of how this could be achieved, see: Edejer TTT. North-South research partnerships: the ethics of carrying out research in developing countries. *BMJ* 1999;319:438-41.

33 See note 32, Edejer 1999:440.

34 A similar example relates to the action of the AIDS Healthcare Foundation, one of the largest providers of specialized AIDS care in the United States. It says that it will bar GlaxoSmithKline from marketing drugs at its outpatient sites, in protest against the company's pricing policy. The foundation claims that the drug manufacturer still charges twice as much as its competitors for drugs in the developing world. See: Avery S. AIDS group bars Glaxo marketing. *Los Angeles Times* 2002 May 28; home ed. C3.

35 Calhoun C. Standing for something. *Journal of Philosophy* 1995;92(5):235-61.

36 See note 35, Calhoun 1995:260.

37 See note 22, Anderson 1999:288-89.

CHAPTER NINE

GENETICS

Web Links

(1) Link to the Universal Declaration on Bioethics and Human Rights (UNESCO).

http://www.unesco.org/new/en/social-and-human-sciences/themes/bioethics/bioethics-and-human-rights/

UNESCO aims to address the need to promote respect for the intrinsic worth of human beings and the integrity of the human species in an age of rapidly expanding genetic and other biotechnological interventions into human life.

(2) Link to Stem Cell Network.

http://www.stemcellnetwork.ca/

The Stem Cell Network is a not-for-profit corporation that pursues applied stem-cell research in order to create therapies and public policy.

* For an up-to-date list of the web links in this book, please visit:
http://sites.broadviewpress.com/healthcare.

57.
HUMAN GENETIC BANKING:
ALTRUISM, BENEFIT AND CONSENT

Garrath Williams and Doris Schroeder

SOURCE: *New Genetics and Society* 23.1 (2004): 89-103.

Introduction

The frequency and scope of human genetic banking has increased significantly in recent years and is set to expand still further. Here we consider how the key ethical considerations raised by these developments are most usefully framed. Our focus will be upon medical and population research. That is to say, we shall leave to one side a related development of potentially still greater import, that of forensic databases, which promises greatly increased state power to investigate individuals' activity, criminal or otherwise.

There is, however, an interesting disanalogy between these two sorts of databases, in terms of the way ethical discussion tends to be framed. In the case of forensic databases, discussion is overwhelmingly structured by an opposition between the public good and individual rights: the public interest (in detecting and even preventing crime) and civil liberties or privacy considerations, that militate against large-scale state access to genetic samples. In the medical context human genetic banking has attracted a quite different discourse, with individual rights at the forefront: that is, rights concerning the informed consent of actual and potential donors to the database. So far as the public good goes, this has tended to be addressed only by rather weakly supported claims regarding possible health care benefits.

It is not surprising, then, that some recent contributions suggest that informed consent is being asked to play too great a role in our thinking about the ethics of these projects. In this paper, we make such a case explicitly.[1] We stress both how limited the informational aspect of "consent" must be for most

donors, as well as arguing that consent is quite insufficient to legitimise such collective projects. We therefore argue that much more searching scrutiny is required of the organisation and exploitation of these projects, particularly in the light of the commercial forces at work here. The individualistic focus of informed consent needs to be supplemented by proactive forms of ongoing institutional governance. Much more attention must be paid to the duties pertaining to the custodians of gene banks, and to the institutions that fund them.

We structure our discussion into three main sections: a brief consideration of why scientific research now demands large human gene banks; the question of informed consent, and issues which that raises (for instance, confidentiality and impact on third parties); and how to conceptualise the moral issues at stake, given the limitations of a framework oriented solely by informed consent.

Human Genetic Banking for Pharmacogenomics and Population Genetics

By human genetic banking we mean large-scale banks which contain either tissue samples, from which genetic material might be or has been extracted or genetic information, which may be coded and stored in various forms; and, in addition, health and "lifestyle" information pertaining to the sample donors. Two current research areas require human genetic banking in previously unknown dimensions: pharmacogenomics and population genetics (Bell, 2000, p. 2; House of Lords, 2001, Chapter 2, p. 1).

Pharmacogenomics relies on the hypothesis that responses to medication are significantly affected by a patient's genetic make-up. Hence, the aim of research is to ensure "the right medicine for the right patient" (Wolf, 2000, p. 1). The advantages of tailor-made medication are obvious. Patients are not put through futile therapies, or therapies likely to cause them dangerous side-effects; medication is not wasted on those who cannot benefit from it. To correlate genetic make-up with reactions to drugs is, however, a matter of "statistical brute force" (Lowrance, 2001, p. 1009). According to the Medical Research Council (2000, p. 5), most collections existing world-wide "are too small to allow statistically meaningful research."

Population genetics relies on the hypothesis that common diseases can be linked to a complex interplay of genetic predispositions with life style and environmental factors. Researchers are seeking to identify susceptibility genes for diseases such as early onset heart disease, asthma, depression, osteoarthritis, migraine, Alzheimer's, Parkinson's and diabetes (Glaxo Wellcome, 2000, p. 2). Ideally, it will become possible to give tailor-made advice on life-style and environmental issues to people at risk from particular diseases. In addition, new drugs might be developed if the links between genetic make-up and such diseases can be understood.

Human Genetic Banking—Three Examples[2]

The best-known human genetic database suitable for pharmacogenomics and population genetics research is the Icelandic collection of the country's health records. The Icelandic Parliament granted a licence to deCode genetics in December 1998. The database contains tissue samples and identifiable health data from official medical records and is based on "opt-out" consent (records are included in the database unless a citizen takes specific measures requesting non-inclusion[3]). Drawing on a population of 270,000, the database offers enormous potential for genetic research: detailed medical records of every Icelandic inhabitant have been kept for over fifty years, as have tissue samples for many; genealogical data also exists for most Icelanders (cf. Chadwick, 1999, p. 442).

An even larger database is about to be set up in Britain where the Medical Research Council in co-operation with the Wellcome Trust and the National Health Service (NHS) are planning "UK Biobank" (previously referred to as the "UK Population Bio-medical Collection"). DNA, lifestyle and medical information will be sought from approximately 500,000 people between 45 and 64 years old (the average time of onset of several common diseases). Samples will be held in public ownership, and data will be made available to commercial companies (Wellcome News, 2000, p. 11).

A much smaller British database is already in place, the "North Cumbria Community Genetics Project." The database stores umbilical cord blood and tissue from newborn babies and their mothers, in addition to limited personal data (about 5,000 samples by 2000). As there is little population movement in the area, long-term follow-up of clinical outcomes is envisaged. The project was triggered by local concerns about genetic implications of the proximity of British Nuclear Fuels at Sellafield (North Cumbria Community Genetics Project, 2000). Samples and data are taken only following explicit consent by the mother, and the whole project was preceded by extensive community consultation (North Cumbria Community Genetics Project, 2000, p. 3, 2001b).

What the above three banks have in common is that they provide or will provide extensive, centralised, and perhaps even standardised genetic information, together with clinical and personal data. It is the ongoing link between genetic and clinical information that makes these banks suitable for pharmacogenomics and population genetics research, as well as their size. In both fields, the linking of genetic (biological) and clinical (personal) data is essential (Martin, 2000, p. 3). Total anonymisation[4] is of course possible, but would prevent the introduction of health data obtained after anonymisation; in other words, the prospective character of the database would be lost. Arguably, this would compromise its scientific value considerably (Glaxo Wellcome, 2000, p. 11; Medical Research Council, 2000, p. 10).

Informed Consent and Human Genetic Banks

Currently the most prominent ethical issue concerning genetic banking relates to individuals' informed consent for the use both of their tissues and their health care information. The information side of this consent requires the explanation of a medical intervention's purpose, its potential benefits and foreseeable risks, as well as its alternatives—all this in a way that is intelligible to a patient or volunteer (Brody, 2001, pp. 11ff), as well as relevant (O'Neill, 2002, p. 156). The "consent" aspect requires a noncoercive setting to obtain agreement as well as some form of authorisation or documentation. (Clearly, other principles will be relevant as regards emergencies, and the situation of incompetent adults and young children.)

How pressing the issue of informed consent has become to the storage of human biological materials has been amply shown by events at the Alder Hey hospital. According to The Royal Liverpool Children's Inquiry (2001), the hospital did not comply with the Human Tissue Act (1961, Section 1(2)) when removing, retaining and disposing of organs and human tissue from deceased children. Instead, it built up one of the most extensive collections in the world of children's hearts as well as substantial collections of other body parts. In doing so without relevantly informed[5] consent, considerable lack of respect was shown toward parents, who were to discover years later that their child's body had been stripped of some or even all internal organs, and been buried as a "shell" (Department of Health, 2001).

What aspects of human genetic banking are problematic for the informed consent procedure? Clearly, some issues are more than usually straightforward: the absence of immediate therapeutic benefit is clear, as is the negligible risk posed by current medical procedures for taking samples. The fact that prospective donors are usually healthy volunteers means that consent for research is given under less threatening and distressing circumstances, as compared with hospital settings (where, for instance, a patient suffering from a debilitating illness would be more vulnerable to excessive deference to doctors or feelings of intimidation). Nonetheless, there are two especial sources of difficulty: the linking of genetic and clinical data, which in turn poses issues around confidentiality, withdrawing, feedback and recontacting; and that of third party involvement.

Linking genetic data and clinical data raises significant problems for informed consent. As we have seen, in both pharmacogenomics and population genetics, the integration of genetic and clinical data is deemed essential, and donors' health care and/or lifestyle data is to be input into the bank on an ongoing basis. This generates issues about withdrawing, feedback and confidentiality, which do not arise in such a general form in other medical research.

The possibility of withdrawing from a research study is one of the basic principles regulating medical experiments according to both the Nuremberg Code (1947, Standard 9) and the Declaration of Helsinki (1996, Basic Principle 9). It is essential that informed consent procedures explain this basic right to subjects of research in pharmacogenomics and population genetics (cf. Porter, 2000, pp. 53, 81). The North Cumbria bank makes provision for complete withdrawal, so that all data and samples are removed on request, while the Icelandic one has a complicated and arguably unsatisfactory opt-out option (cf. Rose, 2001, p. 25); regulations for UK Biobank have not yet been finalised. Neither the Icelandic Health Sector Database nor the North Cumbria Community Genetics Project make it possible to "opt into" certain research projects and "opt out" of others. Either a person withdraws altogether, or the records can be used for all projects approved by the relevant ethics committee (North Cumbria Community Genetics Project, 2001a; Haraldsdottir, 2000, p. 12).

The genetic component of research into pharmacogenomics and population genetics can offer no therapeutic benefit to volunteers. However, research aims include the identification of people who might or might not benefit from certain medications and who are at risk of developing certain common diseases. Volunteers who understand these objectives might reasonably expect to be given such feedback on the analysis of their samples. This is rightly considered a particularly "tricky issue" amongst human genetic bankers (Wellcome News, 2000, p. 11), and has not yet been resolved for UK Biobank. With the North Cumbria Community Genetics Project (2001b) and the Icelandic Health Sector Database, in general no feedback is given to individual volunteers. There is certainly a major resource consideration here: some have even argued that regular feedback would transform a research project into genetic screening requiring an enormous budget for genetic counselling of all donors (e.g., King, 2000, p. 4). Clearly, given that future developments are so uncertain, there are grave problems in foreseeing what implications feedback might have, both for particular individuals and the management of collections.

The Medical Research Council (2000, p. 10), however, expects feedback to be given on a regular basis and therefore recommends that banks budget for genetic counselling. It might also be noted that the UK study on "Public Perceptions of the Collection of Human Biological Examples" found that most people thought donors should have "the right to feedback on anything that emerged from their own sample" (Porter, 2000, p. 8). This might plausibly be seen as something owed "in return" for a donor's participation. Regardless of which position one supports, so far as informed consent is concerned the crucial point is that research subjects know in advance whether they will receive feedback on their samples (Chadwick, 2001, p. 207; Clarke et al., 2001, pp. 90ff), though just what sort of information may turn out to be available cannot yet be known.

Another major issue concerns what type of consent to obtain, which is bound up with the question of whether research subjects should be recontacted in the case of new studies. Evidently, the collections we have mentioned are suitable for a wide range of research studies. Should donors, when depositing a sample, be asked for narrow or open-ended consent? This could range from consent for material to be used in one, well-defined research study (so that future uses would require new informed consent procedures) to open-ended consent for general research (with the main safeguard against "undesirable" research probably being offered by some relevant research ethics committee). To obtain informed consent from every participant for every research study is, obviously, very time-consuming and even unworkable for researchers, particularly with these large collections. This would imply that some sort of open consent is the only realistic option. Interestingly, the recent report on "Public Perceptions of the Collection of Human Biological Examples" found that most respondents were comfortable with the idea of samples being used for disease-specific work, but not for general research (Porter, 2000, p. 7).

One in-between option, consent for general research approved by an ethics committee, with certain further limitations, has been adopted by the North Cumbria Community Genetics Project. Donors, or rather donors' parents, must to a significant degree trust the judgement of an ethics committee but are assured in advance that samples will only "with extreme caution and subject to rigorous examination" be used for "studies that involve intelligence, behaviour, personality and psychiatric disorders" (North Cumbria Community Genetics Project, 2000, p. 5). Beyond the point of donation, though, donors are unable to influence the direction of ongoing research—except by withdrawing should they disapprove of decisions made by project leaders.

A further complicated issue concerns confidentiality, one of the most fundamental and long-standing principles of medical ethics. As we have seen, confidentiality is threatened by the need to make linking access to health care data, if researchers are to incorporate data on an on-going basis. Coding of samples and data can reduce but not eliminate the possibility of breaches of confidentiality. (By contrast a system of complete data anonymisation makes it almost impossible to link any sample to an identifiable individual.) This formed a particular concern of GPs and nurses about UK Biobank, "given the size of the sample and their own experience of maintaining secure records" (Porter, 2000, p. 10; cf. AstraZeneca, 2000, p. 2).[6]

These worries are surely well founded: confidentiality breaches can occur both accidentally, and on public health or criminological grounds. In the UK, Scottish police seized materials from a clinical study on HIV (Yirrell et al., 1997), in disregard of guarantees of confidentiality given to the subjects when they consented to take part. This led to one subject's conviction for culpable and reckless conduct (knowingly exposing his partner to HIV), and a sentence of five years' imprisonment (Dyer, 2001a; Brown, 2001). The Medical Research Council, the funder of the research, claimed: "Confidentiality has never been an absolute.... The case involved an investigation into a serious crime....There was thus a strong public interest in disclosure ..." (Dyer, 2001b).[7] Thus breaches of confidentiality and respect are both possible and, on occasion, arguably legitimate. As well as the state, two other powerful parties might want to acquire genetic information about individuals— employers and insurance companies (Clarke, 2001, p. 143). Both will want to select individuals who are likely to stay healthy (ibid.), whilst agencies of the state may seek access to genetic information for forensic or "security" reasons, or in case of paternity suits.

So far as informed consent is concerned, two conclusions suggest themselves: that consent procedures might draw research subjects' attention to the potential for data breaches and their consequences; and that the administrators of databases should clearly indicate when they would be prepared, or could be obliged, to release data. Interestingly, the North Cumbria project promises potential donors that samples will "never be available for ... police records" and will "only be used for medical research" (North Cumbria Community Genetics Project, 2001b). Yet it seems clear that, in the UK at least, no researcher is in a position to offer such a guarantee.

Finally, complex issues arise with regard to possible effects on third parties, which arguably should be explained during the informed consent procedure. The first is commercial third party benefit, which raises issues of distributive justice and possible exploitation. The second is indirect third party harm such as unwanted health knowledge or ethnic discrimination.

Human genetic banks, as required for pharmacogenomics and population genetics, "will be driven by demand from the commercial sector" (Womack & Gray, 2000, p. 251). This pressure may be of mutual benefit to biotechnology companies and communal health care systems, if it results in, for instance, better and cheaper pharmaceutical products (ibid., p. 252) or more efficient ways to operate a health service (Department of Health, 2000, p. 1; Haraldsdottir, 2000, p. 12). If forthcoming, benefits will accrue to the population at large, not, in the first instance, to sample donors. Conversely, in this altruistic or "gift" scenario, donors will most directly benefit commercial (profit-making) organisations.

Research participants need to be made aware that there might well be possibilities for commercial exploitation in addition to any humanitarian benefits (Chadwick, 2001, p. 209) and, moreover, should individual samples lead to major new pharmaceutical discoveries, that a share of the profits will not ensue.

Third party harm is another issue, particularly with regard to research in population genetics. "Third parties" in this context are those who share a similar genetic make-up with the research participants. For example, Glaxo Wellcome's (2000, p. 2) programme in population genetics includes research to identify susceptibility genes for Parkinson's disease or Alzheimer's disease. It is possible that one member of a family will agree to take part in this research whilst another declines, or for some other reason is not party to the study. In this case, the unasked or unwanted disclosure of genetic information to non-consenting parties could occur. No definitive solution to this problem is possible; one might, though, attempt to enlighten the family member who is donating (and, as a result, being tested) of his or her consequent responsibilities toward other family members (ibid., p. 68), particularly drawing his or her attention to the complexities of unsolicited disclosure.

Third party harm can also occur outside families, when genetic research is carried out on minority groups who share a similar genetic make-up. In this case it is quite possible that group members who did not take part in research will be affected by its outcome (indeed, those who do participate might be affected in unanticipated ways). For instance, susceptibilities for certain conditions may be found— thus "particular mutations predisposing to breast, ovarian, and colon cancer have been identified through studies of Ashkenazi Jews" (Weijer and Emanuel, 2000, p. 1142). It is conceivable that the community might be discriminated against on this knowledge, for instance by health insurance providers. In this case, research outcomes are disadvantageous for a whole group and not only for those who take part in research. It can certainly be argued that this slight but alarming possible effect of genetic research should also be conveyed during the informed consent process.

The Active Governance
of Human Genetic Banks

As we have seen, human genetic banking is increasingly taking the form of large sample collections, where donors (or their parents) have given broad, though probably not unlimited, consent for future research. Concerns about the idea of informed consent as the sufficient legitimating ground of future use of these samples and associated data are not difficult to envisage.

As the previous section has stressed, the information involved is complicated, especially with regard to possible future uses and benefits. One might expect donors to grasp that use of their samples and health data may help generate various possible benefits, with slight, but complicated, risks of harm to them. But they will neither be allowed, nor arguably capable of, any precise input into the research that will be conducted. At most, they may be able to "opt out," if they disapprove of the way research initiatives are heading. Because of informational constraints, among other factors, one would expect this to be done only by a very few donors. Never mind the limits of most persons' grasp of the research science and the political economics of commercially driven medical research; researchers themselves will only have a tentative grasp of some of the possibilities for future investigation, much less a thorough understanding of the justice or injustices of pharmaceutical companies' interaction with national health systems. Consent may be there, but its basis in "information" will, despite all best efforts, be relatively slight. There is, moreover, very little prospect of short- or medium-term benefit to participants. In other words: sample collections are established on the good will and altruism of individual donors, and donors must invest a significant degree of trust—in those who will manage the database, and with regard to the uses to which it is put.

Even if one is less sceptical than we are, about how "informed" consent can be in these cases, clearly it can only play a limited role in legitimating such projects. Suppose, for example, enough donors were to agree to a collection and corresponding research with worrying eugenicist overtones. Just because enough people provide their informed consent, this is hardly enough to legitimate a collection and its planned uses. Correspondingly, a collection that is badly underused or which, however unintentionally, becomes the dominant preserve of a few pharmaceutical companies, would surely represent a questionable enterprise, not least given the altruistic origin of the data bank.[8]

This consideration only sharpens the question of how far gene banks will really deliver benefits (cf. Chadwick, 1999). The focus on informed consent has, we believe, led to inadequate attention toward those to whom trust is being given, and what would vindicate this trust. Pharmaceutical companies, among others, are provided with an extremely valuable resource for which none of the donors will be financially compensated. This altruism should be matched by a moral responsibility to use the resource, at least in part, for the common good.

Bearing in mind this problem of public benefits, Berg and Chadwick (2001, p. 320) suggest that we should rethink some of the attitudes that surround informed consent, and that an alternative ethical approach might be found in the political notions of solidarity and equity. They believe that it may be appropriate to question the right of research subjects to withdraw from these banking projects, once they have consented to inclusion in the first place, arguing that we have duties of solidarity to contribute to medical research. The suggestion that people may have a duty to participate in research is, of course, not new and, especially where the risks to subjects are slight, quite reasonable—especially where health care systems embody strong elements of solidarity, to ensure that all citizens will benefit from the research, should the need arise. Problems emerge, however, if we think of such a duty as enforceable, given that there is considerable scope for reasonable disagreement as to what constitutes desirable research (or, indeed, acceptable risk). In the case of human genetic banking, the fact that consent cannot be given on the basis of full information, only in terms of the broad aims of future research, means that withdrawal is the only effective way of preserving any sort of choice for individual data subjects as to the fate of their samples and health care data.

Moreover, as the emotive example of Alder Hey has demonstrated, informed consent has become a crucial part of the "political settlement" between researchers and the public. If it were explained to potential research subjects that their one-off consent, based on necessarily partial information about future research possibilities, were final, this would surely be damaging in terms of recruitment and, quite possibly, negative publicity. As O'Neill notes (2002, p. 154), a withdrawal right is important for promoting trust in the governance of such projects.

We believe, then, that informed consent, with the on-going possibility of withdrawal, should not be supplanted by alternative approaches, but rather be supplemented. Whether we think of solidarity and equity, or the trust that donors are investing alongside their samples, it seems to us that the priority must be to ensure that genetic banks are used for worthy, publicly endorsed ends. To get a practical hold on this, we do not need to limit the rights of research subjects, any more than we need insist on an unrealistic level of understanding in the consent process. Instead, we must focus on the duties of those who create and manage genetic banks—duties to ensure their exploitation for real public benefit or, in other words, duties to make notions such as solidarity into working realities.

Kaye and Martin (2000) have rightly drawn attention to a crucial difference between the Icelandic database and UK Biobank. Though the Icelandic proposal seems much more commercially oriented, and considerably less "voluntary" in its inclusion of samples and data, it at least was the subject of vigorous public and political debate. On the other hand, UK Biobank, certainly in its earlier stages, seemed to be proposed with little view to public consultation or independent oversight of the collection's use. Nor, one might add, can opinion sampling (Porter, 2000; People, Science & Policy, 2002) form an adequate substitute for political debate on the desirability and aims of such a genetic bank. We suggest that one important focus, and a possible conclusion, of this debate should concern the public responsibilities involved in the governance of large sample collections.

In the first place, there are a series of "negative responsibilities," which all contributors take for granted. These include a duty to ensure that proper procedures are followed in gathering samples and information—one hopes this may be taken as read, after recent organ storage scandals. There is also a duty to ensure the security of confidential data—which may be a more challenging task, especially given the cavalier attitude to privacy rights shown in the development of the national police database (Bingham, 2001) and, one might argue, in the police seizure of material from the Scottish HIV study, discussed above.

Further, there is an uncontroversial duty to review the ethics of research proposals, via research ethics committees. Such bodies should veto, or help reformulate, research proposals that are unnecessary, scientifically unsound, or ethically undesirable. While it is obvious that research using human genetic banks should be subject to this scrutiny, the problem is that such review is essentially negative: it can only stop unethical or unwanted research from being undertaken, but cannot pro-actively steer the usage of a DNA bank. Such committees are almost wholly dependent on the proposals that come before them, and are in no position to satisfy donors' trust that genetic banks will be well-used and maximally contribute to the public good.

These essentially protective roles are likewise alluded to in the so-far brief comments about the governance of UK Biobank (People, Science & Policy, 2002, pp. 27ff; but cf. Wellcome Trust, 2002, p. 2.3.1).[9] They do not, however, capture what we see as the main concern: structures of research governance that will fulfil a positive duty to ensure that worthwhile research is conducted using the collections. We see such structures, alongside the institutions which fund or support large sample collections, as having a much more onerous positive duty of soliciting and prioritising research that is likely to realise the ends set by public and political debate. In the case of wealthy grant-giving institutions such as the Wellcome Trust and the MRC, moreover, there seems to be a clear imperative to enable such research by funding.

It is here that the limitations of the Icelandic bank are most obvious. While the founding legislation speaks of "a duty to use the data" (quoted and critically discussed by Rose, 2001, p. 17), and while the licensee is indeed in a position to "use the data" fairly extensively, the problem is that this use will be determined by the licensee only, that is, by a private company. Even if this is done within adequate protective and research-ethical safeguards, the research will be primarily driven by commercial imperatives, which have only uncertain and contingent relation to the public good or public priorities. The North Cumbria initiative, by contrast, certainly does not face this problem. Its difficulty, instead, is that it is in no position to enact public research priorities. Though it was created only after extensive public consultation, and carefully publicises the research undertaken using the bank, if proposals are not made, or funding not forthcoming, then nothing can be done.[10] UK Biobank is, potentially, in a much more fortunate situation. The founding partners are extremely powerful in determining research priorities in the UK, being among the relatively few non-profit organisations in the world which compare in spending power with the international pharmaceutical companies. These partners face, we suggest, imperatives not only to publicise research projects and future priorities, but also to be open to public debate regarding these.[11] It may be, for example, that custodians of UK Biobank find that there is pressure for coordinated, systematic research on common, chronic conditions which have attracted only patchy research— perhaps because they are rarely fatal, although they may cause widespread misery (for example, asthma or irritable bowel syndrome). It may be also, as those examples suggest, that there is an imperative for research that does not focus primarily on (potentially) very profitable drug treatments. That is to say, the sponsors and guardians of such large databases will have a duty to direct resources and researchers' attention to areas where pharmaceutical companies have little or no incentive to invest. At the same time, there will be a clear need to monitor and report on commercial exploitation of sample collections. Not least, there will be a need to provide regular public reporting on actual benefits obtained from research upon the collections, and not only the speculated benefits so often emphasised in these debates.

What institutional arrangements will promote the fulfilment of these duties is a further question, and not one that we seek to address in any detail. But if the Icelandic case is a failure in this regard, and the North Cumbria project too small and insufficiently wealthy

to take many active steps in the directions we are advocating, UK Biobank is quite differently situated. Unfortunately, however, current governance proposals do not seem to have been properly thought through, permitting doubt whether the oversight mechanisms will be appropriate for the different purposes that the Biobank is proposing to carry out (cf. Kaye, 2002). But in principle there is no reason why specific bodies or committees or regulators cannot monitor the uses to which the bank is put and the benefits it helps to generate. There is no reason, in principle, why those managing and steering the project should not institute means to consult donors and a wider public about priorities for its use, and means to channel funds toward those priorities. But if the details of how this is to be done are a matter for insiders and funders to debate, we believe one thing is clear: specific responsibilities and accountabilities must be allocated and distributed and enforced, if this or other genetic banks are to realise their promises on a sustained basis.

Conclusion

Human genetic banking for pharmacogenomics or population genetics is likely to increase significantly in the near future, and clearly deserves ethical debate and public scrutiny. However, the issue of informed consent, so often propounded as the main ethical concern in these discussions, constitutes only one small part of the ethical story. The reasons for treating consent as important are undoubted and indisputable. But good reasons for treating consent as the main concern are simply not available.

And the reason for this, in turn, is clear. Genetic banks represent major proposals for collective action, designed to yield public benefits. It is a matter of course that individuals should be protected in this process. Nonetheless, if their trust is to be won, and if that trust is to be well-founded, much more is needed: precisely those public benefits that are being promised in the first place must be energetically pursued and promoted. And donors are in no position to ensure this: unavoidably they entrust this task to one or more institutions. What is therefore required is solid institutional design to coordinate activity in ways that not only avoid harm but actively promote benefits and earn trust.

We have therefore suggested that attention must be devoted to the specific duties of custodians and public sponsors, and to the specific institutional arrangements that will ensure those duties are fulfilled. Only those measures can ensure that samples are used for the public good and for publicly endorsed ends. Given the predominance of commercial research interests, and the often haphazard nature of coordination of researchers' efforts, the grave danger exists that sample collections will be selectively exploited—worse still, exploited on terms set by commercial partners. As the banks rely both on donor altruism and extensive public funding for their existence, such exploitation has to be regarded as inequitable and unacceptable, even if some benefits do indeed emerge. The massive public and charitable or public investments involved in genetic banks call for systematic exploitation of such collections for the benefit of the whole community. Research subjects should not have to consent to anything less than this, and—so we have argued—sponsoring institutions and custodians have a duty to ensure that donors, in fact, do not.

Notes

1 For an explicit and more systematic argument concerning the role and limits of informed consent in the context of several questions in bioethics, see O'Neill (2002). O'Neill's book appeared after this article was submitted for publication, and advances more argumentative detail and ranges much more widely than is possible here. Nonetheless, our arguments and broad views about the limits of consent overlap considerably.

2 These are currently standard examples; they are also discussed, for instance, in Berg and Chadwick (2001).

3 On the problematic nature of this, including doubts as to whether opting out will be a genuine option for any but a very small number of adults in the first years of the study, see Rose (2001, pp. 24ff).

4 Data may be classified in terms of the "degree" of anonymity: 1) Anonymous—no information about the donor available when the data were filed. 2) Anonymised—information about donors destroyed. 3) Encoded—information about donors coded with a serial number and the key held elsewhere. 4) Encrypted—data turned into meaningless strings for commercial security. 5) Identified—information about donor kept with the data, without coding (Spallone & Wilkie, 2000, p. 199; European Society of Human Genetics, 2001).

5 Again cf. O'Neill, 2002, pp. 154ff.

6 Various methods may be used to increase data and sample security, for instance, as in North Cumbria, by storing samples and coding information at separate sites. (North Cumbria Genetics Project, 2000, p. 8)

7 Though we think this "public interest" claim dubious in the case at hand, the point here is only that such cases do occur, and may do so legitimately.

8 As noted above, our argument is entirely congruent with Onora O'Neill's broad case in *Autonomy and Trust in Bioethics* (2002, especially Chapters 5 & 7). O'Neill's argument is that informed consent, a means of protecting individuals, offers only one means among others to promote trust in those providing health care, and only one means among others to ensure that those providing that care act in trustworthy ways. A proposal such as UK Biobank is, however, a proposal for collective action: it poses few harms to specific individuals, and promises wide and indefinite benefits to many.

9 The first version of the UK Biobank draft Ethics and Governance framework (<www.biobankuk.ac.uk/ethics.htm>) was published in 2003, after this article was accepted for publication. Thus we do discuss that document here.

10 Since the collection is on nothing like the same scale as the other two, representing a much smaller investment of public resources and overall donor effort, we stress that we do not mean this as a criticism of the North Cumbria project or other relatively small initiatives.

11 Cf. the list of research hypotheses mentioned in the draft protocol, Wellcome Trust, 2002, p. 214.

References

AstraZeneca (2000) Memorandum: Evidence to the Select Committee on Science and Technology <www.publications.parliament.uk/pa/ld199900/ldselect/ldsctech/115/115we07.htm>.

Bell, J. (2000) Memorandum: Evidence to the Select Committee on Science and Technology <www.publications

.parliament.uk/pa/ld199900/ldselect/ldsctech/115/115we50.htm>.

Berg, K. & Chadwick, R. (2001) Solidarity and equity: new ethical frameworks for genetic databases, *Nature Reviews* 2, pp. 318-21.

Bingham, R. (2001) A database of the innocent?, *Splice*, 7(2-3), pp. 8-9.

Brody, B.A. (2001) A historical introduction to the requirement of obtaining consent from research participants. In Doyal, Len & Tobias, Jeffrey S. (eds) *Informed Consent in Medical Research*, pp. 7-14 (London: BMJ Books).

Brown, A.L. (2001) A confidential con job, *Times Higher Education Supplement* 1489, 1 June.

Chadwick, R. (1999) The Icelandic database: do modern times need modern sagas?, *British Medical Journal*, 319, pp. 441-44.

Chadwick, R. (2001) Informed consent and genetic research. In Doyal, Len & Tobias, Jeffrey S. (eds) *Informed Consent in Medical Research*, pp. 203-10 (London: BMJ Books).

Clarke, A. (2001) Genetic counselling. In Chadwick, Ruth (ed) *Ethics of New Technologies*, pp. 131-46 (San Diego, CA: Academic Press).

Clarke, A., English, V., Harris, H. & Wells, F. (2001) Ethical considerations, *International Journal of Pharmaceutical Medicine*, 15, pp. 89-94.

Department of Health (2000) Memorandum: Evidence to the Select Committee on Science and Technology <www.publications.parliament.uk/pa/ld199900/ldselect/ldsctech/115/115we17.htm>.

Department of Health (2001) Milburn Promises Reforms After Alder Hey Inquiry and Pays Tribute to Parents, News Desk <www.doh.gov.uk/newsdesk/latest/4-naa-30012001.htm>.

Dyer, C. (2001a) Use of confidential data helps convict former prisoner, *British Medical Journal*, 322, p. 633.

Dyer, C. (2001b) Scientists Fear Breach of Confidentiality Will Threaten Research <www.guardian.co.uk/Archive/Article/0,4273,4153840,00.htm>.

European Society of Human Genetics (Public and Professional Policy Committee) (2001) Data Storage and DNA Banking for Biomedical Research: Proposed Recommendations (draft consultation document) <www.eshg.org>.

Glaxo Wellcome (2000) Memorandum: Evidence to the Select Committee on Science and Technology <www.publications.parliament.uk/pa/ld199900/ldselect/ldsctech/115/115we24.htm>.

Haraldsdottir, R. (2000) Fire and fury in Iceland, *Science & Public Affairs*, February, pp. 12-13.

House of Lords (Select Committee on Science and Technology) (2001) Human Genetic Databases: Challenges and Opportunities <www.publications.parliament.uk/pa/ld200001/ldselect/ldsctech/57/5701.htm>.

Kaye, J. (2002) UK Biobank: The Current State of Play. Presentation to the NorFA (Nordic Academy for Advanced Study) network on "The Ethics of Medical and Genetic Information," at its workshop in *Lytham St Annes*, 11 May.

Kaye, J. & Martin, P. (2000) Safeguards for research using large scale DNA collections, *British Medical Journal*, 321, pp. 1146-49.

King, D. (2000) Memorandum: Evidence to the Select Committee on Science and Technology <www.publications.parliament.uk/pa/ld199900/ldselect/ldsctech/115/115we23.htm>.

Lowrance, W.W. (2001) The promise of human genetic databases, *British Medical Journal*, 322, pp. 1009-10.

Martin, P. (2000) Memorandum: Evidence to the Select Committee on Science and Technology <www.publications.parliament.uk/pa/ld199900/ldselect/ldsctech/115/115we52.htm>.

Medical Research Council (2000) Memorandum: Evidence to the Select Committee on Science and Technology <www.publications.parliament.uk/pa/ld199900/ldselect/ldsctech/115/115we32.htm>.

North Cumbria Community Genetics Project (2000) Report 1996-2000 (Westlakes Research Institute).

North Cumbria Community Genetics Project (2001a) Further Information (Westlakes Research Institute).

North Cumbria Community Genetics Project (2001b) Informed Consent Form (Westlakes Research Institute).

O'Neill, O. (2002) *Autonomy and Trust in Bioethics* (Cambridge: Cambridge University Press).

People, Science & Policy Ltd (2002) UK Biobank: A Question of Trust: A Consultation Exploring and Addressing Questions of Public Trust. Report prepared for the Medical Research Council and the Wellcome Trust (London: People, Science & Policy).

Porter, T. (2000) *Public Perceptions of the Collection of Human Biological Samples*. Report prepared for the Medical Research Council and the Wellcome Trust (London: Cragg Ross Dawson).

Rose, H. (2001) *The Commodification of Bioinformation: The Icelandic Health Sector Database* (London: Wellcome Trust).

Spallone, P. & Wilkie, T. (2000) The research agenda in pharmacogenomics and biological sample collections, *New Genetics and Society*, 19, pp. 193-205.

The Royal Liverpool Children's Inquiry (2001) Summary and Recommendations <www.rlcinquiry.org.uk>.

Weijer, C. & Emanuel, E.J. (2000) Protecting communities in biomedical research, *Science*, 289, pp. 1142-44.

Wellcome News (2000) A sample solution, Q3—Wellcome News 24, pp. 10-11.

Wellcome Trust (2002) Draft Protocol for Biobank UK, February <www.welcome.ac.uk/en/1/biovenpop-prt.html>.

Wolf, R. (2000) Made-to-measure-medicine. Quoted at BBC News Online <news.bbc.co.uk/hi/english/health/newsid_704000/704577.stm>.

Womack, C. & Gray, N.M. (2000) Human research tissue banks in the UK. National Health Service: laws, ethics, controls and constraints, *British Journal of Biomedical Science*, 57, pp. 250-53.

Yirrell, D.L., Robertson, P., Goldberg, D.J., McMenamin, J., Cameron, S. & Leigh Brown, A.J. (1997) Molecular investigation into outbreak of HIV in a Scottish prison, *British Medical Journal*, 314, pp. 1446-50.

58.
FURTHERING INJUSTICES AGAINST WOMEN: GENETIC INFORMATION, MORAL OBLIGATIONS, AND GENDER

Inmaculada De Melo-Martin

SOURCE: *Bioethics* 20.6 (2006): 301-06.

Introduction

Reliance on highly abstract, universal principles as the appropriate source of moral guidance is one of the trademarks of the western philosophical tradition. In spite of the many differences between deontologists and utilitarians, these approaches share the view that moral problems are to be solved by the application of these abstract principles to cases. It is true that in bioethical discussions many of those within the utilitarian and deontological traditions do appeal to intermediate rules and principles. Nonetheless, this understanding of moral reasoning tends to overlook the importance of particulars, the relevance of the networks of human relationships, the significance of intimacy, and the import of the broad social and political arrangements in which moral decision making takes place.

During the last few decades a number of criticisms of mainstream ethical theory have appeared.[1] Of these criticisms, the ones coming from a feminist perspective have been especially concerned with the need of attending to context.[2] They have called attention to the inadequacy of the impartial and universalizing character of traditional ethical theories when coming to deal with issues of intimate relationships, situated people, or the influence of gender, race, ethnicity, and class inequalities in ethical decision-making. In spite of these criticisms, the defense of abstract moral rules and the decontextualization of moral problems have not withered.

The purpose of this paper is to show that this decontextualized approach to ethical issues is not just unhelpful for the decision making process of real, situated human beings, but dangerous. This is so, because by neglecting the context in which peo-ple make moral decisions we run the risk of furthering injustices against already disadvantaged groups. If we face social and political institutions that hinder particular groups or individuals and we then propose moral obligations that because of the unjust institutional context would place greater burdens on those groups or individuals, we can contribute to reinforcing such injustices. To show this, I will evaluate three putative moral obligations that our ability to obtain genetic information has made salient: the duty to obtain genetic information about ourselves, the obligation to inform family members about genetic risks, and the duty not to reproduce when we know that there is a high risk of transmitting a serious disease or defect. I will argue here that in ignoring the context in which these moral obligations are put into practice, and in particular the situation of women in our society, a defense of these moral duties might further injustices against women.

Genetic Information and Moral Obligations

We live in the era of genetics. The Human Genome Project promises to offer an immense array of benefits by giving us information about our genetic make up. This knowledge together with the existence of reproductive technologies has sparked a series of concerns about our moral obligations to ourselves and to other people. With few exceptions,[3] discussions of the moral implications of genetic knowledge—including whether there are moral obligations that result from such knowledge—tend to neglect issues about whether and how these obligations might differentially affect women. Given the presence of social, economic, and political institutions related to health and reproduction that systematically disadvantage women, such neglect appears quite troublesome.

A number of authors have argued that under certain circumstances we have a duty to seek information about our genetic endowment,[4] an obligation to inform those members of our family who might also be at risk of carrying harmful genetic mutations,[5] and a duty not to bring affected babies into this world.[6] Autonomy and beneficence have been used as grounds to defend these moral obligations. Thus, to make autonomous decisions people ought to acquire information about their genetic endowment. Similarly, it is argued that a duty to prevent unnecessary harm to third parties requires that we inform family members who might be affected by genetic disorders and that we avoid bringing into the world children who might be affected by a serious disability or disease.

Of course, agreement about the existence of these presumed moral duties is far from universal.[7] Thus, some scholars reject these putative obligations and argue that parents ought to unconditionally commit to any kind of child they can have. Others maintain that autonomy is also grounds for a right not to be informed about one's genetic make up because information about future diseases might be so distressful that it can interfere with our ability to make rational decisions. Similarly, some argue that beneficence can ground our obligation not to inform others about their genetic risks because such information may cause psychological anguish to our family members. These arguments appear even stronger when we take into account the fact that there is no cure or possibility of prevention for many of the diseases for which genetic tests exist. In spite of these disagreements, debates about the existence of the moral duties here discussed are prevalent enough to deserve careful consideration of consequences for women. This is especially so because such consequences often are neglected even by those who reject these putative obligations.

Obligations to obtain and disclose genetic information might affect women differentially for several reasons. First, traditionally women have been responsible for family health. Women bear a disproportionate burden for the health care of children and partners. They tend to them when they are ill, nego-

tiate professional health care for their families, and communicate health care information on their behalf.[8] Thus, although care giving is often framed in gender-neutral terms, in practice women are the ones expected to bear the main responsibility for family care. And, this is the case both in the private and the public realm.[9] Wives and mothers are seen as having a duty to care for their husbands and children, as well as for other family members. Similarly, health care reform in many countries has increased demands on women to take on care giving responsibilities that were previously managed by professionals.[10] Given that women are the primary care givers of children and other family members, an obligation to seek and disclose genetic information about themselves would impose disproportional burdens on them. This obligation would be seen as a natural extension of their care giving duties. Thus, they would be the ones in charge of delivering to their relatives what many might see as bad news. This might produce conflicts with women's perceived duty of giving care because the disclosure of information could result in their relatives being anxious about the possibility of developing particular diseases. Women might then see themselves as causing others harm. Similarly, women would be faced with making decisions about which family members might need to be informed, how to deliver the information, or when the disclosure should occur.[11]

Another reason why obligations to obtain and disclose genetic information might affect women differentially is related to the fact that conceptions of responsibility are influenced by social meanings and practices.[12] In the context of our social practices, we have evidence that suggests that women tend to see the self, not as an atomized, autonomous agent, but as constructed in relation to others, as an interdependent self.[13] They see their lives as interconnected with the lives of others and define themselves in term of their social relationships with others and their obligations to them. In this context, to ignore the effects on women that the moral obligations to inform themselves or others might have is seriously problematic. Women seem to be prepared to undergo potentially risky medical interventions to fulfil their perceived obligation of caring for others.[14] Some studies on women undergoing genetic testing or attending genetic counseling indicate that women see the search for genetic information as a way to help their relatives. They tend to see their role in generating genetic information for their relatives as the right thing to do. In many cases they cite the need to preserve others' autonomy, often at the expense of their own, as the justification to obtain information about their own genetic endowments.[15] This raises questions about whether women's search for genetic information might be constrained by their perceived need to care for, and help their relatives, as well as for societies' perceptions that women are more adequate than men to care for others. Moreover, women who are identified as at-risk of suffering some genetic condition also assume responsibility for managing such risks. Thus, some women justify their willingness to adopt potentially harmful risk management, such as prophylactic mastectomies, by appealing to their responsibilities to fulfil their role as mothers or to prevent relatives from seeing them suffer or having to care for them.[16] Similarly, some research shows that women, more so than men, may view any potential risk as a negative appraisal of themselves.[17]

But, if discussing moral obligations to obtain and share genetic information in a decontextualized and gender-neutral fashion is problematic, to defend moral duties not to reproduce when we know that there is a high risk of transmitting a serious disease or defect is even more so. This is so because, as many authors have suggested,[18] women are often seen as more responsible for reproductive decision-making and also because genetic testing is often presented as a way for women to exercise reproductive autonomy.

In order to fulfill the duty not to reproduce when we know that there is a high risk of transmitting a serious disease or defect people might act in several ways. First, they might choose to do carrier testing to determine whether they are at risk of transmitting a harmful genetic mutation. Second, if the pregnancy has already occurred, women might decide to have prenatal testing. Third, if a pregnancy is desired and abortion is not seen as an option, pre-implantation diagnosis might be possible. In all of these cases, a moral obligation not to reproduce when we know that there is a high risk of transmitting a serious disease or defect disproportionately burdens women. Thus, to present such a moral duty in a decontextualized, gender-neutral manner might foster injustices against them.

Although at first glance the decision to undergo carrier testing for reproductive reasons might seem to affect women and men equally, in actuality this is far from being the case. Research indicates that women tend to accept offers of free carrier testing for particular genetic conditions (e.g., cystic fibrosis) more than men in population-based screening programs.[19] Women also tend to be tested initially when there might be a risk of transmitting a genetic mutation to their children. Only if the woman tests positive for a recessive disorder is the male partner involved in the testing.[20] Some have suggested that this might be due to the fact that men see carrier testing as related to reproductive choices and thus more of a women's responsibility.[21] It might also be related to the sense of responsibility for and to others that women tend to have. Other researchers have indicated that the fact that more women than men accept carrier testing might be related to the fact that women tend to use primary health care services more than men.[22] In any case, lack of attention to the context in which we are proposing the fulfillment of moral obligations would neglect that more women than men undergo carrier testing.

Once pregnancy occurs, the fulfillment of a moral duty not to reproduce when we know that there is a high risk of transmitting a serious disease or defect requires that we make use of prenatal testing. Although these tests present different degrees of intrusiveness, obviously, any information about a fetus' genetic condition is mediated through the woman's body. Presenting moral obligations not to reproduce under particular circumstances in a decontextualized fashion neglects the fact that only women can undergo amniocentesis, ultrasound, or any other of these tests. Furthermore, prenatal testing presents the possibility of choosing whether or not to terminate the pregnancy based on the result of the test, and women are the ones who have abortions. To this we must add the difficulty that many women find, in some jurisdictions, of obtaining late termination after detection of a genetic abnormality following amniocentesis. Thus, compared to men, women have to accept more physical invasion and also more responsibility for their fetus and children.

Of course, the fact that women are the only ones who can undergo these kinds of procedures does not make the moral obligation in question problematic. However, there are systemic and structural factors that disadvantage pregnant women and mothers. For example, problems related to lack of maternity leave, childcare services, access to health care, or employment opportunities present women with serious difficulties that men generally do not face. These hindrances do not result from the facts of pregnancy or motherhood, but from social and political choices that necessitate that when women take on the responsibilities associated with pregnancy and motherhood they do so without adequate social and institutional support. Hence a defense of a decontextualized moral duty not to bring particular children into the world, might further injustices against women by increasing the physical and emotional burdens of pregnancy and motherhood.

If a pregnancy is desired but a couple knows, or suspects, that they may transmit a harmful genetic mutation and they don't see abortion as an option, they can fulfill their moral duty not to bring an affected child into the world by using preimplantation genetic diagnoses in conjunction with in vitro fertilization (IVF).[23] Of course, IVF is a set of procedures that can only be undergone by women. Furthermore, IVF involves physical and emotional costs.[24] Women must learn an extraordinary amount of information to adequately prepare for IVF treatment. They must learn how to mix and administer injectable medications, interrupt their daily routines for serial blood tests and ultrasound examinations, and undergo a surgical procedure to retrieve oocytes. Moreover, IVF might pose serious risks to women's health. According to empirical evidence, risks to women undergoing IVF treatment range from simple nausea to death. For example, the hormones that doctors use to stimulate the ovaries are associated with numerous side effects. Some studies assert that ovulation induction may be a risk factor for certain types of hormone-dependent cancers.[25] Women undergoing this procedure are also at an increased risk of suffering from ovarian hyperstimulation syndrome,[26] postoperative infections, punctures of internal organs,[27] and ectopic pregnancies.[28]

Some Objections and Responses

My criticism of a decontextualized defense of moral obligations related to seeking, disclosing, and using genetic information might raise several objections. First, critics might argue that these moral obligations are prima facie obligations. As such, they need to be considered in the context of the full scope of people's responsibilities. This being the case, it seems unnecessary to employ lengthy discussions about the context in which these moral obligations are put into practice. Because these obligations are prima facie, individuals ought to make judgments about their particular situations. To the extent that their evaluations are correct, individuals who refuse to seek genetic information, disclose it to relatives, or use it for reproductive purposes, are fulfilling what they take to be their duties.[29]

This criticism however begs the question. It seems to assume that a decontextualized evaluation of moral obligations related to genetic information is an adequate one, as long as we advise that these are prima facie obligations. My point here has been to argue that such is not the case. When we try to analyze these moral obligations by simply pointing out that other things need to be considered we are implicitly and uncritically sanctioning the status quo. Thus, the philosopher has failed in the traditional role of social gadfly. Considering these obligations in context would draw our attention to the structural problems that must be transformed if we are to fulfill such duties.

Moreover, this objection fails to acknowledge that a defense of moral obligations in a decontextualized fashion carries implications for particular groups. Thus, it seems unclear how an appeal to the prima facie character of these obligations would solve the problem pointed out here, that is, the possibility of increasing injustices against those who already bear the greatest burden of fulfilling these moral duties.

Some might object that social roles often impose differential obligations on people. Hence, we might expect women to have obligations that emanate from their roles as mothers, sisters, or caregivers. This observation seems correct. However, nothing I have said here denies this point. People do, and ought to, have particular obligations that stem from their roles as parents, teachers, government officials, doctors, midwives, gardeners, etc. Meeting these duties can, of course, place different burdens on people and this need not be unjust or unfair. Nevertheless, social choices can either assist people in meeting their obligations or can obstruct their doing so. My goal here is to point out that in an institutional context in which women already face a variety of obstacles to carrying out the duties resulting from their social roles, to propose additional obligations, while ignoring the effects of the social context, can exacerbate existing injustices.

Another possible criticism of the arguments presented here might come from those who are sympathetic to the need of taking context into consideration when dealing with ethical issues. They might argue, however, that my analysis is too narrow and that factors others than gender are essential in any adequate analysis of moral obligations. Moreover, they can also maintain that other aspects of our social context, for example limited support to care for disabled children, also contribute to injustices against women.

I agree that a satisfactory evaluation of possible moral duties related to genetic information must consider many other factors. Thus, I am not claiming that all women might be affected equally by these moral obligations. Nor do I want to maintain that this is the only way in which women are unjustly affected, or that only gender issues are relevant when contextualizing moral duties. Issues of ethnicity and class are, without a doubt, pertinent to genetic information and the obligations associated with such information. Who has access to the technology necessary to fulfill these duties, and whether genetic information can be used to unfairly discriminate against people are just some examples of how particulars influence decision making in ethics.

Conclusion

Although the universalizing character of moral obligations might give us some insights into moral behavior, a strict adherence to an impartial, abstract, unsituated perspective appears not just unhelpful, but dangerous. I have shown here that neglecting the context in which particular moral obligations are implemented might contribute to the burdening of an already disadvantaged group. In particular, I have pointed out that the language of gender-neutrality often used in discussions of moral obligations related to obtaining, disclosing, and using genetic information might further injustices against women. This is so, because such discussions neglect the fact that women are more likely than men to undergo testing, they assume a disproportionate responsibility for disclosing genetic information and they bear the burdens of prenatal testing and preimplantation diagnosis. My arguments here should not be taken as defending the position that because of women's heightened sense of responsibility for care, they should not have access to tests that would give them the opportunity to gain access to information about themselves or about their offspring. On the contrary, my point here is precisely to highlight the fact that a defense of particular moral obligations might demand that we strive to transform those social structures that make the exercise of such moral duties unjustly burdensome to particular groups of people. If we ignore the context in which people make moral decisions, we will do little to ensure the change of those structures that perpetuate injustices against some people.

Acknowledgement

Thanks to Craig Hanks and two anonymous reviewers for helpful comments and suggestions on earlier drafts of this manuscript.

Notes

1   See, for example, M. Nussbaum. 1990. *Love's Knowledge*. Oxford: Oxford University Press; A. Jonsen & S. Toulmin. 1988. *The Abuse of Casuistry*. Berkeley: University of California Press; A. MacIntyre. 1981. *After Virtue. Notre Dame*, IN: University of Notre Dame Press; S. Toulmin. The Tyranny of Principles. *Hastings Cent Rep* 1981; 11: 31-39; P. Foot. 1978. *Virtues and Vices*. Oxford: Blackwell.

2   See, for example, A.L. Carse. Impartial Principle and

Moral Context: Securing a Place for the Particular in Ethical Theory. *J Med Philos* 1998; 23: 153-169; S. Wolf, ed. 1996. *Feminism and Bioethics. Beyond Reproduction*. New York: Oxford University Press; A. Baier. 1994. *Moral Prejudices*. Cambridge: Harvard University Press; S. Sherwin. 1992. *No Longer Patient*. Philadelphia: Temple University Press; V. Held. 1993. *Feminist Morality*. Chicago: University of Chicago Press.

3   See, for example, L. d'Agincourt-Canning. Experiences of Genetic Risk: Disclosure and the Gendering of Responsibility. *Bioethics* 2001; 15(3): 231-247; M.B. Mahowald. 2000. *Genes, Women, Equality*. New York: Oxford University Press; R. Hubbard. Genetics and Women's Health. *J Am Med Womens Assoc* 1997; 52(1): 2-3; A. Asch & G. Geller. 1996. Feminism, Bioethics, and Genetics. In *Feminism and Bioethics: Beyond Reproduction*, S. Wolf. ed. New York: Oxford University Press; M.B. Mahowald. A Feminist Standpoint for Genetics. *J Clin Ethics* 1996; 7(4): 333-340; L. Purdy. What Can Progress in Reproductive Technology Mean for Women? *J Med Philos* 1996; 21(5): 499-514; L.S. Parker. Breast Cancer Genetic Screening and Critical Bioethics' Gaze. *J Med Philos* 1995; 20(3): 313-337; A. Lippman. 1993. Worrying—and Worrying about—the Geneticization of Reproduction and Health. In *Misconceptions: The Social Construction of Choice and the New Reproductive Technologies*. vol 1., G. Basen, M. Eichler & A. Lippman, eds. Ottawa: Voyageur Press: 39-65; A. Lippman. Prenatal Genetic Testing and Screening: Constructing Needs and Reinforcing Inequities. *Am J Law Med* 1991; 17: 15-50.

4   See, for example, W. Glannon. 2001. *Genes and Future People*. Boulder, CO: Westview Press: ch. 2; R. Rhodes. Genetic Links, Family Ties, and Social Bonds: Rights and Responsibilities in the Face of Genetic Knowledge. *J Med Philos* 1998; 23(1): 10-30.

5   See Glannon, op. cit. note 4. See also Rhodes, op. cit. note 4.

6   See, for example, Glannon, op. cit. note 4; A. Buchanan et al. 2000. *From Chance to Choice*. Cambridge: Cambridge University Press: ch. 6; D. Davis. Genetic Dilemmas and the Child's Right to an Open Future. *Hastings Cent Rep* 1997; 27(2): 7-15; C. Cohen. Give Me Children or I Shall Die! New Reproductive Technologies and Harm to Children. *Hastings*

Cent Rep 1996; 26(2): 19-27; L. Purdy. 1996. Genetics and Reproductive Risk: Can Having Children Be Immoral? *In Reproducing Persons: Issues in Feminist Bioethics*. Ithaca: NY, Cornell University Press: 39-49; B. Steinbock & R. McClamrock. When Is Birth Unfair to the Child? *Hastings Cent Rep* 1994; 24(6): 15-21.

7   See, for example, S. Vehmas. Just Ignore It? Parents and Genetic Information. *Theor Med* 2001; 22(5): 473-484; T. Takala & M. Häyry. Genetic Ignorance, Moral Obligations and Social Duties. *J Med Philos* 2000; 25(1): 107-113; T. Takala. The Right to Genetic Ignorance Confirmed. *Bioethics* 1999; 13(3/4): 288-293; A. Huibers and A. van 't Spijker. The Autonomy Paradox: Predictive Genetic Testing and Autonomy: Three Essential Problems. *Patient Educ Couns* 1998; 35(1): 53-62.

8   See, M. Navaie-Waliser, A. Spriggs & P. H. Feldman. Informal Care-Giving: Differential Experiences by Gender. *Med Care* 2002; 40(12): 1249-1259; K. Donelan, M. Falik & C.M. DesRoches. Caregiving: Challenges and Implications for Women's Health. *Women's Health Issues* 2001; 11(3): 185-200; J. Wuest. Repatterning Care: Women's Proactive Management of Family Caregiving Demands. *Health Care Women Int* 2000; 21: 393-411; R.L. Hoffmann & A.M. Mitchell. Caregiver Burden: Historical Development. *Nurse Forum* 1998; 33(4): 5-11.

9   J. Parks. 2003. *No Place like Home?* Bloomington: Indiana University Press; E.F. Kittay. 1999. Love's Labor. New York: Routledge.

10   Wuest, op. cit. note 8.

11   N. Hallowell. Doing the right thing: genetic risk and responsibility. *Sociol Health Illn* 1999; 21(5): 597-621.

12   d'Agincourt-Canning, op. cit. note 3; Held, op. cit. note 2; M. Walker. 1998. *Moral Understandings: A Feminist Study in Ethics*. New York: Routledge.

13   See, for example, C. Mackenzie & N. Stoljar, eds. 2000. *Relational Autonomy. Feminist Perspectives on Autonomy, Agency, and the Social Self*. New York: Oxford University Press; C. Gilligan. 1982. *In a Different Voice: Psychological Theory and Women's Development*. Cambridge: Harvard University Press. See also, Baier, op. cit. note 2; Held, op. cit. note 2.

14   Hallowell, op. cit. note 11.

15   See, N. Hallowell et al. Balancing Autonomy and Responsibility: The Ethics of Generating and Dis-

closing Genetic Information. *J Med Ethics* 2003; 29(2): 74-79; G. Goelen et al. Moral Concerns of Different Types of Patients in Clinical BRCA1/2 Gene Mutation Testing. *Journal of Clinical Oncology* 1999; 17(5): 1595-1600; J. Mason. 1996. Gender, Care and Sensibility in Family and Kin Relationships. In *Sex, Sensibility and the Gendered Body*. J. Holland & L. Adkins, eds. Basingstoke: Macmillan.

16 Hallowell, op. cit. note 11.

17 J.E. Newman et al. Gender Differences in Psychosocial Reactions to Cystic Fibrosis Carrier Testing. *Am J Med Genet* 2002; 113: 155; G. Evers-Kiebooms et al. A Stigmatizing Effect of the Carrier Status for Cystic Fibrosis? *Clin Genet* 1994; 46: 336-343.

18 See, for example, T.M. Marteau et al. Long-term Cognitive and Emotional Impact of Genetic Testing for Carriers of Cystic Fibrosis: The Effects of Test Result and Gender. *J Health Psychol* 1997; 16: 51-62; M. Stacey. 1996. The New Genetics: A Feminist View. In *The Troubled Helix: Social and Psychological Implications of the New Human Genetics*. T.M. Marteau & M.P.M. Richards, eds. Cambridge: Cambridge University Press: 331-349; J.C. Callahan, ed. 1995. *Reproduction, Ethics, and The Law*. Bloomington: Indiana University Press; C. Overall. 1987. *Ethics and Human Reproduction*. Boston: Allen and Unwin; B.K. Rothman. 1986. *The Tentative Pregnancy*. New York: Viking; M. O'Brien. 1981. *Politics of Reproduction*. London: Routledge Kegan and Paul.

19 H. Bekker et al. Uptake of Cystic Fibrosis Testing in Primary Care: Supply Push or Demand Pull? *Br Med J* 1993; 306: 158-586; E.K. Watson et al. Psychological and Social Consequences of Community Carrier Testing Screening for Cystic Fibrosis. *Lancet* 1992; 40: 217-220.

20 Mahowald, op. cit. note 3.

21 Bekker, op. cit. note 19.

22 Watson, op. cit. note 19.

23 D. Wells & D.A. Delhanty. Preimplantation Genetic Diagnosis: Applications for Molecular Medicine. *Trends Mol Med* 2001; 7(1): 23-30.

24 I. De Melo-Martin. 1998. *Making Babies: Biomedical Technologies, Reproductive Ethics, and Public Policy*. Dordercht: Kluwer: ch. 4.

25 See, for example, J.V. Lacey, Jr et al. Menopausal Hormone Replacement Therapy and Risk of Ovarian Cancer. *JAMA* 2002; 288(3): 334-341; C.F. Schairer et al. Menopausal Estrogen and Estrogen-Progestin Replacement Therapy and Breast Cancer Risk. *JAMA* 2000; 283(4): 485-491; A.Venn. Risk of Cancer after Use of Fertility Drugs with In-Vitro Fertilization. *Lancet* 1999; 354(9190): 1586-1890; R.E. Bristow & B.Y. Karlan. The Risk of Ovarian Cancer after Treatment for Infertility. *Current Opinion in Obstetric Gynecology* 1996; 8(1): 32-37; A.F. Berrino et al. Serum Sex Hormone Levels after Menopause and Subsequent Breast Cancer. *J Natl Cancer Inst* 1996; 88(5): 291-296.

26 See, for example, S.Y. Mitchell et al. Ovarian Hyperstimulation Syndrome Associated with Clomiphene Citrate. *West Indian Med J* 2001; 50(3): 227-229; A. Delvigne & S. Rozenberg. Preventive Attitude of Physicians to Avoid OHSS in IVF Patients. *Hum Reprod* 2001; 16(12): 2491-2495; B. McElhinney & N. McClure. Ovarian Hyperstimulation Syndrome. *Baillieres Best Pract Res Clin Obstet Gynaecol* 2000; 14(1): 103-122.

27 See, for example, L. Koch. 1993. Physiological and Psychosocial Risks of the New Reproductive Technologies. In *Tough Choices*. P. Stephenson & M.G. Wagner, eds. Philadelphia: Temple University Press: 122-134; P.J. Taylor & J.V. Kredentser. 1992. Diagnostic and Therapeutic Laparoscopy and Hysteroscopy and Their Relationship to In Vitro Fertilization. In *A Textbook of In Vitro Fertilization and Assisted Reproductive Technology*. P.R. Brinsden & P.A. Rainsbury, eds. Park Ridge, NJ: The Parthenon Publishing Group: 73-92; P.R. Brinsden. 1992. Oocyte Recovery and Embryo Transfer Techniques for In Vitro Fertilization. In P.R. Brinsden & P.A. Rainsbury, eds. Ibid: 139-153.

28 American Society for Reproductive Medicine and Society for Assisted Reproductive Technology. Assisted Reproductive Technology in the United States: 1999 Results Generated from the American Society for Reproductive Medicine/Society for Assisted Reproductive Technology Registry. *Fertil Steril* 2002; 78: 918-931.

29 R. Rhodes. Autonomy, Respect, and Genetic Information Policy: A Reply to Tuija Takala and Matti Häyry. *J Med Philos* 2000; 25(1): 114-120.

59

GENETIC ENHANCEMENT—A THREAT TO HUMAN RIGHTS?

Elizabeth Fenton

SOURCE: *Bioethics* 22.1 (2008): 1-7.

I. Globalism, Bioethics, and Human Rights

The call has been made for global bioethics. In an age of pandemics, international drug trials, and genetic technology, health has gone global, and bioethics must follow suit. George Annas is one among a number of thinkers to recommend that bioethics expand beyond its traditional domain of patient-physician interactions to encompass a broader range of health-related matters. Medicine, Annas argues, must 'develop a global language and a global strategy that can help to improve the health of all of the world's citizens.'[1] Others have identified the need for a lingua franca to address bioethics concerns that transcend national and cultural boundaries.[2] Biotechnology, which potentially affects the whole human species, presents challenges to our moral thinking 'so formidable and far-reaching,' argues Roberto Andorno, that 'individual countries alone cannot address them.'[3]

Individual countries cannot address global health issues, and neither are culturally specific principles adequate for addressing global bioethics concerns. Global issues require global consensus about the grounds from which deliberations on the issues should proceed. This consensus in turn requires a foundation of universally agreed-upon statements about humankind, which will be transcultural yet supportive of moral pluralism. The claim has been made that such a foundation already exists in human rights, and that human rights should, therefore, be the new lingua franca of bioethics.

There are good reasons for advancing this claim. First, global health issues such as disease pandemics are public health issues. Since the adequacy of social conditions is a focus of both public health and human rights practice, human rights language, it is argued, is therefore a fitting articulation of public health ethics. Jonathan Mann has argued for a strong relationship between public health and human rights on the ground that violations of human rights have significant adverse effects on health and well-being.[4] Annas has argued that the Universal Declaration of Human Rights should serve as the code of ethics for public health, since both seek to provide 'the conditions under which humans can flourish.'[5]

Second, human rights discourse, as Robert Baker points out, 'is already the accepted language of international ethics.'[6] As such, it serves as the ubiquitous mode of expressing social criticism, and is a significant framework for addressing social problems. If bioethics is to progress and take part in international debate on social issues, it must take human rights as its starting point.

Third, as part of a legal regime, human rights carry significantly more weight than ethical principles that may be ignored without consequence. Bioethics may benefit from yoking itself to a doctrine with significant legal clout on the global stage.

Fourth, human rights are the currency of an ever-increasing body of nongovernmental organizations (NGOs). Physicians for Human Rights, Médecins sans Frontières, Médecins du Monde, and Annas' own Global Lawyers and Physicians are just some of the many NGOs that form an important and energized political movement focused on promoting human rights. Taking the language of human rights as its foundation could allow bioethics to advance its goals on the wheels of this established political machine.

These four claims indicate the advantages of a strong relationship between bioethics and human rights. But there are also good reasons to be circumspect regarding the potential of human rights to serve as the language of global bioethics. Advocates of a human rights foundation for bioethics, such as George Annas, are placing unreasonable demands on the language and conceptual framework of human rights. A key example of the misplaced use of human rights in bioethical debate is Annas' argument against genetic technology, in which he claims that reproductive cloning and genetic enhancement ought to be classified as a new category of 'crimes against humanity,' and that scientists who develop these technologies are properly considered to be committing terrorist acts.[7] In a similar vein, the European Parliament claims to be convinced that cloning for any reason is 'morally repugnant, contrary to respect for the person, and a grave violation of fundamental human rights.'[8] These claims rely on the language of human rights to argue against biotechnology, but it is unclear whether the human rights framework is the most useful or appropriate basis for such an objection. This paper examines the legitimacy of these claims, both to debunk them as objections to biotechnology, and to illustrate that the language and framework of human rights, while it has much to offer bioethics, must be used judiciously, rather than imported wholesale.[9]

II. Human Nature as the Source of Human Rights

Annas' primary argument against genetic enhancement technology proceeds as follows. First, he assumes that human rights and human equality are grounded in human dignity; and human dignity, in turn, is grounded in a common human nature. Second, he assumes that genetic technology offers possibilities for changing our common human nature, or 'fundamental human characteristics.' For example, it could make some human traits optional (such as sexual reproduction, through cloning), or it could lead to the creation of individuals who did not fit the species definition of Homo sapiens, or who were incapable of sexually reproducing with a member of that species. From these two assumptions Annas concludes that any such changes to our common human nature will undermine the very basis of human rights and human equality:

Because it is the meaning of humanness (our distinctness from other animals) that has given birth to our concepts of both human dignity and human rights, altering our nature threatens to undermine our concepts of both human dignity and human rights. With their loss the fundamental belief in human equality would also be lost.[10]

This argument implicitly assumes that the kinds of changes that biotechnology promises—i.e., changes to genetically based traits or characteristics—are the kinds of changes that threaten human nature. In other words, Annas assumes that the 'human nature' that underpins human rights is essentially biological.

Having concluded that genetic technology threatens human rights and human equality, and making the tacit assumption that human rights and human equality ought to be preserved, Annas argues that human nature, our 'fundamental human characteristics,' should be protected from change. Since human nature is what binds us as a species, his arguments call for protection and preservation of the human species, protection from technology whose use, he believes, constitutes a new category of 'crimes against humanity.'[11] What is really at stake, then, is our very existence as a species. Again, implicit in this argument is the assumption that protecting our existence as a species means protecting the biological traits that currently define the species.

While acknowledging that some genetic enhancements, such as improvements to memory, immunity, or strength, may not change the nature of the species or create individuals who no longer fit the definition of H. sapiens, Annas has serious concerns about the potential of enhancement technology to lead to the creation of a new species of humans, the 'posthumans.' The differences between humans and posthumans, Annas predicts, will be such as to render one species inferior in the eyes of the other, leading to exploitation, enslavement, or even 'genetic genocide.'[12]

In sum: genetic technology endangers our dignity, equality, and rights as human beings; it threatens our existence as a species; and it poses the specter of inter-species warfare.

III. Critique of Annas' Core Argument

(a) Annas' core argument claims that human nature, described in terms of fixed biological traits that define membership in the species Homo sapiens, is the foundation for human rights. This claim implies that fixed biological traits are normatively significant, that their presence or absence determines membership not only in a species, but also in a moral community defined by the notion of human rights.

While remaining agnostic on the question of whether human rights are based on human nature, I reject Annas' assumption that human nature is reducible to biological traits, and his assumption that fixed biological traits are normatively connected to moral status or the notion of human rights. Even if it is the case that human rights are best thought of as founded on commonalities between all humans, biological commonalities are insufficient for this foundation. The moral status of non-human animals, for example, has long been considered by many to depend not on the species to which they belong, but rather on morally relevant characteristics, such as the capacity to feel pain. Some morally relevant characteristics track biological traits, but this is not necessarily so, and it is certainly not the case that the human genome as it is currently constituted, is either necessary or sufficient for membership in the moral community. As Mary Anne Warren argues, 'Genetic humanity ... is at best an indicator, not an independently valid criterion, of moral status.'[13]

The notion that human rights are grounded in the presence of certain biological traits, such as sexual reproduction, obscures the primary function of human rights as equalizing the moral or legal status of human beings, notwithstanding their manifest differences. Moreover, it obscures the notion of the moral community as formed by individuals possessing morally relevant characteristics, such as the capacity to suffer, to experience pain, fear or grief. Biological traits are not in themselves morally relevant: whether a being reproduces sexually or by cloning is irrelevant, just by itself, to the moral status of that being. Such traits cannot therefore be the sole determinants of whether a being is entitled to claim rights or human rights. They may co-exist with or correspond to other features of the being that are morally relevant, as would be the case if it turned out that only sexually reproducing beings are rational, choosing agents. Biological traits like sexual reproduction alone cannot determine moral status or rights claims. Any changes to these traits through genetic engineering cannot, just by themselves, pose a threat to human nature, nor to human rights.

(b) In addition to the claim that human nature is reducible to biology, Annas' argument makes a significant assumption about the foundations of human rights. He claims that human rights have a single foundation, namely human dignity, which, in turn, is grounded in biologically defined human nature. In order to argue successfully that genetic engineering undermines human nature, thereby threatening the foundation of human rights and so the rights themselves, Annas owes us an account of what that foundation is. But further analysis of the concept of dignity is glaringly absent from the argument. I suggest that there are two ways in which Annas' use of 'dignity' can be understood, neither of which advances his argument.

The first possibility is that Annas views dignity as a religious or metaphysical foundation for human rights, perhaps grounded in the claim that human beings are sacred or intrinsically valuable, created in the image of God. But this kind of foundational claim is highly controversial. Since human rights are supposed to be universal in their application—that is, valid for all human beings regardless of their race, religion, gender, and so on—the claim that they are founded on a singular philosophical or theological view of human nature will be problematic. There is widespread religious disagreement among the individuals to whom these rights apply. Atheists will reject the notion that human beings are sacred, since 'sacred' implies a God whose creations are sacred, while non-Christians will reject the notion that humans are sacred in the eyes of a single Christian God. Humans disagree about what kinds of being they are and what makes them special, if anything. To take any single philosophical or religious idea and claim that it is the foundation of a universal doctrine will not only vitiate the doctrine's claim to universality, but will render it illegitimate in the eyes of many of those to whom it is supposed to apply. As Amy Gutmann observes,

> If human rights necessarily rest on a moral or metaphysical foundation that is not in any meaningful sense universal or publicly defensible in the international arena ... then the political legitimacy of human rights talk, human rights covenants, and human rights enforcement is called into question.[14]

In short, this first suggested gloss on Annas' notion of dignity founders on the problem of pluralism. In order to be acceptable to a wide range of people, human rights cannot claim to have a single moral, metaphysical or religious foundation. There is, however, another interpretation of Annas' use of 'dignity' that may be more charitable than the single foundation view. On this gloss, dignity is not a unitary philosophical or religious conception, but rather shorthand, or a placeholder, for a range of concepts that define human rights. For example, 'dignity' could stand in for a single feature of human beings, such as agency. James Griffin argues that dignity is derived from agency; human rights are grounded in the dignity of persons, but the stress is on persons or agents, rather than on dignity.[15] Or it could stand in for the conditions of a fully human or flourishing life. Martha Nussbaum argues that the dignity of a human being consists in the freedom to choose to perform certain functions—i.e., the capability to perform those functions—functions that are 'of central importance to a human life.'[16] For a human being to be free and dignified, she must have the capability to perform these functions in some way guaranteed, whether or not she actually chooses to perform them. On this account human dignity is tethered to humanness per se, since a life without certain basic capabilities is 'too lacking, too impoverished, to be human at all.'[17] When Annas claims that human dignity is the foundation of human rights, he could mean that these capabilities or conditions, or human agency, are what give human rights their meaning and application.

But this interpretation of dignity will not help Annas for two reasons. First, if he wants to claim that dignity is necessarily threatened by genetic technology, Annas would be guilty of begging the fundamental question. If dignity stands in for the conditions of a fully human or flourishing human life, then in claiming that it is threatened by genetic technology, Annas assumes precisely that which he intends to prove, namely that genetic technology can only make life worse, not better. Second, on this interpretation of dignity, Annas loses the thrust behind his claim that dignity is threatened by genetic technology. If dignity is equivalent to agency, then clearly it is not necessarily threatened by genetic technology, since most proposed interventions do not endanger agency, understood as self-determination or the capacity to choose goals and the freedom to pursue them.[18] Enhanced memory or intelligence, for example, would improve capacities that humans already possess. If a student of the future is better able to recall material she was taught years (or even semesters) before, her agency has not been undermined; she is a more efficient agent when it comes to memory recall. Someone who lives to the age of 150 is no less of an agent than someone of the current era who lives only to 85; the extra 65 years would, in fact, actually bestow more time in which to be an agent.

Annas could concede that longevity or better memory does not undermine agency, and still maintain that dignity, standing in for the conditions of a full and flourishing life, is threatened by this technology—i.e., that allowing enhancement will make our society a worse place to live. But this is an empirical claim about the future, one on which Annas could simply be wrong. The conditions of a full and flourishing human life could change as genetic technology proliferates. In listing the capabilities necessary for a fully human life, Nussbaum explicitly claims that the list is 'open-ended' and therefore evolving.[19] Moreover, none of these capabilities (bodily health, imagination, emotion, practical reason, friendship, etc.) are in fact threatened by, for example, enhanced intelligence or athleticism. Even if Annas insists at this point that the technology could have a negative impact on important human institutions or practices, rather than a direct physical or psychological impact on individuals, it is still not necessarily the case that genetic enhancement technology will undermine the conditions for a flourishing life, particularly if those conditions are open-ended. The conditions of a flourishing human life could be met in a society using genetic enhancement technology. If Annas intends dignity to be understood as a placeholder for agency or the conditions of a good life, his objection to genetic technology simply falls flat. This is not to say that genetic technology could never truly threaten human agency or the conditions of a flourishing life, or that there would not be good reasons to oppose technology that does so. Rather, it is to say that wholesale opposition to the technology cannot be supported by the claim that it necessarily threatens either of these.

Annas' appeal to dignity as the foundation for human rights is open to two interpretations, both of which fail to provide any plausible basis for his claim that genetic technology threatens human rights. His attempt to invoke human rights as a means to object to genetic technology doubly fails. It fails in its account of human nature, and in its account of human dignity, and therefore fails to show that either of these is threatened by genetic technology. I thus see no good reason to object to genetic technology on the ground that it threatens human rights.

(c) I turn now to Annas' concern that human use of genetic technology will result in inequalities between individuals, and perhaps even changes so significant as to produce a species of 'posthumans.' Annas is concerned that humans and posthumans would not be equal in the sense required for the applicability of equal human rights. But the only sense in which Annas could surmise that humans and posthumans would not be equal is in the sense that the differences between them, in biological terms, would be significant. Posthumans, for example, may not reproduce sexually, but may reproduce by cloning. As we have already argued, this view is vitiated by the mistaken assumption that the equality necessary for human rights is grounded in shared or common biological traits, but I want here to emphasize a different problem with this view. What Annas fails to acknowledge is that humans, within the species, already vary greatly with respect to their biological characteristics, such as physical strength, intelligence, talents, aptitudes and so on. These differences do not undermine the universality of human rights; in fact, it is the very purpose of human rights

to render all human individuals equal regardless of such differences.[20] The sorts of differences that Annas predicts will cause so much trouble are already with us: humans vary in large degree in terms of their biological makeup. Such differences are the raison d'être of human rights, whose very point is to equalize across differences. The changes most likely to come sooner rather than later from genetic technology (boosts to 'primary goods' such as the immune system, memory, or intelligence)[21] will merely replicate the exact nature of the differences that already exist among individuals protected by human rights. So those rights will continue to protect individuals who may differ from us in significant ways—the differences themselves are morally irrelevant. This point reinforces the argument above, that human rights are not grounded in fixed biological traits, such that individuals who do not share those traits cannot enjoy human rights. Fixed biological traits may ground species distinctions and determine species membership, but if a child born tomorrow lacked, for example, the capacity to reproduce sexually, or had gills instead of normal human breathing apparatus, that child would not be denied human rights, though she may represent the beginning of 'posthumanity.'

Moreover, Annas' attempt to argue for a ban on genetic technology on the grounds that it introduces levels of difference between humans that will be beyond the equalizing power of human rights simply overlooks the potential the technology has for good. At the very beginning of an era of enhancement we should look ahead with a pragmatic optimism, rather than presuming the worst and predicting a future of science fiction horrors.[22] Annas may be exaggerating for rhetorical effect, but exaggeration does not obscure the basic point: although we should proceed with caution, we should do so with an eye for the good outcomes of the technology as well as the bad.

IV. Conclusions

Annas' core argument against genetic technology, in particular enhancement and cloning technology, centers on the claims that human nature is the foundation of human rights, that human nature is threatened by genetic technology, and therefore that human rights are threatened by genetic technology. The appeal to human nature as the foundation of human rights is deeply problematic philosophically. It rests on the dubious claim that human nature is defined by fixed biological traits of the sort that may be altered through genetic technology, and imbues these traits with misplaced normative significance, claiming that the characteristics that determine species membership are also those that determine the applicability of human rights. Not only is Annas mistaken in claiming that human nature can be reduced to biology, he also fails to provide an account of human dignity adequate to justify his claim that it is the foundation of human rights. If he is claiming that dignity is the single, authoritative foundation for human rights, his argument founders on moral pluralism. If instead he is claiming that dignity can stand in for other features of human beings, such as agency, then he begs the question against genetic technology in claiming that it violates human dignity. In this core argument Annas gives no reason to accept that genetic technology threatens either human nature or human rights.

A broader conclusion can also be drawn from this discussion. Annas invokes human rights to justify a ban on genetic technology, in part because he views standard bioethical arguments as 'too weak a reed' on which to base such a ban. Bioethics alone is too weak because the issues at stake concern something grander than medical and scientific practice—viz. 'the nature of humanity and the rights of humans.'[23] But even if human rights talk is not wholly misplaced in the debate over genetic technology, it does not add to the conversation. The ethical problems raised by genetic technology need to be carefully analyzed and thought through, but it is far from clear that human rights are of any help in doing this, particularly since this technology need not violate human rights in any case. Annas' argument against genetic technology is an example of human rights language being deployed as a trump card, an ultimate and unarguable reason to oppose the technology. But as this analysis shows, the deployment of human rights language requires careful thought, and even in the most significant of ethical debates, it may be neither appropriate nor helpful.

The call for a global bioethic is not in itself misguided; bioethics must 'go global' to meet public health challenges that transcend national and cultural boundaries. But the call for human rights to serve as the foundation and lingua franca of the new bioethics is misguided. Human rights form only a part of morality, and so should form only a part of bioethics. The genetic technology debate is a key example of an instance in which it may be better to explore other aspects of our ethical thinking, forsaking human rights talk altogether.

Acknowledgements

I would like to acknowledge the assistance of Professor John D. Arras in developing this argument and making comments on previous drafts. I am thankful to the reviewers of *Bioethics* for their helpful comments.

Notes

1   George Annas. 2005. *American Bioethics: Crossing Human Rights and Health Law Boundaries*. Oxford: Oxford University Press: 24.

2   Lori P. Knowles. The Lingua Franca of Human Rights and the Rise of a Global Bioethic. *Camb Q Healthc Ethics* 2001; 10: 253-263. David C. Thomasma. Proposing a New Agenda: Bioethics and International Human Rights. *Camb Q Healthc Ethics* 2001; 10: 299-310.

3   Roberto Andorno. Biomedicine and International Human Rights Law: In Search of a Global Consensus. *Bull World Health Organ* 2002; 80(12): 959-963.

4   Jonathan M. Mann. Medicine and Public Health, Ethics and Human Rights. *Hastings Cent Rep* 1997; 27(3): 6-14.

5   Annas, op. cit. note 1, p. 24.

6   Robert Baker. Bioethics and Human Rights: A Historical Perspective. *Camb Q Healthc Ethics* 2001; 10: 241-252. Andorno shares this view, calling human rights 'the last expression of a universal ethics,' and 'a "lingua franca" of international relations.' (Andorno, op. cit. note 3, p. 960.)

7   Annas, op. cit. note 1, p. 40.

8   The European Parliament. 1998. Resolution on Human Cloning O.J. (C 34) 164. Available at http://www1.umn.edu/humanrts/instree/cloning2.html [Accessed May 27, 2006].

9   It is important to note that this paper focuses on one particular view of human rights—that emerging in recent criticisms of biotechnology made by George Annas and other 'techno-conservatives' such as Francis Fukuyama and Jürgen Habermas. This view of human rights rests on an account of human nature, and it is to this account that the principle criticisms of the paper are addressed. Other views of human rights reject the human nature account, and so are unlikely to be vulnerable to this critique. Rober Baker, for example, argues in favor of human rights-based global bioethics, but rejects the human nature account of human rights, on the grounds that on such an account rights are so profoundly influenced by culture that they are unable to transcend particular cultural contexts and so serve as an adequate basis of global bioethics. See particularly Robert Baker. A Theory of International Bioethics. *Kennedy Inst Ethics J* 1998; 8(3): 233-274.

10 Annas, op. cit. note 1, p. 37.

11 Ibid: 40.

12 Annas, op. cit. note 1, p. 51.

13 Mary Anne Warren. 1997. *Moral Status: Obligations to Persons and Other Living Things*. Oxford: Clarendon Press: 19.

14 Amy Gutmann, ed. Michael Ignatieff. 2001. *Human Rights as Politics and Idolatry*. Princeton: Princeton University Press: xvii.

15 James Griffin. Discrepancies between the best philosophical account of human rights and the international law of human rights. The Presidential Address, Meeting of the Aristotelian Society, October 9, 2000.

16 Martha C. Nussbaum. 2002. Capabilities and Human Rights. In *Global Justice and Transnational Politics: Essays on the Moral and Political Challenges of Globalization*. Pablo de Greiff and Ciaran Cronin, eds. Cambridge, MA: MIT Press: 127.

17 Martha C. Nussbaum. Social Justice and Universalism: In Defense of an Aristotelian Account of Human Functioning. *Mod Philol* 1993; 90, Supplement: S57.

18 Griffin, op. cit. note 15, p. 4.

19 Martha C. Nussbaum. 1995. Human Capabilities, Female Human Beings. In *Women, Culture, and Development: A Study of Human Capabilities*. Martha C. Nussbaum and Jonathon Glover, eds. Oxford: Clarendon Press: 74.

20 It is important to note that some physical similarity is assumed here. In his discussion of the 'circumstances of justice' Rawls emphasizes the necessity of rough equality of human beings in their physical characteristics, in addition to their moral equality (John Rawls. 1971. *A Theory of Justice*. Cambridge, MA: Harvard University Press: 127; Chapter 3, Section 22.). It is for this reason that animals are not considered in the discussion of the basic principles of justice. But while humans differ from one another much less than they differ from members of other species, individual humans can differ from one another significantly, and the circumstances of justice remain. Enhancement technology will not produce humans so different from us that the circumstances of justice will not obtain. I may be more different from an unenhanced and severely mentally disabled individual than I am from an enhanced individual with a better memory, yet since I recognize the severely disabled person as standing in the relationship of justice to us, then I will also recognize the enhanced individual as a subject of justice.

21 Some very basic characteristics are described as natural primary goods, in the Rawlsian sense of being 'maximally flexible assets,' or goods regardless of one's life plan or vision of the good. Alan Buchanan et al. 2000. From *Chance to Choice: Genetics and Justice*. Cambridge: Cambridge University Press: 80, 174.

22 Dismal fictional accounts of the human future, such as Aldous Huxley's *Brave New World* are often cited in support of arguments against genetic technology. But not all fictional accounts of a genetically engineered future are pessimistic. Perhaps the most apposite science fiction treatment of the subject of enhancement is the X-Men comics and films, which portray the social and political conflicts between humans as presently constituted and 'mutants' endowed with an impressive variety of special powers (e.g., telepathy, teleporting, etc.), who are said to rep-

resent the next stage of human evolution. Importantly, the non-humans and X-characters in these futuristic worlds are portrayed, like the humans, as full
agents; and peaceful co-existence among them all is

viewed as possible and desirable in spite of prejudice
against the mutants on the part of the unmodified
humans.

23   Annas, op. cit. note 1, p. 39.

60.
CLONING, ETHICS, AND RELIGION

Lee M. Silver

SOURCE: *Cambridge Quarterly of Healthcare Ethics* 7.2 (1998): 168-72.

On Sunday morning, 23 February 1997, the world awoke to a technological advance that shook the foundations of biology and philosophy. On that day, we were introduced to Dolly, a 6-month-old lamb that had been cloned directly from a single cell taken from the breast tissue of an adult donor. Perhaps more astonished by this accomplishment than any of their neighbors were the scientists who actually worked in the field of mammalian genetics and embryology. Outside the lab where the cloning had actually taken place, most of us thought it could never happen. Oh, we would say that perhaps at some point in the distant future, cloning might become feasible through the use of sophisticated biotechnologies far beyond those available to us now. But what many of us really believed, deep in our hearts, was that this was one biological feat we could never master. New life—in the special sense of a conscious being—must have its origins in an embryo formed through the merger of gametes from a mother and father. It was impossible, we thought, for a cell from an adult mammal to become reprogrammed, to start all over again, to generate another entire animal or person in the image of the one born earlier. How wrong we were.

Of course, it wasn't the cloning of a sheep that stirred the imaginations of hundreds of millions of people. It was the idea that humans could now be cloned as well, and many people were terrified by the prospect. Ninety percent of Americans polled within the first week after the story broke felt that human cloning should be banned.[1] And while not unanimous, the opinions of many media pundits, ethicists, and policy makers seemed to follow that of the public at large. The idea that humans might be cloned was called "morally despicable," "repugnant," "totally inappropriate," as well as

"ethically wrong, socially misguided and biologically mistaken."[2]

Scientists who work directly in the field of animal genetics and embryology were dismayed by all the attention that now bore down on their research. Most unhappy of all were those associated with the biotechnology industry, which has the most to gain in the short-term from animal applications of the cloning technology.[3] Their fears were not unfounded. In the aftermath of Dolly, polls found that two out of three Americans considered the cloning of animals to be morally unacceptable, while 56% said they would not eat meat from cloned animals.[4]

It should not be surprising, then, that scientists tried to play down the feasibility of human cloning. First they said that it might not be possible at all to transfer the technology to human cells.[5] And even if human cloning is possible in theory, they said, "it would take years of trial and error before it could be applied successfully," so that "cloning in humans is unlikely any time soon."[6] And even if it becomes possible to apply the technology successfully, they said, "there is no clinical reason why you would do this."[7] And even if a person wanted to clone him- or herself or someone else, he or she wouldn't be able to find trained medical professionals who would be willing to do it. Really? That's not what science, history, or human nature suggest to me. The cloning of Dolly broke the technological barrier. There is no reason to expect that the technology couldn't be transferred to human cells. On the contrary, there is every reason to expect that it can be transferred. If nuclear transplantation works in every mammalian species in which it has been seriously tried, then nuclear transplantation will work with human cells as well. It requires only equipment and facilities that are already standard, or easy to obtain by biomedical laboratories and freestanding in vitro fertilization clinics across the world. Although the protocol itself demands the services of highly trained and skilled personnel, there are thousands of people with such skills in dozens of countries. The initial horror elicited by the announcement of Dolly's birth was due in large part to a misunderstanding by the lay public and the media of what biological cloning is and is not. The science critic Jeremy Rifkin exclaimed: "It's a horrendous crime to make a Xerox (copy) of someone,"[8] and the Irvine, California, rabbi Bernard King was seriously frightened when he asked, "Can the cloning create a soul? Can scientists create the soul that would make a being ethical, moral, caring, loving, all the things we attribute humanity to?"[9] The Catholic priest Father Saunders suggested the "cloning would only produce humanoids or androids—soulless replicas of human beings that could be used as slaves."[10] And *New York Times* writer Brent Staples warned us that "synthetic humans would be easy prey for humanity's worst instincts."[11]

Anyone reading this volume already knows that real human clones will simply be later-born identical twins—nothing more and nothing less. Cloned children will be full-fledged human beings, indistinguishable in biological terms from all other members of the species. But even with this understanding, many ethicists, scholars, and scientists are still vehemently opposed to the use of cloning as means of human reproduction under any circumstances whatsoever. Why do they feel this way? Why does this new reproductive technology upset them so?

First, they say, it's a question of "safety." The cloning procedure has not been proven safe and, as a result, its application toward the generation of newborn children could produce deformities and other types of birth defects. Second, they say that even if physical defects can be avoided, there is the psychological well-being of the cloned child to consider. And third, above and beyond each individual child, they are worried about the horrible effect that cloning will have on society as a whole.

What I will argue here is that people who voice any one or more of these concerns are—either consciously or subconsciously—hiding the real reason they oppose cloning. They have latched on to arguments about safety, psychology, and society because they are simply unable to come up with an ethical argument that is not based on the religious notion that by cloning human beings man will be playing God, and it is wrong to play God.

Let us take a look at the safety argument first. Throughout the twentieth century, medical scientists have sought to develop new protocols and drugs for treating disease and alleviating human suffering. The safety of all these new medical protocols was initially unknown. But through experimental testing on animals first, and then volunteer human subjects, safety could be ascertained and governmental agencies—such as the Food and Drug Administration in the United States—could make a decision as to whether the new protocol or drug should be approved for use in standard medical practice. It would be ludicrous to suggest the legislatures should pass laws banning the application of each newly imagined medical protocol before its safety has been determined. Professional ethics committees, institutional review boards, and the individual ethics of each medical practitioner are relied upon to make sure that hundreds of new experimental protocols are tested and used in an appropriate manner each year. And yet the question of unknown safety alone was the single rationale used by the National Bioethics Advisory Board (NBAC) to propose a ban on human cloning in the United States.

Opposition to cloning on the basis of safety alone is almost surely a losing proposition. Although the media have concocted fantasies of dozens of malformed monster lambs paving the way for the birth of Dolly, fantasy is all it was. Of the 277 fused cells created by Wilmut and his colleagues, only 29 developed into embryos. These 29 embryos were placed into 13 ewes, of which 1 become pregnant and gave birth to Dolly.[12] If safety is measured by the percentage of lambs born in good health, then the record, so far, is 100% for nuclear transplantation from an adult cell (albeit with a sample size of 1).

In fact, there is no scientific basis for the belief that cloned children will be any more prone to genetic problems than naturally conceived children. The commonest type of birth defect results from the presence of an abnormal number of chromosomes in the fertilized egg. This birth defect arises during gamete production and, as such, its frequency should be greatly reduced in embryos formed by cloning. The second most common class of birth defects results from the inheritance of two mutant copies of a gene from two parents who are silent carriers. With cloning, any silent mutation in a donor will be silent in the newly formed embryo and child as well. Finally, much less frequently, birth defects can be caused by new mutations; these will occur with the same frequency in embryos derived through conception or cloning. (Although some scientists have suggested that chromosome shortening in the donor cell will cause cloned children to have a shorter lifespan, there is every reason to expect that chromosome repair in the embryo will eliminate this problem.) Surprisingly, what our current scientific understanding suggests is that birth defects in cloned children could occur less frequently than birth defects in naturally conceived ones.

Once safety has been eliminated as an objection to cloning, the next concern voiced is the psychological well-being of the child. Daniel Callahan, the former director of the Hastings Center, argues that "engineering someone's entire genetic makeup would compromise his or her right to a unique identity."[13] But no such "right" has been granted by nature—identical twins are born every day as natural clones of each other. Dr. Callahan would have to concede this fact, but he might still argue that just because twins occur naturally does not mean we should create them on purpose.

Dr. Callahan might ague that a cloned child is harmed by knowledge of her future condition. He might say that it's unfair to go through childhood knowing what you will look like as an adult, or being forced to consider future medical ailments that might befall you. But even in the absence of cloning, many children have some sense of the future possibilities encoded in the genes they got from their parents. Furthermore, genetic screening already provides people with the ability to learn about hundreds of disease predispositions. And as genetic knowledge and technology become more and more sophisticated, it will become possible for any human being to learn even more about his or her genetic future than a cloned child could learn from his or her progenitor's past.

It might also be argued that a cloned child will be harmed by having to live up to unrealistic expectations placed on her by her parents. But there is no reason to believe that her parents will be any more unreasonable than many other parents who expect their children to accomplish in their lives what they were unable to accomplish in their own. No one would argue that parents with such tendencies should be prohibited from having children.

But let's grant that among the many cloned children brought into this world, some will feel badly about the fact that their genetic constitution is not unique. Is this alone a strong enough reason to ban the practice of cloning? Before answering this question, ask yourself another: Is a child having knowledge of an older twin worse off than a child born into poverty? If we ban the former, shouldn't we ban the latter? Why is it that so many politicians seem to care so much about cloning but so little about the welfare of children in general?

Finally, there are those who argue against cloning based on the perception that it will harm society at large in some way. The *New York Times* columnist William Safire expresses the opinion of many others when he says that "cloning's identicality would restrict evolution."[14] This is bad, he argues, because "the continued interplay of genes ... is central to humankind's progress." But Mr. Safire is wrong on both practical and theoretical grounds. On practical grounds, even if human cloning became efficient, legal, and popular among those in the moneyed classes (which is itself highly unlikely), it would still only account for a fraction of a percent of all the children born onto this earth. Furthermore, each of the children born by cloning to different families would be different from each other, so where does the identicality come from?

On the theoretical grounds, Safire is wrong because humankind's progress has nothing to do with unfettered evolution, which is always unpredictable and not necessarily upward bound. H.G. Wells recognized this principle in his 1895 novel *The Time Machine*, which portrays the evolution of humankind into weak and dimwitted but cuddly little creatures. And Kurt Vonnegut follows this same theme in *Galápagos*, where he suggests that our "big brains" will be the cause of our downfall, and future humans with smaller brains and powerful flippers will be the only remnants of a once great species, a million years hence.

As is so often the case with new reproductive technologies, the real reason that people condemn cloning has nothing to do with technical feasibility, child psychology, societal well-being, or the preservation of the human species. The real reason derives from religious beliefs. It is the sense that cloning leaves God out of the process of human creation, and that man is venturing into places he does not belong. Of course, the playing God objection only makes sense in the context of one's definition of God, as a supernatural being who plays a role in the birth of each new member of our species. And even if one holds this particular view of God, it does not necessarily follow that cloning is equivalent to playing God. Some who consider themselves to be religious have argued that if God didn't want man to clone, "he" wouldn't have made it possible.

Should public policy in a pluralist society be based on a narrow religious point of view? Most people would say no, which is why those who hold this point of view are grasping for secular reasons to support their call for an unconditional ban on the cloning of human beings. When the dust clears from the cloning debate, however, the secular reasons will almost certainly have disappeared. And then, only religious objections will remain.

Notes

1   Data extracted from a *Time*/CNN poll taken over the 26th and 27th of February 1997 and reported in *Time* on 10 March 1997; and an ABC Nightline poll taken over the same period, with results reported in the *Chicago Tribune* on 2 March 1997.

2   Quotes from the bioethicist Arthur Caplan in *Denver Post* 1997; Feb 24; the bioethicist Thomas Murrey in *New York Times* 1997; Mar 6; Congressman Vernon [Ehlers] in *New York Times* 1997; Mar 6; and evolutionary biologist Francisco Ayala in *Orange County Register* 1997; Feb 25.

3   James A. Geraghty, president of Genzyme Transgenics Corporation (a Massachusetts biotech company), testified before a Senate committee that "everyone in the biotechnology industry shares the unequivocal conviction that there is no place for the cloning of human beings in our society." *Washington Post* 1997; Mar 13.

4   Data obtained from a Yankelovich poll of 1,005 adults reported in *St. Louis Post-Dispatch* 1997; Mar 9 and a *Time*/CNN poll reported in *New York Times* 1997; Mar 5.

5   Leonard Bell, president and chief executive of Alexion Pharmaceuticals, is quoted as saying, "There is a healthy skepticism whether you can accomplish this efficiently in another species." *New York Times* 1997; Mar 3.

6   Interpretations of the judgments of scientists, reported by Specter M, Kolata G. *New York Times* 1997; Mar 3, and by Herbert W, Sheler JL, Watson T. *U.S. News & World Report* 1997; Mar 10.

7   Quote from Ian Wilmut, the scientist who brought forth Dolly, in Friend T. *USA Today* 1997; Feb 24.

8   Quoted in Kluger J. *Time* 1997; Mar 10.

9   Quoted in McGraw C, Kelleher S. *Orange County Register* 1997; Feb 25.

10 Quoted in the on line version of the *Arlington Catholic Herald* (http://www.catholicherald.com /bissues.htm) 1997; May 16.

11 Staples B. [Editorial]. *New York Times* 1997; Feb 28.

12 Wilmut I, Schnieke AE, McWhir J, Kind AJ, Campbell KHS. Viable offspring derived from fetal and adult mammalian cells. *Nature* 1997; 385: 810-13.

13 Callahan D. [op-ed] *New York Times* 1997; Feb 26.

14 Safire W. [op-ed]. *New York Times* 1997; Feb 27.

61.
ON CLONING HUMAN BEINGS

Inmaculada De Melo-Martin

SOURCE: *Bioethics* 16.3 (2002): 246-65.

[handwritten: my opinion → environmental factor plays a key role]

Introduction

We live in the era of new biotechnological advances. Discussion of the social, legal, ethical, and scientific aspects of genetic therapy, in vitro fertilization, genetically engineered food, or cloning, appear everywhere, from prestigious scientific journals, to television programs, to the tabloids. In a world where the Human Genome Project hoards millions in public and private monies and thousands of scientists, where infertility seems rampant, and where the search for the perfect human baby occupies people's imagination, one might expect to find this focus on biotechnology quite normal and welcomed.

Not only have these discussions captured the public imagination and the interests of scientists, they seem also to have swept many of the members of the bioethics profession away from more mundane issues, such as questions of access to health care, or just distribution of medical resources. Lately, especially since the birth of Dolly, the cloning of human beings seems to be the new kid on the block.[1]

The purpose of this paper is to show that arguments for and against human cloning[2] fail to make their case because of one or both of the following reasons: 1) they take for granted customary beliefs and assumptions that are far from being unquestionable; 2) they tend to ignore the context in which human cloning is developed. In what follows I will analyze some of the assumptions underlying the main arguments that have been offered for and against cloning. Once these assumptions are critically analyzed, arguments both rejecting and supporting human cloning seem to lose weight. I will first briefly present the main arguments that have been proposed against cloning and I will argue that they fail to establish their case. In the next section I will evaluate some of the positive arguments that have been offered supporting such technology. This analysis will show that the case for cloning also fails. Finally, I will maintain that because critics and especially supporters of this technology neglect the context in which human cloning is developed and might be implemented, their arguments are far from compelling.

[handwritten: her view]

Criticizing Cloning: Problematic Assumptions

Most of the arguments that have been offered against cloning can be classified into three major groups: risks of physical harms to the clone; risks of psychological harms to the clone; and harms to society.[3] I will address these arguments in order.

[handwritten: classified into 3 major groups]

Risks of Physical Harms to the Clone *[circled: 1]*

Those who reject cloning often maintain that cloning is morally impermissible because the procedure has not been proven safe.[4] They usually argue that the technique that produced the sheep Dolly was successful in only one of 277 attempts. Thus, this procedure could produce severe developmental abnormalities in any resulting child. It is difficult for this argument to support a total and final ban on cloning. In order to do so, we need to assume that it would be wrong to try to clone humans, unless we can guarantee a healthy baby the first time. The reason for this is that experimentation on humans without their consent is unethical.

Although this argument has more merit than some critics have conceded,[5] still it cannot support a total ban on cloning humans. Of course, proponents of this argument do not need to require the consent of the unborn child. We can obtain the consent of the

[handwritten right margin: - Is not safe - it took a lot of attempts to get Dolly (successful) - So, we need to make sure that when we do clone it will result in healthy baby the first try.]

parents as we do in any other case that involves medical experimentation on children. Now, it is reasonable to argue that, at this point, parents cannot give fully informed consent because they do not have information on the hazards and benefits of cloning. Animal studies are still scarce and the ones that have been done do not show that cloning would be reasonably safe to try on human beings. Lack of, or faulty, information may seriously hinder people's abilities to make informed choices. Obviously, if parents cannot give explicit informed consent, then we cannot assert that they have consented on behalf or their unborn children.

However, there are no good reasons to presuppose that this lack of information will continue forever. At some point, it could be possible for parents to have enough information to allow them to give a freely informed consent. If this is so, then the argument about risks to the child is only an argument for caution. Most reasonable people would agree that at this point, given the knowledge, or the lack of it, that we have on this technique, it would be unethical to try to clone a human being. However, if safety is what we want, we can certainly propose that more research on animals be done,[6] and more investigation completed to establish its safety and effectiveness for humans, before we proceed to use this technique on human beings. Thus, opposition to cloning on the basis of safety fails as an argument against cloning per se.

Risks of Psychological Harms to the Clone

Opposition to cloning is also backed up by arguing that this practice can produce serious psychological harms to the cloned child, such as a possible loss of a sense of individuality or unique identity.[7] The argument, however, seems to presuppose that human individuality or identity is determined by the uniqueness of our genome. This assumption can only be grounded on the crudest genetic determinism. According to genetic determinism, individuals' genetic endowments completely determine who they will be. As a Nobel Laureate put it, soon we will be able to pull a CD with our own mapped genome and say 'here is a human being; It is me.'[8] However, there is no evidence whatsoever that would support this kind of genetic determinism. Whether a particu-

lar trait will be present depends not just on genes but also on biological and environmental factors. Thus, in spite of having practically the same genes, identical twins certainly have unique and distinct personal identities. They develop different interests, relationships; they make different choices. Their individuality does not seem to be threatened by the fact that they do not have unique genetic endowments.

Other scholars have argued that the psychological harm to the clone results from the violation of what Hans Jonas has called 'a right to ignorance,' or what Joel Feinberg has called 'a right to an open future.'[9] Jonas argues that human cloning, in which there is an important time gap between the beginning of the lives of the earlier and later twin, differs essentially from the simultaneous beginning of naturally occurring identical twins. According to Jonas, later twins created by cloning know, or at least they believe they know, too much about themselves. This is so, because there is already in the world another person, who from the same genetic starting point, has made the life choices that are still in the later twin's future. The later twin may feel that her life has already been lived, that her fate has already been determined.

Similarly, Joel Feinberg has argued that a child has a right to an open future. This requires, he says, that others raising a child do not so much close off the future possibilities that the child would otherwise have as to eliminate a reasonable range of opportunities for the child to construct his or her own life. Thus, creating a later twin could violate this right because she will believe that her future has already been set for her by the choices the earlier twin made. As in the case of the arguments about a lack of individuality, these appeals to a right to ignorance or to an open future rest on the questionable assumption that one's genetic endowments completely determine one's entire life path. But, as was said earlier, such an assumption is false because it ignores that genotypes have a range of phenotypic expression, overlooks the importance of the environment, and disregards the significance of one's choices in building a unique and distinctive life. But if the assumption of genetic determinism is rejected, then we have no more reasons to say that a later clone would violate a right to ignorance or to an open future than we have reasons to say that such rights would be violated by an older sibling. After all, brothers and sisters share 50% of their genes. And it may certainly be the case that the life choices of an older sibling influence the kind of choices the younger one will make. If the older sister finds her career choices offered her a meaningful life, then the younger sister might decide to follow her steps; if, on the other hand, the older sibling finds her life wanting because of her decisions, the younger sister may choose to follow some different path. In any case, we do not think that parents violate their younger children's right to an open future or to ignorance when they decide to bring them into the world.

It is true, however, that the falsity of the belief in genetic determinism only shows that a right to ignorance, or a right to an open future, is not being violated by cloning humans.[10] The falsity of this belief, nevertheless, does not show that the possible psychological harms to the clone are nonexistent, especially if the belief in genetic determinism is widespread. Two problems, however, make this argument against cloning not very compelling. First, psychological risks of this kind are presently only speculative, given that we have no experience with human cloning. Second, banning particular practices on the grounds that people's false beliefs can produce individual harms is highly questionable. The argument seems to presuppose that we have to grant weight to shared false beliefs instead of, for example, trying to eliminate those beliefs by educating people.

Harms to Society

Several commentators have argued that cloning humans can also produce social harms.[11] Among these harms I will discuss those created by threatening the stability of the family, and those produced by diminishing our respect for human life.

Appeals to harm to the family are not specific to arguments against cloning. These concerns appeared with the development and use of other reproductive technologies such as in vitro fertilization. Proponents of this type of argument maintain that because cloning allows for the cloned child to be born from a single parent or to have up to seven parents, these kinds of arrangements will threaten the stability of the family. Cloning seems also to promote confusion about who is the mother, the father, the grandparents, or the siblings. For example, if a woman clones herself, it is unclear whether she is mother, or sister, or both. It is also unclear whether the grandfather of the child can be said to be the child's father. This line of argumentation is however problematic for several reasons. First, it seems to assume that by 'family' we can only mean a nuclear family composed of a male, a female and their genetic offspring. Only if we assign priority to genetic relations will we have confusion about whether someone is a sister or a mother. Obviously, if we value highly the social dimensions of parenting these kinds of misunderstanding will likely diminish if not disappear. Second, the argument assumes that the concept of family is constant, unchanging. Third, it appears to presuppose, that our present conception of the family is the best form of human social organization to nurture healthy individuals and to guarantee productive societies. All of these assumptions are problematic for at least two reasons. First, they ignore historical and anthropological evidence that humans have successfully adopted many different kinds of family arrangements.[12] Second, they fail to offer any compelling normative arguments that show that societies built of nuclear families as generally understood are better off than societies with other kinds of family arrangements. This is not to say that conceiving families as mainly characterized by genetic relations has no advantages for human beings. My point is that even if this conception of 'family' is a good one, that in itself makes it neither the only one, nor the best.

Critics of cloning humans also argue that this practice can diminish our respect for human life. This is so, they claim, because cloning allows us to see human beings as replaceable.[13] The problem with this argument is that again it presupposes that genes determine the individuality of persons. Only if this was the case could we say that a later clone is 'replacing' another person. But, as I have said before, there is no evidence to support this kind of genetic determinism. Another reason why cloning might threaten the worth of persons is because this practice invites us to see people as made to order.[14] Opponents of cloning claim that people might produce children with genomes that are of special interest to those doing the cloning. Children thus created

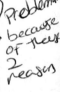

would be valued as means and not ends in themselves. This argument is problematic because it seems to wrongly assume that valuing people as ends is incompatible with valuing their instrumental value.[15] Obviously, we can value Michael Jordan for his instrumental value on a basketball team without diminishing him as a person. The argument is also questionable because it presupposes that cloning people with particular abilities or traits would guarantee that the clones would also have those same abilities or traits. For example, there is no assurance that a clone of Michael Jordan would be an exceptional basketball player. Michael Jordan's abilities as a basketball player depended not only on his genes, but also on the environment in which he developed and on the life choices he made.

Although the arguments I have presented here are not the only ones that critics of human cloning have presented, I think they are the strongest ones. If my analysis of these arguments is correct, then the case against cloning fails. This means neither that these arguments are completely without merit, nor that at some point other possible arguments that would make the practice of cloning impermissible could exist. However, unless we assume anything we can do we must do, absent good reasons not to, then the lack of compelling arguments against cloning is not by itself sufficient reason to proceed with this practice. If this is so, then we need positive arguments in support of cloning human beings.

Defending Cloning: Questionable Assumptions

Proponents of human cloning often use the three following arguments to make their case.[16] First, they claim that this new technology will be an important response to infertility and will allow humans who cannot at present have genetic offspring the opportunity to do so. Second, they argue that cloning will be an important tool in our ongoing battle with genetic diseases. Third, they maintain that cloning will allow some individuals to clone dead loved ones. If these arguments are successful, then not only do we lack compelling arguments against cloning, but we have some reasons to go forward with it. In what follows, however, I will show that these arguments fail. I will discuss these arguments in order.

Solving Infertility

Those who support cloning often defend this practice by arguing that it would benefit infertile couples.[17] For example, human cloning would allow people who suffer from total germ cell failure to have children genetically related to them.

Estimates on the number of people who suffer from infertility vary significantly depending of the definition of infertility. Under one of the most accepted definitions, failure to conceive after twelve months of unprotected intercourse, infertility affects between 7 and 10% of couples with women of childbearing age.[18] Obviously, the larger the number of people who need cloning as the only means to overcome their infertility, the more acceptable cloning appears.

Given the importance that most people attach to having children, and given the serious psychological problems that this impairment might cause to people suffering it, concerns to relieve infertility are certainly admirable. However, in maintaining that cloning of human beings should be permitted because it can solve the problems of infertile people, several assumptions are taken for granted. First, proponents of this argument seem to assume that if something solves infertility, then we should accept it. Second, they also assume that infertility is a medical problem in need of a technological solution. In what follows I will evaluate these two assumptions.

In a world with limited resources and where numerous diseases and impairments affect people, one must ask, what is it about infertility that attracts so much attention. Certainly, the inability to conceive can be stressful, and painful, but this is the case with many other diseases that have not drawn such interest. In spite of supporting cloning as a way to solve infertility, proponents of this argument have neglected to give reasons why solving infertility is a good reason to accept a new technology. In order to understand the importance of this question we need to pay attention to the context in which these arguments appear. Certainly, if we live in a world where most major causes of stress and pain (even if only medical ones) are solved, one might think that if a new technology appears that can solve infertility, then we should support its development. But unfortunately, we are far from living in such a world. First, our resources are limited. Second, human beings are affected by a significant number of diseases, disabilities, and impairments. Some of them are life threatening, or diminish our life opportunities considerably. Some of them do not. In this context, priorities need to be set, and good reasons must be offered for those priorities. Infertility is not a life threatening condition, nor does it seem to significantly reduce our equal opportunities. If this is so, arguments that support cloning on grounds that it will help infertile people are incomplete. They must give good reasons why if something relieves infertility, then it is good and we should do it. Until these reasons are presented, such arguments fail to make their case for cloning.

Another assumption taken for granted by proponents of cloning as a way to solve infertility is that infertility is a medical problem in need of a technological solution. In framing the problem in this way, however, they might be undermining their own attempts to fight infertility.[19] This is so, because in emphasizing technological solutions to the problem of infertility, supporters of cloning might be drawing attention away from the fact that many of the causes of infertility could be prevented. Sexual, contraceptive, and medical practices, occupational health hazards, environmental pollution, and food additives constitute some examples of preventable causes of infertility. Sexually transmitted diseases (STDs) such as chlamydia, gonorrhea, and syphilis are responsible for 20% of the cases of infertility.[20] Thousands of women each year have to deal with procreation problems due to pelvic inflammatory disease (PID) caused by STDs.[21] Hormonal contraceptives such as depoprovera, as well as others such as intrauterine devices, increase the risk of PID and infertility. Also, according to some professionals, iatrogenic or doctor-induced infertility is common. Problems such as infections after childbirth and postoperative infections can cause reproductive difficulties.[22] Likewise social practices such as delaying childbearing may be responsible for reproductive difficulties. Some evidence also suggests environmental pollutants and chemicals can damage the reproductive capability of both women and men. Drugs such as DES can also cause infertility.[23]

Among the poor, inadequate nutrition, poor health, and limited access to health care also contribute to reproductive problems. For example, infertility is higher in poor and minority communities.[24] Black women have an infertility rate one and one half times higher than that of white women.[25] Some of the contributing factors are a higher incidence of STDs, greater use of intrauterine devices, environmental factors (such as occupational hazards affecting reproduction), lack of access to medical treatment, nutritional deficiencies, and complications or infections following childbirth or abortion.

If our concern is with solving infertility, it is certainly the case that other means to relieve the problem might be more effective.[26] Given the low success rates of other reproductive technologies, there is no evidence that cloning will work much better (or that it will work worse). Thus, stressing the importance of developing cloning as a solution to infertility might promote public policies that would result in funds being dedicated mainly to technological solutions rather than also to preventive measures such as stricter controls for environmental pollutants and chemicals, more research funding for safer contraceptives, and educational programs to prevent STDs and for treating them before they cause reproductive difficulties.

Similarly, if we take for granted the assumption that infertility is mainly a medical problem in need of a technological solution, then we might be blinded to the possibility of analyzing infertility as a partly socially generated problem. In doing so, we might restrict possible solutions to reproductive difficulties. It is arguable that there are social factors that make involuntary childlessness a serious problem. Thus, changing those factors could also have a positive effect on the problem of infertility by dissolving it, or making it less onerous. Some of these social elements are pronatalistic pressures on women to reproduce, the strong emphasis of our culture on having genetically related children, and the inextricable ties between womanhood and motherhood. By neglecting these considerations, proponents of cloning as a way to solve infertility have also missed the opportunity to see other solutions to the problem such as implementing social policies that could help to modify the view of motherhood as the primary role of women, encourage an understanding of maternity as a possible but not as a necessary choice, facilitate adoption, or promote different forms of mothering.

Someone might object that those who support cloning because it might help infertile people, might also defend other ways to solve the problem. What is significant, however, is that although many proponents of the infertility argument spend considerable time reflecting on the problem of infertility, they rarely acknowledge nontechnological solutions as a way to solve reproductive difficulties.[27] In fact, I am arguing that advocating these kinds of social solutions would undercut the need for a technological fix such as the cloning of human beings.

Another objection against my analysis of this argument for cloning is that solutions to infertility of the kind I propose here would require unattainable institutional changes.[28] Certainly, some alternatives to the problem of infertility would likely require social transformations such as changes in attitudes toward women and motherhood or alterations in family structures. Prevention would also involve educative programs, social services, legislative changes in occupational health and safety, and environmental legislation. These changes are difficult because of economic pressures and the extensive time period required to obtain results.

Although this criticism raises important concerns, it is incorrect for several reasons. First, if we discard policy options before we adequately evaluate them, it is difficult to see how we can talk about 'unattainable' institutional changes. To affirm that alternatives to the problem of infertility such as prevention require unfeasible changes without giving some evidence for such an argument is then problematic. Moreover, if we only take into account policy options that are highly feasible under the technological status quo, then our evaluations erroneously encourage a self-fulfilling prophecy sanctioning current conditions, regardless of their worth.

Certainly, the argument that the cloning of humans is permissible because it might benefit the infertile could have more strength if the amount of people who will be helped by this technique were significant. However, as even proponents of this argument recognize, there are no reasons to believe that the number of people using this technology will

be large.[29] Thus, unless we want to argue that the good of relieving the suffering of those who cannot have their own children and who have access to expensive technologies such as cloning outweighs the good of justly allocating scarce medical resources, then the development and use of cloning as a solution to infertility is not morally warranted.

Another objection against my analysis is that as long as people who desire to solve their infertility problems by cloning do so with their own money they should be allowed to use their resources as they see fit. Thus, assuming that there is no harm to others, society should not interfere with these people's choices.

This argument, however, presupposes that it is feasible to conduct research on human cloning without making use of any public resources whatsoever. But, even in countries such as the United States, where public money for cloning and associated techniques could be limited, societal interdependencies and professional contracts have created and enhanced doctors' abilities to use this technique. They would employ tools and technologies developed in part through societal resources. Also, public money supports physicians through learning, because virtually no student, even in private schools, pays for the full costs of education; taxes or donations usually supplement that cost.[30]

Furthermore, this objection seems to assume a notion of health care as a business concerned with responding to individuals' desires, as long as they have income available, rather than focused on maximizing public health. It also seems to presuppose a very minimal notion of community, where individuals' main obligations are to their own interests.

In summary, if other means of solving infertility, both through prevention and treatment, are available, and if it is likely that cloning humans will not be used by a large number of people as a way to solve reproductive difficulties, it is hard to see the strength of an argument that uses infertility as one of the main reasons to support cloning.

Fighting Genetic Disease

According to some scholars, the strongest argument for originating a child by NST is that the parents of the child might give him or her a wonderful genetic legacy.[31] Thus, couples at high risk of having offspring with a genetic disease such as cystic fibrosis or Huntington's disease for example, can decide to originate a child by cloning in order to avoid the risks of transmitting the genetic disease.

Supporters of cloning have presented this argument in what I will call the strong and the moderate form. In the strong form, cloning appears as the solution to most of our deadly diseases. Some authors have argued that over 70% of deaths from heart diseases, cancers, and strokes may be from preventable, genetic causes.[32] To these we must also add deaths caused by other genetic diseases such as Huntington's, sickle cell anemia, Tay-Sachs, or muscular dystrophy. Given the existence of all these preventable genetic diseases, originating children by cloning might save the lives of a considerable amount of people by allowing parents to clone a child using genetic material from the nonaffected parent, or from some other 'healthy' relative. Moreover, the argument goes, not only are people permitted to use cloning in order to create children with as much natural talent as possible, with the best genes, and with the best chance at a long, healthy life, they are obligated to do so.[33] This is the case, because it is wrong to choose lives for future people that make them much worse off than they otherwise could have been.

There are several problems with this argument. First, at present there is no scientific evidence showing that the majority of the deaths from cancers, strokes, or heart diseases are from preventable, genetic causes. This is not to say that genetics does not play a role in these diseases at all, but that such a role is not as essential as the argument makes it appear. That is, this argument disregards the fact that, although there are cases in which having a particular gene is sufficient to have a particular disease, these cases are rare. In most cases, particular genes may be necessary for a disease to be present, but such genes are not sufficient. In such instances, other biological or environmental factors must also be present for the disease to be expressed. For example, we know that particular genes are present in phenylketonuria (PKU), an accumulation of phenylalanine that results in mental retardation. However, although the existence of the particular genes helps us to identify the affected individuals, having the genes is not sufficient to have the disease. Thus, a low phenylalanine diet prevents the expression of this disease.

Second, arguing that we are morally obligated to create children with as much natural talent as possible, with the best genes, and with the best chance at a long, healthy life presupposes that the concepts of 'talent,' 'the best genes,' and 'health' have fixed meaning and are clearly unproblematic. However, as the numerous articles and monographs discussing these concepts show, such an assumption is highly questionable. Moreover, this alleged obligation might enter into conflict with the desire to have genetically related children. Thus, assuming that what 'best genes' or 'health' means is clear to everyone, it is certainly the case that some children would be better off if their parents, instead of cloning themselves, would request the help of some other individuals who have better genetic endowments. This, of course, would prevent the parents[34] from having children genetically related to them. I guess, those who propose this argument can also indicate whether this moral obligation to improve our children's genes is or is not outweighed by our desire to have genetically related children.

Some authors, who support cloning on the grounds that it will help parents to avoid the risks of transmitting genetic diseases to their children, propose a more moderate version of this argument.[35] They maintain that cloning can be very helpful in those cases where the existence of a particular gene guarantees the existence of a deadly disease. This moderate form of the argument is immune to the two prior criticisms. However, it shares with the strong version the following problem. It seems to assume that cloning is the best way to avoid hereditary diseases. If other techniques exist that can help us with this endeavor, those who support cloning on this ground need to prove not only that this technology is good but also, that it is better than other techniques. At present, there are certainly other techniques that can be used to avoid the risk of transmitting particular genetic diseases. Parents can decide to use sperm or egg donors (although these methods might be unappealing to those who value a genetic connection to their children); also available to them is preimplantation diagnosis (PID) of embryos created by

IVF. Certainly, IVF and PID are expensive and not very successful procedures, but at present there is no reason to believe that cloning would be either cheaper or more successful. Genetic therapy can also be helpful in the fight against genetic disease, and although it is not very developed, it is no worse off than cloning humans.

Another problem for the moderate version of this argument is that it is unclear that using cloning to prevent genetic disease will help a large number of people. As I said earlier, the cases in which the existence of a particular gene guarantees that a particular disease will appear are rare. In these cases, parents also have other options, such as preimplantation diagnosis or gamete donation. Given the availability of other techniques, and given the fact that we live in a world with limited resources, this argument fails to make a strong case for cloning.

Cloning of Loved Ones

Some authors also support human cloning by arguing that this technique would enable some individuals to clone a person who has special meaning to them.[36] For example, parents might decide to clone their dying children, or other family members. In some cases the examples offered here are highly imaginative.[37] There are several problems with supporting human cloning on this ground. First, although it might be possible that given the chance some people might use cloning for these purposes, there are no reasons to believe that many people would do so. And given, again, a world with limited resources and with other more pressing needs, to support the development and use of a quite likely very expensive technology to help a small number of people seems questionable.

Second, and more importantly, it is unclear what kind of desire we are trying to grant in these cases. There are at least two possibilities. Maybe what people who want to clone dead loved ones desire is to replace those who die with a new copy of the first person. That is, they want to have a baby who would share with the dead one some specific trait, such as strength or interest in music. Or maybe cloning that loved one is a way to accept the loss and move on with their lives.

If what supporters of this argument want is to grant the first kind of desire, then their argument is questionable because it either is grounded on a crude form of genetic determinism for which there is no scientific evidence, or it promotes the granting of desires based on false beliefs. Now, most of those who offer this argument would likely reject the idea that a clone of a loved one will be his or her replacement. They will probably agree that the new cloned child will be a different person with just the same genes. The personalities, interests, traits of the new cloned baby might be very different. But, if supporters of this argument recognize the problems with a crude genetic determinism, and if they still defend the practice of cloning in these cases, then they are endorsing the satisfaction of desires that are based on false beliefs.

On the other hand, people might desire to clone dead loved ones as a way to move on with their lives. We recognize that the pain of losing a loved person, especially because of a premature death, might be unbearable. Thus, attempts to palliate such suffering are laudable. However, it is unclear why encouraging human cloning is better than promoting the support of other siblings, friends, or better than having another child by usual means.

Debates about human cloning make it difficult to believe that one of the jobs of philosophers is, as the mythical gadfly, to awaken people from their complacent dreams. Both those who criticize and those who defend cloning do so in many cases without questioning some of the customary beliefs and assumptions that most people in our society take for granted. Thus, when you read the bibliography against human cloning, you might come to think that genetic determinism has been established beyond any scientific doubt, that the concepts of 'natural,' or 'normal' are beyond discussion; that anything that puts into question our conception of the nuclear family needs to be rejected, as if our conception of 'the family' is not in itself seriously problematic; or that twins suffer irreversible psychological problems because they lack 'individuality.' But, when you read the bibliography supporting the still not possible practice of cloning human beings, things do not get much better. Here you would think that being infertile is one of the most serious menaces to happiness;

that the best way to solve infertility problems is through medical technologies; that the right to procreate is one of the most endangered human rights in our communities; and that cloning people is going to make the world a significantly much better place.

Why Cloning?

Taking for granted assumptions that are far from being unquestionable is not the only problem with most of the arguments that have been offered for and against cloning. These arguments are also problematic because critics and, especially supporters of this technology, neglect the context in which human cloning is developed and might be implemented.

Often, philosophers working in bioethics have a tendency to try to make things general, and simpler, by eliminating context. We hear about doctor-patient relationships, but in many cases those relationships are presented in a decontextualized way: no families, no communities, no institutions. We read about autonomy in ways that picture human beings as completely separated from the environment in which they develop. We hear about the wonderful powers of genetic therapy with its ability to eliminate disease and handicaps from our lives, without considering the actual context in which genetic technologies are implemented. Particulars such as race, economic class, and gender often seem to be lost in this ocean of generality and abstraction. But in losing them, we are neglecting the analysis of serious moral problems, and with it the possibility of offering some kind of solution to such problems. For example, if we ignore gender as a category of analysis we might overlook existing inequalities in access to health care affecting women, gender disparities in access to some of the major diagnostic and therapeutic interventions considered appropriate for certain conditions, and the historical exclusion of women from clinical trials and from positions of authority in the medical profession.

This omission of context is also present in many of the evaluations of human cloning. Thus, when one reads analyses of this technology, one has the impression that we live in a society where our most serious and pressing problems are the pleas of infertile people, or the requests of those who want to replace their dead loved ones; a world where genetic disease is the main cause of preventable deaths, where individuality is threatened, where one of the worst things that can happen to children is that their parents have too many expectations because of their genetic make up, and where resources are all but limited. And, probably, in a world where these are our main worries, the kind of debate about human cloning that is occurring now would make perfect sense.

But that is not the world we live in. Ours is an overpopulated world, where thousands of children are in desperate need of good homes; a world where thousands of mothers who are lucky enough to have children of their own lack access to basic health care for their children or are unable to provide nutritious food, or safe water for them. In our world, preventing most cases of premature death requires not genetic therapy but access to simple vaccinations such as those for measles or tuberculosis, or to basic amounts of food, or to promote social structures that prevent traffic accidents, especially among teenagers. Overbearing parents with high expectations for their offspring do not constitute the main threat to the children of our world, but lack of medical care, food, and education do.

I realize that some proponents of human cloning might see my arguments as controversial attempts to change the world, and that they would prefer for human cloning to be evaluated in its own sphere.[38] This criticism is, however, seriously problematic because it seems to presuppose that a decontextualized evaluation of human cloning is an adequate one. My point here has been to argue that such is not the case. Also, when we try to analyze human cloning 'in its own sphere,' we are implicitly and uncritically sanctioning the status quo. Thus, the philosopher has failed in the traditional role of social gadfly.

When we set our discussion of human cloning in this world of ours, that is, when we do not lose sight of the context in which this technology might be developed and implemented, it seems that deciding how cloning might be legitimately used to relieve the pain of those who cannot have their own children, or of those who request human cloning as a way to have genetically related children without genetic diseases, or of those who solicit this new technology in order to cope with the pain of losing a loved one, is not our most pressing moral and public policy concern.

Let me emphasize that this is not an argument that these kinds of pleas be completely ignored. On the contrary, a contextualized analysis of this technology might indicate better ways to bring relief to people suffering from infertility or coping with the death of loved ones. Neither is this an argument that we put an end to any new technologies until more basic problems are solved. We live in a pluralistic society with competing interests that need to be considered. Nor am I defending that we preclude intellectually stimulating discussions about unlikely scenarios emerging from the use of new techniques. We might learn something from them. This is only an argument to not lose sight of the context in which our new technologies appear. After all, we presumably developed them to improve human existence. This in an argument calling attention to the fact that the assessment of new technologies requires not only discussion of risks and benefits, that is discussions of means, but also a discussion of ends.

Notes

1   See for example P. Lauritzen, ed. 2001. *Cloning and the Future of Human Embryo Research.* New York, NY. Oxford University Press; B. Mackinnon, ed. 2000. *Human Cloning: Science, Ethics, and Public Policy. Champaign,* IL. University of Illinois Press; L. Kass and J. Wilson. 1998. *The Ethics of Cloning.* Washington, DC. American Enterprise Institute; J.M. Humber and R.F. Almeder, eds. 1998. *Human Cloning.* Totowa, NJ. Humana Press; G. McGee, ed. 1998. *The Human Cloning Debate.* Berkeley, CA. Berkeley Hills Books; M.C. Nussbaum and C.R. Sunstein, eds. 1998. *Clones and Clones.* New York. W.W. Norton and Company; G. Pence, ed. 1998. *Flesh of My Flesh.* Lanham, MD. Rowman and Littlefield; G. Pence. 1997. *Who's Afraid of Human Cloning.* Lanham, MD. Rowman and Littlefield (hereafter cited as Pence, Cloning); and US National Bioethics Advisory Commission. 1997. *Cloning Human Beings*: Report and Recommendations of the National Bioethics Advisory Commission. Rockville, MD. The Commission (hereafter cited as NBAC).

2   I will deal in this paper only with cloning techniques,

i.e., nuclear somatic transfer, intended to create a complete human being. Thus, the arguments offered here do not apply to molecular cloning or cellular cloning.

3   See, for example, D.W. Brock. 1998. Cloning Human Beings: An Assessment of the Ethical Issues Pro and Con. In *Clones and Clones,* op. cit. note 1; Pence, Cloning, op. cit. note 1, ch. 9; and NBAC, op. cit. note 1.

4   NBAC, op. cit. note 1; and G. Annas. 1997. Scientific Discoveries and Cloning: Challenges for Public Policy. In *Flesh of My Flesh,* op. cit. note 1, pp. 77-83.

5   See a too quick dismissal of this argument in L.M. Silver. Cloning, Ethics, and Religion. *Cambridge Quarterly of Health Care Ethics* 1998; 7: 168-72; and Pence, Cloning, op. cit. note 1, p. 52.

6   Obviously, experimentation on animals may also need to be justified.

7   L. Kass. 1997. The Wisdom of Repugnance. In *Flesh of My Flesh,* op. cit. note 1, pp. 13-37; NBAC, op. cit. note 1; A.D. Verhey. Cloning: Revisiting an Old Debate. *Kennedy Institute of Ethics Journal* 1994; 4: 227-234; and D. Callahan. Perspective on Cloning: A Threat to Individual Uniqueness. *Los Angeles Times* 1993; November 12: B7.

8   W. Gilbert. 1992. A Vision of the Grail. In *The Code of Codes: Scientific and Social Issues in the Human Genome Project.* D.J. Kevles and L. Hood, eds. Cambridge, MA. Harvard University Press: 83-97.

9   H. Jonas. 1974. *Philosophical Essays: From Ancient Creed to Technological Man.* Englewood Cliffs, NJ. Prentice Hall; and J. Feinberg. 1980. The Child's Right to an Open Future. In *Whose Child? Children's Rights, Parental Authority, and State Power.* W. Aiken and H. LaFollette, eds. Totowa, NJ. Rowman and Littlefield: 124-153.

10   Brock, op. cit. note 3, pp. 153-54.

11   Annas, op. cit. note 4; and NBAC, op. cit. note 1.

12   See, for example, M.C. Bateson. 2000. *Full Circles, Overlapping Lives: Culture and Generation in Transition.* New York, NY. Random House; S. Coontz, M. Parson, and G. Raley, eds. 1998. *American Families: A Multicultural Reader.* New York, NY. Routledge; J. Stacey. 1997. *In the Name of the Family: Rethinking Family Values in the Postmodern Age.* Boston, MA. Beacon Press; L. Holy. 1996. *Anthropological Per-*

spectives on Kinship. London, UK. Pluto Press; S. Coontz. 1992. *The Way We Never Were: American Families and the Nostalgia Trap*. New York, NY. Basic Books; F.K. Goldscheider and L.J. Waite. 1991. *New Families, No Families: The Transformation of the American Home*. Berkeley, CA. University of California Press; and E.R. Service. 1967. *Primitive Social Organization: An Evolutionary Perspective*. New York, NY. Random House.

13 NBAC, op. cit. note 1; and R. Macking. Splitting Embryos on the Slippery Slope: Ethics and Public Policy. *Kennedy Institute of Ethics Journal* 1994; 4: 209-226.

14 Kass, op. cit. note 7; and NBAC, op. cit. note 1.

15 Brock, op. cit. note 3, pp. 158-60.

16 See for example, Pence, Cloning, op. cit. note 1, ch. 8; and J. Robertson. Human Cloning and the Challenge of Regulation. *The New England Journal of Medicine* 1998; 339: 119-122.

17 See for example, R. Winston. The Promise of Cloning for Human Medicine. *British Medical Journal* 1997; 314: 913-14; Pence, Cloning, op. cit. note 1, pp. 106-08; and Robertson, op. cit. note 16.

18 The New York Task Force on Life and the Law. 1998. *Assisted Reproductive Technologies: Analysis and Recommendations for Public Policy*. New York, NY. The Task Force: 10-16 (hereafter cited as NY Task Force).

19 I. De Melo-Martin. 1998. *Making Babies: Biomedical Technologies, Reproductive Ethics, and Public Policy*. Dordrecht. Kluwer: ch. 5.

20 G.B. Ellis. 1990. Infertility and the Role of the Federal Government. In *Beyond Baby M*. D.M. Bartels, R. Priester, D.E. Vawter, and A.L. Caplan, eds. Clifton, NJ. Humana Press: 111-130.

21 R. Jewelewicz and E.E. Wallach. 1994. Evaluation of the Infertile Couple. In *Reproductive Medicine and Surgery*. E.E. Wallach and H.A. Zacur, eds. St. Louis, Missouri. Mosby: 364; and B.A. Mueller and J.R. Daling. 1989. The Epidemiology of Infertility. In

Controversies in Reproductive Endocrinology and Infertility. M.R. Soules, ed. New York, NY. Elsevier.

22 R. Rowland. 1992. Living Laboratories. Bloomington, IN. Indiana University Press: 231, 257.

23 Jewelewicz and Wallach, op. cit. note 21, p. 364; Rowland, op. cit. note 22, pp. 231; and R. Koval and J.A. Scutt. 1988. Genetic and Reproductive Engineering—All for the Infertile. In *Baby Machine. Reproductive Technology and the Commercialization of Motherhood*. J.A. Scutt, ed. Melbourne. McCulloch Publishing: 33-57.

24 NY Task Force, op. cit. note 18; M.S. Henifin. New Reproductive Technologies: Equity and Access to Reproductive Health. *Journal of Social Issues* 1993; 49: 61-74.

25 L. Nsiah-Jefferson. 1989. Reproductive Laws, Women of Color, and Low Income Women. In *Reproductive Laws for the 1990s*. S. Cohen and N. Taub, ed. Clifton, NJ. Humana Press: 23-67.

26 De Melo-Martin, op. cit. note 19.

27 Pence, Cloning, op. cit. note 1, and Robertson, op. cit. note 16.

28 De Melo-Martin, op. cit. note 19.

29 Pence, Cloning, op. cit. note 1, p. 145.

30 De Melo-Martin, op. cit. note 19.

31 J. Robertson. The Question of Human Cloning. *Hastings Center Report* 1994; 24: 6-14; Pence, Cloning, op. cit. note 1, p. 101; and Robertson, op. cit. note 16.

32 Pence, Cloning, op. cit. note 1, p. 103.

33 Pence, Cloning, op. cit. note 1, p. 114.

34 This is the case especially for males, given that females can use their own eggs and thus contribute some (the mitochondrial DNA) to the genetic material of the child.

35 Robertson, op. cit. note 16.

36 Robertson, op. cit. note 31; Pence, Cloning, op. cit. note 1.

37 Pence, Cloning, op. cit. note 1, p. 60.

38 Pence, Cloning, op. cit. note 1, p. 144.

62

PROTECTING THE ENDANGERED HUMAN: TOWARD AN INTERNATIONAL TREATY PROHIBITING CLONING AND INHERITABLE ALTERATIONS

George J. Annas, Lori B. Andrews, and Rosario M. Isasi

SOURCE: *American Journal of Law and Medicine* 28 (2002): 151-78.

I. Introduction

We humans tend to worry first about our own happiness, then about our families, then about our communities. In times of great stress, such as war or natural disaster, we may focus temporarily on our country but we rarely think about Earth as a whole or the human species as a whole. This narrow perspective, perhaps best exemplified by the American consumer, has led to the environmental degradation of our planet, a grossly widening gap in living standards between rich and poor people and nations, and a scientific research agenda that focuses almost exclusively on the needs and desires of the wealthy few. Reversing the worldwide trends toward market-based atomization and increasing indifference to the suffering of others will require a human rights focus, forged by the development of what Vaclav Havel has termed a "species consciousness."[1]

In this article we discuss human cloning and inheritable genetic alterations from the human species perspective, and suggest language for a proposed international "Convention of the Preservation of the Human Species" that would outlaw all efforts to initiate a pregnancy by using either intentionally modified genetic material or human replication cloning, such as through somatic cell nuclear transfer. We summarize international legal action in these areas over the past five years, relate these actions to arguments for and against a treaty and conclude with an action plan.

II. Human Rights and the Human Species

The development of the atomic bomb not only presented to the world for the first time the prospect of total annihilation, but also, paradoxically, led to a renewed emphasis on the "nuclear family," complete with its personal bomb shelter. The conclusion of World War II (with the dropping of the only two atomic bombs ever used in war) led to the recognition that world wars were now suicidal to the entire species and to the formation of the United Nations with the primary goal of preventing such wars.[2] Prevention, of course, must be based on the recognition that all humans are fundamentally the same, rather than on an emphasis on our differences. In the aftermath of the Cuban missile crisis, the closest the world has ever come to nuclear war, President John F. Kennedy, in an address to the former Soviet Union, underscored the necessity for recognizing similarities for our survival:

> Let us not be blind to our differences, but let us also direct attention to our common interests and the means by which those differences can be resolved.... For, in the final analysis, our most basic common link is that we all inhabit this small planet. We all breathe the same air. We all cherish our children's future. And we are all mortal.[3]

That we are all fundamentally the same, all human, all with the same dignity and rights, is at the core of the most important document to come out of World War II, the Universal Declaration of Human Rights, and the two treaties that followed it (together known as the "International Bill of Rights").[4] The recognition of universal human rights, based on human dignity and equality as well as the principle of nondiscrimination, is fundamental to the development of a species consciousness. As Daniel Lev of

Human Rights Watch/Asia said in 1993, shortly before the Vienna Human Rights Conference:

> Whatever else may separate them, human beings belong to a single biological species, the simplest and most fundamental commonality before which the significance of human differences quickly fades.... We are all capable, in exactly the same ways, of feeling pain, hunger, and a hundred kinds of deprivation. Consequently, people nowhere routinely concede that those with enough power to do so ought to be able to kill, torture, imprison, and generally abuse others.... The idea of universal human rights shares the recognition of one common humanity, and provides a minimum solution to deal with its miseries.[5]

Membership in the human species is central to the meaning and enforcement of human rights, and respect for basic human rights is essential for the survival of the human species. The development of the concept of "crimes against humanity" was a milestone for universalizing human rights in that it recognized that there were certain actions, such as slavery and genocide, that implicated the welfare of the entire species and therefore merited universal condemnation.[6] Nuclear weapons were immediately seen as a technology that required international control, as extreme genetic manipulations like cloning and inheritable genetic alterations have come to be seen today. In fact, cloning and inheritable genetic alterations can be seen as crimes against humanity of a unique sort: they are techniques that can alter the essence of humanity itself (and thus threaten to change the foundation of human rights) by taking human evolution into our own hands and directing it toward the development of a new species, sometimes termed the "posthuman."[7] It may be that species-altering techniques, like cloning and inheritable genetic modifications, could provide benefits to the human species in extraordinary circumstances. For example, asexual genetic replication could potentially save humans from extinction if all humans were rendered sterile by some catastrophic event. But no such necessity currently exists or is on the horizon.

As a baseline, if we take human rights and democracy seriously, a decision to alter a fundamental characteristic in the definition of "human" should not be made by any individual or corporation without wide discussion among all members of the affected population. No individual scientist or corporation has the moral warrant to redesign humans (any more than any individual scientist or corporation has the moral warrant to design a new, lethal virus or bacteria that could kill large numbers of humans). Altering the human species is an issue that directly concerns all of us, and should only be decided democratically, by a body that is representative of everyone on the planet.[8] It is the most important decision we will ever make.

The environmental movement has adopted the precautionary principle to help stem the tide of environmental alterations that are detrimental to humans. One version of this principle holds that "when an activity raises threats of harm to human health or the environment ... the proponent of that activity, rather than the public, should bear the burden of proof [that the activity is more likely to be beneficial than harmful]."[9] The only way to shift the burden of proof is to outlaw potentially lethal activities, thus requiring proponents to change the law before proceeding. This can be done nation by nation, but can only be effective (because scientists and laboratories can move from country to country) by an internationally-enforceable ban. The actual text of a treaty banning human replicative cloning and inheritable modifications will be the subject of debate. We suggest the following language, obviously subject to future negotiations as well as added details, as a basis for going forward:

Convention on the Preservation of the Human Species

The Parties to this Convention,

Noting that the Charter of the United Nations affirms human rights, based on the dignity and worth of the human person and on equal rights of all persons;

Noting that the Universal Declaration of Human Rights affirms the right of every person not to be discriminated against;

Realizing that human dignity and human rights derive from our common humanity;

Noting the increased power of genetic science, which opens up vast prospects for improving health, but also has the power to diminish humanity fundamentally by producing a child through human cloning or by intentionally producing an inheritable genetic change;

Concerned that human cloning, which for the first time would produce children with predetermined genotypes, rather than novel genotypes, might cause these children to be deprived of their human rights;

Concerned that by altering fundamental human characteristics to the extent of possibly producing a new human species or subspecies, genetic science will cause the resulting persons to be treated unequally or deprived of their human rights;

Recognizing the history of abuses of human rights in the name of genetic science;

Believing that no individual, nation or corporation has the moral or legal warrant to engage in species-altering procedures, including cloning and genetic alteration of reproductive cells or embryos for the creation of a child;

Believing that the creation of a new species or subspecies of humans could easily lead to genocide or slavery; and

Stressing the need for global cooperation to prevent the misuse of genetic science in ways that undermine human dignity and human rights;

Have agreed on the following:

Article 1

Parties shall take all reasonable action, including the adoption of criminal laws, to prohibit anyone from initiating or attempting to initiate a human pregnancy or other form of gestation using embryos or reproductive cells which have undergone intentional inheritable genetic modification.

Article 2

Parties shall take all reasonable action, including the adoption of criminal laws, to prohibit anyone from utilizing somatic cell nuclear transfer or any other cloning technique for the purpose of initiating or attempting to initiate a human pregnancy or other form of gestation.

Article 3

Parties shall implement systems of national oversight through legislation, executive order, decree or other mechanism to regulate facilities engaged in assisted human reproduction or otherwise using human gametes or embryos for experimental or clinical purposes to ensure that such facilities meet informed consent, safety, and ethical standards.

Article 4

A Conference of the Parties and a Secretariat shall be established to oversee implementation of this Convention.

Article 5

Reservations to this Convention are not permitted.

Article 6

For the purpose of this Convention, the term "somatic cell nuclear transfer" shall mean transferring the nucleus of a human somatic cell into an ovum or oocyte. "Somatic cell" shall mean any cell of a human embryo, fetus, child or adult, other than a reproductive cell. "Embryo" shall include a fertilized egg, zygote (including a blastomere and blastocyst) and preembryo. "Reproductive cell" shall mean a human gamete and its precursors.[10]

Perhaps the most difficult challenge in implementing this treaty is setting up the monitoring and enforcement mechanisms. Article Four would have to address these in detail. Although the specifics are beyond the scope of this article, some general comments are needed. Monitoring and compliance bodies must be broadly representative, possess authority to oversee activities related to human cloning and human genetic modification, and be able to enforce bans by announcing and denouncing potential violators. Moreover, we believe the commission (and the countries themselves) should support, through the Convention and through their national criminal laws, the establishment of two new international crimes: initiation of a pregnancy to create a human clone and initiation of a pregnancy using a genetically-altered embryo.[11]

III. An International Convention: Why Now?

Five years after the announcement of the cloning of Dolly the sheep it is time to ask not *if* cloning and inheritable alterations should be regulated, but *how*. Had a five-year moratorium for further thought and discussion been placed on cloning humans, as the National Bioethics Advisory Commission (NBAC) recommended in 1997, for example, the time would now have expired.[12] What new have we learned in the last five years?

First, virtually every scientist in the world with an opinion believes it is unsafe to attempt a human pregnancy with a cloned embryo.[13] This is, for example, the unanimous conclusion of a 2002 report from the U.S. National Academy of Sciences, which recommended that human "reproductive" cloning be outlawed in the United States following a study that included the viewpoints of the only two scientists in the world who publicly advocate human cloning today.[14] Although scientists seldom like to predict the future without overwhelming data to support them, many believe that human cloning or inheritable genetic alternations at the embryo level will never be safe because they will always be inherently unpredictable in their effects on the children and their offspring. As Stewart Newman has noted, for example, it is unlikely that a human created from the union of "two damaged cells" (an enucleated egg and a nucleus removed from a somatic cell) could ever be healthy.[15] Of course, adding genetic modification to the somatic cell's nucleus just adds another series of events that could go wrong, because genes seldom have a single function, but will usually interact in complex and unpredictable ways with other genes.[16] It is worth underlining that the dangers are not just physical, but also psychological. Whether cloned children could ever overcome the psychological problems associated with their origins is unknown and perhaps unknowable.[17] In short, the safety issues, which inherently make attempts to clone or genetically alter a human being unethical human experiments, provide sufficient scientific justification for the treaty alone.

If and when safety can be assured, assuming this will ever be possible, two primary arguments have been set forth in favor of proceeding with cloning (and its first cousin, inheritable genetic alterations). First, cloning is a type of human reproduction that can help infertile couples have genetically-related children. Second, cloning is a part of human "progress" that could lead to a new type of genetic immortality, therefore, to prevent it is to be anti-scientific.

The infertility argument is made by physiologist Panos Zavos and his former Italian colleague, infertility specialist Severino Antinori. They argue that the inability of a sterile male to have a genetically-related child is such a human tragedy that it justifies human cloning.[18] This view not only ignores the rights and interests of women and children (even if only males are to be cloned, eggs must be procured from a woman, the embryos must be gestated by a woman and the child is the subject of the experiment), but also contains a highly-contested assertion: that asexual genetic replication or duplication should be seen as "human reproduction."[19] In fact, humans are a sexually reproducing species and have never reproduced or replicated themselves asexually.

Asexual replication may or may not be categorized by future courts as a form of human reproduction, but there are strong arguments against it. First, asexual reproduction changes a fundamental characteristic of what it means to be human (i.e., a sexually reproducing species) by making sexual reproduction involving the genetic mixture of male and female gametes optional. Second, the "child" of an asexual replication is also the twin brother of the male "parent," a relationship that has never existed before in human society. The first clone, for example, will be the first human being with a single genetic "parent" (unless the biological grandparents are taken to be the actual "parents" of the clone).[20] Third, the genetic replica of a genetically sterile man would be sterile himself and could only "reproduce" by cloning. This means either that infertility is not a major problem (because if it were, it would be unethical for a physician to intentionally create a child with this problem), or that the desire of existing adults should take precedent over the welfare of children. We find neither conclusion persuasive, and this is probably why, although some ethicists believe that cloning could be considered a form of human reproduction, infertility specialists have not joined Antinori's call for human cloning as a treatment for infertile males. In fact the organization that represents infertility specialists in the United States, and is generally opposed to the regulation of the infertility industry, the American Society of Reproductive Medicine, has nonetheless consistently opposed human cloning.[21]

There are, nonetheless, legal commentators who believe that human cloning should be classified as a form of human reproduction, and protected as such, at least if it is the only way for an individual to have a "genetically-related child." The strongest proponent of this view is probably John Robertson,[22] although Ronald Dworkin[23] shares his enthusiasm as well. Suffice it to say here that it is very unclear that human reproduction or procreation of a kind protected by principles of autonomy and self-fulfillment can be found in a "right to have a genetically-related child." It cannot be just the genetic tie that is important in human reproduction, because if it were, this could be accomplished by having one's twin brother have a child with one's wife[24]—the genetic tie would be identical, yet few, if any, would argue that this method of reproduction should satisfy the twin's right to have a "genetically-related child." Genes are important, but there is more to human reproduction, as protected by the U.S. Constitution, than simple genetic replication.

The second major argument in favor of human cloning is that it can lead to a form of immortality. This is the premise of the Raelian cult that has chartered its own corporation, Clonaid, to engage in human cloning. The leader of the cult, who calls himself Rael (formerly Claude Vorilhon, the editor of a French motor sport magazine), believes that all humans were created in the laboratories of the planet Elohim and that the Elohims have instructed Rael and his followers to develop cloning on Earth to provide earthlings with a form of immortality.[25] The Raelians, of course, can believe whatever they want to; but just as human sacrifice is illegal, experiments that pose a significant danger to women and children can also be outlawed,[26] and the religious beliefs of this cult do not provide a sufficient justification to refrain from outlawing cloning.

Just as two primary arguments in favor of cloning and inheritable genetic alterations have emerged over the past five years, so have two basic arguments about the future regulation of these technologies. The first, exemplified by Lee Silver, is that these technologies, while not necessarily desirable, are unstoppable because the market combined with parental desire will drive scientists and physicians to offer these services to demanding couples.[27] Similar to the way parents now seek early educational enrichment for their children, he believes that parents of the future will seek early genetic enhancement to give them a competitive advantage in life. Silver thinks this will ultimately lead to the creation of two separate species or subspecies, the GenRich and "the naturals."[28]

A related "do nothing" argument is that regulation may not be needed because the technologies will not be widely used. The thought is that humans may muddle through, either because the science of human genetic alterations may never prove possible, or because it will be used by only a handful of humans because most will instinctively reject it. Colin Tudge, a proponent of this argument, also accepts Silver's argument that the market is powerful and often determinative, but nonetheless believes that the three fundamental principles of all religions—personal humility, respect for fellow humans and reverence for the universe as a whole—could lead the vast majority of humans to reject cloning and genetic alterations.[29] In his words:

> The new technologies, taken to extremes, threaten the idea of humanity. We now need to ask as a matter of urgency who we really are and what we really value about ourselves. It could all be changed after all—we ourselves could be changed—perhaps simply by commercial forces that we have allowed to drift beyond our control. If that is not serious, it is hard to see what is.[30]

We agree with Tudge that the issues are serious. We think that they are too serious to be left to religions or human instinct, or even to individual national legislation, to address.

In this regard, we find a second approach, that of a democratically-formed regulatory scheme more reasonable. Indeed, in our view the widespread condemnation of human replicative cloning by governments around the world means that cloning provides a unique opportunity for the world to begin to work together to take some control over the biotechnology that threatens our very existence.[31]

The primary arguments against cloning and inheritable genetic alterations, which we believe make an international treaty the appropriate action, have been summarized in detail elsewhere. In general, the arguments are that these interventions would require massive dangerous and unethical human experimentation,[32] that cloning would inevitably be bad for the resulting children by restricting their right to an "open future,"[33] that cloning would lead to a new eugenics movement for "designer children" (because if an individual could select the entire genome of their future child, it would seem impossible to prohibit individuals from choosing one or more specific genetic characteristics of their future children),[34] and that it would likely lead to the creation of a new species or subspecies of humans, sometimes called the "posthuman."[35] In the context of the species, the last argument has gotten the least attention, and so it is worth exploring.

Specifically, the argument is that cloning will inevitably lead to attempts to modify the somatic cell nucleus not to create genetic duplicates of existing people, but "better" children.[36] If this attempt fails, that is the end of it. If it succeeds, however, something like the scenario envisioned by Silver and others such as Nancy Kress,[37] will unfold: a new species or subspecies of humans will emerge. The new species, or "posthuman," will likely view the old "normal" humans as inferior, even savages, and fit for slavery or slaughter. The normals, on the other hand, may see the posthumans as a threat and if they can, may engage in a preemptive strike by killing the posthumans before they themselves are killed or enslaved by them. It is ultimately this predictable potential for genocide that makes species-altering experiments potential weapons of mass destruction, and makes the unaccountable genetic engineer a potential bioterrorist. It is also why cloning and genetic modification is of species-wide concern and why an international treaty to address it is appropriate.[38] Such a treaty is necessary because existing laws on cloning and inheritable genetic alterations, although often well-intentioned, have serious limitations.

IV. International Restrictions on Cloning and Genetic Modifications

Despite the fact that no children have been born as a result of these species-altering interventions, policymakers around the world have expressed concerns about the use of these technologies. Some countries' lawmakers have enacted bans on these proposed experimental technologies, while others have assumed that existing laws apply to the techniques. However, both categories of laws have shortcomings.

A. Moratoria

Some countries have approached species-altering procedures with caution, instituting moratoria in order to consider the wide range of impacts of the technologies. Israel, for example, has stated that the purpose of such moratoria is to have time "to examine the moral, legal, social and scientific aspects of such types of intervention and their implication on human dignity."[39] In 1998, Israel adopted a five-year moratorium on cloning a human being, defining cloning as "the creation of an entire human being, who is genetically identical to another person or fetus, alive or dead."[40] The same law banned interventions to create a child through the use of reproductive cells that have undergone a permanent intentional genetic modification.[41] Some countries are using that same time period to consider the wealth of issues involved in species-altering procedures.[42] Others, though, have already determined that such technologies are inimical to human values and human dignity.[43]

B. Limitations in Human Cloning Bans

Some countries have attempted to ban human cloning, but have used language that inadvertently creates ambiguities. In other countries, policymakers may believe that their laws ban human cloning, but that may not be the case. Japan, for example, explicitly and clearly bans cloning.[44] Germany bans attempts to bring to birth a human embryo having the same genetic information as another embryo.[45] Spain, Victoria, Australia and Western Australia prohibit cloning and other procedures that bring about the birth of an identical human being.[46] But because cloning includes mitochondrial DNA from the woman whose egg is used, the clone will not have a completely identical genome (unless a woman clones herself and uses her own egg) and thus the practice of cloning may not be adequately banned.

Some countries ban embryo research,[47] but cloning through the Dolly technique of somatic cell nucleus transfer (SCNT) may not be viewed as embryo research. The SCNT technique utilizes an experimental procedure involving an egg to create an embryo.[48] Once the embryo has been created, no experimental technique is necessary. The resulting embryo can be implanted into a woman using the same standard clinical technique as is used in the in vitro fertilization (IVF) process.

British lawmakers thought they had a ban in place to prevent human cloning. The British have created a regulatory structure for IVF and related technology under the Human Fertilisation and Embryology Act of 1990 (HFEA).[49] The statute requires that activities falling within the act, such as the creation, storage, handling and use of human embryos outside of the body, must only be undertaken in licensed facilities.[50] Only activities enumerated in the Act, or approved by the Human Fertilisation and Embryology Authority, may be undertaken.[51] Certain activities, such as placing a human embryo in an animal, are completely prohibited. The British Act defines an "embryo" as a "live human embryo where fertilisation is complete" or "an egg in the process of fertilisation."[52] British lawmakers assumed human reproductive cloning was prohibited under the Act because it was not listed as an allowable activity with human embryos.[53]

In November 2000, the Pro-Life Alliance brought suit claiming that embryos created through cloning are not covered by HFEA. On November 15, 2001, the British High Court of Justice, Queen's Bench Division, Administrative Court, ruled in favor of the Pro-Life Alliance. The judge said, "With some reluctance, since it would leave organisms produced by CNR [cell nuclear replacement] outside the statutory and licensing framework, I have come to the conclusion that to insert these words would involve an

impermissible rewriting and extension of the definition."[54] In response, Parliament passed new legislation just two weeks after the ruling making it an offense, punishable by up to ten years in prison, for a person to place "in a woman a human embryo which has been created otherwise than by fertilisation."[55] Ultimately, a higher court ruled that a human embryo created by cloning was in fact covered by HFEA.[56]

C. Bans on Inheritable Genetic Interventions

Internationally, the bans on inheritable or germline genetic interventions are general enough to reach a wide range of technologies. These laws reflect a profound understanding of the need to avoid the social pressures to engineer a "better" race, as occurred in the Nazi era. German law understandably forbids germline intervention.[57] Victoria, Australia, in its Infertility Treatment Act of 1995, has comprehensive language prohibiting germline genetic alterations.[58] The law prohibits altering the genetic constitution of gametes[59] or altering the genetic, pro-nuclear or nuclear constitution of a zygote.[60] A Western Australia law prohibits the alteration of the genetic structure of an egg in the process of fertilization or an embryo.[61] In Norway, a 1994 law provides that the "human genome may only be altered by means of somatic gene therapy for the purpose of treating serious disease or preventing serious disease from occurring."[62] Sweden prohibits research that attempts to modify the embryo.[63] France, too, prohibits such interventions.[64] Costa Rica bans any manipulation or alteration of an embryo's genetic code.[65]

V. The Legal Status of Human Cloning and Germline Genetic Intervention in the United States

In 1997 President Clinton issued an executive order banning the use of federal funds for human cloning.[66] However, such a ban has little effect on private fertility clinics. For twenty years, the federal government has refused to provide funds for research on IVF, but that has not stopped the hundreds of privately-financed IVF clinics from creating tens of thousands of babies. The ban on federal funding of embryo research and human cloning does not, of course, apply to scientists who wish to undertake either activity with private funds.

A. The Application of U.S. Laws Banning Embryo Research to Human Cloning and Inheritable Genetic Intervention

Existing American laws banning embryo research, dating back in some states to the mid-1970s, could potentially be used to prohibit certain species-altering technologies at the experimental stage.[67] Eleven states have laws regulating research and/or experimentation on conceptuses, embryos, fetuses or unborn children that use broad enough language to apply to early embryos.[68] It should be noted, however, that these bans would not apply once the techniques are no longer considered to be research and instead are thought of as standard practice.

Several arguments could be made to suggest that most of the embryo research statutes should be construed narrowly so as not to apply to cloning. Eight of the eleven states prohibit some form of research on some product of conception, referred to in the statutes as a conceptus,[69] embryo,[70] fetus[71] or unborn child.[72] With cloning, an argument could be made that the experimentation is being done on an egg, not the product of conception, and thus these statutes should not apply.[73] By the time the egg is re-nucleated, the experiment or research has already been completed and the resulting embryo could be implanted under standard practices, as with IVF.

Moreover, two of the eleven states define the object of protection—the conceptus (Minnesota) or unborn child (Pennsylvania)—as the product of fertilization. If transfer of nucleic material is not considered fertilization (as was the case in the initial court decision in England), then these laws would not apply. In addition, at least eight of the states banning embryo research are sufficiently general that they might be struck down as unconstitutionally vague.[74]

Under New Hampshire's embryo research law, a researched-upon pre-embryo may not be transferred to a uterine cavity.[75] Thus, if a re-nucleated oocyte is considered to be a pre-embryo and if cloning is considered to be research, it would be impermissible in

New Hampshire to implant the resulting conceptus to create a child. Possibly as a result of the deficiencies in the embryo research laws, three of the states with embryo research bans have new laws banning cloning.[76]

The embryo research bans could potentially affect the practice of inheritable genetic alterations. Under these laws, research attempts to insert genes into embryos would be prohibited if undertaken strictly to gain scientific knowledge. If the genes were added in an attempt to "cure" a particular embryo that was destined to go to term, however, it is likely to be permissible in most states. Maine might still ban it, because it prohibits "any form of experimentation."[77] But several of the other embryo research bans explicitly allow procedures for the purpose of providing a health benefit to the fetus or embryo, and therefore might not affect gene alterations.[78] In some states, the embryo research bans might forbid the use of evolving or insufficiently-tested therapies if such therapies were not necessary to the preservation of the life of the fetus. However, these laws or related laws generally require the protection and preservation of viable fetuses. Therefore, it seems unlikely that the embryo research laws in these states would be invoked to enforce the withholding of gene therapy as a form of treatment if doctors argued that the procedure held out some actual promise of a health benefit to the embryo and prospective child.

The New Hampshire and Louisiana laws have unique twists. New Hampshire's law might ban creating a child with inheritable alterations because it prohibits the transfer of any embryo donated for research to a uterus.[79] Louisiana's law has the opposite effect, prohibiting farming or culturing embryos solely for research purposes,[80] but apparently allowing research as long as the embryo is implanted.

B. National Implications of Banning Cloning and Inheritable Alterations

We do not believe there is any constitutional prohibition that would limit the legal authority of the federal government to enter into an international treaty banning human cloning and inheritable genetic alterations, although this question has been the subject of wide discussion in the legal literature.[81]

The United States itself currently has no federal law on either cloning or inheritable genetic modification, even though both President George W. Bush and former President Bill Clinton are in favor of outlawing human "reproductive" cloning.[82] In August 2001, the House of Representatives voted to outlaw both research and reproductive cloning, and this proposal, known as the Weldon bill, has reached the Senate.[83] When the Senate takes up the issue, it will have to decide whether to agree with the Weldon bill (in which case it will be signed by the President and become law), or to try to craft a bill that outlaws reproductive cloning, but permits research cloning, as recommended by the National Academy of Sciences. In this case, the Senate bill will be sent to a conference committee where, unless the politics of the issue changes radically, it will likely die.[84] Of course, unless the United States passes legislation outlawing reproductive cloning, it cannot take any meaningful leadership role in the international treaty area on this issue.

VI. Promulgating an International Treaty

The adoption of an international treaty is the most appropriate approach to prohibit species-altering interventions. A rogue doctor or scientist who wishes to offer the procedure can easily move across borders if a particular nation bans the procedure. When the American physicist Richard Seed announced he intended to clone human beings and U.S. lawmakers threatened to clamp down on the procedure, he responded that he would open up a clinic in Mexico[85] or join a Japanese-based project.[86] Restrictions on European biotechnology companies have stimulated some to move to Africa.[87]

Various international declarations and laws already oppose human cloning or inheritable genetic interventions, either directly or indirectly. As summarized above,[88] many of these existing legal documents have shortcomings. Some are mere moratoria, set to expire in 2003. Some are limited in the type of species-altering technologies they ban, covering only cloning and not inheritable genetic interventions, or even just applying to cloning via a limited range of techniques.

Some of the existing laws have also been outpaced by technology and do not comprehensively ban all forms of reproductive cloning and inheritable interventions. Others are ambiguous as to what they cover. In some cases, potentially relevant laws were adopted more than two decades ago to deal with a different set of technologies and concerns; it is unclear whether their expansive prohibitions will be applied to the newer technologies of reproductive cloning and inheritable interventions. Moreover, many of the existing declarations and laws do not include sanctions. Thus, there is a need for an international treaty to encourage participating nations to clarify what is prohibited and have them commit to effective criminal penalties for breaches.

The treaty we propose takes a strong human rights perspective. This approach comports with international human rights traditions because it conceptualizes medical research issues as human rights matters.[89] It also comports with people's concerns about cloning and inheritable intervention. For example, in a survey of 2,700 Japanese doctors and academics, ninety-four percent of respondents found cloning to be ethically unacceptable, primarily because it insulted human dignity.[90] In Portugal, the National Ethics Council for Human Sciences deemed human cloning unacceptable due to concerns about human dignity and about the equilibrium of the human race and social life.[91] Human rights language is also evident in calls for a prohibition on cloning, such as one by the Council of Europe's Parliamentary Assembly, emphasizing that "every individual has a right to his own genetic identity."[92]

Concerns about human cloning run sufficiently deep that even those who would make money on the procedure have come out against it. Ian Wilmut, the scientist whose team cloned Dolly the sheep, might benefit financially if humans were cloned because his group holds a patent on a cloning process. But he has testified around the world against human cloning.[93] Similarly, BIO (the Biotechnology Industry Organization, a U.S. trade association of biotechnology companies) opposes human reproductive cloning.[94]

Numerous entities have called for an enforceable international ban on species-altering interventions. The World Health Organization (WHO) at its fifty-first World Health Assembly reaffirmed that "cloning for replication of human beings is ethically unacceptable and contrary to human dignity and integrity."[95] WHO urges member states to "foster continued and informed debate on these issues and to take appropriate steps, including legal and juridical measures, to prohibit cloning for the purpose of replicating human individuals."[96]

The European Union's Council of Europe adopted the Council of Europe Protocol, prohibiting the cloning of human beings. Twenty-nine countries have signed the treaty.[97] Similarly, the European Parliament has adopted a Resolution on Human Cloning. The Resolution indicates that people have a fundamental human right to their own genetic identity.[98] It states that human cloning is "unethical, morally repugnant, contrary to respect for the person and 'a grave violation of fundamental human rights which cannot under any circumstances be justified or accepted.'"[99] The Resolution calls for member states to enact binding national legislation banning cloning and also urges the United Nations to secure an international ban on cloning.[100]

UNESCO's Universal Declaration on the Human Genome and Human Rights specifically addresses cloning.[101] Like the treaty we propose, the Declaration is based on "universal principles of human rights."[102] The Declaration specifically refers to UNESCO's constitution, which underscores "the democratic principles of the dignity, equality and mutual respect of men."[103] Article 11 of the Declaration states, "Practices which are contrary to human dignity, such as reproductive cloning of human beings, shall not be permitted."[104] However, the Declaration does not have an enforcement mechanism. Rather, it calls upon nations and international organizations to enact national and international policies to prohibit cloning and to identify and prohibit those genetic practices that are contrary to human dignity.[105]

A. The Process for Creating an International Treaty

On August 7, 2001, France and Germany urged the U.N. Secretary-General to add an International Convention against reproductive cloning of human beings to its agenda.[106] The French-German initiative is focused on banning only reproductive cloning apparently because there is an international consensus on this issue. It is worth noting that the laws of both countries ban research cloning and other forms of inheritable genetic interventions as well, and that political leaders in both countries have spoken out publicly in favor of imposing a broader ban. Nonetheless, both of these countries seem content to pursue a two-step process at the United Nations: securing as soon as possible a ban on reproductive cloning, and leaving negotiations on other issues, including inheritable genetic alterations and research cloning, for a second round of international negotiations. This may in fact be the only practicable way to proceed.

In November 2001, the Legal Committee of the United Nations added its support to a ban on reproductive cloning,[107] and the first meeting on the treaty was held in February 2002. There was virtual unanimous support for the treaty among the approximately 80 countries that attended, although the United States took the position that it would only support the treaty if it also outlawed research cloning. The issues of reproductive cloning discussed in this Article can, of course, be separated from those involved in research cloning, and will likely have to be if a treaty on reproductive cloning is to be adopted.[108] Whether the U.S. position will change remains to be seen. It seems likely that this U.N. treaty process is the only way a cloning treaty is likely to be achieved.[109] The treaty we propose is an attempt to provide language that could be used in both stages of a two stage process, or in one process if they are combined. It is drafted in a way to reflect the broad social concerns against species-altering technologies and to close loopholes in existing legal documents and declarations. Like the U.N. Legal Committee, we believe that the time is ripe for a flat-out international ban on human cloning. We also advocate a similar ban on inheritable genetic interventions.

VII. Conclusion

Biotechnology, especially human cloning and inheritable genetic alteration, has the potential to permit us to design our children and to literally change the characteristics of the human species. The movement toward a posthuman world can be characterized as "progress" and enhancement of individual freedom in the area of procreation; but it also can be characterized as a movement down a slippery slope to a neo-eugenics that will result in the creation of one or more subspecies or superspecies of humans. The first vision sees science as our guide and ultimate goal. The second is more firmly based on our human history as it has consistently emphasized differences, and used those differences to justify genocidal actions. It is the prospect of "genetic genocide" that calls for treating cloning and genetic engineering as potential weapons of mass destruction, and the unaccountable genetic researcher as a potential bioterrorist.

The greatest accomplishment of humans has not been our science, but our development of human rights and democracy. Science cannot tell us what we should do, or even what our goals are, therefore, humans must give direction to science. In the area of genetics, this calls for international action to control the techniques that could lead us to commit species suicide. We humans clearly recognized the risk in splitting the atom and developing nuclear weapons; and most humans recognize the risk in using human genes to modify ourselves. Because the risk is to the entire species, it requires a species response. Many countries have already enacted bans, moratoria and strict regulations on various species-altering technologies. The challenge, however, is global, and action on the international level is required to be effective.

We believe that the action called for today is the ratification of an international convention for the preservation of the human species that outlaws human cloning and inheritable genetic alterations. This ban would not only be important in itself; but it would also mark the first time the world worked together to control a biotechnology. Cloning and inheritable genetic alterations are not bioweapons per se, but they could prove just as destructive to the human species if left to the market and individual wants and desires.

We think an international consensus to ban these technologies already exists, and that countries, non-governmental organizations and individual citizens should actively support the treaty process, as they did with the recent Convention on the Prohibition of the Use, Stockpiling, Production and Transfer of Anti-Personnel Mines and their Destruction (Land Mine Treaty).[110]

Cloning may not seem as important as landmines, as no clone has yet been born and thus no children have been harmed by this technique. Nonetheless, cloning has the potential to harm all children, both directly by physically and mentally harming them, and indirectly by devaluing all children—treating them as products of their parents' genetic specifications. Likewise, inheritable genetic alteration carries the prospect of developing a new species of humans that could turn into either destroyers or victims of the human species. Opposition to cloning and inheritable genetic alteration is "conservative" in the strict sense of the word: it seeks to conserve the human species. But it is also liberal in the strict sense of the word: it seeks to preserve democracy, freedom and universal human rights for all members of the human species.

APPENDIX: LEGISLATION IN FORCE RELATED TO HUMAN SPECIES PROTECTION

Asia

Japan
The "Law concerning Regulation Relating to Human Cloning Techniques and Other Similar Techniques," Nov. 2000, in effect since June 2001. English version, *available at* http://www.mext.go.jp/english/shinkou/index.htm.

The Japanese law prohibits the transfer of embryos created by techniques of human cloning, and those created by xenotransplantation. However, it allows the application of these techniques and other similar ones for research purposes as long as the embryo created is not allowed to be transplanted in a human or an animal. It also imposes criminal sanctions.

Guidelines to the "Law concerning Regulation Relating to Human Cloning Techniques and Other Similar Techniques," Dec. 4, 2001, Minister of Education and Science, *available at* http://www.mext.go.jp/a_menu/shinkou/seimei/2001/hai3/17_shishin.pdf (in Japanese).

Commentaries to the Guidelines mentioned above by the Ministry of Education and Science, *available at* http://www.mext.go.jp/a_menu/shinkou/seimei /2001/hai3/20_shishin.pdf (in Japanese).

Europe

Council of Europe
Additional Protocol (Explanatory Report) to the Convention on Human Rights and Biomedicine, 12 January 1998, *available at* http://conventions.coe.int /Treaty/EN/Treaties/Html/168.htm.

Article 1.
Any intervention seeking to create a human being genetically identical to another human being, whether living or dead is prohibited. For the purpose of this article, the term human being 'genetically identical' to another human being means a human being sharing with another the same nuclear gene set.

Convention for the Protection of Human Rights and Dignity of the Human Being with regard to the application of Biology and Medicine - Convention on Human Rights and Biomedicine; Oviedo, Apr. 4, 1997, *available at* http://conventions.coe.int/Treaty /EN/Treaties/Html/164.htm.

Article 13. Interventions on the human genome.
An intervention seeking to modify the human genome may only be undertaken for preventive, diagnostic or therapeutic purposes and only if its aim is not to introduce any modification in the genome of any descendants.

Austria
Federal Law of 1992 (Serial 275) Regulating Medically Assisted Procreation (The Reproductive Medicine Law), and Amending the General Civil Code, The Marriage Law and the Rules of Jurisdiction (1993), *available at* http://www.bmbwk.gv.at/ (in German).

The law does not explicitly prohibit the cloning of human beings, but it limits research on human embryos (defined as "developable cells"). Its central principle is that reproductive medicine is acceptable only within a stable heterosexual relationship for the purpose of reproduction. The law provides that embryos can be used only for implantation in the woman who has donated the oocytes and cannot be used for other purposes. The donation of embryos or gametes is explicitly prohibited.

Denmark
Act No. 460 on Medically Assisted Procreation in connection with medical treatment, diagnosis and research, June 10, 1997, in force Oct. 1, 1997; and Act No. 503 on a Scientific, Ethical Committee System and the Handling of Biomedical Research Projects.

According to § 28 (Act No. 460) research with the following aims is forbidden:

a) research where the aim is to develop human reproductive cloning;

b) research where the aim is to facilitate the creation of a human identity by melting together genetically unidentical embryos or parts of embryos before the implantation in the woman's womb.

Provision § 4 states that it is forbidden to implant identical unfertilized or fertilized ova in one or more women. The Act establishes penalties of fine and imprisonment for the doctor and the authorized health persons that violate its provisions.

Finland
Medical Research Act (No. 488/1999).

The legislation applies to embryo research. Section 15 explicitly prohibits any research which has the objective of modifying the germline, but makes an exception for research done for the purposes of curing or preventing serious hereditary disease.

France
Law No. 94-653 of July 29, 1994, on Respect for the Human Body, *available at* http://www.cnrs.fr/SDV/ loirespectcorps.html (in French).

The law prohibits the invasion into the integrity of the human species, eugenic behaviors intended to organize selection of human beings, and conversion of genetic characteristics leading to any change in descendants of humans (except for studies aiming at prevention and treatment of hereditary diseases) (Article 16-4). The act also amends the Penal Code, prescribing penalties of imprisonment and fine for the implementation of eugenic activities on human beings (Article 511-1).

Law No. 94-654 of July 29, 1994, on the Donation and Use of Elements and Products of the Human Body, Medically Assisted Procreation, and Prenatal Diagnosis, *available at* http://www.cnrs.fr/SDV /loidocorps.html (in French).

The bioethics legislation and its amendments (Law No. 94-653 and Law No. 94-654) specifically prohibit human cloning, creation of hybrids and chimeras, germline gene therapy, the creation of embryos purely for research purposes, and eugenic experiments.

Germany
Gesetz zum Schutz von Embryonen (Embryonen-schutzgesetz), v. 13.12.1990 (BGBI. I S.2747) [Federal Embryo Protection Law], *available at* http://www.bmgesundheit.de/rechts/genfpm/embryo /embryo.htm (in German).

This special criminal law prohibits human reproductive cloning and prescribes criminal penalties (imprisonment or fine) against violations. Regarding germ cells, the act prohibits any artificial changes in the genetic characteristics of human cells and prohibits the use of such altered cells for fertilization.

Hungary
Law No. 154 (1997) on Genetic Research. The law bans germline engineering.

Iceland
Artificial Fertilisation Act No. 55/1996, Regulation No. 568 on Artificial Fertilisation Act, English version, *available at* http://brunnur.stjr.is/interpro/htr /htr.nsf/pages/lawsandregs0002.

Article 12(d): "It is prohibited to perform cloning."

Norway
Law No. 56 of August 5, 1994 on the Medical Use of Biotechnology, (1995) 46 (1), *available at* http://www.stortinget.no/english/index.html.

Article 3-1 prohibits "research on fertilized eggs."

Ministry of Health and Social Affairs, The Act relating to the Application of Biotechnology in Medicine, 1994.

Prohibits germline therapy and prescribes criminal sanctions for its violation.

Russia
Law on Reproductive Human Cloning, Apr. 19, 2002.

The law establishes a moratorium on human reproductive cloning and the importation of cloned embryos for five years.

Spain
Law No. 35/1988, Nov. 22, 1988, on techniques of assisted reproduction, *available at* http://www.geo cities.com/Eureka/9068/SANIDAD/reproduc.html (in Spanish), modified by Organic Law No. 10/995 of 23 November 1995, *available at* http://www.web com.com/kruzes/legislac09.htm (in Spanish).

The law No. 35/1988 establishes in sections § 13.3(d) and 15.2(b) that any therapeutic intervention, investigation or research activity in pre-embryos in vitro, pre-embryos, embryos and fetuses in utero, will be authorized only if such intervention or activity does not alter its genetic make-up (in so far as it does not contain any anomaly), or if it is not aimed to individual or race selection.

The Organic Law introduced in section II of the Penal Code a Title V: Offenses relating to genetic engineering, prescribing criminal and civil sanctions for its violation.

The Spanish Penal Code (Article 16 1,2) prohibits

bringing about the birth of identical human beings as a result of cloning or other procedures aimed at the selection of humans.

Sweden
Law No. 115 of Mar. 14, 1991, Act concerning measures for the purposes of Research or Treatment in connection with Fertilized Human Oocytes (1993). This statute and the *in vitro* Fertilization law of 1988 govern embryo research. Any research, which seeks to genetically modify the embryo, is prohibited.

United Kingdom
Human Reproductive Cloning Act 2001, UK Stat. 2001 c23 &1, in force Dec. 4, 2001.

Makes it an offense for a person to place "in a woman a human embryo which has been created otherwise than by fertilisation."

Middle East

Israel
Prohibition of Genetic Intervention Law No.5759 (cloning on Human Beings and Genetic Modifications for Reproductive Cells) (1998), *available at* http://www.knesset.gov.il/index.html.

The law introduces a five-year moratorium on human reproductive cloning and germline engineering and prescribes criminal sanctions for its violation.

North America

Costa Rica
Decree No.24029-S: A Regulation on Assisted Reproduction, Feb. 3, 1995, *available at* http://www .netsalud.sa.cr/ms/decretos/dec5.htm (in Spanish).

Article 11.
Any manipulation or alteration of an embryo's genetic code is prohibited, as well as any kind of experimentation with embryos.

Oceania

Australia
Victoria Infertility Treatment Act 2000 - No.37/200 (Amendment of the Act No.37/1997, 63/1995), *available at* http://www.dms.dpc.vic.gov.au.

The State of Victoria explicitly bans human reproductive cloning and germline engineering, and prescribes criminal sanctions (fines and imprisonment) for its violation.

South America

Argentina
Decree No.200/97 of Mar. 7, 1997: A Prohibition on Human Cloning Research, *available at* http://infoleg .mecon.gov.ar/txtnorma/42213.htm (in Spanish).

Article 1: Cloning experiments regarding human beings are prohibited.

Brazil
Law No.8974 (1995) on genetically modified organisms, *available at* http://www.mct.gov.br/legis /leis/8974_95.htm (in Portuguese).

Article 8 of the law prohibits the genetic manipulation of the germline as well as the intervention on the human genetic material in vivo, with the exception of the treatment of genetic defects.

Peru
Law No.26842, General Health Law, July 9, 1997, *available at* http://www.congreso.gob.pe.

Article. 7
"The fertilization of a human ovum with an intent other than procreation is prohibited, as well as human cloning." (Unofficial translation.)

Law No. 27636, Criminal Code: Genetic Manipulation.
The genetic manipulation with the purpose of cloning a human being is prohibited. The law establishes criminal sanctions of imprisonment for its violation.

Notes

1 "We still don't know how to put morality ahead of politics, science and economy. We are still incapable of understanding that the only genuine backbone of all our actions, if they are to be moral, is responsibility—responsibility to something higher than my family, my country, my company, my success." Vaclav Havel, Excerpts from Czech Chief's Address to Congress, *N.Y. Times*, Feb. 22, 1990, at A14. See also Amartya Sen, *Development as Freedom* (1999); George J. Annas, Mapping the Human Genome and the Meaning of Monster Mythology, 39 *Emory L.J.* 629, 661-64 (1990).

2 See The Charter of the United Nations: A Commentary 49 (Bruno Simma et al. eds., 1995).

3 Commencement Address at American University in Washington, Pub. *Papers* 459, 462 (June 10, 1963). President George W. Bush echoed Kennedy's words almost forty years later:

> All fathers and mothers, in all societies, want their children to be educated and live free from poverty and violence. No people on earth yearn to be oppressed or aspire to servitude or eagerly await the midnight knock of the secret police.... America will lead by defending liberty and justice because they are right and true and unchanging for all people everywhere. No nation owns these aspirations and no nation is exempt from them. We have no intention of imposing our culture, but America will always stand firm for the non-negotiable demands of human dignity: the rule of law; limits on the power of the state; respect for women; private property; free speech; equal justice; and religious tolerance.

Address Before a Joint Session of the Congress on the State of the Union, 38 *Weekly Comp. Pres. Doc.* 133, 138 (Jan. 29, 2002).

4 See Henry J. Steiner and Philip Alston, *International Human Rights in Context: Law, Politics, Morals* 137-41 (2d ed. 2000).

5 Quoted in Mary Ann Glendon, *A World Made New: Eleanor Roosevelt and the Universal Declaration of Human Rights* 223 (2001).

6 See generally M. Cherif Bassiouni, *Crimes Against Humanity in International Criminal Law* (1992) (exploring the history and evolution of "crimes against humanity"). See also George J. Annas, The Man on the Moon, Immortality, and Other Millennial Myths: The Prospects and Perils of Human Genetic Engineering, 49 *Emory L.J.* 753, 778-80 (2000) (discussing the possibility of species-alteration becoming a new category of "crimes against humanity").

7 See, e.g., Francis Fukuyama, *Our Posthuman Future: Consequences of the Biotechnology Revolution* (2002). Of course, these actions have not yet been recognized as crimes against humanity or any other type of international crime, and this is one reason why some still see these activities as legitimate.

8 Obviously, the only current candidate is the United Nations.

9 *Protecting Public Health and the Environment: Implementing the Precautionary Principle* 354 (Carolyn Raffensperger & Joel A. Tickner eds., 1999).

10 This proposed Convention is the product of many people, including the participants at a September 21-22, 2001 conference at Boston University on "Beyond Cloning: Protecting Humanity from Species-Altering Procedures." The treaty language was the subject of a roundtable that concluded the conference. The authors, together with others, most especially Patricia Baird and Alexander Morgan Capron, had drafted language to be considered at the conference, and revised it after the conference based on the discussion that occurred there and comments on the draft by others. The original draft also included the following codicil to encourage individual countries to examine broader issues as well:

ISSUES FOR NATIONS TO CONSIDER IN FURTHERANCE OF THE CONVENTION ON THE PRESERVATION OF THE HUMAN SPECIES
In the course of discussions about the Convention on the Preservation of the Human Species, countries may desire to expand the provisions to deal in greater detail with other matters. Perhaps there will be a desire to add a moratorium on the creation of cloned human embryos for research. It may also be thought useful to include provisions that deal more comprehensively with assisted reproduction and life-science patents. Such provisions could take into consideration the following issues:

Assisted Human Reproduction

Potential Regulation:
The regulation of the practice of assisted human reproduction could include such provisions as requirements of a license for any healthcare professional who, or healthcare facility that:

- Facilitates assisted human reproduction, e.g., via donor insemination or in vitro fertilization;
- Undertakes research or treatment using an in vitro embryo;
- Collects, stores, transfers, destroys, imports or exports sperm, ova or in vitro embryos for reproduction or research purposes; or
- Undertakes genetic screening on an ex utero embryo.

The regulation of the practice of assisted human reproduction could also include provisions to ensure:

- Free and informed consent of prospective parents and gamete donors as a prerequisite to the use of the techniques;
- Quality assurance and proficiency testing for labs;
- Reporting to a governmental entity the outcomes (including births per attempt and data about morbidity and mortality of the resulting children for the first five years) and disclosure to the public of this information;
- Non-misleading advertising (to the extent that advertising is permitted at all); and
- Confidentiality of individually identifiable health information.

Other prohibitions beyond those on human cloning and germline intervention might include bans on:

- Extracorporeal gestation of a human being;
- Transfer of a human embryo into an animal;
- Creation of embryos solely for research purposes; or
- Transplanting reproductive material (including gametes, ovaries or testes) from animals into humans.

Gene Patents
The purpose of the patent system is to encourage innovation and the development of products by providing the holder of a patent with a twenty-year monopoly over the use of an invention. Patenting genes runs counter to this purpose because gene patents are stifling innovation and impeding access to genetic diagnostic and treatment technologies. Many researchers who are searching for genes that predispose individuals to diseases are reluctant to share information and tissue samples with other researchers because they want to discover the gene themselves and to reap the financial rewards of discovery. These rewards can be high. For example, one particular gene patent in the United States is worth $ 1.5 billion annually.

Once a gene is discovered, the patent holder can prevent any doctor or laboratory from even checking a person's body to see if he or she has a mutation of the gene. Alternatively, the patent holder can collect a very high royalty from the doctors and laboratories that examine the gene. The patent holder can even stop any use of the patented gene. One patent holder, for example, will not permit the use of its gene in prenatal screening because of the controversy surrounding abortion. Another patent holder, a major European pharmaceutical company, will not allow anyone to use its patented gene to develop a test which shows which patients will benefit from one of the company's drugs and which will not. Another biotechnology company has a patent on the genetic sequence of a particular infectious disease and is stopping another company from instituting inexpensive public health screening to determine if people are infected.

On the other hand, patent holders themselves may encourage premature adoption of genetic diagnostic tests and unsafe efforts at gene transfer experiments to benefit the patent holder rather than patients or research subjects. Moreover, special issues are raised in the case of patenting human tissue, including the ethical and legal propriety of ownership of one person's genetic information by another.

Potential regulation:
No patents shall be granted on human genes, parts of human genes or unaltered products of human genes, nor on the genes of bacteria, viruses or other infectious agents that cause disease in humans.

Work on a national regulatory scheme for the new reproductive technologies will, of course, be most relevant to countries that have an in vitro fertilization

(IVF) industry. We also believe that the best existing guidance for approaching such regulation is contained in the final report of Canada's Royal Commission on New Reproductive Technologies. *1 Patricia Baird, Proceed With Care: Final Report of the Royal Commission on New Reproductive Technologies*, 564-76 (1993). Also, to the extent that a country wants to proceed with research cloning (e.g., for the purpose of making stem cells or studying embryonic growth), regulation of the infertility industry will be needed to prevent a cloned embryo from being implanted in a woman's uterus. Such regulation could include, for example, the prohibition of freezing cloned embryos, and the prohibition of any physician or embryologist involved in IVF from making or possessing a cloned embryo.

11   While we believe these crimes should be subject to the jurisdiction of the International Criminal Court, this may not be possible in the near future, and it is more important to establish them as international crimes than to broaden the definition of "crimes against humanity" as it applies to the International Criminal Court at this time.

12   Nat'l Bioethics Advisory Comm'n, Cloning Human Beings 109 (1997), available at http://bioethics .georgetown.edu/nbac/pubs.html.

13   For example, during the 1998 debate on cloning in the U.S. Senate, more than sixteen scientific and medical organizations, including the American Society of Reproductive Medicine and the Federation of American Societies for Experimental Biology (which includes more than sixteen scientific and medical organizations), believed that there should be a moratorium on the creation of humans by cloning. See 144 CONG. REC. S434-38 (1998); 144 CONG. REC. S661 (1998). None of these organizations has since changed their position. See, e.g., Press Release, Am. Soc'y Reproductive Med., ASRM Statement on Attempts at Human Cloning (Apr. 5, 2002) ("We caution policy makers not to be rushed into approving over-reaching legislation that will criminalize valid scientific and medical research and the therapies they might lead to.") available at http://www .asrm.org/Media/Press/cloningstatement4-02; Letter from Carl B. Feldbaum, President, Biotechnology Ind. Org., to President George W. Bush (Feb. 1, 2002) ("The current moratorium on cloning humans

should remain until our nation has had time to fully explore the impact of such cloning."), available at http://www.bio.org/bioethics/cloning_letter_bush.ht ml. See also Rudolf Jaenisch & Ian Wilmut, Don't Clone Humans!, 291 *Science* 2552 (2001) ("We believe attempts to clone human beings at a time when the scientific issues of nuclear cloning have not been clarified are dangerous and irresponsible."); Editorial, Reasons to be Cloned, 414 *Nature* 567 (2001) ("The health risks to mother and child inherent in [cloning] ... demand that it be banned.").

14   Nat'l Research Council, Scientific and Medical Aspects of Human Reproductive Cloning 1 (2002).

Human reproductive cloning ... is dangerous and likely to fail. The panel therefore unanimously supports the proposal that there should be a legally enforceable ban on the practice of human reproductive cloning.... The scientific and medical considerations related to this ban should be reviewed within 5 years. The ban should be reconsidered only if at least two conditions are met: (1) a new scientific and medical review indicates that the procedures are likely to be safe and effective and (2) a broad national dialogue on the societal, religious, and ethical issues suggests that a reconsideration of the ban is warranted.

Id. at ES-1 to ES-2. See also Nat'l Research Council, Stem Cells and the Future of Regenerative Medicine (2001).

15   Stuart A. Newman, Speech at the "Beyond Cloning" Conference, Boston University (Sept. 21, 2001).

16   See, e.g., Jon W. Gordon, Genetic Enhancement in Humans, 283 *Science* 2023, 2023 (1999).

17   Hans Jonas, for example, argued that it is a crime against the clone by depriving the cloned child of his or her "existential right to certain subjective terms of being." Hans Jonas, *Philosophical Essays: From Ancient Creed to Technological Man* 160 (1974). Jonas believes that a clone will not have a "right to ignorance" or the "right ... to a unique genotype." Id. Instead, a clone knows:

Altogether too much about himself and is known ... altogether too well by others. Both facts are paralyzing for the spontaneity of becoming himself .... The clone is antecedently robbed of the freedom which only under the protection of ignorance can thrive: and to rob a human-to-be of that freedom deliberately is an inexplicable crime that must not be committed even once.

Id. at 161. Human reproductive cloning poses both physical and psychological risks to children who might be conceived using this technique. In animals, cloning currently only results in a successful pregnancy three to five percent of the time. And, even in those rare instances, many of the resulting offspring suffer—one-third die shortly before or right after birth. Other cloned animals seem perfectly healthy at first and then suffer heart and blood vessel problems, underdeveloped lungs, diabetes, immune system deficiencies and severe growth abnormalities. The mothers who gestate clones are also at risk, due to the often abnormally large size of the offspring produced—some cattle clones for example, are born up to twice the normal weight expected for calves.

18 Tim Adams, Interview: The Clone Arranger, *The Observer*, Dec. 2, 2001, at 3 (comments of Severino Antinori).

    Male infertility grows.... My invention of ICSI has helped. I have helped men whose sperm are misformed or too slow. I have helped men whose sperm does not come out from their testes! And the next step [cloning] is to help men who—traumatico!—have lost their ability to produce any sperm at all. Through war or accident or cancer. I will help only stable, loving couples. Some doctors say this is a step too far, but those same doctors have said that about all the other steps too. Very few doctors are pioneers! Very few have both the knowledge and the, the, the ... courage. Id. See also Robert Winston, The Promise of Cloning for Human Medicine, 314 *Brit. Med. J.* 913 (1997) (advocating for the use of cloning to help infertile men have genetically-related children). Zavos and Antinori dissolved their partnership in 2002. David Brown, Human Clone's Birth Predicted, *Wash. Post*, May 16, 2002, at A8.

19 See generally, Michael H. Shapiro, I Want a Girl (Boy) Just Like the Girl (Boy) that Married Dear Old Dad (Mom): Cloning Lives, 9 S. *Cal. Interdisk. L.J.* 1 (arguing, in part, that cloning should be considered reproduction, for the essence of reproduction is the creation of a new person).

    A variety of personal desires may interest people in creating a child through cloning or germline genetic engineering. The NBAC report suggests it would be "understandable, or even, as some have argued, desirable" to create a cloned child from one adult if both members of the couple have a lethal recessive gene; from a dying infant if his father is dead and the mother wants an offspring from her late husband; or from a terminally ill child to create a bone marrow donor. *Cloning Human Beings*, supra note 12, at 78-80. Some of the experts testifying before the NBAC suggested that cloning should be appropriate in exceptional circumstances. Rabbi Elliot Dorff opined that it would be "legitimate from a moral and a Jewish point of view" to clone a second child to act as a bone marrow donor so long as the "parents" raise that second child as they would any other. Id. at 55. Rabbi Moshe Tendler raised the scenario of a person who was the last in his genetic line and whose family was wiped out in the Holocaust. "I would certainly clone him," said Tendler. Id. For other Jewish perspectives supporting cloning, see Peter Hirschberg, Be Fruitful and Multiply and Multiply and Multiply, *Jerusalem Rep.*, Apr. 16, 1998, at 33. In contrast, the Catholic viewpoint is that cloning "is entirely unsuitable for human procreation even for exceptional circumstances." *Cloning Human Beings*, supra note 12, at 55.

20 Before a U.S. Senate Committee, which also heard from Ian Wilmut shortly after he had announced the birth of Dolly, one of us made the argument that a human clone would be the first human being with one genetic parent. Testimony on Scientific Discoveries and Cloning: Challenges for Public Policy, Before the Sen. Subcomm. on Public Health and Safety, Sen. Comm. on Labor and Human Resources, 105th Cong. 25 (1997) (statement of George J. Annas), available at http://www.bumc.bu.edu/www/sph/lw/pvl/Clonetest.htm. Population geneticist Richard Lewontin challenged this assertion, writing:

    A child by cloning has a full set of chromosomes like anyone else, half of which were derived from a mother and half from a father. It happens that these chromosomes were passed through another individual, the cloning donor, on the way to the child. The donor is certainly not the child's "parent" in any biological sense, but simply an earlier offspring of the original parents.

R.C. Lewontin, Confusion over Cloning, *N.Y. Rev. Books*, Oct. 23, 1997, at 20.

It should be noted that Lewontin's position takes

genetic reductionism to its extreme: people become no more than containers of their parent's genes, and their parents have the "right" to treat them not as individual human beings, but rather like embryos—entities that they can "split" or "replicate" without consideration of the child's choice or welfare. Children, even adult children, under this view have no say as to whether or not they are replicated because it is their "parents," not them, who are "reproducing." This radical redefinition of reproduction and the denial to children of the choice to procreate or not turns out to be an even stronger argument against cloning children than its biological novelty. George J. Annas, *Some Choice: Law, Medicine & The Market* 13 (1998).

21 See, e.g., Ethics Comm., Am. Soc'y Reproductive Med., Human Somatic Cell Nuclear Transfer (Cloning), 74 *Fertility & Sterility* 873, 873-76 (2000).

22 John A. Robertson, Two Models of Human Cloning, 27 *Hofstra L. Rev.* 609 (1999).

23 Ronald Dworkin, *Sovereign Virtue: The Theory and Practice of Equality* 437-42 (1997).

24 Leon Kass made this point in another context. Leon R. Kass, *Toward a More Natural Science: Biology and Human Affairs* 110-111 (1985).

25 See Rael, *The True Face of God* (Int'l Raelian Movement 1998).

26 See Jay Katz, *Experimentation With Human Beings* (Russell Sage Found. 1972).

27 Lee Silver, *Remaking Eden: Cloning and Beyond in a Brave New World* 123 (1997).

28 Id. at 4.

29 Colin Tudge, *The Impact of the Gene: From Mendel's Peas to Designer Babies* 4 (2000).

30 Id. at 342. See also Ian Wilmut et al., *The Second Creation: Dolly and the Age of Biological Control* 267-98 (2000) (discussing the implications of cloning for humankind).

31 See the appendix to this Article for current national laws on human cloning and inheritable modifications.

32 See generally *The Nazi Doctors and the Nuremberg Code* 3 (George J. Annas & Michael A. Grodin eds., 1992) (exploring the "history, context, and implications of the Doctor's Trial at Nuremberg and the impact of the Nuremberg Code on subsequent codes of research ethics and international human rights").

33 Jonas, supra note 17, at 161-62.

34 It is in this sense that children become "manufactured" products. See Kass, supra note 24, at 71-73.

35 See Annas, supra note 6, at 776-780; Fukuyama, supra note 7, at 22; Francis Fukuyama, Natural Rights and Human History, *Nat'l Interest*, Summer 2001, at 19, 30. For arguments favoring inheritable genetic modifications, see, for example, *Engineering the Human Germline* (Gregory Stock & John Campbell eds., 2000); Gregory Stock, *Redesigning Humans* (2002) (arguing, among other things, that it is inherent in our human nature to want to change our human nature, and that an international treaty would be unenforceable because every nation would have an economic incentive to defect and capture the market for inheritable modifications).

36 See, e.g., Wilmut et al., supra note 30, at 5-6 (discussing how the post-Dolly experiments were designed to use cloning techniques to make "better animals," which was always Ian Wilmut's and Keith Campbell's plan for cloning technology). See also Angelika E. Shnieke et al., Human Factor IX Trans-genic Sheep Produced by Transfer of Nuclei from Transplanted Fetal Fibroblasts, 278 *Science* 2130 (1997).

37 See, for example, Nancy Kress's Beggars series: *Beggars in Spain* (1993); *Beggars and Choosers* (1994); and *Beggar's Ride* (1996).

38 See Annas, supra note 6, at 778-81. An alternative scenario, that sees equal access to genetic "improvement" by all seems like pie in the sky to us in a world where fewer than ten percent of the population has access to contemporary medical care, and even in the world's richest country, more than forty million people lack health insurance. We do not think it is reasonable to even discuss equal access to genetic alterations until all members of the species have access to current medical technologies as a matter of right.

39 Prohibition of Genetic Intervention Law No. 5759 (1998).

40 Id. § 3(1).

41 Id. § 3(2).

42 See Ania Lichtarowicz, Scientist Warns on Human Cloning, *BBC NEWS*, at http://news.bbc.co.uk/hi /English/world/Europe/newsid_1719000- /1719195.stm (Dec. 21, 2001) (noting that Spain and Belgium are still considering different types of legislation for adoption).

43 Britain to Ban Human Cloning, CNN.COM, at

http://www.cnn.com/2001/WORLD/europe/UK/04/1 9/cloning.legislation/index.html (Apr. 19, 2001). See also Human Reproductive Cloning Act 2001, U.K. Stat. 2001, ch. 23, Enactment Clause (Eng.). (stating that the law "prohibit[s] the placing in a woman of a human embryo which has been created otherwise than by fertilization").

44 Ministry Bans Cloning Technology for Humans, *Daily Yomiuri*, July 29, 1998, at 2.

45 Gesetz zum Schutz von Embryonen (Embryonen-schutzgesetz), v. 13.12.1990 (BGBI. I S.2747). [Federal Embryo Protection Law.]

46 Manipulacion Gentica y Reproduccion [Genetic Manipulation and Reproduction]; Victoria Infertility Treatment Act, 2000; Human Reproductive Technology Act, 1991, § 7(1)(d)(i) (W. Austl.).

47 See, e.g., The Logical Next Step? An International Perspective on the Issues of Human Cloning and Genetic Technology, 4 *Ilsa J. Int'l & Comp.L.* 697, 721-25 (1998).

48 See, e.g., Valerie S. Rup, Human Somatic Cell Nuclear Transfer Cloning, the Race to Regulate, and the Constitutionality of the Proposed Regulations, 76 *U. Det. Mercy L. Rev.* 1135, 1138-39 (1999); Christine Willgoos, Note, FDA Regulation: An Answer to the Questions of Human Cloning and Germline Gene Therapy, 27 *Am. J.L. & Med.* 101, 103 (2001).

49 Human Fertilisation and Embryology Act, 1990, ch. 37, Enactment Clause (Eng.). See generally Ruth Deech, The Legal Regulation of Infertility Treatment in Britain, in *Crosscurrents: Family Law and Policy in the U.S. and England* 165-86 (Sanford Katz et al., eds, 2000).

50 Human Fertilisation and Embryology Act. ch. 27, §§ 3, 12.

51 Id. ch. 37, § 41.

52 Id. ch. 37, Enactment Clause.

53 The Act also had a ban, predating Dolly, on the replacement of the nucleus of a human embryo cell with that of any person or embryo, but that prohibition does not cover somatic cell nucleus transfer into a human egg.

54 Pro-Life Alliance v. Sec'y State for Health, CO/4095/2000 (Q.B. 2001), available at 2001 WL 1347031.

55 Human Reproductive Cloning Act, 2001, U.K. Stat. 2001 ch. 23, § 1.

56 R (Quintavalle) v. Sec'y of State for Health, 2 WLR 550 (C.A. 2002), reprinted at Cell Nuclear Replacement Organism is "Embryo," *The Times* (London), Jan. 25, 2002.

57 Federal Embryo Protection Law, 1990 (Eng.).

58 Victoria Infertility Treatment Act, 1995.

59 Federal Embryo Protection Law, 1990 (Eng.), at Part 5, § 39(1).

60 Federal Embryo Protection Law, 1990 (Eng.), at Part 5, § 39(2).

61 Human Reproductive Technology, 1991, § 7(1)(j) (Austl.).

62 The Act Relating to the Application of Biotechnology in Medicine, ch. 7.

63 Law No. 115 of March 14, 1991, Act Concerning Measures for the Purposes of Research or Treatment in Connection with Fertilized Human Oocytes (1993).

64 Law No. 94-654 of July 29, 1994, on the Donation and Use of Elements and Products of the Human Body, Medically Assisted Procreation, and Prenatal Diagnosis.

65 Decree No. 24029-S: A Regulation on Assisted Reproduction, Feb. 3, 1995.

66 See Memorandum on the Prohibition on Federal Funding for Cloning of Human Beings, 33 *Weekly Comp. Press. Doc.* 281 (Mar. 4, 1997); see also Transcript of Clinton Remarks on Cloning, *U.S. Newswire*, Mar. 4, 1997, available at 1997 WL 5711155.

67 Yet despite the risks, only six states—California, Iowa, Louisiana, Michigan, Rhode Island and Virginia—have passed legislation that prohibits human reproductive cloning. CAL. HEALTH & SAFETY CODE ANN. § 24185 (West 2002); IOWA CODE § 707B, CSB 218 (S.F. 2118) (2002); LA. REV. STAT. 40:1299.36.2 (West 2002); MICH. COMP. LAWS ANN. § 750.430a (West 2001); R.I. GEN. LAWS § 23-16.4 (2001); VA. CODE ANN. §§ 32.1-162.21, 162.22 (Michie 2002). In addition, Missouri prohibits the use of any state funds to bring about the birth of a child via cloning techniques. MO. ANN. STAT. § 1.217 (West 2002). The U.S. House of Representatives in July 2001 voted to ban human cloning. See The Human Cloning Prohibition Act of 2001, H.R. 2505, 107th Cong. (2001). See also Sheryl Gay Stolberg, House Backs Ban on Human Cloning for any

Objective, *N.Y. Times*, Aug. 1, 2001, at A1. At the time of this writing, the U.S. Senate was scheduled to consider this issue in 2002.

68   FLA. STAT. ANN. § 390.0111(6) (West 2002); LA. REV. STAT. ANN. § 9:121-129 (West 2002); ME. REV. STAT. ANN. tit. 22, § 1593 (2002); MASS. GEN. LAWS ANN. ch. 112, § 12J West (2002); MICH. COMP. LAWS ANN. § 333.2685-.2692 (West 2002); MINN. STAT. § 145.421 (2001); N.D. CENT. CODE § 14-02.2-01 (2001); N.H. REV. STAT. ANN. § 168-B:15 (2002); 18 PA. CONS. STAT. § 3216 (2001); R.I. GEN. LAWS § 11-54-1 (2001). A South Dakota law bans research that destroys an embryo, when such research has not been undertaken to preserve the life and health of the particular embryo. S.D. CODIFIED LAWS § 34-14-18 (Michie 2001).

69   MINN. STAT. ANN. § 145.421.

70   MICH. COMP. LAWS ANN. § 333.2685.

71   FLA. STAT. ANN. § 390.0111(6); ME. REV. STAT. ANN. tit. 22, § 1593; MASS. GEN. LAWS ANN. ch. 112, § 12J; MICH. COMP. LAWS ANN. § 333.2685-.2692; N.D. CENT. CODE § 14-02.2-01; R.I. GEN. LAWS § 11-54-1.

72   18 PA. CONS. STAT. § 3216.

73   See Ronald M. Green, The Ethical Considerations, 286 *Scientific Am.* 4850, 4850 (Jan. 2002) (arguing that when Advanced Cell Technology created what the company called the "world's first human cloned embryo," all it had really done was create an "activated egg"). The company's president, Michael West, had previously argued that the company's work did not violate the Massachusetts Federal Research statute, and we believe he is correct in this argument.

74   Four states' fetal research bans—those of Arizona, Illinois, Louisiana, and Utah—have already been struck down on those grounds. Forbes v. Napolitano, 236 F.3d 1009 (9th Cir. 2000); Margaret S. v. Edwards, 794 F.2d 994, 998-99 (5th Cir. 1996); Jane L. v. Bangerter, 61 F.3d 1493, 1499-1502 (10th Cir. 1995); Lifchez v. Hartigan, 735 F. Supp. 1361, 1363-66 (N.D. Ill. 1990).

75   N.H. REV. STAT. ANN. § 168-B:15(II) (2002).

76   LA. REV. STAT. ANN. § 40:1299.36.2 (West 2002); MICH. COMP. LAWS ANN. §§ 333.16275, 750.430(a) (West 2001); R.I. GEN. LAWS § 23-16.4-2 (2001).

77   ME. REV. STAT. ANN. tit. 22, § 1593 (2002).

78   See, e.g., FLA. STAT. ANN. § 390.0111(6) (West 2002); MASS. GEN. LAWS ANN. ch. 112, § 12J (West 2002); MICH. COMP. LAWS ANN. § 333.2685-.2692 (West 2002); MINN. STAT. § 145.421 (2001); N.D. CENT. CODE § 14-02.2-01 (2001); 18 PA. CONS. STAT. § 3216 (2001); R.I. GEN. LAWS § 11-54-1.

79   N.H. REV. STAT. ANN. § 168-B:15(II).

80   LA. REV. STAT. ANN. § 9:122 (West 2002).

81   The right to make decisions about whether or not to bear children is constitutionally protected under the constitutional right to privacy. See, e.g., Eisenstadt v. Baird, 405 U.S. 438 (1972); Griswold v. Connecticut, 381 U.S. 479 (1965). The constitutional right to liberty also affords such protection. See Planned Parenthood of S.E. Pa. v. Casey, 505 U.S. 833, 857 (1992). The U.S. Supreme Court in 1992 reaffirmed the "recognized protection accorded to liberty relating to intimate relationships, the family, and decisions about whether to bear and beget a child." Id. at 857. Early decisions held that the right to privacy protected married couples' ability to make procreative decisions, but later decisions focused on individuals' rights as well. The U.S. Supreme Court has stated, "If the right of privacy means anything, it is the right of the individual, married or single, to be free from unwarranted governmental intrusion into matters so fundamentally affecting a person as the decision whether to bear or beget a child." Eisenstadt, 405 U.S. at 453.

A federal district court has indicated that the right to make procreative decisions encompasses the right of an infertile couple to undergo medically-assisted reproduction, including IVF and the use of a donated embryo. Lifchez v. Hartigan, 735 F. Supp. 1361, 1367-69. (N.D. Ill. 1990). Lifchez held that a ban on research on conceptuses was unconstitutional because it impermissibly infringed upon a woman's fundamental right to privacy. Id. at 1363. Although the Illinois statute banning embryo and fetal research at issue in the case permitted IVF, it did not allow embryo donation, embryo freezing or experimental prenatal diagnostic procedures. Id. at 1365-70. The court stated, "It takes no great leap of logic to see that within the cluster of constitutionally protected choices that includes the right to have access to contraceptives, there must be included within that cluster the right to submit to a medical procedure that may bring about, rather than prevent, pregnancy." Id. at 1377. The court also held that the statute was impermissibly vague because of its failure to define "experiment" or "therapeutic." Id. at 1376.

Some commentators argue that the Constitution similarly protects the right to create a child through cloning. See John Robertson, Views on Cloning: Possible Benefits, Address Before the National Bioethics Advisory Commission (Mar. 14, 1997), available at http://bioethics.georgetown.edu/nbac/transcripts/index.html. This seems to be a reversal of Robertson's earlier position that cloning "may deviate too far from the prevailing conception of what is valuable about reproduction to count as a protected reproductive experience. At some point attempts to control the entire genome of a new person pass beyond the central experiences of identity and meaning that make reproduction a valued experience." John Robertson, *Children of Choice: Freedom and the New Reproductive Technologies* 169 (1994).

However, cloning is sufficiently different from normal reproduction and the types of assisted reproduction protected by the Lifchez case that constitutional protections should not apply. In even the most high-tech reproductive technologies available, a mix of genes occurs to create an individual with a genotype that has never before existed. In the case of twins, two such individuals are created. Their futures are open and the distinction between themselves and their parents is acknowledged. In the case of cloning, however, the genotype already exists. Even though it is clear that the individual will develop into a person with different traits because of different social, environmental and generational influences, there is evidence that the fact that he or she possesses an existing genotype will affect how the resulting clone is treated by himself, his family and social institutions.

In that sense, cloning is sufficiently distinct from traditional reproduction or alternative reproduction to not be considered constitutionally protected. It is not a process of genetic mix, but of genetic duplication. It is not reproduction, but a sort of recycling, where a single individual's genome is made into someone else. This change in kind in the fundamental way in which humans can "reproduce" represents such a challenge to human dignity and the potential devalu-

ation of human life (even comparing the "original" to the "copy" in terms of which is to be more valued) that even the search for an analogy has come up empty handed. Testimony on Scientific Discoveries and Cloning: Challenges for Public Policy, Before the Sen. Subcomm. on Public Health and Safety, Sen. Comm. on Labor and Human Resources, 105th Cong. 25 (1997) (statement of George J. Annas), available at http://www.bumc.bu.edu/www/sph/lw/pvl/Clonetest.htm. Gilbert Meilaender, in testifying before NBAC, pointed out the social importance of children's genetic independence from their parents: "They replicate neither their father nor their mother. That is a reminder of the independence that we must eventually grant to them and for which it is our duty to prepare them." *Cloning Human Beings*, supra note 12, at 81.

Even if a constitutional right to clone were to be recognized, any legislation which would infringe unduly upon this fundamental right would be permissible if it furthered a compelling interest in the least restrictive manner possible in order to survive this standard of review. See Lifchez, 735 F. Supp. at 1377. Along those lines, the NBAC raised concerns about physical and psychological risks to the offspring, as well as about "a degradation of the quality of parenting, and family if parents are tempted to seek excessive control over their children's characteristics, to value children according to how well they meet every detailed parental expectation, and to undermine the acceptance and openness that typify loving families." *Cloning Human Beings*, supra note 12, at 77. The NBAC also noted how cloning might undermine important social values, such as opening the door to a form of eugenics, or by tempting some to manipulate others as if they were objects instead of persons, and exceeding the moral boundaries of the human condition. Id.

The potential physical and psychological risks of cloning an entire individual are sufficiently compelling to justify banning the procedure. The notion of replicating existing humans seems to fundamentally conflict with our legal system, which emphatically protects individuality and uniqueness. Banning procreation through nuclear transplantation is justifiable in light of common law and constitutional protection of the sanctity of the individual and personal privacy.

Francis C. Pizzulli, Note, Asexual Reproduction and Genetic Engineering: A Constitutional Assessment of the Technology of Cloning, 47 *S. Cal. L. Rev.* 476, 502 (1974).

In the United States, couples' constitutional arguments regarding a privacy right or liberty right to use inheritable genetic interventions would appear to be stronger than those regarding access to cloning. In decisions construing the Americans with Disabilities Act, including one before the U.S. Supreme Court, individuals with AIDS were judged to be disabled because their disease was seen as interfering with a major life function—reproduction. Bragdon v. Abbott, 524 U.S. 624, 631 (1998). The argument seems to be that "normal" reproduction involves the creation of children without diseases.

Couples who both have sickle cell anemia or some other recessive genetic disorder might argue that a ban on germline interventions deprives them of reproductive liberty because it is the only way they can have healthy children. (There are several fallacies in that argument. The children born may have other diseases. And the genetic modification intervention itself might harm the children or be ineffective.) Forbidding the use of the techniques, it would be argued, forces them to go childless.

The couple might bolster their argument with a reference to another aspect of the Lifchez holding. The court in that case also held the ban on embryo research unconstitutional because it forbade parents from using experimental diagnostic techniques to learn the genetic status of their fetus. See Lifchez, 735 F. Supp. at 1366-67. The court reasoned that, if the woman has a constitutional right to abort, she has a right to genetic information upon which to make the decision. See id. Using an expansive interpretation, Lifchez could be understood as saying that it was understandable that couples would choose to have only children of a certain genetic makeup and that such a decision was constitutionally protected. However, even if there were a constitutional right to use inheritable genetic interventions, such interventions could be banned if they posed compelling physical, psychological or social risks. To be constitutional, the ban would also need to be narrowly focused to operate in the least restrictive manner possible.

82   See Kaiser Family Found., Lawmakers Vow to Introduce Cloning Restrictions, Bush Signals He Will "Work to Pass" Ban, *Kaiser Daily Reprod. Health Rep.*, Mar. 29, 2001, available at http://report.kff.org/archive/repro/2001/3/kr010329.2.htm.

83   As of June, 2002, the Senate had three bills to consider. S. 790, introduced by Senator Brownback of Kansas, is substantially the same as the Weldon bill passed by the House of Representatives in August, 2001. Human Cloning Prohibition Act, S. 790, 107th Cong. (2001). It would ban both the creation of human embryos by cloning as well as attempts to create a human child by cloning. Id. at § 3. S. 1758, introduced by Senator Dianne Feinstein of California bans attempts at human cloning, defined as "asexual reproduction by implanting or attempting to implant the product of nuclear transplantation into a uterus." Human Cloning Prohibition Act, S. 1758, 107th Cong. (2001). It also specifically permits certain activities, including "nuclear transplantation to produce human stem cells." Id. at § 4. It was slightly modified on May 1 and reintroduced as S. 2439 with the endorsement of Senator Orin Hatch. 148 Cong. Rec. S36,633 (2002). Finally, S. 1893, introduced in late January, 2002 by Senator Harkin of Iowa would simply ban cloning as defined as "asexual human reproduction by implanting or attempting to implant the product of nuclear transplantation [defined as 'introducing the nuclear material of a human somatic cell into a fertilized or unfertilized oocyte from which the nucleus has been or will be removed or inactivated'] into a woman's uterus or a substitute for a woman's uterus." S. 1893, 107th Cong. § 498C (2002). For more details, see George J. Annas, Cloning and the U.S. Congress, 346 *New Eng. J. Med.* 1599 (2002).

84   The outstanding question is whether abortion politics will permit members of Congress to outlaw so-called reproductive cloning (which they all agree should be done) without also outlawing research cloning (a prohibition included in the Weldon and Brownback bills because some supporters object to any creation of human embryos in the laboratory, and others believe that once created by cloning, it is inevitable that a cloned human embryo will be introduced into a woman's uterus and eventually result in the birth of a cloned child). The slippery slope from research to reproductive cloning is real, of course, but could be

made much less likely by adding restrictions to what physicians involved in infertility treatment could do (e.g., no creation or use of cloned embryos by infertility specialists). Three further steps would virtually eliminate the danger: creation of a federal oversight panel that would have to approve any research projects involving the creation of cloned embryos; outlawing the purchase and sale of human eggs (as is done now for organs and tissues for transplant); and outlawing the freezing or storage of cloned human embryos, eliminating the potential for stockpiling human embryos, and making it almost impossible for a research embryo to be used for reproduction in practice. George J. Annas, Cell Division, *Boston Globe*, Apr. 21, 2002, E1.

85   Gene Weingarten, Strange Egg, *Wash. Post*, Jan. 25, 1998, at F1.

86   Radical Scientist to Help Open Cloning Clinics in Japan, *Japan Sci. Scan*, Dec. 7, 1998, available at 1998 WL 8029927.

87   Thomas Hirenee Atenga, Africa: Biotech Firms Have Their Eyes on Africa, Euro MPS Say, *Int'l Press Serv.*, Oct. 14, 1998.

88   See supra notes 39 to 56 and accompanying text.

89   Brit. Med. Ass'n, *the Medical Profession and Human Rights* 205-40 (2001), see also sources cited supra note 32.

90   Most Doctors, Academics Oppose Human Cloning, *Japan Econ. Newswire*, Nov. 7, 1998.

91   Conselho Nacional de Etica para as Ciencias de Vida [National Council on Ethics for the Life Sciences], Opinion on Embryo Research and the Ethical Implications of Cloning, No. 21/CNEV/97 (1997).

92   Resolution on Human Cloning, European Parliament, Jan. 15, 1998, O.J. (C 34) 164 (1998).

93   See Ian Wilmut, Cloning for Medicine, *Scientific Am.*, Dec. 1998, at 58:

> None of the suggested uses of cloning for making copies of existing people is ethically acceptable to my way of thinking, because they are not in the interests of the resulting child. It should go without saying that I strongly oppose allowing cloned human embryos to develop so that they can be tissue donors.

Id. Wilmut has testified around the world against human cloning. See, e.g., Christine Corcos et al., Double-Take: A Second Look at Cloning, Science

Fiction and Law, 59 *LA. L. Rev.* 1041, 1051 (denouncing cloning human beings at a talk at Princeton University); Creator of Dolly Stresses Benefits of Further Research on Cloning, Daily Yomiuri, June 7, 1997, available at 19997 WL 1211052 (advocating a worldwide prohibition against human cloning); Cult in the First Bid to Clone Human, *Express*, Oct. 11, 2000, available at 2000 WL 24217743 (responding to a British couple's plan to clone their deceased daughter, stating that "it is absolutely criminal to try this [cloning] in a human."); Curt Suplee, Top Scientists Warn Against Cloning Panic; Recreating Humans Would Be Unethical Experts Say, *Wash. Post*, Mar. 13, 1997, at A03 (testifying against human cloning before the NBAC).

94   Press Release, Biotechnology Ind. org., BIO Reiterates Unequivocal Opposition to Reproductive Cloning; Support for Therapeutic Applications, Nov. 25, 2001, available at http://www.bio.org/news room/news.asp. See also Frances Bishop, 11th Annual Bio Conference: Ethical Issues in Genetics Create Challenges for Biotech Industry, 8 *Bioworld Today* 112 (1997), available at 1997 WL 11130296.

95   Press Release, W.H.O., *World Health Assembly*, World Health Assembly States its Position on Cloning Human Reproduction (May 14, 1997), available at http://www.who.int/archives/inf-pr-1997/en/97wha9.html.

96   W.H.O., *World Health Assembly*, 51st Sess., Ethical, Scientific and Social Implications of Cloning in Human Health, WHA51.10, (1998).

97   1) Croatia, 2) Cyprus, 3) Czech Republic, 4) Denmark, 5) Estonia, 6) Finland, 7) France, 8) Georgia, 9) Greece, 10) Hungary, 11) Iceland, 12) Italy, 13) Latvia, 14) Lithuania, 15) Luxembourg, 16) Moldova, 17) Netherlands, 18) Norway, 19) Poland, 20) Portugal, 21) Romania, 22) San Marino, 23) Slovenia, 24) Slovenia, 25) Spain, 26) Sweden, 27) Switzerland, 28) the former Yugoslav Republic of Macedonia and 29) Turkey. See also *Additional Protocol (Explanatory Report) to the Convention on Human Rights and Biomedicine*, Jan. 12, 1998, available at http://conventions.coe.int/Treaty/en/Reports/Html/168.htm.

98   Resolution on Human Cloning, Eur. Parliament, Jan. 15, 1998 *O.J.* (C34) 164 (1998).

99   Id.

100 Id.

101 U.N.E.S.C.O., *Universal Declaration on the Human Genome and Human Rights*, 29th Sess., 29 C/Res. 16 (1997), available at http://www.unesco.org/human _rights/hrbc.htm. The declaration was adopted by the General Assembly in 1999. G.A. Res. 152, U.N. GAOR, 53rd Sess., U.N. Doc. A/53/152 (1999).

102 *Universal Declaration on the Human Genome and Human Rights*, Introduction.

103 Id.

104 Id. art. 11.

105 Id.

106 Request for the Inclusion of a Supplementary Item in the Agenda of the 56th Session, International Convention Against the Reproductive Cloning of Human Beings, U.N. GAOR, 56th Sess., U.N. Doc. A/56/192 (2001).

107 United Nations Calls for a Treaty to Ban Human Cloning, *Birmingham Post*, Nov. 21, 2001, at 8.

108 See supra note 84. The next meeting of the ad hoc committee is scheduled at the United Nations for September 23-27, 2002. It is anticipated that the mandate to guide subsequent treaty negotiations will be adopted at this meeting, and that treaty language may be agreed upon a year or so later.

109 Stephen P. Marks, Tying Prometheus Down: The International Law of Human Genetic Manipulation, 3 *Chi. J. Int'l L.* (forthcoming 2002). The other U.N. treaty method is known as a framework convention, which is used when countries agree that a particular field needs to be regulated (such as the environment), but do not yet agree on the specifics of how the regulation should work. Because there is basic international agreement on human reproductive cloning, the framework convention is inappropriate. See, e.g., Daniel Bodansky, The United Nations Framework Convention on Climate Change: A Commentary, 18 *Yale J. Int'l L.* 451, 494 (1993). See also Anthony Aust, *Modern Treaty Law and Practice* 97 (2000); Donald M. Goldberg, Negotiating the Framework Convention on Climate Change, 4 *Touro J. Transnat'l L.* 149 (1993); Lee A. Kimball, The Biodiversity Convention: How to Make It Work, 28 Vand. J. *Transnat'l L.* 763 (1995).

110 Convention on the Prohibition of the Use, Stockpiling, Production and Transfer of Anti-Personnel Mines and on Their Destruction, G.A. res. 47/39, 47 U.N. GAOR Supp. (No. 49) at 54, U.N. Doc. A/47/49 (1992).

63.
IN DEFENSE OF POSTHUMAN DIGNITY

Nick Bostrom

Source: *Bioethics* 19.3 (2005): 202-14.

❧

Transhumanists vs. Bioconservatives

Transhumanism is a loosely defined movement that has developed gradually over the past two decades, and can be viewed as an outgrowth of secular humanism and the Enlightenment. It holds that current human nature is improvable through the use of applied science and other rational methods, which may make it possible to increase human health-span, extend our intellectual and physical capacities, and give us increased control over our own mental states and moods.[1] Technologies of concern include not only current ones, like genetic engineering and information technology, but also anticipated future developments such as fully immersive virtual reality, machine-phase nanotechnology, and artificial intelligence.

Transhumanists promote the view that human enhancement technologies should be made widely available, and that individuals should have broad discretion over which of these technologies to apply to themselves (morphological freedom), and that parents should normally get to decide which reproductive technologies to use when having children (reproductive freedom).[2] Transhumanists believe that, while there are hazards that need to be identified and avoided, human enhancement technologies will offer enormous potential for deeply valuable and humanly beneficial uses. Ultimately, it is possible that such enhancements may make us, or our descendants, 'posthuman,' beings who may have indefinite health-spans, much greater intellectual faculties than any current human being—and perhaps entirely new sensibilities or modalities—as well as the ability to control their own emotions. The wisest approach vis-à-vis these prospects, argue transhumanists, is to embrace technological progress, while strongly defending human rights and individual choice, and taking action specifically against concrete threats, such as military or terrorist abuse of bioweapons, and against unwanted environmental or social side-effects.

In opposition to this transhumanist view stands a bioconservative camp that argues against the use of technology to modify human nature. Prominent bioconservative writers include Leon Kass, Francis Fukuyama, George Annas, Wesley Smith, Jeremy Rifkin, and Bill McKibben. One of the central concerns of the bioconservatives is that human enhancement technologies might be 'dehumanizing.' The worry, which has been variously expressed, is that these technologies might undermine our human dignity or inadvertently erode something that is deeply valuable about being human but that is difficult to put into words or to factor into a cost-benefit analysis. In some cases (for example, Leon Kass) the unease seems to derive from religious or crypto-religious sentiments, whereas for others (for example, Francis Fukuyama) it stems from secular grounds. The best approach, these bioconservatives argue, is to implement global bans on swathes of promising human enhancement technologies to forestall a slide down a slippery slope towards an ultimately debased, posthuman state.

While any brief description necessarily skirts significant nuances that differentiate between the writers within the two camps, I believe the above characterization nevertheless highlights a principal fault line in one of the great debates of our times: how we should look at the future of humankind and whether we should attempt to use technology to make ourselves 'more than human.' This paper will distinguish two common fears about the posthuman and argue that they are partly unfounded and that, to the extent that they correspond to real risks, there are better responses than trying to implement broad bans on technology. I will make some remarks on the concept of dignity, which bioconservatives believe to be imperiled by coming human enhancement technologies, and suggest that we need to recognize that not only humans in their current form, but posthumans too could have dignity.

Two Fears about the Posthuman

The prospect of posthumanity is feared for at least two reasons. One is that the state of being posthuman might in itself be degrading, so that by becoming posthuman we might be harming ourselves. Another is that posthumans might pose a threat to 'ordinary' humans. (I shall set aside a third possible reason, that the development of posthumans might offend some supernatural being.)

The most prominent bioethicist to focus on the first fear is Leon Kass:

> Most of the given bestowals of nature have their given species- specified natures: they are each and all of a given sort. Cockroaches and humans are equally bestowed but differently natured. To turn a man into a cockroach—as we don't need Kafka to show us—would be dehumanizing. To try to turn a man into more than a man might be so as well. We need more than generalized appreciation for nature's gifts. We need a particular regard and respect for the special gift that is our own given nature.[3]

Transhumanists counter that nature's gifts are sometimes poisoned and should not always be accepted. Cancer, malaria, dementia, aging, starvation, unnecessary suffering, and cognitive shortcomings are all among the presents that we would wisely refuse. Our own species-specified natures are a rich source of much of the thoroughly unrespectable and unacceptable—susceptibility for disease, murder, rape, genocide, cheating, torture, racism. The horrors of nature in general, and of our own nature in particular, are so well documented[4] that it is astonishing that somebody as distinguished as Leon Kass should still in this day and age be tempted to rely on

the natural as a guide as to what is desirable or normatively right. We should be grateful that our ancestors were not swept away by the Kassian sentiment, or we would still be picking lice off each other's backs. Rather than deferring to the natural order, transhumanists maintain that we can legitimately reform ourselves and our natures in accordance with humane values and personal aspirations.

If one rejects nature as a general criterion of the good, as most thoughtful people nowadays do, one can of course still acknowledge that particular ways of modifying human nature would be debasing. Not all change is progress. Not even all well-intentioned technological intervention in human nature would be on balance beneficial. Kass goes far beyond these truisms, however, when he declares that utter dehumanization lies in store for us as the inevitable result of our obtaining technical mastery over our own nature:

> The final technical conquest of his own nature would almost certainly leave mankind utterly enfeebled. This form of mastery would be identical with utter dehumanization. Read Huxley's *Brave New World*, read C.S. Lewis's *Abolition of Man*, read Nietzsche's account of the last man, and then read the newspapers. Homogenization, mediocrity, pacification, drug-induced contentment, debasement of taste, souls without loves and longings—these are the inevitable results of making the essence of human nature the last project of technical mastery. In his moment of triumph, Promethean man will become a contented cow.[5]

The fictional inhabitants of *Brave New World*, to pick the best known of Kass's examples, are admittedly short on dignity (in at least one sense of the word). But the claim that this is the inevitable consequence of our obtaining technological mastery over human nature is exceedingly pessimistic—and unsupported—if understood as a futuristic prediction, and false if construed as a claim about metaphysical necessity.

There are many things wrong with the fictional society that Huxley described. It is static, totalitarian, caste-bound; its culture is a wasteland. The brave new worlders themselves are a dehumanized and undignified lot. Yet posthumans they are not. Their capacities are not super-human but in many respects substantially inferior to our own. Their life expectancy and physique are quite normal, but their intellectual, emotional, moral, and spiritual faculties are stunted. The majority of the brave new worlders have various degrees of engineered mental retardation. And everyone, save the ten world controllers (along with a miscellany of primitives and social outcasts who are confined to fenced preservations or isolated islands), are barred or discouraged from developing individuality, independent thinking, and initiative, and are conditioned not to desire these traits in the first place. *Brave New World* is not a tale of human enhancement gone amok, but is rather a tragedy of technology and social engineering being deliberately used to cripple moral and intellectual capacities—the exact antithesis of the transhumanist proposal.

Transhumanists argue that the best way to avoid a Brave New World is by vigorously defending morphological and reproductive freedoms against any would-be world controllers. History has shown the dangers in letting governments curtail these freedoms. The last century's government-sponsored coercive eugenics programs, once favored by both the left and the right, have been thoroughly discredited. Because people are likely to differ profoundly in their attitudes towards human enhancement technologies, it is crucial that no single solution be imposed on everyone from above, but that individuals get to consult their own consciences as to what is right for themselves and their families. Information, public debate, and education are the appropriate means by which to encourage others to make wise choices, not a global ban on a broad range of potentially beneficial medical and other enhancement options.

The second fear is that there might be an eruption of violence between unaugmented humans and posthumans. George Annas, Lori Andrews, and Rosario Isasi have argued that we should view human cloning and all inheritable genetic modifications as 'crimes against humanity' in order to reduce the probability that a posthuman species will arise, on grounds that such a species would pose an existential threat to the old human species:

The new species, or 'posthuman,' will likely view the old 'normal' humans as inferior, even savages, and fit for slavery or slaughter. The normals, on the other hand, may see the posthumans as a threat and if they can, may engage in a preemptive strike by killing the posthumans before they themselves are killed or enslaved by them. It is ultimately this predictable potential for genocide that makes species-altering experiments potential weapons of mass destruction, and makes the unaccountable genetic engineer a potential bioterrorist.[6]

There is no denying that bioterrorism and unaccountable genetic engineers developing increasingly potent weapons of mass destruction pose a serious threat to our civilization. But using the rhetoric of bioterrorism and weapons of mass destruction to cast aspersions on therapeutic uses of biotechnology to improve health, longevity, and other human capacities is unhelpful. The issues are quite distinct. Reasonable people can be in favor of strict regulation of bioweapons, while promoting beneficial medical uses of genetics and other human enhancement technologies, including inheritable and 'species-altering' modifications.

Human society is always at risk of some group deciding to view another group of humans as being fit for slavery or slaughter. To counteract such tendencies, modern societies have created laws and institutions, and endowed them with powers of enforcement, that act to prevent groups of citizens from enslaving or slaughtering one another. The efficacy of these institutions does not depend on all citizens having equal capacities. Modern, peaceful societies can have large numbers of people with diminished physical or mental capacities along with many other people who may be exceptionally physically strong or healthy or intellectually talented in various ways. Adding people with technologically enhanced capacities to this already broad distribution of ability would not need to rip society apart or trigger genocide or enslavement.

The assumption that inheritable genetic modifications or other human enhancement technologies would lead to two distinct and separate species should also be questioned. It seems much more likely that there would be a continuum of differently modified or enhanced individuals, which would overlap with the continuum of as-yet unenhanced humans. The scenario in which 'the enhanced' form a pact and then attack 'the naturals' makes for exciting science fiction, but is not necessarily the most plausible outcome. Even today, the segment containing the tallest ninety percent of the population could, in principle, get together and kill or enslave the shorter decile. That this does not happen suggests that a well-organized society can hold together even if it contains many possible coalitions of people sharing some attribute such that, if they ganged up, they would be capable of exterminating the rest.

To note that the extreme case of a war between humans and posthumans is not the most likely scenario is not to say that there are no legitimate social concerns about the steps that may take us closer to posthumanity. Inequity, discrimination, and stigmatization—against, or on behalf of, modified people—could become serious issues. Transhumanists would argue that these (potential) social problems call for social remedies. One example of how contemporary technology can change important aspects of someone's identity is sex reassignment. The experiences of transsexuals show that Western culture still has work to do in becoming more accepting of diversity. This is a task that we can begin to tackle today by fostering a climate of tolerance and acceptance towards those who are different from ourselves. Painting alarmist pictures of the threat from future technologically modified people, or hurling preemptive condemnations of their necessarily debased nature, is not the best way to go about it.

What about the hypothetical case in which someone intends to create, or turn themselves into, a being of such radically enhanced capacities that a single one or a small group of such individuals would be capable of taking over the planet? This is clearly not a situation that is likely to arise in the imminent future, but one can imagine that, perhaps in a few decades, the prospective creation of superintelligent machines could raise this kind of concern. The would-be creator of a new life form with such surpassing capabilities would have an obligation to ensure that the proposed being is free from psychopathic tendencies and, more generally, that it has humane inclinations. For example, a future artificial intelligence programmer should be required to make a strong case that launching a purportedly human-friendly superintelligence would be safer than the alternative. Again, however, this (currently) science fiction scenario must be clearly distinguished from our present situation and our more immediate concern with taking effective steps towards incrementally improving human capacities and health-span.

Is Human Dignity Incompatible with Posthuman Dignity?

Human dignity is sometimes invoked as a polemical substitute for clear ideas. This is not to say that there are no important moral issues relating to dignity, but it does mean that there is a need to define what one has in mind when one uses the term. Here, we shall consider two different senses of dignity:

1. Dignity as moral status, in particular the inalienable right to be treated with a basic level of respect.
2. Dignity as the quality of being worthy or honorable; worthiness, worth, nobleness, excellence.[7]

On both these definitions, dignity is something that a posthuman could possess. Francis Fukuyama, however, seems to deny this and warns that giving up on the idea that dignity is unique to human beings—defined as those possessing a mysterious essential human quality he calls 'Factor X'[8]—would invite disaster:

> Denial of the concept of human dignity—that is, of the idea that there is something unique about the human race that entitles every member of the species to a higher moral status than the rest of the natural world—leads us down a very perilous path. We may be compelled ultimately to take this path, but we should do so only with our eyes open. Nietzsche is a much better guide to what lies down that road than the legions of bioethicists and casual academic Darwinians that today are prone to give us moral advice on this subject.[9]

What appears to worry Fukuyama is that introducing new kinds of enhanced person into the world might cause some individuals (perhaps infants, or the mentally handicapped, or unenhanced humans in general) to lose some of the moral status that they currently possess, and that a fundamental precondition of liberal democracy, the principle of equal dignity for all, would be destroyed.

The underlying intuition seems to be that instead of the famed 'expanding moral circle,' what we have is more like an oval, whose shape we can change but whose area must remain constant. Thankfully, this purported conservation law of moral recognition lacks empirical support. The set of individuals accorded full moral status by Western societies has actually increased, to include men without property or noble decent, women, and non-white peoples. It would seem feasible to extend this set further to include future posthumans, or, for that matter, some of the higher primates or human-animal chimaeras, should such be created—and to do so without causing any compensating shrinkage in another direction. (The moral status of problematic borderline cases, such as foetuses or late-stage Alzheimer patients, or the brain-dead, should perhaps be decided separately from the issue of technologically modified humans or novel artificial life forms.) Our own role in this process need not be that of passive bystanders. We can work to create more inclusive social structures that accord appropriate moral recognition and legal rights to all who need them, be they male or female, black or white, flesh or silicon.

Dignity in the second sense, as referring to a special excellence or moral worthiness, is something that current human beings possess to widely differing degrees. Some excel far more than others do. Some are morally admirable; others are base and vicious. There is no reason for supposing that posthuman beings could not also have dignity in this second sense. They may even be able to attain higher levels of moral and other excellence than any of us humans. The fictional brave new worlders, who were subhuman rather than posthuman, would have scored low on this kind of dignity, and partly for that reason they would be awful role models for us to emulate. But surely we can create more uplifting and appealing

visions of what we may aspire to become. There may be some who would transform themselves into degraded posthumans—but then some people today do not live very worthy human lives. This is regrettable, but the fact that some people make bad choices is not generally a sufficient ground for rescinding people's right to choose. And legitimate countermeasures are available: education, encouragement, persuasion, social and cultural reform. These, not a blanket prohibition of all posthuman ways of being, are the measures to which those bothered by the prospect of debased posthumans should resort. A liberal democracy should normally permit incursions into morphological and reproductive freedoms only in cases where somebody is abusing these freedoms to harm another person.

The principle that parents should have broad discretion to decide on genetic enhancements for their children has been attacked on the grounds that this form of reproductive freedom would constitute a kind of parental tyranny that would undermine the child's dignity and capacity for autonomous choice; for instance, by Hans Jonas:

> Technological mastered nature now again includes man who (up to now) had, in technology, set himself against it as its master ... But whose power is this—and over whom or over what? Obviously the power of those living today over those coming after them, who will be the defenseless other side of prior choices made by the planners of today. The other side of the power of today is the future bondage of the living to the dead.[10]

Jonas is relying on the assumption that our descendants, who will presumably be far more technologically advanced than we are, would nevertheless be defenseless against our machinations to expand their capacities. This is almost certainly incorrect. If, for some inscrutable reason, they decided that they would prefer to be less intelligent, less healthy, and lead shorter lives, they would not lack the means to achieve these objectives and frustrate our designs.

In any case, if the alternative to parental choice in determining the basic capacities of new people is entrusting the child's welfare to nature, that is blind chance, then the decision should be easy. Had Mother Nature been a real parent, she would have been in jail for child abuse and murder. And transhumanists can accept, of course, that just as society may in exceptional circumstances override parental autonomy, such as in cases of neglect or abuse, so too may society impose regulations to protect the child-to-be from genuinely harmful genetic interventions—but not because they represent choice rather than chance.

Jürgen Habermas, in a recent work, echoes Jonas' concern and worries that even the mere knowledge of having been intentionally made by another could have ruinous consequences:

> We cannot rule out that knowledge of one's own hereditary features as programmed may prove to restrict the choice of an individual's life, and to undermine the essentially symmetrical relations between free and equal human beings.[11]

A transhumanist could reply that it would be a mistake for an individual to believe that she has no choice over her own life just because some (or all) of her genes were selected by her parents. She would, in fact, have as much choice as if her genetic constitution had been selected by chance. It could even be that she would enjoy significantly more choice and autonomy in her life, if the modifications were such as to expand her basic capability set. Being healthy, smarter, having a wide range of talents, or possessing greater powers of self-control are blessings that tend to open more life paths than they block.

Why We Need Posthuman Dignity

Similarly ominous forecasts were made in the seventies about the severe psychological damage that children conceived through in vitro fertilization would suffer upon learning that they originated from a test tube—a prediction that turned out to be entirely false. It is hard to avoid the impression that some bias or philosophical prejudice is responsible for the readiness with which many bioconservatives seize on even the flimsiest of empirical justifications for banning human enhancement technologies of certain types but not others. Suppose it turned out that play-ing Mozart to pregnant mothers improved the child's subsequent musical talent. Nobody would argue for a ban on Mozart-in-the-womb on grounds that we cannot rule out that some psychological woe might befall the child once she discovers that her facility with the violin had been prenatally 'programmed' by her parents. Yet when, for example, it comes to genetic enhancements, eminent bioconservative writers often put forward arguments that are not so very different from this parody as weighty, if not conclusive, objections. To transhumanists, this looks like doublethink. How can it be that to bioconservatives almost any anticipated downside, predicted perhaps on the basis of the shakiest pop-psychological theory, so readily achieves that status of deep philosophical insight and knockdown objection against the transhumanist project?

Perhaps a part of the answer can be found in the different attitudes that transhumanists and bioconservatives have towards posthuman dignity. Bioconservatives tend to deny posthuman dignity and view posthumanity as a threat to human dignity. They are therefore tempted to look for ways to denigrate interventions that are thought to be pointing in the direction of more radical future modifications that may eventually lead to the emergence of those detestable posthumans. But unless this fundamental opposition to the posthuman is openly declared as a premise of their argument, this then forces them to use a double standard of assessment whenever particular cases are considered in isolation: for example, one standard for germ-line genetic interventions and another for improvements in maternal nutrition (an intervention presumably not seen as heralding a posthuman era).

Transhumanists, by contrast, see human and posthuman dignity as compatible and complementary. They insist that dignity, in its modern sense, consists in what we are and what we have the potential to become, not in our pedigree or our causal origin. What we are is not a function solely of our DNA but also of our technological and social context. Human nature in this broader sense is dynamic, partially human-made, and improvable. Our current extended phenotypes (and the lives that we lead) are markedly different from those of our hunter-gatherer ancestors. We read and write, we wear clothes, we live in cities, we earn money and buy food from the supermarket, we call people on the telephone, watch television, read newspapers, drive cars, file taxes, vote in national elections, women give birth in hospitals, life-expectancy is three times longer than in the Pleistocene, we know that the Earth is round and that stars are large gas clouds lit from inside by nuclear fusion, and that the universe is approximately 13.7 billion years old and enormously big. In the eyes of a hunter-gatherer, we might already appear 'posthuman.' Yet these radical extensions of human capabilities—some of them biological, others external—have not divested us of moral status or dehumanized us in the sense of making us generally unworthy and base. Similarly, should we or our descendants one day succeed in becoming what relative to current standards we may refer to as posthuman, this need not entail a loss dignity either.

From the transhumanist standpoint, there is no need to behave as if there were a deep moral difference between technological and other means of enhancing human lives. By defending posthuman dignity we promote a more inclusive and humane ethics, one that will embrace future technologically modified people as well as humans of the contemporary kind. We also remove a distortive double standard from the field of our moral vision, allowing us to perceive more clearly the opportunities that exist for further human progress.[12]

Notes

1 N. Bostrom. 2003. The Transhumanist FAQ, v. 2.1. *World Transhumanist Association*. Webpage: www .transhumanism.org/resources/FAQv21.pdf.

2 N. Bostrom. Human Genetic Enhancements: A Transhumanist Perspective. *Journal of Value Inquiry*, Vol. 37, No. 4, pp. 493-506.

3 L. Kass. Ageless Bodies, Happy Souls: Biotechnology and the Pursuit of Perfection. *The New Atlantis* 2003; 1.

4 See e.g., J. Glover. 2001. *Humanity: A Moral History of the Twentieth Century*. New Haven. Yale University Press.

5 L. Kass. 2002. *Life, Liberty, and Defense of Dignity: The Challenge for Bioethics*. San Francisco. Encounter Books: p. 48.

6 G. Annas, L. Andrews & R. Isasi. Protecting the Endangered Human: Toward an International Treaty Prohibiting Cloning and Inheritable Alterations. *American Journal of Law and Medicine* 2002; 28, 2&3: p. 162.

7 J.A. Simpson and E. Weiner, eds. 1989. *The Oxford English Dictionary*, 2nd ed. Oxford. Oxford University Press.

8 F. Fukuyama. 2002. *Our Posthuman Future: Consequences of the Biotechnology Revolution*. New York. Farrar, Straus and Giroux: p. 149.

9 Fukuyama, op cit. note 8, p. 160.

10 H. Jonas. 1985. *Technik, Medizin und Ethik: Zur Praxis des Prinzips Verantwortung*. Frankfurt am Main. Suhrkamp.

11 J. Habermas. 2003. *The Future of Human Nature*. Oxford. Blackwell: p. 23.

12 For their comments I am grateful to Heather Bradshaw, John Brooke, Aubrey de Grey, Robin Hanson, Matthew Liao, Julian Savulescu, Eliezer Yudkowsky, Nick Zangwill, and to the audiences at the Ian Ramsey Centre seminar of June 6th in Oxford 2003, the Transvision 2003 conference at Yale, and the 2003 European Science Foundation Workshop on Science and Human Values, where earlier versions of this paper were presented, and to two anonymous referees.

64.
PRÉCIS OF *AGING, DEATH, AND HUMAN LONGEVITY: A PHILOSOPHICAL INQUIRY*

Christine Overall

SOURCE: *Dialogue: Canadian Philosophical Review/Revue canadienne de philosophie* 45.3 (2006): 537-48.

To die at 70 or 80 or 90 seems better than dying at 30 or 40 or 50. If so, could it be even better to die at 110, 120, or 130?

The past 200 years have witnessed dramatic increases in the average life expectancy in the Western world, and a small but increasing number of people living past the age of 100. Because of these changes, and because of the prospect of new medical and scientific means of deliberately increasing the human life span, it is important to examine the normative question of whether prolonged life *should* be sought.

In considering the possibility of extending human life, I am not referring to mere biological survival: I mean the continuation of life with the human capacities for emotion, perception, thought, and action intact to at least some minimal degree. In *Aging, Death, and Human Longevity* I discuss the normative question of whether increases in the length of human life are good or bad, and whether they should be taken as a goal either individually or as a matter of social policy (or both). The exploration of this issue raises central questions about the nature, value, and meaning of human life itself and the social and cultural context in which it is lived. Is wanting to live longer a rational desire? I argue that, other things being equal, it is. The social policy question is whether the extension of human longevity would be good for and in the interests of the greater community, indeed for the collectivity of human beings. Would it be rational for a society to devote resources to scientific investigation, welfare and social assistance, and the development of health care in order to increase average life expectancy or to extend maximum life span? I answer affirmatively, while identifying some important strictures on the steps societies should take.

Throughout much of the history of Western thought, there are two very different perspectives upon deliberate efforts to prolong human life, perspectives that I call, following Gerald Gruman, apologism and prolongevitism.

In general, apologism accepts the earthly conditions that are humanity's lot and condemns efforts to change them (Gruman 1977, p. 10). In regard to the duration of human life, apologism is "the belief that the prolongation of life is neither possible nor desirable" (ibid., p. 6). Apologism accepts old age and death as inevitable occurrences within human life, and, while not attempting to change them, tries to provide satisfactory explanations for them (ibid., p. 10). Gruman uses the label "prolongevist" to describe "anyone foreseeing [and striving for] an extension of life much beyond [the age of 110]" (ibid., p. 8), but I use the term to describe any individuals or theories that advocate the extension of the human life span significantly beyond its current typical length. The prolongevist seeks "not merely an increase in time *per se* but an extension of the healthy and productive period of life" (ibid.).

What are the arguments for apologism and prolongevitism? I first discuss and assess four main historically dominant groups of arguments against apologism and show that each one is inadequate.

Against Apologism

First, apologists argue that death should not be dreaded. In his long philosophical poem *On the Nature of Things*, Lucretius writes: "[W]e may be assured that in death there is nothing to be dreaded by us; that he who does not exist, cannot become miserable; and that it makes not the least difference to a man, when immortal death has ended his mortal life, that he was ever born at all" (Lucretius 1997, p. 137). But prolongevists wish to extend human life not because they dread the state of being dead, but because they value the state of being alive (Nagel 1975, p. 403). True, the state of death itself ought not to be dreaded and death is the final end of every human life no matter how long it may be; nevertheless, neither of these facts gives us any reason not to resist our death and to want to prolong the brief lives that we do have.

Second, apologists such as Philippe Ariès (1974) argue for apologism on the basis of what they take to be the rhythm of life. They laud people in medieval times who allegedly accepted the course of nature and did not resist death. Apologists believe not only that our current life limits have a basis in biology, but also—just as important—that they have moral significance. Bioethicist Daniel Callahan, for example, says that the existing human life cycle in the Western world serves as "a foundation for living within the boundaries of nature" and a basis for a sustainable medicine (1998, p. 130). Similarly, philosopher John Hardwig writes, "We are mortal beings, and death is not only the end result of life, but its *telos*—the aim or purpose for which we are headed biologically.... Our natural rhythms are cyclical; we are structured to live and then to die. The question is not if, but when and how" (2000, p. 160).

But prolongevitism need not be committed to an irrational denial of the reality and inevitability of death; it is committed only to the promotion of the postponement of death. It is indeed true that death is and probably always will be inevitable for human beings, and, because it is inevitable, we must recognize and acknowledge it. However, I do not think it follows that we must *like* or passively accept this aspect of being human. The assumption that current biological restrictions on the human life span have, in themselves, a normative force for personal decision-making and social policy formation is unjustified. Indeed, it may even be immoral to accept as a given the so-called "natural" course of many life events. In scientific research, social policy formation, and individual decision-making, human beings have not acquiesced in existing biological limits in areas such as reproduction, disease management, and infant and maternal mortality. Instead, through disease prevention, health promotion, and extensive medical care, human beings have sought, successfully, to modify nature's dictates in order to limit the numbers who are born, reduce illnesses, enhance the quality of our lives, and eliminate premature death. I see no reason, based on the "rhythm of life," to cease doing so.

The third argument by apologists is intended to show why the present human life span is already long enough. Callahan argues that the average life expectancy that is now achieved in developed nations is sufficient to constitute a full life (1998, p. 253). The existing life-span framework that is provided by "nature," he says, is "perfectly adequate for human life, both collectively and individually" (ibid., p. 134) to accomplish all that is important for us. Anything longer could result in boredom and ennui, a futile repetition of activities that we already know only too well.

Such fears may be justified if we imagine that a prolonged life must necessarily be spent in mindless drudgery or severely limited by lack of health, education, resources, and opportunities. But, in evaluating the benefits and liabilities of a prolonged life, it is an error to take as one's standard the lives of the poorest, most diseased, or most miserable and deprived human beings. Instead, the debate about prolongevitism and apologism should motivate us to rethink human social arrangements and the limits now placed on the development of human potential.

A further error in this third argument is to let one's views of long life be biased by the notion that being old necessarily involves misery. The error is generated by ageism—unjustified bias, stereotyping, and discrimination on grounds of age, usually (although not always) on grounds of old age. If we reject unwarranted assumptions about the quality of prolonged life and the nature of elderly persons' existence, there are good reasons for repudiating the apologists' pessimism about the absence of novelty in individual lives. Extra years can be devoted to spending time with family, friends, colleagues, and lovers, meeting new people, creating or enjoying music, books, art, films, and plays, playing sports and games, indulging in games and hobbies, and exploring foreign countries, the local parks, or one's own backyard. All these things provide very good reasons for one to want a longer life.

Norah Kizer Bell suggests that there is also a gender bias involved in the third apologist argument: The existence of gendered expectations about women's biological and cultural roles makes it less likely that women will have had a full human life than have men, and more likely that the quality of their lives may be lower than those of men (1992, p. 86). But, with sufficient resources, a longer life gives individuals of either sex a chance to extend and expand their sense of what is worth experiencing and doing, so that not all our lives need be spent in survival activities.

The fourth argument put forward by apologists concerns the social costs of prolonging human life. The vigour and vitality of the human species are renewed, it is claimed, through the ongoing deaths of the old and the births of new human beings. Even more fundamentally, it is necessary that each generation grow old and die simply in order to make room for a new cohort, a claim readily reinforced by the last two centuries of increasing global overpopulation. In a context of finite or even diminishing resources, populations must be contained and the balance between the generations preserved. If elderly people live longer, it will become harder and harder for younger generations to support them.

But, while there are indeed serious costs of overpopulation in the contemporary human species, and it is possible that these problems may be exacerbated by the fact that human beings live longer than they did in past times, it is not self-evident that we must let people die for the sake of alleviating overpopulation, and certainly not that the burden of so doing should fall disproportionately and necessarily upon older people. It is outrageous to expect people of 75 or 80 years to accept death for the sake of alleviating the burdens of population pressures, opening up jobs, or reducing medical costs. Moreover, since the large majority of elderly people are women, apologist claims that the prolongation of elderly people's lives creates a burden are really claims about the burden that elderly women (not persons in general) supposedly constitute.

A particularly worrying form of apologism is expressed in the views of some contemporary philosophers and bioethicists, such as Hardwig, who argues that human beings have a duty to die. One has a duty to die—even if one does not want to die—"when continuing to live will impose significant burdens—emotional burdens, extensive caregiving, destruction of life plans, and ... financial hardship—on [one's] family and loved ones" (1997, p. 38). But Hardwig misconstrues the idea of burdensomeness. Living and working with other human beings inevitably generates burdens that are imposed by some and adopted by others: both being the burden and caring for the burden are roles that we may enter into or adopt at various times during our lives. In particular, there is no evidence that caregivers simply want their elderly relatives to die; indeed, they would find it a repugnant betrayal of their moral commitment. Instead, what they need is sufficient social support to permit the care of dependent elderly people to be undertaken without sacrifice.

In Favour of Prolongevitism

Arguments based on the claim that longevity has intrinsic value or that life itself has intrinsic value are not successful. Alternatively, prolongevitism might be defended on the basis of the right to life. Because there is no duty to die, every human being has a liberty right to life; that is, we all have the right not to have our lives terminated by the activities of other human beings. But the idea of a welfare right to life—the entitlement to all possible assistance to preserve, enhance, and extend life—is more complex. It is sometimes assumed young people have a welfare right to life whereas old ones do not. I suggest that the issue, however, is not simply how long a person has already lived, but, rather, the degree to which the person has had the opportunity to enjoy the goods of human life. James Lindemann Nelson (1999) argues that death is gendered and has no single fixed meaning in the context of lives that differ in gender, race, or class. Many women, along with poor people and people of colour, have had fewer such opportunities than more privileged human beings and therefore have more of a welfare right to life. Hence, I support a limited welfare right to life, but caution that such a right needs to be approached carefully in policy terms.

The fact that death brings an unequivocal end to the chance to enjoy the goods of experience and action is the strongest argument for prolongevitism. Therefore, the burden of proof rests on those who would end life, not on those who would prolong it. This is not to say, however, that we always have a *de facto* obligation to prolong lives, whether of human or non-human beings. I advocate prolongevitism because many people in fact want to live longer, because this life is the only one we have, because many old people have been deprived of life's goods, because continuing to live offers the prospect of ongoing opportunities for further experience and action, and because the apologist alternatives to prolongevitism are morally untenable.

Immortality

If one agrees that apologism is inadequate and that there are good grounds for extending human life because of the ongoing opportunities for experiencing and doing that greater longevity offers, difficult questions arise of just how much life is enough. If prolonging life is, *ceteris paribus*, desirable, is there any reasonable limit to the length of a good life? Is there an upper limit to the human life span that is compatible with being human? The latter is not a question primarily about biology, but is rather about what it means to be human. I explore these issues by examining immortality, defined as the absence of any permanent end to individual personal life, and the unending and eternal persistence of individual awareness, perception, thought, emotion, and activity through infinite temporal duration.

The desire for immortality is a form of prolongevitism. The apparent problem with immortality is that a life that has no temporal limit seems not recognizably *human* (Williams 1975). Many philosophers argue that it is our limits and limitations— material, temporal, and psychological—that help make us human in the moral and social sense. On the other hand, if a person is reasonably healthy, both mentally and physically, then, given the previous arguments against apologism, there do not seem to be good reasons why any particular span of life will necessarily or inevitably be enough.

Some objections to a life of immortality are based not upon the nature of unending life itself, but rather upon such things as the conditions under which immortality is achieved or the impossibility of surrendering immortality once it is achieved. For purposes of evaluating immortality, therefore, I make a few assumptions. First, in a world where immortality is possible, people would not be born immortal. Rather, they would have the opportunity of achieving immortality at some point during their life, through some recognized medical process, operation, or formula. Second, people would have good grounds for believing they were immortal, and could assess its desirability in a realistic way. Third, everyone would have the opportunity to opt for immortality. Fourth, individuals who choose immortality would be reasonably healthy and energetic as immortals. Fifth, having attained immortality, people would still have the opportunity to opt out of it.

The "burden" argument standardly used against the finite prolongation of human life arises in spades with respect to immortality. Assuming that a substantial number of people, though perhaps not everyone, would choose everlasting life, then, unless we also assume that people who live forever would be intelligent enough to figure out how, in material and social terms, to accommodate the needs and wants of an immortal population, the planet would soon be overwhelmed by overpowering resource depletion and waste generation occasioned by the permanent survival requirements of the immortal population.

However, the argument from burdens to society is not sufficient to show that immortality is undesirable from the point of view of an individual, for it is possible that so few individuals would choose immortality that the immortal minority would not necessarily tax the world's resources. I therefore turn to a consideration of the value of unending life from the point of view of the individual.

Some arguments against the value of immortality for individuals are unsuccessful. For example, those who raise concerns about losing all that one knows and outliving one's relatives and friends falsely assume that one could not make new connections with younger people. I point out an analogy to the experience of immigrants to North American in the nineteenth century who gave up all they knew to come here, but nonetheless found the experience worthwhile. A more serious problem, emphasized by Bernard Williams (1975), is the potential for boredom. He suggests that the immortal person would run out of short-term objectives and could have no indefinitely long-term goal, no "categorical" desires that exist independently of the mere desire to continue to survive. But the claim is not convincing. As in a non-mortal life, the immortal person might be bored some of the time, but not necessarily all the time. After all, the immortal would benefit from infinite possibilities for new experiences and relationships, and could undertake projects, moral, spiritual, or intellectual, that do not necessarily have an end. Moreover, boredom is not even the inevitable result of the repetition of experiences: witness our present human lives, where people happily engage in some experiences—eating, sex, and watching hockey come to mind—without growing tired of them.

Nonetheless, the prospect of immortality raises hard questions about identity. The very possibilities of learning, moral development, and the acquisition of wisdom, which I have argued would have the potential to stave off boredom or psychological dormancy, ensure, according to Williams, that one cannot remain the same person if one is immortal. Over great reaches of time, future states of the immortal self would have no relationship to "aims I now have in wanting to survive" (Williams 1975, p. 421). Yet, even in our mortal lives, some human beings make profound personal transformations without losing their identity. In what way does the same person persist throughout these transformations? She persists insofar as each transformed self is desired and actively sought by the previous one, so that the transformed self grows out of the previous self, is causally generated by the previous self, and can be understood in terms of characteristics of the previous self (Nozick 1981, p. 35).

But, although the personal transformations made possible by immortality do not preclude constancy of identity, the physical limitations of the human body create other difficulties. As immortals exhaust all the possibilities of their current bodies, they could perhaps replace their limbs and organs with artificial or cloned substitutes. Eventually, however, through infinite time, the physical capacities even of a cyborg

or cloned body and brain would be exhausted, and it would be necessary to keep amplifying them, perhaps through the much-touted development of nanotechnology, in which molecule-sized robots would repair, rebuild, replace, and enhance parts of the human body indefinitely (Holt 1999, p. 76). Yet, even if it were possible to make replacements of parts of the brain, it seems implausible, given all eternity, that an immortal individual could receive finite brain replacements sufficiently like her own to enable her to maintain at least some minimal continuity as a person while also affording an open-ended range of possible experiences, thoughts, and feelings. In the end, sustaining an eternal life and avoiding the prospect of using up one's capacities appear to require the possession of a body and a brain with capacities that are in principle unlimited. Thus, it may be that to want to be immortal and never run out of the potential for novelty requires giving up the attachment to being human. Could it nonetheless make sense, in these conditions, to want to be immortal? Only if it makes sense to want to be a god, or at least godlike, for that is what one would have to be if one were to live forever and not be limited by one's material being.

My investigation suggests that a life that has no limit, a life that would not entail the prospect of exhausting one's capacities, might not be a recognizably *human* life because it appears to require both the loss of personal human identity and the attainment of godlike abilities. Yet, if a person is reasonably healthy, both mentally and physically, there still appears to be no good reason to regard a finite life of any *particular* length as a good thing. Perhaps the quandaries for identity and the need for change that are generated by imagining immortality arise only because of the assumptions about selfhood that they presuppose. Following Margaret Urban Walker and James Lindemann Nelson, I distinguish between two concepts of selfhood: the career self and the seriatim self. They represent a distinction between, on the one hand, the development and exploitation of talents and abilities in pursuit of long-range goals, and, on the other hand, the sheer immersion in and enjoyment of experiences for their own sake. The career self is expected to create, follow through on, and control the course of a narrative plot or project that governs the unfolding of her life and is the expression of the individual's individual autonomy (Walker 1999, p. 103). By contrast, "the seriatim self may see her life as made up of many jobs, lots of them quite big enough, thank you, but none necessarily life-defining, nor especially valued for the particular role they play in contributing to the achievement of a 'rational plan' for the whole" (Nelson 1999, p. 123). This self might derive value from "the goods of relationships" rather than achievement. I suggest that both sorts of selves may have good reasons to value a long life. At the same time, the argument that immortality is undesirable because one eventually comes to the limits of what is possibly achievable in a material human body may depend on which sort of self one regards as desirable.

Social Policy

I conclude the book [*Aging, Death, and Human Longevity: A Philosophical Inquiry* (Berkeley, CA: University of California Press, 2003)] by considering the pragmatic implications of adopting a prolongevist perspective and recognizing a circumscribed welfare right to life. Are there ways of acting upon prolongevist values that are both fair and beneficent for the whole culture, that do not entail inappropriate sacrifices from any segment of the society, and that are consistent with a vision of social justice and improved welfare for everyone? To raise such questions is imperative, for much of the cultural distrust of prolongevitism has arisen from fears of a prolongevist culture run amuck, in which unreasonable and unjustified practices are implemented solely for the sake of extending the human life span beyond any acceptable limits.

Nelson argues that health care resources should be allocated in ways that not only promote health but also contribute to justice (1996, p. 60). I agree, and I would add that creating just policies may also contribute to health promotion. I therefore advocate a perspective that I call "affirmative prolongevitism."

Affirmative prolongevitism entails

- directing resources, research, and services toward boosting life expectancy, ultimately so that it approaches that of the maximum human

life span, and compressing morbidity, that is, enabling people to remain healthy right up to the end of life, by eliminating or ameliorating negative symptoms of aging and confining illness to the last few years or even months of life;

- recognizing that, because not every person has enjoyed fair and equal opportunities, it is false to assume that all elderly persons—and especially those who are female, who have disabilities, who are poor, or who are racially identified—have already experienced all of life's goods and should be ready to die, therefore placing a special emphasis on improving the life expectancy of members of disadvantaged groups with current low life expectancy; and

- adopting a life-course approach to policy with respect to elderly people that recognizes that it is in people's interests to support elderly people and not regard them as a burden both because elderly people are not some "other" group, but one's own parents, grandparents, friends, coworkers, etc., and because it is very likely that one will oneself some day be elderly and in need of support.

As I have argued, prolonging life creates prospects for self-transformation, for enjoying relationships, and for pursuing new goals. Many human beings, perhaps the vast majority, never have the chance fully to explore and express all their potential as physical/emotional/moral/intellectual beings. A more prolonged life would provide at least some of that missed opportunity. Given the resources and the opportunities, human beings are capable of changing their lives, often even in the face of oppressive or debilitating circumstances. I therefore reject both the arguments for apologism that are based upon classist, racist, sexist, ableist arguments about the alleged burdens constituted by elderly people, and apologism itself, because it disproportionately disadvantages members of groups who have had less access to social goods such as health, education, meaningful work, and comfortable living conditions.

Nonetheless, my rejection of apologism does not mean that human life should be preserved at all costs, or that it is never good for a human life to come to an end. I am not saying that individual human lives *must* be extended or that all persons ought, on pain of irrationality, to desire to extend their lives. As a normative issue, the prolongation of life should be a matter of individual human choice. So, in arguing against apologism, I am not seeking to undermine the legitimate goals of citizens and ethicists who are concerned about developing and preserving a right to die. As an advocate of pro-longevitism, I am not arguing for the creation of an environment in which human life is prolonged at all costs and people live out their last months or years in misery, desperately wishing they could die. Nor do I want to substitute social pressure to go on living for current pressures to accept the end of one's life.

In his famous poem, "Do Not Go Gentle into That Good Night," Dylan Thomas rejects his chronically ill father's growing acquiescence in death and presents a forthright declaration of the significance of life, even into old age, right up until death:

> Do not go gentle into that good night, Old
> age should burn and rave at close of day;
> Rage, rage against the dying of the light.
> (Thomas 1952, p. 116)

In *Aging, Death, and Human Longevity* I do not argue, and would not want to argue, that rage is always a desirable reaction to "the dying of the light." Instead I try to show that *resistance* to "the dying of the light" is not difficult to understand. Other things being equal, a long life is a better life, and a social policy that promotes the extension of human life is amply justified.

References

Ariès, Philippe 1974 *Western Attitudes Toward Death: From the Middle Ages to the Present.* Translated by Patricia M. Ranum. Baltimore, MD: Johns Hopkins University Press.

Bell, Nora Kizer 1992 "If Age Becomes a Standard for Rationing Health Care...." In *Feminist Perspectives in Medical Ethics.* Edited by Helen Bequaert Holmes and Laura M. Purdy. Bloomington, IN: Indiana University Press, pp. 82-90.

Callahan, Daniel 1998 *False Hopes: Why America's Quest for Perfect Health Is a Recipe for Failure.* New York: Simon & Schuster.

Gruman, Gerald J. 1977 *A History of Ideas about the Prolongation of Life: The Evolution of Prolongevity Theses to 1800.* New York: Arno Press. Reprint of Vol. 56, Pt. 9 of the Transactions of the American Philosophical Society, 1966.

Hardwig, John 1997 "Is There a Duty to Die?" *Hastings Center Report*, 27, 2: 34-42. 2000 *Is There a Duty to Die? And Other Essays in Medical Ethics.* With Nat Hentoff, Dan Callahan, Larry Churchill, Felicia Cohn, and Joanne Lynn. New York: Routledge.

Holt, Jim 1999 "Staying Alive." *Lingua Franca*, 8, 9: 76.

Lucretius 1997 *On the Nature of Things.* Translated by John Selby Watson. Amherst, NY: Prometheus Books.

Nagel, Thomas 1975 "Death." In *Moral Problems: A Collection of Philosophical Essays.* 2nd ed. Edited by James Rachels. New York: Harper & Row, pp. 401-09.

Nelson, James Lindemann 1996 "Measured Fairness, Situated Justice: Feminist Reflections on Health Care Rationing." *Kennedy Institute of Ethics Journal*, 6, 1: 53-68. 1999 "Death's Gender." In *Mother Time: Women, Aging, and Ethics.* Edited by Margaret Urban Walker. Lanham, MD: Rowman & Littlefield, pp. 113-29.

Nozick, Robert 1981 *Philosophical Explanations.* Cambridge, MA: Belknap Press.

Thomas, Dylan 1952 "Do Not Go Gentle into That Good Night." In *Collected Poems 1934-1952.* London: J.M. Dent & Sons, p. 116.

Walker, Margaret Urban 1999 "Getting Out of Line: Alternatives to Life as a Career." In *Mother Time: Women, Aging, and Ethics.* Edited by Margaret Urban Walker. Lanham, MD: Rowman & Littlefield, pp. 97-111.

Williams, Bernard 1975 "The Makropulos Case: Reflections on the Tedium of Immortality." In *Moral Problems: A Collection of Philosophical Essays.* 2nd ed. Edited by James Rachels. New York: Harper & Row, pp. 410-28.

ACKNOWLEDGEMENTS

Alward, Peter. "Ignorance, Indeterminacy, and Abortion Policy." *The Journal of Value Inquiry* 41.2-4 (2007): 183-200. With kind permission from Springer Science+Business Media.

Angell, Marcia. "Privatizing Health Care is Not the Answer: Lessons from the United States." *Canadian Medical Association Journal* 179.9, copyright © 2008. This work is protected by copyright and the making of this copy was with the permission of Access Copyright. Any alteration of its content or further copying in any form whatsoever is strictly prohibited unless otherwise permitted by law.

Annas, George J. "The Prostitute, the Playboy and the Poet: Rationing Schemes for Organ Transplantation." *American Journal of Public Health* 75.2 (1985): 187-89. Reprinted with permission of The Sheridan Press.

Annas, George J., et al. "Protecting the Endangered Human: Toward an International Treaty Prohibiting Cloning and Inheritable Alterations." *American Journal of Law and Medicine* 28, Nos. 2&3 (2002): 151-78. Reprinted with permission.

Battin, Margaret. "Euthanasia: The Fundamental Issues." Donald VanDeVeer and Tom Regan (eds.), *Health Care Ethics: An Introduction* (Philadelphia: Temple University Press, 1987). Reprinted by permission of Margaret Battin.

Baylis, Françoise, et al. "Reframing Research Involving Humans." From *The Politics of Women's Health: Exploring Agency and Autonomy* by Susan Sherwin and The Feminist Health Care Research Network. Used by permission of Temple University Press. Copyright © 1998 by Temple University. All rights reserved.

Bernal, Ellen W. "The Nurse as Patient Advocate." *Hastings Center Report* 22.4 (1992): 18-23. Reprinted with permission of The Hastings Center; permission conveyed through Copyright Clearance Center, Inc.

Bostrom, Nick. "In Defense of Posthuman Dignity." *Bioethics* 19.3 (June 2005): 202-14. Reprinted by permission of John Wiley and Sons.

Brody, Howard and Eric N. Avery. "Medicine's Duty to Treat Pandemic Illness: Solidarity and Vulnerability." *Hastings Center Report* 39.1 (January-February 2009): 40-48. Reprinted with permission of The Hastings Center; permission conveyed through Copyright Clearance Center, Inc.

Brown, Barry F. "Proxy Consent for Research on the Incompetent Elderly." From *Ethics & Aging*, James E. Thornton and Earl R. Winkler (eds.). Reprinted with permission of the Publisher. Copyright © University of British Columbia Press 1988. All rights reserved by the Publisher.

Callahan, Daniel. "When Self-Determination Runs Amok." *Hastings Center Report* 22.2 (1992): 52-55. Reprinted with permission of The Hastings Center; permission conveyed through Copyright Clearance Center, Inc.

Caplan, Arthur L., et al. "Moving the Womb." *Hastings Center Report* 37.3 (May-June 2007): 18-20. Reprinted with permission of The Hastings Center; permission conveyed through Copyright Clearance Center, Inc.

Chaoulli v. Quebec, 2005 (Case Summary: C. Morano). http://scc.lexum.org/en/2005/2005scc35/2005scc35.html.

De Melo-Martin, Inmaculada. "Furthering Injustices against Women: Genetic Information, Moral Obligations, and Gender." *Bioethics* 20.6 (November 2006): 301-06. Reprinted by permission of John Wiley and Sons.

De Melo-Martin, Inmaculada. "On Cloning Human Beings." *Bioethics* 16.3 (June 2002): 246-65. Reprinted by permission of the publisher (Taylor & Francis Ltd., http://www.tandf.co.uk/journals).

De Vries, Raymond G., et al. "Choosing Surgical Birth: Desire and the Nature of Bioethical Advice." From *Naturalized Bioethics*, Hilde Lindemann, Marian Ververk, and Margaret Urban Walker (eds.). Cambridge University Press (2009): 42-64. Reprinted with the permission of Cambridge University Press.

Miller, F.G. "Death and Organ Donation: Back to the Future." *Journal of Medical Ethics* 35:10 (October 2009): 616-20. Reproduced with permission from BMJ Publishing Group Ltd.

Miller, Franklin G. and Howard Brody. "A Critique of Clinical Equipoise: Therapeutic Misconception in the Ethics of Clinical Trials." *Hastings Center Report* 33.3 (May-June 2003): 19-31. Reprinted with permission of The Hastings Center; permission conveyed through Copyright Clearance Center, Inc.

Murray, Thomas H. "Moral Obligations to the Not-Yet Born: The Fetus as Patient." From *The Worth of a Child*. Berkeley: University of California Press, 1996: 96-114. Reprinted by permission of the University of California Press.

Overall, Christine. "Précis of *Aging, Death, and Human Longevity: A Philosophical Inquiry.*" *Dialogue: Canadian Philosophical Review/Revue canadienne de philosophie* 45.3 (2006): 537-48. Reproduced with permission of Cambridge University Press.

Overall, Christine. "Reflections on Reproductive Rights in Canada." From *Human Reproduction: Principles, Practices, Policies*. Copyright © Oxford University Press Canada, 1993. Reprinted by permission of the publisher.

Parks, Jennifer A. "Why Gender Matters to the Euthanasia Debate: On Decisional Capacity and the Rejection of Women's Death Requests." *Hastings Center Report* 30.1 (January-February 2000): 30-36. Reprinted with permission of The Hastings Center; permission conveyed through Copyright Clearance Center, Inc.

Peterson, M.M. "Assisted Reproductive Technologies and Equity of Access Issues." *Journal of Medical Ethics* 31.5 (May 2005): 280-85. Reproduced with permission from BMJ Publishing Group Ltd.

Reibl v. Hughes, 1980 (Case Summary: C. Morano). http://csc.lexum.org/en/1980/1980scr2-880/1980scr2-880.html.

Reid, Lynette. "Diminishing Returns? Risk and the Duty to Care in the SARS Epidemic." *Bioethics* 19.4 (August 2005): 348-61. Reprinted by permission of John Wiley and Sons.

Reiss, Michael J. "The Ethics of Xenotransplantation." *Journal of Applied Philosophy* 17.3 (2000): 253-62. Reproduced with permission of John Wiley and Sons.

Robertson, John A. "Class, Feminist and Communitarian Critiques of Procreative Liberty." Chapter 10 of *Children of Choice: Freedom and the New Reproductive Technologies*. Copyright © 1994, Princeton University Press. Reprinted by permission of Princeton University Press.

Rodriguez v. British Columbia, 1993 (Case Summary: C. Morano). http://scc.lexum.org/en/1993/1993scr3-519/1993scr3-519.html.

Rogers, Wendy. "Evidence-Based Medicine and Women: Do the Principles and Practice of EBM Further Women's Health?" *Bioethics* 18.1 (February 2004): 50-71. Reprinted by permission of Taylor & Francis Ltd., http://www.tandf.co.uk/journals.

Schüklenk, Udo, et al. "The Ethics of Genetic Research on Sexual Orientation." *Hastings Center Report* 27.4 (July-August 1997): 6-13. Reprinted with permission of The Hastings Center; permission conveyed through Copyright Clearance Center, Inc.

Seavilleklein, Victoria. "Challenging the Rhetoric of Choice in Prenatal Screening." *Bioethics* 23.1 (January 2009): 68-77. Reprinted by permission of John Wiley and Sons.

Selgelid, M.J. "Pandethics." *Public Health* 123.3 (March 2009): 255-59. Copyright © 2009, with permission from Elsevier.

Sheldon, S. and S. Wilkinson. "Should Selecting Saviour Siblings Be Banned?" *Journal of Medical Ethics* 30.6 (December 2004): 533-37. Reproduced with permission from BMJ Publishing Group Ltd.

Sherwin, Susan. "Abortion through a Feminist Ethics Lens." *Dialogue* 30.3 (1991): 327-42. Reproduced with permission of Cambridge University Press.

Sherwin, Susan. "A Relational Approach to Autonomy in Health Care." From *The Politics of Women's Health: Exploring Agency and Autonomy* by Susan Sherwin and The Feminist Health Care Research Network. Used by permission of Temple University Press. Copyright © 1998 by Temple University. All rights reserved.

Silver, Lee M. "Cloning, Ethics, and Religion." *Cam-

bridge Quarterly of Healthcare Ethics 7.2 (April 1998): 168-72. Reprinted with the permission of Cambridge University Press.

Smith v. Jones, 1999 (Case Summary: C. Morano). http://scc.lexum.org/en/1999/1999scr1-455/1999scr1-455.html.

Spital, Aaron. "Conscription of Cadaveric Organs for Transplantation: A Stimulating Idea Whose Time Has Not Yet Come." *Cambridge Quarterly of Healthcare Ethics* 14.1 (January 2005): 107-12. Reproduced with permission of Cambridge University Press.

Stingl, Michael. "Equality and Efficiency as Basic Social Values." From *Efficiency versus Equality*, Michael Stingl (ed.). Fernwood Publishing (1996). Used by permission of the author.

Thomas, John E. "The Physician as Therapist and Investigator." From *Medical Ethics and Human Life*. Copyright © 1983 John E. Thomas. Reprinted with permission from Dundurn Press Limited.

Truog, Robert D. "Is It Time to Abandon Brain Death?" *Hastings Center Report* 27.1 (January-February 1997): 29-37. Reprinted with permission of The Hastings Center; permission conveyed through Copyright Clearance Center, Inc.

Warren, Mary Anne. "The Moral Significance of Birth." *Hypatia* 4.3 (1989): 46-65. Reprinted by permission of John Wiley and Sons.

Williams, Garrath and Doris Schroeder. "Human Genetic Banking: Altruism, Benefit and Consent." *New Genetics and Society* 23.1 (2004): 89-103. Reprinted by permission of the publisher (Taylor & Francis Ltd., http://www.tandf.co.uk/journals).

Winnipeg Child and Family Services v. D.F.G, 1997 (Case Summary: C. Morano). http://scc.lexum.org/en/1997/1997scr3-925/1997scr3-925.html.

Wolf, Susan M. "Gender, Feminism, and Death: Physician-Assisted Suicide and Euthanasia." Susan M. Wolf (ed.), *Feminism and Bioethics: Beyond Reproduction*. Copyright © 1996 by Oxford University Press, Inc. Reprinted by permission of Oxford University Press, Inc.

Zion, Deborah. "HIV/AIDS Clinical Research, and the Claims of Beneficence, Justice, and Integrity." *Cambridge Quarterly of Healthcare Ethics* 13.4 (October 2004): 404-13. Reprinted with the permission of Cambridge University Press.

The publisher has made every attempt to locate the authors of the copyrighted material or their heirs and assigns, and would be grateful for information that would allow correction of any errors or omissions in subsequent editions of the work.